Travel Medicine

Content Strategist: Belinda Kuhn
Content Development Specialist: Nani Clansey
Content Coordinator: Sam Crowe/Trinity Hutton
Project Manager: Vinod Kumar Iyyappan
Design: Stewart Larking
Illustration Manager: Jennifer Rose
Marketing Manager(s) (UK/USA): Carla Holloway

Travel Medicine

THIRD EDITION

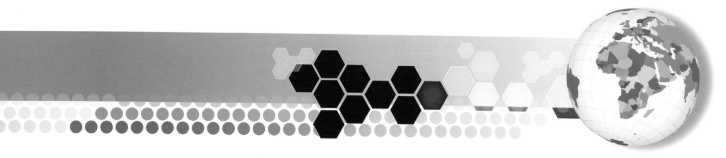

Jay S. Keystone MD, MSc (CTM), FRCPC
Professor of Medicine
University of Toronto
Senior Staff physician, Tropical Disease Unit
Toronto General Hospital;
Director, Medisys Travel Health clinic
Toronto, ON, Canada

David O. Freedman MD
Professor
Director, UAB Travelers Health Clinic
The University of Alabama at Birmingham
Birmingham, AL, USA

Phyllis E. Kozarsky MD
Professor of Medicine
Department of Medicine and Infectious Diseases
Co-Director Tropical and Travel Medicine
Emory University School of Medicine
Atlanta, GA, USA

Bradley A. Connor MD
Clinical Professor of Medicine
Division of Gastroenterology and Hepatology
Weill Medical College of Cornell University
Medical Director, The New York Center for Travel and Tropical Medicine
New York, NY, USA

Hans D. Nothdurft MD
Professor
Department of Infectious Diseases and Tropical Medicine
Head, University Travel Clinic
University of Munich
Munich, Germany

For additional online content visit
expertconsult website

Expert | CONSULT

ELSEVIER
SAUNDERS

SAUNDERS an imprint of Elsevier Inc.
© 2013, Elsevier Inc All rights reserved.

First edition 2004
Second edition 2008

Notices
Knowledge and best practice in this field are constantly changing. As new research and experience broaden our understanding, changes in research methods, professional practices, or medical treatment may become necessary.

Practitioners and researchers must always rely on their own experience and knowledge in evaluating and using any information, methods, compounds, or experiments described herein. In using such information or methods they should be mindful of their own safety and the safety of others, including parties for whom they have a professional responsibility.

With respect to any drug or pharmaceutical products identified, readers are advised to check the most current information provided (i) on procedures featured or (ii) by the manufacturer of each product to be administered, to verify the recommended dose or formula, the method and duration of administration, and contraindications. It is the responsibility of practitioners, relying on their own experience and knowledge of their patients, to make diagnoses, to determine dosages and the best treatment for each individual patient, and to take all appropriate safety precautions.

To the fullest extent of the law, neither the Publisher nor the authors, contributors, or editors, assume any liability for any injury and/or damage to persons or property as a matter of products liability, negligence or otherwise, or from any use or operation of any methods, products, instructions, or ideas contained in the material herein.

ISBN: 978-1-4557-1076-8
Ebook ISBN: 978-1-4557-4543-2

Printed in China
Last digit is the print number: 9 8 7 6 5 4 3 2 1

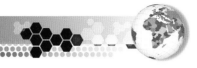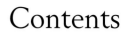

Contents

Section 1: The Practice of Travel Medicine

Chapter 1	Introduction to Travel Medicine	1
Chapter 2	Epidemiology: Morbidity and Mortality in Travelers	5
Chapter 3	Starting, Organizing, and Marketing a Travel Clinic	13
Chapter 4	Sources of Travel Medicine Information	25

Section 2: The Pre-travel Consultation

Chapter 5	Pre-Travel Consultation	31
Chapter 6	Water Disinfection for International Travelers	37
Chapter 7	Insect Protection	51
Chapter 8	Travel Medical Kits	63

Section 3: Immunization

Chapter 9	Principles of Immunization	67
Chapter 10	Routine Adult Vaccines and Boosters	77
Chapter 11	Routine Travel Vaccines: Hepatitis A and B, Typhoid, Influenza	87
Chapter 12	Special Adult Travel Vaccines: Yellow Fever, Meningococcal, Japanese Encephalitis, TBE, Rabies, Polio, Cholera	101
Chapter 13	Pediatric Travel Vaccinations	125

Section 4: Malaria

Chapter 14	Malaria: Epidemiology and Risk to the Traveler	135
Chapter 15	Malaria Chemoprophylaxis	143
Chapter 16	Self-diagnosis and Self-treatment of Malaria by the Traveler	163
Chapter 17	Approach to the Patient with Malaria	173

Section 5: Travelers' Diarrhea

Chapter 18	Epidemiology of Travelers' Diarrhea	179
Chapter 19	Prevention of Travelers' Diarrhea	191
Chapter 20	Clinical Presentation and Management of Travelers' Diarrhea	197
Chapter 21	Persistent Travelers' Diarrhea	207

Section 6: Travelers with Special Needs

Chapter 22	The Pregnant and Breastfeeding Traveler	219
Chapter 23	The Pediatric and Adolescent Traveler	231
Chapter 24	The Older Traveler	241
Chapter 25	The Physically Challenged Traveler	249
Chapter 26	The Travelers with Pre-existing Disease	257
Chapter 27	The Immunocompromised Traveler	265
Chapter 28	The Traveler with HIV	273

Chapter 29 The Corporate and Executive Traveler 283
Chapter 30 International Adoption 291
Chapter 31 Visiting Friends and Relatives 297

Section 7: Travelers with Special Itineraries

Chapter 32 Expatriates 305
Chapter 33 The Migrant Patient 317
Chapter 34 Humanitarian Aid Workers 321
Chapter 35 Expedition Medicine 327
Chapter 36 Medical Tourism 343
Chapter 37 Cruise Ship Travel 349
Chapter 38 Mass Gatherings 357

Section 8: Environmental Aspects of Travel Medicine

Chapter 39 High-Altitude Medicine 361
Chapter 40 Diving Medicine 373
Chapter 41 Extremes of Temperature and Hydration 381
Chapter 42 Jet Lag 391
Chapter 43 Motion Sickness 397
Chapter 44 The Aircraft Cabin Environment 405

Section 9: Health Problems while Traveling

Chapter 45 Bites, Stings, and Envenoming Injuries 413
Chapter 46 Food-borne Illness 425
Chapter 47 Injuries and Injury Prevention 433
Chapter 48 Psychiatric Disorders of Travel 439
Chapter 49 Travelers' Thrombosis 449
Chapter 50 Healthcare Abroad 455
Chapter 51 Personal Security and Crime Avoidance 463

Section 10: Post-travel Care

Chapter 52 Post-travel Screening 467
Chapter 53 Fever in Returned Travelers 475
Chapter 54 Skin Diseases 487
Chapter 55 Eosinophilia 501
Chapter 56 Respiratory Infections 511
                  Appendix: Popular Destinations 523
                  Index 537

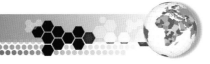

'We live in a wonderful world that is full of beauty, charm and adventure. There is no end to the adventures we can have if only we seek them with our eyes open.'

– Jawaharlal Nehru

'Stop worrying about the potholes in the road and celebrate the journey.'

– Fitzhugh Mullan

Mullan mentions the 'potholes in the road' as a metaphor for the challenges associated with travel, which not infrequently include health issues. Nehru was likely referring to the need to keep an open mind as one experiences the often overwhelming sights, sounds and smells of adventures in the developing world. On the other hand, with some liberties as a travel medicine practitioner, one could interpret his remarks as indicating the need to be prepared to face the rigors of travel. There is little doubt that physical and emotional challenges face us when we venture outside of our 'comfort-zones,' and that the optimal way of dealing with these challenges is to educate ourselves in advance.

In recent years, travel medicine has become a unique specialty that owes its origins to the marked increase in global travel for tourism, business, education, family reunification and migration, and the health risks posed by these population movements. Knowledge of travel medicine is no longer limited to tropical and travel medicine practitioners; it needs greater incorporation into family medicine, internal medicine, pediatrics, emergency medicine, occupational medicine, and the specialty of infectious disease. With the success of the previous two editions of this book, we felt the need to provide both the novice and the more experienced travel medicine practitioner with the most up-to-date knowledge in this burgeoning field.

This edition of Travel Medicine, like its predecessors, was designed to be a 'how to' book that can be read from beginning to end as a complete course in travel medicine. In addition, it is meant to be a reference textbook for those looking for the latest information in the field.

This text is designed to enable practitioners to easily access information that might be required on a day-to-day basis, while at the same time providing them with an approach to the most frequent problems facing the ill returned traveler. Each chapter contains a list of key points that summarize the most important issues discussed within the chapter. We have selected authors from several continents in order to provide the reader with different points of view. We have added chapters that deal with special groups such as those attending mass gatherings, cruise ship travelers, displaced persons, as well as healthcare and disaster workers.

It is hoped that by using both a practical and evidence-based approach our experienced international authors have made this book an essential resource for all travel health providers to keep close at hand.

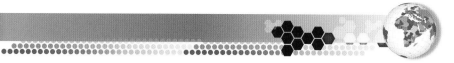

List of Contributors

Martin Alberer MD
Department of Tropical Medicine and
Infectious Diseases
Ludwig-Maximilians-University
Munich, Germany

Susan A. Anderson MD
Clinical Assistant Professor of Medicine/
GeoSentinel Site Director CDC/ITSM
Urgent Care and Travel Medicine
Palo Alto Medical Foundation
Palo Alto, CA, USA

Vernon Ansdell MD, FRCP, DTM&H
Associate Clinical Professor
Department of Public Health Sciences and
Epidemiology
University of Hawaii
Director, Tropical and Travel Medicine
Kaiser Permanente Hawaii
Honolulu, HI, USA

Paul M. Arguin MD
Medical Epidemiologist
Centers for Disease Control
Mailstop G-13
Atlanta, GA, USA

James Aw MD
Medical Director
Medcan Clinic
Toronto, ON, Canada

Howard Backer MD, MPH
Director
California Emergency Management Services
Authority (EMSA)
Rancho Cordova, CA, USA

**Michael Bagshaw MB, MRCS, FFOM,
DAvMed**
Visiting Professor of Aviation Medicine
King's College
London, UK

Roger A. Band MD
Assistant Professor
Department of Emergency Medicine
Hospital of The University of Pennsylvania
Department of Emergency Medicine
Philadelphia, PA, USA

Deborah N. Barbeau MD, MSPH
Clinical Assistant Professor of Medicine
Department of Medicine
Division of Infectious Diseases
Tulane University
New Orleans, LA, USA

Elizabeth D. Barnett MD
Professor of Pediatrics
Boston University School of Medicine
Director, International Clinic
Boston Medical Center
Boston, MA, USA

Trish Batchelor MD
Medical Officer CIWEC Clinic
Former National Medical Director
The Travel Doctor TMVC
(Austrialia & New Zealand)
C/O CIWEC Clinic
Kathmandu, Nepal

Ronald H. Behrens MB, ChB, MD, FRCP
Senior Lecturer
Faculty of Infectious and Tropical Diseases
London School of Hygiene and Tropical
Medicine
Consultant Physician
Hospital for Tropical Diseases London
London, UK

Jiri Beran MD
Head
Department for Tropical and Travel
Medicine
Institute for Postgraduate Medical
Education in Prague
Director
Vaccination and Travel Medicine Centre
Poliklinika II
Hradec Kralove, Czech Republic

Gerd D. Burchard MD, Phd
Professor
Department Tropical Medicine / Infectious
Diseases
University Medical Center Hamburg
Hamburg, Germany

**Michael Callahan MD, MSPH, DTM&H,
DMCC**
Clinical Associate Physician
Division of Infectious Diseases
Massachusetts General Hospital
Harvard Medical School
Boston, MA, USA

Suzanne C. Cannegieter MD, PhD
Clinical Epidemiologist
Leiden University Medical Center
Leiden, The Netherlands

Francesco Castelli MD, FRCP, FFTM RCPS
Professor of Infectious Diseases
Institute for Infectious and Tropical
Diseases
University of Brescia
Brescia, Italy

Eric Caumes MD
Professor
University Pierre et Marie Curie
Department of Infectious and Tropical
Diseases
Teaching Hospital Pitie Salpetriere
Paris, France

Lin Hwei Chen MD
Director
Travel Medicine Center
Mount Auburn Hospital
Cambridge, MA, USA

Jean-Francois Chicoine MD, FRCPC
Paediatrician
Associate Professor
Department of Paediatrics
Adoption and International Health Clinic
CHU Sainte-Justine
Scientific Director, Le monde est ailleurs
Montreal, QC, Canada

Jan Clerinx MD
Consultant
Department of Clinical Sciences
Institute of Tropical Medicine
Antwerp, Belgium

Bradley A. Connor MD
Clinical Professor of Medicine
Division of Gastroenterology and
Hepatology
Weill Medical College of Cornell University
Medical Director, The New York Center for
Travel and Tropical Medicine
New York, NY, USA

Gregory A. Deye MD
Investigator
Division of Experimental Therapeutics
Walter Reed Army Institute of Research
Military Malaria Research Program
Silver Spring, MD, USA

Thomas E. Dietz MD
Affiliate Assistant Professor
Department of Family Medicine
Oregon Health & Science University
Portland, OR, USA

Yoram Epstein PhD
Professor of Physiology
Heller Institute of Medical Research
Sheba Medical Center
Tel Hashomer
Sackler Faculty of Medicine
Tel Aviv University
Tel Aviv, Israel

Charles D. Ericsson MD
Professor of Medicine
Head, Clinical Infectious Diseases
Director, Travel Medicine Clinic
Director, Infectious Disease Fellowship
Program
University of Texas Medical School at
Houston
Houston, TX, USA

Philip R. Fischer MD
Professor of Pediatrics
Pediatric and Adolescent Medicine
Mayo Clinic
Rochester, MN, USA

Mark S. Fradin MD
Adjunct Clinical Associate Professor of
Dermatology
Department of Dermatology
University of North Carolina at Chapel Hill
Chapel Hill, NC, USA

Tifany Frazer MPH
Global Health Program Manager
Institute for Health and Society
Medical College of Wisconsin
Milwaukee, WI, USA

David O. Freedman MD
Professor
Director, UAB Travelers Health Clinic
The University of Alabama at Birmingham
Birmingham, AL, USA

Kenneth L. Gamble MD
Lecturer
University of Toronto
President, Missionary Health Institute
Toronto, ON, Canada

Pier F. Giorgetti MD
Institute for Infectious Diseases
University of Brescia
Brescia, Italy

Jeff Goad PharmD, MPH
Associate Professor of Clinical Pharmacy
University of Southern California School of
Pharmacy
Titus Family Department of Clinical
Pharmacy and Pharmaceutical Economics
and Policy
Los Angeles, CA, USA

Alfons Van Gompel MD
Associate Professor
Department of Clinical Sciences
Institute of Tropical Medicine
Antwerp, Belgium

Larry Goodyer MPharmS, PhD
Professor
Head of the Leicester School of Pharmacy
Faculty of Health and Life Sciences
De Montfort University
Leicester, UK

**Sandra Grieve RGN, RM, BSc (Hons), Dip
Trav Med, FFTM, RCPS (Glasg.)**
Independent Travel Health Specialist Nurse
Alcester, Warwickshire, UK

**Martin P. Grobusch MD, MSc (Lond),
FRCP (Lond), DTM&H (Lond)**
Full Professor (Chair) of Tropical Medicine
Head, Tropencentrum
Division of Infectious Diseases, Tropical
Medicine and AIDS
Department of Medicine
Amsterdam Medical Center
University of Amsterdam
Amsterdam, The Netherlands
Visiting Professor, Institute of Tropical
Diseases
University of Tuebingen, Germany
Visiting Professor, Division of Infectious
Diseases
Department of Internal Medicine
University of the Witwatersrand
Johannesburg, South Africa

Peter H. Hackett MD
Clinical Professor
Department of Emergency Medicine
University of Colorado, Denver
Director
Institute for Altitude Medicine,
Telluride, CO, USA

Davidson H. Hamer MD
Professor of International Health and
Medicine
Schools of Public Health and Medicine
Director, Travel Clinic Boston Medical
Center
Center for Global Health and
Development,
Boston University
Boston, MA, USA

Stephen Hargarten MD, MPH
Professor and Chair
Emergency Medicine
Director, Injury Research Center
Medical College of Wisconsin
Milwaukee, WI, USA

Christoph F. R. Hatz MD
Professor
Department of Medicine and Diagnostics
Swiss Tropical and Public Health Institute
Basel, Switzerland
Division of Communicable Diseases
Institute for Social and Preventive Medicine
University of Zurich
Zurich, Switzerland

Deborah M. Hawker PhD, DClinPsy
Clinical Psychologist
Psychological Health
InterHealth
London, UK

Carter D. Hill MD
Clinical Associate Professor
Department of Medicine
University of Washington
Medical Director
Holland America Line
Emergency Physician
Highline Medical Center
Seattle, WA, USA

**David R. Hill MD, DTM&H, FRCP, FFTM,
FASTM**
Professor of Medical Sciences
Director of Global Public Health
Frank H. Netter MD, School of Medicine
Quinnipiac University
Hamden, CT, USA

Kevin C. Kain MD, FRCPC
Professor of Medicine
University of Toronto
Canada Research Chair in Molecular
Parasitology
Director, SAR Labs, Sandra Rotman Centre
for Global Health
University Health Network-Toronto
General Hospital
Toronto, ON, Canada

Jay S. Keystone MD, MSc (CTM), FRCPC
Professor
Tropical Disease Unit
The Toronto General Hospital
Toronto, ON, Canada

Amy D. Klion MD
Investigator
Eosinophil Pathology Unit
Laboratory of Parasitic Diseases
Bethesda, MD, USA

Herwig Kollaritsch MD
Institute of Specific Prophylaxis and
Tropical Medicine
Center for Pathophysiology, Infectiology
and Immunology
Medical University of Vienna
Vienna, Austria

Phyllis E. Kozarsky MD
Professor of Medicine
Department of Medicine and Infectious
Diseases
Co-Director, Tropical and Travel Medicine
Emory University School of Medicine
Atlanta, GA, USA

**Susan M. Kuhn MD, MSc, DTM&H,
FRCPC**
Associate Professor
Departments of Pediatrics and Medicine
University of Calgary
Alberta Children's Hospital
Calgary, AB, Canada

Beth Lange MB, ChB
Otolaryngologist
Alberta Health Care Services
Calgary, AB, Canada

William L. Lang MD
Senior Medical Director
BioMarin Pharmaceuticals
Arlington, VA, USA

**Ted Lankester MB, Chir, MRCGP, FFTM,
RCPSG**
Director of Health Services
InterHealth
London, UK

**Karin Leder MBBS, FRACP, PhD, MPH,
DTM&H**
Associate Professor
Head of Infectious Disease Epidemiology
Unit
Department of Epidemiology and
Preventive Medicine
School of Public Health and Preventive
Medicine
Monash University
Melbourne, VIC, Australia

C. Virginia Lee MD, MPH, MA
Travelers Health Branch
Division of Global Migration &
Quarantine (DGMQ)
National Center for Emerging & Zoonotic
Infectious Diseases (NCEZID), CDC
Atlanta, USA

Thomas Löscher MD, DTM&H
Professor of Internal Medicine
Director
Department of Infectious Diseases and
Tropical Medicine
University of Munich
Munich, Germany

Sheila M. Mackell MD
Pediatrician & Travel Medicine Consultant
Mountain View Pediatrics
Flagstaff Medical Centre
Flagstaff, AZ, USA

Alan J. Magill MD, FACP, FIDSA, FASTMH
Program Manager
Division of Experimental Therapeutics
Walter Reed Army Institute of Research
COL U.S. Army (retired)
Defense Advanced Research Projects
Agency (DARPA)
Silver Spring, MD, USA

Karen J. Marienau MD, MPH
Centers for Disease Control and Prevention
Center for Emerging and Zoonotic
Infectious Diseases
Division of Global Migration and
Quarantine
St Paul, MN, USA

Alberto Matteelli MD
Head, Unit of Community Infections
Department of Infectious Diseases
Brescia University Hospital
Brescia, Italy

**Marc Mendelson BSc, MBBS, PhD, FRCP,
DTM&H**
Associate Professor
Head of Division of Infectious DIseases and
HIV Medicine
Department of Medicine
University of Cape Town
Cape Town, South Africa

Maria D. Mileno MD
Associate Professor of Medicine
Brown University
Director, Travel Medicine Service
The Miriam Hospital
Providence, RI, USA

Daniel S. Moran PhD
Associate Professor Faculty of Health
Sciences
Ariel University Center
Ariel, Israel

Anne E. McCarthy MD FRCPC, DTM&H
Associate Professor of Medicine
Division of Infectious Diseases
Director, Office of Global Health
Faculty of Medicine
Director, Tropical Medicine and
International Health Clinic
University of Ottawa
Ottawa, ON, Canada

Susan L. F. McLellan MD, MPH
Associate Professor of Medicine
Infectious Diseases Section
School of Medicine
Department of Tropical Medicine, SPHTM
Tulane University Health Sciences Center
New Orleans, LA, USA

Hans D. Nothdurft MD
Associate Professor
Department of Infectious Diseases and
Tropical Medicine
Head, University Travel Clinic
University of Munich
Munich, Germany

Philippe Parola MD, PhD
Professor of Infectious Diseases and Tropical
Medicine
Faculty of Medicine
Aix-Marseille University
Marseille, France

Susanne M. Pechel MD
Director
Fit for Travel – Editorial Department
InterMEDIS GmbH
Munich, Germany

Yoram A. Puius MD, PhD
Assistant Professor
Department of Medicine
Albert Einstein College of Medicine
Attending Physician
Division of Infectious Diseases
Montefiore Medical Center
Bronx, NY, USA

Veronica Del Punta MD
Resident Physician
Post-Graduate Specialization School in
Tropical Medicine
Institute of Infectious and Tropical Diseases
University of Brescia
Brescia, Italy

Pamela Rendi-Wagner MD, MSc, DTM&H
Associate Professor
Institute of Specific Prophylaxis and
Tropical Medicine
Medical University Vienna
Vienna, Austria

Mark S. Riddle MD, MPH&TM, DrPH
Deputy Head
Enteric Diseases Department NMRC
Silver Spring, MD, USA

Frits Rosendaal MD
Department of Clinical Epidemiology
Leiden University Medical Center
Leiden, The Netherlands

Gail A. Rosselot NP, MPH, COHN-S, FAANP
President
Travel Well of Westchester Inc.
Briarcliff Manor
New York, NY, USA

Edward T. Ryan MD, DTM&H
Director
Tropical Medicine
Division of Infectious Diseases
Massachusetts General Hospital
Professor of Medicine
Harvard Medical School
Boston, MA, USA

Nuccia Saleri MD, PhD
Professor
Appropriated Methodologies and
Techniques
International Cooperation for Development
University of Brescia
Institute of Infectious and Tropical Diseases
Brescia, Italy

John W. Sanders MD
Commanding Officer
Naval Medical Research Unit Six
Lima, Peru;
Assistant Professor
Infectious Disease Division
Uniformed Services University
Bethesda, MD, USA

Patricia Schlagenhauf PhD, PD
Senior Lecturer, Research Scientist
University of Zürich Centre for Travel
Medicine
WHO Collaborating Centre for Travelers'
Health
Zürich, Switzerland

Eli Schwartz MD, DTM&H
Professor (clinical) of Medicine
Head of The Center for Geographic
Medicine and Tropical Diseases
Chaim Sheba Medical Center
Tel Hashomer
Sackler School of Medicine
Tel Aviv University
Tel Aviv, Israel

Evelyn Sharpe MB BCh MRCPsych, MFTM RCPSGlasg
Consultant Psychiatrist
Psychological Health Services
InterHealth
London, UK

David R. Shlim MD
Medical Director
Jackson Hole Travel and Tropical Medicine
Kelly, WY, USA

Gerard J.B. Sonder MD, PhD
Director National Co-ordination
Center for Travelers Health Advice (LCR)
Department of Infectious Diseases
Public Health Service Amsterdam
Amsterdam, The Netherlands

Mike Starr MBBS, FRACP
Paediatrician, Infectious Diseases Physician
Consultant in Emergency Medicine
Director of Paediatric Physician Training
Head of Travel Clinic
Royal Children's Hospital
Melbourne, Australia

Robert Steffen MD
Emeritus Professor
University of Zurich
Institute of Social and Preventive Medicine
Division of Epidemiology and Prevention
of Communicable Diseases
WHO Collaborating Centre for Travellers'
Health
Zurich, Switzerland
Adjunct Professor, Epidemiology and
Disease Prevention Division
University of Texas School of Public Health
Houston, TX, USA

Kathryn N. Suh MD, FRCPC
Associate Professor of Medicine
University of Ottawa
Division of Infectious Diseases
The Ottawa Hospital Civic Campus
Ottawa, ON, Canada

Andrea P. Summer MD MSCR
Assistant Professor of Pediatrics
Department of Pediatrics
Medical University of South Carolina
Charleston, SC, USA

Linda R. Taggart MD, FRCPC
Fellow
Division of Infectious Diseases
University of Toronto
Toronto, ON, Canada

David N. Taylor MD, MS
Chief Medical Officer
Vaxlnnate Corporation
Cranbury, NJ, USA

Shiri Tenenboim MD, MSc Int'l Health (MIH), DTM&H
Medical Doctor (Dr.), Cancer Center
Chaim Sheba Medical Center,
Tel Hashomer, Israel

Dominique Tessier MD, CCFP, FCFP
Co-President
Bleu, Réseau d'experts
Medical Director
Clinique santé voyage of the Family
Medicine group Quartier Latin
Associate Professor
Family Medicine Department
University of Montreal
Montreal, QC, Canada

Joseph Torresi MBBS, B.Med.Sci, FRACP, PhD
Associate Professor
Department of Infectious Diseases
Austin Hospital
The University of Melbourne
Heidelberg, VIC, Australia

Thomas H. Valk MD, MPH
President
VEI, Incorporated
Marshall, VA, USA

Eric L. Weiss MD, DTM&H
Associate Clinical Professor
Emergency Medicine & Infectious Diseases
Stanford University School of Medicine
Stanford, USA

Ursula Wiedermann MD, PhD
Professor
Head of Institute of Specific Prophylaxis
and Tropical Medicine
Medical University of Vienna
Vienna, Austria

Annelies Wilder-Smith MD, PhD, MIH, DTM&H
Mercator Professor
Director of Teaching
Institute of Public Health
University of Heidelberg
Heidelberg, Germany

Mary E. Wilson MD
Associate Professor
Department of Global Health and
Population
Harvard School of Public Health
Boston, MA, USA

Acknowledgements

The authors wish to thank Deborah Russell and Louise Cook from Elsevier, whose vision, enthusiasm, and dedication helped to bring the first edition of this book to fruition. Similarly, we wish to thank Nani Clansey, also from Elsevier, who with humor and thoughtfulness has faithfully remained our continuous connection throughout all the editions of this book, and Vinod Kumar Iyyappan, who has been so helpful in the preparation of this edition.

Above all, we wish to thank our families and our partners for their everlasting patience and understanding that have allowed us to put in the time and effort to make this textbook a success.

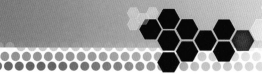
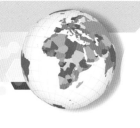

1

Introduction to Travel Medicine

Phyllis E. Kozarsky and Jay S. Keystone

Key points

- Despite the global economic situation, international travel is predicated to increase steadily in the coming decade, especially to E Asia and SE Asia
- No longer is international travel focused only on business and pleasure. It has greatly expanded to include volunteering, medical tourism and visiting friends and relatives
- Never has the need been greater for primary care practitioners to understand the health issues of their traveling patients before travel and upon their return
- Knowledge of the epidemiology and clinical presentation of travel-related infectious diseases has been greatly enhanced by global and regional scientific networks studying many thousands of travelers before departure and those ill on return

Travel medicine, though flourishing, remains a nascent medical field with inputs from many others, such as tropical medicine, preventive medicine, infectious diseases, occupational, pediatric and emergency medicine, and migrant and military medicine. As such, most travel health practitioners do not merely practice travel health, but busy themselves daily trying to remain up to date with ever-changing issues that affect their patients. Providers have little time to attend to issues such as the changing demographics of our communities or the magnitude of world travel and migration. These are just a sample of such statistics.

In 2010 there were 940 million international tourist arrivals, up 6.6% from the previous year, when there had been an economic downturn. Meanwhile, international tourist receipts reached US $919 billion (610 billion euros). The emerging economies saw increases of almost 9% (www.unwto.org/facts, accessed 12/19/11).

Over the last 6 decades, tourism has experienced continued expansion, becoming one of the largest and fastest-growing economic sectors in the world, with many new destinations emerging. In spite of occasional challenges due to epidemics such as SARS or influenza, or the economy, there has been almost uninterrupted growth: 25 million international arrivals in 1950, 277 million in 1980, 675 million in 2000 and now 940 million (Figure 1.1 and Table 1.1, accessed from www.unto.org/facts 12/19/11).

In 2010 travel for leisure accounted for about 51% of travel; business and professional reasons, 15%; and 27% for travel related to religious reasons, pilgrimages, health treatments and visiting friends and relatives. Seven percent of travel was unspecified. For the first time, China rose to third position in tourist destinations, behind France and the United States. Countries such as Malaysia, Turkey and Mexico are in the top 10. The forecast is for East Asia, the Pacific, the Middle East and Africa to experience growth rates >5% per year in tourist arrivals through 2020, with long-haul travel growing faster than intraregional travel.

Why are these numbers relevant to the practitioner, and particularly to the primary care provider?

1. Because their patients are traveling internationally not only for business and pleasure, but also to volunteer (teenage voluntourists), to receive less expensive medical care abroad (medical tourists), and to visit family and friends (VFRs). We know statistically that this latter group of travelers is at the highest risk for serious diseases such as malaria and typhoid, and for hospitalization related to these illnesses.[1-3]

2. Because their patients who travel develop ailments related to their travel, and develop exacerbations of their chronic diseases while traveling.

3. Because travel medicine is preventive medicine: by learning something about travel health, one can help prevent both infectious and non-infection problems that may otherwise contribute substantially to morbidity and mortality.

In recent years, major outbreaks of mosquito-borne Chikungunya virus have led to prolonged arthritis in returned travelers from Asia;[4] drug-resistant strains of enteric bacteria in Asia and SE Asia have reduced the utility of fluoroquinolones for the management of typhoid fever and travelers' diarrhea;[5] and those receiving medical care in hospitals on the Indian subcontinent have become increasingly at risk for the acquisition of novel multidrug-resistant Enterobacteriaceae.[6] Not only are the travelers changing, so are the infections that they acquire.

The message is clear. It is important for all healthcare providers to know something of travel medicine. This textbook, now in its third edition, is not only for use by the travel clinician, but also for use by any primary care practitioner, whether family doctor or general internist. Educating providers to ask patients 'When are you traveling and to where?' is critical in order to ensure that appropriate preventive measures are taken. It may be a bit too hopeful to assume that all

©2012 Elsevier Inc
DOI: 10.1016/B978-1-4557-1076-8.00001-6

Table 1.1 World Tourism Organization Tourist Arrivals

	Base Year	Forecasts		Market share (%)		Average annual growth rate (%)
	1995	2010	2020	1995	2020	1995-2020
		(Million)				
World	565	1006	1561	100	100	4.1
Africa	20	47	77	3.6	5	5.5
Americas	110	190	282	19.3	18.1	3.8
East Asia and the Pacific	81	195	397	14.4	25.4	6.5
Europe	336	527	717	59.8	45.9	3.1
Middle East	14	36	69	2.2	4.4	6.7
South Asia	4	11	19	0.7	1.2	6.2

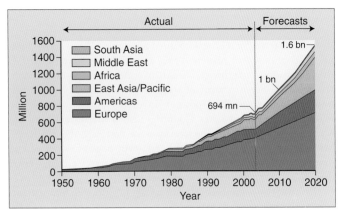

Figure 1.1 Forecast of international tourist arrivals: 2020.

primary care providers could jump into counseling their patients about the many details that can be found in this text. On the other hand, this book represents a standard reference for practitioners. They may choose to use it frequently or occasionally, and may choose to refer patients with more complex medical problems or itineraries to the ever-increasing numbers of travel clinics available (see www.istm.org for listing). Also, the question 'Did you travel, and if so, where?' should be asked of every patient. It is astounding how many individuals return from travel with medical problems that they do not realize were acquired abroad. Again, some practitioners will choose to evaluate patients who have post-travel problems; others will refer. This book is not concerned with tropical diseases, but does shed light on the triage of patients with a variety of common problems encountered following travel.

Since the first edition of this book in 2003, there have been many changes in the field. Resources are increasing and opportunities for training and practicing are increasing. The International Society of Travel Medicine (ISTM), started in 1991, has grown to more than 2500 members worldwide, including physicians, nurses, public health practitioners, and an increasing number of pharmacists. They sponsor their own as well as co-sponsoring conferences with a variety of geographic sites, speakers and participants. National and regional societies have emerged, grown, and support smaller conferences. Opportunities for education have increased both within travel clinics for individuals and within conferences that focus on other aspects in medicine and nursing. Experts in travel medicine host their own courses around the globe and degree programs have developed. The ISTM now administers the examination leading to the Certificate in Travel Health (CTH)

annually, and the Society has developed a mandatory CTH maintenance structured around a 10-year cycle of continuous professional development. The *Journal of Travel Medicine* has developed its niche as a focus for publication of this unique body of information. The listserv TravelMed is remarkably active in bringing together new providers and experts in a low-key format where all aspects of the field are discussed. Authoritative bodies such as the World Health Organization (WHO), the National Travel Health Network and Center in Great Britain (NaTHNaC), the US Centers for Disease Control and Prevention (CDC), and others publish their own health guidance, both in book form and electronically. Information is shared in ways that it has not been previously, resulting in, for example, harmonization of yellow fever vaccine recommendations.

In order to improve the evidence base in travel medicine, sophisticated surveillance networks have matured and have been publishing trends in travel-related infections. GeoSentinel, funded primarily by a cooperative agreement between the ISTM and CDC, currently has over 50 surveillance sites around the world and works collaboratively with EuroTravNet, a group in partnership with the European Centre for Disease Prevention and Control (ECDC). Together and with others, their networking and research capacity continually increases.

In response to the growth of the field and the expansion in the kinds of practitioners, this edition of *Travel Medicine* has been enhanced in a number of ways. Chapters on standard topics contained in the body of knowledge and the key points beginning each chapter remain, though the chapters have been significantly updated. There is still an effort to use graphs, pictorials, and algorithms to amplify learning. New to the book are sections on displaced persons and healthcare and disaster relief workers. Chapters on medical tourism and mass gatherings, both gaining in importance, have been added. Travelers' thrombosis, serious and unfortunately not uncommon in association with long flights, is addressed as well. To simplify reading, the section on vaccination was divided differently so that routine adult vaccines are separated from special adult travel vaccines, and all chapters have been strengthened by the addition of websites that may be accessed for further reading, clarification or updating of information. In addition, for the new travel medicine practitioner we have provided checklists to assist in risk assessment, as well as websites that supply examples of handouts for travelers themselves.

Although the field is growing and there is greater awareness of travel medicine, the importance of education of the healthcare provider and the public cannot be underestimated. Statistics continue to show that only about 50% of people traveling to developing countries access pre-travel health advice. Efforts to educate at every level of medical training are ongoing. Nurses' coalitions are working to advance their education, and so are pharmacists. The 2012 edition of *Travel Medicine* is an essential tool for all healthcare providers – for those in public health and for those in practice, whether they see many patients or few. It may be one of the more important texts remaining on the shrinking book shelf.

References

1. Jones CA, Keith LG. Medical tourism and reproductive outsourcing: the dawning of a new paradigm for healthcare. Int J Fertil Womens Med 2006;51:251–5.

2. Leder K, Tong L, Weld L, et al, for the GeoSentinel Surveillance Network. Illness in travelers visiting friends and relatives: A review of the GeoSentinel Surveillance Network. Clin Infect Dis 2006;43:1185–93.

3. Snyder J, Dharamsi S, Crooks VA. Fly-By medical care: Conceptualizing the global and local social responsibilities of medical tourists and physician voluntourists. Global Health 2011;7(1):6.

4. Taubitz W, Cramer JP, Kapaun A, et al. Chikungunya fever in travelers: Clinical presentation and course. Clin Infect Dis 2007;45:e1–4.

5. Lindgren MM, Kotilainen P, Huovinen P, et al. Reduced fluoroquinolone susceptibility in salmonella enterica isolates from travelers. Finland Emerging Infectious Diseases 2009;15:809–12.

6. Moellering Jr RC. NDM-1—a cause for worldwide concern. N Engl J Med 2010;363:2377–79.

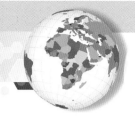

2

Epidemiology: Morbidity and Mortality in Travelers

Robert Steffen and Sandra Grieve

Key points

- Travel health risks are dependent on the itinerary, duration and season of travel, purpose of travel, lifestyle, and host characteristics
- Motor vehicle injuries and drowning are the major causes of preventable deaths in travelers, while malaria remains the most frequent cause of infectious disease deaths
- Complications of cardiovascular conditions are a major cause of death in travelers, particularly when senior citizens spend the winter in southern destinations
- Travelers' diarrhea (TD) remains the most frequent illness among travelers; the risk of TD can be divided into three risk categories based on destination
- Casual sex without the regular use of condom protection continues to be common practice by travelers

Introduction

Compared to staying at home, mortality and morbidity are increased in those who travel, especially when their destination is a developing country. Travel health risks vary greatly according to:

Where

- industrialized versus developing countries
- city or highly developed resort versus off-the-tourist-trail

When

- season of travel, e.g., rainy versus dry

How long

- duration of stay abroad

For what purpose

- tourism versus business versus rural work versus visiting friends or relatives (VFR)
- other (military, airline crew layover, adoption, etc.)

Style

- hygiene standard expected: high (e.g., multistar hotels) versus low (e.g., low-budget backpackers)
- special activities: high-altitude trekking, diving, hunting, camping, etc.

Host characteristics

- healthy versus pre-existing condition, non-immune versus (semi)-immune
- age, e.g., infants, senior travelers.

This chapter will concentrate on the available epidemiological data associated with travel health risks in general; it will not describe the epidemiology of individual diseases at the destinations. Such data are often unsatisfactory because they are incomplete, old, or were generated in studies that may have been biased. Lastly, visitors often experience far less exposure to pathogens than the native population, e.g., with respect to hepatitis B, typhoid. Thus, seroepidemiological data from destination countries are usually of little relevance when assessing the risk in travelers. Among the infectious health risks, only those about which travel-related incidence rates have been published will be mentioned. The reader should consult current websites and tropical medicine textbooks for information about less common travel-related infections, such as trypanosomiasis.

Cornerstones of Travel Health Epidemiology

As shown in Figure 2.1, health problems in travelers are frequent. Three out of four Swiss travelers to developing countries had some health impairment, defined as having taken any therapeutic medication, or having reported being ill. At first glance, this proportion is alarming, but 50% of short-term travelers who crossed the North Atlantic had health impairments, most often constipation.[1] According to other surveys, 22–64% of Finnish, Scottish or American travelers reported some health problem, usually dependent on the destination, and sometimes the season. A larger follow-up study shows that only a few of these self-reported health problems were severe. Less than 10% of travelers to developing countries consulted a doctor either abroad or after returning home, or were confined to bed due to travel-related illness or an accident; <1% were hospitalized, usually only for a few days.[1] However, it remains disturbing that >14% of such travelers are incapacitated. The most tragic consequence of travel is death abroad, which occurs in approximately 1/100 000. Sudden cardiac death, defined as an 'unexpected, non-traumatic death that occurs within 24 h of the onset of symptoms', has been shown to account for up to 52% of deaths during downhill skiing and 30% of mountain hiking fatalities[2] (Fig. 2.2).

©2012 Elsevier Inc
DOI: 10.1016/B978-1-4557-1076-8.00002-8

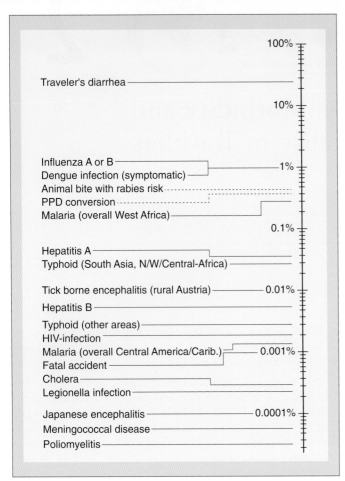

Figure 2.1 Incidence rates/month of health problems during a stay in developing countries – 2011. *(Updated 2011 from materials published in 2008.)*

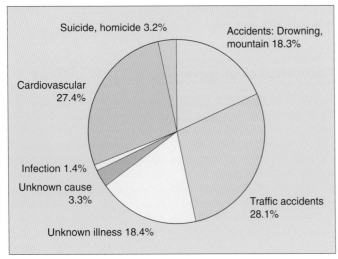

Figure 2.2 Fatalities among French abroad 2000 – 2004. *(Jeannel D, Allain-loos S, Bonmarin I, et al. Bull Epid Heb 2006/no 23–24/p166–8.)*

A study based on medical insurance claims among World Bank staff and consultants demonstrates that business travel may also pose health risks beyond exposure to infectious diseases, and that medical claims are increasing with the increasing frequency of travel.[3] Such data illustrate how non-infectious problems also play a significant role.

Mortality

At first sight, data on the primary cause of deaths abroad appear contradictory. While some studies claim that accidents are the leading cause of death, others demonstrate the predominance of cardiovascular events.[4] These differences are due primarily to the varied examined populations and destinations. Southern Europe, Florida and parts of the Caribbean are favorite destinations for senior travelers, in whom elevated mortality rates due to a variety of natural causes are to be expected, whereas in developing destinations the risk of fatal accidents is clearly higher. In the 13 years between 1999 and 2011 there were 104 recorded deaths in the GeoSentinel global network, which captures trends in travel related morbidity. Similar to Steffen's data, malaria is prominent, along with sepsis, pulmonary syndromes including pneumonia and tuberculosis, and acute encephalitis. Underlying illnesses are also significant cofactors, such as cardiovascular disease, AIDS, diabetes mellitus and cancers (personal communication, Pauline Han, September 2011). One of the limitations of GeoSentinel data is that the providers are generally experts in tropical and travel medicine and thus would not typically be in a position to see patients following trauma, motor vehicle accidents or other ailments unrelated to infectious diseases; thus, infectious diseases would be over-represented.

Accidents

Deaths abroad due to injuries are two to three times higher in 15–44-year-old travelers than in the same age group in industrialized countries.[4] Fatal accidents are primarily due to motor vehicle injury. There are fewer than 20 deaths per 100 000 motor vehicles[5] per annum reported in most Western European countries, compared to 15 in the US, 20–71 in Eastern Europe, 9–67 in Asia and 20–118 in Africa. Motorbikes are frequently implicated (partly because in many countries there is no obligation to wear a helmet), and alcohol often plays a role. Tourists are reported to be several times more likely than local drivers are to be involved in accidents.[6]

Drowning is also a major cause of death and accounts for 16% of all deaths (due to injuries) among US travelers. Reasons include alcohol intoxication, the presence of unrecognized currents or undertow, and being swept out to sea.

Kidnapping and homicides have been increasing, but these are usually limited to employees of international and non-governmental organizations. Fatal assaults on tourists and terrorism may occur anywhere, not only in developing countries.

Animals are a relatively uncommon cause of death among travelers. There are now some 50 annual confirmed shark attacks worldwide and the number is rising, possibly due to neoprene wetsuits, which allow the wearer to stay longer in colder water where the risk is greater.[7] Among safari tourists in South Africa, three tourists were killed by wild mammals in a 10-year period, two by lions after the individuals left their vehicle to approach them. The number of fatal snakebites is estimated to be 40 000 worldwide (mainly in Nigeria and India), but few victims are travelers.

A broad variety of toxins may also be a risk to travelers. Ciguatoxin leading to ciguatera syndrome after the consumption of tropical reef fish is a major risk: the case fatality is 0.1–12%. 'Body-packing' of heroin, cocaine and other illicit drugs in the gastrointestinal tract or in the vagina may result in the death of travelers when the condoms or other packages break. Fatal toxic reactions and life-threatening neurological symptoms after the inappropriate and frequent application of highly concentrated N, N-diethyl-m-toluamide (DEET, now called N, N-diethyl-3-methylbenzamide) in small children have rarely been observed. Lead-glazed ceramics purchased abroad may result in lead poisoning and could remain undetected for a long period of time.

Infectious Diseases

Malaria is the most frequent cause of infectious death among travelers. Between 1989 and 1995, 373 fatalities due to malaria were reported in nine European countries, with 25 deaths in the US.[8] This was almost exclusively due to *P. falciparum*, the case fatality rate ranging from 0% to 3.6%, depending on the country.

Among deaths due to infectious diseases, HIV previously held a prominent place, although it did not appear in the statistics as it is a late consequence of infection abroad and may not be recognized as having been acquired during previous travel. With modern treatment options and post-exposure prophylaxis, mortality associated with HIV infection abroad has decreased. HIV patients have a higher risk of complications while traveling, which ultimately may be fatal.[9]

There is a multitude of other infections that may result in the death of a traveler. There are anecdotal reports about fatal influenza, mainly among older adults participating in cruises. Rabies, if untreated, has a case fatality rate of almost 100%. Overall, however, fatal infections in the traveler can be quite effectively prevented. Two cases of West Nile virus (WNV) were reported in Dutch travelers returning from Israel [10] and one Canadian traveler died of WNV infection after a visit to New York, but not a single traveler's death has been documented as having been associated with bioterrorism or Creutzfeld–Jakob disease acquired abroad.

Non-Infectious Diseases

Senior travelers in particular may experience a new illness, or complications of a pre-existing illness. Of particular concern are cardiovascular conditions.[4] Evidence has also been generated to support the fact that pulmonary embolism associated with deep vein thrombosis occurs after long-distance air travel at a rate of about 5 per million travelers, and many of these cases are fatal. Severe symptomatic pulmonary embolism in the period immediately after travel is extremely rare after flights of less than 8 hours. In flights over 12 hours the rate is 5 per million. Risk factors for this have been clearly identified.[11]

Aeromedical Evacuation

Accounts on repatriation are instructive, as they are a mirror of serious health problems, many of which are not reported otherwise. Some 50% of aeromedical evacuations are due to accidents, often involving the head and spine, and 50% are due to illness. In the latter group, cardio- or cerebrovascular and gastrointestinal problems are the most frequent causes. Psychiatric problems have decreased as a reason for air evacuation. The reason is unknown, but it may be that worldwide communication has improved dramatically, so emotional assistance from home is more easily accessed.

Morbidity

Travelers' Diarrhea

Classic travelers' diarrhea (TD) is defined as three or more unformed stools per 24 h, with at least one accompanying symptom, such as fecal urgency, abdominal cramps, nausea, vomiting, fever, etc. Also milder forms of TD may result in incapacitation.[12]

There are three levels of risk for TD (Fig. 2.3): (1) low incidence rates (up to 8%) are seen in travelers from industrialized countries

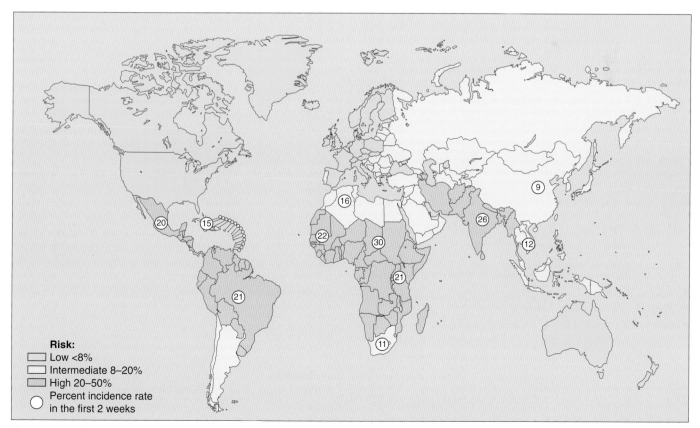

Figure 2.3 Incidence rates of travelers' diarrhea 2006–2008 (n = 2800) *(Pitzurra R. BMC Infect Dis 2010;10:231.)*

who stay for 2 weeks in Canada, the USA, most parts of Europe, or Australia and New Zealand; (2) intermediate incidence rates (8–20%) are experienced by travelers to most destinations in the Caribbean, some southern and eastern European countries, Japan and South Africa; and (3) higher incidence rates (20–66%) of TD are seen in journeys to developing countries during the first 2 weeks of stay.[12] Travelers' diarrhea is still the most frequent illness among travelers who originate from industrialized countries and visit developing countries (Fig. 2.1), whereas those who live in areas of high endemicity have a lower risk as a result of acquired immunity. Groups at particularly high risk of illness include infants, young adults, and persons with impaired gastric acid barrier; some have a genetic predisposition. TD often has a particularly severe and long-lasting course in small children. Men and women present with different profiles of travel-related morbidity. Women are proportionately more likely than men to present with urinary tract infection.[13]

Over the first decade of the 21st century the rates of TD have decreased, mainly in the developing economy countries.[14] The symptoms of TD in tourists frequently start on the third day of the stay abroad, with second episodes in 20% of cases beginning about 1 week after arrival. Untreated, the mean duration of TD is 4 days (median 2 days), and in 1% the symptoms may persist over 1 month. A total of 22% of patients show signs of mucosal invasive or inflammatory disease with fever and/or blood in the stools. Fecal leukocytes and occult blood are found positive in such feces. TD is usually caused by fecal contamination of food and beverages. The pathogens responsible for TD are described elsewhere in this volume (Chs. 18 and 20). In 1.5–10% of TD patients post-infectious irritable bowel syndrome (pIBS) may develop.[15]

Malaria

Some 20 000 malaria infections are imported annually by travelers and immigrants to industrialized nations.[8] Recently the risk has decreased in India, Latin America, and also slightly in Western Africa. Patients treated abroad are typically not included in reporting data. The proportion of *P. falciparum* infection varies depending on the destination. As shown in Figure 2.1, malaria would be a frequent diagnosis among travelers to tropical Africa if they failed to use appropriate prophylactic medication. Using existing surveillance data and the numbers of travelers to the respective destinations, the relative risk of malaria in travelers visiting such countries can be estimated. Such data will only indicate a risk per country, and not a precise destination. In the UK the majority of imported malaria occurs in VFRs who have visited West Africa.[16] The annual entomological inoculation rate clearly demonstrates broad differences within a country. This is illustrated in Kenya, with rates from 0 to 416 (at the coast locally exceeding 200), or within a city and its suburbs, such as Kinshasa, 3–612 (equivalent to two infective bites each night).[17,18]

Risk of infection is influenced not only by destination but also by:

- number of vectors
- *Anopheles* species (infected vector density)
- population density (infected population density)
- infrastructure condition (housing, water management, mosquito control)
- resistance to insecticides
- seasonality, particularly rainfall
- duration of exposure (the cumulative risk of contracting malaria is proportional to the length of stay in the transmission area)
- compliance (personal protection measures, chemoprophylaxis)

- style of travel (camping versus staying in air conditioned or well-screened urban hotel)
- host factors (such as semi-immunity, pregnancy).

These variables illustrate that it is impossible to predict the risk of malaria transmission by more than a rough order of magnitude in any specific traveler. The travel health advisor and even the traveler will often ignore at least some of these parameters. Finally, old data may have become obsolete in view of global warming: in Nairobi, in an area previously free of transmission at an elevation of 1700 m, an increasing risk of malaria is reported. Nevertheless, one can at least estimate whether a traveler will be at high or low risk.

A more detailed account of malaria epidemiology, with maps, is found in Chapter 14, where the adverse events due to prophylactic medication against malaria are discussed.

Vaccine-Preventable Infections

Updated morbidity and mortality data (Fig. 2.1) have recently been generated for vaccine-preventable diseases. It is uncertain as to what degree an observed decrease in the risk of hepatitis A is due to improved hygienic conditions at the destinations or to greater immunization rates.[14] Travel-related vaccine-preventable diseases are often divided into those that are required, routine, and recommended (see also Chs. 9 to 13). Below is a list of those as well as some of the recent epidemiology relating to the illnesses in travelers.

Required Immunizations

Yellow fever occurs only in tropical Africa and northern South America. Usually a few hundred cases are reported to WHO annually, but it is estimated that more than 100 000 cases occur. Yellow fever has never occurred in Asia, although the vectors, *Aedes* (now *Stegomyia*) and *Haemagogus*, have been observed there. Yellow fever is extremely rare in travelers, but nevertheless, cases in unvaccinated travelers have been reported in the last 10 years, despite the fact that these travelers should have been immunized.[19] Also, a number of travelers have recently been reported who died from yellow fever. Sometimes, countries will require a yellow fever vaccine certificate even though there is no risk at the destination, because the traveler has just transited (even staying in the aircraft) a yellow fever zone. Travel health advisors and travelers alike need to remain vigilant about checking on regulations through the WHO website or national guidelines that are updated frequently. Even so, countries have the capacity to alter their policies as they feel necessary.[20]

Until the early 2000s meningococcal disease was frequently observed during or after the *hajj* or *umrah* pilgrimage to Mecca (200/100 000), but this problem has been resolved by public health measures issued by the Saudi authorities. The disease is rare even in travelers staying in countries where the infection is highly endemic (0.04/100 000). The case fatality rate among travelers slightly exceeds 20%. Rarely, *Neisseria meningitidis* may be transmitted during air travel of at least 8 hours' duration.[21]

Polio vaccine for certain populations has also been recently required by the Saudi government for pilgrims to the *hajj*.

Routine Immunizations

To the authors' knowledge, a single case of tetanus was reported in a traveler several decades ago, but such cases may be hidden in national surveillance data.

As demonstrated by a large epidemic in the former Soviet Union during 1990–1997, diphtheria may flare up under specific circumstances.[22] This epidemic resulted in dozens of importations to Western Europe and North America; some travelers died while still in Russia.

Far less serious forms of cutaneous diphtheria are occasionally imported, mainly from developing countries.

Poliomyelitis has continued to be a problem in the past few years, mainly in South Asia, from where it has been exported to Central Asia, and in various countries of tropical Africa. In typical travelers, poliomyelitis has in the past decade been observed in a single VFR student returning from Pakistan to Australia. Despite the lack of documented transmission in travelers, an adult booster is recommended for travel to a number of areas where outbreaks continue to occur (www.polioeradication.org/Dataandmonitoring/Poliothisweek.aspx and www.polioeradication.org/Dataandmonitoring/Poliothisweek/Polioinfecteddistricts.aspx). In fact, the disease is being seen in countries that previously had reported no cases. Thus, WHO has developed an interactive map with the countries or areas for which it recommends polio immunization or boosting (http://apps.who.int/ithmap/).

Very few data exist on pertussis, *Haemophilus influenzae* B, measles, mumps and rubella in travelers. In view of suboptimal compliance with measles vaccination, European, African, and Asian travelers are responsible for outbreaks on the American continent, where vaccine uptake is far superior.[23] Recent reports showed a sharp rise in the number of measles cases reported in EU/EEA countries, five times more than the annual average for the preceding 5 years. These cases may be linked to travel to and from Europe, where unimmunized or non-immune travelers have come into contact with the disease or transported it.[24] Pertussis is a re-emerging disease in many areas and immunity has waned. New vaccine availability in some areas allows boosting of adults to tetanus, diphtheria, and pertussis in a single injection. Hepatitis B, now a routine immunization in most industrialized countries, is mainly a problem for expatriates living close to the local population and for travelers breaking the most basic hygiene rules; the monthly incidence is 25/100 000 for symptomatic infections; 80–420/100 000 for all infections.[25] The estimated incidence in travelers from Amsterdam to HBV-endemic countries is 4.5/100 000 travelers. While minute quantities of the virus are sufficient for transmission and the exact mode of transmission may remain undetected in many individuals, clear risk factors, such as casual unprotected sex, nosocomial transmission, etc., have often been suspected. Behavioral surveys have shown that 10–15% of travelers voluntarily or involuntarily expose themselves to blood and body fluids while abroad in high-risk countries. Besides the risk factors mentioned above, such persons have also visited dental hygienists, had acupuncture, cosmetic surgery, tattooing, ear piercing, or scarification. Travel specifically for surgical procedures abroad (medical tourism) is increasing and is highlighting the emergence of a new antibiotic resistance mechanism and associated consequences for creating a global public health problem.[26]

Recommended Immunizations

The most frequent vaccine-preventable infection in non-immune travelers to developing countries is influenza. Various outbreaks on cruise ships have been described (the usual risk groups are at risk of complications). Hepatitis A is now third, with a current average incidence rate of 30/100 000 per month. It is also the case that 'luxury' tourists staying at multistar resorts may be at risk of infection.

Typhoid fever is diagnosed with an incidence rate of 30/100 000 per month among travelers to South Asia (Pakistan, Nepal, India); elsewhere (except probably in Central and West Africa), this rate is 10 times lower. Those visiting friends and relatives import a fair proportion of these infections, but tourists originating in industrialized countries are also affected. The case fatality rate among travelers is 0–1%.

A recent paper reviewing the morbidity seen in >37 000 travelers revealed that 580 presented with vaccine-preventable diseases. Of those, the most common seen were enteric fever, acute viral hepatitis and influenza. Hospitalizations occurred with greater frequency in those diagnosed with VPD, and deaths also occurred.[27]

The risk of rabies is high in Asia (particularly in India), from where 90% of all human rabies deaths are reported, but there may be underreporting in other parts of the world. Bat rabies may occur in areas that are thought to be rabies free, such as Australia and Europe. Many among the monthly 0.2–0.4% who experience an animal bite in developing countries are at risk of rabies. Rabies is a particular risk in those who are in close contact with indigenous populations over a prolonged time, e.g., missionaries, those traveling by bicycle, those working with animals, or those who explore caves, and also children (because of their attraction to animals and their lack of reporting of bites).

Based on post-travel skin tests, the incidence rate of *M. tuberculosis* infection is 3000/100 000 person-months of travel, and 60/100 000 developed active tuberculosis. Transmission during long-haul flights and also during prolonged train and bus rides has only rarely been reported and outdoor transmission can be neglected, except if there is repeated exposure, as may occur particularly among long-term, low-budget travelers or expatriates. Bacille Calmette–Guérin vaccine is not recommended for travelers; it is still administered in some countries routinely and its major use is for the prevention of disseminated tuberculosis in children.

The risk of cholera is approximately 0.2/100 000, although asymptomatic and oligosymptomatic infections may be more frequent, as demonstrated in Japanese travelers. But as a public health issue this is irrelevant, as secondary infections do not occur.[19] The case fatality rate among travelers is <2%.

For several potentially vaccine-preventable diseases the risk of infection is <1 per million. Although a few dozen cases of Japanese encephalitis have been diagnosed in civilian travelers during the last 25 years, the attack rate in civilians is estimated to be 1 per 400 000 to <1 per million. Sixty percent of these cases occurred in tourists, including some short-term travelers to Bali and Thailand.[28,29] Only two international travelers have been diagnosed with plague since 1966. Few anecdotal reports have documented tick-borne encephalitis in international travelers, although they certainly occur in persons hiking or camping in endemic areas. Changes in climate and habitation are altering the epidemiology of tick-borne encephalitis, and the disease is now being reported from areas previously not known to be endemic.[30,31]

Other Infections

Only a few selected infections will be mentioned in this section. Those about which no more than anecdotal reports have been published will be omitted.

Sexually Transmitted Diseases

According to most surveys, casual sex, in almost 50% of cases without regular condom protection, is practiced by 4–19% of travelers while they are abroad, resulting in HIV infection and other sexually transmitted diseases (STD).[32] In Switzerland, it is estimated that 10% of HIV infections are acquired abroad. In the UK, the risk of acquiring HIV is considered to be 300 times higher while abroad, compared to staying at home. A third of heterosexuals acquired their infection in the UK; the remaining two-thirds are thought to have been acquired in sub-Saharan Africa.[33,34]

The WHO estimates that 75% of all HIV infections worldwide are sexually transmitted, and that the efficiency of transmission per sexual contact ranges from 0.1% to 1%. The transmission probability of HIV is greatly enhanced by the presence of other STD and genital lesions, as is often the case in female commercial sex workers and other infected persons in developing countries. Typically, 14–25% of cases of gonorrhea and syphilis diagnosed in Europe were imported from abroad. The first campaign targeting those over 50 years of age was launched to highlight rising STIs and poor sexual health in this age group, many of whom indulge in casual sexual activity abroad.[35]

Common Cold

This is one of the most frequent health problems, with an attack rate of 13% in short-term travelers; among them, 40% are incapacitated for an average of 2.6 days. From interviews in Chinese hospitals, there is anecdotal evidence that lower respiratory tract infections occur particularly often in this country.

Dengue

In SE Asia, the seroconversion rate of dengue in travelers is 200/100 000; this risk is clearly greater than for malaria.[36] Clearly, dengue is a re-emerging illness in many tropical and subtropical parts of the world, and surveillance systems are documenting larger numbers of returning travelers with dengue from most endemic regions.

Legionella

With easier means of diagnosis the rate of *Legionella* infections reported to Euro surveillance is continuously increasing, reaching 289 in 1999. The highest rate found among British travelers was after a stay in Turkey: 1/100 000, compared to 10 times fewer when the destination was the USA, for example.[37]

Leishmaniasis

This has frequently been described in travelers, with those infected with HIV being at particularly high risk, but to the authors' knowledge no systematic review with data has been published.

Schistosomiasis

Using newer serological tests, there are data to suggest that schistosomiasis is an infection that both long- and short-term travelers, but particularly missionaries and volunteers, acquire in endemic areas.[38] However, it is currently unknown whether or not most of these exposed travelers would ever develop the typical signs and symptoms of the disease.

Trypanosomiasis

Trypanosomiasis, in its African form, was reported in only 29 cases in the US in the 20th century, but the risk seems to be increasing.

Non-Infectious Health Problems

This covers a broad variety of problems, accidents, and illnesses, which can be divided into environment or host related.

Environmental

Travel may result in stress, particularly fear of flying – most prominent during take-off and landing – and flight delays, which are frequent causes for anxiety.[39] Motion sickness may affect up to 80% of passengers in small vessels in rough seas, but also affects passengers (albeit fewer) on jet flights. In-flight emergencies occur in 1/11 000 passengers, the most frequent ones being gastrointestinal, cardiac, neurological, vasovagal, and respiratory.

Changes in climate and altitude also create problems. In particular, high-altitude sickness (described in Ch. 39) will affect every passenger if ascent to high altitudes is rapid. Health impairments related to diving are described in Chapter 40. Other environmental issues occasionally come into play. For example, consideration should be given to long-term travelers or expatriates with chronic heart or lung disease planning on staying in regions where there is excessive air pollution.

In addition to the accidents described in the mortality section, small bruises acquired while swimming, and other marine hazards or lacerations due to sporting activities, may take longer to heal in view of supra-infection. Sprained ankles and other sports injuries are frequent, particularly among senior travelers, who tend to fall, for example, in dimly lit hotels and on stairs.

Host

Persons with pre-existing medical conditions may experience some exacerbations. This is particularly common in those with immunosuppressive illnesses, chronic constipation, diarrhea or other gastrointestinal ailments, whereas others, such as dermatological conditions or degenerative joint pain, may improve in a sunny, warm climate.[40]

Conclusion and Prioritization

In conclusion, health professionals who advise travelers need to keep the described epidemiological facts in mind when determining what preventive measures are needed. Ultimately, the decision regarding to what degree one wishes to protect future travelers is an arbitrary one; no-one should give the illusion that 'complete protection' is possible.

Prioritization, e.g., with respect to vaccines, is possible, but one ought to have concrete goals to reduce just morbidity. Immunization against influenza would be number 1 and against hepatitis A might be number 2 if there are time and financial constraints. However, even when prioritization is necessary, consideration should be given to the specific individual, his or her medical history and travel circumstances. For travelers to malaria-intense regions, despite financial limitations, chemoprophylaxis should still be strongly encouraged and doxycycline is quite inexpensive. Similarly, medication for the management of travelers' diarrhea is inexpensive, whether the choice is loperamide for treatment of symptoms or an antibiotic. In fact, some antibiotics are provided free of charge in the US. Despite the need for prioritization, educational needs do not change and efforts to provide as much information as possible are always imperative. Although these measures can certainly mitigate health problems, travel will always have some inherent additional risks compared to staying at home.

References

1. Steffen R, DeBernardis C, Banos A. Travel epidemiology – a global perspective. Int J Antimicrob Agents 2003;21:89–95.
2. Windsor JS, Firth PG, Grocott MP, et al. Mountain mortality: a review of deaths that occur during recreational activities in the mountains. Postgrad Med J 2009;85:316–21.
3. Liese B, Mundt KA, Dell LD, et al. Medical insurance claims associated with international business travel. Occup Environ Med 1997;54:499–503.
4. Tonellato DJ, Guse CE, Hargarten SW. Injury deaths of US citizens abroad: New data source, old travel problem. J Travel Med 2009;16(5):304–10.
5. Kopits E, Croper M. Traffic fatalities and economic growth. Accid Anal Prev 2005;37:169–78.
6. Dinh-Zarr TB, Hargarten SW. Road crash deaths of American travelers: the make roads safe report. An analysis of US State Department Data on Unnatural Causes of Death to US Citizens Abroad (2004–6). Chapter 6 Conveyance and Transportation issues; CDC Health Information for International Travel 2010. Atlanta: US Department of Health and Human Services, Public Health Service; 2009.
7. Woolgar JD, Cliff G, Nair R, et al. Shark attack: review of 86 consecutive cases. J Trauma 2001;50(5):887–91.
8. Muentener P, Schlagenhauf P, Steffen R. Imported malaria (1985–1995): trends and perspectives. Bull World Health Organ 1999;77(7):560–6.

9. Furrer H, Chan P, Weber R, et al. Increased risk of wasting syndrome in HIV-infected travelers: prospective multicentre study. Trans R Soc Trop Med Hyg 2001;95:484–6.

10. Aboutaleb N, Beersma M, Wunderink H, et al. Case Report: West Nile Virus infection in two Dutch travellers returning from Israel. Eurosurveillance 26 August 2010;15(34):Article 4.

11. Watson HG, Baglin TP. Guidelines on travel-related venous thrombosis. Brit J Haematol 2010;152:31–4. http://www.bcshguidelines.com/documents/travel_related_vte_bjh_2011.pdf.

12. Pitzurra R, Steffen R, Tschopp A, et al. Diarrhoea in a large cohort of European travellers to resource-limited destinations. BMC Infectious Diseases 2010;4 August;10:231 http://www.biomedcentral.com/1471–2334/10/231/abstract.

13. Schlagenhauf P, Chen LH, Wilson ME, et al. Sex and gender differences in travel-associated disease. Clini Infect Dis 2010;50:826–32.

14. Baaten GG, Sonder GJB, Schim Van Der Loeff MF, et al. 2010. Fecal-orally transmitted diseases among travelers are decreasing due to better hygienic standards at travel destination. J Travel Med Sept/Oct 2010;17(5):322–8.

15. Pitzurra R, Fried M, Rogler G, et al. Irritable bowel syndrome among a cohort of European travelers to resource-limited destinations. J Travel Med 2011 Jul;18(4):250–6.

16. Health Protection Agency. Imported malaria cases by species and reason for travel 2006–2010 2011 http://www.hpa.org.uk/web/HPAweb&HPAwebStandard/HPAweb_C/1195733783966

17. Hay SI, Rogers DJ, Toomer JF, et al. Annual Plasmodium falciparum entomological inoculation rates (EIR) across Africa: literature survey, Internet access and review. Trans R Soc Trop Med Hyg 2000;94:113–27.

18. Behrens RH, Carroll B, Hellgren U, et al. The incidence of malaria in travellers to South-East Asia: is local malaria transmission a useful risk indicator? Malar J 2010 Oct 4;9:266.

19. Steffen R, Connor B. Vaccines in travel health: from risk assessment to priorities. J Travel Med 2005;12:26–35.

20. Jentes ES, Poumerol G, Gershman MD, et al. The revised global yellow fever risk map and recommendations for vaccination, 2010: consensus of the Informal WHO Working Group on Geographic Risk for Yellow Fever. Lancet Infect Dis 2011;11(8):622–32.

21. Steffen R. The risk of meningococcal disease in travelers and current recommendations for prevention. J Travel Med 2010;17(Issue Supplement S1):9–17.

22. Cameron C, White J, Power D, et al. Diphtheria boosters for adults: balancing risks. Travel Med Infect Dis 2007;5 (1):35–9.

23. CDC. Notes from the Field: Measles Transmission Associated with International Air Travel – Massachusetts and New York, July–August 2010. MMWR 2010 August 27;59(33):1073. http://www.cdc.gov/mmwr/preview/mmwrhtml/mm5933a4.htm?s_cid=mm5933a4_w

24. European Monthly Surveillance Report Volume 1. June 2011. European Centre for Disease Prevention and Control (ECDC). http://www.ecdc.europa.eu/en/publications/Publications/Forms/ECDC_DispForm.aspx?ID=699

25. Sonder GJ, Van Rijckevorsel GG, Van Den Hoek A. Risk of Hepatitis B for travelers: Is vaccination for all travelers really necessary? J Travel Med 2009;16:18–22. doi: 10.1111/j.1708–8305.2008.00268.x

26. Kumarasamy KK, Toleman MA, Walsh TR. Emergence of a new antibiotic resistance mechanism in India, Pakistan, and the UK: a molecular, biological, and epidemiological study. Lancet Infect Dis September 2010;10(9):597–602.

27. Boggild AK, Castelli F, Gautret P, et al; GeoSentinel Surveillance Network. Vaccine preventable diseases in returned international travelers: results from the GeoSentinel Surveillance Network. Vaccine 2010 Oct 28;28(46):7389–95.

28. Hills SL, Griggs AC, Fischer M. Japanese encephalitis in travelers from non-endemic countries, 1973-2008. Am J Trop Med Hyg 2010;82(5):930–6.

29. Tappe D, Nemecek A, Zipp F, et al. Two laboratory-confirmed cases of Japanese encephalitis imported to Germany by travelers returning from Southeast Asia. J Clin Virol. 2012;54(3):282–5.

30. Suss J, Klaus C, Gerstengarbe FW, Werner PC. 2008. What makes ticks tick? Climate change, ticks, and tick-borne diseases. J Travel Med 2008 Jan-Feb;15(1):39–45.

31. Vaccines against tick-borne encephalitis: WHO position paper. 10 June 2011 WER No 24 2011;86:241–56 http://www.who.int/wer

32. Richen J. Sexually transmitted infections and HIV among travellers: A review. Travel Med Infect Dis 2006;4:184–95.

33. Health Protection Agency. Table 4: Number of selected STI diagnoses made at genitourinary medicine clinics in the UK and England: 2000–2009 http://www.hpa.org.uk/web/HPAwebFile/HPAweb_C/1215589013442

34. Health Protection Agency. HIV in the United Kingdom: 2010 Report. Health Protection Report 2010;4(47). http://www.hpa.org.uk/web/HPAwebFile/HPAweb_C/1287145367237

35. Family Planning. Association (FPA) warns of rising STIs and poor sexual health in the over 50s. http://www.fpa.org.uk/pressarea/pressreleases/2010/september/fpa-warns-of-rising-stis-and-poor-sexual-health-in-the-over-50s

36. Freedman DO, Weld LH, Kozarsky PE, et al. Spectrum of disease and relation to place of exposure among ill returned travelers. N Engl J Med 2006;354:119–30.

37. Joseph CA, Ricketts KD, Yadav R, et al, on behalf of the European Working Group for Legionella Infections. Travel-associated Legionnaires disease in Europe in 2009. Eurosurveillance 14 October 2010;15(41). http://www.eurosurveillance.org/ViewArticle.aspx?ArticleId=19683

38. Nicolls DJ, Weld LH, Schwartz E, et al, for the GeoSentinel Surveillance Network. Characteristics of schistosomiasis in travelers reported to the GeoSentinel Surveillance Network 1997–2008. Am J Trop Med Hyg 2008 Nov;79(5):729–34.

39. Oakes M, Bor R. The psychology of fear of flying (part I): A critical evaluation of current perspectives on the nature, prevalence and etiology of fear of flying. Travel Med Infect Dis 2010;8(6):327–38.

40. Carroll B, Daniel A, Behrens RH. Travel Health part 1: Preparing the tropical traveller. Brit J Nursing 2008;17(16):1046–51.

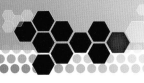
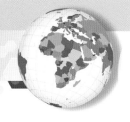

Starting, Organizing, and Marketing a Travel Clinic

David R. Hill and Gail Rosselot

Key points

- Whether a travel health program is standalone or part of another practice, it requires trained personnel and specialized supplies and equipment to provide such services
- Keeping up to date with country-specific health information that may change rapidly is key to providing pre-travel healthcare
- Depending upon the country or individual states within the US, nurses and nurse practitioners, as well as pharmacists, may be able to be primary providers of pre-travel healthcare. Ensure compliance with professional regulations.
- A travel clinic needs to determine whether or not to provide post-travel services. If not, then it is important to be aware of specialist health providers that can handle referrals
- Even with good foresight, the provision of telephone consultations, e-mail services, imminent travel and appropriate fees for service provision remain challenges

Introduction

The delivery of travel medicine services has evolved over the past 30 years. Traditionally, it has occurred in primary care or in specialized travel clinics. However, in the last decade there has been an expansion into other healthcare settings, such as occupational health, college health, walk-in clinics, emergency departments, supermarkets and pharmacies.[1] This chapter will outline the key steps necessary to establish a travel medicine practice. The principles outlined can be applied by practitioners to a variety of settings throughout the world.

The body of knowledge in travel medicine is sufficiently different from general medicine, infectious diseases and tropical medicine, that it is best practiced by healthcare personnel who have been trained in the field, who are seeing travelers on a regular basis, are constantly updating their knowledge, and who have the information and resources to provide pre-travel care.[2]

Those who provide travel medicine need to have up-to-date information on the geography of illness, be able to administer a full panel of immunizations against both common and uncommon vaccine-preventable diseases, and access recommendations of the World Health Organization (WHO), or national bodies such as the United States

(US) Centers for Disease Control and Prevention (CDC), and the United Kingdom National Travel Health Network and Centre (NaTHNaC). If a travel health service can provide this level of expert care, it will distinguish itself from a generalist's office and increase the value of the service to the traveling public (Table 3.1).

Administering immunizations without undertaking a complete risk assessment of the traveler and their planned activities, and not giving other comprehensive preventive advice, is not providing an appropriate level of service.[2] All travelers should receive up-to-date advice on avoiding travel-related illness, health counseling for self-care of any chronic medical conditions, required or recommended immunizations for their trip, and information about health and safety resources at their destination (Table 3.2). Those who provide a travel health service can follow the guidance as outlined in this chapter and book.

The Practice of Travel Medicine

An examination of the practice of travel medicine can help define those elements that are necessary for the establishment of a new travel clinic. There has been no comprehensive survey of travel medicine practice throughout the world since a 1994 survey of the membership of the International Society of Travel Medicine.[3] This survey demonstrated that, even in 1994, travel medicine was practiced in a variety of settings by professionals with a wide range of training and experience in the discipline. A few themes emerged. Nearly all clinics were from North America, Western Europe and Australia (94%). Most clinics saw only a modest number of patients: fewer than 20 patients/week were seen by 61% of clinics (14% saw less than two patients/week), and only 13% saw more than 100 patients/week.

Nearly all clinics provided advice about malaria, insect avoidance, and the prevention and treatment of travelers' diarrhea, and most administered a wide range of vaccines. Although clinics were usually directed by physicians at that time, advice and care were rendered nearly equally by physicians and nurses. In many countries today, nurses provide the majority of pre-travel care. For example, in the UK most pre-travel care is delivered in general practice and the practice nurse is usually the sole provider, giving advice under the direction of specific protocols.[4,5]

Where are travelers going (Fig. 3.1)? Data from the World Tourism Organization indicate that for the 940 million international arrivals during the year 2010, Europe continued to be the most frequent destination (50.7%), but China was the third most visited country,

DOI: 10.1016/B978-1-4557-1076-8.00003-X

Table 3.1 Benefits of a Travel Medicine Service

Comprehensive pre-travel care (see Table 3.2)

Knowledgeable and experienced providers (see Table 3.3)

Up-to-date advice (in verbal and written form) on a wide range of travel-related health risks

Access to current epidemiologic resources and opinion of expert bodies

Availability of immunizations against all vaccine-preventable illnesses

Provision of medications/prescriptions for self-treatment/ prevention of travelers' diarrhea, malaria and environmental illness

Post-travel screening and referral

Table 3.2 Elements of a Travel Medicine Practice: Services

Assessing the health of the traveler[a]
    Underlying medical conditions and allergies
    Immunization history
Assessing the health risk of travel
    Itinerary
    Duration
    Reason for travel
    Planned activities
Preventive advice[b]
    Vaccine-preventable illness
    Travelers' diarrhea prevention and self-treatment
    Malaria prevention
    Other vector-borne and water-borne illness
    Personal safety and behavior
    Environmental illness: altitude, heat, cold
    Animal bites and rabies avoidance
    Management of special health needs during travel
    Travel medical kits
    Travel health and medical evacuation insurance
    Access to medical care overseas
Vaccination
Post-travel assessment

[a]Permanent records should be maintained.
[b]Advice should be given both verbally and in brief written form to reinforce concepts and aid in the recall of information. Referral to authoritative online resources is also helpful.

and many new destinations emerged in Asia, the Pacific and the Middle East.[6]

Starting a Travel Health Program

Frequently Asked Questions

Who Is Qualified to Offer Travel Health Services?

All providers should be trained in travel medicine (Table 3.3). There is ample evidence that healthcare practitioners who are not familiar with the field of travel medicine make errors in judgment and advice, particularly about the prevention of malaria.[7–11] These errors can lead to adverse outcomes for travelers, such as malaria cases and deaths in travelers who were advised to take no or incorrect chemoprophylaxis.[12,13]

Training includes education and experience. A study of general practitioners who provided travel medicine care in Germany

Table 3.3 Elements of a Travel Medicine Practice: Provider Qualifications

Knowledge[a]
Geography
    Travel-associated infectious diseases: epidemiology, transmission, prevention
    Travel-related drugs and vaccines: indications, contraindications, pharmacology, drug interactions, adverse events
    Non-infectious travel risks both medical and environmental: prevention and management
    Recognition of major syndromes in returned travelers: e.g., fever, diarrhea, rash, and respiratory illness
    Access to travel medicine resources: texts, articles, internet resources
Experience
    6 months in a travel clinic with at least 10–20 pre-travel consultations/week
Initial training and continuing education
    Short or long courses in travel medicine
    Membership in specialty society dealing with travel and tropical medicine, e.g., the International Society of Travel Medicine and national societies
    Attendance at national and international travel medicine meetings

[a]Knowledge can be formally assessed by the ISTM Certificate of Knowledge exam or by examination in Diploma or Masters level travel medicine courses.

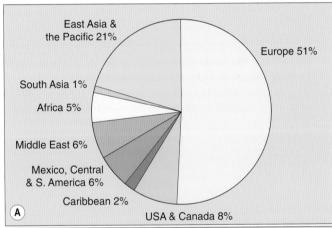

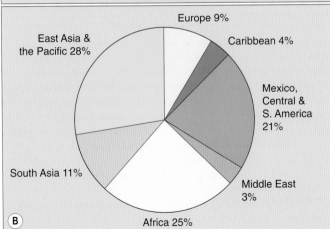

Figure 3.1 **(A)** International arrivals for all world travelers for the year 2010 (n = 940 million). Data from the World Tourism Organization (http://www.unwto.org/facts/menu.html). **(B)** Destinations for travelers receiving pre-travel care at the International Traveler's Medical Service at the University of Connecticut, USA, from January, 1984 through December, 2002 (n = 14,718 travelers).

demonstrated a correlation between giving preventive advice on important topics with specific training in the discipline.[14] The Dutch National Coordination Center for Traveler's Health Advice (LCR) found that the quality of providers improved when they were registered with a national body, took courses and followed national guidelines.[15] Although there is an international exam that certifies knowledge in the field of travel medicine (the International Society of Travel Medicine (ISTM) Certificate of Knowledge exam), as well as a Faculty that recognizes expertise and accomplishment (Faculty of Travel Medicine, Royal College of Physicians and Surgeons, Glasgow: http://www.rcpsg.ac.uk/Travel%20Medicine/Pages/mem_spweltravmed.aspx), there is currently no requirement that those who practice in the field have such qualifications or recognition.

What Can Healthcare Professionals Do to Develop Expertise in Travel Health?

The Canadian Committee to Advise on Tropical Medicine and Travel (CATMAT) and the Infectious Diseases Society of America (IDSA) have defined the important elements of a travel health consultation in their respective guidelines on the practice of travel medicine.[2,16] Travel health providers should have the requisite knowledge, training and experience to deliver these key components of the visit: risk assessment of the traveler and their trip, provision of advice about prevention and management of travel-related disease (both infectious and non-infectious), the administration of vaccines, and recognition of key syndromes in returned travelers (Table 3.2). In order to develop the necessary knowledge, clinicians can attend travel health conferences, enroll in short courses, or pursue a certificate or degree in travel medicine. The ISTM (http://www.istm.org/) and American Travel Health Nurses Association (ATHNA) (http://www.athna.org/) publish calendars of courses and conferences on their websites.

CDC offers free online training programs. The Royal College of Physicians and Surgeons (Glasgow) runs a diploma level course in travel medicine (http://www.rcpsg.ac.uk/Travel%20Medicine/Pages/Foundation_and%20_Diploma_in_Travel_Medicine_%20Courses.aspx), and there are several Masters' level training courses offered in Europe. In addition to the ISTM certificate of knowledge in travel medicine the American Society of Tropical Medicine and Hygiene (ASTMH) administers an examination leading to a certificate of knowledge in tropical and travel medicine.[17,18]

Experience in a travel clinic setting is the other component leading to competence in travel medicine. It is only with regular assessment of travelers who have multiple health conditions, and are planning a wide variety of travel destinations and activities, that one can gain broad competence in the field. Spending time in an established clinic can be invaluable, and competency maintained by regularly performing pre-travel consultations.

Providers are also encouraged to join national societies that are devoted to travel medicine. These will often provide courses, publish newsletters with travel medicine alerts, and link members through discussion groups. Most importantly, anyone working in this specialty must make a personal commitment to ongoing learning, as global health risks are always changing. See Chapter 4: Resources for additional professional development opportunities.

Are There Different Models of Care Delivery?

Most practices of travel medicine have both physicians and nurses participating in the care of patients. The specialty of travel medicine is ideally suited to the involvement of nurses, nurse practitioners, and physician assistants. Increasingly, pharmacists are providing these services, although the pathways toward recognition of pharmacists are not well delineated.[20] Given the variety of providers,

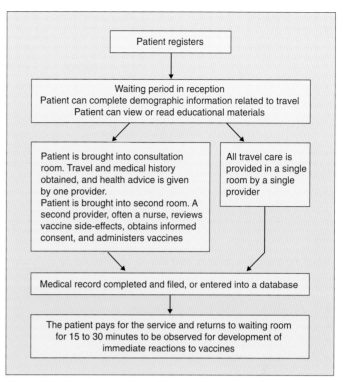

Figure 3.2 A flow diagram for patient care in a travel medicine clinic. Two options are presented: two-provider or single-provider care.

each practice will need to decide how to divide the responsibilities.

For clinics in which both physicians and nurses provide care, there are two general models (Fig. 3.2). In the first, the physician obtains the travel itinerary, planned activities, and the patient's medical and immunization history. The physician then gives the health advice, and decisions are made in conjunction with the travelers as to recommended immunizations. The care of the patient is then transferred to a nurse (or to a person who has competency to administer vaccines), who reviews vaccine adverse events, obtains informed consent, and administers the vaccines. After giving the vaccines, they record vaccine administration information in either a paper or electronic medical record (EMR).

In the second model, the nurse, nurse practitioner, or physician assistant provides the complete pre-travel care, from the medical and travel history, to preventive advice, to administration, and recording of vaccines.

In the UK, this model of independent care rendered by nurses is supported by a legal framework known as Patient Group Directions (PGD). These require a clear and detailed written protocol that is agreed and signed by doctors, nurses, and pharmacists. The document details the indications and situations when a nurse can select, prescribe and administer a prescription-only medication (e.g., vaccine or antimalarial) without recourse to a physician. The PGD requires that the nurse receive appropriate training, updating, and audit of practice.

In US practices where a health professional without prescribing privileges, such as a registered nurse, is the sole provider of care, it is necessary to develop detailed protocols to follow. These should be clinic specific (reflecting the standard of care within the region) and in written form with standing orders for administering vaccines and obtaining prescriptions.[19]

In the future it is anticipated that another model of care will be pharmacy based as pharmacists in the UK, US, Canada, and other countries expand their training and professional role in pre-travel care.[21]

Are There Specific Laws, Health Regulations, and Standards that Affect Travel Healthcare?

Regulations that apply to travel clinics and personnel have increased in recent years. These may include health professional licensing laws, malpractice issues, national, state or provincial regulations, and organizational or institutional requirements. For example, can a nurse provide both patient assessment and vaccinations? Does the clinic need an on-site physician? How is yellow fever (YF) vaccination status certified? Are pharmacists allowed to immunize in your community? This is more fully discussed under 'Legal Issues' later in this chapter.

What Policies, Procedures and Resources Should Be in Place?

Before a clinic schedules its first patient, certain protocols and support services should be in place:

- Anaphylaxis and management of vaccine adverse events
- Emergency vaccine storage: in the event of a power failure
- Needlestick and HIV post-exposure prophylaxis
- Immunization documentation
- Infection control and hazardous waste disposal
- Vaccine Information Statements (US CDC publications), or equivalent) (http://www.cdc.gov/vaccines/pubs/vis/)
- Use of consents and waivers
- Vaccine adverse event reporting systems
- Standing orders (or equivalent) for vaccinations
  - Over time, the clinic will need to add to these protocols and develop a full policy and procedure manual. A resource for travel clinic protocols in the US is the ATHNA Clinic Manual available at www.ATHNA.org and Immunization Action Coalition (IAC) at www.immunize.org
- A dedicated vaccine-grade refrigerator
- An individual who is identified as the Immunization Coordinator.

Is Special Documentation Required?

There may be national, local or institutional regulations that apply to immunization records. The US National Childhood Vaccine Injury Act (NCVIA) and CDC mandate certain vaccination documentation.[22,23] For efficiency, completeness, and to meet current quality standards, it is advisable to use pre-printed documents (or EMR equivalent) when offering pre-travel care.

What Support Services Are Needed?

In some settings, healthcare professionals provide all the services of a pre-travel consultation, including ordering and stocking supplies, taking phone calls, appointment-making, billing, and providing the full range of clinical care. In most practices, however, clinicians provide clinical care, and administrative staff manage other aspects of the service, such as processing the required documents and payment requests from insurance companies.

Should A Clinic Offer Travel Health Services Full-Time? What Are the Best Times for Clinical Sessions?

When starting a clinic it can take time to build patient volume. It may be advisable to start by incorporating a few visits per week and then adding appointments as clinician expertise and patient demand increase. Many travelers will seek care at the last minute and during non-working or non-school hours. If they can be covered, early morning, late afternoon, evening, and weekend appointments are popular.

What Vaccines Should Be Provided? Should the Clinic Offer YF Vaccine?

Many clinicians are knowledgeable about routine adult and childhood vaccines but are not familiar with travel vaccines. Some clinicians will start by offering only a few vaccines, such as influenza, hepatitis A and B, tetanus, polio and typhoid. Others will want to offer comprehensive care and provide all the travel immunizations licensed in their country. Regarding YF vaccination, under International Health Regulations (2005) 'State parties shall designate specific YF vaccination centres within their territories in order to assure the quality and safety of the procedures and materials employed'.[24] Many countries have a specific procedure that must be followed before becoming a YF vaccinating center. See Legal Issues for more information about this process.

How Much Time Should Be Set Aside for Appointments?

Ideally, a pre-travel risk assessment, counseling and vaccine appointment would be allotted 45–60 minutes. In reality, most appointments do not exceed 30 minutes, and when a travel medicine service is integrated into primary care or a pharmacy setting, it may be less. Two-thirds of visits to UK YF vaccination clinics are allotted only 11–20 minutes.[25] If possible, scheduling can be based on the complexity of the itinerary and traveler. Some travelers need multiple visits for further assessment, extended counseling (e.g., families with young children moving abroad), or when multi-dose vaccines are administered.

How Should A Clinic Determine Service Charges?

Around the world charges are handled in different ways. In the US, few private insurers fully reimburse travel healthcare services, and therefore many clinics operate on a fee-for-service basis, with considerable variation in visit and vaccination charges. In order to avoid potential conflicts with managed care contracts, US clinics will need to learn about applicable billing rules. Many clinics issue three charges for a visit: the consultation fee or visit charge, the vaccine charge, and a vaccine administration charge. In primary care settings in the UK, the consultation is not billable as it is considered a free NHS service; however, charges can be made for certain vaccines. Retail sales of travel items such as repellent and mosquito nets can generate additional income.

What Is It Going to Cost to Establish a Travel Health Program?

Travel services that operate within an existing clinic or primary care service can be established with minimal additional investments. The vaccine refrigerator and vaccine supply are two of the largest costs, but careful equipment selection and maintaining a small vaccine inventory can keep these costs to a minimum. Many services will already have a vaccine refrigerator. Each consultation room should have computer access. Subscription to a commercial travel medicine database is also popular.

Organizing a Clinic: Facilities, Equipment, Supplies

Travel health clinics can often function with the same space, equipment, and supplies as for any setting that offers immunizations. The ISTM, ATHNA, and IAC can provide additional guidance to prepare an office to provide travel healthcare.[26]

Facilities

At a minimum, clinics need an area for reception, a private room for consultation and vaccine administration that has a computer with internet access, space for a refrigerator, and storage areas for supplies and clinic records. Busy clinics will have dedicated space with separate consultation and vaccine administration rooms. Travel clinics that are located in hospitals or within a medical school or group practice will typically have access to on-site laboratory testing.

Equipment

Refrigerator and Freezer: A dedicated vaccine refrigerator capable of maintaining vaccines at storage temperatures of 2–8°C (optimal 5°C) is essential.[27] If frozen vaccines are stocked (e.g., varicella), a freezer with a separate door that can sustain temperatures to at least −15°C is needed. Each unit should have 24-hour monitoring, and a calibrated thermometer that can detect temperatures outside the acceptable range. Ideally, the unit should be connected to a back-up generator and an alarm system to alert the clinic if proper temperatures are not maintained. Signage and plug locks can help prevent inadvertent unplugging of the unit.

Temperature monitoring charts should be maintained twice daily and kept for a minimum of 3 years, or as dictated by site policy. The IAC has temperature charts for downloading at: www.immunize.org/news.d/celsius.pdf, as well as immunization sheets. The CDC has a web-based training program describing how to select and organize the clinic refrigerator at: http://www2a.cdc.gov/vaccines/ed/shtoolkit. The Australian Immunization Handbook and Public Health Agency of Canada's National Vaccine Storage and Handling Guidelines for Immunization Providers (2007) provide similar information.[28–30]

Computer: Each consultation room should have a computer with internet access. The computer should have the EMR and the travel medicine database, if the clinic uses them. Providers can consult web-based information services when questions arise about such issues as the status of an outbreak.

Supplies

Vaccine supply: Vaccines can be ordered directly from the manufacturer, a wholesaler, or from a hospital or centralized pharmacy, depending upon where the service is located. Hospital pharmacies usually have purchasing contracts with agreed price structures. Initially, a clinic can store a minimum supply of vaccines and then track weekly usage to anticipate the need for reordering. Vaccines should not be ordered until the clinic refrigerator can adequately and consistently maintain proper temperatures over a period of 1 week. Cold chain maintenance is a management priority, with careful attention paid to vaccine storage and handling best practices.[31]

Vaccination supplies: The clinic will need to stock gloves (can be used when the provider has a hand lesion or the traveler has a skin infection), syringes of multiple sizes, needles of different lengths and gauge (for intramuscular, subcutaneous and intradermal use with patients of different size and weight), bandages, alcohol pads, and cotton gauze. Some clinics use a topical anesthetic such as EMLA cream (AstraZeneca) that can be applied to the immunization site in children approximately 1 hour before injection. The IAC has published a supply list for practices that provide vaccinations: www.immunize.org/catg.d/p3046chk.pdf.[32]

Medications and supplies to manage adverse events: All clinics need procedures for the management of anaphylactic reactions following vaccination. Adrenaline (epinephrine) compounds and antihistamines need to be readily available. Emergency equipment such as blood pressure cuffs should be properly sized for the population served. Some hospital-based clinics have the advantage of on-site emergency medical care in the event of rare, severe adverse reactions. IAC publishes a list of these supplies and a management policy.[33]

Infection control and hazardous waste supplies: Every clinic must comply with regulations concerning infection control and the disposal of hazardous waste. 'Sharps receptacles' should be readily available, and mounted in a convenient location that reduces the risk of needle-stick injuries.

Other patient supplies: Clinics may find it useful to have pregnancy tests and a scale for weights.

Documentation

Travel clinics will need prescription pads, clinic letterheads for correspondence and for providing letters of medical exemption from YF vaccination, a supply of International Certificate of Vaccination or Prophylaxis (ICVP), and chart documents (or EMR). The use of standard documents, forms and patient hand-outs helps to insure comprehensive and consistent pre-travel care. Clinic documents may require legal review and medical director approval. Helpful documents are: pre-travel consultation record, patient immunization record, vaccine inventory log or database, vaccination consents and waivers.

The travel clinic form should become part of the permanent medical record. For insurance companies, a permanent medical record documents the level of care that has been provided. For the traveler, it is a record of the immunizations and advice they received and is useful if they lose their immunization card at some time in the future. For the travel clinic, it can be accessed to create a database (if not already entered directly into an EMR) of each traveler, and their preventive measures.

There should be a complete and accurate immunization record that includes: vaccine type (generic abbreviation and/or trade name), dose, date of administration, manufacturer and lot number, site of administration, and name and title of administrator. In the event of a vaccine recall, having this information in a computerized database will make the task of identifying patients much easier, since records can be searched by patient name, vaccine type, and lot number. An electronic record also allows rapid access to the information in a patient's chart if the traveler calls some months or years after the visit.

Information Resources for the Clinician

Clinicians require access to up-to-date information to determine destination risks and to learn about risk reduction measures. This is best achieved through online authoritative information sources, or frequently updated commercial travel medicine databases. Access to web-based information resources has moved travel medicine to a specialty that can respond daily to changes in the epidemiology, resistance patterns and outbreaks of infectious diseases. Authoritative sources of advice are WHO, CDC, the European Centres for Disease Control and Prevention (ECDC), and national resources such as those provided in Australia, New Zealand, Canada, France, Germany, Switzerland, The Netherlands, and the UK. Travel clinics will most likely use both national and international resources. All of these sources have their own websites that provide information. Of note, the travel health site of the UK has a list of fact sheets for the provider available for downloading (NaTHNaC; www.nathnac.org/pro/factsheets/index.htm).

A limited number of print resources are also useful: a textbook of travel medicine and tropical medicine, and professional journals that focus on these fields. For a complete list, see Chapter 4.

Subscription to a commercial database can provide health professionals with country-specific recommendations and travelers with customized information, disease risk maps, and other prevention recommendations. A hard-copy or electronic world atlas is also useful.

In travel medicine there are communication forums, termed 'listservs', that engage in discussion about emerging infections, outbreaks, or tropical and travel medicine related cases. The ASTM&H and ISTM listservs require membership of the organization; the listserv of the ISTM is active daily, airing problems and solutions that are helpful for the travel medicine provider. ProMed-mail (http://www.promedmail.org/), an open-access program of the International Society for Infectious Diseases, is a moderated reporting system for outbreaks of emerging infectious diseases. Some listservs are not moderated and the information shared may be anecdotal or not comply with national standards or practices.

Each clinic will need to decide how these resources are put into practice to help standardize care in the clinic. While the use of a travel clinic form (or EMR) allows standardization of the intake information, it is more difficult to standardize the advice and vaccines administered. In travel medicine there are frequent differences of opinion whether to give a particular immunization or which antimalarial to prescribe. Despite this, clinics should avoid giving different advice, vaccines and medications to travelers who are going on the same trip and have the same medical circumstances, but who come into the clinic at different times and are seen by different providers. To prevent this, protocols can be written that match the practice standard of the region, province, or country in which the travel clinic is located, or national guidance can be consulted to determine the interventions. Regular conferences and continuing education can build consistency among clinic staff.

Information Resources for the Traveler: Patient Education

In the US, CDC mandates that every clinician must provide vaccine recipients with information about the risks and benefits of immunizations. These are in the form of Vaccine Information Statements (VIS) (www.cdc.gov/vaccines). It is good practice for clinics in all countries to give recipients similar information.

An atlas, world map, and/or globe can help with destination counseling. Information on travel medical evacuation insurance, and demonstration samples of travel supplies and equipment, e.g., sample repellents, mosquito netting, travel medical kits, and water treatment equipment, are also helpful.

As education is the mainstay of pre-travel care, the clinician will need to counsel the traveler on a number of health and safety issues. Many clinics provide the traveler with a customized report generated by a commercial database to reinforce prevention advice. Clinicians may also want to direct travelers to internet sites that have excellent traveler-oriented information, e.g., the CDC (http://www.cdc.gov/travel), Fit for Travel (Health Protection Scotland) (http://www.fitfortravel.nhs.uk/home.aspx), NaTHNaC (http://www.nathnac.org/travel/index.htm), and Public Health Agency of Canada (http://www.phac-aspc.gc.ca/tmp-pmv/index-eng.php) websites. Other resources are discussed more completely in Chapter 4.

Reinforcement of verbal messages can help travelers apply pre-travel recommendations. Most travel health advisors provide the traveler with written materials that summarize and highlight the information. The traveler can review this material when they are under less pressure. Clinics may also provide medication instruction sheets or first aid booklets.

Travel clinics should be able to provide advice about topics more specialized than malaria and diarrhea prevention (see Tables 3.2 and 3.3). These topics include health issues for special needs travelers, such

as pregnant women, the elderly, those with diabetes or HIV/AIDS, or those with chronic cardiac or pulmonary disease. Knowledge of how to access safe and reliable medical care overseas is a key topic for all travelers, but particularly for the long-term or expatriate traveler. Clinics can direct travelers to online travel clinic directories such as those of ISTM or the International Association for Medical Assistance to Travelers (IAMAT, www.iamat.org), and to specialty resources such as the Divers Alert Network (www.diversalertnetwork.org/). Travel clinics that provide this complete range of health resources will further distinguish themselves from a generalist's office and enhance their level of care.[26]

Despite these educational efforts for travelers, it is difficult to measure the acquisition of knowledge during the pre-travel visit,[34,35] and equally difficult to assess whether or not this knowledge is acted upon during travel.[36,37] Airport surveys of travelers departing to regions considered at risk for malaria and/or vaccine-preventable disease document that despite travelers having some knowledge of the diseases, they often neither take antimalarial chemoprophylaxis nor receive vaccines that are indicated.[38,39] This is especially true for travelers who are visiting friends and relatives (VFR travelers).[38–43]

Even though there remain challenges in conveying knowledge and changing behavior, it is important to provide travelers with the tools to be safe and healthy during their trip. Providing travelers with consistent and clear advice about malaria and allowing them to discuss their concerns about chemoprophylaxis can lead to improved compliance with antimalarials.[36,44,45]

Legal Issues

Although travel health services can be subject to a number of regulations, most clinicians practice in settings that already meet most regulatory requirements. Therefore, little or no change may be necessary to insure full compliance with local, national, or institutional guidelines. In the US there are several federal laws that apply to the provision of travel health services, such as the National Childhood Vaccine Injury Act,[46] which provides for the reporting of adverse events through the Vaccine Adverse Event Reporting System (VAERS), the Needlestick Prevention and Safety Act,[47] and the Vaccines for Children Program.

In addition to federal laws, US state laws impact aspects of travel health practice such as the appropriate use in the clinic of nurse practitioners, registered nurses, and pharmacists, including what they are permitted to do with and without physician supervision. Issues regarding standing orders and the validity of a clinic's informed consent letters or waivers should also be clarified.

Each country will have its own regulations and standards for clinical practice, including for travel medicine. For instance, the need for signed consent varies, and in many countries in Europe and Africa, after the provision of relevant information, a verbal agreement to receive vaccinations is acceptable. Clinics must confirm full compliance prior to opening, and ensure ongoing compliance, as rules and regulations can change.

Professional Standards

Several professional groups have developed written standards for the practice of travel health. IDSA and ATHNA have guidelines posted on their websites.[2,48] The Royal College of Nursing in the UK has developed competencies for travel health nursing, and Canada has issued competencies for immunization care.[49,50] Travel clinics that operate in settings such as occupational health, university health, or community health should comply with standards set for those specialties.

Financial Considerations

Fees and Revenue for a Travel Health Practice

There is wide variation in the fee structure and reimbursement for travel health services. In the US, travel clinics range from being entirely private, fee-for-service facilities in which the providers do not join any third-party insurance plans, to hospital or medical school-based clinics in which fees are set by the hospital or university practice plan and all providers participate in insurance programs. In addition, there is wide variability in the reimbursement levels for travel medicine by insurance carriers, with some carriers not covering vaccines and medications prescribed for travel. In other areas, such as Canada, the travel visit and vaccine charges are usually not covered by provincial health plans. In general practice in the UK, some vaccines (such as typhoid, hepatitis A, and polio) are covered under the National Health Service, whereas others are charged to the traveler (e.g., YF, rabies, and Japanese encephalitis), and there is no additional reimbursement for providing advice.

Fee-for-Service Care

Travel clinics that charge on a fee-for-service basis expect payment in full at the time of the visit. Fee-for-service avoids many costly administrative processes involved with enrolling in different insurance plans, billing insurance for services, and billing patients for uncovered charges. Clinics should inform travelers about specific payment arrangements when they book their appointments. If a travel health program is on a fee-for-service basis, but operates within a hospital or medical center that accepts insurance for other services, the clinic may need to create a separate legal identity to avoid potential conflicts.

When a Clinic Participates in Insurance Plans

In the US, travel medicine specialists who are participating providers for third-party insurance carriers are required to accept the terms of reimbursement of those carriers. The clinic cannot request that the traveler pay more than the insurance company's level of reimbursement for a covered service. This frequently leads to underpayment, particularly for vaccines that may cost the provider more than the amount of the insurance company payment. For uncovered services, the travel clinic can request a cash payment. A waiver that indicates to the traveler that they are responsible for payment for uncovered services will need to be agreed and signed before the traveler can be billed, and should be obtained from all patients as they register for their appointments.

In US clinics that participate with insurance plans, a physician must be physically present in the clinic when care is rendered by a registered nurse in order for the nurse to bill for the visit. In this case, the nurse is billing 'incident to' the physician. Nurses can bill independently in entirely private clinics that are fee-for-service.

US Medicaid does not cover any services related to travel, so Medicaid patients have to pay cash for the advice and vaccines that they receive. Medicare will cover routinely recommended vaccines for adults: e.g., influenza, pneumococcal vaccine, tetanus, and hepatitis B.

In many settings, patients will require a referral from their primary care physician in order for the clinic to bill the patient's insurance company. These referrals are best initiated when the appointment is booked.

Clinic Charges

Fees that may be reimbursable or charged in a travel medicine service are the consultation fee (visit fee), vaccine fees, and vaccine administration charges. Providers in some countries charge for writing prescriptions, for completing an ICVP, and for completing other documents.

Profitability: Adding Additional Services

To expand services and enhance revenues, many clinics have extended their care beyond the basic provision of advice, vaccines, and prevention and self-treatment prescriptions. This includes selling travel-related items and rendering in-travel or post-travel care. Some have combined their travel clinic with a general vaccination clinic. The range of potential services is defined in Table 3.4.

Selling Travel-Related Products

Selling travel-related health items can increase revenue, and benefits the traveler by allowing them to immediately purchase items that are useful and may be difficult to locate elsewhere. Several companies sell products specifically tailored to international travelers and clinics can make arrangements to retail these items. Some travel clinics will sell pre-packaged antimalarial drugs, standby treatment for travelers' diarrhea or malaria, and drugs to prevent acute mountain sickness. Having these items on hand allows the provider to explain proper use of the medications.

Vaccination and Tuberculosis Testing Clinics

Combining a travel clinic and a vaccine clinic is a natural association. The vaccines are available, and the expertise of the staff is immediately at hand. This association may already be in place for occupational health or student health services. Vaccine clinics can immunize employee or community groups, migrants who need immunizations to obtain entry visas, students who need immunizations for schooling, and veterinarians and animal handlers who require rabies vaccination. The clinic can also be open to others who require a vaccine but do not have access to a physician who can provide it. Vaccine clinic visits are usually an efficient use of resources, and lead to increased productivity. A separate vaccine clinic form that contains patient demographic data, pertinent medical, immunization and medication history, and the reason for the vaccine, should be generated.

In some cases, for example migrants or veterinarians, it is necessary to use laboratory services to check serology for proof of immunity to measles or varicella, as examples, or whether the titer of rabies

---

Table 3.4 Additional Travel Clinic Services

Sale of travel-related items, e.g., repellents, netting, rehydration salts, first-aid kits
Pre-travel health screening/ fitness-to-fly examinations
Contracts with the private sector and schools or universities
Health advice for corporate, NGO or education clients during travel
Telephone or e-mail advice to physicians and the traveling public
Evaluation and screening for post-travel illness
General vaccination clinic
Pharmacy services
Clinical laboratory testing

antibody in previously immunized persons is sufficient to preclude a booster dose of rabies vaccine.

Pre-Travel Physical Examinations and Post-Travel Care

The setting, expertise, and interests of the travel medicine providers in a clinic will determine whether or not pre-travel physical examinations or post-travel evaluation and care are performed. Clinics that are part of a general medicine practice, a university student health service or an occupational health unit with contracts with corporations or other organizations might perform physical examinations as part of visa or program requirements.

The consensus statement on travel medicine by Canadian travel medicine experts,[16] the IDSA guidelines,[2] as well as the body of knowledge developed by the ISTM,[17] do not indicate that an extensive knowledge of tropical disease is necessary for travel medicine specialists. The Canadians recommend that 'all post-travel consultations should be managed by a physician and should include the following: recognition of any travel-related illness, and timely medical assessment, with referral if required, for the management of travel-related illnesses.'[16] All travel medicine specialists should be able to recognize key syndromes in the returned traveler and know how to refer them for adequate care.[51–54] These key syndromes include fever, skin disorders, acute and chronic diarrhea, and respiratory complaints.[55] For clinics with personnel having expertise in infectious diseases and tropical medicine, it is appropriate to evaluate and treat ill returned travelers without referral. In these settings, there needs to be adequate laboratory assistance to diagnose or confirm suspected illness.

Services to Travelers During Their Journeys

Clinics with contracts with businesses, NGOs or educational institutions may provide health advice for ill clients during their trips via e-mail, Skype, or communication with local health providers.[56] There should be provider expertise in tropical and emergency medicine, availability during off hours, technical capacity to receive, process and transmit information, and protocols for handling different clinical scenarios. This is something that only a few clinics would be able to provide.

Off-Site Services

Travel clinics may be asked to come to a workplace or school setting to provide pre-travel advice and immunization to individuals or groups. This can be a valued service in some communities and an opportunity to generate additional revenue and goodwill. Clear protocols will need to be followed to ensure vaccine cold chain compliance, appropriate care for any adverse events, documentation and handling of medical records, confidentiality, and proper disposal of hazardous waste.

Running a Travel Health Program

Staff and Administrative Issues

Clinical and administrative personnel should be trained to deliver services efficiently and effectively during the three phases of the visit: before the visit when an appointment is arranged, during the visit when the traveler assessment is made and a risk management strategy is developed, and after the consultation is completed, when either follow-up care is scheduled or the traveler calls with post-visit questions.

Before the Visit, Preparation of Reception Staff

Travelers frequently ask administrative staff questions about vaccines, destinations, vaccine charges, insurance coverage, and more. Staff should be prepared for these types of questions, and counseled not to answer risk management queries. Travelers can be advised to wait for their appointment with a healthcare professional or to visit an authoritative website to deal with non-administrative queries.

The following can help facilitate the appointment:

- Obtain traveler-related information: age, date of birth, gender, medical conditions, country of birth, native language
- Have patients bring in any immunization records, medication lists, and a complete itinerary including dates and durations at each destination
- Determine the purpose of trip: holiday, business, study, VFR (visiting friends and relatives), humanitarian work, medical care abroad
- Schedule a consultation length appropriate to the traveler and their trip. Sufficient time will be needed for complex journeys, or multiple family members
- Provide instructions to the traveler about the visit, helping them to anticipate what to expect during the consultation
- Explain any terms of payment
- Try to confirm all appointments 24–48 hours before the visit
- Ensure that sufficient quantities of vaccine are available.

Key Issues During the Pre-Travel Consultation

The key feature of the provider–traveler encounter is a risk assessment that allows the advice and interventions to be individually matched to the traveler. See Chapter 5 for a detailed description of the pre-travel visit.

- Step I: Assessment of the traveler: a focused health history to document critical demographic and medical information. Using a pre-printed questionnaire or EMR will lend consistency, completeness, and efficiency
- Step II: Assessment of the trip: reason for travel, destination, duration, accommodation, planned activities, departure date
- Step III: Itinerary and risk: research internet databases for destination hazards and risk reduction strategies
- Step IV: Implementation of a customized care plan: priority listing of trip health and safety risks, strategies for risk reduction and management; immunizations, travel medications, patient counseling, consults and referrals, self-care guidance, travel health insurance, access to medical care overseas, customized printed report, maps and patient education handouts.

Following the Consultation

Documentation should be completed and clinicians and administrative staff prepared to handle any calls concerning clarification of prescriptions or prevention guidance.

Reporting Vaccine Adverse Events

All administrators of vaccines in the US are required to report adverse events via VAERS.[46] The methods and forms for reporting can be obtained by calling 800-822-7967 or accessing http://vaers.hhs.gov/index. The Division of Immunization in Canada has a similar reporting system and can be reached by calling 866-234-2345, or accessing http://www.hc-sc.gc.ca/dhp-mps/medeff/index_e.html. In the UK, suspected adverse event reports are made to the Medicines Healthcare products Regulatory Agency through the 'Yellow Card Scheme' at http://www.mhra.gov.uk/Safetyinformation/Reportingsafetyproblems/index.htm. Other countries and regions may have their own reporting systems.

Service Evaluation

The hallmark of a quality travel health service is an ongoing commitment to quality improvement. It is important to implement patient satisfaction surveys at the time of the visit as well as post-travel outcome evaluations. Regular chart reviews and competency based training evaluations should be built into the clinic's professional development plan.

After the Trip

Most travelers will not need post-trip evaluation or care. However, certain travelers should schedule a post-travel consultation. Reasons for a post-travel visit include: a traveler to a malaria area who develops a fever after return; travelers who have been ill abroad (with more than a short bout of travelers' diarrhea) or are ill upon return; long-stay travelers; and travelers who worked in healthcare or other 'at risk' occupations.

Many travel health clinics will just focus on pre-travel care. Clinics that are part of general practice, a medical school practice or other multi-specialty group may have expertise in assessing travelers who need evaluation after return. Clinicians should understand the issues of post-travel triage and be ready to refer returned patients to specialists, such as infectious disease and tropical medicine specialists and dermatologists with expertise in tropical disease.

Marketing and Promoting A Travel Health Program

Despite the growth in international travel, it is estimated that only 10–50% of travelers seek pre-travel care.[16,38,39,57] The reasons for this are varied: many travelers and health professionals are unaware of the specialty of travel medicine or the value of specialized travel healthcare. A travel clinic has many opportunities to attract patients. When creating a marketing plan thought should be given to persons who travel in the local community, including businesses, schools, non-profit groups, missionary groups, adoption agencies, and tour operators, to identify these potential travelers (Table 3.5).

Word of Mouth

The value of a 'satisfied customer' should never be underestimated. Communication among travelers who have had a good experience at your service can increase awareness of a clinic and lead to referrals. It is important to make clear to the traveler the advantages of a visit to a travel clinic: provider knowledge of disease epidemiology and prevention, availability of all vaccines necessary for travel, provision of advice and prevention strategies on uncommon diseases, and access to written and online resources on disease epidemiology and prevention (Table 3.1). Travelers will recognize the value of clinics that can deliver this level of service and will share their enthusiasm with family and friends.

Referrals

Physicians and other health providers will refer patients to a clinic if they perceive that their patient has received excellent care in a timely

Table 3.5 Marketing a Travel Medicine Service
Development of clinic website
Word of mouth among travelers, referral physicians, health agencies, community businesses and travel agencies
News releases to web, print, radio, or television media concerning travel medicine care
Direct advertising in:
Internet/print media
Regional/state medical journals, speciality newsletters (adoption groups, student travel, alumni magazines)
Development of a clinic brochure with mailings to:
Physicians and other health professionals
Retail travel agencies
Regional/state health departments
Businesses, schools, universities and non-profit groups that travel, such as churches and museums
Letters to referring providers that detail vaccines administered and medications prescribed
Education sessions for health professionals and lay public

fashion and are provided with information about their patient's visit. All referral physicians should be sent a letter that details which vaccines were administered and which medications were prescribed. This provides the physician with a written record that can be filed with their patient's chart. A clinic can also take this opportunity to include a brochure that describes the clinic and its services. Many generalist offices do not want to stock costly and infrequently used vaccines, and find it difficult to keep up with changing global patterns of disease and prevention strategies. Therefore, if they are pleased with your service they will be willing to let your clinic provide the care.

Direct Marketing Methods: Internet, Print, and Media

Many marketing measures can be employed, including use of the internet (Table 3.5). Clinics should develop websites that explain and promote their service. Some clinics will create elaborate sites that include destination information and links to other travel information resources as well as essential content: office location, hours of operation, personnel, directions to the facility, and telephone number. Clinics that offer YF vaccine can be listed in the CDC Yellow Fever Clinic online directory for US designated centers, or on the NaTHNaC website for UK-based centers. The ISTM website maintains a listing of travel clinics that are directed by members of the society. Accessing these sites is particularly useful when either a provider or traveler is trying to locate a clinic in another part of the country or the world. These lists have also been incorporated into some of the commercial travel information sites.

News releases can generate publicity in newspapers, television, and radio. These releases are timely around the summer months and other holiday periods, or when world health events provide an opportunity to describe the advantages of pre-travel care. If one is practicing travel medicine in a private office, it may be difficult to develop publicity for the press. Hospital- and medical school-based practices can, however, take advantage of their facility's marketing departments. These departments can make public service announcements for radio, arrange interviews, and promote news items for television. Clinic healthcare providers can also give talks to lay groups on the topic of health and travel, or more formal educational sessions (e.g., Grand Rounds) to the medical community.

Table 3.6 Top 10 Problems Encountered in Travel Clinics[a]

1	Insufficient space, time, and staff to meet demands
2	Travelers presenting with a short time interval before departure
3	Telephone calls for advice
4	Need for standardized, up-to-date advice for clinic personnel
5	Conflicting and unreliable advice provided to travelers
6	Patient concern about the cost of service and vaccines
7	Difficulty in assessing patient compliance with and understanding of advice
8	Difficulty in accessing new medications and vaccines
9	Failure of insurance carriers to pay for services
10	Travelers having preconceived ideas about their travel health needs

[a]Adapted from Hill DR and Behrens RH.[3]

Mailings

Direct mailings with a clinic brochure can be employed. Targets for these mailings include local physicians' offices, schools and universities, and local and regional businesses that have international markets. Sending brochures to travel agencies that specialize in international or adventure travel can lead to referrals when they book tours and travel. To generate business from these sources, it may be helpful to visit the sites directly and present what your travel service has to offer. Meeting with the directors of travel agencies, student health center staff and with human resource personnel in corporations, can effectively inform them of the advantages of having their client, students, or employees visit your service.

Contract Services

Establishing contracts with the private sector is an excellent way to guarantee patient volume and income. Under contracts, the clinic agrees to provide certain services, and the corporation or other facility agrees to have all of their travel healthcare administered through your clinic. Many businesses will be happy to establish a relationship with a travel medicine service if it helps provide an expert level of care for their personnel.[58–61] The clinic can seek an annual retainer or a set fee for each visit and service that is provided (such as vaccines, travel health portfolios, on-site services, or post-travel screening). If the travel clinic also has a vaccine clinic, contracts can be established with veterinary offices to provide rabies vaccine, or state or provincial health departments to provide hepatitis B vaccine, as examples.

Brochures

In addition to a website, a clinic can develop a brochure that contains information detailing reasons to obtain pre-travel care, what care will be provided, the hours of operation, directions to the facility, contact numbers, and a web address. Inclusion of statistics about the travel population served by your clinic and pictures of travel destinations can enhance its appeal. These can be mailed to target groups for distribution.

Management Challenges

The 1994 survey of travel clinics identified several challenges to the practice of travel medicine.[3] The Top 10 cited by practitioners are listed in Table 3.6; these represent more than 80% of all of the problems listed by clinics. These concerns remain a challenge today, and if those who are developing a clinic anticipate them during the planning stages, then it is likely that the clinic will be able to deal with them more effectively.

Telephone and E-Mail Advice

Giving travel advice over the telephone is controversial. Most clinics are willing to provide advice to clinicians, but fewer are willing to provide it to the general public. Clinics that have agreements with businesses, non-governmental organizations (NGOs), or schools and universities may choose to provide e-mail advice for their clients. To give advice appropriately takes both time and expertise, and this effort for public enquiries may not translate into patient visits to the clinic. Travel clinics can consider charging for advice given by telephone.

If a clinic chooses to provide telephone or e-mail advice, it should be clear who will respond to the requests, and when the response will be made. Setting aside a certain time each day to deal with the queries is more efficient. The advice given should be from standard protocols; this helps to ensure that answers are consistent between questions and providers. A method should also be developed that records both the query and the advice given. For e-mails, this will happen automatically, but for telephone calls, a standard form should be completed during the call. Additionally, a clinic that handles many telephone requests may wish to develop a voice recording system. Having these procedures in place will help with the queries and provide documentation in the event of medico-legal issues. Some larger travel medicine practices have developed automated telephone response lines that usually charge for the service. These are complex to develop, however, and need constant updating to remain current.

A clinic will need to decide how detailed to make their advice. Giving general rather than specific advice to public inquiries is best because the clinic has not established a formal physician–patient relationship, and all of the medical and itinerary information usually cannot be obtained over the telephone or via e-mail to properly assess health risks. Thus, specific recommendations would be based on incomplete data, and if these were acted upon with a deleterious outcome, the clinic could become legally responsible. If advice is given to another healthcare provider, it should be made clear that they assume responsibility for applying the advice to their traveler.

The following is a suggested way to respond to a request from a traveler for medical advice about a safari to Kenya:

There are several health issues to consider when traveling to Kenya. These involve protecting yourself against insect carriers of disease, receiving vaccines against some diseases, being careful about what you eat and drink to avoid diarrhea, and exercising responsible behavior. The following immunizations can be considered depending upon your planned activities, whether or not you have any medical conditions, and which vaccines you may have previously received: tetanus, diphtheria, hepatitis A, hepatitis B, polio, typhoid, and yellow fever. Malaria is a common and very serious problem in Kenya, and you should take care to avoid the mosquitoes transmitting infection as well as take malaria preventive medication. There are several medicines to choose from; you should discuss with your doctor which one would be best for you. You should also know how to obtain medical care during your trip if you need it, and obtain travel medical insurance before you travel. A visit to a travel medicine specialist can help you to determine which preventive measures are best for you and you will be able to discuss these and other issues in more detail.

Short-Notice Travel

Clinics should try to have all travelers come in for care, even those who are departing within a few days. A last-minute consultation can still address the major risks associated with international travel. Single-dose vaccines can be provided, and prevention counseling for important travel health hazards including malaria and dengue, food- and water-borne illness, accidents, and rabies can be delivered. Clinicians can advise travelers about travel medical insurance, how to access healthcare at their destination, and recommend items for a travel medical kit.

Professional Development

Travel healthcare is not 'just giving shots', and clinicians need initial training and ongoing education to provide comprehensive, quality care that is based on current standards. Physicians, nurses, pharmacists, and other health professionals who may be experienced in immunizations are not automatically qualified to provide the other components of a pre-travel consultation. Traveler and trip assessment and prevention counseling are separate skill sets and all clinicians should be trained and competency tested to provide appropriate care and to avoid clinical liability. ISTM, ASTMH, and ATHNA as well as other national organizations post travel medicine courses and conferences on their websites. CDC offers regular, free training opportunities through the CDC Learning Center: www.cdc.gov/learning. Other countries, including the UK, Australia, and Canada, offer educational programs. Building in regular continuing education opportunities in travel medicine should be standard practice.

Conclusions

As travel medicine has developed into a recognized specialty, the importance of a travel medicine service has become evident. Advantages of this service include provision of care by a health professional that has training and experience and has access to information and resources from expert bodies to provide the highest level of care based on current recommendations. In a travel clinic, the traveler should be given advice on a wide range of topics; be administered required or recommended vaccines; and prescribed medication for prevention or self-treatment of problems such as malaria, diarrhea, and high altitude illness. Providing pre-travel care at this level will establish the service as an important link in the care of international travelers.[62]

References

1. Schlagenhauf P, Santos-O'Connor S, Parola P. The practice of travel medicine in Europe. Clin Microbiol Infect 2010;16:203–8.
2. Hill DR, Ericsson CD, Pearson RD, et al. The practice of travel medicine: guidelines by the Infectious Diseases Society of America. Clin Infect Dis 2006;43:1499–539. Available at: http://cid.oxfordjournals.org/content/43/12/1499.full
3. Hill DR, Behrens RH. A survey of travel clinics throughout the world. J Travel Med 1996;3:46–51.
4. Carroll B, Behrens RH, Crichton D. Primary healthcare needs for travel medicine training in Britain. J Travel Med 1998;5:3–6.
5. Hoveyda N, McDonald P, Behrens RH. A description of travel medicine in general practice: a postal questionnaire survey. J Travel Med 2004;11:295–8.
6. World Tourism Organization. UNTWO Tourism Highlights 2011 Edition. World Tourism Organization. July 2011. Available at: http://mkt.unwto.org/sites/all/files/docpdf/unwtohighlights11enhr.pdf
7. Demeter SJ. An evaluation of sources of information in health and travel. Can J Public Health 1989;80:20–2.
8. Keystone JS, Dismukes R, Sawyer L, et al. Inadequacies in health recommendations provided for international travelers by North American travel health advisors. J Travel Med 1994;1:72–8.
9. Hatz C, Krause E, Grundmann H. Travel advice: a study among Swiss and German general practitioners. Trop Med Int Health 1997;2:6–12.
10. Blair DC. A week in the life of a travel clinic. Clin Micro Rev 1997;10:650–73.
11. Leggat PA. Sources of health advice given to travelers. J Travel Med 2000;7:85–8.
12. Kain KC, MacPherson DW, Kelton T, et al. Malaria deaths in visitors to Canada and in Canadian travellers: a case series. Can Med Assoc J 2001;164:654–9.
13. Newman RD, Parise ME, Barber AM, et al. Malaria-related deaths among U.S. travelers, 1963–2001. Ann Intern Med 2004;141:547–55.
14. Ropers G, Krause G, Tiemann F, et al. Nationwide survey of the role of travel medicine in primary care in Germany. J Travel Med 2004;11:287–94.
15. Ruis JR, Van Rijckevorsel GG, van den Hoek A, et al. Does registration of professionals improve the quality of traveller's health advice? J Travel Med 2009;16:263–6.
16. Committee to Advise on Tropical Medicine and Travel (CATMAT). Guidelines for the practice of travel medicine. An Advisory Committee Statement (ACS). Can Commun Dis Rep 1999;25:1–6.
17. Kozarsky PE, Keystone JS. Body of knowledge for the practice of travel medicine. J Travel Med 2006;13:251–4.
18. Barry M, Maguire JH, Weller PF. The American Society of Tropical Medicine and Hygiene initiative to stimulate educational programs to enhance medical expertise in tropical diseases. Am J Trop Med Hyg 1999;61:681–8.
19. Sofarelli TA, Ricks JH, Anand R, et al. Standardized training in nurse model travel clinics. J Travel Med 2011;18:39–43.
20. Durham MJ, Goad JA, Neinstein LS, et al. A comparison of pharmacist travel health specialists; versus primary care providers' recommendations for travel-related medications, vaccinations, and patient compliance in a college health setting. J Travel Med 2011;18:20–5.
21. Jackson AB, Humphries TL, Nelson KM, et al. Clinical pharmacy travel medicine services: a new frontier. Ann Pharmacother 2004;38:2160–5.
22. Immunization Action Coalition. Adults only vaccination: A step-by-step guide. Available at: www.immunize.org/guide/aov07_documents.pdf
23. Centers for Disease Control and Prevention. Fact Sheet for Vaccine Information Statements. Available at: www.cdc.gov/vaccines/pubs/vis/vis-facts.htm#provider
24. World Health Organization. International Health Regulations (2005). Geneva: World Health Organization; 2005. Available at: www.who.int/ihr/en/
25. Boddington NJ, Simons H, Launders N, et al. Evaluation of travel medicine practice by Yellow Fever Vaccination Centres in England, Wales and Northern Ireland. J Travel Med 2012;19:84–91.
26. International Society of Travel Medicine. Resources for beginning and operating a travelers' health clinic. Available at: www.istm.org/webforms/Members/MemberActivities/VolunteerActivities/standing_committees/profeducation.aspx
27. Centers for Disease Control and Prevention. General recommendations on immunization: recommendations of the Advisory Committee on Immunization Practices (ACIP) MMWR Recomm Rep 2011;60(RR02):1–60. Available at: www.cdc.gov/mmwr/preview/mmwrhtml/rr6002a1.htm
28. Immunization Action Coalition. Vaccine Handling Tips. Available at: www.immunize.org/catg.d/p3048.pdf
29. Australian Technical Advisory Group on Immunization. The Australian Immunisation Handbook 9th ed. 2008. Available at: http://www.health.gov.au/internet/immunise/publishing.nsf/content/handbook-home
30. Public Health Agency of Canada. National Vaccine Storage and Handling Guidelines for Immunization Providers (2007). Available at: www.phac-aspc.gc.ca/publicat/2007/nvshglp-ldemv/index-eng.php
31. Centers for Disease Control and Prevention. Vaccine Storage and Handling Guide. Available at: www.cdc.gov/vaccines/recs/storage/guide/vaccine-storage-handling.pdf
32. Immunization Action Coalition. Supplies Checklist. Available at: http://www.immunize.org/handouts/vaccine-clinic-supplies.asp
33. Immunization Action Coalition. Medical Management of Vaccine Reactions in Adult Patients. 2011. Available at: http://www.immunize.org/catg.d/p3082.pdf
34. Genton B, Behrens RH. Specialized travel consultation. Part II: acquiring knowledge. J Travel Med 1994;1:13–5.

35. Packman CJ. A survey of notified travel-associated infections: implications for travel health advice. J Pub Health Med 1995;17:217–22.

36. Farquharson L, Noble LM, Barker C, et al. Health beliefs and communication in the travel clinic consultation as predictors of adherence to malaria chemoprophylaxis. Br J Health Psychol 2004;9:201–17.

37. Landry P, Iorillo D, Darioli R, et al. Do travelers really take their mefloquine malaria chemoprophylaxis? Estimation of adherence by an electronic pillbox. J Travel Med 2006;13:8–14.

38. Van Herck K, Van Damme P, Castelli F, et al. Knowledge, attitudes and practices in travel-related infectious diseases: the European airport survey. J Travel Med 2004;11:3–8.

39. Hamer DH, Connor BA. Travel health knowledge, attitudes and practices among United States travelers. J Travel Med 2004;11:23–6.

40. Hill DR. The burden of illness in international travelers. N Engl J Med 2006;354:115–7.

41. Bacaner N, Stauffer B, Boulware DR, et al. Travel medicine considerations for North American immigrants visiting friends and relatives. JAMA 2004;291:2856–64.

42. Angell SY, Cetron MS. Health disparities among travelers visiting friends and relatives abroad. Ann Intern Med 2005;142:67–72.

43. Leder K, Tong S, Weld L, et al. Illness in travelers visiting friends and relatives; a review of the GeoSentinal Surveillance Network. Clin Infect Dis 2006;43:185–93.

44. Hill DR. Health problems in a large cohort of Americans traveling to developing countries. J Travel Med 2000;7:259–66.

45. Horvath LL, Murray CK, Dooley DP. Effect of maximizing a travel medicine clinic's prevention strategies. J Travel Med 2005;12:332–7.

46. Centers for Disease Control and Prevention. National childhood vaccine injury act: Requirements for permanent vaccination records and for reporting of selected events after vaccination. MMWR 1988;37:197–200.

47. Occupational Safety and Health Administration. Bloodborne Pathogens and Needlestick Prevention. Available at: www.osha.gov/SLTC/bloodbornepathogens/index.html

48. American Travel Health Nurses Association. Scope of Practice and Standards of Travel Health Nursing. Available at: www.athna.org/menu-standards/standards-default.asp

49. Royal College of Nursing. Competencies: an integrated career and competency framework for nurses in travel health medicine. 2007. Available at: www.rcn.org.uk/__data/assets/pdf_file/0006/78747/003146.pdf

50. Public Health Agency of Canada. Immunization Competencies for Health Professionals. 2008. Available at: www.phac-aspc.gc.ca/im/ic-ci-eng.php

51. Ryan ET, Wilson ME, Kain KC. Illness after international travel. N Engl J Med 2002;347:505–16.

52. Spira A. Assessment of travellers who return home ill. Lancet 2003;361:1459–69.

53. D'Acremont V, Ambresin AE, Burnand B, et al. Practice guidelines for evaluation of fever in returning travelers and migrants. J Travel Med 2003;10: S25–52.

54. Field V, Ford L, Hill DR. Health Information for Overseas Travel. Prevention of Illness in Travellers from the UK. National Travel Health Network and Centre; 2010.

55. Freedman DO, Weld LH, Kozarsky PE, et al. Spectrum of disease and relation to place of exposure among ill returned travelers. N Engl J Med 2006;354:119–30.

56. Callahan MV, Hamer DH. On the medical edge: preparation of expatriates, refugee and disaster relief workers, and Peace Corps volunteers. Infect Dis Clin North Am 2005;19:85–101.

57. Duval B, De Serre G, Shadmani R, et al. A population-based comparison between travelers who consulted travel clinics and those who did not. J Travel Med 2003;10:4–10.

58. Kemmerer TP, Cetron M, Harper L, et al. Health problems of corporate travelers: risk factors and management. J Travel Med 1998;5:184–7.

59. Bunn WB, Bank L. The health of frequent business travellers. Occup Med (Lond) 2002;52:2–3.

60. Weber R, Schlagenhauf P, Amsler L, et al. Knowledge, attitudes and practices of business travelers regarding malaria risk and prevention. J Travel Med 2003;10:219–24.

61. Prince TS, Spengler SE, Collins TR, Corporate travel medicine: benefit analysis of on-site services. J Travel Med 2001;8:163–7.

62. Powell B, Ford C. Risks of travel, benefits of a specialist consult. Clev Clin J Med 2010;77:246–54.

4

Sources of Travel Medicine Information

David O. Freedman

Key points

- Authoritative bodies such as the World Health Organization (WHO) and the Centers for Disease Control and Prevention (CDC) host websites that contain comprehensive travel health and some outbreak information. Numerous national bodies as well as commercial organizations also provide excellent travel health information on public or membership-only websites
- Itinerary-driven databases that generate comprehensive reports for use in travel health counseling can be accessed in real time over the internet via a web-browser on a PC or mobile device
- Broad reference texts in travel medicine can be supplemented from a list of specialized texts for uncommon patient situations
- TravelMed is an important electronic discussion forum of issues related to the practice of travel medicine (www.istm.org/WebForms/Members/MemberActivities/listserve.aspx)

Introduction

Travel medicine is concerned with keeping international travelers alive and healthy. To an extent beyond that in most other disciplines, travel medicine providers need to keep constantly current with changing disease risk patterns in over 220 different countries. The knowledge base upon which preventative and therapeutic interventions are based continues to change rapidly. An increasingly online world allows for frequent and detailed dissemination of disease incidence patterns, information on new outbreaks, the description of new diseases affecting travelers, as well as data on new drug resistance patterns in old diseases. Travelers are going to ever more exotic and previously unvisited locales. In addition, travelers are increasingly online and are bringing ever more sophisticated and updated information with them at the time of the pre-travel medical encounter. Electronic media are now the major source of updated information for travel medicine providers. Many printed publications, manuals and detailed textbooks listed in previous editions of this book no longer exist, or exist only in electronic format. Essentially, all the most important authoritative national and international surveillance bulletins, outbreak information, and official governmental recommendations are available on the internet.

This chapter will provide, mostly in tabular form, information on key travel medicine-oriented information resources targeted to travel medicine professionals. The electronic resources discussed below were current at the time of writing, but some information may be outdated by the time this chapter is in the hands of the reader.

Reference Texts

The first section of Table 4.1 lists selected core reference texts whose primary emphasis is a comprehensive approach to travel medicine and to keeping travelers alive and healthy. Any of these high-quality resources is certainly sufficient to cover completely the practical aspects of caring for those to be seen in a travel medicine practice. The next sections list, by category, large reference texts that contain detailed discussions, factual tables, and primary references that would be helpful in dealing with select or uncommon situations. Web-based, mobile and e-reader editions of these books are increasingly available and over the next years will be progressively formatted on a topical basis rather than a traditional chapter basis.

Journals

Table 4.2 lists selected English-language journals that consistently and frequently feature articles on travel medicine. Most of these journals have their complete contents available electronically in a format that is restricted to their own subscribers.

Travel Medicine Websites

Only selected websites that have data of generally high quality and of a broader international interest to travel medicine providers are referenced in Table 4.3. Checking more than one authoritative site on a specific issue is always recommended. First, authoritative recommendations still contain some element of opinion. Thus, even major sources such as the WHO, CDC, and Nathnac can disagree on some issues. Second, because of changing disease patterns, what was accurate yesterday may not be accurate today, and some sites are more timely in updating than others. Fortunately, most sites put an indicator at

©2012 Elsevier Inc
DOI: 10.1016/B978-1-4557-1076-8.00004-1

Table 4.1 Books

Comprehensive Travel Medicine Resources

CDC Health Information for International Travel 2012. (The 'CDC Yellow Book'). http://www.oup.com/us/catalog/general/subject/Medicine/PublicHealth/?view=usa&ci=9780199769018

WHO International Travel and Health 2012. (WHO 'Green' Book). http://www.who.int/ith/en/

Health Information for Overseas Travel. UK NaTHNaC. http://www.nathnac.org/yellow_book/YBmainpage.htm

Walker PF, Barnett ED, eds. Immigrant Medicine. Philadelphia: Saunders; 2007. http://www.elsevier.com/wps/find/bookdescription.cws_home/711192/description#description

The Travel and Tropical Medicine Manual. 4th edn. Jong EC, Sanford CA, eds. http://www.us.elsevierhealth.com/Medicine/Infectious-Disease/book/9781416026136/The-Travel-and-Tropical-Medicine-Manual/

Comprehensive Immunization Resources

Vaccines, 6th edn. Plotkin SA, Orenstein WA, Offit PA. Philadelphia: W.B. Saunders; 2013. http://www.us.elsevierhealth.com/product.jsp?isbn=9781455700905&navAction=&navCount=2

Epidemiology and Prevention of Vaccine Preventable Diseases ('The Pink Book'). 12th edn. Atlanta, CDC; 2011. http://www.cdc.gov/vaccines/pubs/pinkbook/index.html

Travel and Routine Immunizations. Shoreland; 2012. Annual editions. http://www.shoreland.com/services/travel-routine-immunizations

Pharmacopeias

Martindale, the Complete Drug Reference. 37th edn. Sweetman S, ed. London: Pharmaceutical Press; 2011. http://www.pharmpress.com/product/9780853699330/martindale

British National Formulary. 54th edn. Mehta DK, ed. London: Pharmaceutical Press; 2007. www.pharmpress.com (ISBN: 978 0 85369 7367).

Specialized Resource Texts (in-depth coverage of important areas)

Tropical Infectious Diseases, 3rd edn. Guerrant RL, Walker DH, Weller PF. http://www.us.elsevierhealth.com/Medicine/Infectious-Disease/book/9780702039355/Tropical-Infectious-Diseases-Principles-Pathogens-and-Practice/

Hunter's Tropical Medicine and Emerging Infectious Disease, 9th Edition 2013. Magill AJ, Ryan ET, Solomon T, Hill DR eds. http://www.us.elsevierhealth.com/product.jsp?isbn=9781416043904&navAction=&navCount=4

Manson's Tropical Diseases. 22nd edn. Cook G, Zumla A, eds.2008. http://www.elsevier.com/wps/find/bookdescription.cws_home/716702/description#description

Control of Communicable Disease Manual. 19th edn. Washington DC: Heymann D, ed. American Public Health Association; 2008. www.apha.org

Red Book. 2009 Report of the Committee on Infectious Diseases. 28th edn. Elk Grove, IL: American Academy of Pediatrics; 2009. http://aapredbook.aappublications.org/

Wilderness Medicine. 6th edn. Auerbach PS. 2012 http://www.us.elsevierhealth.com/product.jsp?isbn=9781437716788

Infectious Diseases: A Geographic Guide. Petersen E, Chen LH, Schlagenhauf eds. Wiley-Blackwell. 2011. http://www.wiley.com/WileyCDA/WileyTitle/productCd-0470655291.html

Table 4.2 Journals Frequently Publishing Papers on Travel Medicine

American Journal of Tropical Medicine and Hygiene
Aviation Space and Environmental Medicine
British Medical Journal
Bulletin of the World Health Organization
Clinical Infectious Diseases
Emerging Infectious Diseases Journal
Eurosurveillance
Journal of Infectious Diseases
Journal of Occupational and Environmental Medicine
Journal of Travel Medicine
The Lancet
Lancet Infectious Diseases
Military Medicine
Morbidity and Mortality Weekly Report
Pediatric Infectious Diseases Journal
PLOS Neglected Tropical Diseases
Transactions of the Royal Society of Tropical Medicine and Hygiene
Travel Medicine and Infectious Diseases
Tropical Medicine and International Health
Vaccine
Weekly Epidemiological Record
Wilderness and Environmental Medicine

the bottom of each page stating the date of the last update. Always be suspicious of information on a web page that carries no date.

Point-of-Care Travel Clinic Destination Resources

Since the early 1990s, electronic information systems for travel health counseling have become widely used and increasingly sophisticated. These systems allow the user to query large electronic databases containing information on disease risk, epidemiology, and vaccine recommendations across more than 220 countries. These systems allow a rapid, convenient means of accessing a large body of changing information.

With the advent of database-driven technology, these databases can be accessed in real time over the internet via a web-browser interface at the user's end. All the major English-language vendors of query-driven travel clinic software now make their products available only via the internet. Thus, the most widely used English-language packages are all listed in Table 4.3 under the heading 'Country-Specific Travel Medicine Database (non-governmental)'.

Most high-quality systems have at least two major components: (1) displays of information including country-by-country information on health risks within a given country, country-by-country vaccine recommendations, and disease-by-disease fact sheets for major diseases; (2) an itinerary-maker feature which, after input of a complete traveler itinerary, prints out summary recommendations for the entire itinerary in the order of travel. These printouts generally include a vaccination plan, malaria recommendations, destination risks, in-country resources, and are individualized with the name of the patient and the clinic. In addition, detailed country-by-country disease maps, especially for malaria or yellow fever, are important features to consider in evaluating a system. Printouts of these can be important in educating

Table 4.3 Travel Medicine Websites (Many Provide Twitter, Facebook, RSS, and Linkedin Feeds)

Governmental Travel Medicine Recommendations				
CDC Travelers Health Homepage	http://wwwn.cdc.gov/travel/default.aspx	WHO Global Response and Alert Outbreak News	http://www.who.int/csr/don/en/
CDC YellowBook (Health Information for International Travel)	http://wwwn.cdc.gov/travel/contentYellowBook.aspx	WHO Global Response and Alert Disease Links	http://www.who.int/csr/disease/en/
WHO Green Book (International Travel and Health)	http://www.who.int/ith/	European Centre for Disease Prevention & Control (ECDC)	http://www.ecdc.europa.eu/en/Pages/home.aspx
Public Health Agency of Canada – Travel Health	http://www.phac-aspc.gc.ca/tmp-pmv/index.html	ProMed Mail	http://www.promed.org
UK Nathnac Homepage	http://www.nathnac.org/pro/index.htm	GeoSentinel Surveillance Network of ISTM and CDC	http://www.geosentinel.org
UK YellowBook (Health Information for Overseas Travel)	http://www.nathnac.org/yellow_book/YBmainpage.htm	HealthMap	http://www.healthmap.org
		Canada-ID News Brief	http://www.phac-aspc.gc.ca/bid-bmi/dsd-dsm/nb-ab/index.html
US DOT Disinsection	http://ostpxweb.dot.gov/policy/safetyenergyenv/disinsection.htm	University of Minnestoa CIDRAP	http://www.cidrap.umn.edu/cidrap/index.html
Health Protection Scotland Fit for Travel	http://www.fitfortravel.scot.nhs.uk/	CDC Health Alert Network	http://www2a.cdc.gov/HAN/ArchiveSys/
Health Protection Scotland Travax[a] ('Scottish Travax')	http://www.travax.nhs.uk/	**Surveillance and Epidemiological Bulletins**	
		CDC MMWR Weekly and Summaries	http://www.cdc.gov/mmwr
Australia Travel Guidelines	http://www.smartraveller.gov.au/	WHO Weekly Epidemiological Record	http://www.who.int/wer/
Country Specific Travel Medicine Databases (Non-governmental)		Eurosurveillance	http://www.eurosurveillance.org/
Travax[a] ('International Travax')	www.travax.com	UN ReliefWeb – Humanitarian Agencies	http://www.reliefweb.int
Tropimed[a]	www.tropimed.com	UK Health Protection Report	http://www.hpa.org.uk/hpr/
International SOS Assistance[a]	http://www.internationalsos.com/en/traveler-management.htm	PAHO Ministries of Health Links	http://www.paho.org/English/PAHO/MOHs.htm
GIDEON[a]	www.gideononline.com	PAHO National Bulletins Links	http://www.paho.org/English/SHA/shavsp.htm
Worldwise[a]	www.worldwise.co.nz/	Canada Communicable Diseases Report	http://www.phac-aspc.gc.ca/publicat/ccdr-rmtc/
Shorelands Travel Health Online	www.tripprep.com	Australia Commun Dis Intellig	http://www.health.gov.au/internet/main/publishing.nsf/Content/cda-pubs-cdi-cdicur.htm
SafeTravel Switzerland (French and German)	www.safetravel.ch		
German Fit for Travel (English and German)	www.fit-for-travel.de/	Japanese Surveillance Center	http://idsc.nih.go.jp/index.html
IAMAT	www.iamat.org	US Military Surveillance	http://afhsc.mil/home
MDTravelHealth	www.mdtravelhealth.com	Caribbean Epidemiology Centre	http://www.carec.org
Travel Medicine Inc	www.travmed.com	EpiNorth Europe	http://www.epinorth.org/
MASTA	http://www.masta.org/	EpiSouth Europe	http://www.episouthnetwork.org/
Travel Warnings and Consular Information		**Vaccine Resources**	
US State Department Advisories	http://travel.state.gov/travel/travel_1744.html	US ACIP Statements	http://www.cdc.gov/vaccines/pubs/ACIP-list.htm
UK FCO Warnings	http://www.fco.gov.uk/en/travel-and-living-abroad/travel-advice-by-country/	US Vaccine Information Statements	http://www.cdc.gov/vaccines/pubs/vis/default.htm
		CDCPinkBook on Vaccines	http://www.cdc.gov/vaccines/pubs/pinkbook/index.html
Foreign Affairs Canada Travel Reports and Warnings	http://www.voyage.gc.ca/countries_pays/menu-eng.asp	CDCPinkBkAppendices	http://www.cdc.gov/vaccines/pubs/pinkbook/index.html#appendices
Australia Consular Sheets	http://www.smartraveller.gov.au/zw-cgi/view/Advice/Index	Canadian Immunization Guide	http://www.phac-aspc.gc.ca/im/index.html
France Consular Bulletins	http://www.diplomatie.gouv.fr/fr/les-francais-etranger_1296/voyager-etranger_1341/index.html	Australia Immunization Guide	http://immunise.health.gov.au/internet/immunise/publishing.nsf/Content/Handbook-home
Swiss Consular Bulletins	http://www.eda.admin.ch/eda/fr/home/travad/travel.html	Vaccines and Biologics in US and Other Countries	http://www.immunize.org/
Emerging Diseases and Outbreaks			
WHO Global Response and Alert	http://www.who.int/csr/en	Vaccine Information from the Vaccine Action Coalition	http://www.vaccineinformation.org/

Continued

Table 4.3 Travel Medicine Websites (Many Provide Twitter, Facebook, RSS, and Linkedin Feeds)—cont'd

WHO Vaccine Schedules in All Countries	http://www.who.int/vaccines/GlobalSummary/Immunization/ScheduleSelect.cfm	**Overseas Assistance**	
WHO Vaccines	http://www.who.int/immunization/en/	Blue Cross/Blue Shield Worldwide Providers	https://international.mondialusa.com/bcbsa/index.asp?page=login
WHO Vaccine Links	http://www.who.int/immunization/links/en/	DOS Medical Info Abroad	http://travel.state.gov/travel/tips/brochures/brochures_1215.html
WHO Pre-Qualified Vaccines	http://www.who.int/immunization_standards/vaccine_quality/PQ_vaccine_list_en/en/index.html	IAMAT	http://www.iamat.org/
		International SOS	http://www.internationalsos.com/en/
sanofiWorldCorporateSite	http://www.sanofipasteur.com/sanofi-pasteur2/front/index.jsp?siteCode=SP_CORP&codeRubrique=1&lang=EN	Trav Emerg Net (TEN)	http://www.tenweb.com/
		MedEx Insurance	http://www.medexassist.com/
		Maps and Non-Medical Country Information	
GSKVaccines	http://www.gsk.com/products/vaccines/index.htm	CIA – The World Factbook	https://www.cia.gov/cia/publications/factbook/
Merck Vaccines	http://www.merckvaccines.com/	US State Dept Background Notes	http://www.state.gov/r/pa/ei/bgn/
Baxter Vaccines-TBE	http://www.baxter.com/press_room/factsheets/vaccines/index.html	UN Maps	http://www.un.org/Depts/Cartographic/english/htmain.htm
sanofiUS	http://www.sanofipasteur.us/sanofi-pasteur2/front/index.jsp?siteCode=SP_US	Google Maps	http://maps.google.com/maps?hl=en&tab=wl
sanofiCanada	http://www.sanofipasteur.ca/sanofi-pasteur2/front/index.jsp?siteCode=SP_CA	Falling Rain Global Gazetteer and Altitude Finder	http://www.fallingrain.com/world/
sanofiMSDEurope	http://www.spmsd.com/index.asp?lang=1	Geographic Names Database	http://www.geonames.org
Novartis Vaccines	http://www.novartisvaccines.com/us/portfolio/us_portfolio.shtml	Perry Castaneda Map-Related Web Sites	http://www.lib.utexas.edu/Libs/PCL/Map_collection/map_sites/map_sites.html
Berna	http://www.bernaproducts.com/	**Security and Safety**	
US Vaccine PIs – Vaccine Safety Institute	http://www.vaccinesafety.edu/package_inserts.htm	OSAC	http://www.osac.gov/
International Agencies		Kroll Associates	http://www.krollworldwide.com/
WHO PAHO	http://www.paho.org/	Control Risks Group	http://www.crg.com/
WHO Africa	http://www.afro.who.int/	Road Safety by Country	http://www.asirt.org/
WHO Southeast Asia	http://www.searo.who.int/	EU Air Safety Portal	http://ec.europa.eu/transport/air/index_en.htm
WHO Europe	http://www.euro.who.int/	FAA Air Safety Standards in All Countries	http://www.faa.gov/about/initiatives/iasa/
WHO Eastern Mediterranean	http://www.emro.who.int/	**Professional Societies**	
WHO Western Pacific	http://www.wpro.who.int/	International Society of Travel Medicine	http://www.istm.org
WHO Health Topics A–Z	http://www.who.int/topics/en/		
WHO Fact Sheets	http://www.who.int/inf-fs/en/index.html	American Society of Tropical Medicine and Hygiene	http://www.astmh.org/
World Tourism Organization	http://www.world-tourism.org/	Infectious Diseases Society of America	http://www.idsociety.org/
International Civil Aviation Organization (Regulatory)	http://www.icao.int/	Royal Society of Tropical Medicine and Hygiene	http://www.rstmh.org/
International Air Transport Association (Airline Industry)	http://www.iata.org/	British Travel Health Association	http://www.btha.org/
Disability Resources		Divers Alert Network	http://www.diversalertnetwork.org/
MossRehab ResourceNet	http://www.mossresourcenet.org/travel.htm	Wilderness Medical Society	http://www.wms.org/
Aviation Consumer Protection Home Page	http://airconsumer.ost.dot.gov/publications/disabled.htm	Undersea and Hyperbaric Medicine Society	http://www.uhms.org/
European Civil Aviation	http://www.ecac-ceac.org/index.php	American Travel Health Nurses Association	http://www.athna.org/
American Diabetes Association	http://www.diabetes.org/	Glasgow Faculty of Travel Medicine	http://www.rcpsg.ac.uk/Travel%20Medicine/Pages/mem_spweltravmed.aspx
Society for Accessible Travel and Hospitality	http://www.sath.org/	German Society of Tropical Medicine and International Health (DTG)	http://www.dtg.org
Mobility International	http://www.miusa.org/		

Table 4.3 Travel Medicine Websites (Many Provide Twitter, Facebook, RSS, and Linkedin Feeds)—cont'd

French Travel Medicine Society	http://www.medecine-voyages.org/	**Drug Resources**	
		WHO Drug Information	http://www.who.int/druginformation/
Federation of European Societies of Tropical Medicine	http://www.festmih.eu/Page/WebObjects/PageFestE.woa/wa/displayPage?name=Home	Micromedex Drug Databases	http://www.micromedex.com
South African Society of Travel Medicine	http://www.sastm.org.za/	Sanford Guide to Antimicrobial Therapy	http://webedition.sanfordguide.com/
Latin American Travel Medicine Society (SLAMVI)	http://www.slamviweb.org/es/	Medline Drug Information for Patients	http://www.nlm.nih.gov/medlineplus/druginformation.html
Travel Medicine Society of Ireland	http://tmsi.ie	Up to Date	http://www.uptodate.com
Disease Pages		HIV Drug Interactions	http://www.hiv-druginteractions.org/
WHO – Global Health Atlas	http://www.who.int/GlobalAtlas/	**Training and Academic Institutions**	
WHO Global Malaria Program	http://www.who.int/malaria/en/	The Gorgas Course in Clinical Tropical Medicine	http://www.gorgas.org
WHO AFRO Malaria	http://www.afro.who.int/malaria/index.html	Global Health Education Consortium	http://globalhealtheducation.org/SitePages/Home.aspx
ACT Malaria – Asia	http://www.actmalaria.net/	HealthTraining.org	http://www.healthtraining.org/
WHO Southeast Asia Malaria	http://www.searo.who.int/EN/Section10/Section21/Section340_4015.htm	TropEd Europ Website	http://www.troped.org/
		London School of Hygiene & Tropical Medicine	http://www.lshtm.ac.uk/
National Malaria Treatment Guidelines for All Countries	http://www.who.int/malaria/am_drug_policies_by_region_amro/en/index.html	Liverpool School of Tropical Medicine	http://www.liv.ac.uk/study/postgraduate/
Oxford Malaria Atlas Project	http://www.map.ox.ac.uk/	James Cook Univ	http://www.jcu.edu.au/phtmrs/
PAHO Malaria	http://www.paho.org/english/ad/dpc/cd/malaria.htm	Mahidol Tropical Medicine	http://www.tm.mahidol.ac.th/
		Swiss Tropical Institute	http://www.swisstph.ch/en/teaching-and-training.html
CDC – Influenza	http://www.cdc.gov/flu/		
Europe Influenza	http://ecdc.europa.eu/en/healthtopics/seasonal_influenza/epidemiological_data/Pages/Weekly_Influenza_Surveillance_Overview.aspx	Tulane Tropical Medicine	http://www.sph.tulane.edu/tropmed/
		University of Minnesota	http://www.globalhealth.umn.edu/
		Institute Pasteur	http://www.pasteur.fr/english.html
OIE Zoonoses Reports	http://www.oie.int/hs2/report.asp	Prince Leopold Institute	http://www.itg.be/itg/
Europe Rabies Bulletin	http://www.who-rabies-bulletin.org/	Bernhard Nocht Institute	http://www.bni.uni-hamburg.de/
Global Polio Eradication	http://www.polioeradication.org/	TrainingFinder PHF	https://www.train.org/DesktopShell.aspx?tabid=1
CDC TB	http://www.cdc.gov/tb/default.htm		
WHO TB	http://www.who.int/gtb/	**General Travel Aids**	
WHO Cholera	http://www.who.int/topics/cholera/en/	Times Around the World	http://www.timeanddate.com/
		Embassies in the US	http://www.state.gov/s/cpr/rls/
Reeder Tropical Radiology Atlas	http://tmcr.usuhs.mil/toc.htm#	Embassies in the US Web Links	http://www.embassy.org/embassies/index.html
PAHO Dengue	http://www.paho.org/english/ad/dpc/cd/dengue.htm	Airlines of the Web	http://flyaow.com/airlinehomepages.htm
WHO	Global Schistosomiasis Atlas	http://www.who.int/schistosomiasis/epidemiology/global_atlas/en/index.html	Tourism Offices Worldwide	http://www.towd.com/
		Visa PLUS-ATM Locator	http://visa.via.infonow.net/locator/global/jsp/SearchPage.jsp
CDC DPD Parasitology Diagnostic Atlas	http://www.dpd.cdc.gov/dpdx/	Mastercard Cirrus ATM Locator	http://www.mastercard.com/cardholderservices/atm/
Photo Thumbnails – ASTMH-Zaiman Slide Library	http://www.astmh.org/source/ZaimanSlides/index.cfm?event=thumbnails	International Dialing Codes	http://kropla.com/dialcode.htm
		JAMA Career Center	Volunteer Opportunities	http://www.jamacareercenter.com/volunteer_opportunities.cfm

^aSubscription fees required.

patients who may have indefinite or changeable itineraries. Many software packages also now include global distribution maps for a number of important tropical diseases. As described individually in Table 4.3, a number of other important and useful features are included in many of the available packages.

The quality and timeliness of the information contained in the vendor's database should be the premier consideration. The listed databases all contain high-quality information and the recommendations generated consistently represent a distillation of those of authoritative national or international bodies. In case of discrepancy between WHO, CDC and national bodies, many of the software packages highlight these differences, and allow for selection of one or the other in generating a final report.

Electronic Discussion Forums and Listservs

'Listservs' are electronic distribution lists that function using e-mail with or without a browser-based interface. Anyone who has joined a particular listserv group can e-mail a posting to a central server. The posting is then disseminated to all members who have subscribed to the same list. Several formats exist to join one of these listservs: 1) an e-mail message is sent to the server; 2) an online form is filled out; 3) a menu of available groups or forums is provided by a social networking service such as LinkedIn or Facebook. Once a person is accepted as a list member, the sponsor will generate, by e-mail or onscreen, a list of instructions on how to participate in the discussion for that group.

TravelMed is an unmoderated discussion of clinical issues related to the practice of Travel Medicine (www.istm.org/WebForms/Members/MemberActivities/listserve.aspx) that is restricted to members of the International Society of Travel Medicine. The ISTM Travel Medicine Forum (www.linkedin.com/groups?gid=3538254&trk=myg_ugrp_ovr) is an open group that allows professional and social interaction among those interested in travel medicine. LinkedIn is the most professionally oriented of the social networks and all those who join (free) must post at least brief professional résumés.

Electronic Notifications and Feeds

Many websites, including those in Table 4.3, provide short messages or 'feeds' that instantly inform subscribers when updates are made; usually a direct link back to the complete text is included. One common form of electronic notification is RSS (really simple syndication). To receive these feeds, users must have an RSS reader, either as free-standing software or embedded in a web-browser, e-mail client, or on a mobile device. Users can customize notification settings to send multiple feeds to their different devices. Many websites also provide feeds that can be read via Twitter (www.twitter.com), Facebook (www.facebook.com), or LinkedIn (www.linkedin.com) for those that have accounts on these social networking services. Some websites simply provide a sign-up form to receive regular e-mailed updates or tables of contents of regular publications.

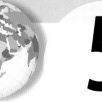

5

Pre-Travel Consultation

Christoph Hatz and Lin H. Chen

Key points

- Consider the 3 major elements of pre-travel medical advice: (1) individual risk assessment based on itinerary, style, and duration of travel; (2) supplemental written educational materials, including links to reliable internet sites to complement oral advice; (3) specialized guidance on health management abroad (self-treatment, seeking medical help)
- Provide travelers with clear and concise information from reliable sources, focused on relevant health issues
- Discuss and administer appropriate vaccinations and prescribe medications for prevention and self-treatment
- Review preventive measures against injuries, arthropod-borne diseases, diarrheal, respiratory tract, and sexually transmitted infections, and cardiopulmonary complications for persons with pre-existing conditions

Introduction

Travelers to distant countries, including the tropics, are exposed to health risks, both non-infectious and infectious. Some of these risks are destination specific whereas others are widely distributed. There is a growing body of evidence with regard to true risks to travelers and this should be considered when counseling an individual.[1,2,3] It is recognized that infants, children, pregnant women, and older adults encounter specific risks. Certain populations of travelers, such as persons with immune suppression or underlying health problems, face additional challenges. Some types of travelers, for example students studying abroad, or travelers visiting friends and relatives (VFR), may have broader risk exposures but inaccurate perceptions of risk.[4,5] Women may have different patterns of health disturbance from men, possibly reflecting behavioral and exposure differences.[6] Some of the anticipated disorders are potentially fatal; many are dangerous, and others may have long-term sequelae. A few can also be transmitted to other people when returning from endemic areas. However, the majority of health disturbances are of limited duration and mild in character. About a third of travelers to tropical and subtropical countries are estimated to suffer from mild diarrheal disturbances, which usually do not lead to severe consequences. Surprisingly, travelers are often more concerned with diarrhea than with upper respiratory disorders, although influenza may be as frequently encountered while traveling. Still, many need to adjust their travel plans at least temporarily due to diarrhea, and even the mild course of an ailment may impair a leisurely atmosphere or seriously interrupt a business transaction.

The pre-travel consultation therefore fulfills three main goals: (i) assessment of the client's fitness for travel, based on their medical history and an understanding of the purpose and type of travel; (ii) analysis of the anticipated and real health risks; and (iii) translation of the findings into a tailored counseling of prophylactic measures. Furthermore, the counseling session should include suggestions for appropriate behavior and self-management, and instruction about seeking medical care when health problems arise during travel. Personal experience positively influences the credibility of the person providing advice. Informing but not frightening travelers is a key function of the advisor.

Logistics and Mechanics of Pre-Travel Consultation

It is ideal if the family or primary care physician who is acquainted with the traveler from the longitudinal care standpoint can provide personalized and relevant tips for safe travel. Their insights into a patient's compliance are relevant, especially for malaria chemoprophylaxis. They are also more likely to have the best approach to address sexual adventures and their consequences with their own patients. In many circumstances, however, this will be relegated to a travel health advisor – even for management of 'routine' developing world travel.

A comprehensive pre-travel consultation may easily span more than an hour, and applies to selected cases such as extended trips, multiple destinations, or a special host. Most consultations, however, may only be allotted 30 minutes or even less. The advisor must therefore concentrate on the most important health risks and their prevention. This requires sound knowledge of the epidemiology in the targeted destinations, and knowledge about the destination. Any personal experience of the advisor is an invaluable asset.

The content of pre-travel advice may be defined by checklists as suggested in Tables 5.1 and 5.2, or may be offered in electronic modules. Referral to travel medicine experts with broad experience is always optimal for more complex situations requiring detailed epidemiological knowledge, special health risks, or advice for immunocompromised travelers.[7]

DOI: 10.1016/B978-1-4557-1076-8.00005-3

Table 5.1 Relevant Questions in Pre-Travel Counseling

Itinerary	Where? Standards of accommodation and food hygiene standards?
Duration	How long?
Travel style	Independent travel or package tour? Business trip? Adventure trip? Pilgrimage? High risk VFR in rural areas with poor hygienic standards? Refugees? Expatriates or long-term travelers?
Time of travel	What season? How long until departure?
Special activities	Hiking? Diving? Rafting? Biking?
Health status	Chronic diseases? Allergies? Regular medications?
Vaccination status	Basic vaccinations up to date? Special (travel) vaccinations up to date?
Previous travel experience	Tolerated (malaria) medication? Problems with high altitude?
Special situations	Pregnancy/breastfeeding? Disability? Physical or psychological problems?

The impact and influence of pre-travel consultation are difficult to measure, but are likely related to the expertise and communications skills of the advisor. Limited data suggest that a face-to-face interview by trained staff is an effective method of delivering counseling.[8] Some studies have shown improved travelers' knowledge regarding malaria risk and prevention following pre-travel consultations,[8,9,10] although the travelers' health beliefs greatly influence adherence. Moreover, data regarding the benefits of counseling on safe sex, road traffic accidents, drowning, and many other topics are lacking.

Components of Pre-Travel Consultation and Order of Importance

Good travel consultations should start with emphasizing the positive aspects of travel, not with enumerating risks and problems while traveling. The advisor should also approach the travelers as 'clients' rather than 'patients.' If compliance is the goal, then it appears logical that the traveler should be convinced by fact rather than threatened by dramatic descriptions of negative events. Conveying a message that translates into a change of behaviour is an art.

Fit for Travel?

Ideally, overseas travelers should be stable in their physical and mental health. Acute disorders are indications for trip cancellation. Special risks for small children, pregnant women, senior travelers or people with chronic disorders require careful advice and balancing the positive and negative consequences of a trip. For example, the pre-travel counseling for a pregnant woman who is obligated to travel to Africa for family reasons should aim to minimize potential health dangers. Ultimately, the travelers need to decide for themselves, but the advisor may also actively advise against a trip if the risks are deemed too high. Cardiovascular problems and injuries are the most common causes of deaths during travel.[11,12,13] The destination and the type of travel influence the magnitude of health risks for particular groups. Physical stress accompanies activities such as mountain trekking and diving, as well as destinations with climatic challenges (temperature, humidity, altitude, and pollution in large cities).

Table 5.2 Key Points of Pre-Travel Advice Practice

Food

Eat freshly prepared food. Whenever possible, avoid raw, un- and undercooked vegetables, salads, and meat. Try to peel the fruit yourself. Try to check that prepared meals are not contaminated by dirty plates and cups, by water, or by insects.

Be aware that the recommendation 'Peel it, cook it, boil it, or forget it!' is correct in principle, but few travelers comply with it.

Water

Drink industrially bottled water (properly sealed; carbonated), hot tea in clean cups. Avoid ice cubes, fresh milk of unknown quality. If no safe water is available, disinfect with respective means (filters are heavy!), iodine, or boil it (see Ch. 6).

Mosquitoes

Prevention of mosquito bites esp. relevant in areas endemic for malaria. Note that a good number of arthropod-borne infections occur in some countries. Discussing them together and making the point of the importance of repellents, protective (insecticide-treated) clothing and mosquito nets emphasizes the importance of those measures.

Hydration/Dehydration

Adequate (lots of fluid intake is essential in hot climates). Thirst is not a good indicator for adequate fluid intake.

Rule of thumb: 'Urine should have a light yellow color'.

Sun

Sun exposure can be dangerous, esp. for children. Adequate protection is required: hat, cap, sunglasses, sunscreen.

Walking Barefoot

Several parasites can enter the intact or damaged skin: larvae of worms (hookworm, *Strongyloides*), jigger fleas.

Even small skin lesions (scratched mosquito bites) can develop into suprainfected ulcers. Wearing shoes or at least sandals helps reduce the risk.

Venomous and Poisonous Animals

Do not touch and do not step on anything that you cannot see. This reduces the risk of snake, scorpion and spider injuries where such animals prevail. Use a torch when going for a walk at night. Robust shoes and long trousers are important preventive measures. Carrying antisera on trips to endemic areas is discouraged (problems of cooling, safe administration).

Sexual Contacts

Casual contacts are best avoided. Carry condoms at all times, just in case.

Accidents

Motor vehicle and cycle accidents, sports and other leisure injuries, violence and aggression, drowning, animal bites are unwanted but relatively common incidents during travel. Alcohol and drugs are often cofactors in such accidents.

Check travel insurance needs prior to departing.

Altitude

High mountain hiking and trekking require individual counseling. Medication to prevent high-altitude sickness may be required.

High fluid intake and avoiding alcohol and drugs are necessary.

A priority in the pre-travel consultation is to minimize unnecessary exposures, particularly in vulnerable persons. Therefore, tourist travel to remote and tropical destinations is typically discouraged for pregnant women and very young children, as they are at risk for various reasons ranging from infectious diseases to general stress, dehydration, and lack of appropriate medical care in remote areas. The travel health expert may need to recommend trip postponement until the traveler's health status is considered to be reasonably stable. Immunocompromised travelers (HIV/AIDS, chronic diseases, medical conditions requiring corticosteroids or immune modulators) also need special attention and preparation. Likewise, stabilization before air travel is desirable because of the increased risk for complications for certain travelers:[1]

- with unstable or recently deteriorated angina pectoris CCSIII
- within 3 weeks after uncomplicated and 6 weeks after complicated cardiac infarction
- within 2 weeks after ACBP (aorto-coronary bypass) surgery
- with congenital defects, including Eisenmenger syndrome and severe symptomatic valvulopathy
- within 2 weeks after stroke
- with lung disorders with dyspnea at minimal effort
- within 10 days after surgical operations of thorax or abdomen
- within 24 hours after diving and after diving accidents.

Analysis of Expected Health Risks in Travelers

Major considerations in the pre-travel consultation are travel style and duration. Individual risks are assessed and discussed with the traveler during pre-travel counseling.[14] Both infectious and non-infectious health risks need tailored attention. Advice must be relevant, feasible, and adapted to the individual client. An athlete flying to Johannesburg will have different risks from a student traveling 3 months through Southern Africa on an overland truck. The following sections suggest ways to address relevant issues which merit mention or in-depth discussion.

General Considerations

Communicating the prevention of potentially serious health problems such as malaria is critical. At the same time, succinct discussion of frequently encountered 'ordinary' health problems is fundamental, but often bypassed due to time constraints. Some common health problems triggered by motion, climate, and different socioeconomic conditions warrant discussion with respect to prevention and self-management. Acute, often benign respiratory and flu-like infections, urinary tract infections, dental problems, gynecological problems, headaches or nausea, and injuries are not routinely mentioned, although these are common and potentially hazardous during travel. The threshold at which signs and symptoms should lead to medical evaluation may depend on the individual traveler and on the available medical facilities in the destination country. The advisor has to choose between issues that the traveler 'needs to know' and what is 'nice to know'. The latter may include Ebola, dangerous influenza viruses, cholera or alleged outbreaks of plague. These diseases will rarely be a true risk to the overwhelming majority of travelers, but media sensation may fuel unnecessary concern.

Specific, Commonly Occurring Topics to be Discussed

Gastrointestinal disturbances do not only occur in countries with lower hygienic standards, but they are also more frequently encountered in the south than in northern industrialized countries.[15,16] Simple preventive and management measures, such as good hydration and reasonable use of medications, are key elements. 'Peel it, cook it, boil it, or forget it' is a rational and catchy phrase, although its practice and efficacy are debated.[17,18] Experience indicates that few travelers adhere to this adage.[17] Sophisticated and individualized advice is required to achieve the essence of the information and translate it into practice. The use of emergency standby antibiotic medication may be useful for certain travelers. Experts vary on their opinion as to whether such self-treatment is recommended: treatment-related adverse events are always a concern. The development of antimicrobial resistance is another reason why some do not prescribe broad use of antibiotics for many travelers.

Cardiovascular problems are reported in association with dehydration, high blood pressure or pre-existing heart disease. There is a growing complexity of relevant advice in an increasingly diverse traveler community that includes older adults, persons with rheumatologic diseases, immune suppression, and other underlying conditions. Pre-existing diseases frequently raise concern regarding one's fitness to travel.

Travel medicine experts should recognize that **neuropsychological problems** may be repressed or misinterpreted. These diagnoses comprise a wide spectrum from mild sleeping disorders to depressive states. The abrupt change from workaday life to holiday may trigger mood oscillations that could be attenuated by a smooth transition phase. Finding out about the destination country and the lifestyle that one will encounter prior to traveling will help adjustment.

Finally, travelers often need recommendations regarding a **travel medical kit** (see Ch. 8). Generally the kits focus on first-aid items (injuries, skin and eye care) and some drugs with broad indications such as paracetamol, loperamide, antihistamine, but should also include specific medication for the traveler with pre-existing conditions or for special risks such as malaria. The further away from tourist routes, the more medications and first-aid items may be necessary.

Inattention, whether stress-related or due to a relaxed state, leads to **accidents**. Road traffic accidents are an important risk worldwide, especially in low-income countries and especially at night. An estimated 3500 traffic-related deaths occur every day.[19] Assessment of fatal accidents among travelers is fragmentary. More than 250 fatal road traffic accidents are reported among US citizens abroad per year, making it the 'leading cause of death to healthy US travelers';[1] at least 15 Swiss travelers die every year abroad in traffic accidents (personal communication, Swiss Federal Office of Statistics). Such figures, however, indicate that road accidents account for more deaths than any vaccine-preventable infectious disease. Indeed, the well-known nursery school motto (modified) becomes useful for surviving a trip to Thailand or other countries with left-hand traffic: 'First look right, then look left, then look right again before crossing a road'. Also remind travelers that wearing helmets when riding bicycles and motorcycles while abroad may save more lives than being vaccinated against a rare, exotic disease. The advice to check the safety equipment of transport vehicles is appropriate but sometimes difficult to implement. More easily followed are tips to request a spirited driver to kindly slow down, or to stop and exit the vehicle to avoid reckless driving.

Caution regarding other exposures is an important component of travel advice, for example excessive **sun exposure** and its possible sequelae of dermatological cancers. The topic of **sexually transmitted infections** is sometimes awkward but should be addressed. Studies have shown that 5–10% of tourists have unplanned sexual contact with new partners.[20,21,22] At least one-third do not use condoms regularly owing to their unavailability, and it is known that alcohol use increases this risk. Simple questions such as 'Do you know the most frequent mode of transmission of HIV?' or skilful exploration of the traveler's openness for new experiences and foreign cultures may help to prevent clumsy or offensive discussion about sexual risks. Incidental mention of unplanned sexual contacts, or only mentioning condoms, may only impair the advisor's credibility.

Health problems triggered almost exclusively by **mobility include motion sickness, jet lag and other situations in an aircraft, ship or motor vehicle**. Dry air and increased pressure in the middle ear in the aircraft cabin, the risk of thromboembolism associated with prolonged immobility or dehydration, and fear of flying are additional topics that concern some travelers. Motion sickness can sometimes be mitigated by medication.[23] To respond to jet lag, travelers can initiate adjustments to the time zone changes even before departure by gradually changing their sleeping time at home.[24] Travelers suffering from fear of flying may be too embarrassed to admit it, but openly discussing the condition and providing resources (courses offered by airlines, autogenic training, medication) will greatly help the concerned traveler.[25,26] Finally, appropriate hydration during flight helps to maintain the sense of wellbeing. The boosted diuresis, leading to modest ambulation from frequenting the toilets, could lower the risk of thromboembolism (see Ch. 49).

Potential health risks related to particular activities or exposures on a trip should be discussed. A tourist going river rafting in Africa should be informed about potential exposure to schistosomiasis. The agricultural consultant spending 6 weeks with peasants in Southeast Asia should be informed about protective measures against various mosquito-borne infections, and also be offered a vaccination against Japanese encephalitis. The trans-Africa biker should be provided an understanding of rabies exposure and transmission, and the cave explorer in East Africa should be informed about the risk of Marburg virus and other diseases transmitted by bats.

Highlighting some positive influences of travel to various climatic zones can balance the caution raised with risk discussions. A stay on the seaside usually improves the skin condition of psoriasis. Joint pains can ameliorate in warm dry climates, and allergic reactions can decrease at higher altitudes.

Application of Preventive Measures

Besides assessing and discussing behavioural aspects concerning preventive measures for the above issues, counseling on chemoprophylaxis and vaccinations is a crucial element of the pre-travel consultation. Communicating the importance of preventive measures against malaria is challenging (see Ch. 15). Information should be evidence based, and supplemented with written material. The advice should balance the benefit of chemoprophylaxis with the risk of possible adverse effects from the medication.

Vaccine recommendations and requirements should also be determined by risk. Vaccine contraindications and the time available to complete vaccinations before departure should be considered. The pre-travel consultation is often the only time to update routine vaccinations for adults (e.g., tetanus/diphtheria/pertussis, measles) who may not see their physicians for immunizations.

Travel health advisors also need to consider the cost of the visit, vaccines, and antimalarial medications. Sometimes this will necessitate prioritization – again weighing the risks against the benefits.

Health Problems During and After Travel

The general rule during and after travel to tropical and subtropical countries is to investigate (i) every fever which lasts more than 24 hours, and (ii) every diarrheal episode with fever, abdominal cramps and bloody stool. Certain travelers with a history of diarrhea may need a follow-up visit after travel to rule out invasive amebiasis even if symptoms have resolved, although typical short-term travelers have low likelihood for this diagnosis. Long-term travelers to tropical areas,

even when asymptomatic, may still benefit from medical screening.[27] In such cases an investigation is recommended, including exposure history and physical examination, blood chemistry and hematology, stool parasitology, as well as selective screening of urine parasitology, and other serologies depending upon exposures (e.g., HIV).[28] Unless overt symptoms exist, some of these investigations may be performed about 3 months after return to account for the incubation periods of most potential pathogens. Despite the fact that most infectious diseases may become symptomatic within weeks, the possibility of a prolonged incubation period must be borne in mind. Falciparum malaria usually appears within 1 month after return, but manifestations after 1 year and longer have rarely been reported.[29,30] Late-onset or recurrent diarrhea may be a manifestation of giardiasis, amebiasis, or post-infectious irritable bowel syndrome; pruritus with skin swellings can be due to filariasis. When in doubt, a specialist in tropical diseases should be consulted for such cases.

People spending longer or having repeated stays in tropical countries should have targeted investigations every 2–3 years to identify silent infections which may cause organ damage if not recognized (e.g., schistosomiasis, echinococcosis, strongyloidiasis).

Challenges Regarding Travel Advice

A considerable amount of time and effort is needed to remain up to date with the growing body of knowledge in travel medicine (Table 5.2). The regular provision of advice is necessary to *obtain* and *maintain* the routine. If such practice is not possible, it may be advisable to work with checklists for standard travel advice, and to refer clients to more experienced colleagues for complex itineraries or special health considerations.

The advisor should be aware of the information sources that their clients use. Some travelers obtain information from travel agencies, which naturally emphasize the positive aspects of travel. Some travelers receive information from friends and relatives; others visit pharmacies for advice. The media publish abundantly about travel destinations as well. A wide range of inadequate or conflicting information from different perspectives often creates confusion rather than clarity. Contradictory information unsettles travelers and raises their skepticism about preventive measures, leading to poor compliance with recommendations.[31] Clear, accurate, and up-to-date information must therefore be conveyed.

The client is often overwhelmed with abundant information and is likely to forget most of it. Thus, there are four key suggestions that may help with all consultations:

1. Advise the traveler in a personal, individualized conversation that responds to their needs and allows for questions. The assessment should always include details regarding travel itinerary and style, previous travel experience and vaccinations as well as existing health problems. Offering concise information is best, but elaborate on areas of concern to the traveler. Administering vaccinations is straightforward and does not require much compliance, but convincing the client of the need to comply with antimalarial medication during travel and continuing after return is more of a challenge. The concept of malaria suppression usually takes time to convey, and many travelers mistake chemoprophylaxis for some sort of vaccination. This is one of the reasons why they discontinue taking the drugs after leaving the endemic area.[32] Shorter regimens after return appear to favour compliance.[33]

2. Provide written material as additional information. This allows the traveler to quietly go through guidebooks or leaflets after the

consultation, or even in the plane before arriving at the destination. Such information must be consistent with the oral advice given and should not replace the consultation.

3. Provide links to reliable internet sources (WHO, CDC, national recommendations) to guide the traveler through the plethora of available information and to guarantee reliable guidance.

4. Provide required, necessary documents (Box 5.1).

One possible structure for the discussion of vaccines and other risks is shown in Figure 5.1.

Discussion of the combination vaccine against hepatitis A and B allows the provider to steer the discussion elegantly from uncontroversial hepatitis A to the sensitive, sexually transmitted hepatitis B.

BOX 5.1

Documents to be Carried by Travelers

The advisor should check:

Certificate of vaccination (yellow card, if necessary: exemption letter)

Scanned copies (carried on laptop, iPad) or photocopies of original documents should be carried in a place separate from originals

Travel insurance card

Medical reports (appropriate, in English or other language), recent ECG (scanned, on laptop or mobile devices)

List of allergies

Blood type and group

Name, address, telephone number and fax or e-mail of emergency rescue organization, personal physician

Name, address, telephone number of family members

Responsibility of traveler:

Passport, visa, extra passport photos

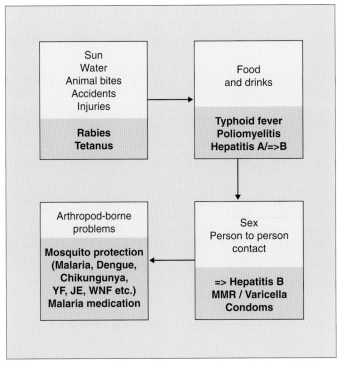

Figure 5.1 Discussion of the combination vaccine against hepatitis A and B allows the provider to elegantly steer the discussion from uncontroversial hepatitis A to the sensitive, sexually transmitted hepatitis B. *(Adapted from Furrer HJ, University Hospital, Berne, Switzerland.)*

Bear in mind that controversial information must be discussed, otherwise there may be confusion and eventual non-compliance. Addressing discrepancies between different sources of information may be illustrative of controversies that travelers may encounter. Many clients will have consulted other (mainly electronic) information sources or received advice from non-professionals. Recognize the fact that only limited evidence exists on certain issues, leading to arguably different advice from different advisors. One way to achieve an impact on health behavior is to combine individualized advice, based on scientific evidence (body of knowledge), and enriched with personal experience.

Acknowledgments

The authors thank Professors Robert Steffen and Hansjakob Furrer for their valuable suggestions.

References

1. CDC Health Information of International Travel 2012. The Yellow Book, pp 96–103.

2. World Health Organisation. International travel and health. Geneva, 2011 Available at: www.who.int/ith. Accessed August 1, 2011.

3. Hatz C, Nothdurft HD. Reisemedizinische Beratung. In: Löscher T, Burchard GD, editors: Tropenmedizin in Klinik und Praxis. New York: Georg Thieme Verlag Stuttgart; 2010:914–22.

4. Hartjes LB, Baumann LC, Henriques JB. Travel health risk perceptions and prevention behaviors of US study abroad students. J Travel Med 2009;16(5):338–43.

5. LaRoque RC, Rao SR, Tsibris A, et al. Pre-travel health advice-seeking behavior among US international travelers departing from Boston Logan International Airport. J Travel Med 2010;17:387–91.

6. Schlagenhauf P, Chen LH, Wilson ME, et al; GeoSentinel Surveillance Network. Sex and gender differences in travel-associated disease.

7. Hill DR, Ericsson CD, Pearson RD, et al; Infectious Diseases Society of America. The practice of travel medicine: guidelines by the Infectious Diseases Society of America. Clin Infect Dis 2006;43(12):1499–1539.

8. Genton B, Behrens RH. Specialized Travel Consultation Part II: Acquiring knowledge. J Travel Med 1994;1(1):13–15.

9. Farquharson L, Noble LM, Barker C, et al. Health beliefs and communication in the travel clinic consultation as predictors of adherence to malaria chemoprophylaxis. Br J Health Psychol 2004;9(Pt 2):201–17.

10. Teodósio R, Gonçalves L, Atouguia J, et al. Quality assessment in a travel clinic: a study of travelers' knowledge about malaria. J Travel Med 2006;13(5):288–93.

11. Groenheide AC, van Genderen PJ, Overbosch D. East and west, home is best? A questionnaire-based survey on mortality of Dutch travelers abroad. J Travel Med 2011;18(2):141–4.

12. Redman CA, MacLennan A, Walker E. Causes of death abroad: analysis of data on bodies returned for cremation to Scotland. J Travel Med 2011;18(2):96–101.

13. Tonellato DJ, Guse CE, Hargarten SW. Injury deaths of US citizens abroad: new data source, old travel problem. J Travel Med 2009;16(5):304–10.

14. Hatz C, Krause E, Grundmann H. Travel advice – a study among Swiss and German general practitioners. Trop Med Int Health 1997;2:6–12.

15. McIntosh IB, Reed JM, Power KG. Travellers' diarrhea and the effect of pre-travel health advice in general practice. Br J Gen Pract 1997;47(415):71–5.

16. Pitzurra R, Steffen R, Tschopp A, et al. Diarrhea in a large prospective cohort of European travellers to resource-limited destinations. BMC Infect Dis 2010;10:231.

17. Shlim DR. Looking for evidence that personal hygiene precautions prevent traveler's diarrhea. Clin Infect Dis 2005;41(Suppl 8):S531–S535.

18. Kozicki M, Steffen R, Schär M. 'Boil it, cook it, peel it or forget it': does this rule prevent travellers' diarrhea? Int J Epidemiol 1985;14(1):169–72.

19. World Health Organisation. Global status report on road safety. Geneva, 2009. Available at: www.who.int/violence_injury_prevention/road_safety_status/2009. Accessed August 1, 2011.

20. Gagneux O, Blöchliger C, Tanner M, et al. Malaria/Casual Sex: What travellers know and what they do. J Travel Med 1996;3:14–21.

21. Cabada MM, Montoya M, Echevarria JI, et al. Sexual behavior in travelers visiting Cuzco. J Travel Med 2003;10(4):214–18.

22. Nielsen US, Petersen E, Larsen CS. Hepatitis B immunization coverage and risk behaviour among Danish travellers: are immunization strategies based on single journey itineraries rational? J Infect 2009;59(5):353–9.

23. Spinks A, Wasiak J. Scopolamine (hyoscine) for preventing and treating motion sickness. Cochrane Database Syst Rev 2011(6):CD002851.

24. Sack RL. Clinical practice. Jet lag. N Engl J Med 2010;362(5):440–7.

25. Rothbaum BO, Anderson P, Zimand E, et al. Virtual reality exposure therapy and standard (in vivo) exposure therapy in the treatment of fear of flying. Behav Ther 2006;37(1):80–90.

26. Tortella-Feliu M, Botella C, Llabrés J, et al. Virtual reality versus computer-aided exposure treatments for fear of flying. Behav Modif 2011;35(1):3–30.

27. Chen LH, Wilson ME, Davis X, et al; GeoSentinel Surveillance Network. Illness in long-term travelers visiting GeoSentinel clinics. Emerg Infect Dis 2009;15(11):1773–82.

28. Franco-Paredes C. Chapter 5: Post-Travel Evaluation. Asymptomatic post-travel screening. In: Centers for Disease Control and Prevention. CDC Health Information for International Travel 2012. New York: Oxford University Press; 2012.

29. Leder K, Black J, O'Brien D, et al. Malaria in travelers: a review of the GeoSentinel surveillance network. Clin Infect Dis 2004;39(8): 1104–12.

30. Skarbinski J, James EM, Causer LM, et al. Malaria surveillance-United States, 2004. MMWR Surveill Summ 2006;55(4):23–37.

31. Chen LH, Wilson ME, Schlagenhauf P. Controversies and misconceptions in malaria chemoprophylaxis for travelers. JAMA 2007;297(20): 2251–63.

32. Landry P, Iorillo D, Darioli R, et al. Do travelers really take their mefloquine malaria chemoprophylaxis? Estimation of adherence by an electronic pillbox. J Travel Med 2006 Jan-Feb;13(1):8–14.

33. Goodyer L, Rice L, Martin A. Choice of and adherence to prophylactic antimalarials. J Travel Med 2011 Jul;18(4):245–9.

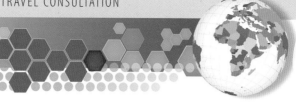

6

Water Disinfection for International Travelers

Howard Backer

Key points

- Potable water is one of the most important factors in ensuring the health of travelers and local populations in developing areas
- The risk of water-borne illness depends on the number of organisms consumed, volume of water, concentration of organisms, host factors, and the efficacy of the treatment system
- Methods of water treatment include the use of heat, ultraviolet light, clarification, filtration and chemical disinfection. The choices for the traveler or international worker are increasing as new technology is applied to field applications
- Different microorganisms have varying susceptibilities to these methods

Introduction

Safe and efficient treatment of drinking water is among the major public health advances of the 20th century. Without it, water-borne disease would spread rapidly in most public water systems served by surface water.[1,2] However, worldwide, more than one billion people have no access to potable water, and 2.4 billion do not have adequate sanitation. This results in billions of cases of diarrhea every year and a reservoir of enteric pathogens for travelers to these areas.[3] In certain tropical countries the influence of high-density population, rampant pollution, and absence of sanitation systems means that available raw water is virtually wastewater. Contamination of tap water commonly occurs because of antiquated and inadequately monitored disposal, water treatment, and distribution systems.[4] Testing of improved water sources in 13 developing countries showed that only 5/22 of these urban water sources had any detectable free chlorine residual.[5]

Travelers have no reliable resources to evaluate local water system quality. Less information is available for remote surface water sources. As a result, travelers should take appropriate steps to ensure that the water they drink does not contain infectious agents. Look, smell, and taste are not reliable indicators to estimate water safety. Even in developed countries with low rates of diarrhea illness, regular water-borne disease outbreaks indicate that the microbiologic quality of the water, especially surface water, is not assured.[6] In both developed and

developing countries, after natural disasters such as hurricanes, tsunamis, and earthquakes, one of the most immediate public health problems is a lack of potable water.

Etiology and Risk of Water-Borne Infection

Infectious agents with the potential for water-borne transmission include bacteria, viruses, protozoa, and non-protozoan parasites (Table 6.1). Although the primary reason for disinfecting drinking water is to destroy microorganisms from animal and human biologic wastes, water may also be contaminated with industrial chemical pollutants, organic or inorganic material from land and vegetation, biologic organisms from animals, or organisms that reside in soil and water. *Escherichia coli* and *Vibrio cholerae* may be capable of surviving indefinitely in tropical water. Most enteric organisms, including *Shigella* spp., *Salmonella enteria* serotype *typhi*, hepatitis A, and *Cryptosporidium* spp., can retain viability for long periods in cold water and can even survive for weeks to months when frozen in water. Survival of enteric bacterial and viral pathogens in temperate water is generally only several days; however, *E. coli* O157: H7 can survive 12 weeks at 25°C.[7]

The risk of water-borne illness depends on the number of organisms consumed, which is in turn determined by the volume of water, concentration of organisms, and treatment system efficiency.[8,9] Additional factors include virulence of the organism and defenses of the host. Microorganisms with a small infectious dose (e.g., *Giardia*, *Cryptosporidia*, *Shigella* spp., hepatitis A, enteric viruses, enterohemorrhagic *E. coli*) may cause illness even from inadvertent drinking during water-based recreational activities.[10] Because total immunity does not develop for most enteric pathogens, reinfection may occur. Most diarrhea among travelers is probably food-borne; however, the capacity for water-borne transmission must not be underestimated.

The combined roles of safe water, hygiene, and adequate sanitation in reducing diarrhea and other diseases are clear and well documented. The WHO estimates that 94% of diarrheal cases globally are preventable through modifications to the environment, including access to safe water.[1] Recent studies of simple water interventions in households of developing countries clearly document improved microbiological quality of water, a 30–60% reduced incidence of diarrheal illness, enhanced childhood survival, and reduction of parasitic diseases, many of which are independent of other measures to improve sanitation.[11–15]

©2012 Elsevier Inc
DOI: 10.1016/B978-1-4557-1076-8.00006-5

Table 6.1 Water-borne Pathogens[9,62,63]

Bacterial	Viral	Protozoan	Other parasites[a]
Enterotoxigenic *E. coli* E. coli O157: H7	Hepatitis A	*Giardia intestinalis*	*Ascaris lumbricoides*
Shigella species	Hepatitis E	*Entamoeba histolytica*	*Ancylostoma duodenale*
Campylobacter species	Norovirus	*Cryptosporidium parvum*	Fasciola hepatica
Vibrio cholerae	Poliovirus	*Blastocystis hominis*	*Dracunculus medinensis*
Salmonella spp. (primarily *enterica* serotype Typhi)	Miscellaneous enteric viruses (more than 100 types)	Isospora belli	*Strongyloides stercoralis*
Yersinia enterocolitica		*Balantidium coli*	*Trichuris trichiura*
Aeromonas		*Acanthamoeba*	*Clonorchis sinensis*
		Cyclospora	*Paragonimus westermani*
			Diphyllobothrium latum
			Echinococcus granulosus

[a]Water-borne transmission is possible but uncommon for all these parasites except *D. medinesis*.

Table 6.2 Methods of Water Treatment that Can be Applied by Travelers

Heat
Clarification
   Sedimentation
   Coagulation–flocculation
   Granular-activated charcoal
Filtration
   Microfiltration, ultrafiltration, nanofiltration
Halogens
   Chlorine
   Iodine
   Iodine resins
Miscellaneous chemical
   Chlorine dioxide and mixed species
   Silver
Solar photocatalytic
Ultraviolet and SODIS

Water Treatment Methods for Travelers and Aid/Relief Workers

Multiple techniques for improving the microbiologic quality of water are available to individuals and small groups who encounter questionable water supplies while traveling or working (Table 6.2). For more detailed discussion of these techniques, please refer to the chapter in Auerbach's *Wilderness Medicine*.[16] As with all advice in travel medicine, the specific recommendation for any traveler depends on the destination and the style and purpose of travel. Those working in areas without adequate sanitation and water treatment may encounter highly contaminated water sources. Adventurous travelers may stay in hotels at night and explore remote villages or wilderness parks during the day, which requires an understanding of more than one method of water treatment for a spectrum of conditions. Bottled water may be a convenient and popular solution but creates ecological problems in countries that do not recycle the plastic.

The term **disinfection**, the desired result of field water treatment, is used here to indicate the removal or destruction of harmful microorganisms, which reduces the risk of illness. This is sometimes used interchangeably with **purification**, but this term is used here to refer to improving the esthetics of water, such as clarity, taste, and smell. **Potable** implies 'drinkable' water, but technically means that a water source, on average, over a period of time, contains a 'minimal microbial hazard,' so that the statistical likelihood of illness is acceptable. All standards, including water regulations in the US, acknowledge the impracticality of trying to eliminate all microorganisms from drinking water. Generally the goal is a 3–5 log reduction (99.9–99.999%), allowing a small risk of enteric infection.[17–19]

Heat

Heat is the oldest and most reliable means of water disinfection (Table 6.3). Heat inactivation of microorganisms is a function of time and temperature (exponential function of first-order kinetics). Thus, the thermal death point is reached in a shorter time at higher temperatures, while lower temperatures are effective if applied for a longer time. Pasteurization uses this principle to kill enteric food pathogens and spoiling organisms at temperatures between 60°°C (140 F) and 70°C (158 F), well below boiling, for up to 30 minutes.[20]

All common enteric pathogens are readily inactivated by heat, though microorganisms vary in heat sensitivity.[21,22] Protozoal cysts, including *Giardia* and *Entamoeba histolytica*, are very susceptible to heat. *Cryptosporidia* are also inactivated at these lower pasteurization levels. Parasitic eggs, larvae, and cercariae are all susceptible to heat. For most helminth eggs and larvae the critical lethal temperature is 50–55° C (122–131° F).[23] Common bacterial enteric pathogens (*E. coli, Salmonella, Shigella*) are killed by standard pasteurization temperatures of 55°C (131°F) for 30 minutes or 65°C (149°F) for < 1 minute.[20,24] Viruses are more closely related to vegetative bacteria than to spore-bearing organisms and are generally inactivated at 56–60°C (132.8–140°F) in less than 20–40 minutes.[25] A review of data from food industry studies confirms the susceptibility of hepatitis A virus and other enteric viruses to heat at pasteurization temperatures.[26]

As enteric pathogens are killed within seconds by boiling water, and rapidly at temperatures >60°C (140°F), the traditional advice to boil water for 10 minutes to ensure potable water is excessive. The time required to heat water from 55°C (131°F) to a boil works toward disinfection; therefore, any water brought to a boil should be adequately disinfected. Boiling for 1 minute, or keeping the water covered and allowing it to cool slowly after boiling, will add an extra margin

Table 6.3 Advantages and Disadvantages of Water Disinfection Methods

Advantages	Disadvantages
Heat	
Relative susceptibility of microorganisms to heat: Protozoa > Bacteria > Viruses	
Does not impart additional taste or color to water	Does not improve the taste, smell or appearance of poor quality water
Can pasteurize water without sustained boiling	Fuel sources may be scarce, expensive, or unavailable
Single-step process that inactivates all enteric pathogens	
Efficacy is not compromised by contaminants or particles in the water, as with halogenation and filtration	
Coagulation–Flocculation (C-F)	
Relative susceptibility of microorganisms to coagulation-flocculation: Protozoa > Bacteria = Viruses	
Highly effective to clarify water and remove many microorganisms	Unfamiliar technique and substances to most travelers
Improves efficacy of filtration and chemical disinfection	Adds extra step unless combined flocculent-disinfectant tablet
Inexpensive and widely available	
Simple process with no toxicity	
Filtration	
Susceptibility of microorganisms to filtration: Protozoa > Bacteria > Viruses	
Simple to operate	Adds bulk and weight to baggage
Mechanical filters require no holding time for treatment (water is treated as it passes through the filter	Most filters not reliable for sufficient removal of viruses
Large choice of commercial products	Expensive relative to halogens
Adds no unpleasant taste and often improves taste and appearance of water	Channeling of water or high pressure can force microorganisms through the filter
Rationally combined with halogens for removal or destruction of all microorganisms	Filters eventually clog from suspended particulate matter; may require some maintenance or repair in field
Inexpensive	
Halogens	
Relative susceptibility of microorganisms to halogens: Bacteria > Viruses > Protozoa	
Iodine and chlorine are widely available	Corrosive, stains clothing
Very effective for bacteria, viruses, and *Giardia*	Not effective for *Cryptosporidia*
Taste can be removed	Imparts taste and odor
Flexible dosing	Flexibility requires understanding of disinfection principles
As easily applied to large quantities as small quantities	Potential toxicity (especially iodine)
Chlorine Dioxide	
Relative susceptibility of microorganisms to chlorine dioxide: Bacteria > Viruses > Protozoa	
Effective against all microorganisms, including *Cryptosporidia*	Volatile, so do not expose tablets to air and use generated solutions rapidly
Low doses have no taste or color	
More potent than equivalent doses of chlorine	No persistent residual, so does not prevent recontamination during storage
Less affected by nitrogenous wastes	Sensitive to sunlight, so keep bottle shaded or in pack during treatment
SODIS and Ultraviolet (UV)	
Relative susceptibility of microorganisms: Protozoa > Bacteria > Viruses	
Effective against all microorganisms	Requires clear water
Imparts no taste	Does not improve water esthetics
Simple to use	No residual effect – does not prevent recontamination during storage
Portable device now available for individual and small group field use	Expensive
	Requires power source

of safety. The boiling point decreases with increasing altitude, but this is not significant compared with the time required for thermal death at these temperatures.

Although attaining boiling temperature is not necessary, boiling is the only easily recognizable endpoint without using a thermometer. Hot tap water temperature and the temperature of water perceived to be too hot to touch vary too widely to be reliable measures for pasteurization of water. Nevertheless, if no reliable method of water treatment is available, tap water that has been kept hot in a tank for at least 30 minutes and is too hot to keep a finger immersed for 5 seconds (estimated 55–65°C; 131–149°F) is a reasonable alternative. Travelers with access to electricity can boil water with either a small electric heating coil or a lightweight electric beverage warmer brought from home. In very austere and desperate situations with hot, sunny climate, adequate pasteurization temperature can be achieved with a solar oven or simple reflectors[27] (see UV–SODIS).

Clarification

Clarification refers to techniques that reduce the turbidity or cloudiness of surface water caused by natural organic and inorganic material. These techniques can markedly improve the appearance and taste of water and are properly considered purification methods. Frequently used interchangeably with 'disinfection,' purification is more accurately used to indicate the removal of organic or inorganic chemicals and particulate matter to improve color, taste and odor. It may reduce the number of microorganisms, but not enough to ensure potable water; however, clarifying the water facilitates disinfection by filtration or chemical treatment. Cloudy water can rapidly clog microfilters. Moreover, cloudy water requires increased levels of chemical treatment, and the combined effects of the water contaminants plus chemical disinfectants can be quite unpleasant to taste.

Sedimentation

Sedimentation is the separation of suspended particles such as sand and silt that are large enough to settle rapidly by gravity. Microorganisms, especially protozoan cysts, also settle eventually, but this takes much longer. Simply allow the water to sit undisturbed for about 1 hour or until sediment has formed on the bottom of the container, then decant or filter the clear water from the top through a coffee filter or finely woven cloth. A second method of disinfection must then be used.

Coagulation–Flocculation

Coagulation–flocculation (C-F), a technique in use since 2000 BC, can remove smaller suspended particles and chemical complexes too small to settle by gravity (colloids).[28] Coagulation is achieved with the addition of a chemical that causes particles to stick together by electrostatic and ionic forces. Flocculation is a physical process that promotes the formation of larger particles by gentle mixing. Alum (an aluminum salt), lime (alkaline chemicals principally containing calcium or magnesium with oxygen), or iron salts are commonly used coagulants. Alum is non-toxic and used in the food industry for pickling. It is readily available in any chemical supply store. In an emergency, baking powder or even the fine white ash from a campfire can be used as a coagulant. Other natural substances are used in various parts of the world. C-F removes 60–98% of microorganisms, heavy metals, and some chemicals and minerals (Table 6.3).

The amount of alum added in the field – approximately a large pinch (one-eighth teaspoon) per gallon (approximately 4 L) of water – need not be precise. Stir or shake briskly for 1 min to mix, and then agitate gently and frequently for at least 5 min to assist flocculation. If the water is still cloudy, add more flocculent and repeat mixing. After at least 30 min for settling, pour the water through a fine-woven cloth or paper filter. Although most microorganisms are removed with the floc, a final process of filtration or halogenation should be completed to ensure disinfection. Several products combine coagulation–flocculation with halogen disinfection.[29]

Granular-Activated Carbon

Granular-activated carbon (GAC) purifies water by adsorbing organic and inorganic chemicals, thereby improving odor and taste. GAC is a common component of field filters. It may trap but does not kill organisms; in fact, non-pathogenic bacteria readily colonize GAC.[30] In field water treatment, GAC is best used after chemical disinfection to make water safer and more palatable by removing disinfection byproducts and pesticides, as well as many other organic chemicals

Table 6.4 Microorganism Susceptibility to Filtration

Organism	Approximate Size (μm)	Recommended filter rating (μm)[1]
Viruses	0.03	Ultrafilter or nanofilter
Escherichia coli	0.5 by 3–8	0.2–0.4 (microfilter)
Campylobacter	0.2–0.4 by 1.5–3.5	
V. cholerae	0.5 by 1.5–3.0	
Cryptosporidium oocyst	2–6	1
Giardia cyst	6-10 by 8–15	3–5
Entamoeba histolytica cyst	5–30 (average 10)	
Nematode eggs	30–40 by 50–80	20
Schistosome cercariae	50 by 100	Coffee filter or fine cloth, or double thickness closely woven cloth
Dracunculus larvae	20 by 500	

[1]Microfilters (includes most filters with pore size of 0.1–0.2 μm) can filter bacteria and protozoal cysts, but rely on electrostatic trapping of viruses or viral clumping with larger particles. Hollow fiber tubule filters with 0.02 μm (Sawyer) and reverse osmosis filters are capable of filtering viruses.

and some heavy metals. It removes the taste of iodine and chlorine (see Halogens).

Filtration

Filtration is both a physical and a chemical process influenced by characteristics of filter media, water, and flow rate. The primary determinant of a microorganism's susceptibility to filtration is its size (Table 6.4 and Fig. 6.1). Portable microfilters can readily remove protozoan cysts and bacteria, but may not remove all viruses, which are much smaller than the pore size of most field filters.[31] However, viruses often clump together or to other larger particles or organisms, and electrochemical attraction may cause viruses to adhere to the filter surface. Through these mechanisms, mechanical filters using ceramic elements with a pore size of 0.2 μm, can reduce viral loads by 2–3 logs (99–99.9%), but should not be considered adequate for complete removal of viruses. Two portable filters have been able to meet the US EPA standards for water purifiers, which include 4-log removal of viruses: First Need filter (General Ecology, Exton, PA), which functions through a combination of filtration and electrostatic attraction, and Sawyer Biologic viral filter (Sawyer Products, Safety Harbor, FL), which is composed of microtubules with an absolute pore size of 0.02 μm (ultrafiltration).

There are a large number of filters available commercially for individuals and for small groups, and their ease of use is attractive to many travelers (Table 6.5). Most of the filters sold for field water treatment are microfilters that remove particles down to about 0.1 μm. Recently hollow-fiber technology has been adapted for field use, which uses bundles of tubules whose port size can be engineered to achieve nanofiltration and viral removal. The large surface area allows these hollow-fiber tubule filters to have high flow rates at low pressure. Most filters incorporate a pre-filter on the intake tubing to remove large particles, protecting the inner microfilter; if this is lacking, a fine-mesh cloth or coffee filter can be used (see clarification techniques for cloudy water).

In pristine protected watersheds where human activity (and viral contamination) is minimal and the main concerns are bacteria and cysts, microfiltration alone can provide adequate disinfection.

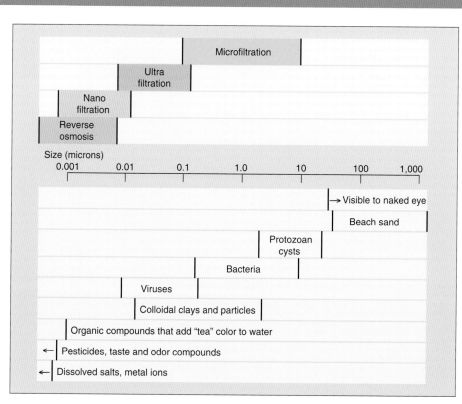

Figure 6.1 Levels of filtration required relative to the size of microorganisms and other water contaminants. *Used with permission from Auerbach PS, Editor, Wilderness Medicine, 6th ed. Philadephia: Elsevier; 2011.*

Table 6.5 Examples of Commercial Devices for Field Water Disinfection[1]

Product, Manufacturer	Microbial Claims[1]	Description and Comments[2]	Capacity and suggested use	Retail Price[3]
Aquarain www.aquarain.com				
AquaRain 200/400	P, B	Gravity drip Stacked stainless steel bucket filter with 1–4 ceramic elements and carbon core. Price depends on size and number of filter elements	Small group (Model 200) or large group (400)	$160–320
British Berkfeld www.jamesfilter.com				
Big Berkey SS-4 Multiple other models	P, B	Gravity drip Stainless steel or lexan bucket filter, up to ceramic elements with carbon matrix. Also available with compressed carbon elements, but ceramic performs better than pure carbon element	Small to large group Base camp, expatriate household	$220–260
General Ecology www.generalecology.com		Claims for viral removal are based on electrostatic attraction in structured matrix compressed carbon block filter. Variety of sizes and configurations also available for in-line use and electric powered units		
First-Need XL	P, B, V	Hand pump Compressed charcoal element	Small group in domestic or international settings	$100
Base Camp	P, B, V	Hand pump or electric Compressed Charcoal element similar to First Need. High flow, high capacity. Stainless steel housing	Large group in most settings	$650
Trav-L-Pure	P, B	Hand pump Same compressed charcoal filter element as First Need in plastic housing	Small group (same as XL)	$200

Continued

Table 6.5 Examples of Commercial Devices for Field Water Disinfection—cont'd

Product, Manufacturer	Microbial Claims[1]	Description and Comments[2]	Capacity and suggested use	Retail Price[3]
Hydro-Photon www.steripen.com		Hand-held ultraviolet purifier uses batteries with timer. Active end of unit is held in bottle or other small container of water	1–2 persons	$50
Steri-Pen Classic, Traveler, Adventurer, Journey, Freedom	P, B, V	Multiple units differ in type of battery (AA or CR123 or rechargeable), size, LCD display	Individual or several persons. Any water quality, but must be clear	$50–120
Katadyn www.katadyn.com		Katadyn filters contain either a 0.2 μm ceramic filter or 0.3 μm glass-fiber filter. Ceramic filters provide high level of micro filtration and can be cleaned to restore flow	Useful in any setting, but if highly polluted water, treat with chlorine or iodine for viruses before or after filtration	
Pocket	P, B	Hand pump ceramic filter with prefilter	Small group	$250
Combi	P, B	Hand Pump ceramic filter and activated carbon cartridge; Combi can be converted for in-line faucet use	Small group	$130
Mini			Mini for 1–2 persons	$90
Expedition	P, B	Large stainless steel pump with ceramic filter	Large group	$1200
Ceradyn Gravidyn	P, B	Gravity drip bucket filter, 3 ceramic candles; optional activated carbon core filters with Gravidyn	Small-large group Similar to Berkfeld and Aquarain above	$200–250
Hiker Hiker Pro	P	Hand pump Pleated glass-fiber 0.3 μm filter with granular-activated charcoal core and prefilter; for high-quality source water, removes 'most' bacteria	1–2 persons Limited use for developing countries	$60–80
Exstream MyBottle	P, B, V	Sport bottle Iodine resin with filter for protozoan cysts, and granular activated charcoal. Drink-through filters have limitations	1–2 person. Iodine resin and filter allow use in most settings	$50
Survivor 06 Survivor 35	P, B, V	Hand pump reverse osmosis filter that desalinates as well as disinfects. Power units available	1–2 person Because of very low flow rate and high cost, these are generally reserved for survival at sea	$900 $1900
Cascadia Designs/MSR www.msrcorp.com/filters		Ceramic filters provide high level of micro filtration and can be cleaned to restore flow. Carbon element removes chlorine pretreatment during filtration Hollow fiber filters are recent application of advanced technology to field disinfection	Useful in any setting, but if highly polluted water, treat with chlorine or iodine for viruses before or after filtration	
Miniworks EX	P, B	Hand pump with ceramic filter and activated carbon core	Small group	$90
Sweetwater MicroFilter	P, B	Hand pump with 0.2 μm borosilicate fiber filter and granular activated carbon Purifier solution (chlorine) as pretreatment to kill viruses	Small group	$90
Hyperflow Autoflow	P, B	Hand pump or gravity drip (Autoflow) units containing 0.2 μm hollow-fiber filter	Small group	$100
Miox Purifier	P, B. V	Chemical purifier, battery operated 1' × 6' device that produces disinfectant through electrolysis of water and salt. Active disinfectant hypochlorite and chlorine dioxide	Small group Useful in any setting, since broad microbiologic efficacy	$140

Table 6.5 Examples of Commercial Devices for Field Water Disinfection—cont'd

Product, Manufacturer	Microbial Claims[1]	Description and Comments[2]	Capacity and suggested use	Retail Price[3]
Sawyer www.sawyerproducts.com		Versatile filter cartridges using hollow fiber technology that can be used as in-line gravity drip from reservoir bag, as bucket adapter, faucet or in-line attachment, squeeze bags, or drink-through water bottle		
PointOne Water Treatment System	P, B	Filter cartridge containing hollow fiber 0.1 μm filter. Price varies depending on system application	Small to large size group Settings without viral contamination or pretreat with chlorine	$60–230
Point Zero Two Water Purifier	P, B, V	Gravity drip cartridges with hollow fiber filter 0.02 μm membrane; in-line gravity drip from reservoir bag, or bucket adaptor	Small group Capable of removing viruses, so useful in situations with any water quality	$145
Puralytics www.puralytics.com		Photocatalytic chemical oxidation kills all microorganisms and breaks down organic and heavy metal contaminants	Useful in any situation including poor quality source water	
SolarBag	P, B, V	Reservoir bag with coating of titanium oxide on one side activated by sunlight UV	Individual or small group	$80
Shield 500	P, B, V	High volume unit uses UV LEDs to activate photocatalyst; requires power source	Large group or facility	
Global Hydration Water Treatment Systems www.globalhydration.com		Large, high volume systems that require vehicle for transport	Large group or facility Can be used for emergency and disaster relief	
Can Pure Water Purification System	P, B, V	Dual-process purification system with microfiltration and UV disinfection; requires power source		
First Water Systems www.firstwaterinc.com		UV disinfection that can be run off generator, battery or solar power. Can be supplemented with residual chlorination system	Large group Used for emergency, disaster or humanitarian relief	
Responder Outpost-4	P, B, V	Portable and vehicle transported units that circulate water twice through UV source. Prefilter removes particulates		

[1]P = protozoa, B = bacteria, V = viruses.
[2]Consider additional features, such as flow rate, filter capacity, size, and filter weight.
[3]Prices vary.

However, for developing world travel and for surface water with heavy levels of fecal or sewage contamination, higher levels of filtration may be needed to remove viruses. Alternatively, additional treatment with halogens before or after filtration guarantees effective virus removal.

Several factors influence the decision of which filter to buy: (1) how many persons are to use the filter; (2) what microbiologic demands will be put on the filter (claims); and (3) what is the preferred means of operation (function). Cost may also be an important consideration.

Reverse Osmosis

Reverse osmosis filtration uses high pressure (100–800 psi) to force water through a semi-permeable membrane that filters out dissolved ions, molecules, and solids (nanofiltration). This process can both remove microbiologic contamination and desalinate water. Although small hand pump reverse osmosis units have been developed, their high price and slow output currently prohibit use by land-based travelers. They are, however, important survival aids for ocean voyagers and the preferred field method for large military operations.

Forward Osmosis

Instead of high pump pressure, osmotic pressure also can be used to draw water through a membrane to create highly purified drinking water from low-quality source water, including brackish water. These products use a double-chamber bag or container with the membrane in between. A high-osmotic substance is added to the clean side that draws water from the dirty side (Hydration Technology Innovations, Albany, OR). Since some form of sugar and/or salt is often used to create osmotic pressure, this may result in a sweetened solution similar to a sports-electrolyte drink.

Filter Testing and EPA Registration

The United States Environmental Protection Agency (EPA) has developed consensus-based performance standards as a guideline for testing and evaluation of portable water treatment devices.[32] Many companies now use these standards as their testing guidelines. Challenge water at specified temperatures, turbidity, and numbers of microorganisms is pumped through the filter at given intervals within the claimed volume capacity. Filter or chemical methods that claim to remove, kill, or inactivate all types of disease-causing microorganisms from the water, including bacteria, viruses, and protozoan cysts, are designated 'microbiologic water purifiers.' They must demonstrate that they meet the testing guidelines, which require a 3-log (99.9%) reduction for cysts, 4-log (99.99%) for viruses and 5–6-log reduction for bacteria. Filters can make limited claims to serve a definable environmental need, for example removal of protozoan cysts, or cysts and bacteria only. The EPA does not endorse, test, or approve mechanical filters: it merely assigns registration numbers. Testing is done or contracted by the manufacturer.

Halogens

Worldwide, chemical disinfection with halogens, chiefly chlorine and iodine, is the most commonly used method for improving and maintaining the microbiologic quality of drinking water and can be used by individuals and groups in the field (Table 6.3). The germicidal activity of halogens results from oxidation of essential cellular structures and enzymes, and a wealth of data support their effectiveness.[33–40] Hypochlorite, the major chlorine disinfectant, is currently the preferred means of municipal water disinfection worldwide. Both calcium hypochlorite ($Ca[OCl]_2$) and sodium hypochlorite ($NaOCl$) readily dissociate in water to form hypochlorite, the active disinfectant. Iodine is effective in low concentrations for killing bacteria, viruses, and cysts, and in higher concentration against fungi and even bacterial spores; however, it is a poor algaecide. Elemental (diatomic) iodine (I_2) and hypoiodous acid (HOI) are the major germicides in an aqueous solution. Disinfection effectiveness is determined by characteristics of the disinfectant, the microorganism, and environmental factors.

Given adequate concentrations and contact times, both iodine and chlorine are effective disinfectants with similar biocidal activity under most conditions. Of the halogens, iodine reacts least readily with organic compounds and is less affected by pH, indicating that low iodine residuals should be more stable and persistent than corresponding concentrations of chlorine. Taste preference is individual. Common sources and doses of iodine and chlorine are given in Table 6.6. Chlorine is still advocated by the World Health Organization and the Centers for Disease Control and Prevention as a mainstay of large-scale community, individual household, and emergency use.[41] There are extensive data on its effectiveness in remote settings.[42] Another advantage is the ease of adjusting the dose for large volumes of water.[5,43] The CDC/WHO Safe Water System for household disinfection in developing countries provides a dosage of 1.875 or 3.75 mg/L of sodium hypochlorite with a contact time of 30 minutes, sufficient to inactivate most bacteria, viruses, and some protozoa that cause waterborne diseases.[5,44]

Vegetative bacteria (non-spore forming) are very sensitive to halogens; viruses have intermediate sensitivity, requiring higher concentrations or longer contact times. Protozoal cysts are more resistant than enteric bacteria and enteric viruses, but can be inactivated by field doses of halogens.[36–40,45,46] Cryptosporidium oocysts, however, are much more resistant to halogens and inactivation is not practical with common doses of iodine and chlorine used in field water disinfection.[47] Little is known about Cyclospora, but it is assumed to be similar to Cryptosporidium. Certain parasitic eggs, such as those of Ascaris, are also resistant, but these are not commonly spread by water. All these resistant cysts and eggs are susceptible to heat or

filtration. Relative resistance between organisms is similar for iodine and chlorine.

The Disinfection Reaction

Understanding factors that influence the disinfection reaction allows flexibility with greater reassurance. The primary factors of the first-order chemical disinfection reaction are concentration and contact time.[34,35] Concentrations of 1–16 mg/L for 10–60 minutes are generally effective. Even clear surface water often has at least 1 mg/L of halogen demand, so it is prudent to use 4 mg/L as a target halogen concentration for clear water. Lower concentrations (e.g., 2 mg/L) can be used for back-up treatment of questionable tap water. The need for prolonged contact times with low halogen concentrations in cold water is suggested by (1) data suggesting that extended contact times are required for 99.9% kill of Giardia in very cold water;[36,46] and (2) uncertainty about residual concentration.

Iodine Resins

Iodine resins are considered demand disinfectants. The resin has low solubility, so that as water passes through, little iodine is released into aqueous solutions. On the other hand, when microorganisms contact the resin, iodine is transferred and binds to the microorganisms, apparently aided by electrostatic forces.[48] Bacteria and cysts are effectively exposed to high iodine concentrations, which allow reduced contact time compared with dilute iodine solutions. However, some contact time is necessary, especially for cysts. Resins have demonstrated effectiveness against bacteria, viruses, and cysts, but not against C. parvum oocysts or bacterial spores.

Iodine resins are effective disinfectants that can be engineered into attractive field products, but the effectiveness of the resin is highly dependent on the product design and function. Most incorporate a 1 μm cyst filter to remove Cryptosporidium, Giardia, and other halogen-resistant parasitic eggs or larvae, in an attempt to avoid prolonged contact time. Carbon, which removes residual dissolved iodine, preventing excessive iodine ingestion in long-term users, may not allow sufficient contact time for cyst destruction. However, when residual iodine is not controlled, high levels of iodine have been reported in effluent water in very hot climates.[49] Cloudy or sediment-laden water may clog the resin, as it would any filter, or coat the resin, thereby inhibiting iodine transfer. Several companies have abandoned iodine resin-containing portable hand-pump filters due to repeat testing that demonstrated viral breakthrough, despite initial pre-marketing testing that passed the EPA protocol. Only one drink-through bottle remains on the US market, but other products may still be available outside the US. Iodine resins may prove useful for small communities in undeveloped and rural areas where chlorine disinfection is technically and economically unfeasible.

Improving Halogen Taste

Objectionable taste and smell limit the acceptance of halogens, but taste can be improved by several means. One method is to use the minimum necessary dose with a longer contact time. Several chemical means are available to reduce free iodine to iodide, or chlorine to chloride, that have no color, smell, or taste. These chemical species also have no disinfection action, and so these techniques should be used only after the required contact time. The best and most readily available agent is ascorbic acid (vitamin C), available in crystalline or powder form. A common ingredient of flavored drink mixes, it accounts for their effectiveness in removing the taste of halogens.

Table 6.6 Chemical Products for Field Water Disinfection

Product	Application	Comments
Iodine	See text for discussion of efficacy, toxicity, and improving taste. Use extended contact times in very cold water.	
Iodine tabs tetraglycine hydroperiodide EDWGT (emergency drinking water germicidal tablet) Potable Aqua (Wisconsin Pharmacal Co, Jackson, WI) Globaline	1/2 tab per liter provides 4 ppm iodine; 1 tab yields 8 ppm.	Developed by the military for individual field use because of broad-spectrum disinfection effect, ease of handling and rapid dissolution. Taste more acceptable at 4ppm. Limited shelf-life after opening.
2% iodine solution (tincture)	0.2 ml (5 gtts[a])/L water yields 4 ppm iodine.	Widely available as topical disinfectant, but contains iodide, which is not an active disinfectant, but biologically active.
10% povidone-iodine solution[b]	0.35 ml (8 gtts)/L water yields 4 ppm iodine.	Widely available as topical disinfectant. In aqueous solution, provides a sustained-release reservoir of halogen (normally, 2 to 10 ppm is present in solution).
Saturated solution: iodine crystals in water Polar Pure (Polar Equipment, Inc, Saratoga, CA)	13 ml/L water yields 4 ppm (use capful as measure, or can use syringe).	A small amount of elemental iodine goes into solution (no significant iodide is present); the saturated solution is used to disinfect drinking water. Water can be added to the crystals hundreds of times before they are completely dissolved.
Chlorine	See text for discussion of efficacy and improving taste. Simple field test kits or swimming pool test kits with color strips are widely available to assure adequate residual chlorine. Can easily be adapted to large or small quantities of water.	
Sodium hypochlorite Household bleach 5% CDC-WHO Safe Water System (1% hypochlorite)	(5%) 0.1 ml (2 gtts)/L water yields 5 ppm hypochlorite.	Inexpensive and widely available. Safe Water System dosage provides about 2–4 ppm hypochlorite/L. Generally designed to use capful as measure.
Calcium Hypochlorite Redi Chlor (1/10 gm tab) (Gripo Laboratories, Delhi, India) HTH (Arch Water Products Castleford, West Yorkshire, UK)	¼ tab/ 2 quarts water yields 10 ppm hypochlorite.	Stable, concentrated (70%), dry source of hypochlorite that is commonly used for chlorination of swimming pools. Multiple products available in various size tablets or granular form.
Sodium dichloroisocyanurate Aquatabs (Medentech, Wexford, Ireland) Kintabs (Bioman Products Mottram, Cheshire, U.K.) NaDCC (Gripo laboratories, Delhi, India) Global Hydration (Global Hydration Water Treatment Systems, Kakabeka Falls, Ontario, Canada)	1 tab (8.5 mg NaDCC)/L water yields 10 ppm active disinfectant.	Stable, non-toxic chlorine compound that releases free active chlorine with additional available chlorine that remains in compound.
Halazone Aquazone (Gripo Laboratories, Delhi, India)	Each tablet releases 2.3 to 2.5 ppm of titratable chlorine.	Tablets contain a mixture of monochloraminobenzoic and dichloraminobenzoic acids. Limited use given other available chlorine products.
Chlorine plus flocculating agent Chlor-floc PUR Purifier sachets (Proctor and Gamble Corp, Cincinnati, OH)	One 600-mg tablet yields 8 mg/L of free chlorine. PUR sachet is added to 10L water.	Contain 1.4% available chlorine (sodium dichloro-s-triazinetrione) with flocculating agents (alum or ferric sulfate). Flocculant clarifies cloudy water while residual chlorine provides disinfection. Useful for humanitarian disasters where available surface water is often highly turbid.
Chlorine Dioxide	Several new chemical methods for generating chlorine dioxide on-site can now be applied in the field for water treatment. Advantages of chlorine dioxide are greater effectiveness than chlorine at equivalent doses and the ability to inactivate *Cryptosporidium* oocysts with reasonable doses and contact times.	
Micropur MP-1 (Katadyn Corp, Wallisellen, Switzerland) AquaMira (McNett Outdoor, Bellingham, WA) Pristine (Advanced Chemicals Ltd., Vancouver, BC) Potable Aqua Aquarius Bulk Water Treatment	1 tablet/L water. Follow product instructions.	Available in tablets or liquid (two solutions that are mixed to activate prior to use).
Silver	Although widely used in some countries for disinfection, silver is approved in U.S. only for preserving stored water.	
MicroPur Classic (Katadyn Corp., Wallisellen, Switzerland)	Available in tablets, liquid, or crystals.	Releases silver ions. Not recommended for primary water treatment.
MicroPur Forte (Katadyn Corp)	Available in tablets, liquid, or crystals.	Tablets contain silver chloride 0.1% and NaDCC 2.5%. The chlorine kills viruses, bacteria, and *Giardia*. The silver prevents recontamination for up to 6 months, if water is stored.

[a]Measure with dropper (1 drop = 0.05 mL) or small syringe.

[b]Povidone-iodine solutions release free iodine in levels adequate for disinfection, but few data are available.

Other safe and effective means of chemical reduction are sodium thiosulfate and hydrogen peroxide. GAC will remove the taste of iodine and chlorine, partially by adsorption and partially by chemical reduction. Finally, alternative techniques such as filtration or heat that do not affect taste can be used in many situations.

Halogen Toxicity

Chlorine has no known toxicity when used for water disinfection. Sodium hypochlorite is not carcinogenic; however, reactions of chlorine with certain organic contaminants yield chlorinated hydrocarbons, chloroform, and other trihalomethanes, which are considered carcinogenic. Nevertheless, the risk of severe illness or even death from infectious diseases if disinfection is not used is far greater than any risk from byproducts of chlorine disinfection.

There is much more concern with iodine because of its physiologic activity, potential toxicity, and allergenicity. Data reviewed by Backer and Hollowell[50] suggest the following guidelines as appropriate:

- High levels of iodine (16–32 mg/day), such as those produced by recommended doses of iodine tablets, should be limited to short periods of 1 month or less.
- Iodine treatments that produce a low residual ≤1–2 mg/L appear safe, even for long periods of time, in people with normal thyroid glands.
- Anyone planning to use iodine for prolonged periods should have their thyroid examined and thyroid function tests done to assure that they are initially euthyroid. Optimally, repeat thyroid function test and examine for iodine goiter after 3–6 months of continuous iodine ingestion and monitor occasionally for iodine-induced goiter thereafter. If this is not feasible, ensure low-level iodine consumption (see above) or use a different technique.

Certain groups should not use iodine for water treatment:

- Pregnant women (because of concerns of neonatal goiter);
- Those with known hypersensitivity to iodine;
- Persons with a history of thyroid disease, even if controlled on medication;
- Persons with a strong family history of thyroid disease (thyroiditis);
- Persons from countries with chronic iodine deficiency.

Miscellaneous Disinfectants

Ozone and chlorine dioxide are both effective disinfectants that are widely used in municipal water treatment plants, but until recently were not available in stable form for field use. These disinfectants have been demonstrated effective against *Cryptosporidia* in commonly used concentrations.[51]

New products enable chlorine dioxide generation for use in an array of small-scale, on-site applications, including solutions, and tablets (Tables 6.3 and 6.6). MicroPur and Aquamira tablets are US EPA registered as a 'water purifier,' (see Filter testing and EPA registration). Aquamira solution is currently approved for sale in the USA under more limited bactericidal claims. Pristine solution and tablets, the equivalent product sold in Canada, makes full claims for protozoa, including *Cryptosporidia*.

A portable product developed for military use and transferred to the civilian market uses an electrochemical process to convert simple salt into a mixed-oxidant disinfectant containing free chlorine, chlorine dioxide and ozone.[52] The Miox purifier has been reduced to a cigar-sized unit that operates on camera batteries (MSR Inc, Seattle, WA) (Table 6.5). Larger units for field use and small communities are also available (Miox Corp, Albuquerque, NM).

Silver

Silver ion has bactericidal effects in low doses and some attractive features, including absence of color, taste and odor. However, the concentrations are strongly affected by adsorption onto the surface of any container as well as common substances in water, and scant data for disinfection of viruses and cysts indicate limited effect, even at high doses. The use of silver as a drinking water disinfectant has been much more popular in Europe, where silver tablets are sold widely for field water disinfection. The EPA has not approved them for this purpose in the USA, but they were approved as a water preservative, to prevent bacterial growth in previously treated and stored water. There is also a combined chlorine solution with the silver (Micropur Forte) to provide water disinfection plus preservation (Table 6.6).

Ultraviolet

Ultraviolet (UV) radiation is widely used to sterilize water used in beverages and food products, for secondary treatment of waste-water, and to disinfect drinking water at the community and household level (Table 6.3). In sufficient doses of energy, all water-borne enteric pathogens are inactivated by UV radiation. The ultraviolet waves must actually strike the organism, so the water must be free of particles that could act as a shield. The UV rays do not alter the water, but they also do not provide any residual disinfecting power. The requirement for power has limited its adaptation for field use, but a portable, battery-operated unit is available for disinfection of small quantities (Hydro-Photon Inc, Blue Hill, ME) (Table 6.5). Although previous data suggested limited ability of monochromatic UV rays to inactivate protozoan cysts, company product testing appears solid and shows effectiveness against important water-borne pathogens, including *Cryptosporidia*. Simple, table-sized UV units with low power requirements (WaterHealth, Lake Forest, CA) and larger units that use various power sources (Global Hydration Water Treatment Systems Inc., Ontario Canada; First Water Systems, Inc., Suwanee, GA) are available for international and disaster relief applications.

Solar UV Disinfection (SODIS)

UV irradiation by sunlight can substantially improve the microbiologic quality of water and reduce diarrheal illness in developing countries. Recent work has confirmed the efficacy and optimal procedures of the SODIS technique. Transparent bottles (e.g., clear plastic beverage bottles), preferably lying on a dark surface, are exposed to sunlight for a minimum of 4 hours with intermittent agitation.[53] UV and thermal inactivation are strongly synergistic for the solar disinfection of drinking water.[54]

Photocatalytic Disinfection

Advanced oxidation processes use sunlight to catalyze the production of hydroxyl radicals (OH⁻) and free electrons, which are potent oxidizers.[55] Various materials can be used, but the most efficacious is titanium dioxide (TiO_2). High-energy short-wavelength photons from sunlight promote the photochemical reactions. In addition to being an excellent disinfectant for various microorganisms, this process is unique in its ability to break down complex organic contaminants and most heavy metals into carbon dioxide, water, and inorganics, which is driving considerable research for industrial processes and large-scale water treatment. For field water disinfection, nanoparticles coated with TiO_2 can be integrated into a plastic bag and remain active for hundreds of uses (Puralytics, Beaverton, OR) (Table 6.5).

Table 6.7 Summary of Field Water Disinfection Techniques

	Bacteria	Viruses	*Giardia*/Ameba	*Cryptosporidium*	Nematodes/Cercarea
Heat	+	+	+	+	+
Filtration	+	+/–*	+	+	+
Halogens	+	+	+	–	+/–†
Chlorine dioxide and photocatalytic	+	+	+	+	DNA†

*Most filters make no claims for viruses. Reverse osmosis is effective. (see Table 6.5).
†Eggs are not very susceptible to halogens but very low risk of water-borne transmission. No data available for photocatalytic.
DNA, Data Not Available.

Table 6.8 Choice of Method for Various Source Water

Source Water	'Pristine' wilderness water with little human or domestic animal activity	Tap water in developing country	Developed or developing country	
			Clear surface water near human and animal activity[1]	Cloudy water
Primary concern	*Giardia*, enteric bacteria	Bacteria, *Giardia*, small numbers of viruses	All enteric pathogens, including *Cryptosporidium*	All enteric pathogens
Effective methods	Any single-step method[2]	Any single-step method	1) Heat 2) Microfiltration plus halogen (can be done in either order); iodine resin filters 3) Ultra- or nanofiltration 4) Chlorine dioxide 5) Ultraviolet (commercial product, not sunlight)	CF[3] followed by second step (heat, filtration or halogen)

[1]Includes agricultural run-off with cattle grazing, or sewage treatment effluent from upstream villages or towns.
[2]Includes heat, filtration, or chemical methods.
[3]CF – coagulation-flocculation.

Citrus and Potassium Permanganate

Both citrus juice and potassium permanganate have some demonstrated antibacterial effects in an aqueous solution. However, data are few and not available for effect on cysts. Either could be used in an emergency to reduce bacterial and viral contamination, but cannot be recommended as a primary means of water disinfection.

Preferred Technique

The optimal water treatment technique for an individual or group will depend on the number of persons to be served, space and weight accommodations, quality of source water, personal taste preferences, and fuel availability. Since halogens do not kill *Cryptosporidia* and filtration misses some viruses, optimal protection for all situations may require a two-step process of (1) filtration or coagulation–flocculation, followed by (2) halogenation (Tables 6.7 and 6.8).[56,57] Heat is effective as a one-step process in all situations, but will not improve the esthetics of the water. Chlorine dioxide generating techniques can be used as single-step processes. Iodine resins, combined with microfiltration to remove resistant cysts, are also a viable one-step process, but questions have recently surfaced of product effectiveness under all conditions, so few products are available.

Expatriates or persons engaged in community projects or international relief activities are at higher risk that the average international traveler. Sobsey reviewed data for point-of-use methods for household disinfection in developing countries.[13]

On long-distance ocean-going boats where water must be desalinated as well as disinfected during the voyage, only reverse osmosis membrane filters are adequate. Water storage also requires consideration. Iodine will work for short periods only (i.e., weeks) because it is a poor algaecide. For prolonged storage, water should be chlorinated and kept in a tightly sealed container to reduce the risk of contamination.[58] Narrow-mouthed jars or containers with water spigots prevent contamination from repeated contact with hands or utensils.[59]

Sanitation

Studies in developing countries have demonstrated a clear benefit in the reduction of diarrheal illness and other infections from safe drinking water, hygiene, and adequate sanitation. The benefit is greater when all are applied together, especially with appropriate education.[11,60] Personal hygiene, particularly hand-washing, prevents spread of infection from food contamination during preparation of meals. Disinfection of dishes and utensils is accomplished by rinsing in water containing enough household bleach to achieve a distinct chlorine odor. Use of halogen solutions or potassium permanganate solutions to soak vegetables and fruits can reduce microbial contamination, especially if the surface is scrubbed to remove dirt or other particulates. Neither method reaches organisms that are embedded in surface crevices or protected by other particulate matter.[61] The sanitation challenge for wilderness and rural travelers is proper waste disposal to prevent additional contamination of water supplies. Human waste should be buried 8–12 inches deep, at least 100 ft from any water, and at a location from which water run-off is not likely to wash organisms into nearby water sources. Groups of three persons or more should dig a common latrine to avoid numerous individual potholes and inadequate disposal.

Conclusion

Although food-borne illnesses probably account for most enteric problems that affect travelers, nearly all causes of travelers' diarrhea can also be water-borne. It is not possible for travelers to judge the microbiologic quality of surface water, and it is not prudent to assume the potability of tap water in many areas. Many simple and effective field techniques to improve microbiologic water quality are available to travelers. It is important to learn the basic principles and limitations of heat, filtration, and chemical disinfection, and then to become familiar with at least one technique appropriate for the destination, water source, and group composition.

References

1. World Health Organization. Combating waterborne disease at the household level. 2007.
2. World Health Organization. The Global Water Supply and Sanitation Assessment 2000. Geneva: WHO and UNICEF Joint Monitoring Programme for Water Supply and Sanitation; 2000.
3. Pruss A, Kay D, Fewtrell L, et al. Estimating the burden of disease from water, sanitation, and hygiene at a global level. Environ Health Perspect 2002;110(5):537–42.
4. Wright J, Gundry S, Conroy R. Household drinking water in developing countries: a systematic review of microbiological contamination between source and point-of-use. Trop Med Int Health 2004;9(1):106–17.
5. Lantange D. Sodium hypochlorite dosage for household and emergency water treatment. J Am Water Works Assoc 2008;100(8):106–19.
6. Yoder J, Roberts V, Craun GF, et al. Surveillance for waterborne disease and outbreaks associated with drinking water and water not intended for drinking – United States, 2005–2006. MMWR Surveill Summ 2008;57(9):39–62.
7. Wang G, Doyle M. Survival of enterohemorrhagic *Escherichia coli* O157: H7 in water. J Food Protection 1998;61:662–7.
8. Hurst C, Clark R, Regli S. Estimating the risk of acquiring infectious disease from ingestion of water. In: Hurst C, editor. Modeling Disease Transmission and its Prevention by Disinfection. Melbourne: Cambridge University Press; 1996. p. 99–139.
9. Ford TE. Microbiological safety of drinking water: United States and global perspectives. Environ Health Perspect 1999;107(Suppl. 1):191–206.
10. Yoder JS, Hlavsa MC, Craun GF, et al. Surveillance for waterborne disease and outbreaks associated with recreational water use and other aquatic facility-associated health events – United States, 2005–2006. MMWR Surveill Summ 2008;57(9):1–29.
11. Sobsey M, Handzel T, Venczel L. Chlorination and safe storage of household drinking water in developing countries to reduce waterborne disease. Water Sci Technol 2003;47(3):221–8.
12. Fewtrell L, Colford JM Jr. Water, sanitation and hygiene in developing countries: interventions and diarrhoea – a review. Water Sci Technol 2005;52(8):133–42.
13. Sobsey MD, Stauber CE, Casanova LM, et al. Point of use household drinking water filtration: A practical, effective solution for providing sustained access to safe drinking water in the developing world. Environ Sci Technol 2008;42(12):4261–7.
14. Clasen T, Roberts I, Rabie T, et al. Interventions to improve water quality for preventing diarrhoea. Cochrane Database Syst Rev 2006;3: CD004794.
15. Lule JR, Mermin J, Ekwaru JP, et al. Effect of home-based water chlorination and safe storage on diarrhea among persons with human immunodeficiency virus in Uganda. Am J Trop Med Hyg 2005;73(5):926–33.
16. Backer H. Field Water Disinfection. In: Auerbach P, editor. Wilderness Medicine. 6th ed. Philadelphia: Elsevier; 2011. p. 1324–59.
17. Sobsey M. Enteric viruses and drinking water supplies. J Am Water Works Assoc 1975;67:414–8.
18. Reynolds KA, Mena KD, Gerba CP. Risk of waterborne illness via drinking water in the United States. Rev Environ Contam Toxicol 2008;192:117–58.
19. Guidelines for Canadian Drinking Water Quality. (Accessed 1/3, 2010, at http://www.hc-sc.gc.ca/ewh-semt/pubs/water-eau/protozoa/chap_9-eng. php.)
20. Frazier W, Westhoff D. Preservation by Use of High Temperatures. New York: McGraw-Hill; 1978.
21. Fayer R. Effect of high temperature on infectivity of *Cryptosporidium parvum* oocysts in water. Appl Environ Microbiol 1994;60:273–5.
22. Bandres J, Mathewson J, DuPont H. Heat susceptibility of bacterial enteropathogens. Arch Intern Med 1988;148:2261–3.
23. Shephart M. Helminthological aspects of sewage treatment. In: Feachem R, McGarry M, Mara D, editors. Water, Wastes and Health in Hot Climates. New York: John Wiley and Sons; 1977. p. 299–310.
24. Neumann H. Bacteriological safety of hot tapwater in developing countries. Public Health Rep 1969;84:812–4.
25. Perkins J. Thermal destruction of microorganisms: Heat inactivation of viruses. In: Thomas C, editor. Principles and Methods of Sterilization in Health Sciences. Springfield; 1969. p. 63–94.
26. Baert L, Debevere J, Uyttendaele M. The efficacy of preservation methods to inactivate foodborne viruses. Int J Food Microbiol 2009;131(2–3):83–94.
27. McGuigan KG. Solar disinfection: use of sunlight to decontaminate drinking water in developing countries. J Med Microbiol 1999;48:785–7.
28. Binnie C, Kimber M, Smethurst G. Basic Water Treatment. 3rd ed. London: IWA; 2002.
29. Powers E, Boutros C, Harper B. Biocidal efficacy of a flocculating emergency water purification tablet. Appl Environ Microbiology 1994;60:2316–23.
30. Le Chevallier M, McFeters G. Microbiology of activated carbon. In: McFeters G, editor. Drinking Water Microbiology. New York: Springer-Verlag; 1990. p. 104–20.
31. Environmental Health Directorate Health Protection Branch. Assessing the effectiveness of small filtration systems for point-of-use disinfection of drinking water supplies. Ottawa: Department of National Health and Welfare; 1980. Report No.: 80-EHD-54.
32. US Environmental Protection Agency. Report to Task Force: Guide standard and protocol for testing microbiological water purifiers. Cincinnati: USEPA; 1987 (Revision).
33. National Academy of Sciences Safe Drinking Water Committee. The Disinfection of drinking water. Drinking Water and Health 1980;2:5–139.
34. White G. Handbook of Chlorination. 3rd ed. New York: Van Nostrand Reinhold; 1992.
35. Hoff J. Inactivation of microbial agents by chemical disinfectants. Cincinnati: US Environmental Protection Agency; 1986 July. Report No.: EPA/600/2–86/067.
36. Hibler C, Hancock C, Perger L, et al. Inactivation of *Giardia* cysts with chlorine at 0.5C to 5.0C. Denver: AWWA Research Foundation; 1987.
37. Powers E. Efficacy of flocculating and other emergency water purification tablets. Natick, MA: United States Army Natick Research, Development and Engineering Center; 1993. Report No.: Report Natick/TR-93/033.
38. Rogers M, Vitaliano J. Military and small group water disinfecting systems: an assessment. Milit Med 1979;7:267–77.
39. Powers E. Inactivation of *Giardia* cysts by iodine with special reference to Globaline: a review. Natick, MA: United States Army Natick Research, Development and Engineering Center; 1993. Report No.: Technical report natick/TR-91/022.
40. Gerba C, Johnson D, Hasan M. Efficacy of iodine water purification tablets against *Cryptosporidium* oocysts and *Giardia* cysts. Wilderness Environ Med 1997;8:96–100.
41. Prevention CfDCa. Safe Water Systems for the Developing World: a handbook for implementing household-based water treatment and safe storage projects. Atlanta, GA: Centers for Disease Control and Prevention; 2001.
42. Arnold BF, Colford JM Jr. Treating water with chlorine at point-of-use to improve water quality and reduce child diarrhea in developing countries: a systematic review and meta-analysis. Am J Trop Med Hyg 2007;76(2):354–64.
43. U.S. Army. Sanitary control and surveillance of field water supplies. Washington, DC: Departments of the Army, Navy, and Air Force; 2005 Dec 15. Report No.: Dept. of Army Technical Bulletin (TB Med 577).
44. Kotlarz N, Lantange D, Preston K, et al. Turbidity and chlorine demand reduction using locally available physical water clarification mechanisms

before household chlorination in developing countries. J Water Health 2009;7(3):497–506.

45. Ongerth J, Johnson R, MacDonald S, et al. Backcountry water treatment to prevent giardiasis. Am J Public Health 1989;79:1633–7.

46. Fraker L, Gentile D, Krivoy D, et al. *Giardia* cyst inactivation by iodine. J Wilderness Med 1992;3:351–8.

47. Carpenter C, Fayer R, Trout J, et al. Chlorine disinfection of recreational water for *Cryptosporidium parvum*. Emerg Infect Dis 1999;5(4):579–84.

48. Marchin G, Fina L. Contact and demand-release disinfectants. Crit Rev Environ Control 1989;19:227–90.

49. Kettel-Khan L, Li R, Gootnick D, et al. Thyroid abnormalities related to iodine excess from water purification units. Lancet 1998;352:1519.

50. Backer H, Hollowell J. Use of iodine for water disinfection: iodine toxicity and maximum recommended dose. Environ Health Perspectives 2000;108(8):679–84.

51. Clark RM, Sivagnesan M, Rice EW, et al. Development of a Ct equation for the inactivation of *Cryptosporidium* occysts with chlorine dioxide. Water Res 2003;37:2773–83.

52. Venczel L, Arrowood M, Hurd M, et al. Inactivation of *Cryptosporidium parvum* oocysts and *Clostridium perfringens* spores by a mixed-oxidant disinfectant and by free chlorine. Appl Environ Microbiol 1997;63:1598–601.

53. Meierhofer R, Wegelin M, SODIS Manual. Gallen: Department of water and sanitation in developing countries, Swiss Federal Institute of envirnomental science and technology; 2002.

54. McGuigan K, Joyce T, Conroy R, et al. Solar disinfection of drinking water contained in transparent plastic bottles: characterizing the bacterial inactivation process. J Appl Microbiol 1998;84:1138–48.

55. Blanco-Galvez J, Fernandez-Ibanez P, Malato-Rodriguez S. Solar photocatalytic detoxification and disinfection of water: recent overview. J Solar Energy Engin 2006.

56. U.S. Army. Preventive medicine concerns of hand held water treatment devices. Aberdeen Proving Ground, Maryland: U.S. Army Center for Health Promotion and Preventive Medicine; 2003 March 10. Report No.: Water Quality Information Paper No 31–032.

57. Schlosser O, Robert C, Bourderioux C, et al. Bacterial removal from inexpensive portable water treatment systems for travelers. J Travel Med 2001;8:12–8.

58. Lantagne DS. Viability of commercially available bleach for water treatment in developing countries. Am J Public Health 2009;99(11):1975–8.

59. Sobel J, Mahon B, Mendoza C, et al. Reduction of fecal contamination of street-vended beverages in Guatemala by a simple system for water purification and storage, handwashing, and beverage storage. Am J Trop Med Hyg 1998;59:380–7.

60. Quick RE, Kimura A, Thevos A, et al. Diarrhea prevention through household-level water disinfection and safe storage in Zambia. Am J Trop Med Hyg 2002;66(5):584–9.

61. Ortega YR, Roxas CR, Gilman RH, et al. Isolation of *Cryptosporidium parvum* and *Cyclospora cayetanensis* from vegetables collected in markets of an endemic region in Peru. Am J Trop Med Hyg 1997;57(6):683–6.

62. Schoenen D. Role of disinfection in suppressing the spread of pathogens with drinking water: possibilities and limitations. Water Res 2002;36:3874–88.

63. Theron J, Cloete TE. Emerging waterborne infections: contributing factors, agents, and detection tools. Crit Rev Microbiol 2002;28(1):1–26.

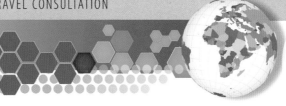

Insect Protection

Mark S. Fradin

Key points

- Personal protection measures include habitat avoidance, and the use of insect repellents, protective clothing and bed-nets. Many of these items can be accessed through websites
- With DEET-based repellents each 10°C increase in ambient temperature can cause as much as a 50% reduction in protection
- Despite common beliefs, DEET toxicity is minimal, with rare cases of encephalopathy reported over the last half century of use (and in most circumstances the product had been misused)
- It is important to carefully read the directions on all insecticides and repellents, particularly regarding reapplication timing
- A variety of options are now available as insect repellents, one being picaridin, which is available in many countries

Introduction

In preparation for travel to many tropical and subtropical locations, the well-informed traveler needs to be aware of the potential risks of arthropod-transmitted disease. Mosquitoes, flies, ticks, midges, chiggers, and fleas are capable of transmitting multiple bacterial, viral, protozoan, parasitic and rickettsial infections to humans (Table 7.1). A multi-pronged approach is necessary to prevent becoming a victim of insect-borne disease: protection from insect bites is best achieved through avoiding infected habitats, wearing protective clothing, and applying insect repellents. This chapter will review all available techniques for preventing arthropod bites, and will provide practical information to the traveler that will make it possible to distinguish between effective and ineffective methods of protection. A summary of the topics covered in this chapter is shown in Figure 7.1.

Stimuli that Attract Insects

Scientists have not yet elucidated the exact mechanism by which arthropods are attracted to their hosts. The stimuli that attract mosquitoes have been best studied. Mosquitoes use visual, thermal, and olfactory stimuli to locate a bloodmeal.[1,2] For mosquitoes that feed during the daytime, host movement and the wearing of dark-colored clothing may initiate orientation towards an individual. Visual stimuli appear to be important for in-flight orientation, particularly over long ranges. As a mosquito nears its host, olfactory stimuli then help guide the mosquito to its host. Carbon dioxide, released from breath and skin, serves as a long-range air-borne attractant, at distances up to 36 m. Lactic acid, skin warmth, and moisture also serve as attractants. Volatile compounds, derived from sebum, eccrine and apocrine sweat, and/or the bacterial action of cutaneous microflora on these secretions, may also act as chemoattractants. Different species of mosquito may show strong biting preferences for different parts of the body, related to local skin temperature and sweat gland activity. Floral fragrances, found in perfumes, lotions, detergents and soaps, may also lure biting arthropods. One study has shown that alcohol ingestion increases the likelihood of being bitten by mosquitoes.

There can be significant variability in the attractiveness of different individuals to the same or different species of mosquitoes – a point that travelers should keep in mind when visiting new areas. In some studies, men have been found to be bitten more readily than women, and adults are more likely to be bitten than children. Adults tend to be bitten less as they get older. Heavyset individuals tend to attract more mosquitoes, perhaps due to their greater relative heat or carbon dioxide output.

Personal Protection

Personal protection against arthropod bites is best achieved by avoiding infested habitats, using protective clothing and shelters, and applying insect repellents.[3,4]

Habitat Avoidance

It is obvious that avoiding arthropods' breeding and resting places, when feasible, will reduce the risk of being bitten. Many species of mosquito and other blood-sucking arthropods are particularly active at dusk, making this a good time to remain indoors. To avoid the usual resting places of biting arthropods, campsites should ideally be situated in areas that are high, dry, open, and as free from vegetation as possible. Any area with standing or stagnant water should be avoided, as these are ideal breeding grounds for mosquitoes.

DOI: 10.1016/B978-1-4557-1076-8.00007-7

Table 7.1 Diseases Transmitted to Humans by Biting Arthropods

Mosquitoes

Eastern equine encephalitis
Western equine encephalitis
St Louis encephalitis
La Cross encephalitis
West Nile virus
Japanese encephalitis
Venezuelan equine encephalitis
Malaria
Yellow fever
Dengue
Lymphatic filariasis
Epidemic polyarthritis (Ross River virus)
Chikungunya fever
Rift Valley fever

Ticks

Lyme disease
Southern tick-associated rash illness (STARI)
Rocky mountain spotted fever
Colorado tick fever
Relapsing fever
Ehrlichiosis/Anaplasmosis
Babesiosis
Tularemia
Tick paralysis
Tick typhus
Rickettsial pox
Taiga encephalitis
Tick-borne relapsing fever
364D rickettsiosis

Flies

Tularemia
Leishmaniasis
African trypanosomiasis (sleeping sickness)
Onchocerciasis
Bartonellosis
Loiasis

Chigger Mites

Scrub typhus (tsutsugamushi fever)
Rickettsial pox

Fleas

Plague
Murine (endemic) typhus

Lice

Epidemic typhus
Relapsing fever

Kissing Bugs

American trypanosomiasis (Chagas' disease)

Table 7.2 Sampling of Manufacturers of Protective Clothing, Protective Shelters, and Insect Nets

Protective Clothing (Includes Hooded Jackets, Pants, Head Nets, Ankle Guards, Gaiters, and Mittens)

Bug Baffler, Inc.
　PO Box 444
　Goffstown, NH 03045
　(800) 662–8411
　www.bugbaffler.com
Skeeta
　19706 77th Avenue East
　Bradenton, FL 34202
　(941) 322–9739
　www.skeeta.com
The Original Bug Shirt Company
　60 Industrial Parkway
　Cheektowaga, NY 14227
　(888) 998–9096
　www.bugshirt.com
Shannon Outdoor Bug Tamer
　P.O.Box 444
　Louisville, GA 30434
　(800) 852–8058
　www.bugtamer.com
Nomad Travelers Store
　www.nomadtravel.co.uk
Protective Shelters and Insect Nets
　Long Road Travel Supplies
　111 Avenida Drive
　Berkeley, CA 94708
　(800) 359–6040
　www.longroad.com
Wisconsin Pharmacal Co.
　1 Repel Road
　Jackson, WI 53037
　(800) 558–6614
　www.wpcbrands.com
Travel Medicine, Inc.
　369 Pleasant Street
　Northampton, MA 01060
　(800) 872–8633
　www.travmed.com
GearZone
　www.gearzone.co.uk
Nomad Travelers Store
　www.nomadtravel.co.uk

Physical Protection

By blocking arthropods' access to the skin, physical barriers can be very effective in preventing insect bites. A long-sleeved shirt, socks, full-length pants, and a hat will readily protect most of the skin surface. Ticks and chigger mites usually gain access to the skin around the ankle area, so tucking pant legs into socks or (ideally rubber) boots will reduce the risk of being bitten. Loose-fitting shirts made of tightly woven fabric and worn over a tucked-in undershirt will effectively reduce bites to the upper body. Light-colored clothing will attract fewer mosquitoes and biting flies, and will make it easier to see any ticks that might have crawled on to the fabric. A broad-brimmed, preferably light-colored, hat will also help protect the head and neck and reduce the chance of being bitten by mosquitoes, deerflies, black-flies and biting midges.

Mesh overgarments, or garments made of tightly woven material, can block ready access to the skin surface, thereby reducing the risks of being bitten. Hooded jackets, pants, mittens and head nets are available from several manufacturers in a wide range of styles for both adults and children (Table 7.2). With a mesh size of < 0.3 mm, these

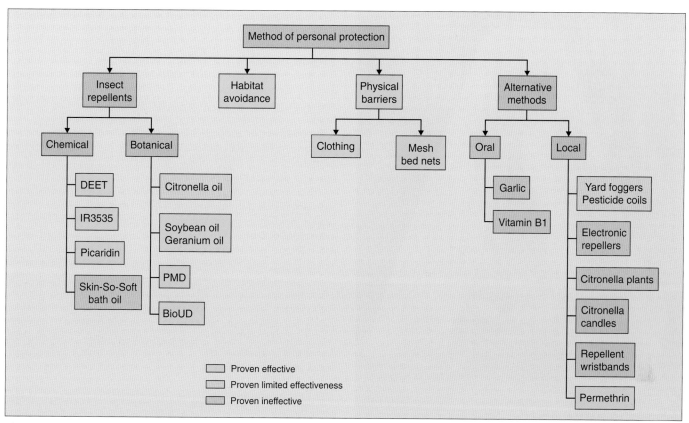

Figure 7.1 Methods of personal protection

garments are woven tightly enough to exclude even biting midges and immature ticks. The main limitation of these garments is that, as with any clothing, bending or sitting may pull the garments close enough to the skin to enable insects to bite through the fabric. Some people may also find mesh garments to be uncomfortable to wear during vigorous activity or in hot weather.

Lightweight insect nets and mesh shelters are also available to protect travelers while they sleep (Table 7.2 and Fig. 7.2). The simplest net is a large piece of mesh fabric suspended above and draped over a bed or sleeping bag to protect the occupant. More complex free-standing, tent-like shelters are also available, made with flexible hoops that support the protective mesh over the occupant. The efficacy of insect nets or shelters can be greatly enhanced by spraying them with a permethrin-based contact insecticide, which can provide weeks of protection following a single application.

Insect Repellents

For many people, applying a topical insect repellent may be the most effective and easiest way to prevent arthropod bites. The search for the 'perfect' insect repellent has been ongoing for decades and has yet to be achieved. The ideal agent would repel multiple species of biting arthropod, remain effective for at least 8 h, cause no irritation to skin or mucous membranes, possess no systemic toxicity, be resistant to abrasion and washoff, and be greaseless and odorless. No currently available insect repellent meets all of these criteria. Efforts to find such a compound have been hampered by the multiplicity of variables that affect the inherent repellency of any chemical. Repellents do not all share a single mode of action, and different species of insect may react differently to the same repellent.

Many chemicals that are capable of repelling biting arthropods evaporate or absorb into the skin too quickly to maintain their repellent effect. To be effective as an insect repellent, a chemical must be volatile enough to maintain an effective repellent vapor concentration at the skin surface, but not evaporate so rapidly that it quickly loses its effectiveness. Multiple factors play a role in effectiveness, including concentration, frequency and uniformity of application, the user's activity level and inherent attractiveness to blood-sucking arthropods, and the number and species of the organisms trying to bite. Gender may also play a role in how well a repellent works – one study has shown that DEET-based repellents work less well on women than on men.[5] The effectiveness of any repellent is reduced by abrasion from clothing; evaporation and absorption from the skin surface; washoff from sweat, rain, or water; physical activity; and a windy environment.[2] Each 10°C increase in ambient temperature can lead to as much as 50% reduction in protection time, owing to greater evaporative loss of the repellent from the skin surface. One of the greatest limitations of insect repellents is that they do not 'cloak' the user in a chemical veil of protection – any untreated exposed skin will be readily bitten by hungry arthropods.

Chemical Repellents
DEET

N,N-diethyl-*m*-toluamide (also called *N,N*-diethyl-3-methylbenzamide), or DEET, has been the gold standard of insect repellents for several decades. Only recently have other repellents come to market that show comparable broad-spectrum efficacy (discussed below). In the United States, DEET has been registered for use by the general public since 1957. It is effective against many species of crawling and flying insects, including mosquitoes, biting flies, midges, chiggers, fleas, and ticks.

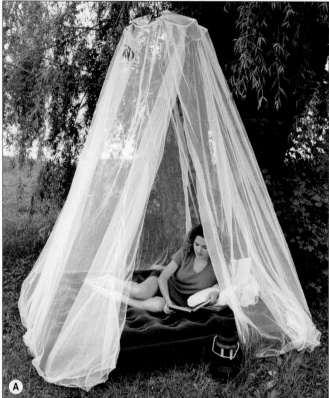

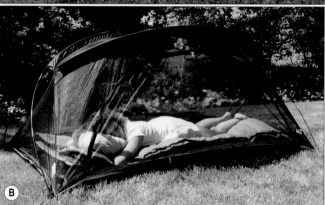

Figure 7.2 Protective mesh garments. (A) Bed-net. **(B)** Protective shelter *(courtesy of Wisconsin Pharmacal Co.)*

The United States Environmental Protection Agency estimates that about 30% of the US population uses a DEET-based product every year; worldwide use exceeds 200 million people annually.[6] More than 50 years of empirical testing of more than 20 000 other compounds have not yet led to the release of a clearly superior repellent.[7–9]

DEET may be applied to skin, clothing, mesh insect nets or shelters, window screens, tents, or sleeping bags. Care should be taken to avoid inadvertent contact with plastics (such as watch crystals and spectacle frames, lenses, or other optics), rayon, spandex, leather, or painted and varnished surfaces, since DEET may damage these. DEET does not damage natural fibers such as wool and cotton.

Choosing a DEET Formulation DEET is sold worldwide in concentrations of 5–100%. DEET is available in lotion, solution, towelette, gel, solid stick, and spray forms. As a general rule, higher concentrations of DEET will provide longer-lasting protection. Mathematical models of repellent effectiveness show that the protection is proportional to the logarithm of the concentration of the product. This curve

tends to plateau out at higher repellent concentrations, providing relatively less additional protection for each incremental dose of DEET >50%. Hence, for most activities, 10–35% DEET will usually provide adequate protection; 100% DEET formulations are rarely needed. The higher strengths of DEET repellent are appropriate to use under circumstances in which the wearer will be in an environment with a very high density of insects (e.g., a rain forest, tundra in the early summer), where there is a high risk of disease transmission from arthropod bites, or under circumstances where there may be rapid loss of repellent from the skin surface, such as high temperature and humidity, or rain. Under these circumstances, reapplication of the repellent will still likely be necessary to maintain its effectiveness.

Two companies (3M, and Sawyer Products) currently manufacture extended-release formulations of DEET that make it possible to deliver long-lasting protection without requiring the use of high concentrations of DEET. 3M's product, Ultrathon, was developed for the US military. This acrylate polymer 35% DEET formulation, when tested under multiple different environmental/climatic field conditions, was as effective as 75% DEET, providing up to 12 h of >95% protection against mosquito bites.[2] Sawyer Products' controlled-release 20% DEET lotion traps the chemical in a protein particle which slowly releases it to the skin surface, providing repellency equivalent to a standard 50% DEET preparation, lasting about 5 h. About 50% less of this encapsulated DEET is absorbed than from a 20% ethanol-based preparation of DEET.

DEET Safety and Toxicity Given its use by millions of people worldwide for over 50 years, DEET continues to show a remarkable safety profile. In 1980, to comply with more current standards for repellent safety, the US EPA issued an updated Registration Standard for DEET.[6] As a result, 30 new animal studies were conducted to assess acute, chronic, and subchronic toxicity; mutagenicity; oncogenicity; and developmental, reproductive, and neurological toxicity.[10] The results of these studies neither led to any product changes to comply with current EPA safety standards, nor indicated any new toxicities under normal usage. The EPA's Reregistration Eligibility Decision (RED) released in 1998 confirmed the Agency position that 'normal use of DEET does not present a health concern to the general US population'.[11]

Case reports of potential DEET toxicity exist in the medical literature, and have been summarized in several medical literature reviews.[2,12] Fewer than 50 cases of significant toxicity from DEET exposure have been documented in the medical literature over the last five decades; over three-quarters of these resolved without sequelae. Many of these cases involved long-term, excessive, or inappropriate use of DEET repellents; the details of exposure were frequently poorly documented, making causal relationships difficult to establish. These cases have not shown any correlation between the risk of toxicity and the concentration of the DEET product used or the age of user.

The reports of DEET toxicity that raise the greatest concern involve 16 cases of encephalopathy, 13 in children under age 8 years.[2,12] Three of these children died, one of whom had ornithine carbamoyl transferase deficiency, which might have predisposed her to DEET-induced toxicity. The other children recovered without sequelae. The EPA's analysis of these cases concluded that they 'do not support a direct link between exposure to DEET and seizure incidence'.[11] Animal studies in rats and mice show that DEET is not a selective neurotoxin.[6] According to the EPA, even if a link between DEET use and seizures does exist, the observed risk, based on DEET usage patterns, would be <1 per 100 million users.[11] Other studies have confirmed that children under 6 years old are not at greater risk for developing adverse effects from DEET than older individuals.[13–16]

A review of adverse events reported to the DEET Registry from 1995 to 2001 concluded that individuals with underlying neurological disorders were not predisposed to a greater risk for DEET toxicity. There was no evidence that using higher concentrations of DEET increases the risk of adverse events.[17]

Consumers applying both a DEET-based repellent and a sunscreen should be aware that the repellent might reduce the sunscreen's effectiveness. In a study of 14 patients who sequentially applied a 33% DEET repellent and an SPF 15 sunscreen, the sunscreen SPF was decreased by a mean of 33%, although the repellent maintained its potency.[18] Another study showed a decreased protection time of DEET when there was reapplication of sunscreen 2 hours after the repellent was applied.[19] There has been some concern that DEET and the sunscreen oxybenzone act synergistically to enhance the percutaneous absorption of the other chemical.[20] Combination sunscreen/DEET products are available, and will deliver the SPF as stated on the label. However, these products are generally not the best choice, as it is rare that sunscreen and repellent need to be reapplied at exactly the same time. In an effort to maintain adequate sun protection, consumers applying combination products will often apply more repellent than they would otherwise have needed. For these reasons, in 2000 Health Canada decided to discontinue the approval of combination sunscreen and insect repellent products. In 2007, the US EPA issued a request for information regarding the proper regulation of combination products, given the conflicting issues regarding proper application frequency.

There are always special concerns about the use of insect repellents during pregnancy. Most repellents are not tested in pregnant women. One published study followed 450 Thai women who used 20% DEET daily during the second and third trimesters of pregnancy to reduce the risk of contracting malaria.[21] Four percent of these women had detectable levels of DEET in umbilical cord blood at the time of delivery. However, no differences in survival, growth, or neurological development could be detected in the infants born to mothers who used DEET, compared to an equal number of mothers treated with a daily placebo cream during their pregnancies.

Guidelines for the safe use of repellents are shown in Table 7.3 (adapted from the EPA).[22] Careful product choice and common-sense application will greatly reduce the possibility of toxicity. The American Academy of Pediatrics' current recommendations are that children over the age of 2 months can safely use up to 30% DEET.[23] For consumers who choose to use the lower-concentration DEET products, reapplication of the repellent can compensate for their inherent shorter duration of protection. Individuals averse to applying DEET directly to their skin may get long-lasting repellency by applying DEET only to their clothing. DEET-treated garments, stored in a plastic bag between wearings, will maintain their repellency for several weeks. Questions regarding the safety of DEET may be addressed to the EPA-sponsored National Pesticide Telecommunications Network, available every day from 6:30 am to 4:30 pm PST at (800) 858-7378 or via their website at http://npic.orst.edu/.

IR3535 (Ethyl-Butylacetylaminoproprionate)

IR3535 (butylacetylaminopropionate) is an analog of the amino acid β-alanine, and has been used in Europe for over 20 years. In the United States, this compound is classified by the EPA as a biopesticide, effective against mosquitoes, ticks, and flies. IR3535 was brought to the US market in 1999 and is sold by Avon Products, Inc. and Sawyer Products in concentrations from 7.5% to 20%, with and without sunscreen. Depending on the concentration of the tested product, the species of mosquito, and the testing methodology, this repellent has demonstrated widely variable effectiveness, with complete protection

Table 7.3 Guidelines for Safe and Effective Use of Insect Repellents[22]

- For casual use, choose a repellent with no more than 35% DEET. Repellents with 30% DEET or less are most appropriate for use in children
- Use just enough repellent to lightly cover the skin; do not saturate the skin
- Repellents should be applied only to exposed skin and/or clothing – do not use under clothing
- For maximum effectiveness, apply to all exposed areas of skin
- To apply to the face, dispense into palms, rub hands together, and then apply thin layer to face
- Avoid contact with eyes and mouth – do not apply to children's hands to prevent possible subsequent contact with mucous membranes
- After applying, wipe repellent from the palmar surfaces to prevent inadvertent contact with eyes, mouth and genitals
- Never use repellents over cuts, wounds, inflamed, irritated or eczematous skin
- Do not inhale aerosol formulations or get in eyes
- Frequent reapplication is rarely necessary, unless the repellent seems to have lost its effectiveness. Reapplication may be necessary in very hot, wet environments, due to rapid loss of repellent from the skin surface
- Once inside, wash off treated areas with soap and water. Washing the repellent from the skin surface is particularly important under circumstances where a repellent is likely to be applied for several consecutive days

times ranging from 23 minutes to over 10 hours.[24–26] IR3535 can provide up to 12 hours of protection against black-legged ticks.[26] Higher concentrations of IR3535 give longer protection times, but in general do not match the efficacy of high-concentration DEET repellents. IR3535 is non-greasy, nearly odorless, will not dissolve plastics, and has a superior safety profile. In 2008, the Centers for Disease Control and Prevention (CDC) released a statement adding IR3535 to the list of approved repellents that could be used effectively to prevent mosquito-borne diseases.

Although Avon never marketed its *Skin-So-Soft* Bath Oil as a mosquito repellent, and although it is not effective as such, there remains widespread belief among consumers that it is. When tested under laboratory conditions against *Aedes aegypti* mosquitoes, Skin-So-Soft Bath Oil's effective half-life was found to be 0.51 hours.[2] In one study, against *Aedes albopictus*, Skin-So-Soft oil provided 0.64 hours of protection from bites, 10 times *less* effective than 12.5% DEET.[2] Skin-So-Soft oil has been found to be somewhat effective against biting midges, but this effect is likely due to its trapping the insects in an oily film on the skin surface. It has been proposed that the limited mosquito repellent effect of Skin-So-Soft oil could be due to its fragrance, or to the other chemicals used in its formulation.

Picaridin

Picaridin is the newest repellent active ingredient to become available in the US. Picaridin-based insect repellents have been sold in Europe since 1998, under the brand names Autan and Bayrepel. Picaridin is a synthetic repellent, derived from piperidine, which was originally isolated from pepper. Picaridin-based repellents are currently sold in many countries, including in the US, where concentrations from 5% to 20% are available (Table 7.4). It is effective against mosquitoes, biting flies, and ticks. When tested at the higher concentration, studies show that picaridin repellents offer comparable efficacy to DEET.[27–31]

Table 7.4 Biopesticide Repellents

Manufacturer	Product Name	Form(s)	Active Ingredients
S.C. Johnson Wax Racine, WI (800) 558-5566	OFF! Family Care Insect Repellent II	Spray pump	Picaridin 5%
Spectrum Brands Alpharetta, GA (800) 336-1372	Cutter Advanced Cutter Advanced Sport Cutter Skinsations Ultra Light	Spray pump, wipes Aerosol spray Aerosol spray	Picardin 5.75% Picaridin 15% Picaridin 15%
Tender Corp. Littleton, NH (800) 258-4696	Natrapel	Pump spray, aerosol spray, wipes	Picaridin 20%
Sawyer Products Safety Harbor, FL (800) 940-4664	Picaridin Insect Repellent	Pump spray	Picaridin 20%
Avon Products, Inc. New York, NY (800)367-2866	Skin-So-Soft Bug Guard Plus Picaridin	Pump spray, aerosol spray, wipes	Picaridin 10%
Avon Products, Inc. Suffern, NY (800) 367-2866	Skin So Soft Bug Guard Plus IR3535 SPF 30 Skin So Soft Bug Guard Plus IR3535 Skin So Soft Bug Guard Plus IR3535 Expedition	Lotion Aerosol spray Pump spray, aerosol spray	IR3535 7.5% IR3535 10% IR3535 20%
Sawyer Products Tampa, FL (800) 940-4664	Sunblock Insect Repellent IR3535 (SPF30)	Pump spray	IR3535 20%
HOMS, LLC Pittsboro, NC (800) 270-5721	BiteBlocker BioUD	Lotion, pump spray	2-Undecanone 7.75%

Table 7.5 Botanical Insect Repellents

Manufacturer	Product Name	Form(s)	Active Ingredient
Spectrum Brands St. Louis, MO (800) 874-8892	Cutter Lemon Eucalyptus Repel Lemon Eucalyptus	Pump spray Pump spray	Oil of lemon eucalyptus 40% Oil of lemon eucalyptus 40%
Vifor Pharma Potters Ltd. Manchester, UK	Mosi-Guard Natural	Lotion, pump spray, cream, stick	Oil of lemon eucalyptus 30%–40%
HOMS, Inc. Pittsboro, NC (888)270-5721	BiteBlocker Xtreme Sportsman BiteBlocker Herbal	Lotion & pump spray Pump spray	Soybean oil 3%, geranium oil 6%, castor oil 8% Soybean oil 2%, geranium oil 5%
Quantum, Inc. Eugene, OR (800) 448-1448	Buzz Away Extreme	Towelette & pump spray	Soybean oil 3%, geranium oil 6%, castor oil 8%, cedarwood oil 1.5%, citronella oil 1%
All Terrain Co. Sunapee, NH (800) 246-7328	Herbal Armor Herbal Armor SPF 15 Herbal Armor	Lotion Lotion Pump spray	Citronella oil 12%, oils of cedar, peppermint oil 2.5%, cedar oil 2%, lemongrass oil 1%, geranium oil 0.05%, in a slow-release encapsulated formula

The chemical is esthetically pleasant, and, unlike DEET, shows no detrimental effects on contact with plastics. The EPA states that picaridin did not show any toxicologically significant effects in animal studies. In April 2005, the CDC released a statement adding picaridin to the list of approved repellents that could be effectively used to prevent mosquito-borne diseases.

Botanical Repellents

Thousands of plants have been tested as sources of insect repellents. Although none of the plant-derived chemicals tested to date demonstrate the broad effectiveness and duration of DEET, a few show repellent activity. Plants with essential oils that have been reported to possess repellent activity include citronella, cedar, eucalyptus, verbena, pennyroyal, geranium, lavender, pine, cajeput, cinnamon, rosemary, basil, thyme, allspice, garlic, and peppermint.[8,32,33] Unlike DEET-based repellents, botanical repellents have been relatively poorly studied. When tested, most of these essential oils tended to show short-lasting protection, lasting minutes to 2 hours. A summary of readily available plant-derived insect repellents is shown in Table 7.5.

Citronella

Oil of citronella was initially registered as an insect repellent by the United States EPA in 1948. It is the most common active ingredient found in 'natural' or 'herbal' insect repellents. Originally extracted from the grass plant *Cymbopogon nardus*, oil of citronella has a lemony scent.

Data on the efficacy of citronella-based products are conflicting, varying greatly depending on the study methodology, location, species of biting insect tested, and the formulation of the tested repellent. One citronella-based repellent was found to provide no repellency when tested in the laboratory against *Aedes aegypti* mosquitoes.[34] Another study of the same product, however, conducted in the field, showed an average of 88% repellency over a 2-hour exposure. The product's effectiveness was greatest within the first 40 minutes after application, and then decreased with time over the remainder of the test period.[35] In a comparative laboratory study of the efficacy of insect repellents, no tested citronella-based product (concentration range 0.1–12%) completely repelled mosquitoes for more than 19 minutes.[25]

Oil of citronella tends to evaporate quickly from the skin surface, causing rapid loss of activity. To maintain the vapor concentration on the skin surface longer, some manufacturers mix the essential citronella oil with a large molecule such as vanillin, which slows the loss of the repellent from the skin. Another strategy has been to use nano-emulsions to slow the release rate of the citronella oil, which prolongs its protection time.[36] Many citronella repellents on the market now incorporate geranium oil and/or soybean oil to increase the product's repellent effect.

The short duration of action of citronella can be partially overcome by frequent reapplications. In 1997, after analyzing the available data on the repellent effect of citronella, the EPA concluded that citronella-based insect repellents must contain the following statement on their labels: 'For maximum repellent effectiveness of this product, repeat applications at 1-hour intervals.'[37]

Citronella candles have been promoted as an effective way to repel mosquitoes from one's local environment. One study compared the efficacy of commercially available 3% citronella candles, 5% citronella incense, and plain candles to prevent bites by *Aedes* species mosquitoes under field conditions.[2] Subjects near the citronella candles had 42% fewer bites than controls who had no protection (a statistically significant difference). However, burning ordinary candles reduced the number of bites by 23%. There was no difference in efficacy between citronella incense and plain candles. The ability of plain candles to reduce biting may be due to their serving as a 'decoy' source of warmth, moisture, and carbon dioxide.

The citrosa plant (*Pelargonium citrosum* Van Leenii) has been marketed as being able to repel mosquitoes through the continuous release of citronella oils. Unfortunately, when tested, these plants offered no protection against bites, and mosquitoes were found to readily alight on the leaves of the plant themselves.[2] In contrast, in experimental hut trials in Africa, potted live plants of *O. americanum, L. camara, L. uckambensis* repelled an average of 40%, 32%, and 33% of mosquitoes, respectively.[38]

BiteBlocker

Although available in Europe for several years, BiteBlocker, a 'natural' repellent, was not released to the US market until 1997. It is currently distributed by HOMS (Pittsboro, NC). BiteBlocker's formula combines soybean oil, geranium oil, and castor oil into lotion and spray forms. Studies conducted at the University of Guelph (Ontario, Canada) showed that this product was capable of providing >97% protection against *Aedes* species mosquitoes under field conditions, even after 3.5 hours of application. During the same time period, a 6.65% DEET-based spray gave 86% protection.[2] A second study showed that Blocker provided a mean of 200 (SD 30) minutes of complete protection from mosquito bites.[2] Blocker also provided about 10 hours of protection against biting black flies; in the same test, 20% DEET offered 6.5 hours of complete protection.[2]

BioUD (2-Undecanone)

HOMS is the sole distributor in the US of another repellent, BioUD (2-undecanone). This repellent was derived from the wild tomato plant and registered by the US EPA in 2007 as a biopesticide for use against mosquitoes and ticks. In field studies against mosquitoes, 7.75% BioUD provided comparable repellency to 25% DEET.[39] BioUD repelled the American dog tick, *Dermacentor variabilis,* from human skin for > 2.5 hours and was still effective 8 days after its application to cotton fabric.[40] Laboratory testing demonstrated that BioUD was 2–4 times more effective than 98% DEET at repelling *Amblyomma americanum, Dermacentor variabilis* and *Ixodes scapularis*.[41] BioUD was significantly better than either IR3535 or PMD (see below) at repelling *A. americanum*.[41]

Eucalyptus

A derivative (*p*-menthane-3,8-diol, or PMD) isolated from waste distillate of the essential oil of the lemon eucalyptus plant has shown promise as an effective 'natural' repellent. This menthol-like repellent has been very popular in China for years, and is currently available in Europe under the brand name Mosi-Guard. PMD was registered as a biopesticide by the US EPA and licensed for sale in the United States in March 2000.[42] In the US it is currently available as Repel Lemon Eucalyptus Insect Repellent and Cutter Lemon Eucalyptus Insect Repellent (Table 7.5). In a laboratory study against *Anopheles* mosquitoes, 30% PMD showed efficacy comparable to 20% DEET, but required more frequent reapplication to maintain its potency.[43] Field tests of this repellent have shown mean complete protection times ranging from 4 to 7.5 hours, depending on the mosquito species.[44,45] Oil of eucalyptus-based repellents can cause significant ocular irritation, so care must be taken to keep them away from the eyes and not to use them in children under 3 years of age. In 2005, the CDC added oil of eucalyptus-based repellents to its list of approved products that can be effectively used to prevent mosquito-borne disease.

Efficacy of DEET vs Botanical Repellents

Few data are available from studies that directly compare plant-derived repellents to DEET-based products. Available data proving the efficacy of botanical-derived repellents are often sparse, and there is no uniformly accepted standard for testing these products. As a result, different studies often yield varied results, depending on how and where the tests were conducted.

Studies comparing plant-derived repellents to low-strength DEET products, conducted under carefully controlled laboratory conditions with caged mosquitoes, typically demonstrate dramatic differences in effectiveness among currently marketed insect repellents. Citronella-based insect repellents usually provide the shortest protection, often lasting only a few minutes. Low-concentration DEET lotions (<7%) typically prove to be more effective than citronella-based repellents in their ability to prevent mosquito bites, and can generally be expected to provide about 1.5–2 hours of complete protection.[25] Reapplication of these low-concentration DEET products can compensate for their shorter duration of action. Since DEET repellents show a clear dose–response relationship, higher concentrations of DEET can be used to provide proportionately longer complete protection times – up to 6–8 hours after a single application.

Wristbands impregnated with either DEET or citronella offered no spatial protective 'cloaking' against bites.[25]

Table 7.6 Permethrin Insecticides

Manufacturer	Product Name	Form(s)	Active Ingredient
Coulston Products Easton, PA (610) 253-0167	Duranon Perma-Kill	Aerosol & pump sprays Liquid concentrate	Permethrin 0.5% Permethrin 13.3%
Sawyer Products Tampa, FL (800) 940-4464	Permethrin Tick Repellent	Aerosol & pump sprays	Permethrin 0.5%
Spectrum Brands St. Louis, MO (800) 874-8892	Cutter Outdoorsman Gear Guard	Aerosol spray	Permethrin 0.5%
3M St Paul, MN (888) 364-3577	Ultrathon Clothing and Gear Insect Repellent	Pump spray	Permethrin 0.5%
LifeSystems www.lifesystems.co.uk	AntiMosquito Fabric Treatment	Pump spray	Permethrin 0.49%

For people who choose to use 'natural' repellents, reapplication of the repellent on a frequent basis, preferable hourly, will help to compensate for the short duration of action of these repellents. Travelers in areas of the world where insect-borne disease is a considerable threat would be better protected by using a DEET, oil of eucalyptus (PMD), IR3535, or a picaridin-based repellent. Depending on the product chosen, and the circumstances in which it is being used, these repellents can provide 4–12 hours of complete protection following a single application.

Alternative Repellents

There has always been great interest in finding an oral insect repellent. Oral repellents would be convenient and would eliminate the need to apply sprays or lotions to the skin or put on protective clothing. Unfortunately, no effective oral repellent has been discovered. For decades, the lay literature has made the claim that vitamin B$_1$ (thiamine) works as a systemic mosquito repellent. When subjected to scientific scrutiny, however, thiamine has not been found to have any repellent effect on mosquitoes.[46] In 1983 the United States FDA, prompted by misleading consumer advertising, issued the following statement: 'There is a lack of adequate data to establish the effectiveness of thiamine or any other ingredient for OTC (over the counter) internal use as an insect repellent. Labeling claims for OTC orally administered insect repellent drug products are either false, misleading, or unsupported by scientific data.'[47] Tests of over 100 ingested drugs, including other vitamins, failed to reveal any that worked well against mosquitoes.[2] Ingested garlic has also never proved to be an effective arthropod deterrent.

Insecticides

Permethrin

Pyrethrum is a powerful, rapidly acting insecticide originally derived from the crushed dried flowers of the daisy *Chrysanthemum cinerariifolium*. Permethrin is a manmade synthetic pyrethroid. It does not repel insects, but instead works as a contact insecticide, causing nervous system toxicity, leading to death, or 'knockdown', of the insect. The chemical is effective against mosquitoes, flies, ticks, fleas, lice, and chiggers. Permethrin has low mammalian toxicity, is poorly absorbed by the skin, and is rapidly metabolized by skin and blood esterases.[48]

Permethrin should be applied directly to clothing or to other fabrics (tent walls, mosquito nets), not to skin. Permethrins are non-staining, nearly odorless, resistant to degradation by heat or sun, and will maintain their effectiveness for at least 2 weeks, through several launderings.[2]

The combination of permethrin-treated clothing and skin application of a DEET-based repellent creates a formidable barrier against biting insects. In an Alaskan field trial against mosquitoes, subjects wearing permethrin-treated uniforms and a polymer-based 35% DEET product had >99.9% protection (1 bite/h) over 8 hours; unprotected subjects were bitten an average of 1188 bites/h.[49]

Permethrin-sprayed clothing also proved very effective against ticks: 100% of *D. occidentalis* ticks (which carry Rocky Mountain Spotted Fever) died within 3 hours of touching permethrin-treated cloth.[3] Permethrin-sprayed pants and jackets also provided 100% protection from all three life stages of ticks, one of the vectors of Lyme disease.[3] Permethrin-sprayed sneakers and socks can reduce the likelihood of being bitten more than 73-fold.[50] In contrast, DEET alone (applied to the skin) provided 85% repellency at the time of application; this protection deteriorated to 55% repellency at 6 hours, when tested against the Lone Star tick *Amblyomma americanum*.[3] *Ixodes scapularis* Say ticks, which may transmit Lyme disease, also seem to be less sensitive to the repellent effect of DEET.[51]

Permethrin-based insecticides available in the US are listed in Table 7.6. To apply to clothing, spray each side of the fabric (outdoors) for 30–45 seconds, just enough to moisten. Allow to dry for 2–4 hours before wearing. Permethrin solution is also available for soak-treating large items, such as mesh bed-nets, or for treating batches of clothing. For those who would prefer the convenience of purchasing shirts and pants already treated with permethrin, Buzz Off Insect Repellent Apparel is available in many sporting goods stores, and from online retailers.

Reducing Local Mosquito Populations

Consumers may still find advertisements for small ultrasonic electronic devices meant to be carried on the body and that claim to repulse mosquitoes by emitting 'repellent' sounds, such as that of a dragonfly (claimed to be the 'natural enemy' of the mosquito), male mosquito, or bat. Multiple studies, conducted both in the field and laboratory, show that these devices do not work.[52] One study even showed that electronic mosquito repellents increased the biting rates of *A. aegypti*.[53] Pyrethrin-containing 'yard foggers' set off before an outdoor event can temporarily reduce the number of biting arthropods in a local environment. These products should be dispensed before any food is brought outside, and should be kept away from animals or fishponds. Burning coils that contain natural pyrethrins or synthetic pyrethroids (such as D-allethrin or D-transallethrin) can also temporarily reduce local populations of biting insects.[35] Some concerns have been raised about the long-term cumulative safety of use of these coils in an indoor environment. Wood smoke from campfires can also reduce the likelihood of being bitten by mosquitoes.

Relief From Mosquito Bites

Cutaneous responses to mosquito bites range from the common localized wheal-and-flare reaction to delayed bite papules, 'skeeter syndrome' (which mimics cellulitis), rare systemic Arthus-type reactions, and even anaphylaxis.[2] Bite reactions are the result of sensitization to mosquito salivary antigens, which lead to the formation of both specific IgE and IgG antibodies. Immediate-type reactions are mediated by IgE and histamine, whereas cell-mediated immunity is responsible for the delayed reactions.

Several strategies exist for relieving the itch of mosquito bites. Topical corticosteroids can reduce the associated erythema, itching, and induration; a short, rapidly tapering course of oral prednisone can also be very effective in reducing extensive bite reactions. Topical diphenhydramine and ester-type topical anesthetics should be avoided, owing to concerns about inducing allergic contact sensitivity. Oral antihistamines can be effective in reducing the symptoms of mosquito bites. In a 2-week double-blind placebo-controlled crossover trial cetirizine was given prophylactically to 18 individuals who had previously experienced dramatic cutaneous reactions to mosquito bites.[54] Subjects given the active drug had a statistically significant 40% decrease in both the size of the wheal response at 15 minutes and the size of the 24-hour bite papule. The mean pruritus score, measured 0.25, 1, 12, and 24 hours after being bitten, was 67% less than that of the untreated controls. Similar results have been found with ebastine, loratadine, and levocetirizine.[55,56] In highly sensitized individuals, prophylactic treatment with non-sedating antihistamines may safely reduce the cutaneous reactions to mosquito bites.

AfterBite, a 3.6% ammonium solution, has been found to relieve type I hypersensitivity symptoms associated with mosquito bites. In a double-blind placebo-controlled trial, 64% of mosquito-bitten subjects experienced complete relief of symptoms after a single application of the ammonium solution; the remaining 36% experienced partial relief, lasting 15–90 minutes after a single application. No subjects treated with placebo reported complete symptom relief.[57]

Summary – A Comprehensive Approach to Personal Protection

An integrated approach to personal protection is the most effective way to prevent arthropod bites, regardless of where one is in the world and which species of insects may be biting. Maximum protection is best achieved through avoiding infested habitats, and using protective clothing, topical insect repellents, and permethrin-treated garments.[9] When appropriate, mesh bed-nets or tents should be used to prevent nocturnal insect bites.[9]

For more than 50 years DEET-containing insect repellents have been the most effective products on the market, providing the most broad-spectrum, longest-lasting repellency against multiple arthropod species. Based on strong scientific support for their safety and efficacy, the CDC has now approved picaridin, IR3535, and oil of eucalyptus (PMD) as alternatives to DEET that may be used to reduce the likelihood of contracting a vector-borne disease. Of the 'botanical' repellents BiteBlocker and oil of eucalyptus repellents offer the best protection, but some consumers may object to their odor; the more neutral esthetic qualities of IR3535 and picaridin may be better choices for those sensitive individuals. Picaridin repellents, especially at the higher concentrations, can provide comparable efficacy to DEET, and also offer the benefit of being more esthetically pleasing to users. BioUD also shows promise as an effective alternative to DEET in repelling both mosquitoes and ticks.

Insect repellents alone, however, should not be relied upon to provide complete protection. Mosquitoes, for example, can find and bite any untreated skin, and may even bite through thin clothing. Deerflies, biting midges, and some blackflies prefer to bite around the head, and will readily crawl into the hair to bite where there is no protection. Wearing protective clothing, including a hat, will reduce the chances of being bitten. Treating one's clothes and hat with permethrin will maximize their effectiveness, by causing 'knockdown' of any insect that crawls or lands on the treated clothing. To prevent chiggers or ticks from crawling up the legs, pants should also be tucked into the boots or stockings. Wearing smooth, closely woven fabrics, such as nylon, will make it more difficult for ticks to cling to the fabric. After returning indoors, the skin should be inspected for the presence of ticks. Any ticks found attached to the skin should be removed to reduce the potential risk of disease transmission. Most ticks require over 48 hours of attachment to transmit Lyme disease.[58] The best method of tick removal is to simply grasp the tick with a forceps as close to the skin surface as possible, and pull upwards, with a steady, even force.

The US military relies on this integrated approach to protect troops deployed in areas where arthropods constitute either a significant nuisance or a medical risk. The Department of Defense's Insect Repellent System consists of DEET applied to exposed areas of skin, and permethrin-treated uniforms, worn with the pant legs tucked into boots, and the undershirt tucked into the pants' waistband. This system has been proven to dramatically reduce the likelihood of being bitten by arthropods.

Travelers visiting parts of the world where insect-borne disease is a potential threat will be best able to protect themselves if they learn about indigenous insects and the diseases they might transmit. Protective clothing, mesh insect tents or bedding, insect repellent, and permethrin spray should be carried. Travelers would be wise to check the most current World Health Organization (www.who.int/en), Centers for Disease Control and Prevention (www.cdc.gov/travel/index.htm), or national authorities' recommendations about traveling to countries where immunizations (e.g., against yellow fever), or chemoprophylaxis (e.g., against malaria) should be considered.

References

1. Bock GR, Cardew G, editors. Olfaction in Mosquito-Host Interactions. New York: J Wiley; 1996.
2. Fradin MS. Mosquitoes and mosquito repellents: a clinician's guide. Ann Int Med 1998;128(11):931–40.

3. Fradin MS. Protection from blood-feeding arthropods. In: Auerbach PS, editor. Wilderness Medicine. 5th ed. St. Louis: Mosby Press, 2007. p. 892–904.

4. Curtis CF. Personal protection methods against vectors of disease. Rev Med Vet Entomol 1992;80(10):543–53.

5. Golenda CF, Solberg VB, Burge R, et al. Gender-related efficacy difference to an extended duration formulation of topical N,N-diethyl-m-toluamide (DEET). Am J Trop Med Hyg 1999;60(4):654–7.

6. US Environmental Protection Agency. Office of Pesticides and Toxic Substances. Special Pesticide Review Division. N,N-diethyl-m-toluamide (DEET) Pesticide Registration Standard (EPA 540/RS-81–004). Washington D.C.: US Environmental Protection Agency; 1980.

7. King WV. Chemicals evaluated as insecticides and repellents at Orlando, Fla. USDA Agric Handb 1954;69:1–397.

8. Maia MF, Moore SJ. Plant-based insect repellents: a review of their efficacy, development and testing. Malaria Journal 2011;10:S11.

9. Goodyer LI, Croft AM, Frances SP, et al. Expert review of the evidence base for arthropod avoidance. J Travel Med 2010;17:182–92.

10. Completed studies for the DEET Toxicology Data Development Program. Washington, DC: The DEET Joint Venture Group, Chemical Specialties Manufacturers Association; 1996.

11. US Environmental Protection Agency. Office of Pesticide Programs, Prevention, Pesticides and Toxic Substances Division. Reregistration Eligibility Decision (RED): DEET (EPA 738-F-95-010). Washington, D.C.: US Environmental Protection Agency; 1998.

12. Osimitz TG, Grothaus RH. The present safety assessment of DEET. J Am Mosq Control Assoc 1995;11(2):274–8.

13. Veltri JC, Osimitz TG, Bradford DC, et al. Retrospective analysis of calls to poison control centers resulting from exposure to the insect repellent N,N-diethyl-m-toluamide (DEET) from 1985–1989. J Toxicol Clin Toxicol 1994;32(1):1–16.

14. Bell JW, Veltri JC, Page BC. Human exposures to N, N-diethyl-m-toluamide insect repellents reported to the American Association of Poison Control Centers 1993–1997. Int J Toxicol 2002;21:341.

15. Sudakin DL, Trevathan WR. DEET: A review and update of safety and risk in the general population. Clin Toxicol 2003;41:831.

16. Koren G, Matsui D, Bailey B. DEET-based insect repellents: safety implications for children and pregnant and lactating women. CMAJ 2003;169:209.

17. Osimitz TG, Murphy JV, Fell LA, et al. Adverse events associated with the use of insect repellents containing N,N-diethyl-m-toluamide (DEET). Regul Toxicol Pharmacol 2010;56:93–9.

18. Murphy ME, Montemarano AD, Debboun M, et al. The effect of sunscreen on the efficacy of insect repellent: A clinical trial. J Am Acad Dermatol 2000;43:219–22.

19. Webb CE, Russell RC. Insect repellents and sunscreen: implications for personal protection strategies against mosquito-borne disease. Aust N Z J Public Health 2009;33(5):485–90.

20. Kasichayanula S, House JD, Wang T, et al. Percutaneous characterization of the insect repellent DEET and sunscreen oxybenzone from topical skin application. Toxicol Appl Pharmacol 2007;223:187-94.

21. McGready R, Hamilton KA, Simpson JA, et al. Safety of the insect repellent N, N-dietyyl-m-toluamide (DEET) in pregnancy. Am J Trop Med Hyg 2001;65:285–9.

22. Using insect repellents safely. Office of Pesticide Programs, United States Environmental Protection Agency (EPA-735/F-93–052R); 1998.

23. Weil WB. New information leads to changes in DEET recommendations. AAP News 2001;19:52.

24. Comparative efficacy of IR3535 and DEET as repellents against adult Aedes aegypti and Culex quinquefasciatus. J Am Mosq Control Assn 2004;20:299–304.

25. Fradin MS, Day JF. Comparative efficacy of insect repellents. N Engl J Med 2002;347:13–18.

26. Carroll SP. Prolonged efficacy of IR3535 repellents against mosquitoes and blacklegged ticks in North America. J Med Entomol 2008;45(4):706–14.

27. Badolo A, Ilboudo-Sanogo E, Ouedraogo AP, et al. Evaluation of the sensitivity of Aedes aegypti and Anopheles gambiae complex mosquitoes to two insect repellents: DEET and KBR 3023. Trop Med Int Health 2004;9:330.

28. Frances SP, Van Dung N, Beebe NW, et al. Field evaluation of repellent formulations against daytime and nighttime biting mosquitoes in a tropical rainforest in northern Australia. J Med Entomol 2002;39:541.

29. Debboun M, Strickman D, Solberg VB, et al. Field evaluation of DEET and a piperidine repellent against Aedes communis (Diptera: Culicidae) and Simulium venustum (Diptera: Simuliidae) in the Adirondack Mountains of New York. J Med Entomol 2000;37:919.

30. Frances SP, Waterson DGE, Beebe NW, et al. Field evaluation of repellent formulations containing DEET and picaridin against mosquitoes in Northern Territory, Australia. J Med Entomol 2004;41:414–7.

31. Carroll JF, Benante JP, Kramer M, et al. Formulations of DEET, picaridin, and IR3535 applied to skin repel nymphs of the lone star tick (Aari: Ixodidae) for 12 hours. J Med Entomol 2010;47:699–704.

32. Quarles W. Botanical mosquito repellents. Common Sense Pest Control 1996;12(4):12–19.

33. Duke J. USDA-Agricultural Research Service Phytochemical and Ethnobotanical Databases http://www.ars-grin.gov/~ngrlsb/.

34. Chou JT, Rossignol PA, Ayres JW. Evaluation of commercial insect repellents on human skin against Aedes aegypti (Diptera: Culicidae). J Med Entomol 1997;34:624–30.

35. Fradin MS. Insect repellents. In: Wolverton S, Comprehensive Dermatologic Drug Therapy. 2nd ed. Philadelphia, PA: WB Saunders; 2007. p. 785–801.

36. Sakulku U, Nuchuchua O, Uawongyart N, et al. Characterization and mosquito repellent activity of citronella oil nanoemulsion. Int J Pharm 2009;372:105–11.

37. United States Environmental Protection Agency, Office of Pesticide Programs, Prevention, Pesticides and Toxic Substances Division: Reregistration eligibility decision (RED) for oil of citronella (EPA-738-F-97-002) Washington DC, 1997.

38. Seyoum A, Kabiru EW, Wnade WL, et al. Repellency of live potted plants against Anopheles gambiae from human baits in semi-field experimental huts. Am J Trop Med Hyg 2002;67:191–5.

39. Bissinger BW, Stumpf CF, Donohue KV, et al. Novel arthropod repellent, BioUD, is an efficacious alternative to DEET. J Med Entomol 2008;45(5):891–8.

40. Bissinger BW, Apperson CS, Sonenshine DE, et al. Efficacy of the new repellent BioUD against three species of ixodid ticks. Exp Appl Acarol 2009;48:239–50.

41. Bissinger BW, Zhu J, Apperson CS, et al. Comparative efficacy of BioUD to other commercially available arthropod repellents against ticks Amblyomma americanum and Dermacentor variabilis on cotton cloth. Am J Trop Med Hyg 2009;81:685–90.

42. United States Environmental Protection Agency, Office of Pesticide Programs. p-Menthane-3,8-diol. Washington, DC 2000: www.epa.gov/pesticides/biopesticides/factsheets/fs011550e.htm.

43. Trigg JK, Hill N. Laboratory evaluation of a eucalyptus-based repellent against four biting arthropods. Phytotherapy Research 1996;10:313–6.

44. Barnard DR, Xue RD. Laboratory evaluation of mosquito repellents against Aedes albopictus, Culex nigripalpus, and Ochlerotatus triseriatus (Diptera: Culicidae). J Med Entomol 2004;41:726–30.

45. Moore SJ, Lenglet A, Hill N. Field evaluation of three plant-based insect repellents against malaria vectors in Vaca Diez Province, the Bolivian Amazon. J Am Mosq Control Assoc 2002;18:107-10.

46. Ives AR, Paskewitz SM. Testing vitamin B as a home remedy against mosquitoes. J Am Mosq Control Assoc 2005;21:213–7.

47. Food and Drug Administration. Drug products containing active ingredients offered over-the-counter (OTC) for oral use as insect repellents. Fed Red 1983;48:26987.

48. Insect repellents. Med Lett Drugs Ther 1989;31:45–47.

49. Lillie TH, Schreck CE, Rahe AJ. Effectiveness of personal protection against mosquitoes in Alaska. J Med Entomol 1988;25(6):475–8.

50. Miller NJ, Rainone EE, Dyer MC, et al. Tick bite prevention with permethrin-treated summer-weight clothing. J Med Entomol 2011;48:327-33.

51. Schreck CE, Fish D, McGovern TP. Activity of repellents applied to skin for protection against Amblyomma americanum and Ixodes scapularis ticks (Acari: Ixodidae). J Am Mosq Control Assoc 1995;11:136–40.

52. Coro F, Suarez S. Review and history of electronic mosquito repellers. Wing Beats 2000;Summer 2000:6–32.
53. Andrade CFS, Cabrini I. Electronic mosquito repellers induce increased biting rates in *Aedes aegypti* mosquitoes (Diptera: Culicidae). J Vector Ecol 2010;35:75–8.
54. Reunala T, Brummer-Korvenkontio H, Karppinen A, et al. Treatment of mosquito bites with cetirizine. Clin Exp Allergy 1993;23:72–5.
55. Karppinen A, Kautiainen H, Petman L, et al. Comparison of cetirizine, ebastine and loratadine in the treatment of immediate mosquito-bite allergy. Allergy 2002;57:534–7.
56. Karppinen A, Brummer-Korvenkontio H, Petman L, et al. Levocetirizine for treatment of immediate and delayed mosquito bites. Acta Derm Venereol (Stockh) 2006;86:329–31.
57. Zhai H, Packman EW, Maibach HI. Effectiveness of ammonium solution in relieving type I mosquito bite symptoms: a double-blind, placebo-controlled study. Acta Derm Venereol (Stockh) 1998;78:297–8.
58. Sood SK, Salzman MB, Johnson BJ, et al. Duration of tick attachment as a predictor of the risk of Lyme disease in an area in which Lyme disease is endemic. J Infect Dis 1997;175(4):996–9.

Travel Medical Kits

Larry Goodyer

Key points

- Travelers should purchase medical and health-related items prior to departure
- The contents of a medical kit should be determined by a risk assessment – consider destination, type and duration of travel, and activities
- Travelers should be aware of the legal restrictions on carrying certain medicines, particularly narcotics and psychotropics, into certain countries
- Items should be packaged appropriately for the travel environment
- A kit should be constructed in a stepwise manner, building up from the most essential items used in all travel situations to those required in specific circumstances

Introduction

A central function of the pre-travel consultation is to provide the necessary prophylaxis together with appropriate verbal and written advice. If a traveler should become ill or injured overseas there are two choices that need to be made: whether to self-treat or to seek the advice of a healthcare practitioner. In either case it is likely that first aid or medication will be needed to manage the condition. This chapter addresses the issue of the range of such items that could be considered for inclusion into a first-aid/medical kit for personal use as well as the potential range of items suitable for groups of travelers and expeditions. In addition, for completeness there are a range of health-related items such as sunscreens, hand-washes and repellents that should also be carried in many travel situations.

The extent to which travelers carry or use items for self-treatment has not been well investigated. One small study identified the items used by a cohort of longer-term travelers, mostly backpackers, and concluded that the range of items frequently used was relatively limited.[1] Surveys of trekkers in the Khumbu region of Nepal from 1995 to 1997 revealed that only 18% of respondents carried a comprehensive kit.[2] A few other studies have described the use of medical kits in a variety of situations.[3,4,5]

There are a number of compelling reasons why the traveler should try to purchase all medical and health-related items before departure rather than at destination, even though the latter may involve a considerable financial saving:

- **Availability**. In many developing countries the required products may simply not be available, and this is difficult to anticipate before arrival. This may also apply to other health products, such as certain types of insect repellent.
- **Equivalence.** If the product is available it may be difficult to explain to the health professional precisely what is required in another language. Both the names of the ingredients and the instructions may also not be in the traveler's own language.
- **Quality.** There is wide recognition that in some developing and emerging countries there may be poor drug regulatory systems, and along with that, high levels of either forged or poor-quality pharmaceuticals. In some developing countries more than 30% of all medications available for sale could be counterfeit.[6]

Summary of Factors Determining Medical and First-Aid Kit Construction

Risk assessment is at the heart of all pre-travel preparation, and this should inform the contents of any medical kit that might be carried. Below are the standard questions that contribute to a risk assessment, with an indication of how they influence medical kit construction:

- Destination
  - Diseases endemic to area – Awareness of outbreaks and endemic diseases may warrant carrying specific medications, e.g., malaria emergency standby
  - Quality of medical facilities – Poor facilities would imply carrying a greater range of items if these are not available locally
  - Environmental extreme – Preparation for coping with the treatment of illness relating to the environment, acute mountain sickness or heat exhaustion/stroke are prime examples
  - Security – Those venturing to areas of very poor security such as war zones may need to consider more extensive emergency first-aid items
- Type of travel
  - **Tourists** on shorter-term holidays to popular destinations may only require the most basic of items, whereas **backpackers**

who might be visiting more remote destinations should consider a broader range, but may be constrained in the amount that can be carried

- **Business travelers** may well need very little if staying for short periods in major urban areas, but quite extensive kits if traveling long-term and with family
- **Those visiting friends and relatives (VFRs) in their countries of birth (typically developing countries)** should be aware of the importance of carrying a medical kit as described above
- **Wilderness travel** demands particular attention to self-sufficiency in treating any likely medical issue or emergency. Frequently this is undertaken as a group or **expedition,** where a very comprehensive kit is required with sufficient supply to treat a range of people. Such a kit may be difficult to transport, so is often viewed as a 'Base camp' unit, with a smaller individualized kit being carried when away from base. **Overland groups** traveling for long periods in truck transportation visiting many different regions will also carry a group medical and first-aid kit as well as individual kits

- Activities will help determine the range of first-aid items required
- Duration of travel and time at destination will determine the quantities of each item
- Pre-existing medical conditions also inform quantity and type of prescribed medication
- Legal restrictions on importation. The medications that cause the most problems when carried across borders are those defined as narcotic and psychotropic. Many countries will allow travelers to carry a supply for personal use of less than 1 month, but there are others where such items either require special permits or are completely banned under any circumstances. The International Narcotics Control Board (INCB) website[3,7] contains country-specific information on regulations for carrying such items, though they can be difficult to interpret in some cases. Obtaining consistent and reliable advice from embassies can also be difficult, and it is not always easy to identify the relevant information on the official country websites. There are some destinations, such as the United Arab Emirates, which have long lists of banned items, some falling outside the category of narcotic and psychotropic. Box 8.1 describes the general advice

regarding carrying medicines for personal use across borders. If larger quantities need to be carried then importation licences may be required

- Type of packaging able to be transported. Packaging of items for travel should be considered, particularly if backpacks are being used for groups or in camping/wilderness situations. In these types of travel loose tablets in bottles can become broken, and cardboard boxes holding blister packs will quickly deteriorate and instruction leaflets get lost. It is sometimes appropriate to repackage into sealable plastic bags with the information leaflet, or use individually labeled blisters (Fig. 8.1). All items should be stored in a well-organized pouch or bag which has PVC pockets for easy identification (Fig. 8.2); a number of companies now supply such bags, and also ready-made kits (Table 8.1).

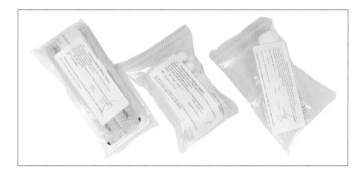

Figure 8.1 Appropriate packaging of tablets for travel.

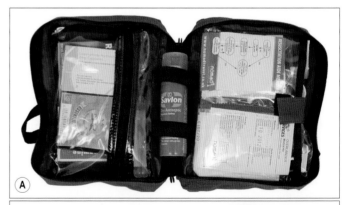

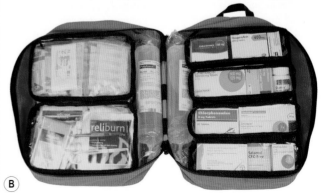

Figure 8.2 Personal travel medical kits.

BOX 8.1

General Advice Regarding Carrying Medicines Overseas

- The International Narcotics Control Board website (www.incb.org) and official government sites should be checked for requirements and regulations regarding traveling with narcotic or psychotropic medications
- Check regulations regarding traveling with medications that have a high potential for abuse, such as anabolic steroids
- Check regulations regarding the carrying of any questionable medication, as some countries permit taking only a 30-day supply and require carrying a prescription or an import license certificate
- Keep tablets together with the original packaging and information leaflet
- Carry copies of prescriptions for those that act on the central nervous system

Table 8.1 A Sample of Specialist Providers of Medical Kits for Travelers

Nomad Travelstore Ltd – UK	www.Nomadtravel.co.uk
Chinook Medical Gear Inc – US	www.Chinookmed.com
Travmed Products – US	www.medexassist.com
Lifesystems UK	www.lifesystems.co.uk
Travel Clinics Australia	www.travelclinic.com.au
Tropicaire (Netherlands)	www.tropenzorg.nl

BOX 8.2

The Basic Medical Kit for All Classes of Travel

Analgesic
Antidiarrrheal
Cough or cold medication
Motion sickness medication
Insect repellent
Insect bite treatment
Antiseptic/wipes
Sticking plaster
Soothing cream or gel
Scissors/tweezers
Sunscreens
Water purification tablets/purifier
Digital thermometer
Condoms

BOX 8.3

Comprehensive Personal Medical Kit

Items in Box 8.2 as well as:
Non-adherent dressing/tape
Blister plasters
Burn dressings
Support bandage
Wound bandage and gauze swabs
Wound closure
Protection for mouth to mouth resuscitation
Gloves
Lip balm
Cotton buds
Antacid
Laxative
Temporary fillings
Antihistamine
Antifungal
Artificial tears
Sterile kit of syringes, needles and cannula
Emergency tooth repair kit
Prescription items
    Broad-spectrum oral antibiotic
    Antibiotic eye and ear drops
    Antiemetic
Additional items for particular situations, e.g.:
Healing (hydrocolloid) plasters and dressings
Antibiotic creams and powders
Malaria emergency standby treatment
Acetazolamide

Contents of Medical and First-Aid Kits

Designing a medical and first-aid kit should be approached in a step-wise manner as described in Boxes 8.2 to 8.4. The majority of travelers should consider carrying the items listed in Box 8.2. Those in higher-risk situations, such as independent longer-term travelers, should consider those in Boxes 8.2 and 8.3. For group travel the items in both Boxes 8.2, 8.3 and 8.4 should be considered for the large base camp or truck kit.

The Basic Medical and First-Aid Kit

In the basic medical kit a simple analgesic such as an NSAID and/or acetaminophen should always be carried. For many destinations an agent to treat travelers' diarrhea will also be a basic component (see Chapter 20). Motion sickness prevention may be required by some (see Chapter 43). Local reactions to mosquitoes and other biting insects are also a common source of minor but troublesome problems for travelers; topical corticosteroids and oral antihistamines are useful treatments (see Chapter 45). Simple first-aid items should also be carried for treatment of minor injuries such as cuts and grazes. For most situations sticking plasters or small bandages are all that is required. Antiseptic impregnated towelettes are useful for cleaning minor wounds. Among the most effective of antiseptic solutions are those containing povidone-iodine, dry powder sprays and tinctures being suitable for travel. These may be preferred over tubes of antiseptic cream, where the sterility of the product may be lost with repeated use. Other health-related products are also advised, such as high protection factor sunscreens (SPF >15 and a UVA protection

---

BOX 8.4

Medical Kit Contents if Caring for Others

Analgesic for severe pain, e.g., Tramadol, nalbuphine IM, diclofenac IM

Extended range of oral antimicrobials, such as metronidazole, macrolides, mebendazole, injectable third-generation cephalosporin

Corticosteroids: prednisolone, IV hydrocortisone
Rectal diazepam
Normal saline eye-wash
Surface anesthetic eye drops
Fluorescein strips for eye examination
Intravenous sets
Intravenous fluids – colloids and crystalloids
Anesthetic for local injection
Suturing equipment
Adrenaline injection 1:1000
Silver sulfadiazine for burns
Airway various sizes
Sterile equipment for minor procedures

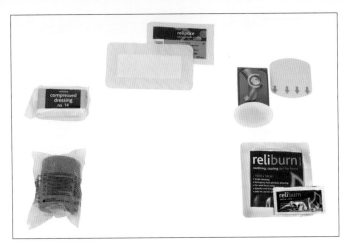

Figure 8.3 A range of wound dressings for travel kits. From top left clockwise: non-adherent dressing with adhesive edging, foot blister plaster, burn dressing, conforming support bandage, field wound dressing. *(All pictures courtesy of Nomad Travel store.)*

rating), mosquito bite avoidance products (See Chapter 7) and water purification (see chapter 6).

More Comprehensive Kits

For those who fall into higher-risk categories, such as backpackers on independent longer trips to developing countries, additional items as described in Box 8.3 should be considered. The list of potential first-aid items may be more extensive depending on the type of activity being undertaken. For instance, a range of wound dressings should be included (Fig. 8.3) when intensive outdoor activities are being pursued: non-adherent wound dressings are standard, and those that combine an adhesive outer rim are more convenient than applying with surgical tape. Foot blister plasters which incorporate a hydrogel are essential for trekkers and walkers, as are support bandages for sprains and joint injuries. If first aid to treat more major injury is anticipated then a larger wound field dressing and wound closure items may be advised. For the latter, suturing requires access to a person trained in its use; adhesive Steristips are useful, but sometimes not as effective. The new wound closure glues are more user-friendly but extremely expensive.

Higher-risk travelers should consider carrying a range of sterile equipment such as needles, syringes and cannulae, as sterile equipment may be unavailable or in short supply.

Depending on individual requirements, a range of preparations to treat minor ailments such as dyspepsia and upper respiratory tract infections can be included. An antiemetic is quite useful, and buccal prochlorperazine or promethazine suppositories can avoid the use of injectable drugs. An antifungal cream or powder preparation would be useful in the hot and wet conditions of the rainforest. Other useful items might include those for treating conjunctivitis (an antibiotic eye

drop or ointment) or outer ear infection, the latter particularly common if undertaking a great deal of swimming or diving activities. Somewhat contentious is providing travelers with a cadre of broad-spectrum antibiotics to treat conditions such as cellulitis, urinary tract infections and pneumonia. Certainly for wilderness conditions these may be essential and life-saving. There is also an argument that in some countries where the quality of medicines is poor, carrying a personal supply is warranted. In the study by Goodyer, 16% of longer-term travelers used or obtained antibiotics while away.[1]

There are also situations where particular items might be necessary, such as acetazolamide and dexamethasone for the prevention or treatment of mountain sickness (see Chapter 39) and malaria chemoprophylaxis and standby treatment (see Chapter 16). In the rainforest, where wound healing is problematic, a hydrogel dressing is advised to provide a good healing environment that can be left undisturbed for a long period of time. Topical antibiotic creams and ointments are also preferred by some to aid healing of wounds that are likely to be contaminated when trekking in jungle environments.

Expedition and Group Kits

For groups and expeditions sufficient quantities of items described in Boxes 8.2, 8.3 and 8.4 will need consideration. There are a range of items that may be included which require trained individuals caring for the members of the group. It is beyond the scope of this chapter to discuss in detail the specialist requirements of expedition and wilderness travel, but those items listed would form an important core for the expedition medical officer. Some specialist overland groups may also require certain of those listed even if no medical personnel are present, if the regions of travel are likely to have a poor supply of medical items. For more detailed information, see wilderness and expedition texts.[8,9]

References

1. Goodyer LI, Gibbs J. Medical supplies for travellers to developing countries. J Travel Med 2004;11:208–12.
2. His Majesty's Government of Nepal. Nepal tourism statistics, 1996. Kathmandu, Nepal: Asian Printing Press; 1996.
3. Sakmar TP. The traveler's medical kit. Infect Dis Clin North Am 1992;6:355–70.
4. Deacon SP, McCulloch WJ. Medical kits for business travellers. J Soc Occupational Med 1990;40;103–4.
5. Harper LH, Bettinger J, Dismukes R, et al. The evaluation of the Coca-Cola Company travel health kit. J Travel Med 2002;9:244–66.
6. IMPACT. Counterfeit Medicines: an update on estimates. 2006. (http://www.who.int/medicines/services/counterfeit/impact/TheNewEstimatesCounterfeit.pdf). Accessed 12 September 2011.
7. The International Narcotics Control Board (INCB) www.incb.org/incb/guidelines_travellers.html
8. Weiss EA. Wilderness 911 – A Step-by-step Guide for Medical Emergencies and Improvised Care in the Backcountry. Seattle: The Mountaineers; 1998.
9. Warrell D, Anderson S, editors. Expedition Medicine. London: Profile Books; 1998. p. 73–9.

9

Principles of Immunization

Herwig Kollaritsch and Pamela Rendi-Wagner

Key points

- In travel medicine both live and killed vaccines are used. Both types have specific effects with respect to immune induction, long-term response and memory, and adverse reactions
- Vaccines can be administered via several routes: oral and parenteral, the latter being subdivided into intradermal (lower amount of antigen, non-adjuvanted vaccines), subcutaneous (live vaccines) and intramuscular (adjuvanted vaccines). Administration route depends on antigen, but also on preferred location of induced immunity
- Killed vaccines are often adjuvanted. These substances are immunomodulating and can trigger the immune response in a number of different ways. Adjuvants are potentially irritating and should only be administered intramuscularly
- There are strict guidelines for body site, route of administration and length of needle for each vaccine, and they should be adhered to. Separate recommendations for children and adults should be followed
- Adverse reactions after vaccinations should be documented meticulously and reported to national pharmacovigilance systems
- All vaccines can be administered concomitantly, unless otherwise stated in the product information: no overload of the immune system occurs. If live vaccines are not given simultaneously, they should be separated by at least 4 weeks to avoid interference
- Vaccines have to be stored correctly and their use must be documented in the patient's vaccination record. The consent of the vaccinee must be obtained. Vaccinees have to be examined with respect to possible contraindications and detailed medical history, including allergies and hypersensitivity reactions

Introduction

Recent decades have provided the indisputable insight that the control of major infectious diseases is less effective by therapeutic than by preventive means, in particular by well-targeted use of vaccines. The global eradication of smallpox in 1977 serves as the primary example

for effective disease control through immunization. The application of modern biotechnological tools has resulted in an array of vaccine candidates arising from various sources, creating the promise of effective prevention (and treatment) of many more diseases associated with high mortality and morbidity. There are many online sources concerned with vaccines and vaccinations which are regularly updated, e.g., www.immunize.org, www.vaccineinfo.org or the CDC Pink Book (http://www.cdc.gov/vaccines/pubs/pinkbook/index.html).

Immunology of Vaccination

Active Immunization

Generally, active immunization represents a harmless, yet highly effective active interaction between the host's immune system and specific pathogens. Details may be also obtained via http://www.cdc.gov/vaccines/pubs/pinkbook/prinvac.html. The main requirement of a successful vaccine is the induction of a sufficiently high titer of protective antibody/T cells and induction of immunological memory, both memory T and B cells (seroprotection), enabling the organism to respond effectively to a repeated exposure to the same pathogen by enhanced and accelerated recruitment of protective antibodies (Table 9.1).

Three main categories of vaccine can be defined:

- Live
- Killed
- Genetically engineered (DNA, RNA vaccines, transgenic plants).

Active immunization involves the administration of either killed (inactivated) or live (attenuated) whole pathogens, parts of inactivated microorganisms, or modified pathogen's product (e.g., tetanus toxoid), by either the oral or the parenteral route. The induction of antibodies of antitoxin, anti-invasive, or neutralizing activity usually represents an indirect measure of protection (immunogenicity).[1] However, in some cases, such as pertussis vaccine, serum antibody titers are not necessarily predictive of protection, but may be used as a surrogate marker for induced T-cell immunity (Table 9.1). If so, reliance can only be placed on quantifying the protection rate against natural infection in the field (efficacy, Table 9.2).

Live Vaccines

Live vaccines contain live attenuated microorganisms which are still capable of replicating within the host (vaccinee). The microorganisms

Table 9.1 Degree of Correlation between Different Immune Mechanisms and Clinical Protection Induced by Vaccines

Vaccine Type	Humoral Immune Response	Cell-mediated Immunity	Comments
Diphtheria	++		Protective titer ELISA >0.01 IU/mL. Serology indicated in the case of unclear vaccination status and lack of documentation
Hib	++	+	Precise minimal protective Ab titer not known; possibly 0.15–1.0 μg anti-PRP Ab. Test not routinely used
Hepatitis A	++		Pre-vaccination serology might be cost-effective for persons with likely prior natural infection. (ELISA >10 mIU: protective titer)
Hepatitis B	++		Post-vaccination serology indicated in high-risk persons (protective ELISA titer >10 mIU/mL, except UK: ≥100 mIU/mL)
Influenza (inact.)	++	+	Protective anti-hemagglutinin titer: 1/40. Immunity rarely exceeds 1 year. Concomitant CTL induction? Testing recommended in the immunocompromised
JEV (mouse brain)	++	+	Mouse brain: No international standard for protective Ab titer established. Cave: Cross-reactive antibodies (flavivirus)
JE (Vero-cell)	++		Vero-cell: Plaque Reduction Neutralization Test considered good correlate for protection (no routinely used test, no international standard)
Measles	++	+	Protective titer: NT >1:4; induction of important cellular immune response?
Meningococcus	++		Correlation between post-vaccination ELISA titers and vaccine efficacy suggests that >2 μg of antibody is protective
Mumps	++		Post-vaccination serology (ELISA) correlates with protection. Precise minimal protective Ab titer not known
Pertussis (acellular)	+	+	Precise minimal protective Ab titer not known. Routine tests not available. Efficacy tested in controlled field trials
Pneumococcus	++		23 subtypes, determination of Ab titer not feasible for routine use
Polio[b]	++		IPV: protective Ab titer NT >1:8. Correlated with immunity. OPV: serum+ mucosal Ab response. NT does not necessarily correlate with immunity
Rabies	++	+	Protective Ab titer: RFFIT: >0.5 IU/mL or NT: 1:25
Rubella	++		Protective Ab titer: >1:32 (hemagglutination-inhibition-test) or ELISA. Tests correlate with protection. Mucosal Ab involved in protection
Tick-borne encephalitis	++		ELISA tests give surrogate markers for immunity. Cave at: cross-reactivity of antibodies (flavivirus) – NT required!
Tetanus	++		Protective Ab titer: ELISA >0.01IU/mL but usually >0.1IU/mL (more reliable). See also under diphtheria
Tuberculosis (BCG)	–	++	No easily measurable correlate of immunity to tuberculosis
Typhoid[b]	+		Testing almost impossible. Mucosal antibodies following live typhoid vaccine (oral)
Varicella	+	+	Regular antibody testing indicated for leukemia patients
Yellow fever	++		Cave at: cross-reactive antibodies (flavivirus). Neutralization test only available at the CDC

+, low correlation; ++, high correlation.

are 'weakened', meaning that they have lost most of their disease-causing capacity but are still in possession of their immunogenic properties. In most cases, live vaccines show a significantly higher immunogenicity (Table 9.2) than inactivated vaccines, since natural infection is imitated almost perfectly by eliciting a wider range of immunologic responses, both humoral (B cells) and cellular (CD8+ and CD4+ T cells). A single vaccine administration is usually sufficient to induce long-term, sometimes even lifelong, protection.

However, the main disadvantages of this vaccine category are safety concerns: in particular, older live vaccines such as oral polio vaccine (OPV) carry the risk of reversion to natural virulence via back-mutations of the attenuated organism and the possibility of causing a symptomatic affection similar to wild-virus infection in the recipient or in unprotected contacts (e.g., vaccine-associated paralytic poliomyelitis after oral poliovirus vaccine, OPV). New generations of live vaccines, especially those that are stable genetic mutants, e.g., typhoid 21a vaccine, carry no enhanced risk of back-mutations.

Killed Vaccine

Most vaccines against viruses and bacteria are inactivated (killed) whole cell or subunit preparations (Table 9.2), which are incapable of replicating within the vaccinee. These types of vaccine may need to contain a higher antigenic content than live vaccines to induce an adequate immunologic response, usually including B-cell and CD4+ T-cell response. Therefore, many of the killed pathogens or their products need immunomodulators – so-called adjuvants – mostly aluminum hydroxide or aluminum phosphate, to improve antigen presentation and prolong the stimulatory effect by the formation of

Table 9.2 Major Terms to Aid Perusal of Clinical Vaccine Literature

Acellular vaccines	Purified component vaccines
ACIP	Advisory Committee on Immunization Practices of the US CDC
Adjuvant	Constituent particularly of killed vaccines to increase immunogenicity and prolong the stimulatory effect (e.g., aluminum salt)
Adverse reaction	Post vaccination events which may result in permanent sequelae or be life-threatening. Occurrence does not necessarily prove causality
Antigenicity	(Syn: Immunogenicity) The ability of an agent(s) to elicit systemic or local immunologic response
Booster	Repeated immunizations in defined intervals to generate further antibody secreting cells and memory B cells to provide long-term immunity
CMI	Cell mediated immunity (T-cell response)
Conjugate vaccine	Chemical linking of polysaccharide antigen to a carrier protein which converts the polysaccharide from a T-cell independent into a T-cell dependent antigen
Efficacy of vaccines	(Syn: Protective efficacy) Proportion of subjects in the placebo group of a vaccine trial who would not have become ill if they had received the vaccine
GMT	Geometric Mean Titer
Immunity	Resistance developed in response to a stimulus by an antigen (infecting agent or vaccine) and usually characterized by the presence of antibodies
Immunogenicity	The ability of an infectious agent or vaccine antigen to induce specific immunity
Immunologic memory	Ability of the immune system (B-cell and T-cell memory) to recognize antigens and respond in a reinforced manner after reinfection or booster
Inactivated vaccines	Vaccines containing killed whole cell, subunit, or toxoid preparations of the pathogen which are incapable of replicating within the vaccinee
Live attenuated vaccines	Vaccines containing live attenuated (weakened) microorganisms, which are still capable of replicating within the vaccinee
Priming	Stimulation of adequate humoral immune response including immunologic memory to be accelerated by follow-up booster inoculations
Recombinant vaccine	Vaccine containing antigens (e.g., HBs Antigen) attained by expression of a gene encoding for a specific protein in a heterologous host
Seroconversion	Detectable humoral immune response after natural infection or vaccination
Seroprotection	Specific serum antibody titer predictive of protection
Side-effect	Unavoidable reactions intrinsic to the antigen or other vaccine components are mild to moderate in severity without permanent sequelae
Subunit vaccine	Active vaccines merely containing purified protective epitopes and their corresponding polypeptides
Toxoid	Active vaccines containing detoxified bacterial toxins (e.g., tetanus, diphtheria) as immunogenic agent
Vaccination	Procedure for immunization against infectious diseases
Vaccine	Immunobiologic substance used for active immunization
Vaccine coverage	Proportion of vaccinated individuals within a group or population
Whole cell vaccine	Vaccines containing inactivated whole bacteria or whole viruses

an antigen depot.[2] More recently, various other potent adjuvant systems, such as virosomes, biodegradable microspheres or novel adjuvant substances such as MF59 or MPLA, have been introduced.

The maintenance of long-term immunity with some vaccines, including toxoids, recombinant subunit and polysaccharide conjugate vaccines (Table 9.2), requires multidose courses consisting of two to three inoculations, followed by periodic administration of booster (Table 9.2) doses. Doses administered at intervals less than the minimum can lead to a suboptimal immune response. In clinical practice, however, it is recommended that vaccine doses administered 4 days or less before the minimum interval may be counted as valid (except rabies vaccine).

Unconjugated polysaccharide vaccines, however, do not require multiple doses. In general, bacterial antigens do not induce long-term immunity irrespective of the route of vaccination. Because of immunological memory, delays in recommended booster intervals or interruption of primary immunization courses are usually negligible and never require reinstitution of the complete vaccination series.

However, some inactivated vaccines are incapable of eliciting immunological memory, and are thus booster-incompetent. These vaccines include all preparations that use capsular polysaccharides as vaccine antigens. Yet another shortcoming of carbohydrate vaccines is that capsular polysaccharides, being T-cell-independent immunogens, are poorly immunogenic in vaccinees under 2 years of age, owing to the immature status of their immune systems. However, coupling of those antigens with protein carriers renders the polysaccharides visible to T cells, which assist the antibody response, including stimulation of B-cell memory, also induced in the young (e.g., conjugated Hib, pneumococcus vaccines and conjugated meningococcal vaccines).

The main advantage, regardless of the type, of inactivated vaccines lies in their superior safety profile owing to the incapacity of antigen multiplication and reversion to pathogenicity within the host.

Passive Immunization

In some circumstances, immediate protection against a specific infection is necessary. As active immunization does not elicit protective antibodies until 1–2 weeks after inoculation, the administration of specific preformed antibodies, such as hepatitis B immunoglobulin (HBIg), rabies Ig, tetanus Ig, varicella-zoster Ig and hepatitis A Ig, seems to be indicated if potential disease exposure is given in the recent past or near future. These specific hyperimmunoglobulins, derived from adult donors with high titers of the desired antibodies (95% IgG, trace amounts of IgA and IgM), stimulated by immunization or recent natural infection, are not known to transmit viruses such as HIV-1, or any other infectious agent. Hyperimmunoglobulins are usually recommended for i.m. administration followed by peak serum antibody levels about 48–72 h after administration.

Vaccine Handling and Administration

Personnel administering vaccines should take necessary precautions to minimize the risk of spreading disease. Hands should be washed before and after each patient contact. Gloves are not required unless the person vaccinating has a lesion on their hands; is likely to come into contact with potentially infectious body fluids; or as long as hand contact with blood or other potentially infectious materials is not reasonably anticipated. To prevent contamination, syringes and needles must be sterile and a separate needle and syringe should be used for each injection. The needle used for drawing the vaccine should not be used for injection, not because of risk of contamination but because the needle top may be blunted. Unless specifically licensed, different vaccines should never be mixed in the same syringe.

To prevent needle-stick injury, needles should never be recapped after use and should be discarded promptly in puncture-proof, specifically labeled containers. In the USA, federal regulations require safer injection devices (needle-free injectors) to be used if commercially available and medically appropriate. Additional information concerning this regulation may be obtained at: http://www.immunize.org/genr.d/needle.htm

Anesthetic Techniques

Anxiety about vaccinations is widespread. Some local anesthetic agents, such as 5% lidocaine-prilocaine emulsion (EMLA, manufactured by AstraZeneca), applied 30–60 minutes before injection, may relieve discomfort during vaccination without interfering with the immune response. Because of the risk of methemoglobinemia, such lidocaine-prilocaine treatment should not be used in infants younger than 12 months old under treatment with methemoglobin-inducing agents. A topical refrigerant spray may be administered shortly before vaccination to reduce short-term pain. Moreover, in newborn infants, sucrose placed on the tongue immediately before injection may have a calming effect.

Techniques of Vaccine Administration (http://www.cdc.gov/vaccines/pubs/pinkbook/genrec.html)

Route of Immunization[3]

The route of vaccination is generally determined in pre-licensure studies. Intramuscular vaccinations are used for adjuvant-containing, potentially irritating antigens (e.g., tetanus/diphtheria vaccine). Administration by subcutaneous injection is preferred for live viral vaccines, to lessen the discomfort due to local inflammation (e.g., yellow fever vaccine). Intradermal injection, such as for BCG vaccine, requires careful technique to avoid inadvertent subcutaneous antigen injection and consequent diminished immunologic response. The oral route of administration is used for certain vaccines where the stimulation of intestinal IgA and other mucosal immune mechanisms defend against the pathogenesis of infection (e.g., oral polio vaccine, oral typhoid vaccine, oral cholera vaccine). Nasal immunization with LAIV against influenza is a well-established method.[4] Vaccines for rectal and vaginal administration are under investigation.

Table 9.3 How to Administer Vaccines via the Intramuscular Route. Needle Length and Injection Site of Intramuscular Injections[10]

Age	Needle Length	Injection Site
≤18 years		
Newborn[a]	⅝ in (16 mm)[b]	Anterolateral thigh
Infant 1–12 months	1 in (25 mm)	Anterolateral thigh
Toddler 1–2 years	⅝ in[b]–1 in (16–25 mm)	Anterolateral thigh[c]
	1 in–1¼' (25–32 mm)	Deltoid muscle of the arm
Child/adolescent 3–18 years	⅝ in[b]–1 in (16–25 mm)	Deltoid muscle of the arm[c]
	1 in –1¼ in (25–32 mm)	Anterolateral thigh
≥19 years		
Sex/weight		
Male and female <60 kg (130 lb)	1 in (25 mm)	Deltoid muscle of the arm
Female 60–90 kg (130–200) Male 60–118 (130–260 lb)	1–1½ in (25–38 mm)	
Female >90 kg (200 lb) Male >118 (260 lb)	1½ in (38 mm)	

[a]First 28 days of life.
[b]If skin stretched tight, subcutaneous tissues not bunched.
[c]Preferred site.

Local pain and swelling at the injection site are the most common side-effects of all vaccines given by injection. The severity of the symptoms and number of patients experiencing them may vary from vaccine to vaccine, depending on the components of the vaccine. However, it is advisable to use only the administration technique and site of injection recommended by the manufacturer, unless data are available to support using alternative sites. Using unapproved alternate sites could reduce the immune response to the vaccine.

Intramuscular Route

The choice of site for i.m. administration (Table 9.3) is based on the volume of injected material and the size of the muscle. For infants younger than 18 months of age the preferred site for i.m. injections is the musculus vastus lateralis in the anterolateral aspect of the thigh (Figure 9.1). In older children and adults, the deltoid muscle provides the ideal site for i.m. injections (Figure 9.2). The needle length used for i.m. injections depends on age for infants and children and weight in adults (Table 9.3). A 22–25-gauge needle is appropriate for administration of most i.m. vaccinations (Figure 9.3).

Owing to the thickness of overlying subcutaneous fat and the consequentially decreased immune response, and because of the possibility of damaging the nearby sciatic nerve, the gluteal region should be avoided for active i.m. vaccinations. However, the gluteal site is often used for i.m. administration of large volumes of immunoglobulin preparations. At this injection site caution should be used to avoid nerve injury, which is most perfectly done by injecting in the center of a triangle bordered by the anterior superior iliac spine, the tubercle of the iliac crest, and the upper border of the greater trochanter of the femur.

Many experts recommend 'aspiration' by pulling back the syringe plunger before injection, although there are no data to document the

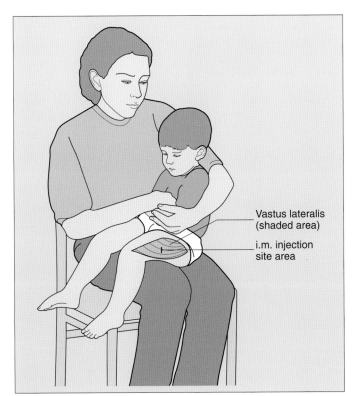

Figure 9.1 Intramuscular injection site for infants and toddlers (birth to 36 months of age). Insert needle at a 90° angle into vastus lateralis muscle in anterolateral aspect of middle or upper thigh.

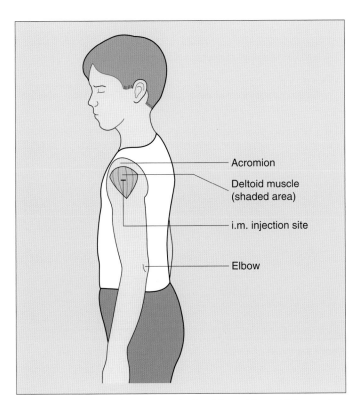

Figure 9.2 Intramuscular injection site for older toddlers, children and adults. Insert needle at a 90° angle into the densest portion of deltoid muscle – above armpit and below acromion.

- Use a needle long enough to reach deep into the muscle. Insert the needle at an 90° angle to the skin with a quick thrust.

- Retain pressure on the skin around injection site with thumb and index finger while needle is inserted.

- There are no data to document the necessity of aspiration; however, if performed and blood appears after negative pressure, the needle should be withdrawn and a new site selected.

- Multiple injections given in the same extremity should be separated as far as possible (preferably 1" to 1½" with minimum of 1" apart).

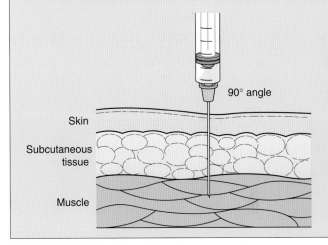

Figure 9.3 Angle of needle insertion for intramuscular injection.

Table 9.4 How to Administer Vaccines via the Subcutaneous Route

Age	Needle Size	Injection Site
Infants (≤12 months)	⅞–1 in, 23–25 gauge	Vastus lateralis muscle in anterolateral
Toddlers (1–3 years)	⅝–¾ in, 23–25 gauge	Fatty area of the thigh or outer aspect of upper arm
Children and adults	⅝–¾ in, 23–25 gauge	Outer aspect of arm

Adapted from: American Academy of Pediatrics, Red Book, 2006.

necessity for this procedure and in the USA, CDC guidelines do not require it. However, if blood appears after aspiration, the needle should be withdrawn and a new site selected.

In patients with bleeding disorders, the risk of bleeding after i.m. injection can be reduced by the application of firm pressure to the site of inoculation, vaccinating shortly after application of clotting factor replacement, or using smaller needles (23-gauge or smaller). Moreover, some vaccines recommended for i.m. application may exceptionally be given subcutaneously (s.c.) to persons at risk for bleeding. If a patient with bleeding diathesis must receive an IM injection, using a smaller-gauge needle, placing steady pressure over the injection site for at least 2 minutes and limiting the movement of the extremity for a few hours may reduce the development of bleeding complications.

Subcutaneous Route
Subcutaneous injections (Table 9.4) can be administered in the antero-lateral aspect of the thigh or the upper arm by inserting the needle at

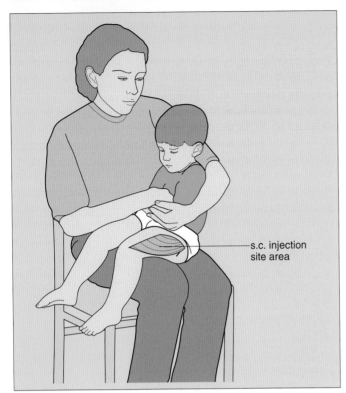

Figure 9.4 Subcutaneous injection site for infants and toddlers (birth to 36 months of age). Insert needle at a 45° angle into the fatty area of anterolateral thigh. Make sure subcutaneous tissue is pinched, to prevent injection into muscle.

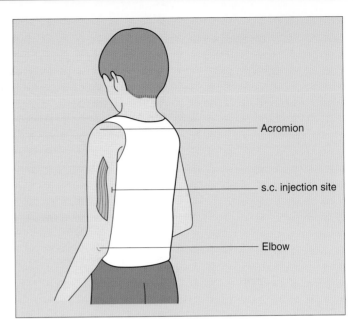

Figure 9.5 Subcutaneous injection site for injection of toddlers, children and adults. Insert needle at a 45° angle into the outer aspect of upper arm. Make sure subcutaneous tissue is pinched, to prevent injection into muscle.

about 45° in a pinched-up skinfold. A ⅝ in, 23–25-gauge needle is recommended (Figures 9.4–9.6).

Intradermal Route

Intradermal injections are usually administered on the volar surface of the forearm or the deltoid region by inserting the needle parallel to the long axis of the arm and raising a small bleb with the injection material. A ⅜–¾ in, 25- or 27-gauge needle is optimal (Figures 9.7 and 9.8).

Needle-Free Application of Vaccines

Numerous methods of needle-free application have been developed to reduce the risks of needle-stick injuries and to prevent reuse of syringes and needles. However, except for influenza and (technically) MMR vaccine, none of these devices are on the market, but may become more popular during the next few years. Details may be obtained through: http://www.hhs.gov/nvpo/meetings/dec2003/Contents/ThursdayPM/Weniger.pdf

Oral Application

Vaccines given orally, such as OPV or live typhoid vaccine, should be swallowed and retained. The dose should be repeated if the person fails to retain the vaccine longer than 10 minutes after the first application.

Simultaneous Administration of Different Vaccines[5]

Simultaneous administration of different vaccines is of particular importance when preparing for international travel. Moreover, simultaneous administration of vaccines is critical for childhood immunization programs. Since combination vaccines increase the probability that a child will be fully immunized at the appropriate age,

- Insert the needle at 45° angle to the skin.

- Pinch up on s.c. tissue to prevent injection into muscle.

- There are no data to document the necessity of aspiration; however, if performed and blood appears after negative pressure, the needle should be withdrawn and a new site selected.

- Multiple injections given in the same extremity should be separated as far as possible (preferably 1" to 1½" with minimum of 1" apart).

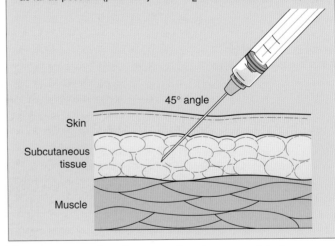

Figure 9.6 Angle of needle insertion for subcutaneous injection.

immunization rates are raised significantly. Usually, most widely used live and inactivated vaccines can be safely and effectively (in terms of seroconversion rates) administered at the same time (Table 9.5).

With the exception of live vaccines administered within an interval of 4 weeks of each other, vaccines can be administered at any time before or after a different vaccine. Because of the potential

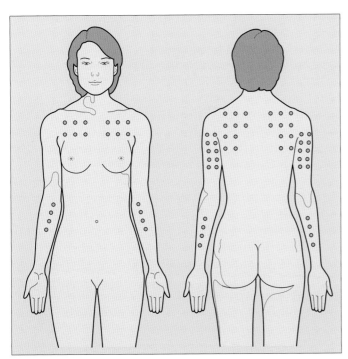

Figure 9.7 Intradermal injection sites. The most common intradermal injection site is the ventral forearm. Other sites (indicated by dotted areas) include the upper chest, upper arm, and shoulder blades. Skin in these areas is usually lightly pigmented, thinly keratinized, and relatively hairless, facilitating detection of adverse reactions.

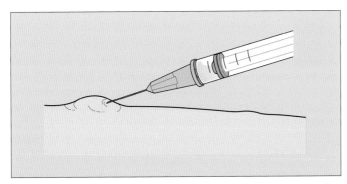

Figure 9.8 Angle of insertion for intradermal injection. Insert the needle at a 10–15° angle, so it punctures the skin's surface. When injected, the drug should raise a small wheal.

Table 9.5 Recommended Spacing of Different Vaccines

Combination of Different Vaccine Antigens	Minimum Interval
Killed – Killed	None
Live – Killed	None
Killed – Live	None
Live – Live	≈4 weeks, if not given simultaneously (except OPV – MMR – oral typhoid vaccines: no interval required)
Killed – Immunoglobulin	None
Immunoglobulin – Killed	None; if simultaneously: at different sites
Live – Immunoglobulin	≈2–3 weeks (except OPV, yellow fever, oral typhoid: no interval required)
Immunoglobulin – Live	≈3–5[a] months (except OPV, yellow fever, oral typhoid: no interval required)

[a]Dose-dependent.

of pre- or post-exposure prophylaxis has not been demonstrated to cause inhibition of the immune response, yet provides immediate and long-term protection. The combined administration of hepatitis A vaccine and Ig has been observed to negligibly reduce serum antibody titers, but not impair seroconversion rates.

Interchangeability of Vaccine Products

Although precise data concerning safety, immunogenicity, and efficacy are lacking, vaccines against the same diseases with similar antigens from different manufacturers are usually considered interchangeable when used according to their licensed indication. Available data indicate that all brands of diphtheria, tetanus toxoids, live and inactivated polio, hepatitis A, hepatitis B, tick-borne encephalitis, and rabies vaccines can be used interchangeably within a vaccine series. Owing to lack of a correlate for *Bordetella pertussis* infection, the interchangeability of acellular pertussis vaccines is difficult to assess. Therefore, whenever feasible, the same brand of DTaP should be used. Vaccination series should never be interrupted if the same brand is not available.

Special caution is indicated when using vaccines of the same brand and vaccine name obtained in different countries, as there may be differences in their formulation.

Serologic Testing Before and After Immunizations[1]

Apart from BCG, vaccination may be undertaken regardless of prior knowledge of the immune status of the vaccinee. This is particularly true for low-priced vaccines such as polio, diphtheria and tetanus vaccines, whereas in the case of high-priced vaccines (e.g., hepatitis A or B) it may be more cost-effective to test immune status prior to vaccination, particularly if acquisition of immunity via natural infection in the past is very likely. Moreover, serologic testing may be reasonable in the case of unclear immunization status due to incomplete or lack of documentation of vaccination courses.

Checking post-vaccination antibody titer in healthy vaccinees is medically merely indicated after hepatitis B (for persons with occupational risk of hepatitis B and – only recommended by some national vaccination advisory boards – also for travelers) and rubella vaccine. Unresponsiveness to the hepatitis B vaccine poses a serious problem,

immunological interference, some live vaccines, if not given simultaneously, should be separated by at least 4 weeks. There is no evidence, however, that OPV and Ty21a interfere with other parenterally administered live vaccines when administered concurrently or within 4 weeks.

The administration of immunoglobulin (Ig)-containing preparations shortly before or simultaneously with certain vaccines may also adversely affect the immune response of the active immunizations (e.g., measles and rubella vaccine), depending on the dose of Ig. The immune response following yellow fever and oral polio vaccine seems not to be influenced by co-administration of immunoglobulin.[7] Similarly, Ty21a can be administered at any time with respect to Ig. The interference with inactivated vaccines is far less pronounced than with attenuated vaccines. For example, concurrent administration of HBIg, or tetanus Ig and the corresponding vaccine or toxoid in the course since more than 10% of healthy immunocompetent adults fail to develop protective antibody levels after the recommended three-dose i.m. vaccination course (non-responders).[6] In the chronic dialysis population, current hepatitis B vaccination regimens result in a disappointing 50–75% rate of development of anti-HBs.[7] In addition, all women of child-bearing age need to be protected adequately against rubella infection. Owing to similar potential unresponsiveness to rubella vaccine, it appears most reasonable to check antibody titer after vaccination.

Seroconversion rates and antibody levels after vaccines may also be reduced in immunocompromised subjects, who should be considered for post-vaccination serologic testing.

However, when interpreting serological results by employing specific antibody titers as surrogate markers for level of protection, it must be borne in mind that assessed serum antibodies, such as after pertussis vaccination, are not reliably neutralizing and therefore may not be necessarily predictive of protection. Thus, we may not always rely on serology as the standard means of measuring post-vaccination clinical protection (Table 9.1).[1] Although specific methods to measure cellular immunity exist, they are unsuitable for routine application.

Vaccination in Those with Impaired Immunity[8, 9]

In the case of impaired immunocompetence, including congenital immune deficiencies, HIV infection, malignant neoplasm, or recipients of immunosuppressive therapy, cautious consideration of the risks and benefits of vaccinations is needed. In general, patients with uncertain or severely impaired immune status should not receive live vaccines because of the risk of disease from the vaccine strains after administration of attenuated viral or bacterial vaccine. One exception, however, is delivery of the combined measles/mumps/rubella (MMR) vaccine to individuals with asymptomatic HIV infection or symptomatic HIV infection without severe immunosuppression.

Because decreased immunity results in reduced immunogenicity of vaccines reflected by significantly diminished seroconversion rates and antibody levels, these patients should be considered for post-vaccination serologic testing.

Detailed management of specific risk groups will be covered elsewhere.

Management of Adverse Reactions

It is beyond doubt that currently licensed modern vaccines are safe and effective, having undergone extensive and strictly controlled preclinical and clinical safety trials before being licensed for routine use by public health authorities. However, despite all sorts of safety precautions one cannot absolutely exclude sporadic cases of undesirable vaccine-associated adverse reactions (Table 9.6). Therefore, vaccine recommendations should always be made on the basis of careful evaluation of their benefits and safety weighed against the risk of vaccine-preventable disease.

Vaccine-associated side-effects (Table 9.2) are usually mild and harmless. On average, about 5–10% of all vaccinees complain about post-vaccination problems, mostly moderate and local (redness, swelling and pain of the limb), or systemic (fever, headache) in nature, occurring shortly after vaccination (6–48 h).

Vaccine-associated anaphylactic reaction resulting in cutaneous, respiratory, cardiovascular, and/or gastrointestinal signs and symptoms is an extremely rare event. Vaccine components that may cause allergic reactions include the vaccine antigen (e.g., tetanus toxoid), animal protein (e.g., gelatin), and antibiotics (e.g., neomycin). A history of anaphylaxis to a vaccine component is a contraindication to receipt

Table 9.6 Potential Hypersensitivity Reactions to Common Vaccine Components

Vaccine Component	Contained in the Vaccine Against	Hypersensitivity Reaction
Egg protein	Yellow fever[c] Influenza[b] Measles[a] Mumps[a] Rabies[a] TBE[a]	Mostly in traces (μg), only in YF-vaccine mg. On rare occasions, anaphylaxis or immediate hypersensitivity reaction; dose-dependent risk
Antibiotics (gentamicin, neomycin etc.)	Measles Mumps Rubella TBE Rabies	In traces only; mostly delayed-type (cell-mediated) local contact dermatitis; no contraindication to vaccinations
Mercury compounds (Merthiolate)	Almost eliminated from modern vaccines	Mostly delayed-type local contact dermatitis; no contraindication to vaccinations
Phenol	Pneumococcus (PS vaccine only)	Delayed-type local contact dermatitis; no contraindication
Gelatin	Measles, mumps, rubella (lyophilized vaccines only!)	Very rarely anaphylaxis or immediate hypersensitivity reaction

[a]Very low risk.
[b]Moderate risk.
[c]High risk.

of that vaccine. Latex used in vial stoppers and syringe plungers may also be a cause of vaccine-associated anaphylaxis. For latex allergies other than anaphylactic allergies (e.g., a history of contact allergy to latex gloves), vaccines supplied in vials or syringes that contain dry natural rubber or rubber latex may be administered. Vaccine packaging increasingly indicates the material used in stoppers and plungers. A recent study, however, suggests that the frequency of anaphylaxis after vaccination is very low, estimating a risk of 1.5 cases/million doses.[10] Nonetheless, immediate facilities (epinephrine and equipment for maintaining an airway) and personnel should always be available for treating such allergy emergencies.

Very rarely, unpredictable serious life-threatening adverse reactions may occur. However, occurrence does not necessarily prove causality. Association of such an event is only considered if there is timely and symptomatic correlation between vaccination and adverse reaction, and if other diseases with similar symptomatic appearance can be excluded. For most attenuated virus vaccines a definite causative association is established by isolation of the vaccine strain from the vaccinee or their contacts.

If there is strong suspicion of such a serious adverse reaction, official reporting to the national health authority is of the utmost importance, since in the context of other similar reports, further clues about this incidence may be detected.

Contraindications to Vaccinations

Vaccine contraindications and precautions are described in the manufacturer's product labeling.

Table 9.7 Invalid Contraindications to Vaccination

- Mild illness (e.g., low-grade fever < 38°; mild diarrhea)
- Antimicrobial therapy (except for oral typhoid Ty21a)
- Topical or inhaled application of steroids
- Anticoagulant therapy (injection technique may be altered)
- Allergy (except to products present in the vaccine)
- Preterm birth
- Breastfeeding (except for yellow fever).
- Disease exposure or convalescence
- Family history of adverse events
- Pregnant or immunocompromised person in the household
- Chronic stable and non-inflammatory diseases (e.g., hypertension, coronary heart disease)
- Multiple vaccines

Absolute contraindications to the administration of vaccines are most uncommon. Except for severe hypersensitivity to vaccine constituents, no further contraindications exist against killed vaccines. Administration of live vaccines, however, may be contraindicated in specific situations such as pregnancy and impaired immunity.

Hypersensitivity reactions can vary in severity from mild local symptoms to severe anaphylaxis (Table 9.6). However, allergic reactions occurring immediately after vaccination are very suggestive of an anaphylactic reaction and act as a contraindication to follow-up vaccinations. However, persons with a history of systemic anaphylactic-like symptoms after egg ingestion needing yellow fever vaccine may be skin tested before vaccination and desensitized. Local delayed-type hypersensitivity reactions, such as allergic response to neomycin, are not a contraindication to vaccination. If a person reports an anaphylactic reaction to latex, vaccines supplied in vials containing natural rubber should be avoided unless the benefit of the vaccination outweighs the risk of an allergic reaction.

No evidence indicates any influence on vaccine-associated reactogenicity or efficacy if vaccine is administered during minor illness (≤38°C, ≤100°F). However, if fever (≥38°C, ≥100°F) or clinical symptoms suggest serious illness, immunizations should be delayed until after recovery.

Vaccinations are not recommended during pregnancy unless specifically indicated.[11] However, there is no doubt that licensed killed vaccines given by chance during pregnancy will never be harmful.[12,13] Live vaccines, particularly rubella and varicella vaccine, are contraindicated 3 months before and during pregnancy, although there is no evidence for increased side-effects.[14] However, in non-immune women at imminent risk for yellow fever exposure, vaccination is indicated. Breastfeeding poses no contraindication for either vaccine.

Numerous invalid contraindications to vaccination do exist (Table 9.7) and therefore the vaccinee's history must be evaluated very carefully and in detail.

Legal Issues

Documentation and Risk Counseling

Vaccinees or parents of underage children need to be counseled by the person responsible for vaccine administration about the benefits of disease prevention as well as the risk of preventive and therapeutic options, including vaccinations. In the USA, the National Childhood Vaccine Injury Act of 1986 requires that the person administering a vaccine covered by this Act must provide a copy of the relevant, current edition of the vaccine information material provided by the Centers for Disease Control and Prevention (CDC). It is recommended to document consent, but vaccinees do not need to sign a consent form.

In addition, the liable physician is obliged to keep a record about the exact date of vaccination; any adverse reactions; vaccine manufacturer; lot number; site and route of administration; date of risk–benefit counseling; and vaccine type and date, in case of rejection of a recommended vaccination by the patient. Moreover, mentioned vaccination details need to be documented in an official vaccination document. Such data are essential for surveillance and studies of vaccine safety, efficacy, and coverage.

Vaccinations currently regulated by the World Health Organization (WHO), such as yellow fever vaccine, need to be documented in an international valid immunization certificate.

Mercury Preservatives in Vaccines

Thimerosal, which contains 49% ethylmercury, has been used as a preservative in vaccines since the 1930s. Preservatives are not required for single-dose vials. Thimerosal is added at the end of the production process to prevent contamination of multi-dose vials after they are opened. Thimerosal may also be used in the early stages of manufacturing for a few vaccines but is removed during processing, with only trace (insignificant) amounts remaining. Vaccines can be classified into three groups: (1) thimerosal-free; (2) containing a trace (<0.3 µg) of mercury (considered by the US FDA to be equivalent to thimerosal-free products); (3) containing thimerosal as a preservative (25 µg of mercury/0.5 mL dose).

Recently, concerns have been raised about the use of thimerosal in vaccines and other products even though both the US FDA and the US Institute of Medicine have found no harm from the use of thimerosal other than local hypersensitivity reactions. Nevertheless, since the late 1990s most countries have mandated the removal of thimerosal from all pediatric vaccines as a precautionary measure, and very few vaccines are currently produced in multi-dose vials. For travelers, the vaccines that still contain 25 µg of thimerosal are quadrivalent polysaccharide meningococcal vaccine in multi-dose vials, and a few brands of influenza vaccine. An updated list of the thimerosal content of all vaccines available in the USA can be found at: http://www.fda.gov/cber/vaccine/thimerosal.htm. Many of these vaccines are the same preparations that are available internationally.

Vaccine Stocking and Storing

Vaccines need to be suitably stored and handled to avoid vaccine failure. Once opened, the remaining doses from a multi-dose vial that does not require any reconstitution may be used until the expiration date printed on the vial, providing that the vial has been stored correctly. For vaccines requiring reconstitution, the manufacturer's guidelines need to be followed.

Regular temperature monitoring and control (by a 'minimum–maximum' thermometer) is essential to guarantee stable temperature. It may be advisable to designate a single person as a vaccine coordinator, responsible for accounting, purchasing, and safe and careful handling of vaccines. A temperature data logger with continuous recording is considered state of the art for temperature recording and controlling.

Recommendations for handling regulations are usually given in the manufacturers' product information and in publications by the

Advisory Committee on Immunization Practices (ACIP) of the Centers for Disease Control and Prevention (http://www.cdc.gov/vaccines/pubs/pinkbook/vac-storage.html).[12]

Immunizations in Travelers

Besides eradication of disease, immunizations can reduce the risk of vaccine-preventable diseases in individuals, including travelers. The risk for travelers of contracting infections abroad is variable, depending mostly on well-known risk factors such as destination, travel season, duration of stay, and individual travel conditions.

Since most travelers seeking pre-travel health advice often just refer to vaccinations officially required for entry, it appears most reasonable to point out the differentiation between official vaccination regulations and individual vaccination recommendations for the travelers' safety:

- Yellow fever vaccination, the only vaccination currently regulated by the WHO, is required for all travelers to certain endemic countries that have established this requirement under the International Health Regulations. In addition, many countries outside the endemic zone require proof of immunization from travelers arriving from or via an infected country (see Ch. 12).
- Saudi Arabia requires proof of vaccination against meningococcal meningitis (and influenza) in order to procure a *Hajj* or *Umrah* visa. This is a frequently encountered situation in travel medicine practice, although not recognized under the International Health Regulations.

To compile an individually tailored immunization schedule, selection of travel vaccinations is based on various critical factors, including:

- *The epidemiological trends in the country of destination*: which vaccine-preventable diseases stand for risk to the traveler? What is the disease incidence? Detailed updated information about disease epidemiology and immunization requirements can be obtained from the Centers for Disease Control and Prevention (CDC; http://wwwnc.cdc.gov/travel/page/yellowbook-2012-home.htm) and the WHO (http://www.who.int/ihr/en/index.html). In addition, many countries regularly publish national guidelines regarding travel vaccinations and health requirements
- *Style of travel*: detailed itinerary, duration of travel, timing of departure, type of accommodation, adventure travel or luxury tour
- *Purpose of travel*: tourism, work, visiting relatives, etc.
- *Vaccinations officially required for entry* (e.g., yellow fever vaccination)
- *Cost–benefit of vaccinations*: prioritization of certain immunizations by ability to pay and frequency of traveling

- *Individual contraindications to vaccinations*: hypersensitivity, concomitant disease, medication, pregnancy, medical history
- *Personal history of immunizations*: including primary and booster doses of routine and travel vaccinations.

Conclusion

By assisting health professionals obtain a deeper understanding of major immunologic as well as practical issues of vaccination, this chapter contributes to the elimination of potential malevolent prejudices concerning vaccine-associated harm. It is beyond doubt that the benefit of immunization, if used correctly, far outweighs any vaccine-associated risk. Immunization prevents disease. However, the best vaccine will have little impact unless promoted and delivered by motivated health professionals and taken up by individuals.

References

1. Plotkin SA. Correlates of protection induced by vaccination. Clin Vaccine Immunol 2010;17:1055–65.
2. Coffman RL, Sher A, Seder RA. Vaccine adjuvants: putting innate immunity to work. Immunity 2010;33:492–503.
3. Petousis-Harris H. Vaccine injection technique and reactogenicity–evidence for practice. Vaccine 2008;26:6299–304.
4. Ambrose CS, Luke C, Coelingh K. Current status of live attenuated influenza vaccine in the United States for seasonal and pandemic influenza. Influenza Other Respi Viruses 2008;2:193–202.
5. Kroger AT, Atkinson WL, Marcuse EK, et al. General recommendations on immunization: recommendations of the Advisory Committee on Immunization Practices (ACIP). MMWR Recomm Rep 2006;55:1–48.
6. Rendi-Wagner P, Kundi M, Stemberger H, et al. Antibody-response to three recombinant hepatitis B vaccines: comparative evaluation of multicenter travel-clinic based experience. Vaccine 2001;19:2055–60.
7. Roukens AH, Visser LG. Hepatitis B vaccination strategy in vaccine low and non-responders: A matter of quantity of quality? Hum Vaccin 2011;7.
8. Ljungman P, Cordonnier C, Einsele H, et al. Vaccination of hematopoietic cell transplant recipients. Bone Marrow Transplant 2009;44:521–6.
9. Jong E, Freedman D. Immunocompromised travelers. In: CDC Health Information for International Travel 2012: Centers for Disease Control, United States; 2011.
10. Bohlke K, Davis RL, Marcy SM, et al. Risk of anaphylaxis after vaccination of children and adolescents. Pediatrics 2003;112:815–20.
11. Moro PL, Broder K, Zheteyeva Y, et al. Adverse events in pregnant women following administration of trivalent inactivated influenza vaccine and live attenuated influenza vaccine in the Vaccine Adverse Event Reporting System, 1990–2009. Am J Obstet Gynecol 2012;204:146 e1–7.
12. Gruslin A, Steben M, Halperin S, et al. Immunization in pregnancy. J Obstet Gynaecol Can 2009;31:1085–101.
13. D'Acremont V, Tremblay S, Genton B. Impact of vaccines given during pregnancy on the offspring of women consulting a travel clinic: a longitudinal study. J Travel Med 2008;15:77–81.
14. Bar-Oz B, Levichek Z, Moretti ME, et al. Pregnancy outcome following rubella vaccination: a prospective controlled study. Am J Med Genet A 2004;130A:52–4.

10

Routine Adult Vaccines and Boosters

Ursula Wiedermann

Key points

- Advice on routine adult vaccines for international travel including Tdap, MMR, Varicella-zoster, pneumococcal, HPV
- Recommendations for adult vaccinations in different European countries and US according to the national vaccination boards
- Internet links in the text to current recommendations of CDC and ECDC
- Information on newly licensed adult vaccines
- Overview of most common trade names of vaccines, indications, dosing, and contraindications for adult vaccines

Tetanus, Diphtheria, Pertussis

Tetanus is ubiquitous worldwide, and therefore tetanus vaccination should be up to date regardless of travel. However, adequate protection is particularly important for travelers, since injuries, insect and animal bites occur quite frequently in travelers.[1,2]

Diphtheria transmission is likely to be increased in areas of the world where immunization programs have not yet reached coverage goals and socioeconomic conditions favor disease transmission. Diphtheria remains endemic in Africa, Latin America, Asia, Albania, Russia and countries of the former Soviet Union. Therefore, diphtheria vaccination is particularly important for travelers who plan to live or work in such endemic areas.[3]

Pertussis (whooping cough) is increasingly recognized as a cause of significant morbidity in adults in both developed and developing countries, even if they were properly immunized as children. Data on pertussis incidence in travelers are scarce, and therefore it is not known whether travelers belong to a particular risk group. Among Hajj pilgrims, though, the incidence of pertussis has been shown to be higher than of other travel-associated vaccine-preventable diseases, and therefore this subgroup of travelers should be informed in detail about the importance of this vaccine prior to departure.[4]

Regardless of travel plans, adults who have completed an adequate primary series of diphtheria, pertussis, and tetanus vaccines but who have not received a previous dose of an acellular pertussis-containing vaccine should receive a dose of Tdap vaccine (combination tetanus toxoid, reduced diphtheria toxoid and acellular pertussis, adsorbed), at least once, in place of the regular every-10-year Td alone booster as soon as is feasible, regardless of interval from the last Td dose. In some European countries (e.g., Austria) Tdap booster vaccinations are recommended every 10 years for adults until 60 years of age; thereafter booster vaccination every 5 years is recommended due to immunosenescence[5] and significant decline of antibody titers.[6] Tdap can be administered regardless of how much time has elapsed since the most recent Td-containing vaccine. Tdap vaccine (Adacel, Sanofi Pasteur) contains less diphtheria toxoid than the pediatric DTaP, DTP or DT and the acellular pertussis component is antigenically different from the pediatric DTaP. Adacel (Sanofi Pasteur) is licensed for use from ages 11–65 in most countries, but off-label use in those over 65 is recognized by most national vaccine programs. Another Tdap preparation, Boostrix (GlaxoSmithKline), can be used in individuals 4 years of age and older. This vaccine is licensed for booster vaccinations but not for primary immunization. DTaP vaccines combined with polio are also available, e.g., Boostrix-Polio (GSK) or Repevax (Sanofi).

Similarly, the diphtheria toxoid content in Td vaccine (many brands worldwide) is lower than in the pediatric DTaP, DTP or DT vaccines. In some countries the Td combination vaccine is not available, and monovalent tetanus toxoid vaccine is used to booster adult immunity against tetanus. Travelers receiving tetanus-only boosters would be unprotected against diphtheria and pertussis.

In unvaccinated adults primary vaccination should be performed irrespective of travel plans. Those who have incomplete immunization or whose immunity is uncertain should follow a catch-up schedule with DT/DTaP, in which DTaP can be substituted for any DT dose.

Indications

All adults, whether they are traveling or not, should be up to date on tetanus, diphtheria, and pertussis immunizations appropriate for age[3] (Table 10.1 and see 10.5).

Contraindications

- Severe allergic reaction (e.g., anaphylaxis) after a previous vaccine dose or to a vaccine component
- Encephalopathy not attributable to another cause within 7 days of administration of a previous dose of DTP, DTaP or Tdap (see Table 10.4).

Precautions

- Moderate or severe acute illness with or without fever
- Guillain–Barré syndrome within 6 weeks after a previous dose of a tetanus toxoid-containing vaccine

DOI: 10.1016/B978-1-4557-1076-8.00010-7

Table 10.1 Recommended Minimum Ages and Intervals between Vaccine Doses

Vaccine and Dose Number	Recommended Age for This Dose	Minimum Age for This Dose	Recommended Interval to Next Dose	Minimum Interval to Next Dose
HPV1	11–12 years	9 years	2 months	4 weeks
HPV2	11–12 years (+2 months) –	109 months	4 months	12 weeks
HPV3	11–12 years (+6 months)	112 months	–	–
Pneumococcal conjugate vaccine (PCV)1	2 months	6 weeks	2 months	4 weeks
PCV2	4 months	10 weeks	2 months	4 weeks
PCV3 (some European countries recommend only a 2+1 schedule	6 months	14 weeks	6 months	8 weeks
PCV4 (3)	12–15 months	12 months	–	–
Measles, mumps, and rubella (MMR)1	12–15 months (and at any age in seronegative/ unvaccinated persons)	12 months	3–5 years (most European countries: minimum 4 weeks)	4 weeks
MMR2	4–6 years (in certain European countries: 2nd year of life); minimum interval to MMRI: 4 weeks	13 months	–	–
Varicella1 (Var1)	12–15 months	12 months	3–5 years	12 weeks (in Europe 6 weeks)
Var2	4–6 years (in certain European countries: 2nd year of life); minimum interval from Var1 6 weeks	15 months	–	–
Tetanus–diphtheria (Td)	11–12 years	7 years	10 years	5 years
Tetanus–diphtheria– acellular pertussis (Tdap)	>11 years	10 years	–	–
Pneumococcal polysaccharide (PPV)1	–	2 years	5 years	5 years
PPV2	–	7 years	–	–
PCV conjugated 13-valent for adults	>50 years in Europe and USA	50 years	–	–
Zoster	>50 yrs (>60 yrs in USA)	>50 yrs	–	–

- History of Arthus-type reaction following a previous dose of a tetanus toxoid-containing vaccine.

Dosing Schedules

Adults who completed an adequate primary series of DTP as children and who have not received a previous dose of an acellular pertussis-containing vaccine (either as Tdap or the pediatric DTaP) at some point during their life, should receive a dose of Tdap vaccine, at least once, in place of the next scheduled 10-year Td booster as soon as is feasible, regardless of interval from the last Td dose. Subsequent 10-year boosters should be with Td. Healthcare workers, postpartum women and others expected to have very close contact with local populations in developing countries are high priority and a dose of Tdap regardless of interval since the last Td booster, in order to afford better protection against pertussis in a high-risk situation. Some clinicians offer Td or Tdap if 5 years have elapsed since the last booster in order to eliminate the need for a tetanus toxoid or Td booster in a developing country should the traveler sustain a dirt-contaminated wound during the trip, a situation that normally mandates a booster if more than 5 years have elapsed since the previous tetanus-containing vaccine.

Adults without a history of an adequate primary series should begin (or complete) a three-dose primary series. The preferred schedule is a single dose of Tdap followed by a dose of Td at least 4 weeks after the Tdap dose, and a second dose of Td 6–12 months after the previous Td dose. However, Tdap may be substituted for any one of the three doses of the series. As many doses as possible should be completed prior to travel (Tables 10.2 and 10.3).

Measures of Immune Response and Duration of Immunity/Protection

Tests to measure serum antibody levels against tetanus and diphtheria are available, but not routinely for pertussis. Data on correlates of protection and duration of protection of the pertussis component of Tdap are not available.

Adverse Effects

Local adverse effects, including injection site redness, swelling, tenderness, and/or induration, are common. Painful swelling from elbow to shoulder 2–8 h after injection has been reported with Td but not Tdap. Rarely, anaphylaxis, generalized rash/itching, fever, systemic symptoms, occurrences of brachial neuritis and Guillain–Barré syndrome have been reported with Td. Experience with Tdap is limited, but in the principal initial safety study significant adverse events occurred in 0.9% of recipients (Table 10.4).

Table 10.2 Trade Names of Important Adult Travel-Related Vaccines Worldwide

Diphtheria–tetanus	Diphtheria & Tetanus Toxoids Adsorbed, Td-pur; Td-Rix; DiTeBooster, Ditanrix; Anatoxal
Diphtheria–tetanus–pertussis (Tdap)	Adacel, Boostrix, Revaxis
Diphtheria–tetanus–pertussis–polio	Boostrix-Polio; Repevax
Human papilloma virus	Gardasil (quadrivalent), Cervarix (bivalent)
Measles–mumps–rubella	MMR-II, Priorix, Vaccine-Priorix
Pneumococcal (polysaccharide, unconjugated)	Pneumovax, Pneumo23
Pneumococcal conjugated	Prevenar 13, Prevnar 13
Varicella	Varivax III, Varilrix, Varicela Biken, Okavax,
Zoster	Zostervax

Most widely distributed trade names listed first. Vaccines are parenteral unless specified.

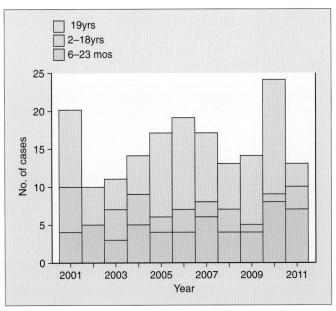

Figure 10.1 Number of imported measles cases in US residents (n = 172), by age group, January 2001–February 2011. (CDC, MMWR April 8, 2011/60 (13); 397–400. Measles imported by returning US travelers aged 6–23 months, 2001–2011.)[8]

Measles, Mumps, and Rubella Vaccine (MMR)

Measles remain common in most developing countries, and outbreaks continue to occur in some industrialized countries with falling MMR vaccination coverage due to anti-vaccine movements. Measles, which has a higher complication rate in adults, is highly contagious and all travelers need to be immune to measles as well as to mumps and rubella.

In the USA, persons born before 1957 are presumed to have immunity against measles and do not require vaccination prior to travel. Because the epidemiology of measles differs between countries, the presumptive cutoff year for measles immunity varies from country to country. For example, 1970 is the cutoff year for presumed measles immunity in Canada. Prior to 1967, inactivated measles vaccine preparations were in use, and long-lasting immunity was not assured from these immunizations. Many recipients of these inactivated measles vaccines developed a severe syndrome called atypical measles when subsequently exposed to natural measles infection. Vaccines employing live attenuated measles virus came into use in 1963, but were not used in routine childhood vaccination practice until the 1970s. In some European countries persons born between 1966 and 1976 were vaccinated with an inactivated measles vaccine (as a single or a combined vaccine, Qintovirelon). In these countries (e.g., Switzerland, Austria) the cutoff year is 1964/1965 and persons born thereafter with uncertain vaccination status, no, or only one measles vaccination (particularly with inactivated vaccine), should be vaccinated with two doses of MMR.

Mumps component: Persons vaccinated before 1979 with either killed mumps vaccine or mumps vaccine of unknown origin should be vaccinated with two doses of MMR. The two-dose schedule should be followed because only about 80% of recipients of a single dose of MMR vaccine respond to the mumps component, even though current vaccines are highly immunogenic. For this reason, in many countries, including the USA, Canada and Europe, a second dose of measles vaccine is recommended at the time of primary school entry (in several countries in Europe the recommendation is to give both MMR vaccines in the second year of life, with a minimum interval of 1 month:[7] http://ecdc.europa.eu/EN/ACTIVITIES/SURVEILLANCE/EUVAC/Pages/index.aspx), secondary school or college entry if not previously received and documented. Similarly,

adult international travelers who are often going into risk situations should have had at least two lifetime doses of modern MMR vaccine spaced at least 1 month apart.

Although persons born before 1957 are presumed to be immune to mumps, one dose of MMR or single-antigen mumps vaccine (in Europe only the combined MMR vaccine is available) should be considered for persons without specific other evidence of mumps immunity who were born before 1957 (in the USA) and are traveling for purposes of healthcare or humanitarian work potentially entailing close contact with persons who are ill.

Rubella component: Rubella immunity should be determined in women of childbearing age, regardless of birth year, who should be vaccinated with two doses of MMR if no immunity is evident. Seronegative pregnant women should be vaccinated after delivery, ideally before discharge from hospital.

Individuals with documented physician-diagnosed measles, mumps or rubella or laboratory evidence of measles, mumps, and rubella immunity do not need vaccination. Persons seronegative only for one MMR component should also be vaccinated as indicated with two doses of MMR.

The importance of MMR vaccination in travelers has been reported by the CDC, showing that during 2001–2010 87% of 692 reported measles cases were import-associated: 54% of the imported cases were in US residents; 30% were children, of whom only 6% were vaccinated against MMR before departure (Figure 10.1).

A recent publication from Canada documented that 36% of immigrants and refugees tested for MMR immunity (n=1480), were susceptible to measles, mumps or rubella. In particular, in women < 35 years coming from Southeast Asia, South Asia, or Latin America seronegativity to one of the vaccine components was high (41%).[9] Therefore, catch-up programs for adult immigrants/refugees are recommended.

In Europe a dramatic increase in indigenous measles cases has been reported, beginning in 2010 and reaching over 30 000 cases during 2011. France, Italy, Romania, Spain and Belgium have notified the

Table 10.3 Summary of Routine Adult Vaccines

Disease	Vaccine Type; Commercial Name (Manufacturer)	Efficacy	Primary Course – Adult	Boosters	Accelerated Schedule	Pregnancy or Lactation	Comments
Diphtheria, tetanus, pertussis	Diphtheria & Tetanus Toxoid Adsorbed, Adacel, Boostrix, Revaxis	Diphtheria: 87–98%; Tetanus: 94%; Pertussis: 92%	3 doses in unvaccinated; Booster every 10 years (at least once with pertussis component-ACIP)	Every ten years (>60 yrs every 5 yrs in some countries)		Possible	Irrespective of travel immunizations should be up to date for age
Human papilloma virus	Gardasil (quadrivalent), Cervarix (bivalent)	Studies ongoing	Females: 9–45 years; Males: 9–26 years: 3 doses: 0–1(2)–6 months i.m.	Not known yet	None	Not recommended	Vaccination of both females and males to reduce virus transmission
Measles, mumps, and rubella	MMR, live attenuated virus vaccine (many brands)	95% response rate per dose	Adults over 18 years: 0.5 mL s.c. 1 or 2 doses at least 1 month apart to complete a documented 2-dose series with attenuated live virus vaccine	None	None	Category C. Not recommended during pregnancy and for 1 month prior to onset of pregnancy because of theoretical risk to the fetus. Inadvertent vaccination not an indication for pregnancy termination. Some risk of transmission via breast milk. Patient should be advised not to breast-feed for 1 month after vaccination	Give on same day as PPD skin test or separate by 28 days
Pneumococcal disease	Pneumovax (unconjugated, 23 valent); Prevnar/ Prevenar 13 (conjugated)	Pneumovax: 50–70%; Efficacy studies in adults with Prevenar13 currently ongoing	Pneumovax. 1 single dose i.m. or s.c.; PCV-13 i.m.	Not in immunocompetent persons	None	Pneumovax may be used in pregnancy if indicated. PCV-13: no data available	Regardless of travel plans: people >60/65 yrs (Pneumovax); >50 years. Prevenar 13
Varicella	Live attenuated viral vaccine; Varivax III (Merck); Varilrix (GlaxoSmithKline)		For non-immune adults) 0.5 mL at 0 and 4–8 weeks	Unknown. May be as little as 10 years	None	Category C. Not recommended during pregnancy and for 1 month prior to onset of pregnancy because of theoretical risk to the fetus. Inadvertent vaccination not an indication for pregnancy termination. Some risk of transmission via breast milk. Patient should be advised not to breast-feed for 1 month after vaccination	Breakthrough disease increases dramatically at 6–8 years post vaccination in those receiving only a single dose
Zoster	Live attenuated viral vaccine; Zostervax (Merck, Sanofi)	51–63% reduction of herpes zoster; 66% reduction of postherpectic neuralgia; 61–65% reduced burden of disease	Adults >50 years with previous episode of chickenpox infection In the US FDA approved for >50 years but ACIP recommended >60 years of age	Not known	None	Not applicable	Regardless of travel plan advisable (upon vaccine availability)

Table 10.4 Estimated Risk from Disease and Sequelae Versus Risk from Vaccines

Disease	Risk of Acquiring Disease or Complications from Disease	Risk from Vaccine
Diphtheria	Case fatality rate: 1 in 20	Tetanus/diphtheria/pertussis (Tdap) vaccine
Tetanus	Case fatality rate: 3 in 100	Local pain, swelling, and induration at the site of injection are common
Pertussis	Pneumonia: 1 in 8 Encephalitis: 1 in 20 Case fatality rate: 1 in 200	Local pain, swelling, induration possible
Measles	Pneumonia: 1 in 20 Encephalitis: 1 in 2000 Thrombocytopenia 1/30 000–100 000 Death: 1 in 3000	MMR vaccine: Encephalitis or severe allergic reaction: 1 in 1 000 000 In 2–6% rash, fever, flu-like symptoms possible
Mumps	Encephalitis: 1 in 300	Same as for measles vaccine
Rubella	Congenital rubella syndrome (in newborn to a woman with infection in early pregnancy): 1 in 4	Very rare risk for rubella-vaccine associated arthritis in adult women
Pneumococcal diseases	Invasive disease in adults: 80% bacteremic pneumonia, meningitis, sepsis	Pain, redness, swelling at injection site, rarely fever or severe systemic effects
Varicella	Encephalitis: 1.8 in 10 000 Death: 1 in 60 000 cases Age-related case fatality rate: 　1–14 years: 1 in 100 000 　15–19 years: 2.7 in 100 000 　30–49 years: 25.2 in 100 000	Generalized varicella-like rash: 4–6% of vaccine recipients
Zoster	10–20% of persons with previous chickenpox infection develop H.Z: H. Z. in 45–50% of >65; 25% of >50 post-herpetic syndrome	Local reactions (pain, swelling, redness), fever, very rare varicella-like rash

highest numbers of cases as of 2011, but almost all countries have been affected. Travelers to Europe should be immune to measles by virtue of age, documented disease, serology, or previous adequate vaccination. Non-immune persons should be vaccinated[10] (Figure 10.2).

Indications

All non-immune adult travelers should be immunized against measles, mumps and rubella, especially those traveling to developing countries or other countries with recent outbreaks. Immigrants who return to their home countries and have no documentation of the disease or clear clinical history may have their serologies tested and managed according to the immune status; immunity should not be assumed in this population (Tables 10.1 and 10.5).

Contraindications

- Severe allergic reaction (e.g., anaphylaxis) to gelatin or neomycin or after a previous vaccine dose or to a vaccine component. MMR vaccine contains neomycin. MMR vaccines can be given to people who are allergic to eggs without prior skin testing or changes in vaccination protocols
- Pregnancy, or those planning to become pregnant within 1 month
- Immunocompromised hosts, including HIV patients with severe compromise (see Table 10.4).

Precautions

Moderate or severe acute illness with or without fever. History of thrombocytopenia (primary vaccination can be performed, as the benefit of vaccination overwhelms the potential risk of thrombocytopenia; a second dose should be avoided, though, if an episode of

thrombocytopenia occurred within 6 weeks after the first dose). The immune response to the measles component of the vaccine is diminished for a variable period after administering Ig. MMR should be deferred for 3 months after post-exposure prophylaxis for hepatitis A, and for a longer, undefined interval after higher doses used in other disease states. If Ig is used for travel, the MMR should be given at least 2 weeks before Ig. MMR may suppress the immune response and cause a false negative result to the tuberculin skin tests. A PPD skin test can be reliably given concurrently or 4 weeks after immunization with MMR.

Dosing Schedule

In previously non-immunized adults without other evidence of immunity, two doses of the measles vaccine separated by at least 1 month are used for primary immunization. A single MMR vaccine dose should be given to complete the two-dose series, if an initial MMR immunization dose with a live attenuated measles vaccine after 1970 is documented. Not all national authorities recognize the use of a two-dose series in routine or travel-related immunization schedules. A combination MMR-varicella vaccine (ProQuad, Merck, Priorix tetra, GSK) is available in some countries and can be used in children from 9–12 months to 12 years of age for either the first or second MMR dose when varicella vaccination is also indicated. MMRV is not tested or approved for use in adults (see Tables 10.2 and 10.3).

Adverse Effects

Between 10 and 14 days after vaccination 1 in 15 recipients can develop a red maculopapular, often confluent rash, fever, and a flu-like syndrome, with fever lasting 1–2 days, due to the vaccination. These persons are not contagious for measles. Side effects from the second dose are less frequent than with the first dose. There is a rare risk of

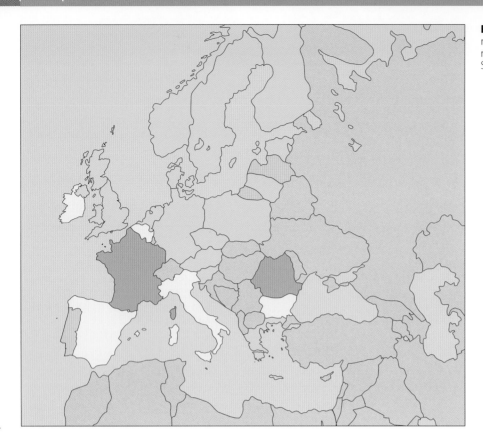

Figure 10.2 Distribution of measles notification rate (cases per 100 000 population) by country reported through EU or EEA countries, January–September 2011. www.ecdc.europa.eu

Notification rate
- >3.0 Very high
- 2.0–3.0 High
- 0.1–1 Intermediate
- <0.1 Low

Table 10.5 Routine Adult Vaccines: Sample Immunization Schedule for Adults According to CDC Recommendations and Recommendations of National Boards of Immunization in Europe (e.g. Austria) 2011/2012

Vaccines	19–26 years	27–49 years	50–59 years	60–64 years	>65 years
Tetanus Diphtheria (Td) Pertussis (Tdap)*	Substitute 1 time dose of Tdap for Td booster; Td (US)/Tdap (A) every 10 years				Td/Tdap booster every 5–10 years;
Polio	No routine vaccination; only when traveling in endemic countries				
MMR	1 or 2 doses, if seronegative		1 dose, if some risk factor is present (medical; occupational; life style; other indications)		
Pneumococcal vaccine**			1 dose		
Zoster***			1 dose	in US: 1 dose >60 yrs	
HPV****	3 doses female and male	3 doses females			
Influenza	1 dose annually				
Hepatitis A (particular for travelers*)	2 doses, if not previously vaccinated				
Hepatitis B	3 doses, if not previously vaccinated				
Meninogococcal (quadrivalent)	1 or 2 doses (in adolescence; for travellers in endemic areas for A, C, Y, W135)				

Pneumococcal polysaccharide vaccine (US): >65 years 1 vaccination in immunocompetent persons; in adults with comorbidities, immunocompromised patients a single revaccination dose in a minimum interval of 5 years.

The FDA now approves the quadrivalent HPV vaccine also as an anal cancer vaccine (additional to cervical cancer and condyloma)). The licensure also includes vaccination of boys and young men between ages 9–26.

*Td, TdaP: A dose of Tdap should be given at least once in place of the regular 10 year Td vaccination. In some countries in Europe Tdap every 10 years until 60 years, thereafter booster every 5 years.

**Pneumococcal conjugate vaccine: >50 years 1 vaccination according to licensure in immunocompetent persons; Previously unimmunized asplenic, HIV-infected, and immunocompromised adults aged ≥19 years should receive 1 dose of 13-valent pneumococcal conjugate vaccine (PCV13) followed by 1 dose of pneumococcal polysaccharide vaccine (PPSV23) ≥8 weeks later. People with these conditions previously immunized with PPSV23 should follow catch-up guidelines per ACIP.

***Zoster: 1 dose with Zoster vaccine in adults >50 (according to licensure, upon availability); 1 dose >60 according to ACIP (US).

****HPV: Licensure for HPV vaccine now includes vaccination of females aged 9–45.

rubella vaccine-associated arthritis reported among women of reproductive age (see Table 10.4).

Measures of Immune Response and Duration of Immunity/Protection

Serum antibody tests for measles, mumps, and rubella are used to measure immunity to each individual disease, and are widely available through public and private laboratories. Duration of immunity and seroconversion rates are discussed above.

Varicella and Herpes Zoster Vaccines

Acute varicella infection (chickenpox) is highly contagious and endemic in most countries. Varicella is a disease of adolescents and young adults in tropical, non-industrialized countries, as opposed to being a disease of childhood in temperate climates. Although there are no data on the incidence of varicella infection in travelers, the susceptible traveling adult may be at increased risk when traveling in tropical environments. Non-immune traveling adults should strongly consider vaccination, as disease can be severe in adults and varicella pneumonia is a relatively common complication. Evidence of varicella immunity in adults includes: being born in the USA before 1980 (US criteria only), two doses of varicella vaccine given at least 6 weeks apart, physician-diagnosed acute varicella or herpes zoster, or laboratory evidence of immunity.

In many European countries a recommendation for adult vaccination exists for all persons without evidence of varicella infection, particularly for women of childbearing age, as well as for all healthcare workers (particularly those working in obstetric or pediatric units). Where status is uncertain, immunity should be determined. If indicated, two doses of varicella vaccine should be given with a minimum interval of 6 weeks, regardless of age. Pregnant women who have no evidence of varicella immunity should receive the first dose after delivery; the second dose should be given 4–8 weeks after the first.

In the USA, where an aggressive varicella elimination strategy is in place, varicella vaccine has been a routinely recommended immunization for all non-immune adults, regardless of travel plans, since 2007. To date, most other countries have opted to focus on control of pediatric disease. Two varicella vaccines are generally available in many countries: Varivax III (Merck) and Varilrix (GlaxoSmithKline). Each consists of a lyophilized, live attenuated varicella virus designated the Oka strain, which was developed in Japan in the mid-1970s. (Since 2005/06 combined MMRV vaccines (Proquad, Sanofi, Priorix tetra, GSK) have also been available, but are only licensed for vaccination in those under 12 years of age.)

Herpes zoster represents a reactivation of varicella virus after years of dormancy in nerve roots in those with a previous episode of chickenpox. Zostavax (Merck, Sanofi), a live zoster vaccine, has been available since 2006. Live zoster vaccine is a varicella virus-containing vaccine that reduces the risk of herpes zoster ('shingles') and leads particularly to reduction of post-herpetic neuralgia.[11,12] The vaccine is licensed to be given to persons over 50 years of age. It is administered as 0.7 mL subcutaneously as a single dose; duration of protection is not known. It is not a travel vaccine and will likely continue to be administered as a single dose, mainly in primary care practice. It is important to note, however, that Zostavax contains 14 times more varicella virus than Varivax III or Varilrix, and should therefore not be used to prevent varicella infection in seronegative individuals. On the other hand, Varivax III and Varilrix are ineffective in shingles and not licensed for its prevention; they should only be used for prevention of a primary varicella infection.

As of late 2011, supply shortfalls of Zostavax have precluded routine use of this vaccine in persons over 50 in Europe, and recommendations for routine use in the USA have been limited to those aged 60 or older. Expected increased production capacity should eventually result in increased usage. Limited data on long-term duration of the immune response and on the possible need for a booster 20–30 years after the initial vaccine[13] will shape future recommendations. Persons with chronic medical conditions may be vaccinated unless their condition constitutes a contraindication.

Indications for Varicella and Zoster Vaccination

All healthy, non-pregnant international travelers without evidence of varicella immunity, particularly those who plan to have close personal contact with local populations and who are traveling for more than short vacations, should consider immunization against varicella.

In contrast, vaccination against herpes zoster is not particularly recommended for persons with travel plans, but might be generally indicated (upon availability) in those over 50 (60 years according to ACIP) with a history of previous chickenpox infection. Persons with a reported history of zoster can be vaccinated. Although the safety and efficacy of zoster vaccine have not been assessed in persons with a history of zoster, different safety concerns are not expected in this group[14] (http://www.cdc.gov/mmwr/pdf/rr/rr5705.pd) (see Tables 10.1 and 10.5).

Contraindications: Varicella and Zoster Vaccination

- Severe allergic reaction (e.g., anaphylaxis) after a previous vaccine dose or to a vaccine component (gelatin or neomycin)
- Varicella and zoster vaccines are live attenuated virus vaccines, and the usual precautions in pregnant women and compromised hosts apply (see Ch. 22). It is, however, permissible to vaccinate any household members living with a pregnant or lactating woman or an immunocompromised host
- Active, untreated tuberculosis is a contraindication (see Table 10.4).

Precautions

Moderate or severe acute illness with or without fever. Vaccine recipients should not become pregnant for 1–3 months after vaccination. Recent receipt of an antibody-containing blood product.

PPD tests should be done either the same day or 4–6 weeks after administration of varicella or zoster vaccination. Specific antivirals (e.g., aciclovir, famciclovir, valaciclovir) should be received 24 hours before vaccination. If possible, a delay in resumption of the antiviral drugs for 14 days after vaccination should be considered. Vaccine candidates should be asked if there is a family history of immunodeficiency, or if they are living in a household with high-risk persons. Vaccinees should avoid household contact with pregnant women lacking documented immunity to varicella and any immunocompromised individual for 6 weeks after receiving varicella vaccine, especially if a rash develops after the vaccine. Aspirin therapy, particularly in children and adolescents, should be withheld for 6 weeks after immunization.

Upon risk–benefit considerations varicella vaccination might be applied to HIV-infected children, adolescents, or adults according to ACIP, if children are over 12 years and have CD4$^+$ percentages >15%, or in adolescents and adults when CD4$^+$ T cells are >20/mL.

The herpes zoster vaccine is contraindicated in all patients with primary or secondary immunodeficiencies.

Dosing Schedules

The varicella vaccine schedule for adults consists of two doses of 0.5 mL administered by subcutaneous injection in the deltoid area, given 4–8 weeks apart (if more than 8 weeks elapse after the first dose, the second dose can be administered without restarting the schedule).

The zoster vaccine is given as a single dose (0.7 mL) by the subcutaneous route (see Tables 10.2 and 10.3).

Measures of Immune Response and Duration of Immunity/Protection

A single dose of varicella vaccine has an efficacy of 80–85% against any presentation of disease, and about 15% of children given a single dose of vaccine do not develop antibody titers consistent with protection against disease. In addition, protection after a single dose appears to wane after about 5 years, as manifest by a dramatic increase in breakthrough disease more than 5 years after vaccination. The recommendation for a routine second dose has been too recent to ascertain the duration of protection of a two-dose series.

Varicella vaccination is effective in preventing or modifying disease severity if given to a non-immune individual within 72 h (or even within 5 days) of exposure to someone with varicella. The vaccine should be administered on the standard schedule given above.

The effectiveness of the herpes zoster vaccine (in persons aged 60–69 years: 51–63% reduction of incidence of herpes zoster; 66% reduction of incidence of post-herpetic neuralgia; 61–65% reduced burden of illness) is based on the induction/booster of varicella zoster virus-specific cell-mediated immunity.[15] The long-term duration of immunity and protection is currently unknown.

Adverse Events

Side-effects after vaccination against varicella or herpes zoster are reported to be mild and may include redness, induration, swelling and transient pain at the injection site, and fever. A varicella-like rash (local or generalized) may develop in 3–6% of vaccinees and very rarely after herpes zoster vaccination, with the occasional reaction typically noted within 2 days of vaccination and the generalized reaction typically noted within 2–3 weeks of vaccination. Herpes zoster following vaccination in healthy children is a rare occurrence (18/100 000 person-years of follow-up) and has been mild and without complications (see Table 10.4).

Drug and Vaccine Interactions

Varicella vaccine should be delayed by 3 months after having received immunoglobulin for hepatitis A (both 0.02 mL/kg and 0.06 mL/kg doses) (hepatitis A hyperimmunoglobulin is currently not available in Europe, or is rarely in use). Use of salicylates (such as aspirin) should be avoided for 6 weeks after varicella vaccination because of association between aspirin use and Reye syndrome after varicella (however, no adverse reactions have been reported so far after varicella vaccination and aspirin use). Intervals for live attenuated vaccines and PPD testing should be followed.

Pneumococcal Vaccine

Streptococcus pneumoniae, of which more than 91 serotypes exist, is a major cause of mortality and morbidity worldwide, affecting both children (particularly those under 5 years) and adults (50 years and older). In adults it has been shown that age and comorbidities, such as chronic cardiovascular disease, lung diseases including asthma, chronic renal and liver disease, diabetes mellitus, or diseases leading to immunodeprivation, are important risk factors for acquiring invasive pneumococcal infections. Additional risk factors are smoking and alcoholism. The major manifestations of invasive pneumococcal diseases in adults >50 years are bacteremic pneumonia (80%) and meningitis.

The estimated incidence of pneumococcal infections in travelers is not clearly defined. However, after diarrheal disease, respiratory illnesses are one of the most common afflictions related to travel. Although it is probable that most are viral in nature, pneumococcal infections are probably included in such estimates. The global emergence of penicillin or multidrug-resistant *S. pneumoniae*, coupled with potentially limited availability of antimicrobials in numerous countries, also needs to be considered when reviewing the need for pneumococcal vaccination for the traveler.

Indications

The CDC recommends routine vaccination with the 23-valent pneumococcal polysaccharide vaccine (PPV-23) for adults 19–64 years of age with asthma, and for cigarette smokers and all persons aged 65 and older, regardless of travel plans. People over 65 who received the 23-valent vaccine before age 65 for an underlying condition should be revaccinated if at least 5 years have passed since the previous vaccination.[16]

Routine revaccination of immunocompetent persons is not recommended (including those with asthma and cigarette smokers). Vaccination before travel or one-time revaccination 5 years after primary vaccination is recommended for persons with chronic renal failure or nephrotic syndrome, functional or anatomic asplenia (e.g., sickle cell disease or splenectomy), chronic liver disease, diabetes mellitus, and for patients with immunocompromising conditions. Multiple revaccinations are not recommended because of uncertainty about clinical benefit and safety.

The vaccine may be considered for healthy persons 2–64 years of age if they are planning to expatriate for a prolonged duration to a country with high rates of drug-resistant pneumococci.

In many European countries, a single vaccination with the polyvalent polysaccharide vaccine has been recommended for adults 60 years and over without comorbiditities[17] (e.g., Germany) or 65 years and over (e.g., Austria, Sweden, Switzerland). In adults with existing comorbidities revaccination within at least 5 years of the previous vaccination is recommended.

In October 2011 the conjugated 13-valent pneumococcal vaccine (PCV-13, Prevenar/Prevnar 13, Pfizer), previously licensed for infants and children from 7 months to 5 years of age, was approved by the EMA (European Medical Agency) also for adults ≥ 50 years[18] (SmPC Prevenar13). The current recommendation for adults according to the licensure allots a single vaccination. The necessity for revaccination is currently unknown, and ongoing studies will be clarified within the next few years whether, and for which risk groups, additional vaccination doses might be indicated. In cases of pre-existing pneumococcal vaccination with PPV-23, immunization with PCV-13 should be administered not earlier than 5 years after the previous vaccination according to European guidelines. Currently the benefit of sequential immunization with PPV-23 is unknown, particularly for adult risk patients, but in case sequential immunization is planned, vaccination with PCV-13 should be given first (according to licensure). A recent trial of combined pneumococcal conjugate and polysaccharide vaccination schedules over a 1-year period did not demonstrate improved immunogenicity over a single use of either of the vaccines but further studies are forthcoming.[19]

In immunocompromised adults (e.g., HIV, cancer patients) immunization with the 7-valent pneumococcal vaccine has shown that the conjugate vaccine protects against recurrent invasive pneumococcal disease.[20,21]

PCV-13 for adults in the US was licensed in early 2012. The US ACIP recommends that previously unimmunized asplenic, HIV-infected, and immunocompromised adults aged ≥19 years should receive 1 dose of 13-valent pneumococcal conjugate vaccine (PCV13) followed by 1 dose of pneumococcal polysaccharide vaccine (PPSV23) ≥8 weeks later. People with these conditions previously immunized with PPSV23 should follow the complicated catch-up guidelines per ACIP. At least 1 year should elapse from the last PPSV23 before PCV13 is administered. (see Tables 10.1 and 10.5).

Contraindications

- Severe allergic reaction (e.g., anaphylaxis) after a previous vaccine dose or to a vaccine component
- Pneumococcal vaccine may be used in pregnancy if clearly indicated. For PCV-13 no data on use during pregnancy exist. Nevertheless, no indications for teratogenic effects have been derived from preclinical (animal) studies. No data are available on vaccination during breastfeeding or whether the pneumococcal conjugates might be delivered via breast milk (see Table 10.4).

Precautions

Moderate or severe acute illness with or without fever.

Dosing Schedule

PPV-23: Immunization with PPV-23 consists of a single dose of 0.5 mL given by either i.m. or subcutaneous injection. Revaccination is not routinely recommended for adults, except in the following circumstances:

- For persons aged 65 or over, a revaccination dose of PPV-23 if the patient received vaccine 5 or more years previously and was under 65 at the time
- For persons aged 2–64 years with functional or anatomic asplenia; for persons over 10 years of age, give a revaccination dose 5 or more years after the previous dose
- For immunocompromised persons (e.g., HIV, chronic renal failure and nephrotic syndrome, malignancies, solid organ transplants) give a single revaccination dose if 5 years or more have elapsed since the first dose.

PCV-13: According to the licensure of PCV-13 a single dose administration is recommended for adults 50 years and over[18] (SmPC Prevenar/Prevnar). Previously unimmunized asplenic, HIV-infected, and immunocompromised adults aged ≥19 years should receive 1 dose of 13-valent pneumococcal conjugate vaccine (PCV13) followed by 1 dose of pneumococcal polysaccharide vaccine (PPSV23) ≥8 weeks later. The need for further booster vaccinations, as well as vaccination schedules in risk populations, is currently under investigation. The vaccine should be administered intramuscularly. In patients with thrombocytopenia or other blood coagulation disorders the vaccine can be given subcutaneously.

Measures of Immune Response and Duration of Immunity/Protection

The 23-valent pneumococcal polysaccharide vaccine induces type-specific antibody responses to the capsular polysaccharide antigens of 23 serotypes of *S. pneumoniae*. The type-specific antibodies are induced within 3–4 weeks in >80% of healthy recipients. The vaccine's efficacy is estimated to be 50–70% in case–control studies. Vaccination is associated with a decrease in hospitalization and mortality.[17]

Multiple revaccinations are not recommended because of insufficient data on clinical benefit, in particular with respect to degree and duration of protection and safety.[16]

The immunogenicity studies in PCV-13-immunized adults are based on measurement by a serotype-specific opsonophagocytosis assay (OPA) to determine functional antibody levels against *S. pneumoniae*.[22] One month after vaccination with PCV-13 the antibody levels against the 12 serotypes present with both the 13- and the 23-valent vaccines were not inferior to those after immunization with PPV-23; against nine serotypes the OPA titers were even higher. A head-to-head study with PCV-13 and PPV-23 in adults >70 years who had received a single dose of PPV-23 5 years ago revealed that the immune responses to 10 of 12 common serotypes were significantly higher in PCV-13-immunized subjects[18] (SmPC Prevenar 13). Studies on clinical efficacy and duration of protection are ongoing (see Tables 10.2 and 10.3).

Adverse Events

Injection site pain, redness, swelling; rarely fever, myalgias, or severe systemic effects after application of each of the vaccines PPV-23 or PCV-13.

Human Papilloma Virus Vaccine

Human papilloma viruses (HPV) have worldwide spread and about 70% of the population will contact HPV virus at least once in life. More than 120 different HPV types are known, of which 40 preferably affect the mucosae of the genital tract and the oropharynx. Most infections, transmitted mainly by sexual contact, resolve spontaneously but do not induce a long-lasting immunity; persistence of oncogenic viruses for more than 1 year leads to a risk of neoplasia and invasive carcinoma. The most common oncogenic HPV are 16 and 18, which are responsible for the development of cervical cancer in 75%, but also for other carcinomas such as cancer of the vulva, vagina, anus, larynx and tonsils. HPV 6 and 11 are mainly (90%) responsible for the development of genital warts.[23] A quadrivalent HPV types 6, 11, 16, 18, recombinant vaccine (Gardasil, Merck, Sanofi) and a bivalent HPV type 16/18 vaccine (Cervarix, GlaxoSmithKline) have been licensed. In order to be effective, vaccination should be initiated prior to natural infection with a given HPV type. Many countries have included HPV vaccination of adolescents in their national vaccination programs. A very recent study in Australia showed a decrease in high-grade cervical abnormalities within 3 years after implementation of a population-wide vaccination program.[24] Nevertheless, vaccination is not a substitute for routine cervical cancer screening, and vaccinated women should continue to have cervical cancer screening as recommended.

Indications

The HPV4 vaccine is approved for females and males aged 9–26 years. Very recently HPV4 has been approved also for women aged 25–45 years. HPV2 is approved for girls/women aged 10–25, but not for boys or men. The ACIP and most countries in Europe recommend vaccinating females at age 11 or 12 years (or even at 9 years) or as catch-up vaccination for women aged 13–26. In some countries vaccinations of males aged 9–26 years is also recommended to prevent transmission and – in the case of the quadrivalent vaccine – to prevent genital warts. Routine administration is recommended for sexually active adults, up to 45 years for women[25] and 26 years for men (including men who have sex with men).[26,27] Sexually active women not already infected with any of the HPV vaccine types would receive full benefit, and less but worthwhile benefit would accrue to women already infected with one or more of the four vaccine HPV types.[28,29] Both vaccines can be administered to persons with a history of genital warts or abnormal PAP smears, because these conditions do not indicate an infection with all vaccine HPV types.[30]

Travel has not been demonstrated to increase HPV risk, but there is some evidence of increased sexual activity when people travel, so the pre-travel consultation is an effective opportunity for catch-up vaccination (see Tables 10.1 and 10.5).

Dosing Schedules

Gardasil and Cervarix are administered intramuscularly as three separate 0.5 mL doses. The second dose should be administered 2 months (1 month in case of Cervarix) after the first dose and the third dose 6 months after the first. Ongoing efficacy studies indicate protection to last at least 9.5 years. Booster doses are not recommended so far (see Tables 10.2 and 10.3).

Contraindications and Precautions

Severe allergic reaction (e.g., anaphylaxis) after a previous vaccine dose or to a vaccine component.

Moderate or Severe Acute Illness With or Without Fever Neither HPV vaccine is recommended for use during pregnancy, or should only be administered if clearly indicated. The remaining doses should preferably be delayed until pregnancy is completed for women who become pregnant during the vaccine series. No well-controlled studies in pregnant women exist, but preclinical studies in rats did not reveal any evidence of infertility or harm to the fetus (see Table 10.4).

References

1. Freedman DO, Weld LH, Kozarsky PE, et al. GeoSentinel surveillance network: Spectrum of diseases and relation to place of exposure among ill returned travelers. N Engl J Med 2006;354:119–30.
2. Gautret P, Schwartz E, Shaw M, et al. Animal-associated injuries and related diseases among returned travellers: a review of the GeoSentinel surveillance network. Vaccine 2007;25:2656–63.
3. Gautret P, Wilder-Smith A. Vaccination against tetanus, diphtheria, pertussis and poliomyelitis in adult travellers. Travel Med Infect Dis 2010;8:155–60.
4. Health conditions for travellers to Saudi Arabia for the pilgrimage to Mecca (Hajj). Wkly Epidemiol Rec 2009;84:477–80.
5. Chen W-H, Kozlovsky B, Effros R, et al. Vaccination in the elderly: an immunological perspective. Trends Immunol 2009;30:351–9.
6. Hainz U, Jenwein B, Asch E, et al. Insufficient protection for healthy elderly adults by tetanus and TBE vaccines. Vaccine 2005:3232–5.
7. http://ecdc.europa.eu/EN/ACTIVITIES/SURVEILLANCE/EUVAC/Pages/index.aspx
8. CDC, MMWR April 8, 2011/60 (13); 397–400. Measles imported by returning U.S. travellers aged 6–23 months, 2001–11.
9. Greenaway C, Dongier P, Boivin JF, et al. Susceptibility to measles, mumps, and rubella in newly arrived adult immigrants and refugees. Ann Intern Med 2007;146:20–4.
10. Surveillance report: European monthly measles monitoring (EMMO). Oct. 2011. Vol.5 www.ecdc.europa.eu
11. Oxman MN, Levin MJ. Vaccination against herpes zoster and postherpetic neuralgia. J Infect Dis 2008;197(Suppl 2):S228–236.
12. Simberkoff MS, Arbeit RD, Johnson GR, et al; Shingle Prevention Group. Ann Intern Med 2010;152:545–54.
13. Weaver AB. Update on the Advisory Committee on Immunization Practices' Recommendations for use of herpes zoster vaccine. J Am Osteopath Assoc 2011;111(suppl 6):S32–3.
14. Prevention of Herpes Zoster. Recommendation of the Advisory Committee on Immunization Practises (ACIP). MMWR, June 6, Vol 57/RR-5. http://www.cdc.gov/mmwr/pdf/rr/rr5705.pd
15. Levin MJ, Smith JG, Kaufhold RM, et al. Decline in varicella-zoster virus (VZV)-specific cell mediated immunity with increasing age and boosting with a high-dose VZV vaccine. 2003. J Infect Dis 2003;188:1336–44.
16. CDC, MMWR September 3, 2010/59 (34); 1102–6. Updated recommendations for prevention of invasive pneumococcal disease among adults using the 23-valent pneumococcal polysaccharide vaccine (PPSV23).
17. Fedson D.S, Nicolas-Spony L, Klemets P, et al. Pneumococcal polysaccharide vaccination for adults: a new perspective for Europe. Expert Rev Vaccines 2011 Aug;10(8):1143–67.
18. Summary of Product Characteristics Prevenar 13. http://www.medicines.org.uk/emc/medicine/22689/SPC/Prevenar+13+suspension+for+injection/
19. Lazarus R, Clutterbuck E, Yu LM, et al. A randomized study comparing combined pneumococcal conjugate and polysaccharide vaccination schedules in adults. Clin Infect Dis 2011;15:736–42.
20. French N, Gordon,SB, Mwalukomo T, et al. A trial of a 7-valent conjugate vaccine in HIV-infected adults. N Engl J Med 2010;362:812–22.
21. Chan CY, Molrine DC, George S, et al. Pneumococcal conjugate vaccine primes for antibody responses to polysaccharide pneumococcal vaccine after treatment of Hodgkin's disease. J Infect Dis 1996;173:256–8.
22. Cooper D, Yu X, Sidhu M, et al. The 13-valent pneumococcal conjugate vaccine (PCV13) elicits cross-functional opsonophagocytic killing responses in humans to Streptocccus pneumoniae serotypes 6C and 7A. Vaccine 2011;29:7207–11.
23. Centers for Disease Control and Prevention. Sexually transmitted diseases treatment guidelines, 2010. Atlanta, GA: Centers for Disease Control and Prevention; 2010. Retrieved August 25, 2011.
24. Brotherton J, Fridman M, May C.L et al. Early effect of the HPV vaccination programme on cervical abnormalities in Victoria, Australia: an ecological study. Lancet 2011;377:2085–92.
25. Nubia M, Manalastas R, Pitisuttithum P, et al. Safety, immunogenicity, and efficacy of quadrivalent human papillomavirus (types 6,11, 16,18) recombiant vaccine in women aged 24-45 years: a randomized , double-blind trial. Lancet 2009;373:1949–7.
26. Palefsky JM, Giuliano AR, Goldstone S, et al. HPV vaccine against anal HPV infection and anal intraepithelial neoplasia. N Eng J Med 2011;365:1576–85.
27. Swedish KA, Factor SH, Goldstone SE. Prevention of recurrent high-grade anal neoplasia withj quadrivalent human papillomavirus vaccination of men who have sex with men: a nonconcurrent cohort study. Clin Infect Dis 2012;54:891–8.
28. Olson SE, Kjaer S, Sigurdsson K, et al. Evaluation of quadrivalent HPV 6/11/16/18 vaccine efficicy against cervical and anogenital disease in subjects with serological evidence of prior vaccine HPV types. Human Vaccines 2009;5:696–704.
29. Joura E, Garland SM, Paavonen J, et al. Effect of the human papillomavirus(HPV) quadrivalent vaccine in a subgroup of women with certvical and vulvar disease: retrospective pooled analysis of trial data. BMJ 2012;344:e1401.
30. CDC, MMWR Febr 4, 2011, Vol 60/No4. Recommended adult immunization schedule- United States, 2011.

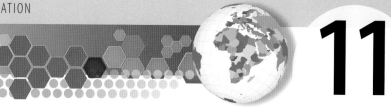

11

Routine Travel Vaccines: Hepatitis A and B, Typhoid, Influenza

Jiri Beran and Jeff Goad

Key points

- On the basis of a risk assessment of the itinerary, the style of travel and the traveler's underlying health, routine travel vaccines (hepatitis A and B, typhoid and influenza vaccines) should be widely considered by healthcare providers in the 'first line' of travelers' vaccine recommendations
- Immunization against hepatitis A should be recommended for all travelers to developing countries where the disease is endemic, especially to rural areas or places with inadequate sanitary facilities
- Hepatitis B immunization should be recommended to travelers who will be residing in areas with high levels of endemic hepatitis B or working in healthcare facilities, and those likely to have contact with blood or to have sexual contact with residents of such areas
- Typhoid vaccine would be recommended for travelers who will have prolonged exposure to potentially contaminated food and water, especially those traveling in rural areas off the usual tourist itineraries in countries with a high incidence of disease
- People at high risk of influenza complications traveling to destinations where influenza is circulating should be immunized with the most current available vaccine

Hepatitis A Vaccine

Hepatitis A (HA) is one of most common vaccine-preventable infections in travelers[1,2] and the most common form of viral hepatitis.[1,3] HA virus (HAV) is a picornavirus, an icosahedral, non-enveloped virus containing positive, single-stranded RNA[4] (http://www.who.int/mediacentre/factsheets/fs328/en/index.html). Virus is shed in large quantities in the stool of infected persons.[1] HAV is transmitted by the fecal–oral route owing to ingestion of contaminated food or water or by close contact with infected individuals,[5] and by occasional transmission through sexual contact and blood transfusions. The incubation period is usually 15–50 days (average 28).[6,7] Childhood infection is generally asymptomatic, but 75 % of adults develop mostly uncomplicated icteric disease.[1] Rare complications include fulminant

hepatitis which is age dependent.[6] Older non-immune travelers are at greater risk of severe disease.[2] The case fatality rate is 27/1000 in those aged 50+ years or with chronic liver disease, but only 0.004/1000 in the 5–14 age group.[1] Approximately 10% of apparently ill individuals have prolonged or relapsing symptoms over 5–9 months.[7] The risk of hepatitis A virus infection in non-immune travelers during travel to developing countries has been estimated to be as high as 1–5/1000/month.[8] More recent data suggest that the overall risk for non-immune travelers has reduced to 6–30/100 000/month in areas of high or intermediate endemicity.[9] This still represents a significant risk of illness. Children of immigrants who were born and grew up in developed countries traveling to visit friends and relatives are at increased risk of HA infection (http://wwwnc.cdc.gov/travel/yellowbook/2012/chapter-3-infectious-diseases-related-to-travel/hepatitis-a.htm).

Indications

All susceptible people aged > 1 year traveling for any purpose, frequency, or duration to countries with high or intermediate hepatitis A endemicity should be vaccinated or receive immune globulin (Ig) before departure.[7] In practice, Ig is rarely used now owing to the long-term protection afforded by active vaccination. In addition, men who have sex with men, illicit drug users, those who have occupational risk, and those with chronic liver disease should be vaccinated regardless of destination. Worldwide, geographic areas are characterized by high, intermediate, low, or very low levels of endemicity (Fig. 11.1). Australia, Canada, western Europe, Japan, New Zealand, and the USA are countries in which HA endemicity is low.[9,10] Several countries, including Argentina, China, Israel, and the United States, have introduced the vaccine into routine childhood immunizations.[4]

Contraindications

'Absolute' contraindications are hypersensitivity after a previous vaccine dose or to any vaccine component. 'Relative' contraindications are in subjects with an acute severe illness with or without fever. For them, HA vaccination should be delayed. Seropositivity against hepatitis A is not a contraindication, but indicates pre-existing immunity.

Precautions

In subjects with an impaired immune system, adequate anti-HAV antibody titers may not be obtained after the primary immunization,

©2012 Elsevier Inc
DOI: 10.1016/B978-1-4557-1076-8.00011-9

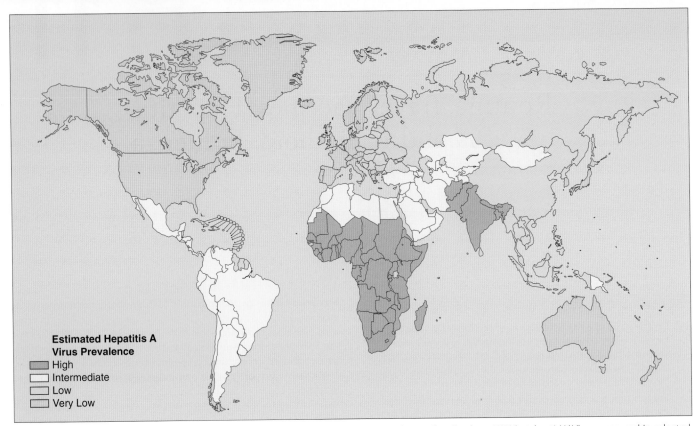

Figure 11.1 Estimated Prevalence of Hepatitis A Virus. The map indicates the seroprevalence of antibody to HAV (total anti-HAV) as measured in selected cross-sectional studies among each country's residents. Vaccination is indicated for all travelers to high- or intermediate-risk areas. *Source: Centers for Disease Control and Prevention. CDC Health Information for International Travel 2012. New York: Oxford University Press; 2012.*

Table 11.1 Recommended Minimum Ages and Intervals Between Vaccine Doses

Vaccine and Dose number	Recommended Age for this Dose	Minimum Age for this Dose	Recommended Interval to Next Dose	Minimum Interval to Next Dose
Hepatitis B1	Birth	Birth	1–4 months	4 weeks
Hepatitis B2	1–2 months	4 weeks	2–17 months	8 weeks
Hepatitis B3	6–18 months	24 weeks	–	–
Hepatitis A1	12–23 months	12 months	6–18 months	6 months
Hepatitis A2	18–41 months	18 months	–	–
Influenza inactivated (Standard dose i.m.)	≥ 6 months	6 months	4 weeks	4 weeks
Influenza live attenuated	2–49 years	2 years	4 weeks	4weeks

and such patients may therefore require additional doses of vaccine. In such cases, it is recommended to measure the antibody (anti-HAV) response to be sure of protection and, if possible, to wait for the end of any suppressive treatment before vaccination. Nevertheless, vaccination of subjects with chronic immunodeficiency, such as HIV infection, is recommended and well tolerated, although the antibody response may be limited.[11]

Dosing Schedules

Several hepatitis A vaccines are available internationally. All are similar in terms of protection and reactogenicity. No HA vaccine is licensed for children younger than 1 year of age (Tables 11.1, 11.2).[7] Primary immunization consists of a single dose of HA vaccine and usually confers protective antibody levels against hepatitis A within 2–4 weeks, though clinical protection appears to occur even if the first dose of vaccine is given after an acute exposure (http://www.cdc.gov/mmwr/preview/mmwrhtml/mm5641a3.htm). Thus, vaccination is indicated regardless of time period before departure, even if the traveler is already en route to the airport. A full vaccination series includes two doses, the second dose 6–12 months (Havrix) or 6–18 months (Vaqta) or 6–36 (Avaxim) after the first. All hepatitis A vaccines should be administered intramuscularly. Using the vaccines according to the licensed schedules is preferable. However, an interrupted series does not need to be restarted. Monovalent HA vaccines are interchangeable.[7] For immunocompetent children and adults who complete the

Table 11.2 Trade Names of the Most Important Adult Travel-Related Vaccines Worldwide

Hepatitis A	Havrix 1440, VAQTA, Avaxim, Epaxal, HAVpur
Hepatitis B	Engerix-B, Recombivax HB, HBVaxPro, H-B-Vax II
Hepatitis A/B combination	Twinrix Adult
Hepatitis A/typhoid combination	Hepatyrix, ViATIM, Vivaxim
Typhoid Vi polysaccharide	Typhim Vi, Typherix, Typhoid Polysaccharide vaccine
Typhoid (oral)	Vivotif, Vivotif L, Vivotif Berna, Typhoral L

Most widely distributed trade names listed first. Vaccines are parenteral unless specified.

EMEA
http://www.ema.europa.eu/ema/index.jsp?curl=/pages/home/Home_Page.jsp
EU – National competent authorities
http://www.ema.europa.eu/ema/index.jsp?curl=pages/medicines/general/general_content_000155.jsp&murl=menus/partners_and_networks/partners_and_networks.jsp&mid=WC0b01ac0580036d63
Regulators outside of EU
http://www.ema.europa.eu/ema/index.jsp?curl=pages/partners_and_networks/general/general_content_000214.jsp&murl=menus/partners_and_networks/partners_and_networks.jsp&mid=WC0b01ac058003176d&jsenabled=true

full series, booster doses of vaccine are not recommended.[7,12] Some authorities, notably the US CDC, state that adjunctive Ig can be considered in addition to vaccine for adults over 40, immunocompromised persons, and persons with chronic liver disease or other chronic medical conditions who are traveling to an endemic area within 2 weeks.[10] Ig (0.02 mL/kg) can be simultaneously administered at a separate anatomic injection site. Screening for natural immunity using anti-HAV IgG to avoid unnecessary vaccination is recommended in those born before 1945,[13] those who spent their childhood in endemic areas, and in those with a past history of unexplained hepatitis or jaundice. If anti-HAV antibodies are present, the individual is immune and does not require vaccination.[1,4] There is no risk of increased rates of adverse events in vaccinating already immune travelers. A combined hepatitis A and hepatitis B vaccine is licensed in many countries and primary immunization consists of three doses, given on a 0-, 1-, and 6-month schedule or on accelerated schedule (see below). Also, combined HA and typhoid fever vaccine is licensed in some countries.

Accepted Accelerated Schedule

Since seroconversion rates and protective antibody titers (total anti-HAV ≥ 20 mIU/mL at 4 or 6 weeks after a single dose of a HA vaccine) uniformly approach 100% for commonly used vaccines (Havrix, Vaqta, Avaxim), there is no need for an accelerated schedule. An accelerated schedule of combined hepatitis A+B vaccine (doses at days 0, 7, and 21–30) for adult travelers has been approved by many regulators; however, in this case, a booster dose should be given at 12 months to promote long-term immunity.

Measures of Immune Response and Duration of Immunity

HA vaccines confer immunity against hepatitis A virus by inducing antibody titers greater than those obtained after passive immunization with immunoglobulin. The lowest protective antibody level against HAV infection has not been clearly defined. Antibody appears shortly after the first injection, and 14 days after vaccination > 90% of immunocompetent subjects are seropositive (titer ≥20 mIU/mL). One month after the first injection, almost 100% of subjects aged 2–18 or adult immunocompetent individuals have antibody titers > 20 mIU/mL. In order to ensure long-term protection, a booster dose should be given between 6 and 12/18/36 months (depending upon formulation) after the primary dose of the particular HA vaccine. However, if the booster dose has not been given between 6 and 36 months after the primary dose, the administration of this booster dose can be delayed. In some trials, a booster dose of HA vaccine given up to several years after the primary dose has been shown to induce similar antibody levels as a booster dose given between 6 and 12–18 months after the primary dose.[14–18] Flexible two-dose vaccination schedules with a delayed second dose are very important, especially for travelers, who often miss the second dose of HA vaccine.[19] Clinical data demonstrate that a humoral response persists for at least 15 years.[20,23] Data available after 15 years allow prediction (by mathematical modeling) that at least 97% of subjects will remain seropositive (≥20 mIU/mL) 25–35 years after vaccination.[21–23] The T-cell-mediated response plays an important role in long-term protection after natural infection as well as after HA vaccination.[24] Based on this demonstrated persistence of protective antibodies for 15 years, HA booster vaccination may be unnecessary.[19,25]

Adverse Events (AE)

Monovalent or combined hepatitis A vaccines are very well tolerated. AEs are usually mild and confined to the first 2–3 days after vaccination. The most common local reactions are injection site pain, erythema and induration. Less common are general symptoms such as headache, fatigue and nausea.

Drug and Vaccine Interactions

When concurrent administration is considered necessary, HA vaccines must not be mixed with other vaccines in the same syringe. Other vaccines or Ig should be administered at different sites with different syringes and needles. Concurrent administration of other vaccines such as hepatitis B, tetanus toxoid, diphtheria toxoid, polio, typhoid vaccines, cholera, Japanese encephalitis, rabies or yellow fever (YF) vaccines is safe and unlikely to reduce the immune response to the HA or the co-administered vaccines. Travelers receiving Ig concurrently with HA vaccine developed similar seroconversion rates at week 4, but both the seroconversion and the titers were significantly lower after 2 years than in the subjects who received the vaccine alone. Responses after second boosters were similar.

Immune Globulin for Hepatitis A Prevention

Immune globulin is concentrated preparation of gamma globulins, predominantly IgG, from a large pool of human donors. It is used for passive immunization against hepatitis A (and also for other infections) and for replacement therapy in patients with immunoglobulin deficiencies. Passive immunization is safe for adults and children, pregnant or lactating women and immunosuppressed persons, but it only provides a limited duration of protection after a single dose.

Indications

Ig may be used to provide pre-exposure, short-term prophylaxis, but its use is discouraged in favor of active immunization with hepatitis A vaccine, which provides long-term immunity. However, immunocompromised people, those over 40 years of age and those with chronic liver disease or other chronic medical conditions planning to depart to an area in <2 weeks should receive the initial dose of HA vaccine along with Ig (0.02 mL/kg) at a separate anatomic injection site.[7] Ig should also be used for post-exposure prophylaxis against HA, but increasing data indicate the utility of hepatitis A vaccine instead for this indication.

Contraindications

Absolute: hypersensitivity after a previous Ig dose or to any Ig component. Ig should not be given to persons with isolated immunoglobulin A (IgA) deficiency due the increased risk of anaphylaxis with repeated administration of blood products that contain IgA. Relative: subjects with an acute severe illness with or without fever.

Dosing Schedules

Travelers aged <12 months or ≥ 40 years, who are allergic or otherwise contraindicated to a vaccine component, or who otherwise elect not to receive vaccine should receive a single dose of Ig (0.02 mL/kg), which provides effective protection against HAV infection for up to 3 months. Those who do not receive vaccination and plan to travel for >3 months should receive an Ig dose of 0.06 mL/kg, which must be repeated if the duration of travel is >5 months.[7]

Adverse Events

Local pain and tenderness at the injection site, urticaria, and angioedema may occur. Anaphylactic reactions, although rare, have been reported following the injection of human immunoglobulin.

Drug and Vaccine Interactions

Ig can interfere with the immune response to live, attenuated vaccines (measles, mumps, rubella (MMR) and varicella). The administration of MMR should be delayed at least 3 months (5 months for varicella) after administration of Ig. On the other hand, Ig should not be administered within 2 weeks after administration of live, attenuated vaccines.

Hepatitis B Vaccine

Hepatitis B (HB) is a viral infection that attacks the liver and can cause both acute and chronic disease[4] (http://www.who.int/mediacentre/factsheets/fs204/en/index.html). Disease is caused by hepatitis B virus (HBV), a small, circular, partially double-stranded DNA virus in the Hepadnaviridae family.[7] The virus is 50–100 times more infectious than HIV and is transmitted through contact with the blood or other body fluids of an infected person[4] (http://www.who.int/immunization_delivery/new_vaccines/hepb/en/index.html). The incubation period is usually 45–160 days (average 120).[26] The overall case-fatality ratio of acute hepatitis B is approximately 1%. Acute hepatitis B progresses to chronic HBV infection in 30–90% of people infected as infants or young children and in <5% of people infected during adolescence or adulthood. Chronic infection with HBV results in chronic liver disease, including cirrhosis and liver cancer.[7] About 2 billion people worldwide have been infected with the virus and about 350 million live with chronic infection. An estimated 600 000 persons die each year due to the acute or chronic consequences of hepatitis B.[4] Figure 11.2 divides the world into high-, intermediate-, and low-prevalence countries based on the prevalence of hepatitis B surface antigen (HBsAg) in the population. The risk for

HBV infection in international travelers is generally low, except for certain travelers to regions where the prevalence of chronic HBV infection is high or intermediate (i.e., hepatitis B surface antigen prevalence ≥2%). Expatriates, missionaries, and long-term aid workers may be at increased risk for HBV infection, and HBV incidence could be up to 240/100 000/month[27] (http://wwwnc.cdc.gov/travel/yellowbook/2012/chapter-3-infectious-diseases-related-to-travel/hepatitis-b.htm). The current widely used vaccines are based on recombinant HBsAg expressed in yeast cells. So far, around 165 countries have integrated hepatitis B vaccine into their routine infant immunization schedules, which gives approximately 50% global coverage.[4]

Indications

Hepatitis B vaccine is indicated for active immunization against HBV infection caused by all known subtypes in non-immune subjects. The most commonly encountered risk factors for travel-related hepatitis B are long-term travel, casual sexual activity with a new partner, potential for medical and dental care abroad, activity in the expatriate community, and adoption of children who are hepatitis B carriers.[28,29] Adventure travelers or those whose activities put them at increased risk for injury requiring medical intervention abroad are also likely at increased risk. The risk of HB infection for short-term travelers is less (only 2–10 times) than that for long-stay (>1 month) travelers, expatriates and long-term workers[8] when traveling to regions with intermediate or high endemicity for hepatitis B, such as Asia, Africa, Latin America, and the Middle East. Thus the WHO recommends HB vaccination for all travelers to high- and intermediate-risk areas, because it is difficult to avoid involuntary unpredictable exposures such as accidents and the need for urgent healthcare with invasive procedures[30] (http://www.cdc.gov/mmwr/preview/mmwrhtml/rr5516a1.htm?s_cid=rr5516a1_e).

Immigrants and their children from high-prevalence countries who are returning home to visit their families should be screened for HB disease before vaccination. Persons adopting children from these higher-prevalence countries should also be vaccinated. Unvaccinated individuals who have usual indications for routine HB vaccination who are traveling to any destination should be vaccinated as part of the pre-travel routine.

Contraindications

Absolute: hypersensitivity after a previous vaccine dose or to any vaccine component including yeast. Relative: subjects with an acute severe illness with or without fever. For them, HB vaccination should be delayed.

Precautions

A number of factors reduce the immune response to hepatitis B vaccines. They include older age, male gender, obesity, smoking, route of administration, and some chronic underlying diseases. In HIV-infected patients, as also in patients with renal insufficiency, including patients undergoing hemodialysis and persons with an impaired immune system, adequate anti-HBs antibody titers may not be obtained after the primary immunization course and such patients may therefore require administration of additional doses of vaccine.

Dosing Schedules

Conventional primary immunization schedule at 0, 1, and 6 months gives optimal protection (>90% individuals) at month 7 and produces high antibody titers in healthy adults aged <40 years.[31,32] Alternative

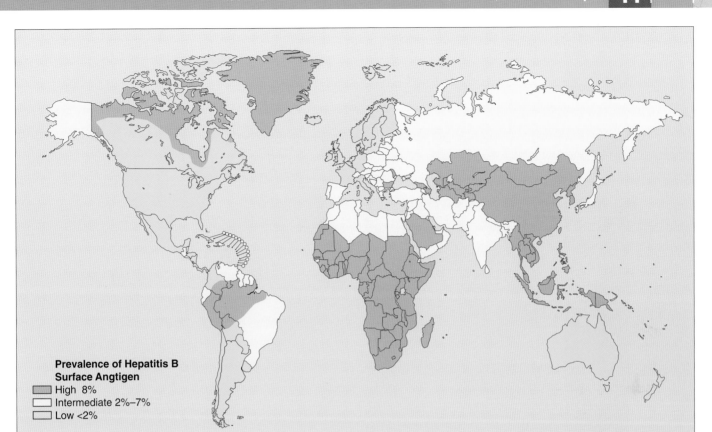

Figure 11.2 Prevalence of HBsAg as Indicator of Chronic Infection with Hepatitis B Virus, 2006. The map shows the prevalence of chronic HBV infection globally. The risk for HBV infection among international travelers is low. However, the risk of HBV infection is considered higher in countries where the prevalence of chronic HBV infection is intermediate or high. Expatriates, missionaries, and long-term aid workers may be at increased risk for HBV infection. *Source: Centers for Disease Control and Prevention. CDC Health Information for International Travel 2012. New York: Oxford University Press; 2012.*

vaccination schedules (e.g., 0, 1, and 4 months or 0, 2, and 4 months) have been demonstrated to elicit dose-specific and final rates of seroprotection similar to those obtained on a 0-, 1-, and 6-month schedule.[33] Minimum intervals between doses should always be respected (Table 11.3), but prolonging the interval does not alter the immunogenicity or necessitate restarting the series.

No differences in immunogenicity are observed when vaccines from different manufacturers are used to complete the vaccine series.[34] HBV booster doses are not required in immunocompetent individuals who have responded to a completed vaccination course.[12,34] However, in immunocompromised subjects (e.g., subjects with chronic renal failure, hemodialysis patients, HIV-positive subjects), boosters should be administered to maintain anti-HBs antibody titer equal to or higher than the accepted protective level of 10 IU/L. For these immunocompromised subjects, post-vaccination testing every 6–12 months is advised.

Accelerated Schedules

Two accelerated schedules are used: the first, with immunization at 0, 1 and 2 months, will confer protection more quickly and is expected to provide better patient compliance. The second one is applied when even more rapid induction of protection is required for persons traveling to areas of high endemicity and who commence a course of vaccination against hepatitis B within 1 month prior to departure. Three doses are given at 0, 7, and 21 days. When both accelerated schedules are applied, a fourth dose is recommended 12 months after the first dose for long-term protection.[5,28,34,35]

Measures of Immune Response and Duration of Immunity/Protection

Anti-HBs antibodies are the only easily measurable correlate of vaccine-induced protection. Immunocompetent persons who achieve anti-HBs concentrations of >10 mIU/mL after vaccination have nearly complete protection against both acute disease and chronic infection, even if anti-HBs concentrations decline subsequently to <10 mIU/mL.[36–39] The mechanism for continued vaccine-induced protection is thought to be the preservation of immune memory through selective expansion and differentiation of clones of antigen-specific B and T lymphocytes.[40] When the conventional 0-, 1-, and 6-month schedule is followed, ≥96 % of vaccinees have seroprotective levels of antibody 7 months after the first dose. When the accelerated 0-, 1-, 2-month (or days 0, 7, and 21) schedules are followed, 15% (65.2%) and 89% (76 %) of vaccinees have seroprotective levels of antibody, respectively 1 month after the first dose (and 1 month after the third dose). When a fourth dose is applied at month 12, then 1 month after the fourth dose, 95.8 % (98.6%) of vaccinees achieve seroprotective levels of antibody. Although serologic testing for immunity is not necessary after routine vaccination of adults, post-vaccination testing is recommended for persons whose subsequent clinical management depends on knowledge of their immune status, including certain healthcare and public safety workers; chronic hemodialysis patients, HIV-infected persons, and other immunocompromised persons; and sex or needle-sharing partners of HBsAg-positive persons.[34]

In high-risk individuals who have had titers checked after primary HB immunization, a small percentage of apparently healthy recipients

Table 11.3 Summary of Adult Routine Travel Vaccines

Disease	Vaccine Type; Commercial Name (Manufacturer)	Efficacy	Primary Course – Adult	Boosters	Accelerated Schedule	Pregnancy or Lactation	Comments
Hepatitis A	Inactivated viral antigen; Havrix (GlaxoSmithKline)	~70–80% in 2 weeks; >95% in 4 weeks	Adult ≥19/>16 years: 1.0 mL (1440 ELISA units) i.m. deltoid. One each at 0 and 6–12 months	None	None	Category C. Not contraindicated during lactation	Can be used interchangeably as a second dose in persons previously vaccinated with Avaxim, Epaxal or Vaqta
Hepatitis A	Inactivated viral antigen; VAQTA (Merck)	~70–80% in 2 weeks; ~95% in 4 weeks	Adult ≥19 years: 1.0 mL (50 units) i.m. deltoid. One each at 0 and 6–18 months	None	None	Category C. Not contraindicated during lactation	Can be used interchangeably as a second dose (booster) in persons previously vaccinated with Avaxim, Epaxal or Havrix
Hepatitis A	Inactivated viral antigen; Avaxim (Sanofi Pasteur)	>90% in 2 weeks; 100% in 4 weeks	Adult: 0.5 mL (160 units) i.m. in the deltoid region at 0 and 6–36 months	None	None	Category C. Not contraindicated during lactation	Can be used interchangeably as a second dose in persons previously vaccinated with Epaxal, Havrix or Vaqta
Hepatitis A	Inactivated virosome-formulated antigen; Epaxal (Berna)	~97% in 2 weeks; 99% in 4 weeks	0.5 mL i.m. in the deltoid region at 0 and 12 months	None	None	Category C. Not contraindicated during lactation	Can be used interchangeably as a second dose (booster) in persons previously vaccinated with Avaxim, Havrix or Vaqta
Hepatitis A	Immune globulin for hepatitis A prophylaxis	85–90% protection	Deep i.m. deltoid muscle. For a stay of <3 months: 0.02 mL/kg. For a stay of 3–5 months: 0.06 mL/kg. Maximum volume in one site: 5 mL for adults, (if 3–5 months >5 mL, give in divided doses in two sites)	Repeat doses are required with continued exposure. Re-dose every initial dose given	None	Considered safe in pregnancy	See text: wait the required interval after receipt of Ig before administration of MMR or Varicella vaccines

Vaccine	Type	Effectiveness	Dose		Schedule	Pregnancy category	Comments
Hepatitis A plus Hepatitis B	Inactivated viral antigen; Twinrix Adult (GlaxoSmithKline)	100% protective Hep A Ab levels, 94% protective Hep B Ab levels after 3 doses	Adult >18/16 years: 1.0 mL i.m. in deltoid (720 units for Hepatitis A and 20 µg B for Hepatitis B). One each at 0, 1 and 6 months	None	0, 7, 21 days plus booster at 1 year	Category C. Not contraindicated during lactation	If 2 doses prior to departure not possible, administer monovalent Hepatitis A and Hepatitis B
Hepatitis B	Inactivated viral antigen; Engerix-B Recombinant vaccine (GlaxoSmithKline)	95% protective Hep B Ab levels after 3 doses	Adult >19/15 years: 1.0 mL (20 µg Hepatitis B surface antigen) i.m. deltoid at 0, 1 and 6 months. Dialysis patients: use Engerix-B 40 µg i.m. at 0, 1, 2, and 6 months	Boosters may be necessary in immuno-compromised patients with anti-HBs titer of <10 mU/mL	0, 1, 2, 12 months or 0,7,21 days and 12 months	Category C. Not contraindicated during lactation	Can be used interchangeably with Recombivax or HBvaxPRO
Hepatitis B	Inactivated viral antigen; Recombivax Recombinant vaccine (Merck)	95% protective Hep B Ab levels after 3 doses	Adult >19 years: 1.0 mL (10 µg Hepatitis B surface antigen) i.m. deltoid at 0, 1 and 6 months. Dialysis patients: use Recombivax 40 µg i.m. at 0, 1, 2, and 6 months	Boosters may be necessary in immuno-compromised patients with anti-HBs titer of <10 mU/mL	0,7,21 days and 12 months	Category C. Not contraindicated during lactation	Can be used interchangeably with Engerix-B doses or HBvaxPro
Typhoid, oral	Live attenuated bacterial vaccine, capsule. Typhoid Ty21a, Vivotif (Berna)	50–80% effective	3 capsules, 1 capsule taken orally every other day on days 0, 2, 4. In North America, the schedule is 4 capsules, 1 capsule taken orally every other day on days 0, 2, 4, 6	3–7 years. Wide variation in package inserts between countries	None	Category C. No clinical studies available in pregnant or lactating women, but live vaccines should be avoided during pregnancy	The capsules must be refrigerated, and taken on an empty stomach (1 h before meals) with a cool liquid
Typhoid, oral	Live attenuated bacterial vaccine, suspension. Typhoid Ty21a, Vivotif L (Berna)	50–70% effective	3 doses of suspension taken orally every other day on days 0, 2, 4	3 years	None	Category C. No clinical studies available in pregnant or lactating women	The vaccine components (sachets of vaccine and buffer) and capsules must be refrigerated: each dose is mixed according to directions immediately before use, and taken on an empty stomach

Continued

Table 11.3 Summary of Adult Routine Travel Vaccines—cont'd

Disease	Vaccine Type; Commercial Name (Manufacturer)	Efficacy	Primary Course – Adult	Boosters	Accelerated Schedule	Pregnancy or Lactation	Comments
Typhoid	Polysaccharide vaccine. Typhoid Injectable. Typhim Vi (Sanofi Pasteur) or Typherix (GlaxoSmithKline)	50–70% effective	0.5 mL (25 μg purified Vi polysaccharide) i.m. deltoid	Every 2–3 years	None	Category C. No clinical studies available in pregnant or lactating women	
Typhoid plus hepatitis A	Vi polysaccharide and inactivated hepatitis A vaccine. Vivaxim (Sanofi Pasteur) or Hepatyrix (GlaxoSmithKline)	See monovalent vaccines	1.0 mL i.m. monovalent hepatitis A vaccine should be used to complete the primary series at 6–12 months	None for hepatitis A. 2–3 years for monovalent typhoid vaccine	None	Category C. No clinical studies available in pregnant or lactating women	
Influenza	Inactivated and live viral vaccine; Influenza (many brands)	Approximately 70–90% effective in healthy persons <65 years of age. Among elderly persons the vaccine is 30–70% effective in preventing hospitalizations and influenza	TIV 0.5 ml i.m. TIV 0.1 ml ID LAIV 0.2 ml intransal	Annually	None	Category C. All who are pregnant or who anticipate pregnancy during the influenza season should be vaccinated with TIV. Breast-feeding is not a contraindication for vaccination	

EMEA

http://www.ema.europa.eu/ema/index.jsp?curl=/pages/home/Home_Page.jsp

EU – National competent authorities

http://www.ema.europa.eu/ema/index.jsp?curl=pages/medicines/general/general_content_000155.jsp&murl=menus/partners_and_networks/partners_and_networks.jsp&mid=WC0b01ac0580036d63

Regulators outside of EU

http://www.ema.europa.eu/ema/index.jsp?curl=pages/partners_and_networks/general/general_content_000214.jsp&murl=menus/partners_and_networks/partners_and_networks.jsp&mid=WC0b01ac05800376d&jsenabled=true

do not mount a detectable response to the vaccine. This failure to respond is related to factors such as age (>40 years), male gender, smoking, obesity, HIV infection, or chronic disease. Persons over the age of 40 years have an immune response <90%, whereas only 65–75% of persons above the age of 65 develop protective anti-HBs antibody levels.[4] For persons with these risk factors and who are at high risk of hepatitis B exposure, a post-vaccination serology 1–6 months after the last dose should be done. Patients without detectable anti-HBs titers after primary series should begin a standard three-dose series and have serology 1 month after each dose for up to three doses until they seroconvert, or may wait until the three additional doses are administered before being tested.

It may be advisable to check titers and boost with a single dose if anti-HBs are undetectable in persons who received HB vaccine more than 10 years ago, who will be at very high risk for hepatitis B exposure (e.g., a surgeon planning to do surgery in a country with high HB prevalence).

Adverse Events

Monovalent or combined hepatitis B vaccines are very well tolerated. AE are usually mild and confined to the first 2–3 days after vaccination. The most common local reactions are injection site pain, erythema and induration. Less common are general symptoms, which include headache (headache is very common in children), malaise, fatigue, gastrointestinal symptoms (such as nausea, vomiting, diarrhoea, abdominal pain). The risk of serious AE from the vaccine against hepatitis B is very small compared to the risk of disease and chronic sequelae (Table 11.4).

Drug and Vaccine Interactions

Concurrent administration of HB immunoglobulin or vaccines such as hepatitis A, tetanus toxoid, diphtheria toxoid, polio, typhoid vaccines, cholera, Japanese encephalitis, rabies or YF vaccines is safe and unlikely to reduce the immune response in HB or co-administered vaccinees, when they are administered at different injection sites and are not mixed in one syringe.

Combined Hepatitis A and Hepatitis B Vaccine

Indication

Hepatitis A/B vaccine (Twinrix Paediatric and Twinrix Adult) are indicated for use in non-immune travelers >1 year of age (≥16 or ≥19, depending on country licensing) (Table 11.3) who are at risk of both hepatitis A and hepatitis B infection. The indications for use of combined HA and HB vaccines are the same as for the use of the monovalent vaccines.

Contraindications

'Absolute' are hypersensitivity after a previous vaccine dose or to any vaccine component, including yeast. 'Relative' is in subjects with an acute severe illness with or without fever. For them, HA + HB vaccination should be delayed.

Precautions

Obesity (defined as BMI ≥30 kg/m²) reduces the immune response to hepatitis A vaccines. Older age, male gender, obesity, smoking, route of administration, and some chronic underlying diseases reduce the immune response to hepatitis B vaccines. Consideration should be

Disease	Risk of Acquiring Disease or Complications from Disease	Risk from Vaccine
Hepatitis A	**Risk of acquiring disease while traveling:** High endemic areas: 1–5/1000/month of travel Low or intermediate endemicity: 6–30/100000/ month of travel **Case fatality rate:** Overall: 0.3% 5–14 age group: 0.04 % (0.004/1000) Over 50 years of age: 2.7 % (27/1000)	No serious attributable adverse event reported in over 20 years of widespread use
Hepatitis B	≥2% prevalence of HBsAg carriage in parts of Asia, Africa, and Latin America Long-term aid workers up to 240/100 000/month	No serious attributable adverse event reported in over 25 years of widespread use
Typhoid fever	**Risk of acquiring disease while traveling** The incidence of typhoid among travelers to the Indian subcontinent is 10–100 times higher (or an estimated 0.3/1000 travelers) than for all other destinations **Case fatality rate:** 12–30% (without therapy)	No serious attributable adverse event reported
Influenza	**Risk of acquiring disease while traveling** 1% per month of travel to tropical and subtropical countries Attack rates: Cruise ships (17–37%), airplane (27–72%), 20% (Hajj pilgrims) (ref 71)	No serious attributable adverse event reported

Table 11.4 Estimated Risk from Disease and Sequelae Versus Risk from Vaccines

CDC – Diseases related to travel
http://wwwnc.cdc.gov/travel/page/diseases.htm
ECDC – Annual epidemiological report on communicable diseases in Europe – 2010
http://www.ecdc.europa.eu/en/publications/Publications/Forms/ECDC_DispForm.aspx?ID=578

given to serological testing of those subjects who may be at risk of not achieving seroprotection following a complete course of Twinrix vaccine.

Dosing Schedules

The adult combination vaccine (Twinrix Adult) contains 720 ELISA units of hepatitis A antigen and 20 µg of recombinant hepatitis B surface antigen (HBsAg) in each 1 mL dose. The pediatric combination vaccine (Twinrix Paediatric) contains 360 ELISA units of hepatitis A antigen and 10 µg of HBsAg in each 0.5 mL dose. The primary conventional immunization schedule consists of three doses of vaccine given on a schedule of 0, 1 and 6 months.[30] It should be noted that two doses of the combined vaccine will protect almost 100% against

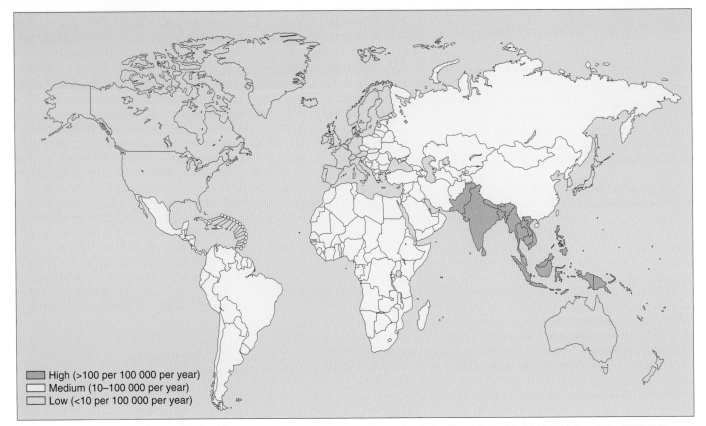

Figure 11.3 Estimated Prevalence of Typhoid Fever. *Crump JA, Luby SP, Mintz ED. The global burden of typhoid fever.* Bulletin of the World Health Organization *82(5):346–53.*

Legend:
- High (>100 per 100 000 per year)
- Medium (10–100 000 per year)
- Low (<10 per 100 000 per year)

hepatitis A but result in protective anti-HBs antibodies levels in 50–95% of individuals. Higher rates of seroprotection may be achieved when three doses of vaccine or accelerated schedule are given to travelers before travel.[41] A single dose of hepatitis A/B vaccine will not provide adequate protection against HAV or HBV.[30] Since hepatitis A is a more significant risk, combined vaccine should not be used in cases where the return of the traveler for a second pre-departure dose is not certain.

Accepted and Possible Accelerated Schedules

For adult travelers who present 21–28 days prior to departure an accelerated schedule of Twinrix Adult of 0, 7 and 21 days plus 12 months is licensed, which has demonstrated good protective antibody levels for both HAV and HBV.[41] Two doses 7 days apart should be given to those with less than 3 weeks prior to departure, as protection against hepatitis A will likely be obtained.

Measures of Immune Response and Duration of Immunity/Protection

Protection against hepatitis A and hepatitis B develops within 2–4 weeks. In clinical studies, specific humoral antibodies against hepatitis A were observed in approximately 94% of adults 1 month after the first dose and in 100% 1 month after the third dose (i.e., month 7). Specific humoral antibodies against hepatitis B were observed in 70% of adults after the first dose and in approximately 99% after the third dose. In situations where a booster dose of both hepatitis A and hepatitis B is desired, hepatitis A/B vaccine can be given. Alternatively, subjects primed with hepatitis A/B vaccine may be administered a booster dose of either of the monovalent vaccines.

Adverse Events

Combined HAB vaccine is very well tolerated. AE are usually mild and confined to the first 2–3 days after vaccination and are similar to those for the monovalent vaccines.[25]

Drug and Vaccine Interactions

Although the concomitant administration of Twinrix vaccine and other vaccines has not specifically been studied, it is anticipated that, if different syringes and other injection sites are used, no interaction will be observed.

Typhoid Vaccine

Typhoid fever, caused by *Salmonella typhi*, is prevalent worldwide, and is a disease associated with poor sanitation and contaminated food and water supplies. Humans with acute or chronic infections serve as the reservoir of infection. The risk of acquiring typhoid is highest during travel to the Indian subcontinent, followed by countries in SE Asia (Fig. 11.3).[42,43] The incidence of typhoid among travelers to the Indian subcontinent is 10–100 times higher (or an estimated 0.3/1000 travelers) than for all other destinations.[44–47] The emergence of quinolone-resistant *Salmonella typhi* in the Indian subcontinent and SE Asia pose a threat to easy oral treatment, as infected individuals now often require hospitalization for intravenous therapy with effective antibiotics.

Two types of typhoid vaccine are currently distributed worldwide: purified Vi capsular polysaccharide vaccines administered by injection, and an oral live attenuated vaccine Ty21a vaccine. Combination vaccines (Hepatyrix, Vivaxim, ViATIM) containing Vi polysaccharide typhoid vaccine and inactivated hepatitis A are available in many countries for the initiation of vaccination against both diseases (Table 11.1).[48–50] Existing typhoid vaccines are not thought to offer significant protection against *Salmonella paratyphi*, which is an emerging cause of enteric fever in travelers.[44]

Indications

Typhoid vaccine is recommended for travelers to developing countries. As the risk of disease acquisition varies with type of travel (e.g., off the usual tourist itinerary and eating in smaller, more remote areas), longer duration, eating behavior (e.g., an adventurous eater) and contact with local populations (e.g., lodging with local people), vaccine recommendations will vary accordingly. Nevertheless, typhoid fever is well reported even in individuals on short, upscale itineraries.[45] Typhoid vaccination should be recommended to all travelers going to very high-risk countries. Short-term travelers to intermediate-risk countries may consider the vaccination if they are at high risk of acquisition because of planned activities, or are risk-averse and prefer maximum protection. Food and water precautions should be followed even if a traveler receives typhoid vaccination, as the vaccines are not fully protective and a large oral inoculum may overwhelm even an optimal antibody response.

Contraindications

Severe allergic reaction (e.g., anaphylaxis) after a previous vaccine dose or to a vaccine component. The live oral typhoid vaccine contains viable organisms of attenuated *Salmonella typhi* Ty21a. The vaccine is contraindicated during pregnancy on theoretical grounds, as there are no data for safety in pregnant women or immunocompromised persons. However, there does not appear to be a risk for an immunocompromised person in the household of a vaccinee, as vaccine strain bacteria cannot be isolated from the stools of vaccinees.

Precautions

Moderate or severe acute illness with or without fever. Oral Ty21a should not be administered in the presence of nausea, vomiting, or diarrhea. The vaccine should be used with caution in persons with inflammatory bowel disease or other ulcerative conditions of the gastrointestinal tract. Although the vaccine should be kept refrigerated at 5°C ±3°C, it maintains its stability even if kept at 25°C for up to 7 days.[51] Shorter (<24 h) exposure to a higher ambient temperature of 37°C also does not affect its potency. If the Ty21a is accidentally frozen it should be thawed in the refrigerator. During the course of the vaccine and for 48–72 h before and afterwards, alcohol and antibiotics should be avoided. Ideally, live antigen vaccines should be given at the same time or separated by 4 weeks. However, if necessary, oral typhoid may be administered simultaneously with or at any interval before or after other live-virus vaccines or immunoglobulin.

Dosing Schedules

Vi Polysaccharide Typhoid Vaccine

The Vi polysaccharide typhoid vaccine is approved for use in adults and children 2 years of age or older. The vaccine is given as a single dose of 0.5 mL by i.m. injection and may be preferred when poor adherence is likely. Unlike the injectable, use of the oral vaccine may result in non-adherence or a suboptimal response, which may result after self-administration at home by the traveler.[52] The i.m. vaccine should be completed at least 2 weeks prior to exposure for optimal immune response. In situations of repeated or continued risk of exposure, the single vaccine dose can be given every 2 (US labeling) to 3 years (labeling in many other countries).

Ty21a Oral Typhoid Vaccine

The Ty21a oral typhoid vaccine is distributed in two forms: an enteric-coated capsule form which is available in the USA and Canada as well as in Europe, and a suspension form, which is not available in the USA. There are two different immunization schedules used for the oral typhoid vaccine in capsule form. In the USA and Canada, a four-dose immunization schedule is followed for adults and children 6 years old and above. In Europe and other countries, a three-dose schedule is mostly used. Irrespective of whether four or three doses are recommended, the schedule consists of one capsule taken on alternate days. The capsules should be taken on an empty stomach with cool or lukewarm (not more than 37°C) water or milk and refrigerated between doses. The capsule form of the vaccine should never be broken open to mix with food and drink. A repeat full four- or three-dose series is advised every 3–7 years (varies by national labeling) for persons with continued or repeated exposure. In two studies, the liquid formulation Ty21a was shown to be significantly more efficacious than the capsules.[53] The last dose should be completed at least 1 week prior to exposure.

There are very limited data to guide situations of interrupted Ty21a oral vaccine courses (see below). A general guideline is to complete the course if the course was interrupted <3 weeks ago. Persons may need to restart the entire course if not completed and >3 weeks have elapsed.

Measures of Immune Response and Duration of Immunity/Protection

Vi Polysaccharide Typhoid Vaccine

Field trials in endemic areas with ongoing exposure to *Salmonella* bacteria show an efficacy of 72%, 17 months after the vaccination. Another study showed 64% efficacy at 21 months and 55% at the 36-month follow-up. A recent study in India showed an overall 61% vaccine efficacy and 80% efficacy in children 2–5 years of age.[54] The repeat doses do not have a booster effect on the primary dose. Efficacy trials in travelers have not been performed. Typhim Vi and Typherix show equivalent immunogenicity.

Ty21a Oral Typhoid Vaccine

Three doses of the enteric-coated capsules provide 67% protection over a 3-year period and 62% over 7 years in individuals with ongoing exposure to environmental salmonella in endemic areas.[53] A four-dose series provided significantly higher protection than the three-dose series. Protective immunity following the four-dose series lasts up to 5–7 years in some vaccines, but may be less in travelers. Prolonging the interval between vaccine doses in an immunization series leaves the patient at risk for disease until the series is completed. Studies have shown that the liquid formulation is significantly more immunogenic than the capsular formulation (three-dose series), showing 78% protection at 5 years. Adequate efficacy trials in travelers have not been performed.

Adverse Events

The injectable Vi polysaccharide vaccine is very well tolerated,[55] with fever or flu-like symptoms reported in <1% of recipients. The most common side-effect associated with the Ty21a is abdominal discomfort; other side-effects include nausea, vomiting, rash, urticaria, or headache (0–5%).

Drug and Vaccine Interactions

Co-administration of other vaccines such as YF, MMR, tetanus, hepatitis A or hepatitis B does not appear to diminish the response to typhoid Vi polysaccharide.

The oral Ty21a vaccine may be administered at the same time or at any other interval as other live viral vaccines such as YF or MMR. When given in conjunction with live oral cholera vaccine, both vaccines maintained their immunogenicity; however, it may be best to separate the two by at least 8 h.

Antibiotics, antimalarials (proguanil, mefloquine and chloroquine) and alcohol may inhibit the Ty21A vaccine if taken concurrently. The patient should be off antibiotics for at least 24–72 h and not receive any antibiotics for 48–72 h after completion of vaccination.

Proguanil may interfere with the immune response, but the data were derived from limited studies using a higher dose of proguanil alone than is contained in the current antimalarial combination drug, atovaquone plus proguanil (Malarone). A study looking at the efficacy of the oral Ty21a vaccine taken at the same time as the combination atovaquone plus proguanil showed no effect of concurrent atovaquone plus proguanil on serum IgA or IgG response to Ty21a, so there should be no limitation to the concurrent use of Malarone and Ty21a vaccine.[56]

Mefloquine hydrochloride inhibits the oral vaccine in vitro and has a long elimination half-life, therefore prophylactic mefloquine should be started at least 72 h after oral typhoid vaccination is complete.

Influenza Vaccine

After diarrhea, respiratory illness is the most common cause of morbidity in travelers, likely due to the close contact travelers have with large numbers of other people in close quarters.[57] Recent data suggest that influenza is the commonest vaccine-preventable disease of travelers (see Ch. 52), occurring in an estimated 1% per month of travel to tropical and subtropical countries.[58,59] Influenza is a wintertime disease in temperate climates, but there is year-round risk of transmission in tropical countries and year-round transmission on cruise ships.[60–62] Influenza season in temperate climates is November–April in the northern hemisphere and April–October in the southern hemisphere.

National influenza guidelines in most countries do not cover complex travel-related issues in sufficient detail to fully orient travel medicine practitioners. Although travelers in traditional risk groups as defined by national authorities in each country should be prioritized for vaccination, all travelers are at increased risk for influenza, so any traveler to a destination during influenza season at that destination should consider influenza vaccination.

Currently, two subtypes of influenza A (H3N2 and H1N1) and one strain of influenza B (B viruses are not subtyped) circulate among humans, so seasonal influenza vaccines are trivalent.[61] Because of the ongoing antigenic drift in influenza viruses, WHO makes two sets of vaccine recommendations annually:[63] (1) in February for the next northern hemisphere winter season (November–April), and (2) in September for the next southern hemisphere winter season (April–October). At each one of those points (February and September), one of two separate 6-month production cycles begins. Even though northern and southern hemisphere vaccines are produced at different times of year in mostly the same plants of multinational manufacturers, southern vaccine is generally not available in northern countries, and vice versa. In some tropical countries the most recently produced vaccine is always available, whether it is the northern or the southern product for that year.

As vaccine seed strains are all supplied and standardized by WHO and produced using similar technology, all brands of influenza vaccine are considered equivalent. In North America, a live attenuated intranasal vaccine (LAIV, Flumist, MedImmune) using the same viral formulation as the parenteral vaccine is produced each year for the northern hemisphere winter and is approved for use only in those between the ages of 2 and 49.[64–66]

Indications

Influenza vaccine is indicated for all travelers 6 months and older, especially travelers with any chronic or compromising conditions, and should be strongly encouraged for travelers wishing to minimize influenza risk who are:[67]

- going to the tropics at any time of year
- going on cruises at any time of year
- traveling to or within temperate climates during the flu (winter) season at that destination.

Influenza vaccine is indicated for all *Hajj* travelers,[68,69] all travelers going with large organized groups, and all travelers going to mass-gathering events, no matter what time of year.

Contraindications

- Severe allergic reaction (e.g., anaphylaxis) after a previous vaccine dose or to a vaccine component
- Patients with a history of anaphylaxis to egg or egg protein, but not for lesser reactions, such as hives[70]
- Live intranasal influenza vaccine should not be given to persons with chronic disorders of the cardiovascular or pulmonary systems, including asthma or reactive airways disease; persons with underlying medical conditions such as metabolic diseases (including diabetes), renal dysfunction, or hemoglobinopathies; or to persons with known or suspected immunodeficiency diseases or who are receiving immunosuppressive therapies
- If a healthcare worker is vaccinated with the live attenuated vaccine, he or she should avoid contact with severely immunosuppressed persons for 7 days following vaccination
- Live vaccine should not be given in pregnancy.

Precautions

Moderate or severe acute illness with or without fever. Past history of Guillain–Barré syndrome within 6 weeks of a previous influenza dose.

Dosing Schedules

Dosing schedules may differ slightly between countries, but are generally similar given that worldwide production is restricted to a small number of manufacturers and a small number of production plants. For those aged 36 months and older, the influenza vaccine schedule consists of a single 0.5 mL dose of the current year's vaccine given as an i.m. injection (trivalent inactivated influenza vaccine, TIV), annually. From 6 months to 35 months, a single 0.25 mL dose is administered i.m. The dose of live intranasal influenza vaccine is 0.2 mL in a prefilled single-use spray divided equally between nostrils for those 2–49 years of age. Children aged 6 months to 8 years receiving influenza vaccination for the first time should receive two age-appropriate doses 1 month apart. In some countries an intradermal (ID) TIV influenza vaccine is available for 18–64-year-olds and contains 9 μg per strain in a 0.1 mL dose. A high-dose antigen (60 μg per strain) containing TIV IM vaccine is available for those over 65. Influenza vaccines adjuvanted with oil-in-water emulsions are available in some countries but have not yet found a separate niche in authoritative guidelines. Such adjuvants have been used as antigen-sparing strategies in the preparation of pandemic vaccines against pH1N1 (2009) and H5N1 strains. If the planned travel is during the influenza season and if the current year's vaccine is available, then that particular vaccine should be used. For travelers from the temperate northern hemisphere going to the southern hemisphere from April to October, the most recent influenza vaccine should be used if the traveler was not vaccinated the previous fall or winter. There is no evidence to support the need to re-vaccinate summer travelers already vaccinated the preceding fall. Temperate-zone travelers to the opposite hemisphere may need to obtain the most current vaccine at their destination if they plan a prolonged stay during influenza season. Tropical travelers should be vaccinated with the most recent vaccine available at the time and place of the encounter if they have not received influenza vaccination during the current year with that vaccine.

Measures of Immune Response and Duration of Immunity/Protection

Although immune correlates such as achievement of certain antibody titers after vaccination correlate well with immunity on a population level, the significance of reaching or failing to reach a certain antibody threshold (typically defined as a hemagglutination titer of 1:32 or 1:40) is not well understood on the individual level. Nevertheless, protective efficacy among healthy adults <65 years of age varies from approximately 70% to 90%, and is lower among persons >65 years.[71] A TIV preparation containing 60 μg (instead of the standard 15 μg) of each of the three strains is licensed for persons ≥65 years and has demonstrated a substantially higher geometric mean hemagglutinin inhibition (HI) titer, but data on clinical influenza protection are lacking.[72] Duration of protection has been shown to be 3–6 months; however, studies have also shown that there is no additional benefit from receiving a second dose of the same vaccine composition during the same 12-month period.

Adverse Events

Most commonly reported side-effects of the influenza vaccine are injection site pain and swelling, which are more common with the high-dose and intradermal TIV. Fever, malaise, or muscle pain infrequently occur 6–12 h after vaccination. Hypersensitivity reactions (hives, angioedema, allergic asthma, and systemic anaphylaxis) are rare, and when they occur may be related to remnant egg protein. Live intranasal influenza vaccine generally has mild side-effects, including runny nose or nasal congestion, cough, headache, sore throat, chills, and a feeling of tiredness or weakness. No increased incidence of Guillain–Barré syndrome has been shown with current vaccines. All multidose vials of influenza vaccine contain 25 μg of thimerosol (0.01% thimerosol) as a preservative, which is of concern to some consumers but no credible data exists to indicate a safety concern. In some countries thimerosol-free single-dose syringes or vials are mandated for very young children.

References

1. Mayer CA, Neilson AA. Hepatitis A – prevention in travelers. Aust Fam Physician 2010;39(12):924–8.
2. Steffen R, Amitirigala I, Mutsch M. Health risks among travelers – need for regular updates. J Travel Med 2008;15:145–6.
3. Luxemburger C, Dutta AK. Overlapping epidemiologies of hepatitis A and typhoid fever: the needs of the traveler. J Travel Med 2005;12:s12–21.
4. World Health Organization. Hepatitis. Available at www.who.int/csr/disease/hepatitis/en/index.html (Accessed 29 July 2011).
5. Centers for Disease Control and Prevention. Hepatitis A. In: Atkinson W, Hamborsky J, McIntyre L, Wolfe S, editors. Epidemiology and Prevention of Vaccine-preventable Diseases. 9th ed. Washington DC: Public Health Foundation; 2006. p. 193–206.
6. National Health and Medical Research Council. The Australian Immunization Handbook. 9th ed. Canberra: National Health and Medical Research Council; 2008.
7. Centers for Disease Control and Prevention. CDC Health Information for International Travel 2012. New York: Oxford University Press; 2012.
8. Steffen R. Changing travel-related global epidemiology of hepatitis A. Am J Med 2005;118:46S–9S.
9. Askling Hh, Rombo L, Andersson Y, et al. Hepatitis A risk in travelers. J Travel Med 2009;16:233–8.
10. Advisory Committee on Immunization Practices (ACIP), Centers for Disease Control and Prevention (CDC). Update: Prevention of hepatitis A after exposure to hepatitis A virus and in international travelers. Updated recommendations of the Advisory Committee on Immunization Practices (ACIP). MMWR Morb Mortal Wkly Rep 2007;56(41):1080–4.
11. Mofenson LM, Brady MT, Danner SP, et al. Guidelines for the prevention and treatment of opportunistic infections among HIV-exposed and HIV-infected children: Recommendations from CDC, The National Institutes of Health, The HIV Medicine Association of The Infectious Diseases Society of America, the Pediatric Infectious Diseases Society, and The American Academy of Pediatrics. MMWR Recomm Rep 2009;58(RR-11):1–166.
12. Van Damme P, Banatvala J, Fay O, et al. Hepatitis A booster vaccination: is there a need? Lancet 2003;362:1065–71.
13. Grabenstein JD. Hepatitis A vaccine. ImmunoFacts 2006:175–85.
14. Landry P, Tremblay S, Darioli R, et al. Inactivated hepatitis A vaccine booster given ≥24 months after the primary dose. Vaccine 2000;19(4–5):399–402.
15. Iwarson S, Lindh M, Widerström L. Excellent booster response 4 to 8 years after a single primary dose of an inactivated hepatitis A vaccine. J Travel Med 2004;11(2):120–1.
16. Williams JL, Bruden DA, Cagle HH, et al. Hepatitis A vaccine: immunogenicity following administration of a delayed immunization schedule in infants, children and adults. Vaccine 2003;21(23):3208–11.
17. Beck BR, Hatz C, Brönnimann R, et al. Successful booster antibody response up to 54 months after single primary vaccination with virosome-formulated, aluminum-free hepatitis A vaccine. Clin Infect Dis 2003;37(9):126–8.
18. Beck BR, Hatz CF, Loutan L, et al. Immunogenicity of booster vaccination with a virosomal hepatitis A vaccine after primary immunization with an aluminum-adsorbed hepatitis A vaccine. J Travel Med 2004;11(4):201–6.
19. Van Damme P, Van Herck K. A review of the long-term protection after hepatitis A and B vaccination. Travel Med Infect Dis 2007;5(2):79–84.
20. Van Herck K, Van Damme P, Lievens M, et al. Hepatitis A vaccine: indirect evidence of immune memory 12 years after the primary course. J Med Virol 2004;72(2):194–6.
21. Bovier PA, Bock J, Ebengo TF, et al. Predicted 30-year protection after vaccination with an aluminum-free virosomal hepatitis A vaccine. J Med Virol 2010;82(10):1629–34.
22. Vidor E, Dumas R, Porteret V, et al. Aventis Pasteur vaccines containing inactivated hepatitis A virus: a compilation of immunogenicity data. Eur J Clin Microbiol Infect Dis 2004;23(4):300–9.
23. Van Herck K, Jacquet JM, Van Damme P. Antibody persistence and immune memory in healthy adults following vaccination with a two-dose inactivated hepatitis A vaccine: Long-term follow-up at 15 years. J Med Virol 2011;83:1885–91.
24. Lemon SM. Immunologic approaches to assessing the response to inactivated hepatitis A vaccine. J Hepatol 1993;18(Suppl 2):S15–9.
25. Zuckerman JN, Connor BA, von Sonnenburg F. Hepatitis A and B booster recommendations: implications for travelers. Clin Infect Dis 2005 Oct 1;41(7):1020–6.
26. Spira AM. A review of combined hepatitis A and hepatitis B vaccination for travelers. Clin Ther 2003;25:2337–51.
27. Zuckerman Jn, Van Damme P, Van Herck K, et al. Vaccination options for last-minute travelers in need of travel-related prophylaxis against hepatitis A and B and typhoid fever: a practical guide. Travel Med Infect Dis 2003;1:219–26.

28. Keystone JS. Travel-related hepatitis B: risk factors and prevention using an accelerated vaccination schedule. Am J Med 2005 Oct;118(Suppl 10A):63S–8S.

29. Connor BA, Jacobs RJ, Meyerhoff AS. Hepatitis B risks and immunization coverage among American travelers. Travel Med 2006;13(5):273–80.

30. Committee to Advise on Tropical Medicine and Travel (CATMAT). Statement on hepatitis vaccines for travelers. An Advisory Committee Statement (ACS). Can Commun Dis Rep 2008;34(ACS-2):1–24.

31. Andre FE. Summary of safety and efficacy data on a yeast-derived hepatitis B vaccine. Am J Med 1989;87(Suppl 3A):S14–20.

32. Zajac BA, West DJ, McAleer WJ, et al. Overview of clinical studies with hepatitis B vaccine made by recombinant DNA. J Infect 1986;13(Suppl A):39–45.

33. Lemon SM, Thomas DL. Vaccines to prevent viral hepatitis. N Engl J Med 1997;336:196–204.

34. Mast EE, Weinbaum CM, Fiore AE, et al. Advisory Committee on Immunization Practices (ACIP) Centers for Disease Control and Prevention (CDC). A comprehensive immunization strategy to eliminate transmission of hepatitis B virus infection in the United States: recommendations of the Advisory Committee on Immunization Practices (ACIP) Part II: immunization of adults. MMWR Recomm Rep 2006;55(RR-16):1–33; Erratum in: MMWR Morb Mortal Wkly Rep 2007;56(42):1114.

35. Keystone JS, Hershey JH. The underestimated risk of hepatitis A and hepatitis B: benefits of an accelerated vaccination schedule. Int J Infect Dis 2008;12(1):3–11.

36. Francis DP, Hadler SC, Thompson SE, et al. The prevention of hepatitis B with vaccine: report of the Centers for Disease Control multi-center efficacy trial among homosexual men. Ann Intern Med 1982;97:362–6.

37. Hadler SC, Francis DP, Maynard JE, et al. Long-term immunogenicity and efficacy of hepatitis B vaccine in homosexual men. N Engl J Med 1986;315:209–14.

38. Jack AD, Hall AJ, Maine N, et al. What level of hepatitis B antibody is protective? J Infect Dis 1999;179:489–92.

39. Szmuness W, Stevens CE, Harley EJ, et al. Hepatitis B vaccine: demonstration of efficacy in a controlled clinical trial in a high-risk population in the United States. N Engl J Med 1980;303:833–41.

40. Banatvala JE, Van Damme P. Hepatitis B vaccine-do we need boosters? J Viral Hepat 2003;10:1–6.

41. Nothdurft HD, Zuckerman J, Stoffel M, et al. Accelerated vaccination schedules provide protection against hepatitis A and B in last-minute travelers. J Travel Med 2004;11:260–2.

42. Crump JA, Luby SP, Mintz ED. The global burden of typhoid fever. Bull World Health Organ 2004;82:346–53.

43. Freedman DO, Weld LH, Kozarsky PE, et al. Spectrum of disease and relation to place of exposure among ill returned travelers. N Engl J Med 2006;354:119–30.

44. Connor BA, Schwartz E. Typhoid and paratyphoid fever in travelers. Lancet Infect Dis 2005;5:623–8.

45. Steinberg EB, Bishop R, Haber P, et al. Typhoid fever in travelers: who should be targeted for prevention? Clin Infect Dis 2004;39:186–91.

46. Mermin JH, Townes JM, Gerber M, et al. Typhoid fever in the United States, 1985–1994: changing risks of international travel and increasing antimicrobial resistance. Arch Intern Med 1998;158:633–8.

47. Meltzer E, Schwartz E. Enteric fever: a travel medicine oriented view. Curr Opin Infect Dis Oct 2010;23(5):432–7.

48. Beran J, Beutels M, Levie K, et al. A single dose, combined vaccine against typhoid fever and hepatitis A: consistency, immunogenicity and reactogenicity. J Travel Med 2000;7:246–52.

49. Guzman CA, Borsutzky S, Griot-Wenk M, et al. Vaccines against typhoid fever. Vaccine 2006;24:3804–11.

50. Loebermann M, Kollaritsch H, Ziegler T, et al. A randomized, open-label study of the immunogenicity and reactogenicity of three lots of a combined typhoid fever/hepatitis A vaccine in healthy adults. Clin Ther 2004;26:1084–91.

51. Cryz Jr SJ, Pasteris O, Varallyay SJ, et al. Factors influencing the stability of live oral attenuated bacterial vaccines. Dev Biol Stand 1996;87:277–81.

52. Kaplan DT, Hill DR. Compliance with live, oral Ty21a typhoid vaccine. JAMA 1992;267:1074.

53. Levine MM, Ferreccio C, Abrego P, et al. Duration of efficacy of Ty21a, attenuated Salmonella typhi live oral vaccine. Vaccine 1999;17(suppl 2):S22–7.

54. Sur D, Ochiai RL, Bhattacharya SK, et al. A cluster-randomized effectiveness trial of Vi typhoid vaccine in India. N Engl J Med Jul 23 2009;361(4):335–44.

55. Begier EM, Burwen DR, Haber P, et al. Postmarketing safety surveillance for typhoid fever vaccines from the Vaccine Adverse Event Reporting System, July 1990 through June 2002. Clin Infect Dis 2004;38:771–9.

56. Faucher JK, Binder R, Missinou MA, et al. Efficacy of Atovaquone/ Proguanil for Malaria Prophylaxis in Children and Its Effect on the Immunogenicity of Live Oral Typhoid and Cholera Vaccines. Clin Infect Dis 2002;35:1147–54.

57. Leder K, Sundararajan V, Weld L, et al. Respiratory tract infections in travelers: a review of the GeoSentinel surveillance network. Clin Infect Dis 2003;36:399–406.

58. Mutsch M, Tavernini M, Marx A, et al. Influenza virus infection in travelers to tropical and subtropical countries. Clin Infect Dis 2005;40:1282–7.

59. Leggat PA, Leder K. Reducing the impact of influenza among travelers. J Travel Med 2010;17:363–6.

60. Miller JM, Tam TW, Maloney S, et al. Cruise ships: high-risk passengers and the global spread of new influenza viruses. Clin Infect Dis 2000;31:433–8.

61. Freedman DO, Leder K. Influenza: changing approaches to prevention and treatment in travelers. J Travel Med 2005;12:36–44.

62. Brotherton JM, Delpech VC, Gilbert GL, et al. A large outbreak of influenza A and B on a cruise ship causing widespread morbidity. Epidemiol Infect 2003;130:263–71.

63. Barr Ig, McCauley J, Cox N, et al. Epidemiological, antigenic and genetic characteristics of seasonal influenza A(H1N1), A(H3N2) and B influenza viruses: basis for the WHO recommendation on the composition of influenza vaccines for use in the 2009–10 Northern Hemisphere season. Vaccine Feb 3 2010;28(5):1156–67.

64. Belshe R, Lee MS, Walker RE, et al. Safety, immunogenicity and efficacy of intranasal, live attenuated influenza vaccine. Expert Rev Vaccines 2004;3:643–54.

65. Sasaki S, Jaimes MC, Holmes TH, et al. Comparison of the influenza virus-specific effector and memory B-cell responses to immunization of children and adults with live attenuated or inactivated influenza virus vaccines. J Virol 2007;81:215–28.

66. Fleming DM, Crovari P, Wahn U, et al. Comparison of the efficacy and safety of live attenuated cold-adapted influenza vaccine, trivalent, with trivalent inactivated influenza virus vaccine in children and adolescents with asthma. Pediatr Infect Dis J 2006;25:860–9.

67. Statement on travel, influenza, and prevention. Can Commun Dis Rep 2005;31:1–8.

68. Balkhy HH, Memish ZA, Bafaqeer S, et al. Influenza a common viral infection among Hajj pilgrims: time for routine surveillance and vaccination. J Travel Med 2004;11:82–6.

69. Mustafa AN, Gessner BD, Ismail R, et al. A case-control study of influenza vaccine effectiveness among Malaysian pilgrims attending the Hajj in Saudi Arabia. Int J Infect Dis 2003;7:210–4.

70. CDC. Prevention and Control of Influenza with Vaccines: Recommendations of the Advisory Committee on Immunization Practices (ACIP), 2011. MMWR – MMWR Aug 26 2011;60:1128–32.

71. Smith NM, Bresee JS, Shay DK, et al. Prevention and Control of Influenza: recommendations of the Advisory Committee on Immunization Practices (ACIP). MMWR Recomm Rep 2006;55:1–42.

72. Falsey AR, Treanor JJ, Tornieporth N, et al. Randomized, double-blind controlled phase 3 trial comparing the immunogenicity of high-dose and standard-dose influenza vaccine in adults 65 years of age and older. J Infect Dis 2009;200:172–80.

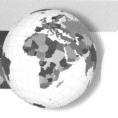

Special Adult Travel Vaccines: Yellow Fever, Meningococcal, Japanese Encephalitis, TBE, Rabies, Polio, Cholera

Joseph Torresi and Herwig Kollaritsch

Key points

- Vaccine recommendations for travelers are based on the anticipated risks of exposure to vaccine-preventable diseases on a given travel itinerary, the severity of the disease if acquired, and any risks of the vaccine itself
- The risk for each vaccine-preventable disease depends on the prevalence of the disease at the destination(s) as well as traveler-dependent risk factors, which include recreational and occupational activities, mode of travel and accommodations, duration of travel, degree of close contact (including sexual relations) with local residents, and time of year the travel is undertaken
- Special travel vaccines to be considered are divided into required, recommended, and special circumstances categories. Required vaccines may on certain itineraries include yellow fever and meningococcal (*Hajj* travel only); recommended vaccines may include Japanese encephalitis, tick-borne encephalitis, rabies, polio and cholera; vaccines for special circumstances include anthrax, smallpox and plague

Introduction

Based on regional patterns of disease transmission, a vaccine considered routine or standard in one country may represent a travel immunization for visitors originating in another country. Examples of this are Japanese encephalitis (JE) virus vaccine, rabies vaccine, and yellow fever vaccine, each of which may be administered routinely to residents of countries where there is a high risk of transmission of the given disease, but which are considered travel vaccines for visitors to those same countries.

Further complicating the consideration of international immunization practices are the variations that exist in travel vaccine product formulations, when more than one vaccine against a particular disease is produced by several manufacturers. Some confusion also arises when a given vaccine produced by a single pharmaceutical manufacturer has been licensed under different brand names, dosing schedules, and booster intervals in different countries. Trade names of the commonly used travel vaccines are given in Table 12.1. Whereas most travelers may be able to complete a recommended primary series for a given vaccine before departure from the home country,

other travelers, especially long-term travelers, expatriates, and immigrants, may start an immunization series in one country and receive additional doses to complete or boost the primary series in another country. When this is necessary, the fact that vaccine products and practices vary from country to country could affect immunization planning. When available, information on accelerated immunization schedules will be provided in this chapter. Most vaccine series have defined minimum ages for the initial doses as well as defined minimum intervals between each of the subsequent doses, which may be shorter than the generally used regimen. In general, if a missed or delayed dose in a vaccine series is identified, it is not necessary to re-start the vaccine series from the beginning. The vaccine dose that is due or overdue should be administered and documented, and the immunization schedule should proceed according to age-appropriate minimal intervals for each subsequent dose in the series from that point on.

The WHO develops and adopts International Health Regulations (IHRs), which were last updated in 2005. These guidelines regarding vaccine requirements for international travelers can be found in the International Travel and Health book published annually by WHO (with electronic access through its website at: www.who.int/ith). IHR 2005 specifies requirements for only one vaccine, yellow fever, but contains language allowing for the rapid introduction of vaccine requirements for other vaccines for international travel in cases of international public health emergencies. WHO also publishes and updates 'Position Papers' for vaccines on a regular basis (http://www.who.int/immunization/documents/positionpapers/en/index.html). These position papers, although not tailored for travel medicine specialists, offer an excellent review of current knowledge about the respective vaccine. In addition, these papers represent an official position of WHO and may therefore be used as a valid reference.

The CDC also develops guidelines and information for international travelers, which are contained in its publication *Health Information for International Travel* (published on a biannual basis, with online access through the CDC website: www.cdc.gov/ travel). Similar information and guidelines are also published for use in other countries such as Canada and Australia. These can be accessed at: http://www.phac-aspc.gc.ca/im/index-eng.php and http://immunize.health.gov.au/internet/immunize/publishing.nsf/Content/handbook03, respectively.

Healthcare providers should consult national public health agencies in the country where they work for current information on the standards of care and vaccine practices appropriate for that country.

©2012 Elsevier Inc

DOI: 10.1016/B978-1-4557-1076-8.00012-0

Table 12.1 Trade names of Important Adult Travel-Related Vaccines Worldwide

Cholera (oral)	Dukoral, Shanchol
Japanese encephalitis	Ixiaro, Jespect, Imojev, Japanese Encephalitis Vaccine (live 14–14–2)
Meningococcal (polysaccharide)	Menomune, Mencevax ACWY, ACWY Vax, MenceACW, Polysaccharide Meningococcal A + C Vaccine, MenAfriVac, Menomune A/C, Meningovax A + C, Vacina Antimeningococic A + C, Meninvact, Vacina Meningococica A + C, Meningokokken-Impfstoff A + C, Imovax Meningo A + C, Mencevax AC, Menpovax A + C, Mengivac A + C, Meningococcal Polysaccharide vaccine, Vaccin Meningoccique Mérieux, MeNZB
Meningococcal (conjugate)	Menactra (ACWY), Menveo (ACWY), Nimenrix (ACWY), Menjugate (C), Neisvac-C, Meningitec (C), Vacina meningococcica conjugada Grupo C
Rabies	Imovax Rabies, Imovax Rabies HT, Rabies Imovax, Immovax Rabbia, RabAvert Rabies Vaccine BP, VeroRab, Rabipur, Rabipur, Rabies Vaccine Adsorbed, Lyssavac, Lyssavac N, Rabies MIRV, Tollwut-Impfstoff (HDC), TRC VeroRab, Rabies Vero; Rabivac, Speeda, Abhayrab
Rabies immune globulin	Imogam, Imogam Rabies HT, Bayrab, HyperRAB, HyperRAB S/D, Berirab, Imogam Rabia, Imogam Rage, Tollwutglobulin, Favirab (equine)
Yellow fever	YF-Vax, Stamaril, Arilvax, Yellow Fever Vaccine (live), Vacina contra Febre Amarela
Tick-borne encephalitis	Encepur, FSME-Immun; Russia and neighbouring countries: TBE vaccine Chumakow, Encevir

Most widely distributed trade names listed first. Vaccines are parenteral unless specified.

Practical Vaccine Considerations

One of the common practical challenges when advising travelers about pre-travel immunizations is that of scheduling the recommended vaccines in the time available before trip departure. An overview of commonly administered vaccines for adult travelers, including dosing schedules, accelerated regimens, efficacy estimates, and interchangeability is presented in Table 12.2.

Adverse Events

Discussions of major vaccine-related adverse events are found below under each individual vaccine. In counseling patients and recommending vaccines, familiarity with numerical data on the risks and benefits of each vaccine is helpful for the provider. Table 12.3 provides a comparison of the estimated risk of acquiring a vaccine-preventable disease or being harmed by a complication of that disease, with an estimate of the risk of the vaccine for that disease.

Attenuated Live Vaccines

Live virus vaccines, such as yellow fever vaccine, are in general contraindicated in pregnant patients and those with congenital, acquired or pharmacologically induced immunodeficient states because of the concern that an attenuated vaccine virus strain may exhibit increased virulence in immunodeficient persons, causing severe disease. When travel to the area of risk cannot be postponed or deferred, decisions regarding vaccination against a particular disease must consider the potential risk of life-threatening illness or death from a disease weighed against the potential risks from the vaccine itself, as well as the possibility of the induction of a suboptimal response to the vaccine itself. See Chapters 27 and 28 for expanded discussion.

Required Vaccines

Yellow Fever Vaccine

Yellow fever is a serious viral hemorrhagic fever that is spread by *Aedes* or *Haemogogus* spp. mosquitoes. Although *Aedes aegypti* mosquitoes are found in all warm climates, yellow fever has only occurred in Africa and South America (Fig. 12.1). The clinical illness follows a short incubation period of 2–5 days. This is followed by an influenza-like illness with fever, myalgias, headache, prostration, nausea and vomiting. Most patients recover, but approximately 15% progress to severe disease with jaundice, multi-organ failure, bleeding and shock. The case fatality rate in severe disease is 25–50%.[1]

Yellow fever has three types of transmission cycle. The first is the jungle or sylvatic cycle, which is an enzootic viral disease transmitted among non-human primate hosts by a variety of mosquito vectors, which may also bite and infect humans. The second is the urban cycle, an epidemic disease of humans transmitted from infected to susceptible persons by the *Aedes aegypti* mosquito. The third is the intermediate or savannah cycle, a mode of transmission that occurs only in Africa and involves transmission of yellow fever virus from *Aedes* spp. to humans living or working in jungle border areas. In this cycle, the virus may be transmitted from monkeys to humans or from human to human via these mosquitoes. Both the sylvatic and the urban transmission cycles occur in Africa, whereas jungle transmission predominates in South America. In South America, peak transmission of YF virus occurs during the months of January to March, while in Africa the period of peak transmission occurs through the months of July to October. WHO estimates that some 200 000 cases occur each year, with almost all of these in sub-Saharan Africa.[1,2]

The risk of yellow fever for travelers is difficult to determine and so far has been based on the risk to indigenous populations.[3,4] For a 2-week stay, the risks for illness and death due to yellow fever for an unvaccinated traveler to an endemic area in West Africa are 50 per 100 000 and 10 per 100 000, respectively; for South America the risks are 5 per 100 000 and 1 per 100 000, respectively.

The vaccine is a live attenuated strain of the YF virus (17D) that was originally developed in 1927.[4] Sub-strains of the WHO-standardized 17D virus seed-lot strains in current use are designated 17DD, 17D-204, and 17D-213, and these three strains share 99.9% sequence homology. WHO currently approves only four manufacturers of YF vaccine: Sanofi Pasteur, France, produces 17D-204 vaccine in France (Stamaril); Institut Pasteur Dakar, Senegal, produces 17D-204 YF vaccine; BioMaguinos, Brazil, produces 17DD vaccine; and Chumakov Institute of Poliomyelitis and Viral Encephalitides produces 17D-204 vaccine in the Russian Federation (Table 12.1). In addition, Sanofi Pasteur produces YF-Vax 17D-204 vaccine in the USA. Updated lists of WHO pre-qualified vaccines are available at: http://www.who.int/immunization_standards/vaccine_quality/PQ_vaccine_list_en/en/index.html.

Table 12.2 Summary of Commonly used Special Travel Vaccines

Disease	Vaccine Type; Commercial Name (Manufacturer)	Efficacy	Primary Course – Adult	Boosters	Accelerated Schedule	Pregnancy or Lactation	Comments
Cholera, oral	Killed whole-cell-recombinant B subunit vaccine; Dukoral (SBL)	85–90%	>6 years of age: 2 doses orally 7–42 days apart	Every 2 years for persons over 6 years of age	None	Category C. Insufficient data about pregnancy or excretion in breast milk	Some cross-protection against heat-labile toxin of enterotoxigenic E. coli (ETEC) (see text). Licensed for travelers' diarrhea protection in some countries
	Killed whole cell (incl. O139) Shanchol (Shanta Biotechnics Ltd. India)	66%	2 doses, 1 week apart	Not known	None	No data available	Available only in India and Indonesia, contains O139
Japanese B encephalitis	IXIARO (IC51; Novartis) JESPECT (AUSTRALIA)	Non-inferior to JE-VAX (mouse-brain vaccine) in seroconversion studies	>18 years old 0.5 ml at 0, 28 days	Booster after 12–24 months, further boosters not defined	Doses spaced by 14 days results in only 40% seroconversion No accelerated schedule available	Category C (add reference)	Pediatric Approval expected in 2012 or 2013
Japanese B encephalitis	IMOJEV (Sanofi Pasteur)	99% seroconversion rate from single dose	Adults over 18 years: 1 dose	None	None	Not recommended during pregnancy	Registered by TGA in Australia 2011
Meningococcal disease	Polysaccharide vaccine. Neisseria meningitidis Groups A, C, Y, W-135. Menomune (Sanofi Pasteur) ACYW Vax (GlaxoSmithKline) and many others	85–90% efficacy after 1–2 weeks	Adults: 0.5 mL s.c. Single dose	Same dose. Re-dose every 3–5 years for adults at continued risk of exposure	None	Category C. No data available during lactation.	Travelers should only receive quadrivalent vaccine (ACYW). A or A + C vaccine is marketed in many countries
Meningococcal disease	Menactra (Sanofi Pasteur) Quadrivalent conjugate Neisseria meningitidis Groups A, C, Y, W-135 Conjugated to D	>97% seroconversion to all four serogroups after 28 days	One single i.m. dose for ≥2 yrs old; children 9–23 mo: 2 doses, 3 months apart, starting at age 9 mo.	Not known at present, likely 3 years	None	Category C. No data available during lactation.	Travelers should only receive quadrivalent vaccine (ACYW). A C conjugate vaccine is marketed in many countries for routine pediatric vaccination but is not appropriate for travelers

Continued

Table 12.2 Summary of Adult Routine Travel Vaccines—cont'd

Disease	Vaccine Type; Commercial Name (Manufacturer)	Efficacy	Primary Course – Adult	Boosters	Accelerated Schedule	Pregnancy or Lactation	Comments
	Menveo (Novartis) Quadrivalent conjugate *Neisseria meningitidis* Groups A, C, Y, W-135. Conjugated to CRM 197	81–95% (serotype-dependent) Seroprotection in hSBA[62] >97% seroconversion to all four serogroups after 28 days[69]	One single i.m. dose for ≥2 yrs old; licensure for smaller children awaited 2012 One single i.m. dose for age 12 months and above	Not known at present	None	Category C. No data available during lactation.	Vaccine licensed in EC for adolescents and adults < 11 yrs–55 yrs; In US <2–55 yrs
	Nimenrix (GlaxoSmith Kline) Quadrivalent conjugate *Neisseria meningitidis* Groups A, C, Y, W-135 Conjugated to TT	82–95% seroconversion to all four serotypes after 1 month		Likely 3 years	None	Category C. No data available during lactation.	Vaccine licensed in EC in 2012
Poliomyelitis	Inactivated viral injectable. IPV (many brands)		0.5 mL s.c. 3 doses at 0, 2, 8–14 months	Same dose. If >10 years since completion of the primary vaccine series, boost once in adult life for travel to a polio endemic area	Primary Series Accelerated: 3 doses at 0, 1, 2 months (minimum 4 weeks apart). Give as many doses as time permits and complete remaining doses as soon as possible thereafter	Category C. If protection required during pregnancy either OPV or IPV can be given. Not contraindicated during lactation	
Rabies	Inactivated viral vaccine, Human Diploid Cell Vaccine (HDCV). Imovax Rabies (Sanofi Pasteur)		1.0 mL i.m. deltoid. Or 0.1 mL intradermal on the forearm. Pre-exposure schedule of 0, 7, and 21 or 28 days	Not needed for typical travelers. Possibly 3 years if persistent high risk. Recommend checking serology before boosting	Days 0, 7, and 21	Category C. No data available during lactation.	Intradermal dosing is endorsed by the WHO and supported by data. Vaccine packaging for 0.1 mL ID dosing is not available from the manufacturer. 1.0 mL vials reconstituted to use for 10 ID doses must be used within 1 h
Rabies	Inactivated viral vaccine, Purified Chick Embryo Cell vaccine (PCECV). Rabavert or Rabipur (Novartis)		1.0 mL i.m. deltoid. Never use gluteal muscle. Pre-exposure schedule of 0, 7, and 21 or 28 days	See remarks above	Days 0, 7, and 21	Category C. No data available during lactation.	See remarks above on ID dosing

Disease	Vaccine	Efficacy/Seroconversion	Dose & schedule	Booster	Schedule	Category	Remarks
Rabies	Inactivated viral vaccine, Verocell vaccine Verorab (Sanofi Pasteur)		0.5 mL i.m. Pre-exposure schedule of 0, 7, and 21 or 28 days	See remarks above	Days 0, 7, and 21	Category C. No data available during lactation	
Tick-borne encephalitis	Inactivated viral vaccine. FSME-immune (Baxter AG) and Encepur (Novartis)	Seroconversion rates of ~100% after 3 doses	FSME-immun: 0.5 mL i.m. deltoid. Given on day 0, 4–12 weeks, and 9–12 months after the second dose. Encepur: 0.5 mL i.m. deltoid. Given on day 0, 4–12 weeks, and 5–12 months after the second dose	Every 3–5 years	FSME Immun: 0.5 mL on days 0 and 14, 3rd dose 6–15 months after second. Encepur: days 0, 7, 21, with a booster 12–18 months later	Category C. Contraindicated in pregnancy and during breastfeeding unless the benefits far outweigh any potential risk	Protects against both European and Far Eastern strains of tick-borne encephalitis
Yellow Fever	Live attenuated viral vaccine. YF-VAX, Stamaril (Sanofi Pasteur), Arilvax		One dose 0.5 mL s.c.	Every 10 years Being re-examined by WHO in 2012	None	Category C. Contraindicated in pregnancy except if exposure is unavoidable. Risk of disease exposure to patient versus risk of vaccine strain disease to fetus must be weighed before vaccination. Two YEL-AND cases have been reported in exclusively breastfed infants whose mothers were vaccinated with yellow fever vaccine. Vaccination should be avoided in nursing mothers if possible	Yellow Fever AND (acute neurotropic disease): 50–400 per 100000 in children <1 yr AVD (acute viscerotropic disease): 60–69 yrs: 1.0 per 100000 70+: 2.3 per 100000[5]

Table 12.3 Estimated Risk from Disease and Sequelae Versus Risk from Vaccines

Disease	Risk of Acquiring Disease or Complications from Disease	Risk from Vaccine
Cholera	Risk of acquiring disease while traveling: 1 in 500 000 travelers	63 adverse reactions in 1 000 000 million doses sold in Scandinavia 1992–2003[93]
Japanese encephalitis	Risk of JE in highly endemic areas: 1: 40 000 -1: 1 000 000 per month of stay Overt encephalitis 1 in 20–1000 cases Case fatality rate: 33% of encephalitis cases Severe neuropsychiatric sequelae: 33% of encephalitis cases	Minimal risk with IC51[45], IMOJEV, or SA-14–14–2 vaccines
Meningococcal disease	Outbreak defined by >100 cases/100 000 per year[94] Rates in endemic areas of Africa during epidemics: up to 1000/100 000 Case fatality rates in industrialized countries: Meningitis: 7% Septicemia: 19% Mortality in developing countries during epidemics: Meningitis: 2–10% Septicemia: 50–70%	Local pain and swelling at the site of injection <5% SAE (conjugated vaccines) very rare, not specified Guillain Barré: slightly increased after ACWY-D (Menactra); no data for ACWY-CRM (Menveo and Nimenrix)[95]
Poliomyelitis	Paralytic cases: 2% of all infections Case fatality rate: Children: 2–5% in clinical cases Adults: 15–30% in clinical cases	Vaccine associated paralytic polio (VAPP): 1 case for every 2–3 million doses of OPV No risk of VAPP with IPV
Rabies	Case fatality rate: 100%	Cell culture vaccines (CCV): No risk of vaccine-associated neurologic adverse side-effects; 20% incidence of minor side-effects HDCV: 6% of booster vaccine recipients experience acute hypersensitivity reactions, 3% as immediate reaction, 3% as delayed type 6–14 days post-boost. Hypersensitivity reactions are extremely rare during primary course[96]
Yellow fever	Case fatality rate: >50% Risk of acquiring disease in endemic regions (2 weeks stay) in Africa: 10–50/100.000 America: 1–5/100.000[5]	Type I hypersensitivity reactions: 1/131 000 doses. Anaphylaxis in 1.8 cases per 100 000 doses. Yellow fever vaccine Associated Neurologic Disease (Yell-AND): 5/1 000 000 Yellow fever vaccine Associated Viscerotrophic Disease (Yel-AVD): 0.9 to 2.5 per 1 000 000 doses overall, 1 in 55 000 for age >60 years; 1 in 30 000 for age >70 years. Case fatality rate 65%.

Recommendations

Under IHR (2005), any country may require a YF vaccination certificate from travelers coming from areas with risk of yellow fever transmission, even if the travelers are only in transit through that country. Only a small number of African countries (Angola, Benin, Burkina Faso, Burundi, Cameroon, Central African Republic, Congo, Cote D'Ivoire, Democratic Republic of Congo, Gabon, Ghana, Guinea-Bissau, Liberia, Mali, Niger, Rwanda, Sao Tome and Principe, Sierra Leone, Togo) and one in South America (French Guiana) require proof of YF vaccination from all arriving travelers.[5]

Although most countries that have YF risk themselves request proof of YF vaccination for at least some arriving travelers as a requirement for entry, certain countries outside risk areas may also designate YF vaccine as required or mandatory. Such YF-free countries have the appropriate climatic and entomologic conditions to initiate and maintain a YF transmission cycle, and the purpose of the vaccine requirement in this case is to prevent importation of YF through the entry of latent viremic infections in travelers arriving from YF endemic countries. Figures 12.1 A & B show maps of vaccine recommendations for countries with at least the potential for YF transmission, although a number of countries with YF requirements understand the IHR to mean that they can establish their own lists of risk countries that may differ from that of the WHO.[5] For potentially receptive countries, WHO recommends that vaccination not be required for travelers arriving from Zambia, Tanzania, Eritrea, and Sao Tome, countries no longer considered to be at risk of yellow fever transmission in Annex 1 of the WHO Publication *International Travel Health*. In general, all countries with any requirement declare their specific requirements to WHO, which maintains a regularly updated list of such requirements at: www.who.int/ith.

YF vaccination is considered valid if the person received a WHO-approved vaccine and it was administered at an approved YF Vaccination Center, with an approved stamp from national authorities. A personal signature cannot substitute for the official stamp. Individual countries control the number and locations of YF Vaccination Center

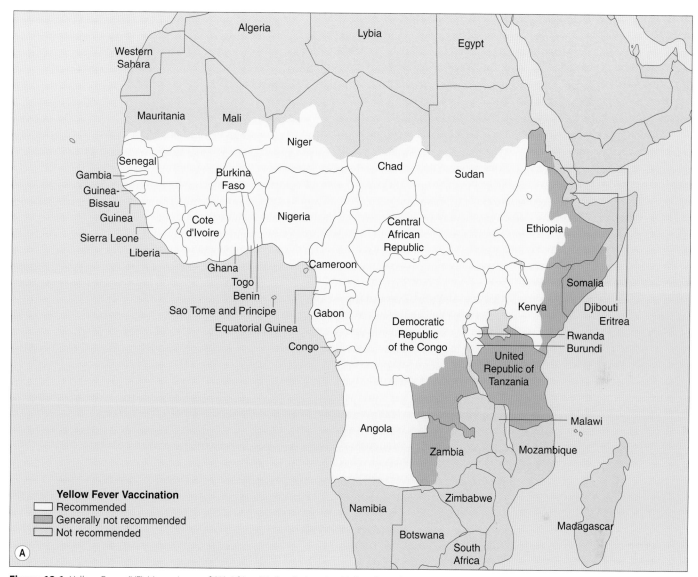

Figure 12.1 Yellow Fever (YF) Maps. Areas of (**A**) Africa (**B**) South America. Yellow fever (YF) vaccination is generally not recommended in areas where there is low potential for YF virus exposure.[5] *(Gershman M, Staples JE. Yellow fever. In: CDC, Health Information for International Travel: The Yellow Book Oxford University Press; 2012.)*

Continued

sites, which may be at either public health clinics or private health centers, depending on the population of the area served, the estimated at-risk population, and national vaccine program priorities. In many countries, especially in Latin America, the YF stamp is obtainable only from government clinics that provide the YF vaccine and not from private clinics, even if they can purchase and administer the vaccine.

The immunization must be given no less than 10 days prior to the planned date of entry to meet official requirements, and is valid for 10 years. Vaccine administration is documented and stamped on the appropriate page of the *International Certificate of Vaccination*. Unlike the IHRs (1969) that specifically exempted travelers making only airport transit stops in YF-risk countries, the IHRs (2005) do not provide this exemption.[5] Thus, at the pre-travel consultation travelers need to provide a full travel itinerary, including transit stops en route, as individual countries may require proof of vaccination for all passengers arriving on an airplane from a risk country even if the passenger only transited that country.

Under the IHR, a letter of waiver can be provided to travelers who have medical or other contraindications for receiving the YF vaccination. The waiver letter must be on an official letterhead, signed by a physician authorized to provide the YF vaccination, and bear the stamp of the authorized center. Acceptance of the waiver letter is at the discretion of the receiving country. Travelers unable to receive the vaccine and using a letter of waiver to meet the YF vaccine entry requirement for a destination in a YF-endemic area need pre-travel counseling about how to reduce the risks of natural disease transmission at destination, through effective use of insect precautions and avoidance of environments where the risk of transmission is likely to be higher.

In the USA, the 2012 CDC vaccination recommendations are based on four categories of risk for YFV transmission that apply to all geographic areas: endemic, transitional, low potential for exposure, and no risk.[5] Yellow fever vaccination is recommended for travel to endemic and transitional areas. Vaccination is generally not

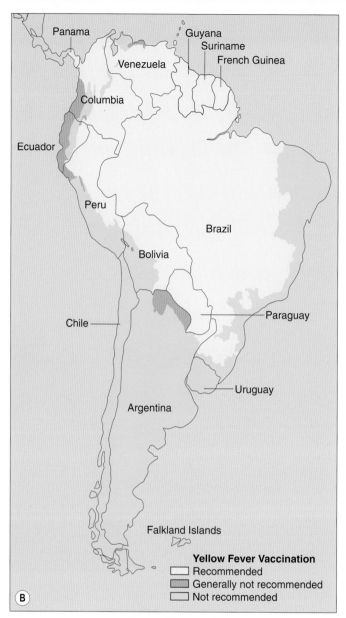

Figure 12.1, cont'd

recommended for travel to areas with low potential for exposure unless traveler-related factors place them at markedly increased risk for exposure to YFV; these are all areas where a case of human yellow fever has never been recorded, so this will rarely include typical travelers. The CDC yellow fever maps and country-specific information now designate three levels of yellow fever vaccine recommendations: recommended, generally not recommended, and not recommended. Countries that contain areas with low potential for exposure to YFV are not included on the official WHO list of countries with risk of YFV transmission. Proof of yellow fever vaccination should therefore not be required if traveling from a country with low potential for exposure to YFV to a country with a vaccination entry requirement, unless that country requires proof of yellow fever vaccination from all arriving travelers.

Travelers to coastal Brazil or Peru, Cuzco and Machu Picchu face no risk and do not need vaccination. It is generally not recommended

for coastal Ecuador or Colombia, and not recommended for travel to Quito or Bogota, which are above the 2300 m above-sea-level transmission threshold.

Indications

The main purpose of vaccination is prevention of disease in individuals at risk. Yellow fever vaccine is approved for use in all persons over 9 months of age who have no YF vaccine contraindication[6] (see Chapter 13 for considerations on immunizing children under the age of 9 months). However, because of uncommon but possible vaccine-associated adverse side-effects (see below), persons who are not at risk of exposure should not receive the vaccine. In countries where there is risk of the disease and there is a YF vaccine requirement for entry, the risk of disease is usually restricted to limited areas of the country. If a traveler has no possibility of visiting that particular area, then YF vaccination may not be warranted on a health risk basis, although YF vaccine certification or an official letter of waiver would be needed to meet the legal requirements for entry. However, if such a traveler then plans to continue travel into another country with YF entry requirements, vaccination would be required to meet the entry requirements of the second country. It is prudent to vaccinate persons who have anything less than a definite fixed itinerary and/or anticipate travel outside urban areas in YF-endemic countries, regardless of whether the YF vaccine is required.

Contraindications and Precautions

Age

Infants **<6 months** of age are more susceptible to serious adverse reactions (for example encephalitis) than older children and **should never be immunized**. The vaccine may be given to children ≥**9 months** of age, if traveling or living in areas of South America and Africa where yellow fever is officially reported, or to countries that require yellow fever immunization.

For adults aged 60 years and over, yellow fever vaccine should be given with a caution because of a greater likelihood of serious adverse event, including both YEL-AND (associated neurologic disease) and YEL-AVD (associated viscerotropic disease). If travel is unavoidable, the decision to vaccinate travelers aged ≥60 years needs to weigh the risks and benefits of the vaccination in the context of their destination-specific risk for exposure to YFV.[5] Provision of medical waivers based solely on age >60 is controversial and not specifically addressed either by the IHR or any WHO-provided advice. Such waivers may be misunderstood by travelers to mean that they are immune for a subsequent trip to a very high-risk area. In addition, waivers do nothing to protect the public health of the receiving country against the introduction of yellow fever virus, so that widespread use in an increasingly aging traveling population may serve to defeat the purpose of the IHR.

Because of the risk of serious adverse events, including vaccine-associated viscerotropic and neurotropic disease that can occur after yellow fever vaccination, only people who (1) are at risk of exposure to YFV or (2) require proof of vaccination to enter a country should be vaccinated.

Pregnancy

Although small studies exist, the safety of yellow fever vaccine during pregnancy has not been established, and the vaccine is contraindicated on theoretical grounds. Avoid vaccination during pregnancy unless travel to very high-risk areas is unavoidable.[6]

Nursing Mothers

Two YEL-AND cases have been reported in exclusively breastfed infants whose mothers were vaccinated with yellow fever vaccine. Vaccination of nursing mothers should be avoided because of the potential risk for transmission of the vaccine virus to the breastfed infant. However, nursing mothers traveling to a yellow fever-endemic area should be vaccinated.

Thymic Disorder or Dysfunction

In view of the four reported cases of yellow fever vaccine-associated viscerotropic disease (YEL-AVD) in persons with thymic disorder, travelers, irrespective of age, with a history of thymic disorder or dysfunction – including myasthenia gravis, thymoma, thymectomy, or DiGeorge syndrome – should not be given this vaccine.[7] This excludes those with post-traumatic thymectomy. If travel to a yellow fever-endemic area cannot be avoided in these individuals a medical waiver should be provided, and counseling on protective measures against mosquito bites should be emphasized.

Altered Immune States

The vaccine is contraindicated in persons with immunodeficiency due to cancer, HIV/AIDS, transplantation, or treatment with immunosuppressive drugs, as prolonged viremia may increase the risk of encephalitis.[5] Persons with asymptomatic HIV infection may be vaccinated if exposure to yellow fever cannot be avoided and the individual's CD4 count is >200×10^9 cells/L.[8] If travel to a yellow fever-endemic area cannot be avoided in these individuals or in those with symptomatic HIV, a medical waiver should be provided, and counseling on protective measures against mosquito bites should be emphasized.

Hypersensitivity to Eggs

Yellow fever vaccine should not be given to those with known anaphylactic hypersensitivity to hens' eggs (manifested as urticaria, swelling of the mouth and throat, difficulty breathing or hypotension).

Dosing Schedules

The primary schedule for YF vaccine in adults is a single 0.5 mL injection given subcutaneously or intramuscularly. A booster dose is recommended for persons with continued risk of exposure 10 years from the last dose (Table 12.2). The YF vaccine contains no preservative and must be administered within 1 h of reconstitution.[6]

Measures of Immune Response and Duration of Immunity/Protection

The vaccine induces neutralizing antibodies in 90% of vaccine recipients within 10 days after inoculation, and in 99% within 30 days.[9] The vaccine mimics natural infection, and a low level of viremia with the vaccine strain virus is noted in 50–60% of vaccinees in the first week after vaccination. Seroprotective neutralizing antibodies to YF develop within 7–10 days of vaccination.

Although the YF certificate is officially valid for 10 years, the true duration of immunity from YF vaccination is probably much longer. The antibodies have been detected in 92–97% of vaccinees 16–19 years after initial vaccination. In another study, approximately 80% of vaccinees were seropositive 30 years after a single dose.[9] A WHO/IHR-convened Expert Panel is scheduled to examine the 10-year rule in 2012, and changes may result.

Adverse Events

Approximately 2–5% of vaccinees will develop mild headache, myalgia, low-grade fever or other minor symptoms 5–10 days after vaccination (most commonly on the sixth or seventh day). Daily activities may be curtailed in up to 1% of vaccinees. Immediate hypersensitivity reactions characterized by rash, urticaria and/or asthma are extremely uncommon (incidence <1 : 1 000 000), and occur principally in persons with a history of egg allergy. Severe hypersensitivity reactions, including anaphylaxis, reported to occur at a rate of 1.8 cases per 100 000 doses of yellow fever vaccine administered (Table 12.3).

Two serious reactions reported to occur following vaccination include yellow fever vaccine-associated neurotropic disease (YF-AND) and yellow fever vaccine-associated viscerotropic disease (YF-AVD) (Table 12.3). A total of 50 cases of YF-AND have been documented; historically, these occurred in infants 7 months of age or younger, predominantly in infants 4 months of age or less. In more recent years, four cases of encephalitis have been reported among adults, with onset 4–28 days after immunization, all following first doses.[9,10] Recovery has generally been rapid and complete. One case of fatal meningoencephalitis has been reported in an immunocompromised HIV-infected man, but prospective surveillance established in 1993 during an immunization campaign in Kenya did not demonstrate more frequent severe reactions in HIV-infected persons. The estimated incidence of YF-AND ranges from four to six cases per 1 000 000 doses (in the United States) to one in 8 million.[9]

YF-AVD has been reported in 59 individuals since 1973 and is associated with severe multiple organ system failure following the administration of the yellow fever vaccine.[9,11–16] This complication has been associated with both the 17D-204 and 17DD yellow fever virus strains. Vaccine recipients generally presented within 2–5 days of vaccination with an illness characterized by fever, myalgia, and gastrointestinal symptoms, followed by a rapid progression to hypotension, liver, renal and respiratory failure, encephalopathy, lymphocytopenia, thrombocytopenia, disseminated intravascular coagulation, and death in the majority. The reported case-fatality ratio for YEL-AVD is 65%. Crude estimates of the reported frequency of YF-AVD range from 0.9 to 2.5 per 1 000 000 doses distributed. The risk is highest in individuals over the age of 60–65. In those over 75 the risk is 12 times higher than in young adults. This syndrome has not been reported in individuals receiving booster doses of the vaccine. Four (17%) of the 23 vaccinees reported with this syndrome had a history of thymus disease (thymectomy and thymic tumour), suggesting that thymic dysfunction is an independent risk factor.[7]

Yellow fever vaccination providers should be fully conversant with the actual infection risk at the traveler's destination, or have resources at hand to determine relative risk. Naturally acquired YF infection in previously non-exposed individuals most often manifests as a life-threatening hemorrhagic fever.

Drug and Vaccine Interactions

Yellow fever vaccine can be administered concurrently with MMR, varicella and smallpox. If this cannot be achieved, they should be given 4 weeks apart. However, if time is limited, the vaccines should be given within whatever time is available. Sabin (OPV) can be given at any time. Immunoglobulin does not affect the immune response to yellow fever vaccine and may be given concomitantly. The antibody response to yellow fever vaccine is not inhibited by simultaneous immunization with BCG, oral cholera vaccine, measles, diphtheria–pertussis–tetanus, meningococcal vaccine, poliomyelitis (OPV and IPV), hepatitis A, hepatitis B, tetanus, typhoid oral and parenteral vaccines.[9,17] There are no data on possible interference between yellow fever and plague, rabies, or Japanese encephalitis vaccines. Experimental data suggest that chloroquine inhibits the replication of YF virus in vitro. However, a study in humans has shown that the antibody responses to the YF vaccine are not affected by routine antimalarial doses of chloroquine.

Recommended Vaccines

Cholera Vaccine

Cholera is a fecal–oral toxin-induced disease, endemic in many countries with poor sanitation and inadequate food and water hygiene, and most often is transmitted in epidemic patterns. The risk of cholera to an average traveler is extremely low (0.01–0.001% per month of stay in a developing country), as most travelers practice proper hygiene when confronted with epidemic situations.[18] Almost all cases of cholera now occur in Africa and Asia and the island of Hispaniola (Haiti and the Dominican Republic). Almost no cases occur in Latin America despite a large outbreak in the 1990s. In Bangladesh and India, a substantial number of cases are also caused by *V. cholerae*

O139, which is covered by Shancol but not Dukoral vaccine (see below).

Dukoral, which is licensed as a cholera vaccine in 60 countries, is a killed whole-cell recombinant B-subunit (WC-rBS) oral vaccine that contains formalin and heat-inactivated whole bacterial cells from the *V. cholerae* O1 Inaba, Ogawa and El Tor strains and a recombinant B subunit of the toxin (Table 12.1).[19] WC-rBS is widely available outside but not in the USA, so may be purchased en route or on arrival by those few travelers for whom it is indicated. A second oral vaccine (Shanchol, bivalent inactivated vaccine against O1 and O139, no recombinant B-subunit) is currently only available in India, Vietnam and Indonesia.[20]

The oral WC-rBS subunit toxin vaccine has some protective efficacy against enterotoxigenic *E. coli* (ETEC) infection, a common cause of travelers' diarrhea. The basis of this is immunologic cross-reactivity between the B-subunit of cholera toxin and the LT toxin (heat labile) of ETEC. Dukoral is registered for protection against travelers' diarrhea in Canada, UK, New Zealand, Sweden, Norway and several other countries.[19] Results on protective efficacy against travelers' diarrhea vary within a broad range and are not conclusive with respect to a clear recommendation.[20,21]

Shanchol (or mORCVAX, other manufacturer and other preparation method, but identical type of vaccine) was licensed in 1997 in Vietnam and since that time more than 20 million doses have been used locally, mainly in children. In 2004 it was reformulated to meet GMP and WHO criteria, and in 2009 was licensed in India as Shanchol and mORCVAX in Vietnam.[22]

Indications

Cholera vaccine is not required for entry into any country under the current IHR (2005). Cholera vaccine is not recommended for the short-term tourist traveling to an endemic country. Indications for travelers are restricted to high-risk populations at immediate risk of cholera. This primarily includes emergency relief workers and healthcare workers in endemic and epidemic areas in proximity to displaced populations, especially in crowded camps and urban slums.

Contraindications and Precautions (Applies for both Vaccines)

- Severe allergic reaction (e.g., anaphylaxis) after a previous vaccine dose or to a vaccine component
- Moderate or severe acute illness with or without fever
- Do not administer WC-rBS in cases of acute febrile illness or acute GI illness
- Postpone in the event of persistent diarrhea or vomiting
- A history of severe local or systemic reactions following a previous dose is a contraindication
- Although the safety of Dukoral has not been studied in pregnant women, the risk is considered to be minimal since this is an inactivated oral vaccine. Depending on the context, administration to a pregnant woman may be considered after careful evaluation of benefits and risks
- WC-rBS vaccine has been shown to be well tolerated in breastfeeding women.

Dosing Schedules

For cholera prevention in adults Dukoral is taken in two doses, separated by 7–42 days. The series should be restarted if more than 42 days elapse. Each dose consists of 1 mg non-toxic subunit B and 10[11] killed *V. cholerae* taken with an alkaline buffer mixed in a glass of water. The acid-labile vaccine is taken on an empty stomach (1 h before or

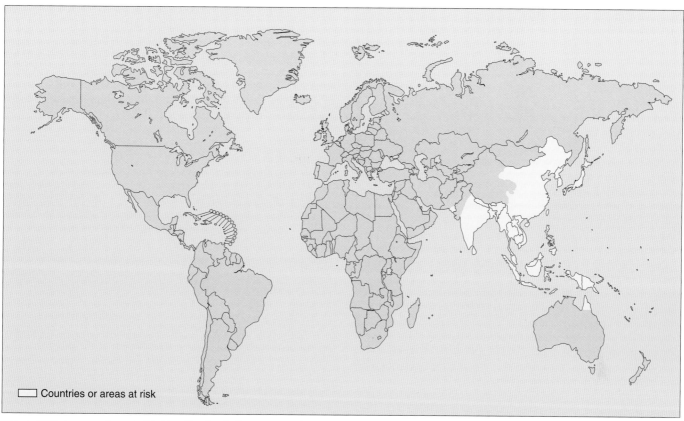

Figure 12.2 Japanese Encephalitis Map. Shading indicates areas where transmission is seasonal, generally May–November with a July–September peak. Consider vaccination for travelers who plan to spend more than short periods in endemic areas, particularly in rural farming areas during the transmission season. Travelers such as cyclists, hikers, and adventure travelers planning extensive unprotected outdoor, evening, and night-time exposure in rural areas may be at risk even if the trip is very short.

1 h after a meal). Vaccination should be completed at least 1 week prior to exposure. A booster of the same dose is recommended every 2 years for repeated exposure to cholera. In countries where WC-rBS has an indication for travelers' diarrhea boosters are required every 3 months for ETEC protection (Table 12.2).

Shanchol: The basic immunization schedule consists of two vaccinations 14 days apart; a booster is recommended after 2 years.

Measures of Immune Response and Duration of Immunity/Protection

Dukoral: The primary immunization series provides short-term protection (6 months) against cholera, with an overall protective efficacy of 85–90% and 50–60% for 2 years.[23] For adults and children >6 years of age, protective efficacy averages 63% over a 3-year period without a booster dose, but drops to <50% after the first year. The protective efficacy against classic and El Tor cholera is similar in the first 6 months. A large oral inoculum of bacteria can overwhelm even an optimal response to vaccine. Travelers should be advised to observe careful food and water precautions, regardless of vaccination status.

Shanchol: Results of clinical trials show a good safety profile, and a large Phase III efficacy trial in India confirmed a clinical efficacy of 67% after 2 years. An ongoing investigation will provide data on 5-year efficacy.

Adverse Events

Both vaccines: Side-effects have been reported as mild gastrointestinal symptoms. Rarely, some individuals have reported diarrhea, abdominal cramps, nausea, or fever (Table 12.3).

Drug and Vaccine Interactions

Because of the different buffers in the WC-rBS vaccine and the oral live attenuated Ty21a typhoid vaccine, it is recommended that the two vaccines be separated by at least 8 h. Limited data suggest that WC-rBS vaccine can be administered concurrently with YF vaccine.

Japanese Encephalitis Vaccine

Japanese encephalitis (JE) is a mosquito (*Culex* species)-transmitted flavivirus infection that is endemic in Asia (Fig. 12.2), with an estimated 67 000 cases each year.[24] There are two main patterns of transmission. In northern temperate regions of China, Siberia, Korea and Japan, transmission occurs in warmer months from April to November with a peak in July–September. Further south, the season extends from March to October. In tropical areas of South-East Asia and India, seasonal transmission is specific to local monsoon rain and bird migration patterns, sometimes with two annual peaks.[24,25] In 1995 JEV was reported in the Torres Strait islands, and in 1998 a case of Japanese encephalitis was reported from the Cape York Peninsula in Australia. Japanese encephalitis is mostly a disease in rural rice farming areas, where an enzootic cycle exists between the mosquitoes and wading birds, with pigs serving as amplification reservoirs. Increased risk is associated with monsoon season. Occasionally, epidemics have been reported in suburban areas of large cities in these countries, such as Hanoi (Vietnam), Lucknow (India), Bangkok (Thailand), Beijing and Shanghai (China). Japanese encephalitis infection is most often asymptomatic and neuroinvasive disease occurs in <1:250 of those infected. Seizures occur in >75% of children, whereas adults more commonly present with headache and meningism. The case-fatality rate of symptomatic cases is 5–30%, and approximately 60% of survivors will have permanent neurological sequelae, with half of these being left with severe neurological damage.[25]

The risk for travelers has been difficult to quantify. However, from 1973 to 2008, 55 cases of JE have been reported among unvaccinated travelers.[26] The majority of cases (60%) occurred in tourists (including persons who were visiting friends and relatives (VFRs) and students), 16% occurred in expatriates, and 11% in soldiers. Two-thirds of the travelers had a duration of travel > 1 month; however, even travel duration of less than 2 weeks was associated with JE infection, highlighting that even travel for short periods may pose a very small but measurable risk for sporadic cases of JE. Thirty-five per cent of travel-related cases were acquired in Thailand (particularly the Chiang Mai valley), 15% from Indonesia, 13% from China; no travel-related cases have been recorded from India. The case-fatality rate was 18%, 44% had neurological sequelae and only 22% recovered completely. The estimate of overall risk for JE for the average tourist to endemic areas is <1 : 1 000 000. In unimmunized intensely exposed soldiers in Asia, rates of 0.005–2.1 per 10 000 per week have been documented. These rates are similar to the rates of 0.1–1 per 10 000 per week for children in hyperendemic areas. Accepting the higher estimate and allowing for transmission in most areas being limited to 5 months of the year, the risk can be estimated as 1 per 200 000 per week of exposure. For long-term travelers and expatriates the rates may be similar to those for children living in hyperendemic areas (Table 12.3).

There are currently three Japanese encephalitis vaccines available and all are based on the SA-14-14-2 strain of JE (Table 12.1). These include an inactivated cell-culture vaccine, a live attenuated JE–yellow fever chimeric vaccine, and a live attenuated SA-14-14-2 vaccine. JE-Vax (Biken), an inactivated mouse brain-derived vaccine with a significant adverse effect profile frequently referenced in the literature, is no longer available anywhere.[27]

Inactivated Cell-Culture Vaccine, IC51

An inactivated cell-culture vaccine, IC51 (Novartis; IXIARO in US and Europe; JESPECT in Australia), made from the SA-14-14-2 strain of JE, has been approved for use in the USA, Europe, and Australia. Vaccination with IC51 is well tolerated.[28] A recent Phase II study in Indian children aged 1–3 years has shown that the vaccine was safe and immunogenic.[29] As of 2011, the vaccine is only approved for use in individuals over the age of 17, but ongoing Phase III pediatric studies are expected to lead to licensure in children. As of 2011, many authorities are sanctioning off-label use of IC-51 in children (see Chapter 13).

Chimeric JE Vaccine (JE-CV)

A chimeric JE vaccine (JE-CV; IMOJEV (Sanofi Pasteur) containing recombinant JE antigen on a backbone of live attenuated YF virus has recently been registered in Australia for use from the age of 12 months[27,30–32] (Table 12.1). As of 2012, there are no immediate plans to introduce this vaccine in either the US or Europe. The reactogenicity profile of JE-CV was comparable to that of placebo in adults[33] and to hepatitis A vaccine in children[34] (Table 12.2).

Live Attenuated SA-14-14-2 JE Vaccine

A single-dose live attenuated SA-14-14-2 JE vaccine is widely used in China and has also been approved for use in Korea, Nepal, Sri Lanka, India, and Thailand. The vaccine has recently been shown to be phenotypically and genotypically stable,[35] and reversion to neurovirulence is considered highly unlikely. WHO technical specifications have now been established for the vaccine's production. Live SA-14-14-2 vaccine

accounts for the majority of the world's production each year and has been administered to over 200 million children to date. The vaccine has been shown to have an efficacy of at least 95% following two doses administered at an interval of 1 year. Extensive use of this vaccine has contributed to a significant reduction in the burden of JE in China, from 2.5/100 000 in 1990 to <0.5/100 000 in 2004.[36] Smaller amounts of mouse brain-derived JEV for local use are also produced in India, Japan, Korea, Thailand, and Vietnam.[24,27,37]

Indications

The risk of JE in persons from non-endemic countries traveling to Asia is very low, with an overall estimated incidence of JE < 1 case per 1 million travelers. However, for expatriates and travelers who stay for prolonged periods in rural areas with active JEV transmission the risk likely reflects that among the susceptible resident population.[26,38] Factors for considering the JE vaccine are the duration of stay in the endemic area, extent of outdoor activities, especially in rural areas, and season of travel.[38] Extremes of age are associated with a higher likelihood of developing symptomatic disease. JE infection in a pregnant woman may potentially cause an intrauterine fetal infection or death.

An average short-term traveler's risk of acquiring JE during travel to endemic countries is low.[3,39] Urban-only itineraries generally present no risk, although there is some transmission at the suburban–rural interface in a few cities such as Beijing and Hanoi. Typical 1–2-week tourist itineraries that include brief trips to sites in rural areas, especially during the daytime, similarly present an insignificant risk. The following itineraries may justify JE vaccination of travelers:

- Persons expatriating to JE-endemic countries
- Consider JEV for travelers who plan to spend more than just a brief period in rural, predominantly farming areas of endemic countries during the transmission season. Travelers planning extensive unprotected outdoor, evening and night-time exposure in rural areas may be at risk even if the trip is very short. Vaccination should therefore be considered for short-term travelers (<1 month) to endemic areas during the JE transmission season if they plan to travel outside an urban area and their activities will increase the risk of exposure to JE.

As there are no clear data on the duration of immune response from natural infection, immigrants returning to their home countries should be vaccinated with the same guidelines as natives of industrialized countries.

Regardless of vaccination status, travelers should be counseled to take precautions against mosquito bites.

Contraindications and Precautions

- Severe allergic reaction (e.g. anaphylaxis) after a previous vaccine dose or to a vaccine component
- Moderate or severe acute illness with or without fever
- JE-CV vaccine is a live attenuated chimeric vaccine and consequently should not be used in immunocompromised individuals. The safety and immunogenicity of the vaccine in pregnancy has not been tested
- Live SA-14–14–2 vaccine should not be used in immunocompromised hosts or pregnant women.

Dosing Schedules

The primary schedule for IC51 consists of two doses intramuscularly at 0 and 28 days. This interval should not be reduced, as the efficacy of the vaccine is markedly reduced by using accelerated regimens. Antibody titers wane over the first 12–24 months after vaccination, and therefore a booster dose is recommended 12–24 months later for those at continued or renewed exposure in high-risk destinations (Table 12.1). Adult travelers who have previously completed a 3-dose primary series of mouse-brain vaccine (eg JE-VAX) require only 1 dose of JE Vero cell vaccine (Ixiaro; Novartis) to boost immunity. No recommendation on subsequent booster intervals is available at the time of publication.[40]

SA-14-14-2 and JE-CV vaccines are single-dose vaccines. Data suggest that a single dose of JE-CV will provide adequate seroprotection for at least 5 years.[41] In contrast, in China an SA-14-14-2 booster is administered to children at 1 year, but data indicate up to 11 years of efficacy after even a single dose[42,43] (Table 12.2).

Measures of Immune Response and Duration of Immunity/Protection

Vaccination with IC51 results in a seroconversion rate of 98% following a primary immunization series of two doses 28 days apart[44,45] (Table 12.2). Antibody titers wane over the first 12–24 months following vaccination.[46] Therefore, if the primary series of vaccine was administered more than 1 year previously, a booster dose should be given for those again traveling to or residing in high-risk destinations. A single-dose regimen for the last-minute traveler is much less effective than the standard two doses administered 28 days apart. At 28 days after receiving one dose of the vaccine only 41% of recipients will have seroconverted. At 56 days after receiving one dose of vaccine only 26% of the subjects who received a single dose will have a protective neutralising antibody level of PRNT50 ≥10, (defined as the serum dilution giving a 50% reduction in plaque count in a plaque reduction neutralistaion test) compared to 97% of subjects who have received two doses.[47] Two doses spaced by 14 days give similarly suboptimal responses compared to the standard 28-day spacing. The immunogenicity and safety of IC51 have not been studied in immunocompromised individuals and pregnant women.

JE-CV vaccine results in high seroconversion rates in both adults (99%)[33] and children (100% in children aged 2–5 years and 96% in infants aged 12–24 months).[34,48] After 1 year the seroprotection rates in the two age groups were 97% and 84%, respectively.[34] In adults the reported 5-year seroprotection rate after one dose of JE-CV vaccine is 93%, increasing to 97% if a second dose is given 6 months after the initial vaccination.[41] This study would support the use of a single dose of JE-CV for primary immunization in adult travelers.

A single dose of the live attenuated SA-14-14-2 JE vaccine results in at least 80% efficacy after a single dose and 97.5% efficacy following two doses administered at 1-year intervals,[37,49–51] and durable neutralizing antibody responses that persist for up to 5 years.[42,43]

Adverse Events

The modern JE vaccines based on the cell culture-derived SA14-14-2 strain of JEV are well tolerated. JE-CV results in injection site redness and pain swelling in <1% of vaccine recipients. Similarly, IC51 produces injection site redness, pain and swelling in 1% of recipients.[28,44] Severe or delayed hypersensitivity reactions have not been reported with either vaccine. In large randomized trials, live SA-14-14-2 has been equivalent to controls without any neurologic, febrile or allergic events.

Drug and Vaccine Interactions

Co-administration of other travel vaccines is not considered a risk factor for increasing adverse reactions to JEV. For JE-CV, prior immunization against yellow fever does not suppress the response to JE-CV. Similarly, prior immunization with JE-CV does not interfere with the immunogenicity of yellow fever vaccine.

Meningococcal Vaccine

Neisseria meningitidis spreads through the air via droplets of contaminated respiratory secretions, or through person-to-person contact (kissing, sharing cigarettes and drinking glasses, etc.). Humans are the only natural reservoir for *N. meningitidis*, and the bacteria may be carried in the nasopharynx of asymptomatic hosts in up to 10% of the population during periods of endemic infection. The carrier prevalence is highest among diverse populations mixing or living in crowded conditions (pilgrims on the *Hajj* and *Umrha* in Saudi Arabia, military recruits, students living in dormitories, campers at youth camps, participants in rave concerts, etc.).

There are at least 13 distinct serogroups of *Neisseria meningitides*, although the majority of human infections are caused by serogroups A, B, C, Y, and W-135. Of the five, serogroups A and C are most often associated with epidemics of meningitis, especially in the sub-Saharan Africa 'meningitis belt' during the dry, winter months from December to June annually.[52–54] In recent years, serogroup W-135 has emerged as an epidemic strain in Africa and the Middle East, although serogroup A still predominates (Fig. 12.3). Although serogroup A caused epidemics of meningococcal disease in China, Mongolia, India, and Nepal in the 1970s, and also was associated with an epidemic in Mongolia in the early 1990s, there is currently no excess travel-related risk. Serogroup B causes the majority of the sporadic invasive meningococcal disease seen in the USA and most other industrialized countries, but no group B vaccine has been licensed apart from a vaccine against a local strain in New Zealand.

Several meningococcal polysaccharide vaccines are in current use. Menomune (Sanofi pasteur) and Mencevax ACWY (GlaxoSmithKline) are A, C, Y, W-135 quadrivalent meningococcal polysaccharide vaccines that have been used in North America and many other industrialized countries since 1981. Bivalent (A+C) meningococcal polysaccharide vaccines are widely available in Europe, the Middle East, and Africa, and A-only as well as ACW vaccines are also available (Table 12.1).

Three quadrivalent conjugate vaccines have now been licensed. Menactra (MCV4) (Sanofi Pasteur), the first quadrivalent (A, C, Y, W-135) protein conjugate vaccine, was introduced in 2005. Menactra contains meningococcal polysaccharide conjugated to a small amount of diphtheria toxoid. Menveo (MenACWY-CRM) (Novartis Vaccines) was licensed in 2010 and consists of meningococcal groups A, C, Y, and W-135 oligosaccharide conjugated to CRM197 (non-toxic diphtheria toxin mutant).[55–59] Nimenrix (MenACWY-TT) (Glaxo Smith Kline) was licensed in 2012 and consists of meningococcal groups A, C, Y, W-135 oligosaccharide conjugated to tetanus toxoid. Oligosaccharide–protein conjugate vaccines produce a long-lived T-cell-dependent response to a polysaccharide that normally induces a less robust T-cell-independent response (Table 12.1).

Indications

Travelers to the classic meningitis-prone areas in equatorial Africa (Fig. 12.3) during the December–June dry season, especially if prolonged contact with the local populace is anticipated, and all long-stay travelers should be vaccinated against meningococcal meningitis with a quadrivalent vaccine. Out-of-season epidemics have been reported in Sudan, Ethiopia, Somalia, and Tanzania, indicating possible changes in epidemiologic trends, perhaps due to climatic changes. Occasionally, meningococcal epidemics may extend to other 'meningitis-prone' sub-Saharan countries, such as Angola, Democratic Republic of Congo, Zambia, Mozambique, Uganda, Rwanda, Burundi, and Tanzania. International agencies and NGOs are increasingly recommending vaccination of staff to these 'meningitis-prone' countries, and especially for travelers to areas with current outbreaks. Healthcare workers traveling to any of the above countries at any time of year

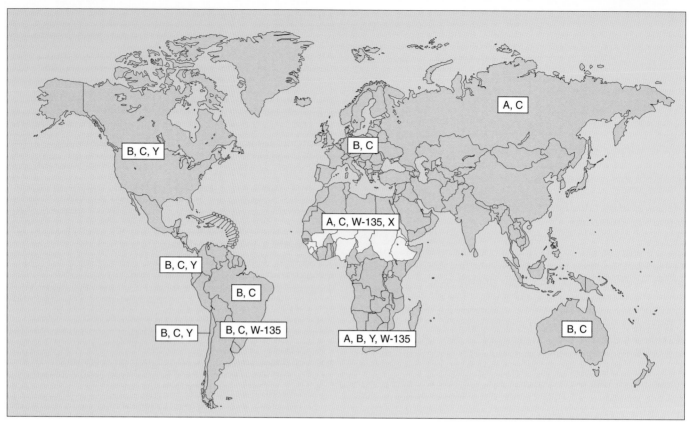

Figure 12.3 Meningococcal Serogroup Global Geographic Distribution. *(Harrison LH, Trotter CL, Ramsay ME. Global epidemiology of meningococcal disease. Vaccine 2009; 27 Suppl 2: B51–63.)*

should be vaccinated. Quadrivalent conjugate vaccines are preferred for these travelers. In the US MCV4 is licensed for use from ages 9 months to 55 years, MenACWY-CRM for use in those from 2 to 55 years old and Nimenrix in those from the age of 12 months and above. Expanded pediatric licensure is expected in 2012 or soon thereafter. The conjugated vaccines are effective in adults over 55 and can be offered in this age group if there is a clear indication for use.[52,54,55,60–66] The Advisory Committee on Immunization Practices (ACIP)[67] in the US recommends quadrivalent meningococcal conjugate vaccine for all persons aged 9 months and over who are at increased risk for meningococcal disease, including travelers to countries where meningococcus is hyperendemic or epidemic.[65]

Polysaccharide meningococcal vaccine containing A + C or A serogroup is less costly, but its use should be discouraged in travelers to the meningitis belt. As of 2002, Saudi Arabia requires proof of vaccination with a quadrivalent vaccine within the previous 3 years (both conjugate and polysaccharide vacines are acceptable) before issuing entry visas for the *Hajj* pilgrimage. Prior immunization with the meningococcal C conjugate vaccine does not substitute for a quadrivalent vaccine for pilgrims requiring these vaccines for travel to the *Hajj*.

The requirement for quadrivalent or C-conjugate or A + C conjugate varies by institution and national government policy. Meningococcal vaccine is also recommended for all travelers with anatomical or functional asplenia, and those with component deficiencies in the terminal common complement pathway (C3, C5–C9), as individuals with these conditions are at increased risk of death from overwhelming sepsis due to meningococcal infections.

Contraindications and Precautions

- Severe allergic reaction (e.g. anaphylaxis) after a previous vaccine dose or to a vaccine component

- Persons with a prior history of Guillain–Barré syndrome and who are not high risk for meningococcal disease should avoid vaccination with MCV4
- Meningococcal vaccine should not be given in pregnancy unless substantial risk exists. Known hypersensitivity to diphtheria toxoid is a contraindication for MCV4 and MenACWY-CRM. Both MCV4 and MPSV4 may be administered in pregnancy if clearly indicated for travel
- Moderate or severe acute illness with or without fever.

Dosing Schedules

The quadrivalent conjugate vaccines are administered as a single 0.5 mL IM dose. The quadrivalent polysaccharide vaccines are administered as a single dose of 0.5 mL by subcutaneous injection. This vaccine should be administered 1–2 weeks before departure to allow maximum antibody response. In adults, a booster every 5 years should be administered if the risk of disease continues (Table 12.2). This interval is based on meningococcal epidemiology in developed countries, and more rapidly waning titers against serogroup A endemic in Africa should lead clinicians to consider boosters after 3 years for high-risk travel.

Measures of Immune Response/Duration of Immunity/ Protection

The efficacy of serogroups A and C polysaccharide vaccines has been estimated at 85–100% among adults. Serogroup Y and W-135 efficacy data do not exist, but the vaccine is highly immunogenic against these serogroups. As the immune response is T-cell independent, long-term immunity does not occur. Multiple doses of serogroup A- and/or C-containing polysaccharide vaccines may induce immune hyporesponsiveness to future doses of these serogroups.

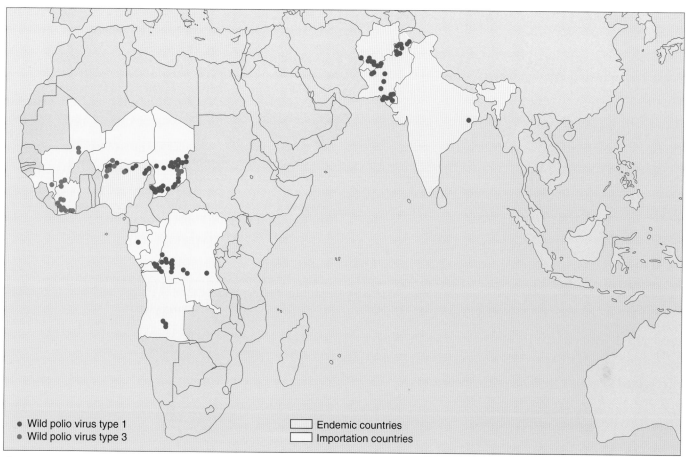

Figure 12.4 Polio Endemic Areas as of June 2011 (WHO).

MenACWY-CRM vaccine was licensed on the basis of non-inferiority in immunogenicity to quadrivalent polysaccharide vaccine.[55–58,68] MenACWY-CRM similarly demonstrated close to 100% 28-day immunogenicity for all four serogroups in adults. At 3 years, antibody titers were significantly higher in those given Men-ACWY-CRM than in those given quadrivalent polysaccharide vaccine.[54,60–64] MenACWY-CRM is also safe and immunogenic in infants and toddlers, in whom the administration of two doses of MenACWY-CRM results in hSBA titers ≥8 in 100% for C, W-135, and Y, 84% for A, and 96% for C.[60,69]

In three comparative studies of the persistence of immune response after a single dose of MenACWY-CRM compared to MCV4 in adults a significantly higher proportion of MenACWY-CRM recipients than MCV4 recipients had persisting hSBA titers ≥8 for serogroups A, W-135 and Y.[63,64] At 1 month after vaccination 95–100% of recipients have SBA titers ≥8 and 91–100% titers ≥ 128. However, these proportions fall significantly with both vaccines after 22 months, with 60–97% having titers ≥ 8 and 49–94% titers ≥ 128.[70]

Adverse Events

The most commonly reported adverse reactions in adolescents and adults are local pain, headache, and fatigue. Except for redness in adults, local reactions were reported more frequently after MCV4 than MPSV4.[69] In the first 18 months of use 17 reports of Guillain–Barré syndrome occurring in teens 2–4 weeks after administration of quadrivalent conjugate vaccine indicated an excess of 1.25 cases per million doses of vaccine over expected incidence rates, which is lower than the attack rate of meningococcal disease in most

settings.[71] At present there is insufficient evidence to suggest a causal effect (Table 12.3).

Drug and Vaccine Interactions

Concomitant administration of MCV4, which contains diphtheria toxoid, with Td did not result in reduced tetanus, diphtheria, or meningococcal antibody responses compared to MCV4 given 28 days after Td. Concomitant administration of MCV4 with Td did not result in increased adverse events such as local pain, redness, and swelling at the injection sites.

Polio Vaccine

Polio is eradicated from most of the world but still circulates in many developing countries, particularly in Africa and the Indian subcontinent (Fig. 12.4). Poliovirus is an enteric virus transmitted by oral–fecal contamination of food and water in areas of poor sanitation. Risk to travelers to endemic areas was minimal even when polio was common worldwide, and is even lower currently in the pre-eradication phase in countries where the polio virus still circulates. However, WHO is emphasizing the public health utility of vaccinating travelers so that they do not act as vectors in transporting polio to a country that has already eradicated the infection. Details of WHO's position on the use of polio vaccines may be accessed through http://www.who.int/wer/2010/wer8523.pdf.

Oral polio vaccine is no longer available in most developed countries for either adult or pediatric immunization. Inactivated polio vaccine (enhanced potency IPV) is produced by a large number of manufacturers worldwide.

Indications for Polio Vaccines

Adults traveling to countries where the polio virus currently circulates or where cases are currently reported should be immune to polio (Fig. 12.4).[72] Travelers who have received three or more doses of either OPV or IPV at any time previously should receive one dose of IPV vaccine before leaving.[72] Non-immunized individuals should receive a complete series of inactivated vaccine. Many clinicians vaccinate travelers to all African countries because of the significant numbers of introduced cases that have occurred in recent years in many non-endemic countries. All *Hajj* travelers should be immune to polio owing to the large number of pilgrims originating in Africa.

Dosing Schedules

The adult booster dose consists of 0.5 mL of IPV administered IM. Adults who completed a primary series after childhood should have the one-time booster dose if more than 10 years has elapsed since completion of the primary series. However, there is strong evidence that IPV protects for much longer, possibly for up to two decades.[73] The primary immunization schedule for adults consists of three doses of 0.5 mL IPV administered by IM injection at 0, 2, and 8–14 months (Table 12.2).

Accelerated Schedules for Primary IPV Immunization

Previously unimmunized travelers and/or those whose immunization status is unknown should complete the primary three-dose IPV series before travel to a polio-endemic or -epidemic area, although even a single primary dose prior to travel is of benefit. The minimum recommended interval between IPV doses is 4 weeks. When the traveler is leaving imminently and time is short, the following schedules can be used: if there is a month before travel, the second dose should be given 1 month after the first; if at least 8 weeks are available three doses of IPV can be given 4 weeks apart.

Contraindications

- Severe allergic reaction (e.g., anaphylaxis) after a previous vaccine dose or to a vaccine component
- IPV should not be given to persons with a history of anaphylactic reaction to neomycin, polymyxin B, or streptomycin.

Precautions

Moderate or severe acute illness with or without fever. Caution should also be exercised if administering polio vaccine to pregnant women.

Side-Effects

Injection site pain, fever; rarely anaphylaxis or other systemic effects.

Rabies Vaccine

Rabies is a viral zoonosis transmitted in most countries of the world. WHO estimates that there are around 55 000 fatal cases per year, although the numbers are likely to be grossly under-reported.[74] The difference among countries is in the degree of endemicity, highest in India, with 2×10^{-5} per population at risk. Countries with higher prevalence of rabies include countries in South Asia (the Indian subcontinent), and SE Asia, especially Thailand. Countries in Central and South America have largely controlled rabies in recent years (Fig. 12.5).

WHO defines a rabies-free country as one with no animal or human cases of rabies in 2 consecutive years. Some rabies-free countries have had no cases in 100 or more years, whereas others have been considered rabies free for much shorter periods of time, so that the list may change slightly on an ongoing basis. Surveillance is better in more developed countries than in less developed countries. Small numbers of fatal human cases of bat *Lyssavirus* infection have occurred in several countries in recent years, including the UK and Australia, both considered rabies free. Bat *Lyssaviruses* and rabies virus are closely related members of the *Lyssavirus* family (11 species in total) and several of them may cause clinical rabies in terrestrial mammals, including humans. European bat *Lyssavirus* is carried by insectivorous bats in several European countries, some of which are considered rabies free, and does not transmit readily to terrestrial species, so that human infection is rare. Risk to travelers from these *Lyssaviruses* is virtually non-existent and rabies pre-exposure immunization is not recommended. Post-exposure rabies prophylaxis may be considered for documented bat bites in rabies-free countries with known endemicity of bat *Lyssaviruses*. Regular occupational exposure to bats might be considered an indication for rabies pre-exposure vaccination even in rabies-free countries.

Dogs are responsible for 99% of rabies transmission in Asia, Africa, and Latin America. However, other animals implicated in transmission of rabies include cats, monkeys, tigers, rabbits, rats, mongoose, and squirrels. Small rodents, although highly susceptible to rabies, transmit rabies poorly to humans and therefore are not major vectors. Bats play an important role in rabies transmission in the USA and increasingly in other parts of the world. Important vectors in Europe, Canada, Alaska, and the former Soviet Union include foxes and the raccoon dog.

There are many different rabies vaccine formulations available throughout the world (Table 12.1). Among all the rabies vaccine products, the modern cell-culture vaccines (CCV) are the safest and most immunogenic. HDCV (human diploid cell vaccine), PCECV (chick embryo cell vaccine) vaccines, and Verocell vaccines are the most widely distributed CCVs. Distribution of RVA (fetal rhesus cell) is more limited. The production cost of these cultured-cell vaccines is high, making the CCV vaccines relatively unaffordable and thus not always easily available in many developing countries.

Rabies vaccine can be used as a pre-exposure vaccination or – in previously unvaccinated persons – as a combined active/passive immunization together with (human) rabies immunoglobulin. Vaccination schedule will depend on either indication; see below.

Indications for Pre-Exposure Vaccination

Rabies is not a common travel-acquired infection but has potentially long latency (up to several months) and uniformly fatal outcome. Advice on avoiding animal contact is essential for pre-travel counseling. Expatriates, so-called 'pet addicts' and young children who are less likely to report animal bites are at higher risk. Pre-exposure prophylaxis (PreP) is recommended for anyone who will be at continual, frequent or increased risk of exposure to rabies virus, especially if travel is to the highest-prevalence countries and the travelers belong to one of the groups below:

- Long-term travelers or expatriates going to a risk country
- Shorter-duration travelers at high risk for exposure during travel, such as those who are very likely to come in contact with animals in dog rabies enzootic areas and where near immediate access to appropriate medical care, including CCV vaccine and rabies immunoglobulin (RIg), might be limited. Risk groups include adventure travelers, bikers, hikers, cave explorers, or business travelers who travel for short but frequent trips and plan to go running outdoors on these trips
- Persons with potential occupational exposure.

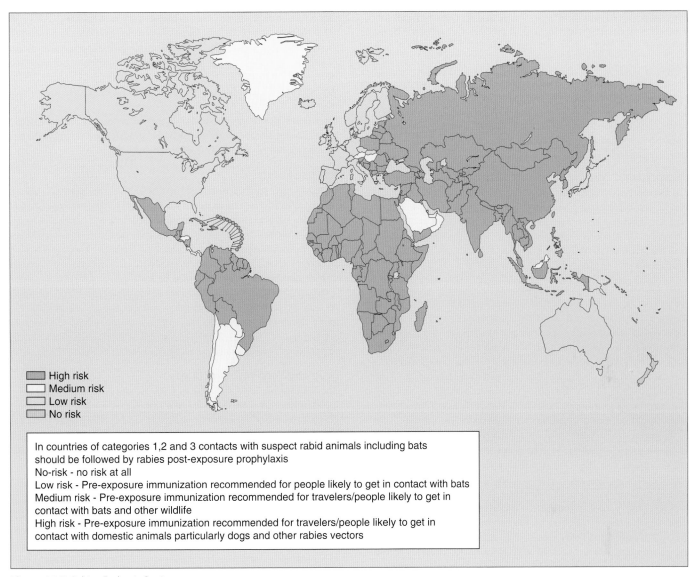

☐ High risk
☐ Medium risk
☐ Low risk
☐ No risk

In countries of categories 1,2 and 3 contacts with suspect rabid animals including bats
should be followed by rabies post-exposure prophylaxis
No-risk - no risk at all
Low risk - Pre-exposure immunization recommended for people likely to get in contact with bats
Medium risk - Pre-exposure immunization recommended for travelers/people likely to get in
contact with bats and other wildlife
High risk - Pre-exposure immunization recommended for travelers/people likely to get in
contact with domestic animals particularly dogs and other rabies vectors

Figure 12.5 Rabies-Endemic Regions.

Contraindications

- Severe allergic reaction (e.g., anaphylaxis) after a previous vaccine dose or to a vaccine component
- Persons with a history of 'immune-complex-like' hypersensitivity from a HDCV rabies vaccine dose should not have more doses of HDCV unless a high-risk bite has occurred and RVA or PCEC vaccines are not available.

Precautions

Moderate or severe acute illness with or without fever. The earlier rabies vaccines were derived from infected brain/neural tissue of animals (Semple vaccines) or cultured in embryonated duck eggs (duck embryo vaccine or DEV). These older vaccines were less efficacious than the modern CCVs and were associated with potentially severe adverse effects. The neural tissue-derived vaccines contained myelin basic protein, which has been associated with the development of myeloencephalitis. Because of cost, the older types of vaccine are available and still used mostly in Asia. Travelers should be specifically advised to avoid these vaccines should post-exposure immunization be required during travel to developing countries, and

to accept a possible delay up to 1 day to achieve immunization with CCV.

Dosing Schedules

Pre-Exposure Vaccination

The widely available CCVs against rabies are considered interchangeable. The standard primary pre-exposure CCV series consists of three doses of 1.0 mL each given intramuscularly in the deltoid on days 0, 7 and 28, but the day 28 dose can be advanced towards day 21 if time is short (Table 12.2).[74]

Intradermal dosing of CCV is highly economical and is endorsed by the WHO as an acceptable alternative. Antibody titers are uniformly adequate, though not as high as after IM dosing.[75] Vaccine packaging for 0.1 mL intradermal dosing at 0, 7, and 21–28 days, which had been in use for many years, is no longer available from any manufacturer. The 1.0 mL vials reconstituted to use for 10 ID doses must be used within 1 h. Because the current 1.0 mL vials are generally not specifically manufactured to specifications for multi-dose vials, use of ID regimens may pose liability issues in some countries. Only individuals highly trained and experienced with intradermal injections should administer vaccine in this way. Inadvertent subcutaneous infiltration of the vaccine will produce an ineffective immune response.

Boosting

Routine boosters are only recommended for persons with continuous (occupational) risk. Preferably, such subjects should be tested for antibodies every 6 months to 2 years and boosters should be given accordingly. Data support that in most cases vaccine-induced immunity will persist for many years, and boosting is possible even 20 years after the primary course.[76]

Accepted and Possible Accelerated Schedules

For persons traveling imminently, the rabies pre-exposure vaccination can be accelerated to a schedule of three injections given on days 0, 7 and 21. Several other accelerated schedules (0–3–7; 0–0–7) are considered to be suitable; however, evidence from studies is lacking and it is unclear how to deal with respect to RIg in such subjects in case of exposure.

Post-Exposure Vaccination (PEP)

All travelers going to rabies-endemic areas should be advised to immediately cleanse the animal bite wounds, scratches or saliva contact by vigorous scrubbing with large amounts of soap and water to remove animal saliva as quickly as possible. If no pre-exposure vaccination course with a CCV is documented such persons should receive as a standard WHO recommendation a full five-dose series of CCV rabies vaccine (0–3–7–14–28) for post-exposure treatment in addition to (human) rabies immunoglobulin ((H)RIg; 20 IU/kg; as much as possible should be administered into or around the wound site).[77]

However, WHO offer also an alternative schedule of active PEP immunization, consisting of four doses instead of five (0–0–7–21) which applies two doses on day 0 in each of the two deltoid sites, followed by one dose each on days 7 and 21. This schedule is closely related to the old Zagreb PEP schedule.[78]

CDC and WHO recommend a four-dose PEP schedule (0–3–7–14) as an alternative in 1) healthy, fully immunocompetent individuals who 2) receive (qualified) wound care and 3) high-quality human rabies immunoglobulin and 4) WHO pre-qualified rabies vaccines. Taking suboptimal PEP conditions for travelers into account, this schedule will mostly not be applicable.[77,79]

Increasingly human RIg (HRIg), which is necessary if there is no history of pre-exposure immunization, is either scarce or only rabies immunoglobulin of equine origin (ERIg) is available. Although the adverse event rate (serum sickness) is low with purified ERIg (e.g., Favirab, Sanofi Pasteur), which is increasingly widely distributed and the potency good, ERIg use should still be restricted to situations where HRIg is unavailable, and should not be used solely to reduce cost. A decision to administer post-exposure rabies vaccine in a previously unimmunized person is also a decision to administer HRIg no matter the length of time since the actual bite. However, if HRIg is not available, vaccine should be immediately started and HRIg only administered if it can be started within 7 days of starting the rabies vaccine series, otherwise the HRIg will interfere with the beneficial effect of the CCV.

In pre-immunized subjects (full basic immunization of three vaccinations at regular intervals is required), in case of potential exposure two additional vaccinations serving as boosters are given on days 0 and 3; no immunoglobulin is required irrespective of the time elapsed since the basic course.

Measures of Immune Response and Duration of Immunity/Protection

There have been no placebo-controlled randomized studies on efficacy. However, three doses given during a 21–28-day schedule induce protective antibody levels (in surrogate tests such as the RFFIT) in 100% of individuals. To date there is no vaccine breakthrough reported in subjects with regular PreP and adequate post-exposure treatment. Minimal intervals between doses in the series should be respected because of the lack of specific data on other than the 0, 7, and 21–28-day regimen and the uniformly fatal outcome of rabies. Individuals who have had fewer than three doses of rabies vaccine or have had three doses at unapproved intervals should be considered completely unvaccinated for the purposes of post-exposure care regimens unless antibodies can be demonstrated by serology.

Adverse Events

Injection site pain is observed in 35–45% of recipients.[74] Other, mostly mild adverse effects noted with the CCV rabies vaccine include headache, nausea, abdominal pain, muscle aches, and dizziness (occurring in approximately 5–15%). Urticaria, pruritus, and malaise or other 'immune-complex-like' illness may be experienced by 6% of persons receiving HDCV booster vaccinations. Urticaria was noted in a small number of recipients of PCECV.[80]

Inactivated nerve tissue vaccines made from the brains of adult animals or suckling mice (Semple vaccines), which are available in many developing countries, may induce neuroparalytic reactions in approximately 1/200–1/2000 persons and 1/8000 persons vaccinated, respectively. Travelers need to avoid these vaccines (Table 12.3).

Drug and Vaccine Interactions

The IM formulations of the rabies CCV do not have any specific drug interactions and there is no known interaction with other vaccines. Concurrent use of chloroquine phosphate and possibly other structurally related antimalarials such as mefloquine may interfere with antibody response to intradermal CCV. In situations where the antimalarials need to be started before travel, IM CCV should be administered.

Tick-Borne Encephalitis Vaccine

Tick-borne encephalitis (TBE) is the most prevalent cause of viral infections of the central nervous system in most Central and Northern European countries and the Russian Federation, and is also endemic in China and Mongolia. The endemic areas cover the southern part of the non-tropical Eurasian forest belt (Fig 12.6). Around 8500 cases are reported every year, but significant under-reporting is suggested. Between 1974 and 2004 a 400% increase in cases was reported in Europe; TBE was found in several new regions and in higher altitudes up to 1.600 m. At present the highest incidence of clinical cases is reported from Russia (regionally), Slovenia, the Baltic states and the Czech Republic.[81] The responsible flavivirus is transmitted by infected ticks (mostly *Ixodes ricinus* and *I. persulcatus*), regionally also by unpasteurized dairy products, particularly goats' milk. Three virus subtypes (European, Siberian, and Far Eastern) are described, being closely related both phylogenetically and antigenically. Clinical manifestation of the disease varies between asymptomatic infection, flu-like disease and characteristic biphasic febrile/neurologic illness. Case-fatality rate is around 1% for the European subtype, 6–8% for the Siberian subtype and up to 20% for the Far Eastern subtype. In ≤40% of encephalitic cases the disease is followed by neurologic sequelae, which are characteristic for postencephalitic syndrome. The disease tends to be more severe with age and there is no treatment available.

Currently there are two cell culture-derived formalin-inactivated TBE vaccines in use in Europe: Encepur (Novartis) and FSME-IMMUN (Baxter), manufactured in Germany and Austria, respectively (Table 12.1).[82] The K23 and Neudoerfl strains used are highly homologous and so are assumed to induce the same immune response.[83] These vaccines are not available in the USA, but the FSME-IMMUN

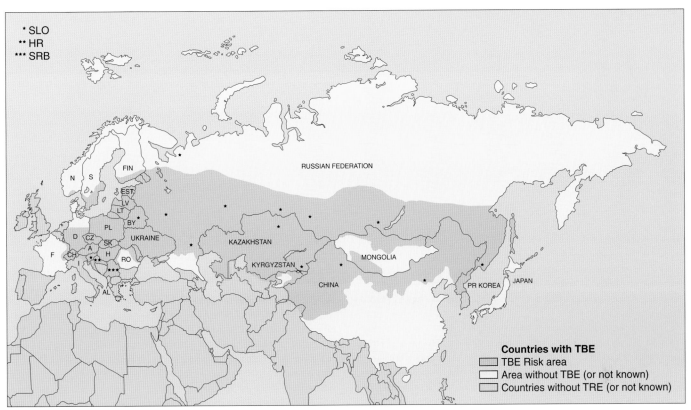

Figure 12.6 Tick-Borne Encephalitis-Endemic Areas. *(Adapted after Solomon T, Dung NM, Kneen R, Gainsborough M, Vaughn DW, Khanh VT. Japanese encephalitis. J Neurol Neurosurg Psychiatry 2000;68:405–15.)*

is available by special release in Canada and both vaccines are available in the UK on a named-patient basis.

Two inactivated TBE vaccines are available locally in the Russian Federation (TBE vaccine Moscow and EnceVir) and some neighbouring countries.[84]

Indications

Risk to travelers is low unless extensive outdoor activities are planned in forested regions of countries where TBE is prevalent. In highly endemic regions such as rural Austria risk is calculated to be 1/10 000 per month during transmission season (April–November), but solid surveillance data on exported TBE cases from endemic countries are missing.[85] The decision to vaccinate travelers should take into account precise itinerary, duration of stay in risk areas, activities, intensity of TBE in the risk areas, and the transmission season. Travelers hiking, camping, or engaging in similar outdoor activities in rural wooded areas in risk regions are at highest risk. Vaccination strategy in endemic countries varies extraordinarily: only Austria has implemented a mass vaccination program of the whole population, resulting in a decrease in yearly cases by 90% in 25 years.[86]

Criteria

- Active immunization with the TBE vaccine is recommended for persons planning to expatriate or live for an extended period of time in endemic countries with ongoing transmission
- Short-term travelers going to work (e.g., farmers, woodcutters, field work) or planning on adventure travel, extensive outdoors exposure, or camping in the forests of the endemic countries during the endemic season.

Contraindications

- Severe allergic reaction (e.g., anaphylaxis) after a previous vaccine dose or to a vaccine component
- Moderate or severe acute illness with or without fever
- TBE vaccine is formally contraindicated in persons with hypersensitivity to eggs
- Pregnant or lactating women, or persons with a history of autoimmune diseases, should undergo vaccination only if the risk of TBE disease is high and the vaccine is considered necessary.

Dosing Schedules (Table 12.4)

All TBE vaccines are whole virus, alum adsorbed and inactivated vaccines. They follow a three-dose conventional schedule (0–(1–3) –(9–12) month) with a first booster after 3 years and consecutive boosters dependent on age after 5 years (subjects under 60 years of age) or after 3 years (over 60 years of age). However, for the Western vaccines 'accelerated' schedules have been licensed, allowing with two (0–14 days) or three (0–7-21 days) vaccinations a faster immunization, consecutive boosters depending on the respective schedule of the primary immunization. Details for immunization schedules may be achieved through: http://www.who.int/wer/2011/wer8624.pdf (WHO position paper)

Measures of Immune Response and Duration of Immunity/Protection

Both European TBE vaccines induce seroconversion rates of nearly 100% after three doses on the conventional schedule. Seroconversion with both Encepur and FSME-IMMUN is close to 100% after two

Table 12.4 There are Several Dosing Schedules Licensed for the European and Russian Vaccines®

Schedule	Encepur®					
	Basic immunization (days)				Boosters (years)	
	First	Second	Third	Fourth	First booster	Subsequent boosters
Conventional	0	28–90	270–365	–	3	5(3*)
Rapid	0	7	21	365–540	5(3*)	5(3*)
FSME-IMMUN®						
Conventional	0	28–90	270–365	–	3	5(3*)
Accelerated	0	14	150–365	–	3	5(3*)

*Boosting every 5 years, 3 years only for persons > 60 years of age.

conventional-schedule doses. On the accelerated schedules Encepur gives 100% seroconversion after three doses, and FSME-IMMUN gives 95% seroconversion after two doses. The antibodies induced are protective towards all strains of TBE.[87] In persons with history of a flavivirus disease or vaccination, antibody tests may be biased (except the neutralization test).[88]

The European TBE vaccines have been proved very effective. Vaccination in regularly vaccinated subjects will confer nearly 100% protection.[89] Vaccination breakthroughs do occur, but are very rare.[84]

Immunity after basic immunization will persist for at least 3 years, and after consecutive boosters for 5 years minimum.[90] In older persons (>60 years of age) there is some evidence that boosters should be given at 3-year intervals.[91] There is little evidence about immunogenicity and efficacy in immunocompromised subjects.[84] No post-exposure prophylaxis (immunoglobulins) is available.

Adverse Events

The European TBE vaccines are considered to be safe.[92] Local reactions can occur with both vaccines. Occasionally fatigue, nausea, lymphadenitis, or headaches occur. Fever and rash may be seen. Rarely, neurological side-effects such as neuritis have been reported, but causal relationship is not clear.

Drug and Vaccine Interactions

The vaccines are interchangeable after the basic immunization course.

Vaccines Used in Special Circumstances

Anthrax Vaccine

Although anthrax is uncommon in industrialized countries and the true global estimate is unknown, it still occurs in rural agricultural parts of many countries. Anthrax is reported from Southern and Eastern Europe, Asia, Africa, the Middle East, Caribbean, Central and South America as an occupational disease among persons who work in close contact with livestock, hides, and wool, and the majority of the cases are cutaneous. In 2001 anthrax spores were used as an agent of bio-terrorism. The risk of anthrax to the international traveler is negligible and never enough to warrant vaccination.

The availability of anthrax vaccine products and their formulation are variable worldwide. In the USA, the vaccine is currently available only through the military and restricted government agencies. Anthrax vaccine absorbed (AVA), licensed in 1965, is prepared from cell-free filtrates of bacterial cultures and contains no live or dead bacteria. It is administered in six doses: one dose subcutaneously at 0, 2, and 4 weeks followed by boosters at 6, 12, and 18 months, with annual boosters thereafter. Approximately 95% of vaccinees demonstrate

antibody response by indirect hemagglutination after three doses. The protective efficacy of the AVA is approximately 92% in preventing disease. Approximately 95% of vaccinees seroconvert after three doses. However, the correlation between antibody titer and protection against infection has not been defined. There are no data on the use of AVA in persons <18 years or >65 years of age. The duration of the efficacy is unknown. Mild local reactions occur in approximately 30% of recipients, moderate local reactions occur in 4%, and severe local reactions (erythema and induration >20 mm) occur in <0.2%. Systemic reactions (fever, chills, myalgia, nausea) following vaccination occur in 5–35% of recipients. In case of known and documented exposure to aerosolized spores, prophylaxis with ciprofloxacin or doxycycline for 60 days should be initiated.

Smallpox

Naturally occurring smallpox, caused by variola virus, was declared eradicated by the WHO in 1979. Global eradication of smallpox followed a successful WHO immunization campaign using vaccinia vaccine in the preceding decades. The last case of naturally occurring smallpox was reported from Somalia in 1977. Currently, smallpox is not considered a risk for international travelers.

Supplies of the vaccinia vaccine and vaccinia immunoglobulin are officially stockpiled and controlled by national governments. Existing stocks of vaccine now consist of newer cell culture-based vaccines. ACAM-2000 is a modern live virus cell-culture vaccine produced in Vero cells by Acambis and Baxter and is derived from the same vaccinia strain as was Dryvax. It was licensed in 2007. It is a clonal vaccine, based on a single type of NYBOH vaccinia virus, which has been well characterized. In 2007 it was licensed by the US FDA. It should not be administered to children under the age of 1 year and is labeled only for emergency use in children from 1 to 17 years of age. The US strategic stockpile now contains 300 million doses of the vaccine, and 30 other national governments currently hold a total of 420 million additional doses. ACAM-2000 is not commercially available but is held by various government authorities.

The vaccine is administered by a unique percutaneous multiple puncture technique with a bifurcated needle. All other possible routes of administration have been proved ineffective. Adverse effects following immunization include the development of a pustule, erythema, induration and tenderness at the vaccine site, and regional lymphadenitis. Inadvertent autoinoculation of the vaccine virus can result in a severe vaccinia virus infection involving the face, eyes, and other body sites. More severe side-effects include myocarditis, eczema vaccinatum, progressive vaccinia (vaccinia necrosum) infection, post-vaccination encephalitis, and keratitis. The vaccine is contraindicated in persons with eczema, pregnancy, or immunodeficient states such as HIV/

AIDS or other. During an outbreak of documented smallpox, the risk of exposure to smallpox versus the risks of vaccine-related complications must be weighed between the vaccine candidate and the healthcare provider.

Two different attenuated viral vaccines have been developed. The first, modified vaccinia Ankara (MVA), developed in Germany (Imvamune (US), Imvanexr (Europe); Bavarian Nordic), is a strain of vaccinia that cannot replicate inside human cells. MVA is therefore unable to cause a severe or spreading infection. As of 2012 fast track approval is underway at FDA, EMA, and the Public Health Agency of Canada. It is given through conventional routes and not via a bifurcated needle (as is the procedure for ACAM2000). The second, LC16m8 was developed in Japan in the 1970s and is now licensed in Japan. The vaccine was tested in 50 000 Japanese children and no significant complications were reported. Both vaccines are considered safer than the conventional smallpox vaccine, particularly for people with weakened immune systems, pregnant women, and children.

Plague Vaccine

Yersinia pestis, the bacterium that causes plague, is prevalent in many countries of Asia, Africa, Central and South America, and in parts of North America and southeastern Europe. Disease transmission can occur through bites of infected rat fleas, direct exposure to body fluids of infected rodents, or rarely by aerosolization. Usual short-term and long-term travelers are at negligible risk of exposure to plague. However, the risk increases with travel to rural, semiarid and mountainous regions by travelers who hike or camp in rural locations, or who handle dead or infected animals as part of their work in countries where plague is enzootic.

Access to plague vaccine is subject to regional availability and product formulations worldwide. Most plague vaccines are formalin-inactivated whole-cell bacterial vaccine. There are limited controlled human studies evaluating vaccine efficacy, and it is not clear whether the vaccine is protective against aerosolized pulmonary infections. Plague vaccine is administered subcutaneously. The initial course of plague vaccine consists of two 0.5 mL doses given 1–3 months apart in adults and adolescents and three doses (0.1–0.3 mL) for children under 12 years of age. Thereafter, boosters can be given every 6 months for 18 months, and every 1–2 years if the person continues to be at high exposure risk. The vaccine, which is not currently being manufactured, is approved for use only in persons 18–61 years of age. Adverse effects include local erythema, lymphadenopathy and pain (~29% of recipients). The vaccine is contraindicated in persons with a previous reaction to a dose or any of the components.

Owing to a lack of clear efficacy, and low risk of exposure for most travelers, plague vaccine is not routinely recommended. In case of a potential exposure, a 7-day course of antibiotics (tetracycline, doxycycline or trimethoprim/sulfamethoxazole) at therapeutic doses against *Yersina pestis* may be prescribed as post-exposure prophylaxis.

References

1. Monath TP. Yellow fever: an update. Lancet Infect Dis 2001;1:11–20.
2. Barnett ED. Yellow fever: epidemiology and prevention. Clin Infect Dis 2007;44:850–6.
3. Marfin AA, Eidex RS, Kozarsky PE, et al. Yellow fever and Japanese encephalitis vaccines: indications and complications. Infect Dis Clin North Am 2005;19:151–68, ix.
4. Monath TP. Yellow fever vaccine. Expert Rev Vaccines 2005;4:553–74.
5. Gershman M, Staples JE. Yellow fever. In: CDC, Health Information for International Travel: The Yellow Book Oxford University Press; 2012.
6. Cetron MS, Marfin AA, Julian KG, et al. Yellow fever vaccine. Recommendations of the Advisory Committee on Immunization Practices (ACIP), 2002. MMWR Recomm Rep 2002;51:1–11; quiz CE1–4.
7. Barwick R. History of thymoma and yellow fever vaccination. Lancet 2004;364:936.
8. Veit O, Niedrig M, Chapuis-Taillard C, et al. Immunogenicity and safety of yellow fever vaccination for 102 HIV-infected patients. Clin Infect Dis 2009;48:659–66.
9. Monath TP, Cetron MS, Teuwen DE. Yellow fever vaccine. In: Plotkin SA, Orenstein WA, Offit P, editors. Vaccines. 5th ed. Philadelphia: Saunders Elsevier; 2008. p. 959–1055.
10. McMahon AW, Eidex RB, Marfin AA, et al. Neurologic disease associated with 17D-204 yellow fever vaccination: a report of 15 cases. Vaccine 2007;25:1727–34.
11. Adverse events associated with 17D-derived yellow fever vaccination–United States, 2001–2002. MMWR Morb Mortal Wkly Rep 2002;51:989–93.
12. Monath TP, Cetron MS, McCarthy K, et al. Yellow fever 17D vaccine safety and immunogenicity in the elderly. Human vaccines 2005;1:207–14.
13. Khromava AY, Eidex RB, Weld LH, et al. Yellow fever vaccine: an updated assessment of advanced age as a risk factor for serious adverse events. Vaccine 2005;23:3256–63.
14. Vellozzi C, Mitchell T, Miller E, et al. Yellow fever vaccine-associated viscerotropic disease (YEL-AVD) and corticosteroid therapy: eleven United States cases, 1996–2004. Am J Trop Med Hyg 2006;75:333–6.
15. Lindsey NP, Schroeder BA, Miller ER, et al. Adverse event reports following yellow fever vaccination. Vaccine 2008;26:6077–82.
16. Monath TP. Suspected yellow fever vaccine-associated viscerotropic adverse events (1973 and 1978), United States. Am J Trop Med Hyg 2010;82:919–21.
17. Kollaritsch H, Que JU, Kunz C, et al. Safety and immunogenicity of live oral cholera and typhoid vaccines administered alone or in combination with antimalarial drugs, oral polio vaccine, or yellow fever vaccine. J Infect Dis 1997;175:871–5.
18. Steffen R, Amitirigala I, Mutsch M. Health risks among travelers–need for regular updates. J Travel Med 2008;15:145–6.
19. Jelinek T, Kollaritsch H. Vaccination with Dukoral against travelers' diarrhea (ETEC) and cholera. Expert Rev Vaccines 2008;7:561–7.
20. Lopez-Gigosos RM, Plaza E, Diez-Diaz RM, et al. Vaccination strategies to combat an infectious globe: oral cholera vaccines. J Glob 2011;3:56–62.
21. Hill DR, Ford L, Lalloo DG. Oral cholera vaccines: use in clinical practice. Lancet Infect Dis 2006;6:361–73.
22. Cholera Vaccines: WHO position paper. accessed 11–29–2011.
23. Sinclair D, Abba K, Zaman K, et al. Oral vaccines for preventing cholera. Cochrane Database Syst Rev 2011;CD008603.
24. Campbell GL, Hills SL, Fischer M, et al. Estimated global incidence of Japanese encephalitis: a systematic review. Bull World Health Organ 2011 Oct 1;89(10):766–74E.
25. Solomon T, Dung NM, Kneen R, et al. Japanese encephalitis. J Neurol Neurosurg Psychiatry 2000;68:405–15.
26. Hills SL, Griggs AC, Fisher M. Japanese encephalitis in travelers from non-endemic countries, 1973–2008. Am J Trop Med Hyg 2010;82:930–6.
27. Halstead SB, Thomas SJ. Japanese encephalitis: new options for active immunization. Clin Infect Dis 2010;50:1155–64.
28. Dubischar-Kastner K, Kaltenboeck A, Klingler A, et al. Safety analysis of a Vero-cell culture derived Japanese encephalitis vaccine, IXIARO (IC51), in 6 months of follow-up. Vaccine 2010;28:6463–9.
29. Kaltenbock A, Dubischar-Kastner K, Schuller E, et al. Immunogenicity and safety of IXIARO (IC51) in a Phase II study in healthy Indian children between 1 and 3 years of age. Vaccine 2010;28:834–9.
30. Monath TP, Guirakhoo F, Nichols R, et al. Chimeric live, attenuated vaccine against Japanese encephalitis (ChimeriVax-JE): phase 2 clinical trials for safety and immunogenicity, effect of vaccine dose and schedule, and memory response to challenge with inactivated Japanese encephalitis antigen. J Infect Dis 2003;188:1213–30.
31. Guy B, Guirakhoo F, Barban V, et al. Preclinical and clinical development of YFV 17D-based chimeric vaccines against dengue, West Nile and Japanese encephalitis viruses. Vaccine 2010;28:632–49.
32. Morrison D, Legg TJ, Billings CW, et al. A novel tetravalent dengue vaccine is well tolerated and immunogenic against all 4 serotypes in flavivirus-naive adults. J Infect Dis 2010;201:370–7.

33. Torresi J, McCarthy K, Feroldi E, et al. Immunogenicity, safety and tolerability in adults of a new single-dose, live-attenuated vaccine against Japanese encephalitis: Randomised controlled phase 3 trials. Vaccine 2010;28:7993–8000.

34. Chokephaibulkit K, Sirivichayakul C, Thisyakorn U, et al. Safety and immunogenicity of a single administration of live-attenuated Japanese encephalitis vaccine in previously primed 2- to 5-year-olds and naive 12- to 24-month-olds: Multicenter Randomized Controlled Trial. Pediatr Infect Dis J 2010;29:1111–7.

35. Yu Y. Phenotypic and genotypic characteristics of Japanese encephalitis attenuated live vaccine virus SA14–14–2 and their stabilities. Vaccine 2010;28:3635–41.

36. Japanese encephalitis vaccines. Releve epidemiologique hebdomadaire / Section d'hygiene du Secretariat de la Societe des Nations = Weekly epidemiological record / Health Section of the Secretariat of the League of Nations 2006;81:331–40.

37. Japanese encephalitis vaccines. Wkly Epidemiol Rec 2006;81:331–40.

38. Fischer M, Lindsey N, Staples JE, et al. Japanese encephalitis vaccines: recommendations of the Advisory Committee on Immunization Practices (ACIP). MMWR Recomm Rep 2010;59:1–27.

39. Shlim DR, Solomon T. Japanese encephalitis vaccine for travelers: exploring the limits of risk. Clin Infect Dis 2002;35:183–8.

40. Erra E, Askling HH, Rombo L, et al. A single dose of Vero cell-derived Japanese encephalitis (JE) vaccine (Ixiaro®) effectively boosts immunity in travellers primed with mouse brain-derived JE vaccines. Clin Infect Dis 2012.

41. Nasveld PE, Ebringer A, Elmes N, et al. Long term immunity to live attenuated Japanese encephalitis chimeric virus vaccine: randomized, double-blind, 5-year phase II study in healthy adults. Human vaccines 2010;6:1038–46.

42. Tandan JB, Ohrr H, Sohn YM, et al. Single dose of SA 14–14–2 vaccine provides long-term protection against Japanese encephalitis: a case-control study in Nepalese children 5 years after immunization. drjbtandan@yahoo.com. Vaccine 2007;25:5041–5.

43. Sohn YM, Tandan JB, Yoksan S, et al. A 5-year follow-up of antibody response in children vaccinated with single dose of live attenuated SA14–14–2 Japanese encephalitis vaccine: immunogenicity and anamnestic responses. Vaccine 2008;26:1638–43.

44. Tauber E, Kollaritsch H, Korinek M, et al. Safety and immunogenicity of a Vero-cell-derived, inactivated Japanese encephalitis vaccine: a non-inferiority, phase III, randomised controlled trial. Lancet 2007;370:1847–53.

45. Schuller E, Jilma B, Voicu V, et al. Long-term immunogenicity of the new Vero cell-derived, inactivated Japanese encephalitis virus vaccine IC51 Six and 12 month results of a multicenter follow-up phase 3 study. Vaccine 2008;26:4328–86.

46. Dubischar-Kastner K, Eder S, Buerger V, et al. Long-term immunity and immune response to a booster dose following vaccination with the inactivated Japanese encephalitis vaccine IXIARO, IC51. Vaccine 2010;28:5197–202.

47. Schuller E, Klade CS, Wolfl G, et al. Comparison of a single, high-dose vaccination regimen to the standard regimen for the investigational Japanese encephalitis vaccine, IC51: a randomized, observer-blind, controlled Phase 3 study. Vaccine 2009;27:2188–93.

48. Chokephaibulkit K, Plipat N, Yoksan S, et al. A comparative study of the serological response to Japanese encephalitis vaccine in HIV-infected and uninfected Thai children. Vaccine 2010;28:3563–6.

49. Hennessy S, Liu Z, Tsai TF, et al. Effectiveness of live-attenuated Japanese encephalitis vaccine (SA14–14–2): a case-control study. Lancet 1996;347:1583–6.

50. Liu ZL, Hennessy S, Strom BL, et al. Short-term safety of live attenuated Japanese encephalitis vaccine (SA14–14–2): results of a randomized trial with 26,239 subjects. J Infect Dis 1997;176:1366–9.

51. Ohrr H, Tandan JB, Sohn YM, et al. Effect of single dose of SA 14–14–2 vaccine 1 year after immunization in Nepalese children with Japanese encephalitis: a case-control study. Lancet 2005;366:1375–8.

52. Meningococcal vaccines: WHO position paper, November 2011. Releve epidemiologique hebdomadaire / Section d'hygiene du Secretariat de la Societe des Nations = Weekly epidemiological record / Health Section of the Secretariat of the League of Nations 2011;86:521–39.

53. Harrison LH, Trotter CL, Ramsay ME. Global epidemiology of meningococcal disease. Vaccine 2009;27(Suppl 2):B51–63.

54. Bilukha OO, Rosenstein N. Prevention and control of meningococcal disease. Recommendations of the Advisory Committee on Immunization Practices (ACIP). MMWR Recommendations and reports: Morbidity and mortality weekly report Recommendations and reports / Centers for Disease Control 2005;54:1–21.

55. Bilukha O, Messonnier N, Fischer M. Use of meningococcal vaccines in the United States. Pediatr Infect Dis J 2007;26:371–6.

56. Girard MP, Preziosi MP, Aguado MT, et al. A review of vaccine research and development: meningococcal disease. Vaccine 2006;24:4692–700.

57. Keyserling H, Papa T, Koranyi K, et al. Safety, immunogenicity, and immune memory of a novel meningococcal (groups A, C, Y, and W-135) polysaccharide diphtheria toxoid conjugate vaccine (MCV-4) in healthy adolescents. Arch Pediatr Adolesc Med 2005;159:907–13.

58. Pichichero M, Casey J, Blatter M, et al. Comparative trial of the safety and immunogenicity of quadrivalent (A, C, Y, W-135) meningococcal polysaccharide-diphtheria conjugate vaccine versus quadrivalent polysaccharide vaccine in two- to ten-year-old children. Pediatr Infect Dis J 2005;24:57–62.

59. Snape MD, Pollard AJ. Meningococcal polysaccharide-protein conjugate vaccines. Lancet Infectious Diseases 2005;5:21–30.

60. Snape MD, Perrett KP, Ford KJ, et al. Immunogenicity of a tetravalent meningococcal glycoconjugate vaccine in infants: a randomized controlled trial. JAMA 2008;299:173–84.

61. Perrett KP, Snape MD, Ford KJ, et al. Immunogenicity and immune memory of a nonadjuvanted quadrivalent meningococcal glycoconjugate vaccine in infants. Pediatr Infect Dis J 2009;28:186–93.

62. Jackson LA, Jacobson RM, Reisinger KS, et al. A randomized trial to determine the tolerability and immunogenicity of a quadrivalent meningococcal glycoconjugate vaccine in healthy adolescents. Pediatr Infect Dis J 2009;28:86–91.

63. Reisinger KS, Baxter R, Block SL, et al. Quadrivalent meningococcal vaccination of adults: phase III comparison of an investigational conjugate vaccine, MenACWY-CRM, with the licensed vaccine, Menactra. Clin Vaccine Immunol 2009;16:1810–5.

64. Stamboulian D, Lopardo G, Lopez P, et al. Safety and immunogenicity of an investigational quadrivalent meningococcal CRM(197) conjugate vaccine, MenACWY-CRM, compared with licensed vaccines in adults in Latin America. Int J Infect Dis 2010;14:e868–75.

65. Licensure of a meningococcal conjugate vaccine (Menveo) and guidance for use – Advisory Committee on Immunization Practices (ACIP), 2010. MMWR Morbidity and mortality weekly report 2010;59:273.

66. Recommendation of the Advisory Committee on Immunization Practices (ACIP) for use of quadrivalent meningococcal conjugate vaccine (MenACWY-D) among children aged 9 through 23 months at increased risk for invasive meningococcal disease. MMWR Morbidity and mortality weekly report 2011;60:1391–2.

67. Updated recommendations for use of meningococcal conjugate vaccines – Advisory Committee on Immunization Practices (ACIP), 2010. MMWR Morbidity and mortality weekly report 2011;60:72–6.

68. Lagos R, Papa T, Munoz A, et al. Safety and immunogenicity of a meningococcal (Groups A, C, Y, W-135) polysaccharide diphtheria toxoid conjugate vaccine in healthy children aged 2 to 10 years in Chile. Human Vaccines 2005;1:228–31.

69. Halperin SA, Diaz-Mitoma F, Dull P, et al. Safety and immunogenicity of an investigational quadrivalent meningococcal conjugate vaccine after one or two doses given to infants and toddlers. European journal of clinical microbiology & infectious diseases: official publication of the European Society of Clinical Microbiology 2010;29:259–67.

70. Gill CJ, Baxter R, Anemona A, et al. Persistence of immune responses after a single dose of Novartis meningococcal serogroup A, C, W-135 and Y CRM-197 conjugate vaccine (Menveo(R)) or Menactra(R) among healthy adolescents. Human Vaccines 2010;6:881–7.

71. Update: Guillain-Barre syndrome among recipients of Menactra meningococcal conjugate vaccine–United States, June 2005-September 2006. MMWR 2006;55:1120–4.

72. Polio vaccines and polio immunization in the pre-eradication era: WHO position paper. Wkly Epidemiol Rec 2010;85:213–28.

73. Bottiger M. Polio immunity to killed vaccine: an 18-year follow-up. Vaccine 1990;8:443–5.

74. Rabies vaccines: WHO position paper–recommendations. Vaccine 2010;28:7140–2.

75. Khawplod P, Wilde H, Benjavongkulchai M, et al. Immunogenicity study of abbreviated rabies preexposure vaccination schedules. J Travel Med 2007;14:173–6.

76. Suwansrinon K, Wilde H, Benjavongkulchai M, et al. Survival of neutralizing antibody in previously rabies vaccinated subjects: a prospective study showing long lasting immunity. Vaccine 2006;24:3878–80.

77. Rabies vaccines: WHO position paper. Weekly Epidemiological Record 2010;85:309–20.

78. Vodopija I, Sureau P, Smerdel S, et al. Interaction of rabies vaccine with human rabies immunoglobulin and reliability of a 2–1-1 schedule application for postexposure treatment. Vaccine 1988;6:283–6.

79. Use of a Reduced (4-Dose) Vaccine Schedule for Postexposure Prophylaxis to Prevent Human Rabies: Recommendations of the Advisory Committee on Immunization Practices. MMWR 2010;59:1–9.

80. Dobardzic A, Izurieta H, Woo EJ, et al. Safety review of the purified chick embryo cell rabies vaccine: Data from the Vaccine Adverse Event Reporting System (VAERS), 1997–2005. Vaccine 2007;25:4244–51.

81. Suss J, Kahl O, Aspock H, et al. Tick-borne encephalitis in the age of general mobility. Wien Med Wochenschr 2010;160:94–100.

82. Zent O, Broker M. Tick-borne encephalitis vaccines: past and present. Expert Rev Vaccines 2005;4:747–55.

83. Broker M, Schondorf I. Are tick-borne encephalitis vaccines interchangeable? Expert Rev Vaccines 2006;5:461–6.

84. Vaccines against tick-borne encephalitis: WHO position paper. Wkly Epidemiol Rec 2011;86:241–56.

85. Rendi-Wagner P. Risk and prevention of tick-borne encephalitis in travelers. J Travel Med 2004;11:307–12.

86. Kollaritsch H, Chmelik V, Dontsenko I, et al. The current perspective on tick-borne encephalitis awareness and prevention in six Central and Eastern European countries: report from a meeting of experts convened to discuss TBE in their region. Vaccine 2011;29:4556–64.

87. Orlinger KK, Hofmeister Y, Fritz R, et al. A tick-borne encephalitis virus vaccine based on the European prototype strain induces broadly reactive cross-neutralizing antibodies in humans. J Infect Dis 2011;203:1556–64.

88. Holzmann H, Kundi M, Stiasny K, et al. Correlation between ELISA, hemagglutination inhibition, and neutralization tests after vaccination against tick-borne encephalitis. J Med Virol 1996;48:102–7.

89. Heinz FX, Holzmann H, Essl A, et al. Field effectiveness of vaccination against tick-borne encephalitis. Vaccine 2007;25:7559–67.

90. Paulke-Korinek M, Rendi-Wagner P, Kundi M, et al. Booster vaccinations against tick-borne encephalitis: 6 years follow-up indicates long-term protection. Vaccine 2009;27:7027–30.

91. Rendi-Wagner P, Zent O, Jilg W, et al. Persistence of antibodies after vaccination against tick-borne encephalitis. IJMM 2006;296(Suppl 40): 202–7.

92. Demicheli V, Debalini MG, Rivetti A. Vaccines for preventing tick-borne encephalitis. Cochrane Database Syst Rev 2009;CD000977.

93. Holmgren J, et al. Oral B-subunit killed whole-cell cholera vaccine. In: Levine M, et al, editor. New Generation Vaccines. New York: Marcel Dekker; 2004. p. 991–1014.

94. Meningococcal Vaccines: WHO position paper. Weekly Epidemiological Record 2011;86:521–39.

95. Global Advisory Committee on Vaccine Safety. Weekly Epidemiological Record 2007;82:245–60.

96. Human Rabies Prevention – United States, 2008. Recommendations of the Advisory Committee on Immunization Practices. MMWR 2008;57.

Pediatric Travel Vaccinations

Sheila M. Mackell and Mike Starr

Key points

- Polysaccharide vaccines (meningococcal, pneumococcal and typhoid) are poorly immunogenic and therefore less effective in children <2 years old
- Routine pediatric vaccinations may be accelerated for last-minute travelers (see Table 13.5)
- Bacille Calmette–Guérin vaccine (BCG) protects against disseminated and severe forms of tuberculosis in young children, who are at greater risk for these complications. BCG should be considered for long-stay infants and children, particularly those visiting friends and relatives
- Yellow fever vaccine is contraindicated below the age of 9 months and tick-borne encephalitis vaccines below the age of 1 year

Introduction

Vaccinating children for travel requires consideration of differences in the pediatric immune response from that of adults, the rationale for vaccine usage or omission at certain ages, and a working knowledge of the current recommendations for routine vaccinations for children. Vaccine considerations that may be unique to infants and children include: adverse event profile, interfering maternal antibody, lack of safety and efficacy data and off-label usage. Recommendations on routine vaccines for children often change yearly. This chapter will address vaccination considerations particular to traveling children compared to the adult recommendations described in Chapters 10, 11 and 12. Recommendations for updating and/or accelerating routine pediatric vaccinations as dictated by specific travel plans will be emphasized. Detailed information on routine recommended childhood schedules by country may be found at: http://apps.who.int/immunization_monitoring/en/globalsummary/CountryProfileSelect.cfm

Vaccine Considerations in Infants and Children

The immune response begins in utero. Immunoglobulins transferred via the placenta during the third trimester form the beginnings of antigen response-recognition. Premature infants lack the late gestational maternal antibodies and thus are incapable of fighting many postnatally acquired infections, yet they are able to respond to vaccine antigens at an acceptable rate. However, schedules for vaccinating former premature infants are identical to those for full-term infants.

The vaccine response in infants and children is characterized by several factors that affect efficacy. The infant immune system is characterized by impaired T-cell function; with decreased collaboration between B and T cells the immunoglobulin repertoire is restricted and the antibody response is of low affinity.[1]

Vaccine responses in infancy are affected by a variety of factors: the nature and dose of antigen, the number of vaccine doses, the age at immunization, and the level of residual maternal antibody at the time of immunization.[2] Maternal antibodies to pertussis, mumps, and polio are present transiently and are generally gone within the first 4–6 months of life. Little or no protection is conferred to hepatitis A, typhoid fever, polio, Japanese encephalitis, yellow fever, pertussis, mumps, rubella, and measles, despite the presence of maternal antibodies to these organisms. Nevertheless, antibody presence interferes with the ability of the infant to respond to vaccine-associated antigens to differing degrees.

Polysaccharide Vaccines

Polysaccharides are T-cell-independent antigens and poorly immunogenic in young children and infants. In addition, children less than 2 years old are unable to make the IgG_2 subclass, the main response elicited by the polysaccharide vaccines.[3] Without T-cell involvement polysaccharide vaccines do not elicit immune memory – the reason why booster doses are less effective. Examples of polysaccharide vaccines include meningococcal (standard A+C or A/C/Y/W-135), pneumococcal (23-valent polysaccharide and typhoid (Vi polysaccharide) vaccines. Age limitations for these vaccines are based on an ineffective response under the licensed age, which is generally 2 years.

Conjugate Vaccines

Oligosaccharide–protein conjugate vaccines, on the other hand, produce a T-cell-dependent response to a polysaccharide that allows children under the age of 2 years to respond to important antigens and also induces immunologic memory, which is important for robust booster responses to future doses. Meningococcal and pneumococcal conjugate vaccines are examples of this advance in vaccinology.

Table 13.1 USA immunization Schedule.
Recommended Immunization Schedule for Persons Aged 0 Through 6 Years—United States · 2012
For those who fall behind or start late, see the catch-up schedule

Vaccine ▼ Age ▶	Birth	1 month	2 months	4 months	6 months	12 months	15 months	18 months	19–23 months	2–3 years	4–6 years	
Hepatitis B[1]	HepB	HepB				HepB						Range of recommended ages for all children
Rotavirus[2]			RV	RV	RV[2]							
Diphtheria, Tetanus, Pertussis[3]			DTaP	DTaP	DTaP	see footnote[3]	DTaP				DTaP	
Haemophilus in-fluenzae type b[4]			Hib	Hib	Hib[4]	Hib						
Pneumococcal[5]			PCV	PCV	PCV	PCV				PPSV		
Inactivated Poliovirus[6]			IPV	IPV		IPV					IPV	
Influenza[7]						Influenza(Yearly)						Range of recommended ages for certain high-risk groups
Measles, Mumps, Rubella[8]						MMR		see footnote[8]			MMR	
Varicella[9]						Varicella		see footnote[9]			Varicella	
Hepatitis A[10]						HepA(2 doses)				HepA series		
Meningococcal[11]											MCV4	

This schedule includes recommendations in effect as of December 21, 2010. Any dose not administered at the recommended age should be administered at a subsequent visit, when indicated and feasible. The use of a combination vaccine generally is preferred over separate injections of its equivalent component vaccines. Considerations should include provider assessment, patient preference, and the potential for adverse events. Providers should consult the relevant Advisory Committee on Immunization Practices statement for detailed recommendations: http://www.cdc.gov/vaccines/pubs/acip-list.htm. Clinically significant adverse events that follow immunization should be reported to the Vaccine Adverse Event Reporting System (VAERS) at http://www.vaers.hhs.gov or by telephone, 800-822-7967. Use of trade names and commercial sources is for identification only and does not imply endorsement by the U.S. Department of Health and Human Services.
(Source: http://www.cdc.gov/vaccines/recs/schedules/child-schedule.htm, for Footnote and Catch-Up Schedule, see Source)

Intercurrent Illness and Vaccination

Minor febrile illnesses are not a contraindication to any of the routine or travel vaccines and should not lead to postponement of indicated doses. Simultaneous administration of vaccines is acceptable and does not diminish antibody response. As with adults, live viral vaccines should be given together or, if separate, at least 30 days apart.

Routine Pediatric Vaccines

Immunization against common vaccine-preventable diseases occurs routinely throughout the first 24 months of life. The current recommendations for routine childhood vaccination in the USA are shown in detail in Table 13.1. Most industrialized countries follow similar schedules, with some variations that are mostly in the timing of each initial and serial dose. A few vaccines, including varicella, rotavirus, and human papilloma virus vaccine, may not be routinely recommended or available in some countries. Combination vaccines containing five or more antigens in a single preparation are available in most industrialized countries. Detailed information on routine recommended childhood schedules by country can be found at: http://apps.who.int/immunization_monitoring/en/globalsummary/CountryProfileSelect.cfm. More relevant to developing countries, the World Health Organization-sponsored Global Alliance for Vaccines and Immunizations (GAVI) focuses on six core vaccine-preventable diseases in formulating recommendations for worldwide childhood vaccination schedules: polio, diphtheria, tuberculosis, pertussis, measles, and tetanus. As additional options, hepatitis B vaccine is recommended globally, *Haemophilus influenzae* B vaccine is recommended in Latin America, the Middle East and where evidence of disease exists, and yellow fever vaccine is recommended in Africa and South America in endemic areas. GAVI recommendations for childhood vaccination are summarized in Table 13.3. Some

member countries are also embracing the second dose of measles vaccine in an attempt to reduce measles morbidity and mortality.

Diphtheria–Tetanus–Acellular Pertussis

The combination of diphtheria, tetanus and pertussis is recommended for all children in the sequence shown in Tables 13.1 and 13.2. Refinements in the pertussis component of the vaccine in the past decade have improved the side-effect profile but diminished immunity may occur in view of recent large outbreaks in children. The acellular pertussis component is minimally reactogenic compared to the whole cell pertussis vaccine and is still the preferred product.

Contraindications to subsequent DTaP vaccination include an immediate anaphylactic reaction or encephalopathy within 7 days of an earlier dose, although a large Canadian study found no evidence of encephalopathy following acellular pertussis vaccines.[4] Adverse events, including a seizure with or without fever within 3 days of the vaccine, persistent, inconsolable crying for ≥3 h, collapse or shock-like state within 48 h, and otherwise unexplained fever ≥40.5°C (104.9°F) are considered precautions, not absolute contraindications to further vaccination. Decisions on further doses of vaccine must be weighed individually. The whole cell pertussis vaccine (DTP) should be avoided in infants and children at increased risk of convulsions and those who have underlying conditions that predispose to seizures.[5]

Adolescent Pertussis Vaccine (Tdap)

Vaccines with reduced doses of diphtheria and pertussis toxins are now available for use in adolescents and adults. The reduced dose of these two components reduces the likelihood of local side-effects at the injection site. Boostrix (GlaxoSmithKline) is licensed for use in anyone over 10 years old for booster doses of tetanus and pertussis. Adacel (Sanofi Pasteur) can be used in 11–64-year-olds. These are the booster

Table 13.2 Recommended Immunization Schedule for Persons Aged 7 Through 18 Years—United States · 2012
For those who fall behind or start late, see the schedule below and the catch-up schedule

Vaccine ▼ Age ▶	7–10 years	11–12 years	13–18years	
Tetanus, Diphtheria, Pertussis[1]		**Tdap**	**Tdap**	Range of recommended ages for all children
Human Papillomavirus[2]	see footnote[2]	**HPV (3 doses)(females)**	**HPV Series**	
Meningococcal[3]	**MCV4**	**MCV4**	**MCV4**	
Influenza[4]	**Influenza(Yearly)**			Range of recommended ages for catch-up immunization
Pneumococcal[5]	**Pneumococcal**			
Hepatitis A[6]	**Hep A Series**			
Hepatitis B[7]	**Hep B Series**			
Inactivated Poliovirus[8]	**IPV series**			Range of recommended ages for certain high-risk groups
Measles, Mumps, Rubella[9]	**MMR Series**			
Varicella[10]	**Varicella Series**			

This schedule includes recommendations in effect as of December 23, 2011. Any dose not administered at the recommended age should be administered at a subsequent visit, when indicated and feasible. The use of a combination vaccine generally is preferred over separate injections of its equivalent component vaccines.
(From US Department of Health and Human Services, Centers for Disease Control and Prevention)

Table 13.3 WHO GAVI Immunization Schedule

Age	Vaccine
Birth	BCG, OPV-0, HBV-1
6 weeks	DPT-1, OPV-1, HBV-2 (HBV-1)[a]
10 weeks	DPT-2, OPV-2 (HBV-2)
14 weeks	DPT-3, OPV-3, HBV-3
9 months	Measles, yellow fever

[a]HBV schedule option.

vaccines of choice in the adolescent population, given their susceptibility and waning immunity to pertussis. Either Tdap product may be given 2 years (or earlier if necessary) after a previous dose of DTaP or Td for high-risk travel to pertussis-endemic areas.[6] Other vaccines can be administered concurrently.

Children >7 years old, but <11 years old should receive Tdap for the first dose in the catch-up series if unimmunized previously, followed by Td.

Measles–Mumps–Rubella

Measles remains the leading cause of vaccine-preventable death in children worldwide and an active WHO initiative for the global eradication of measles is ongoing. Vaccination programs are aimed at protecting young children from the severe consequences of infection. Outbreaks of measles occur in developed as well as developing countries. Child travelers need particular attention to the status of their measles immunity if traveling to developing countries. Under-vaccination in the past decade is thought to be responsible for the 2010–2011 measles outbreak in Europe, where, as of mid-2011, 6500 cases have been reported.

The first dose of measles–mumps–rubella (MMR) vaccine is recommended at 12–15 months of age in most industrialized countries. By this age, the effect of maternal antibody to measles is waning and an adequate immune response to the vaccine is likely. The first dose of the MMR vaccine gives protective immunity in approximately 95% of recipients. The second dose is not a booster dose, but induces immunity in the remainder of those who may not have responded. The second dose can be given as soon as 1 month after the first dose.

In the routine pediatric vaccine schedule in many countries, it is given at 4–5 years old at kindergarten entry.

In view of the risk of measles during travel, infants between the ages of 6 and 12 months traveling to the developing world should be vaccinated with a dose of the monovalent measles vaccine, or, if unavailable, MMR.[7] This will provide immediate protection for several months or more, but not a durable or lasting immune response. Thus, any dose given before the age of 12 months is not considered countable towards the routine immunization schedule and the child still requires the two routine MMR vaccines after the age of 12 months. Any child between the age of 12 months and 4–5 years traveling to measles-endemic areas should receive their second MMR vaccine before departure, as long as it is at least 4 weeks since the first dose. This second dose is a countable dose towards their routine immunization schedule.

The MMR vaccine is well tolerated. At 7–10 days after vaccination 1 in 15 recipients will develop a red maculopapular, often confluent rash, a fever and a flu-like syndrome, with fever lasting 1–2 days. These persons are not contagious for measles. Minor side-effects include local discomfort at the site of injection, headache, and malaise. Side-effects from the second dose are less frequent than with the first dose.

The MMR vaccine should not be given if there has been a serious allergic reaction to a previous dose or if there is a history of anaphylaxis to neomycin. Persons with a history of anaphylactic reactions to gelatin-containing products should be immunized with caution under close supervision. There have been several case reports of persons with gelatin allergy having a severe allergic reaction to the MMR vaccine, which contains a small amount of gelatin in the formulation. Allergy to eggs or egg protein is not a contraindication to receiving the vaccine.

Polio Vaccine

The recommendations for the primary polio vaccine series have been modified in many industrialized countries in recent years. The injectable inactivated polio vaccine is recommended for the primary series instead of the oral polio vaccine (OPV), which is still the standard in the WHO polio eradication program. The relative risk of vaccine-associated poliomyelitis, albeit very low with the oral vaccine, is non-existent with the all-inactivated schedule. The use of the oral polio vaccine is reserved for control programs, for outbreak situations, or recommended when an unimmunized traveler is unable to get two doses of the inactivated vaccine. OPV production has ceased in several countries, including the USA. Traveling infants can begin the IPV series as soon as 6 weeks of age.[8] Maternal antibody presence limits its effectiveness at earlier ages.[9] The second dose of IPV should be given at least 4 weeks later. For infants traveling sooner than 6 weeks, the oral polio vaccine is preferred, if available. The OPV can be started as early as birth, and subsequent doses can be given 4 and 8 weeks later. A single booster dose of the inactivated vaccine is recommended for travelers to polio-endemic regions in the adolescent years. No data exist to indicate the exact waning of polio immunity, but approximately 10 years after the primary series has been suggested as an appropriate interval to administer the IPV booster if indicated for travel.

Pneumococcal Vaccine

The most common cause of otitis media and invasive bacterial disease in children is pneumococcal infection. The 7-valent pneumococcal conjugate vaccine was recently replaced by a 13-valent vaccine (PCV-13). The vaccine is recommended routinely at 2, 4, and 6 months of age, with a single booster dose at 12–18 months of age. Infants and children older than 6 months and under 5 years are vaccinated at the schedule outlined in Table 13.1. The serotypes present in the 13-valent vaccine are those which cause disease in young children and are most commonly resistant to penicillin. The 23-valent polysaccharide pneumococcal vaccine is recommended for children older than 2 years with underlying chronic medical conditions, and adults, as noted in Chapter 10.

Influenza Vaccine

Influenza is the most common travel-related vaccine-preventable infection. Influenza vaccination should be considered in all children >6 months (whether or not they are traveling), especially those traveling during the influenza season, which is year-round in the tropics, December–April in northern hemisphere temperate zones, and April–October in southern hemisphere temperate zones. Infants younger than 6 months do not respond well to the current vaccine.[10]

Injectable influenza vaccine protects against influenza A & B. Infants and children <13 years old should receive the split virus preparation, which is less reactogenic than the whole virus product. Children >13 years can receive the whole cell vaccine. Any child <9 years old receiving the influenza vaccine for the first time should receive two doses of the vaccine, 1 month apart. Children <3 years old should receive 0.25 mL of vaccine, half the dose for older children and adults. Immunization of all children 6 months to 18 years of age is recommended regardless of travel plans, because of a higher incidence of complications and hospitalization associated with influenza infections. Some brands of influenza vaccines still contain 25 μg of thimerosal, but in most countries enough thimerosal-free influenza vaccine is produced to meet the needs of children under 3, if this is a concern to parents. Egg allergy is not a contraindication to this vaccine unless anaphylaxis occurs.

An intranasal influenza vaccine (Flumist, MedImmune) is licensed in the US for use in 2–49-year-olds.[11] It is a live virus vaccine and so is contraindicated for anyone with suspected immune deficiency, a history of Guillain–Barré syndrome or receiving aspirin therapy. It is also contraindicated for any person with asthma or egg allergy. A booster dose, 45–60 days after the first dose, is recommended for those 5–8 years old receiving this preparation for the first time. There are data suggesting that the intranasal vaccine is more effective in children

< 9 years than the injectable vaccine. Egg allergy *is* a contraindication to the intranasal vaccine.

Varicella

According to the Centers for Disease Control, 90% of varicella in the USA occurs in children. Tropical regions have a higher proportion of cases in adults. Child and adult travelers from tropical countries to temperate climates may be at risk of acquiring varicella. If a traveler has no definitive history of the disease, he/she should be tested for immunity, and vaccinated if susceptible.

Varicella vaccine was licensed in the USA in March 1995 and is recommended for all susceptible children and adolescents over 12 months of age.[12] It is also recommended for international travelers, and non-pregnant adults who live in households with children, who work in daycare settings, or are exposed to settings of high transmission risk (colleges, military, or correctional institutions). Susceptible adolescents are strongly encouraged to obtain vaccination, as they are more likely to experience complications of the disease. Two doses of vaccine are required, with routine doses at ages 12–15 months and at school entry at 4–6 years of age. Children from 1 to 12 years old may receive the booster dose 3 months after the primary dose, if necessary. For older children and adolescents, two doses should be given 1 month apart.[12] Varicella or varicella-containing vaccine should not be used by most immunocompromised people. A combination MMR and varicella vaccine is available in the USA for primary or booster dose. The combination product (MMRV) has a higher incidence of febrile seizures in recipients when used for the first dose compared to using the two separate vaccines. This increased risk is not present when used for the second dose. Although either is acceptable, separate administration of MMR and VZ is preferable for the first doses. A personal or family history of seizures is a contraindication against the use of MMRV at either dose.

This vaccine is very well tolerated, and so far no major side-effects have been demonstrated. A total of 7–8% of those vaccinated develop a mild vaccine-associated rash, often consisting of 2–5 chickenpox-like lesions. This vaccine should not be given if there has been a serious allergic reaction to a previous dose, or if there is a history of allergy to gelatin or neomycin.

The manufacturer recommends that salicylates not be administered for 6 weeks after varicella vaccine administration, owing to the association of varicella virus (*not* the vaccine), salicylates and Reye's syndrome. Reye's syndrome was first described in the 1970s as severe brain and liver failure associated with an unknown interaction between salicylates and varicella in children. It has not been reported with the vaccine.

Hepatitis B

Hepatitis B vaccine is increasingly a routine childhood vaccination in many countries and is part of the WHO GAVI recommendations for highly endemic countries. The three-dose series can be started immediately at birth, with a schedule of 0, 1, and 6 months. Alternatively, doses can be given at 2, 4, and 6 months of age, with dose two being at least 1 month after dose one, and dose three being at least 4 months after dose one. The birth dose is favored as opportunities can be missed in those infants lost to follow-up. Pre-term infants should be immunized before hospital discharge if weighing at least 2 kg, or at 2 months of age. The vaccine should be given intramuscularly (i.m.) for the best response. A two-dose schedule (0 and 4–6 months) is in use for adolescents 11–15 years old.[13] As for adults, vaccine efficacy is between 90% and 95%. Routine post-immunization serologic testing is not recommended for the pediatric population. Infants born to hepatitis B surface antigen-positive mothers are recommended to have serology performed 1–2 months after the third dose of vaccine. Side-effects of the hepatitis B vaccine include local pain at the injection site and a low-grade fever. It is estimated that 1–6% of vaccine recipients experience fever. Allergic reactions are rare.

Rotavirus

Rotavirus is the most common cause of severe gastroenteritis in infants and young children worldwide. A live oral pentavalent rotavirus vaccine (Rotateq) has been available in several countries since 2006. It is indicated for routine immunization of children at ages 2, 4, and 6 months. A second vaccine (Rotarix) is licensed as a two-dose series at 2 and 4 months of age. Both vaccines should be started by 14 weeks 6 days of age, and should not be given to children over the age of 32 weeks, even if they have not been fully vaccinated by that time. Current rotavirus vaccines have been associated with an increased risk of intussusception for a short period after administration of the first dose in some populations.[14]

Human Papilloma Virus Vaccine

Human papilloma viruses (HPVs) are transmitted through sexual contact and cause both genital warts and cervical cancer. HPV vaccines have been developed using recombinant DNA technology based on virus-like particles (VLPs), which are not infectious and do not have any cancer-causing potential. There are two HPV vaccines licensed for use in the US: a quadrivalent vaccine (Gardasil, Merck) containing VLPs of HPV genotypes 16, 18, 6 and 11 (6 and 11 prevent genital warts) and a bivalent vaccine containing VLPs of HPV genotypes 16 and 18 vaccine (Cervarix, GlaxoSmithKline). Vaccination must be initiated prior to natural infection with a given HPV type in order to be effective. Vaccination is not a substitute for routine cervical cancer screening, and vaccinated women should have cervical cancer screening as recommended.

Indications

HPV vaccine is recommended in some countries as a routine childhood vaccination prior to sexual debut, and generally at ages 11–12. For adults under the age of 26 not previously vaccinated, the vaccine is recommended even in sexually active women, and even if they have acquired one or more HPV subtypes. Travel has not been demonstrated to increase HPV risk; however, since increased sexual activity has been associated with travel, the pre-travel consult is a reasonable setting to discuss vaccination.

Dosing schedules: Both vaccines are administered i.m. as three separate 0.5 mL doses. The second dose should be administered 1 and 2 months after the first dose for Cervarix and Gardasil, respectively, and the third dose 6 months after the first dose. Booster doses are not currently recommended; duration of immunity after vaccination is not yet known.

The quadrivalent vaccine is licensed for use in males aged 9–15 years.[31] Recent data suggest that vaccination of males can prevent transmission of HPV or provide protection against genital HPV infection, genital warts, anogenital dysplasia or anogenital cancers.[15,16] The bivalent vaccine is not registered for use in males.

Contraindications and Precautions

- Severe allergic reaction (e.g., anaphylaxis) after a previous vaccine dose or to a vaccine component.

Table 13.4 Accelerating Routine Pediatric Vaccinations

	Age	Minimum Interval
DTaP	6 weeks	4 weeks
Hepatitis B	Birth	4 weeks
Hib	6 weeks	4 weeks
IPV	6 weeks	4 weeks
MMR	6–11 months, followed by MMR at 12 months old	4 weeks
OPV	Birth	4 weeks
PCV13	6 weeks	4 weeks
Rotavirus	6 weeks	4 weeks

Table 13.5 Age Limitations to the Use of Yellow Fever Vaccine

Age	Recommendation
<6 months	*Never*
6–9 months	In unusual circumstances (consult with experts)
>9 months	If travel to yellow fever endemic or infected areas

Accelerating Routine Vaccines

Routine pediatric vaccinations may need to be accelerated if the traveling child is departing before the primary series can be completed and he/she will be at high risk. The recommended minimum amount of time between doses is listed in Table 13.4. Earliest ages of vaccination recommendations are derived on the basis of interfering maternal antibodies, lack of effective immune response, or lack of data. The minimum interval noted is required to produce an immunologic response but longer intervals are preferable.[17]

Pediatric Travel Vaccinations

Required Vaccinations

Yellow Fever Vaccine

Itineraries involving travel to sub-Saharan Africa or the Amazonian region of South America may require the yellow fever (YF) vaccine for entry into the country. For most countries in the endemic or infected zone, vaccination is medically recommended on the basis of risk of yellow fever, rather than because of legal requirements (see Chapter 11 for general advice on risk areas). Initial experience with the vaccine revealed an increased incidence of YF encephalitis in young infants, particularly those under 4 months.

The vaccine-associated encephalitis syndrome typically occurs 7–21 days after immunization and is characterized by a reversion to wild-type virus. A brief clinical course with complete recovery is typical. The basis for this increased risk in infants is unknown.

In 1960, an age restriction (9 months) was placed on the use of the vaccine and is generally adhered to internationally. Current advice is for infants <9 months to avoid travel to very high-risk areas or those with ongoing epidemics or current cases. If travel is unavoidable, vaccine can be given above the age of 6 months, but an expert in the current epidemiology of transmission should be consulted to assess the real risk at the particular destination (Table 13.5).[18] The incidence of vaccine-associated encephalitis in young infants has been estimated at 0.5–4/1000.[16] A waiver letter should be given to travelers of any age to relevant regions who are not given YF vaccine for medical reasons.

Booster doses are recommended every 10 years, as for adults.

Recommended Vaccinations

Hepatitis A Vaccine

Hepatitis A in young children is usually a mild disease. Young children can serve as reservoirs and transmit the infection to adults and caregivers, while they shed the virus asymptomatically. Vaccination in this age group is indicated to control the disease in both the child traveler and contacts both during travel and after return.

As for adults, hepatitis A vaccination is recommended for travel to developing countries. In addition, routine vaccination with hepatitis A vaccine is recommended to begin at age 1 year in all children in the USA and several other countries. Older children who have not been vaccinated should consider a catch-up dose regardless of travel plans.[20]

Data exist to show that infants as young as 6 months will respond to hepatitis A vaccination if they do not have an interfering maternal antibody present.[19] Maternal antibody, if present, interferes with seroconversion response for a variable amount of time. Seropositive infants respond well at ≥1 year of age, once the maternal antibody levels decline. At least three pediatric vaccines are available for global use. There is no place for the routine use of human immunoglobulin to prevent hepatitis A in travelers.[20]

Hepatitis A–Hepatitis B Combination Vaccine

A hepatitis A–hepatitis B combination vaccine (Twinrix, GlaxoSmithKline) is now widely used for adults. The adult formulation is licensed for use in adolescents >18 years in North America and >16 years in many other countries. For children 1–17 years, Twinrix-Junior (GlaxoSmithKline) is widely available and licensed for use in many countries.[21,22] It is also administered in a three-dose series at 0, 1, and 6 months. Twinrix is registered for use in an accelerated schedule (0, 7, 21 days, and 1 year) in many countries. Hepatitis A–hepatitis B combination vaccines can be used in a two-dose schedule (day 0, 6–12 months) in children from 1 to 15 years of age in Canada and Europe.[22]

Meningococcal Vaccines

Children traveling to the meningitis-prone areas in equatorial Africa during the December–June dry season, or to the *Hajj* in Saudi Arabia, should receive the vaccination against meningococcal disease. Four vaccines are currently available. The quadrivalent A/C/Y/W-135 polysaccharide vaccine (Menomune) and three quadrivalent A/C/Y/W-135 conjugate vaccines (Menactra, Sanofi Pasteur and Menveo, Novartis; Nimenrix, GSK).

The conjugate vaccine is the preferred product and both are currently licensed in the US for use in 2–55-year-olds as a single dose. Only Menactra is currently licensed for use in 9–23-month-olds, in a two-dose series, 3 months apart. There are data demonstrating safety and efficacy of both quadrivalent conjugate meningococcal vaccines down to 2 months of age.

The polysaccharide vaccine confers little immunity to children <2 years old. Infants as young as 3 months old will respond to serogroup A (the most common serogroup in epidemics) to a limited extent, when two doses of the vaccine are given. Infants are unable to make significant antibody response to serogroup C.[23] The polysaccharide vaccine should be boosted every 2–3 years if risk of disease exists.

A conjugate quadrivalent vaccine (Menactra, Sanofi Pasteur or Menveo, Novartis is recommended for routine vaccination of all children. Nimenrix (GSK) is licensed only in Europe, and can be used in anyone older than 12 months (see Table 13.6). Recommendations for the conjugate vaccines are as follows: routine adolescents, first dose 11–12 years old: booster at age 16 years; first dose 13–15 years: booster between 16 and 18 years.[29] Minimum interval 8 weeks; first dose after 16 years: no booster routinely.

Travelers with continued exposure risk: First vaccine 2–6 years old: revaccinate in 3 years; first dose > 7 years old: revaccinate every 5 years. Side effects of the conjugate vaccine are generally local. Meningococcal serogroups C and Y, W-135 have emerged as significant causes of meningococcal meningitis. Group B remains a serious cause of disease, especially in infants. At this time, vaccines against serogroup B are available in Cuba, Norway, The Netherlands, New Zealand, and Canada, and are made against outer membrane proteins (OMP).

Other Meningococcal Conjugate Vaccines

Protein conjugate vaccines for serogroups A, C, and A/C combination are now available in several countries. The conjugate vaccine produces a T-cell-dependent response and so is immunogenic in infants.[27] The meningococcal conjugate vaccines (e.g., Menjugate, Novartis or NeisVac-C, Baxter) have been licensed for use in infants <2 years in Canada, the UK, and several other countries. Schedules vary from country to country, but many recommend doses at 2, 4, and 6 months of age (three doses, at least 4 weeks apart). A single dose is recommended for children between 1 and 4 years old. College students in the UK (as well as foreign students attending college in the UK) receive the meningococcal A+C conjugate vaccine owing to an incidence (2/100 000) of disease, predominantly serogroup C, twice the national average.

Typhoid Vaccine

Both live attenuated oral Ty21a *S. typhi* and injectable killed Vi polysaccharide vaccines are available for pediatric use. The capsule form of Ty21a is widely licensed for use in children >6 years, who can swallow the capsules whole. The capsules need to be swallowed intact so that the contained liquid suspension of live bacteria passes undisturbed through the acid milieu of the stomach. In many countries, but not the USA, a lyophilized preparation that is reconstituted in water is available in a three-dose regimen for children older than 3 years.

The Vi polysaccharide vaccine is poorly immunogenic in children <2 years old. It can be given as a single injection to children older than 2 years and confers protection for 2–3 years. The oral vaccine provides protection for 4–5 years. Children under 2 years old currently have no available vaccine for protection, therefore recommending meticulous food and water precautions is prudent. Efforts are under way to convert the Vi antigen into a T-cell-dependent antigen and produce an immunogenic vaccine for infants.

Rabies Vaccine

Rabies is highly endemic in many countries worldwide. Given its potentially long latency and uniformly fatal outcome, advice on avoiding animal contact is essential for pre-travel counseling, whether for children or for adults. Pre- and post-exposure algorithms are found in Chapter 11 and do not differ in dose or timing between children and adults. Nevertheless, children appear be more likely to contact animals and may not report encounters,[25] therefore the pre-exposure rabies vaccine series should be considered for ambulatory children who will travel extensively or live in rural villages in countries where rabies is endemic, even when parents refuse it for themselves. High cost is an issue for rabies pre-exposure immunization, so that prioritization for young children is an important consideration. Infants and children

Table 13.6 Summary of Travel Vaccinations for Children. (See Text for Specific Vaccine Details.)

Vaccine	Age	Primary series	Booster interval/comments
Cholera, oral (inactivated WC-rBS)[b]	>2 years	2–6 years: 3 doses at 1 week intervals; >6 years: 2 doses 1 week apart	Optimal interval not established: Mfr recommends 6 months for ages 2–6 years, and 2 years for age >6 years
Hepatitis A	>2 years[a] >1 year >12 years	Havrix (GSK): 2 doses (0.5 mL i.m.) at 0, 6–18 months, later Vaqta (Merck): 2 doses (0.5 mL i.m.) at 0 and 6 months Avaxim (AventisPasteurMerieux) Europe and Canada; Epaxal (Berna Biotech): >1 year old Switzerland	See text Available in combination with hepatitis B vaccine
Immune globulin	Birth	0.02 mL/kg IM	See text
Japanese B encephalitis	>2 months	2 months – 2 years: 0.25 mL i.m. 1 month apart >3 years: 0.5 mL i.m. 1 month apart (2 doses)	Optimum regimen not determined; recommended 1 year after primary series
Menactra (MCV-D)	9 months – 2 years	2 doses at 0, 2 months	If exposure risk boost after 3 years once, then at 5 years
Meningococcal meningitis conjugate vaccine (MCV4)	2–55 years	1 dose	None recommended
Meningococcal meningitis polysaccharide vaccine (ACYW-135)	>2 years	1 dose (0.5 mL s.c.)	Boost annually if first dose was given before 4 years old. (See text for age <2)
Menveo (MCV-CRM)	2–55 years	1 dose	At 5 years
Nimenrix	>2 months	1 dose	At 5 years
Plague vaccine	>18 years	Not for use in children	
Rabies vaccine	Any age	3 doses (1 mL i.m., deltoid/ anterolateral thigh for infants, or 0.1 mL i.d.) at 0, 7, 21, or 28 days	Only HDCV approved for intradermal (i.d.) use
Tick-borne encephalitis[b]	1–11 years	Encepur Kinder (Chiron-Behring): i.m.) at 0, 1–3 months, and 9–12 months FSME-IMMUN junior (Baxter): 3 doses (0.25 mL i.m.) at 0, 1–3 months, and 9–12 months	Booster dose recommended 3 years after the primary series for the standard dosing regimen of either vaccine. (See text for accelerated schedule Encepur Kinder)
Typhoid, oral Ty21a	>3 years[a] >6 years	3 doses: 1 sachet p.o. in 100 mL water every other day 4 doses: 1 capsule p.o. every other day	Liquid vaccine[b] booster: 7 years Capsule vaccine: 5 years
Typhoid, Vi, parenteral	>2 years	1 dose (0.5 mL i.m.)	Boost after 2 years for continued risk of exposure
Yellow fever	>9 months	1 dose (0.5 mL s.c.)	10 years. (See text for <9 months.)

[a]Manufacturer's package insert for recommendations on dosage.
[b]Not approved in the USA. Available in Canada and Europe.

respond well to the vaccine and there are no age limits to its administration. The Vero cell vaccine has been studied in combination with the DTP and IPV vaccines and no interference exists.[30] Limited data exist to support its safety and efficacy when given concurrently with other routine pediatric immunizations.

Japanese B Encephalitis

Japanese encephalitis (JE) is rarely a disease of travelers; however, indications for vaccination exist, as with adults. JE vaccine is primarily indicated for long-stay travel in rural areas of risk. JE primary vaccination in early childhood occurs in many Asian countries, including China, Japan, Taiwan, Korea, and Thailand. Published and true incidence rates for human cases of JE may be low in such countries owing to high vaccination coverage, and will mask a significant risk of infection in rural farming areas.

Two new JE vaccines are available in some countries, although neither is currently licensed for use in children. (IXIARO in US and Europe, JESPECT in Australia; IC51, Intercell, is not licensed for individuals below 17 years of age.) However, at the time of this publication the manufacturer (Novartis) is studying a 6 µg per 0.5 mL dose (adult dose) for children ≥3 years of age and a 3 µg per 0.25 mL dose (half adult dose) for children aged 2 months to 2 years; many practitioners are recommending this off-label regimen in children based on at least one small publication showing safety and good sero-protection.[26,27] Details can be obtained on the above options and current situation at http: //www.cdc.gov/ncidod/dvbid/jencephalitis/children.htm

A live Chinese JE vaccine is widely available in India and Thailand and at expat clinics in China. The SA 14-14-2 JE vaccine is a live attenuated vaccine that has been used for almost 20 years in China in over 200 million children. Several studies have demonstrated an excellent safety and immune response after a single dose, with neutralizing antibody responses produced in 85–100% of non-immune children[28,29] IMOJEV (Sanofi Pasteur) is a live attenuated yellow fever JE chimeric viral vaccine that is registered for use in Australia from 12 months of age, although it is not readily available. In the meantime, families must be reminded to use mosquito avoidance measures.

Tick-Borne Encephalitis Vaccine

Tick-borne encephalitis (TBE) is transmitted by the bite of the *Ixodes runcinus* tick, present in forested areas of central and Eastern Europe. It can also rarely be acquired by consuming unpasteurized milk from infected cows, goats, and sheep. Symptoms of TBE range from meningitis to severe meningoencephalitis with significant residual neurologic sequelae. It is seasonally (summer) acquired in endemic areas (see Chapter 12). In endemic areas, the vaccine is incorporated into the routine pediatric schedule. There are two available vaccines licensed for use in children. Encepur Kinder (Chiron-Behring) is manufactured in Germany. It is an inactivated viral vaccine and can be used in children 1–11 years, but children 12 years and older should receive the adult vaccine. An accelerated schedule of 0.25 mL given on days 0, 7, and 21 is recommended if rapid immunization is required. Seroconversion can be expected no sooner than 14 days after the second vaccination. A booster is recommended 12–18 months later.

Although generalized flu-like symptoms may occur after the first vaccine, an increased incidence of febrile reactions >38°C is reported in children between 1 and 2 years old, therefore vaccination in this age group must be considered on an individual basis.

In some countries FSME-IMMUN junior (Baxter), formulated for children 1–12 years old, is available. The adult formulation is recommended for those >12 years. Dosages are listed in Table 13.6 along with a summary of other pediatric travel vaccines. FSME-IMMUN is available in Canada and by a special release mechanism in the UK. TBE vaccine is not available in the USA or Australia.

BCG

Tuberculosis (TB) is more rapidly progressive and more severe in children. Bacille Calmette–Guérin vaccine (BCG) protects against disseminated and severe forms of the disease in young children, but is only 50% protective against pulmonary TB in older children and adults. BCG is included in the routine immunization schedule in most developing countries. In these countries, infants are immunized at birth with a single dose. BCG is not routinely recommended or used in children in the USA or Canada, where management relies on screening, case identification, and treatment. The vaccine is contraindicated in immunocompromised individuals.

Although there is wide disagreement across national boundaries, BCG should be considered in infants and children under the age of 5 traveling to areas of high TB prevalence, and particularly those visiting friends and relatives (VFR travelers), as this group can be expected to have close contact with the local population.[30] Pre- and post-travel testing for tuberculosis should be done on an individual basis.[18]

Summary

Pediatric travelers require special attention to immunize them appropriately from disease. Advances in vaccine development have led to many recent changes and additions to the routine childhood immunization schedule. Vaccination of a child requires knowledge of the indications and immunologic actions of all available travel vaccines. Published age limits to pediatric vaccination are based on the development of the child's immune system, potential adverse events, the presence of interfering maternal antibodies, and, in some cases, the lack of adequate data on safety and/or efficacy. Informed parental consent is recommended for the use of vaccinations outside of recommended limits and licensure.

References

1. Siegrist CA. Vaccination in the neonatal period and early infancy. Int Rev Immunol 2000;19:195–219.
2. Siegrist CA, Cordova M, Brandt C, et al. Determinants of infant responses to vaccines in presence of maternal antibodies. Vaccine 1998;16:1409–14.
3. Plotkin SA. Immunologic correlates of protection induced by vaccination. Pediatr Infect Dis J 2001;20:63–74.
4. Moore DL, Le Saux N, Scheifele D, et al. Lack of evidence of encephalopathy related to pertussis vaccine: active surveillance by IMPACT, Canada, 1993–2002. Pediatr Infect Dis J 2004;23:568–71.
5. American Academy of Pediatrics. In: Pickering L.K, editor. 2009 Red Book: Report of the Committee on Infectious Diseases. 27th ed. Elk Grove Village: American Academy of Pediatrics; 2009; Pertussis.
6. Centers for Disease Control and Prevention. National Immunization Program. Record of the meeting of the Advisory Committee on Immunization Practices: June 29–30, 2005. Online. Available: http://www.cdc.gov/nip/ACIP/minutes/acip-min-jun05.rtf (accessed Nov 13, 2005).
7. American Academy of Pediatrics. In: Pickering LK, editor. 2006 Red Book: Report of the Committee on Infectious Diseases. 26th ed. Elk Grove Village: American Academy of Pediatrics; 2006; Measles: 441. American Academy of Pediatrics. In: Pickering L.K, ed. 2009 Red Book: Report of the Committee on Infectious Diseases. 27th edn. Elk Grove Village: American Academy of Pediatrics; 2009.
8. American Academy of Pediatrics. In: Pickering LK, editor. 2009 Red Book: Report of the Committee on Infectious Diseases. 27th ed. Elk Grove Village: American Academy of Pediatrics; 2009;Poliovirus Infections: 547.
9. Steffen R. Influenza in travelers: epidemiology, risk, prevention, and control issues. Curr Infect Dis Rep 2010 May; 12(3):181–5.
10. Centers for Disease Control and Prevention. Prevention and Control of Influenza: Recommendations of the Advisory Committee on Immunization Practices (ACIP). MMWR Recomm Rep 2006;55(RR-10):1–42.
11. Influenza Virus Vaccine Live. Intranasal. Online. Available: http://www.flumist.com/pdf/prescribinginfo.pdf (accessed Nov 13, 2005).
12. Centers for Disease Control and Prevention. National Immunization Program. June 2006 ACIP Recommendations Pending MMWR; 2007.
13. Cassidy WM, Watson B, Ioli VA, et al. A randomized trial of alternative two- and three-dose hepatitis B vaccination regimens in adolescents: antibody responses, safety, and immunologic memory. Pediatrics 2001;107:626–31.
14. Wkly Epidemiol Rec 2011 Jul 22; 86(30):317–21. Rotavirus vaccine and intussusception: report from an expert consultation.
15. American Academy of Pediatrics. In: Pickering LK, editor. 2009 Red Book: Report of the Committee on Infectious Diseases. 27th ed. Elk Grove Village: American Academy of Pediatrics; 2009; Active Immunization: p. 9–49.
16. Joel M, Palefsky MD, Anna R, et al. HPV vaccine against anal HPV infection and anal intraepithelial neoplasia. N Engl J Med 2011;365:1576–85.
17. Anna R, Giuliano PhD, Joel M, et al. Efficacy of quadrivalent HPV vaccine against HPV infection and disease in males. N Engl J Med 2011;364:401–11.

18. Arguin P, Kozarsky P, Reed C. CDC Health Information for International Travel, 2008. St Louis: Mosby; 2008.

19. Dagan R, Amir J, Mijalovsky A, et al. Immunization against hepatitis A in the first year of life: priming despite the presence of maternal antibody. Pediatr Infect Dis J 2000;19:1045–52.

20. Fiore AE, Wasley A, Bell BP. Prevention of hepatitis A through active or passive immunization: recommendations of the Advisory Committee on Immunization Practices (ACIP). MMWR Recomm Rep 2006;55(RR-7):1–23.

21. Diaz-Mitoma F. A combined vaccine against hepatitis A and B in children and adolescents. Pediatr Infect Dis J 1999;18:109–14.

22. Kurugol Z, Mutlubas F, Ozacar T. A two-dose schedule for combined hepatitis A and B vaccination in children aged 6–15 years. Vaccine 2005;23:2876–80.

23. Granoff DM, Feavers IM, Borrow R. Meningococcal vaccines; In: Plotkin S.A, Orenstein W, editors. Vaccines. 4th ed. Philadelphia: W.B. Saunders; 2004.

24. Centers for Disease Control and Prevention. Prevention and control of meningococcal disease. Recommendations of the Advisory Committee on Immunization Practices (ACIP). MMWR Recomm Rep 2005;54(RR07):1–21.

25. Castelli ED, Barnett WM. Stauffer and for the GeoSentinelStefan Hagmann, Richard Neugebauer, Eli Schwartz, Cecilia Perret, Francesco Illness in Children After International Travel: Analysis From the GeoSentinel Network. Pediatrics 2010;125:e1072.

26. MMWR 5/27/11;60(20):664–5 Update on JE vaccine for children.

27. Kaltenböck A, Dubischar-Kastnera K, Schuller E, et al. Immunogenicity and safety of IXIARO (IC51) in a Phase II study in healthy Indian children between 1 and 3 years of age. Vaccine 2010;28:834–9.

28. Sohn YM, Park MS, Rho HO, et al. Primary and booster immune responses to SA14–14–2 Japanese encephalitis vaccine in Korean infants. Vaccine 1999;17:2259–64.

29. Xin YY, Ming ZG, Peng GY, et al. Safety of a live-attenuated Japanese encephalitis virus vaccine (SA14–14–2) for children. Am J Trop Med Hyg 1988;39:214–7.

30. Centers for Disease Control and Prevention. The role of BCG vaccine in the prevention and control of tuberculosis in the United States: a joint statement by the Advisory Committee on Immunization Practices and Advisory Council for the Elimination of Tuberculosis. MMWR 1996;45(RR-4):1.

31. Recommendations on the Use of Quadrivalent Human Papillomavirus Vaccine in Males – Advisory Committee on Immunization Practices (ACIP), 2011December 23; 2011 / 60(50):1705–8.

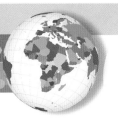

Malaria: Epidemiology and Risk to the Traveler

Gregory A. Deye and Alan J. Magill

Key points

- Travelers to sub-Saharan Africa and Oceania are at the highest risk of acquiring malaria
- Particular special population groups, such as those visiting friends and relatives (VFRs), have a higher risk
- The risk of malaria in endemic populations may not reflect the risk of acquiring malaria in travelers, because activities, behaviors, and sleeping conditions are often different between the two groups
- The geographic distribution of drug resistance restricts the use of suitable antimalarial drugs. Never prescribe chloroquine or chloroquine-containing regimens for travel to sub-Saharan Africa
- Fatal imported malaria is uncommon and preventable. Risk factors are non-immune travelers, older age, travel to East Africa, and absence of chemoprophylaxis

Introduction

Malaria is no longer an endemic infectious disease in the industrialized countries of North America, Europe, Australia, New Zealand, and Japan. However, the marked increase in pleasure and business travelers to malaria-endemic areas, as well as immigration and refugee migrations into non-endemic areas, have led to increasing numbers of imported cases of malaria in industrialized countries. After a temporary slowing associated with the world economy from 2008 to 2009, in 2010 international tourist arrivals to sub-Saharan Africa – the geographic destination at highest risk – saw a 6% increase to 49 million arrivals compared to 2009.[1] Table 14.1 shows reported malaria cases in selected European countries since 2000 as reported to the WHO Regional Office for Europe. Although the reporting methods as well as the accuracy and completeness of surveillance vary between countries,[2] almost 115 000 cases were reported in the 11-year period from 2000 to 2010. There has been a downward trend in the number of cases over this period, possibly exacerbated by reduced travel over the period 2008–2009.[3]

The UK and France alone represented over half the total reported cases, possibly reflecting better surveillance, a large immigrant population who frequently visit their country of birth, and a large traveling population. Over the period 2000–2009, the USA reported 14 103 total cases. Between 1980 and 2009, the number of imported cases in the USA ranged from a low of 803 in 1983 to 1691 in 2010, and has remained over 1000 cases per year since 1993.[4] Between 2000 and 2009, Australia recorded over 6000 cases of imported malaria, with a change from vivax predominant in 2000 to falciparum predominant by 2005 (Australia's notifiable diseases status annual reports of the National Notifiable Diseases Surveillance System; available at: http://www.health.gov.au/internet/main/publishing.nsf/Content/cdi3403–1).

Who is at Risk?

Although any non-immune person not taking efficacious chemoprophylaxis may develop clinical malaria if bitten by an infected mosquito, some groups are at higher risk, based on increased exposure due to behaviors, activities, and sleeping conditions. Travelers who fail to take chemoprophylaxis, use inadequate regimens, or are nonadherent to prevention measures routinely develop clinical symptoms at higher rates than those without these risk factors. Particular groups, such as those returning to homes and families in endemic countries ('visiting friends and relatives' or VFRs), seem to be at much higher risk. Studies from public health agencies in Europe, the USA, and Canada reveal an increasing percentage of cases in immigrants and the foreign-born. In a study from a multinational travel medicine network (GeoSentinel), foreign-born VFRs traveling to sub-Saharan Africa, Latin America, or Asia had odds of being diagnosed with malaria respectively eight times, three times or twice as high as tourist travelers to the same regions.[5] When migrants return to their home countries they often spend more time. They may return to rather simple country villages of their youth, and often bring their children with them, who may be completely nonimmune. Adults may have left their home country, such as India, at a time when malaria transmission was relatively low, only to return years later when transmission is much higher. Many never used chemoprophylaxis in their youth, and are unaware that clinical immunity to malaria wanes over a few years. Table 14.2 shows the primary reason for travel for cases of imported malaria as reported by the US CDC in their annual surveillance summaries between 2006 and 2010. The trend shows cases of imported malaria in VFRs to be fairly stable, whereas other categories have declined, causing VFR to

©2012 Elsevier Inc
DOI: 10.1016/B978-1-4557-1076-8.00014-4

Table 14.1 Reported Malaria Cases in Selected European Countries 2000–2010 as Reported to the WHO Regional Office for Europe (Available at: http://data.euro.who.int/CISID/)

	2000	2001	2002	2003	2004	2005	2006	2007	2008	2009	2010	Total
Austria	62	74	65	74	54	54	50	33	58	44	48	616
Belgium	337	327	113	235	212	259	195	193	181	181	213	2446
Bulgaria	15	15	18	12	10	12	13	4	0	–	5	104
Czech Republic	23	26	21	25	14	18	16	22	20	–	13	198
Denmark	202	154	135	103	106	87	101	80	91	54	61	1174
Finland	38	38	31	22	26	25	30	21	40	34	33	338
France	8056	7370	6846	6392	6107	5300	5267	4403	2239	2218	2438	56636
Germany	732	1040	861	819	708	628	566	540	547	523	617	7581
Greece	28	30	25	43	–	–	31	21	36	45	41	300
Hungary	14	21	14	7	7	6	18	7	5	8	5	112
Ireland	19	11	20	20	25	44	96	71	82	90	82	560
Israel	53		41	40	41	46	38	38	46	40	181	564
Italy	986	984	736	672	661	637	630	573	–	–	–	5879
Netherlands	691	568	395	356	307	299	253	214	226	241	–	3550
Norway	79	78	45	55	49	35	44	28	–	34	37	484
Poland	24	27	22	17	30	20	18	11	22	22	35	248
Russian Federation	752	764	503	461	382	165	132	112	88	107	101	3567
Spain	333	346	341	356	351	307	377	319	295	362	346	3733
Sweden	132	143	132	99	102	112	93	88	90	81	115	1187
Switzerland	317	322	239	230	229	204	189	188	216	–	228	2362
United Kingdom	2069	2050	1945	1722	1660	1754	1758	1548	1370	1495	1761	19132
All Europe	15528	14869	13269	12387	11347	10363	10116	8801	5874	5791	6513	114858

Table 14.2 Number of Imported Malaria Cases among US Civilians by Purpose of Travel at the Time of Acquisition, US 2006–2010

	2006		2007		2008		2009		2010	
Category	n	(%)	n	(%)	n	(%)	n	(%)	n	(%)
Visiting friends or relatives	363	50.9	376	62.8	332	65.3	417	63.3	586	54
Missionary or dependant	53	7.4	51	8.5	40	7.9	65	9.9	75	7
Business representative	41	5.7	47	7.8	36	7.1	40	6.1	65	6
Teacher/student	26	3.6	29	4.8	15	2.9	28	4.2	38	3
Tourist	71	9.9	61	10.2	32	6.3	32	4.8	43	4
Peace corps volunteer	5	0.7	6	1	–	–	–	–	–	–
Sailor/aircrew	4	0.6	1	0.2	2	0.4	–	–	9	1
Unknown/other	150	21	128	21.3	51	10	73	11.1	267	25
Total	713	100	699	117	508	100	655	100	1083	100

make up a greater proportion of cases. Immigrants and VFRs are less likely to be aware of and use effective chemoprophylaxis when returning to their home countries for a visit. In a study of imported cases in Italian travelers from 1989 to 1997, only 4% of foreign-born immigrants or VFRs, mostly Africans, used regular chemoprophylaxis, compared to 36% of all traveling Italian citizens.[6] Similarly, in a comparison of the epidemiology of imported malaria into the UK from 1987 to 2006, patients born in Africa took chemoprophylaxis significantly less frequently than European-born patients (28% vs. 61%).[7] Clearly, the VFR group is at much higher relative risk of acquiring malaria. Furthermore, although case-fatality rates are typically lower in this group (0.25% vs. 1.9% for other travelers), malaria deaths do occur in this population.[7]

Although age itself should not be a risk factor for acquiring malaria, activities in which different age groups may participate could predispose certain age groups to more infections. For example, young backpackers may be at increased risk of infection because of their more exotic destinations and activities, less controlled sleeping arrangements, and longer duration of travel. Activities and sleeping arrangements can dramatically affect infection risk. For example, individual travelers were at almost a nine times greater risk of infection than those on package tours to sub-Saharan Africa.[8] This increased risk seen in German travelers was possibly related to longer stay and less protected travel and sleeping conditions.

Once infection occurs, older travelers are at higher risk of poor clinical outcomes and death. The case-fatality rate of *P. falciparum*

Table 14.3 Relative Risk of Travel-Associated Malaria by Destination

Region Visited	Cases of Malaria	No. of Travelers Visiting Region (Millions)[a]	Risk per 10 Million Travelers of Presenting to a Geosentinel Clinic with Malaria	RR (95% CI)
Very low-risk area[b]	83	1766.9	0.5	1 (0.7–1.4)
Caribbean	9	50.5	1.8	3.8 (1.9–7.5)
North Africa	10	30.8	3.2	6.9 (3.6–13.3)
South America	17	43.8	3.9	8.3 (4.9–13.9)
Southeast Asia	64	118.8	5.4	11.5 (8.3–15.9)
Central America	24	13.5	17.8	37.8 (24.0–59.6)
South Asia	45	17.8	25.3	53.8 (37.4–77.4)
Oceania	31	8.6	36	76.7 (50.8–115.9)
Sub-Saharan Africa	514	52.7	97.5	207.6 (164.7–261.8)

[a]Estimated from World Travel Organization data.
[b]Non-risk/very low-risk areas were Europe, Northeast Asia, Australia/New Zealand, North America, and the Middle East.
From Leder K., Black J., O'Brien D., et al: Malaria in travelers: a review of the GeoSentinel surveillance network. Clin Infect Dis 2004; 39:1104–12. Used with permission.

malaria in US travelers from 1966 to 1987 was 3.8% (66 deaths/1760 cases). The case-fatality rate increased dramatically with age. For persons younger than 19 it was 0.4%; from 20 to 39 years of age it was 2.2%; from 40–69 years of age, it was 5.8%; and for those aged 70–79 it was 30.3% (10 deaths/33 cases).[9] More recent data from Europe also strongly support the notion that increasing age is a risk factor for severe clinical disease and poor outcomes, with death rates in those >60 years of age six times higher than in younger age groups.[10] A review of deaths caused by malaria in Switzerland between 1988 and 2002 showed the mean age of fatal cases to exceed the annual means by 10–15 years.[11] Similar results have also been reported from France in a retrospective review of fatal cases reported between 1996 and 2003 that showed an almost twofold increase in the case-fatality rate for each decade of advancing age.[12] Along with lower Glasgow Coma Score and higher parasitemia, in a retrospective study of French patients admitted to intensive care units with severe *P. falciparum* malaria, older age was found to be predictive of death.[13] Whether older age should be considered a reason to recommend chemoprophylaxis or not is not clear, but there is an abundance of data from multiple sources to conclude that poor outcomes are correlated with advancing age.

Where are Travelers at Risk of Acquiring Malaria?

The impact of the disease on persons who live in endemic areas has increased significantly over the past three decades. From a nadir in the early 1960s following the eradication efforts of the 1950s, malaria, and especially drug-resistant malaria, has reclaimed historic geographic distributions in the Amazon and the Indian subcontinent. However, the geographic locations where persons acquire imported malaria may vary depending on the reason for travel and the preventive measures used by the traveler. Despite these differences in risk between endemic populations and travelers, it is generally true that travel to regions with high transmission intensity represents a higher risk than travel to destinations with much lower transmission rates. Figure 14.1 shows the current intensity of *P. falciparum* transmission worldwide.

Sub-Saharan Africa is the destination where the vast majority of malaria infections are acquired. Without chemoprophylaxis, the risk

of symptomatic malaria is estimated to be 1.2% per month in East Africa.[14] In Italian travelers between 1989 and 1997, a relatively stable incidence of acquiring malaria was calculated as 1.5/1000 in Africa, 0.11/1000 in Asia, and 0.04/1000 in Central-South America, despite a significant increase in travel to Asia and Central-South America.[6] According to data from GeoSentinel, an international network of travel medicine clinics, the incidence associated with travel to Africa was 4–20 times higher than with travel to Asia or the Americas (Table 14.3). Risk varies for specific localities and traveler activities. For many popular tourist destinations outside sub-Saharan Africa the risk of infection is non-existent or extremely low, and chemoprophylaxis is not indicated.

Travel medicine practitioners can access destination risk information from many sources, including national guidelines, the WHO, the internet, and numerous commercial software and hardcopy sources. *Health Information for International Travel 2012* (the CDC yellow book) is a very common source for many USA-based practitioners and available for sale (Oxford University Press). An online version and a free download in pdf format are available at http://wwwnc.cdc.gov/travel/page/yellowbook-2012-home.htm.

There are two types of malaria risk information in the yellow book. Geographic risk is described at the country level, with clarification in some cases of specific risk areas based on elevation above sea level, focal areas within countries, and some popular tourist destinations. This information is limited by the infrequent consideration of seasonal variability and the inherent difficulty in quantifying actual transmission risk to an individual traveler. For example, in much of West Africa transmission of malaria is intense and year round, whereas in the tropical Americas the transmission risk is focal, seasonal, and often very low. Since much of the specific geographic risk information is listed by political boundaries within countries, it is necessary to have access to sufficiently detailed maps in order to locate the travel destinations and the listed risk areas. The addition of selected geographic reference maps showing administrative districts in the 2012 yellow book is welcome and useful. Along with geographic area of risk, specific mention is made of the presence or absence of chloroquine-resistant malaria, knowledge that is no longer very useful as most of the malaria-endemic areas of the world where malaria prophylaxis is indicated are chloroquine resistant. The yellow book also provides malaria-specific recommendations

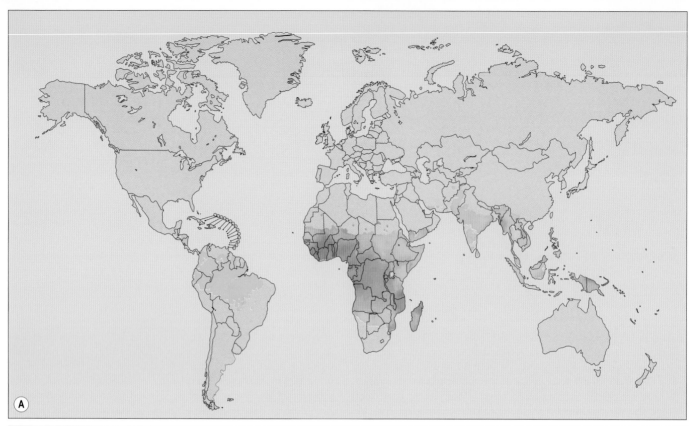

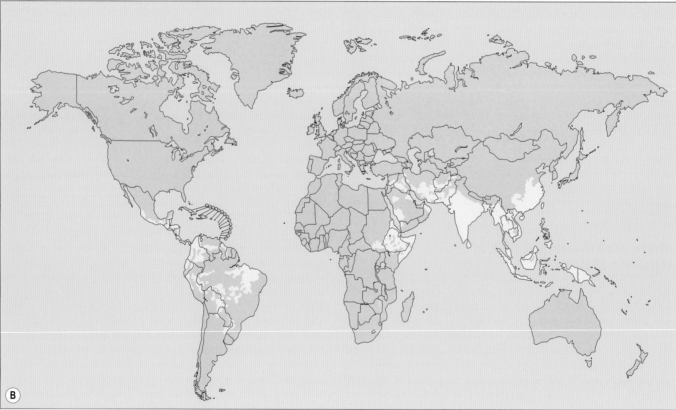

Figure 14.1 Current estimates of transmission intensity of *Plasmodium falciparum* (top) and *Plasmodium vivax* (bottom). *Adapted with permission from Hay SI, Guerra C, Gething PW et al. (2009). A world malaria map: Plasmodium endemnicity in 2007. PLoS Medicine 2009, Mar 6(3) and Guerra CA, Howes RE, Patil AP, et al. (2010) The International Limits and Population at Risk of Plasmodium vivax Transmission in 2009. PLoS Negl Trop Dis 4(8): e774.*

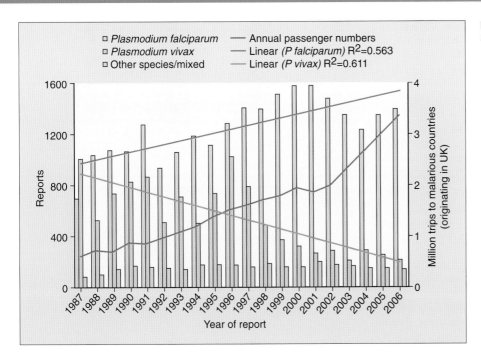

Figure 14.2 Imported malaria cases (with *P. falciparum* cases) into the UK, 1987–2006.[7]

concerning antimalarial drugs for chemoprophylaxis licensed for use in the USA.

Although there are many other sources of geographic risk information, it is challenging for the infrequent or non-expert practitioner of travel medicine to identify and assess the credibility of these sources in a busy practice environment. Malaria destination risk information is also available from the World Health Organization (WHO) International Travel and Health home page (http://www.who.int/ith/chapters/en/index.html), the Canadian Committee to Advise on Tropical Medicine and Travel (CATMAT) Recommendations for the Prevention and Treatment of Malaria Among International Travelers (http://www.phac-aspc.gc.ca/publicat/ccdr-rmtc/09vol35/35s1/index-eng.php), the UK National Travel Health Network and Centre (NaTHNaC) Health Information for Overseas Travel (http://www.nathnac.org/yellow_book/YBmainpage.htm), and several other national level organizations. American readers should note that some recommendations from different authorities may differ from CDC recommendations.

In the last few years, the epidemiology of travelers' malaria has been better defined owing to the formation of traveler-specific surveillance networks such as GeoSentinel (http://www.istm.org/geosentinel/main.html) and the European Network on Imported Infectious Disease Surveillance, also known as TropNet (http://www.tropnet.net/).[15] Recent malaria-specific publications from both groups have better defined the risks of malaria in travelers.[16–20]

Distribution of Malaria Species

The vast majority of imported cases are caused by *P. falciparum* or *P. vivax*. In most countries <5% of cases are caused by *P. ovale* and *P. malariae*. The reported proportions of *Plasmodium* species vary considerably between geographic regions. The proportion of imported malaria cases caused by *P. falciparum* and *P. vivax* seen in individual countries reflects the destinations travelers choose for travel, and to a larger extent the nature of the immigrant communities. For example, historically a relatively large proportion of cases in the UK were caused

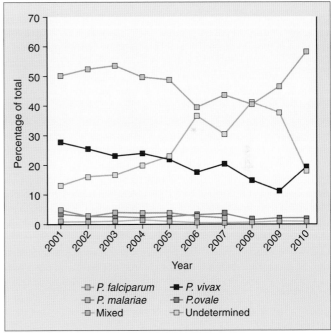

Figure 14.3 Percentage of malaria cases by Plasmodium species (USA, 2000–2009). [CDC Annual report data]

by *P. vivax*, reflecting the large number of immigrants from India and Pakistan, former British colonies.[21] The ratio has changed more recently to predominantly *P. falciparum*, reflecting the change in travel patterns due to an influx of African immigrants who travel back to their country of origin.[7] (Fig. 14.2). This predominance of *P. falciparum* cases is also seen in other countries with large populations of immigrants from Africa, such as France and Italy.[22,23] Figure 14.3 shows the proportion of malaria cases in American travelers by species over the 10 year period 2001–2010. *P. falciparum* malaria has been about 50% of the total for the last few years. The observed steep decline in *P. vivax* cases is consistent with data from Europe and elsewhere. One striking and unfortunate trend in the US data is the dramatic increase in the number of cases reported as undetermined or unspecified, likely reflecting the widespread loss of microscopic diagnostic capabilities in many clinical settings.[24] This loss will endanger surveillance activities if it is not addressed.

Species proportions can also vary at different times of the year. For example, marked increases in *P. falciparum* cases are documented in France and Italy in September, which corresponds to the return of travelers following the August holidays.[25] In Italy, a second peak is seen in January, reflecting Italian tourists returning from a Christmas holiday in a warm tropical locale.[6]

Drug-Resistant Malaria

Chloroquine

Chloroquine (CQ)-resistant *P. falciparum* (CRPf) malaria is now found throughout most malaria-endemic areas, including all of sub-Saharan Africa, South America, the Indian subcontinent, Southeast Asia, and Oceania. CRPf was first recognized in the early 1960s in Colombia,[26] spreading throughout the Amazon Basin within a decade. It was then identified in Cambodia,[27] spreading through South Asia and into East Africa in 1978. By the late 1980s CRPf was widely distributed throughout sub-Saharan Africa.[28–31]

There remain a few countries and destinations in the Americas with CQ-sensitive *P. falciparum* malaria, including Mexico, all countries of Central America west of the Panama Canal, rural areas of Paraguay and northern Argentina, and the island of Hispaniola (Haiti and the Dominican Republic), the only remaining endemic focus in the Caribbean. The risk in these countries is often seasonal, focal, unpredictable, and quite low. Occasionally, small epidemic outbreaks can occur. Many of these risk areas are destinations seldom visited by short-term tourists on holiday, but may be visited by other types of traveler, such as soldiers, construction workers, and aid or relief workers. The risk of acquiring *P. vivax* malaria is much higher than that of *P. falciparum* malaria in many of these countries with CQ-sensitive malaria, especially the Americas.

CQ-resistant *P. vivax* (CRPv) malaria was first described in an Australian soldier returning from Papua New Guinea in 1987.[32] Since that initial recognized case, studies have shown that CRPv is relatively widespread in Indonesia and Papua New Guinea, with more sporadic reports from Borneo, Thailand, Myanmar (Burma), and India in the Old World[33] and Guyana.[34] Therapeutic failures without documentation of therapeutic blood levels for chloroquine have also been seen in Colombia[35] and Brazil. Since all of these areas are also co-endemic with CRPf, this has minimal impact on recommendations for chemoprophylaxis for the traveler, as the chemoprophylaxis choice for these areas is not CQ.

Two cases of CQ-resistant *P. malariae* have been reported from Indonesia, but the clinical significance and distribution of this entity remains undefined.[36]

Mefloquine

At present, significant mefloquine (MQ) resistance is geographically limited to portions of Southeast Asia (Fig. 14.4). The prevalence of MQ resistance in this region in often very high, making MQ a poor choice for chemoprophylaxis for travelers to this area.[37] Sporadic cases of MQ prophylaxis failures have been reported from other locations in Africa[38] and South America, but these few cases do not indicate widespread resistance and do not alter routine travel chemoprophylaxis recommendations.[39]

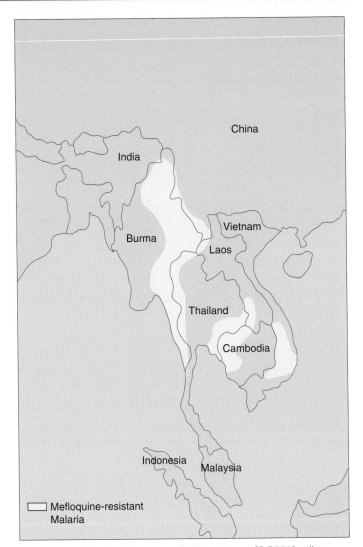

Figure 14.4 Map depicting areas of MQ resistance. CDC 2012 yellow book Ch 3.

Doxycycline

There are no known geographic areas or destinations where doxycycline should not be recommended because of drug resistance. However, decreased in vitro drug susceptibility for some African *P. falciparum* isolates is associated with increased copy numbers and amino acid sequence polymorphisms of transporter genes.[40] The clinical relevance of this observation is not known.

Atovaquone/Proguanil

Resistance to either atovaquone or proguanil is based on single point mutations in the cytochrome B gene or the dihydrofolate reductase (DHFR) gene, respectively. Drug-resistant parasites can emerge rather quickly during treatment when either drug is used separately. In combination, therapeutic failures caused by treatment-emergent drug resistance are much less common. Surveillance of cytochrome B mutations in returning travelers has identified only a very few such mutations, not always associated with therapeutic failure.[41] In these cases, parasite recrudescence observed >3 weeks after initial clinical improvement (late treatment failure) had been reported in returning travelers treated with atovaquone/proguanil. Despite extensive use for over a decade, no confirmed prophylaxis breakthroughs on atovaquone/proguanil have been reported to date. The two prophylaxis breakthroughs described in one of the pre-licensure prophylaxis studies were associated with very low or non-detectable levels of cycloguanil, the primary metabolite of proguanil, suggesting a therapeutic failure due to pharmacokinetic reasons; genetic analysis of the parasite to confirm a drug resistance was not performed.[42]

Primaquine

Primaquine is used as an anti-hypnozoite agent to prevent relapse of *P. vivax* or *P. ovale* malaria. When considering drug resistance and primaquine it is necessary to distinguish acquired drug resistance from therapeutic failures due to other causes. It is also important to distinguish the different indications for which primaquine is used. When used in combination with chloroquine for the radical cure of *P. vivax* malaria in symptomatic patients, it has long been recognized that strains of *P. vivax* from some areas (e.g., Oceania) require higher doses and have higher rates of failure than strains from other regions (e.g., India).[43]

When used as primary prophylaxis, that is, for the prevention of the initial malaria infection in asymptomatic persons, there is no evidence of resistance to primaquine for this indication. Primaquine is not approved by the US FDA for a primary prophylaxis indication, though it is recommended by the US CDC as an alternative agent for short duration travel to areas with transmission of principally *P. vivax*.[44]

References

1. Organization WT. UNWTO World Tourism Barometer. 2011 January.
2. Legros F, Danis M. Surveillance of malaria in European Union countries. Euro Surveill 1998 May;3(5):45–7.
3. UNWTO World Tourism Barometer. 2011.
4. Mali S, Tan KR, Arguin PM. Malaria surveillance–United States, 2009. MMWR Surveill Summ 2011 Apr 22;60(3):1–15.
5. Leder K, Tong S, Weld L, et al. Illness in travelers visiting friends and relatives: a review of the GeoSentinel Surveillance Network. Clin Infect Dis 2006 Nov 1;43(9):1185–93.
6. Romi R, Sabatinelli G, Majori G. Malaria epidemiological situation in Italy and evaluation of malaria incidence in Italian travelers. J Travel Med 2001 Jan-Feb;8(1):6–11.
7. Smith AD, Bradley DJ, Smith V, et al. Imported malaria and high risk groups: observational study using UK surveillance data 1987–2006. BMJ 2008;337:a120.
8. Jelinek T, Loscher T, Nothdurft HD. High prevalence of antibodies against circumsporozoite antigen of Plasmodium falciparum without development of symptomatic malaria in travelers returning from sub-Saharan Africa. J Infect Dis 1996 Dec;174(6):1376–9.
9. Greenberg AE, Lobel HO. Mortality from Plasmodium falciparum malaria in travelers from the United States, 1959 to 1987. Ann Intern Med 1990 Aug 15;113(4):326–7.
10. Muhlberger N, Jelinek T, Behrens RH, et al. Age as a risk factor for severe manifestations and fatal outcome of falciparum malaria in European patients: observations from TropNetEurop and SIMPID Surveillance Data. Clin Infect Dis 2003 Apr 15;36(8):990–5.
11. Christen D, Steffen R, Schlagenhauf P. Deaths caused by malaria in Switzerland 1988–2002. Am J Trop Med Hyg 2006 Dec;75(6):1188–94.
12. Legros F, Bouchaud O, Ancelle T, et al. Risk factors for imported fatal Plasmodium falciparum malaria, France, 1996–2003. Emerg Infect Dis 2007 Jun;13(6):883–8.
13. Bruneel F, Tubach F, Corne P, et al. Severe imported falciparum malaria: a cohort study in 400 critically ill adults. PLoS One 2010;5(10):e13236.
14. Steffen R, Fuchs E, Schildknecht J, et al. Mefloquine compared with other malaria chemoprophylactic regimens in tourists visiting east Africa. Lancet 1993 May 22;341(8856):1299–303.
15. Ross K. Tracking the spread of infectious disease: two networks prove the power of international collaboration. EMBO Rep 2006 Sep;7(9):855–8.
16. Jelinek T. Imported falciparum malaria in Europe: 2007 data from TropNetEurop. Euro Surveill 2008 Jun 5;13(23).
17. Leder K. Travelers as a sentinel population: use of sentinel networks to inform pretravel and posttravel evaluation. Curr Infect Dis Rep 2009 Jan;11(1):51–8.
18. Wilson ME, Weld LH, Boggild A, et al. Fever in returned travelers: results from the GeoSentinel Surveillance Network. Clin Infect Dis 2007 Jun 15;44(12):1560–8.
19. Freedman DO, Weld LH, Kozarsky PE, et al. Spectrum of disease and relation to place of exposure among ill returned travelers. N Engl J Med 2006 Jan 12;354(2):119–30.
20. Leder K, Black J, O'Brien D, et al. Malaria in travelers: a review of the GeoSentinel surveillance network. Clin Infect Dis 2004 Oct 15;39(8):1104–12.
21. Phillips-Howard PA, Bradley DJ, Blaze M, et al. Malaria in Britain: 1977–86. Br Med J (Clin Res Ed) 1988 Jan 23;296(6617):245–8.
22. Talarmin F, Sicard JM, Mounem M, et al. [Imported malaria in Moselle: 75 cases in three years]. Rev Med Interne 2000 Mar;21(3):242–6.
23. Romi R, Boccolini D, D'Amato S, et al. Incidence of malaria and risk factors in Italian travelers to malaria endemic countries. Travel Med Infect Dis 2010 May;8(3):144–54.
24. Abanyie FA, Arguin PM, Gutman J. State of malaria diagnostic testing at clinical laboratories in the United States, 2010: a nationwide survey. Malar J 2011;10:340.
25. Legros F, Gay F, Belkaid M, et al. Imported malaria in continental France in 1996. Euro Surveill 1998 Apr;3(4):37–8.
26. Moore DV, Lanier JE. Observations on two Plasmodium falciparum infections with an abnormal response to chloroquine. Am J Trop Med Hyg 1961 Jan;10:5–9.
27. Eyles DE, Hoo CC, Warren M, et al. Plasmodium falciparum resistant to chloroquine in Cambodia. Am J Trop Med Hyg 1963 Nov;12:840–3.
28. Moran JS, Bernard KW. The spread of chloroquine-resistant malaria in Africa. Implications for travelers. JAMA 1989 Jul 14;262(2):245–8.
29. Moran JS, Bernard KW, Greenberg AE, et al. Failure of chloroquine treatment to prevent malaria in Americans in West Africa. JAMA 1987 Nov 6;258(17):2376–7.
30. Wongsrichanalai C, Pickard AL, Wernsdorfer WH, et al. Epidemiology of drug-resistant malaria. Lancet Infect Dis 2002 Apr;2(4):209–18.
31. Laufer MK, Thesing PC, Eddington ND, et al. Return of chloroquine antimalarial efficacy in Malawi. N Engl J Med 2006 Nov 9;355(19):1959–66.
32. Whitby M, Wood G, Veenendaal JR, et al. Chloroquine-resistant Plasmodium vivax. Lancet 1989 Dec 9;2(8676):1395.
33. Whitby M. Drug resistant Plasmodium vivax malaria. J Antimicrob Chemother 1997 Dec;40(6):749–52.
34. Phillips EJ, Keystone JS, Kain KC. Failure of combined chloroquine and high-dose primaquine therapy for Plasmodium vivax malaria acquired in Guyana, South America. Clin Infect Dis 1996 Nov;23(5):1171–3.
35. Soto J, Toledo J, Gutierrez P, et al. Plasmodium vivax clinically resistant to chloroquine in Colombia. Am J Trop Med Hyg 2001 Aug;65(2):90–3.
36. Maguire JD, Sumawinata IW, Masbar S, et al. Chloroquine-resistant Plasmodium malariae in south Sumatra, Indonesia. Lancet 2002 Jul 6;360(9326):58–60.
37. Khim N, Bouchier C, Ekala MT, et al. Countrywide survey shows very high prevalence of Plasmodium falciparum multilocus resistance genotypes in Cambodia. Antimicrob Agents Chemother 2005 Aug;49(8):3147–52.
38. Wichmann O, Betschart B, Loscher T, et al. Prophylaxis failure due to probable mefloquine resistant P. falciparum from Tanzania. Acta Trop 2003 Apr;86(1):63–5.
39. Lobel HO, Varma JK, Miani M, et al. Monitoring for mefloquine-resistant Plasmodium falciparum in Africa: implications for travelers' health. Am J Trop Med Hyg 1998 Jul;59(1):129–32.
40. Briolant S, Wurtz N, Zettor A, et al. Susceptibility of Plasmodium falciparum isolates to doxycycline is associated with pftetQ sequence polymorphisms and pftetQ and pfmdt copy numbers. J Infect Dis 2010 Jan 1;201(1):153–9.

41. Wichmann O, Muehlberger N, Jelinek T, et al. Screening for mutations related to atovaquone/proguanil resistance in treatment failures and other imported isolates of Plasmodium falciparum in Europe. J Infect Dis 2004 Nov 1;190(9):1541–6.

42. Sukwa TY, Mulenga M, Chisdaka N, et al. A randomized, double-blind, placebo-controlled field trial to determine the efficacy and safety of Malarone (atovaquone/proguanil) for the prophylaxis of malaria in Zambia. Am J Trop Med Hyg 1999 Apr;60(4):521–5.

43. Goller JL, Jolley D, Ringwald P, et al. Regional differences in the response of Plasmodium vivax malaria to primaquine as anti-relapse therapy. Am J Trop Med Hyg 2007 Feb;76(2):203–7.

44. CDC Health Information for International Travel 2012. New York: Oxford University Press, 2012.

15

Malaria Chemoprophylaxis

Patricia Schlagenhauf and Kevin C. Kain

Key points

All travelers to malaria-endemic areas need to:

- Be aware of the risk of malaria and understand that it is a serious, potentially fatal infection
- Know how to best prevent it with insect protection measures and chemoprophylaxis (where appropriate)
- Seek medical attention urgently should they develop a fever during or after travel
- The use of chemoprophylaxis drug regimens should be carefully directed at high-risk travelers where their benefit most clearly outweighs the risk of adverse events
- None of the available regimens is ideal for all travelers, and the travel medicine practitioner should attempt to match the individual's risk of malaria to the appropriate regimen based on drug efficacy, tolerability, safety, and cost

Approach to Malaria Prevention

Protection against malaria can be summarized into four principles.

Assessing Individual Risk

Estimating a traveler's risk is based on a detailed travel itinerary and specific risk behaviors of the traveler. The risk of acquiring malaria will vary according to the geographic area visited (e.g., Africa versus SE Asia), the travel destination within different geographic areas (urban versus rural), type of accommodations (camping versus well-screened or air-conditioned), duration of stay (1-week business travel versus 3-month overland trek), time of travel (high or low malaria transmission season; risk usually is highest during and immediately after the rainy season), efficacy of and compliance with preventive measures used (e.g., treated bed nets, chemoprophylactic drugs), and elevation of destination (malaria transmission is rare above 2000 m).

Despite an overall decline in malaria incidence in certain African countries, there have been recent reports of a resurgence of malaria at higher elevations, particularly in the highlands of East Africa. Although there was initial speculation that this was attributable to climate change, other data have not supported this contention.[1] Escalating drug resistance and population movements are a more plausible explanation for these highland epidemics. Country-specific altitude limitations to malaria can generally be found in destination references.[2-7] It should be noted that the starting points and base camps for many higher altitude hikes, e.g., Mount Kilimanjaro, *are* at altitudes where there may be a high risk for malaria.

Additional information can be obtained from studies that estimate risk of malaria in travelers using malaria surveillance data and the numbers of travelers to specific destinations. These studies demonstrate a higher risk of infection, particularly with *P. falciparum*, in Africa and New Guinea than in Asia or Latin America.[6-9] Several studies have shown that immigrants who are settled in industrialized countries are at particularly high risk of malaria when they return to their home countries to visit friends and relatives (VFR travelers).[7] This particular group of travelers is less likely to seek pre-travel advice, and many are unaware that their pre-existing semi-immunity to malaria wanes over time and is no longer protective. In contrast, many frequently visited tourist destinations in malaria-endemic countries, e.g., Phuket in Thailand or Rio de Janeiro in Brazil, have zero or negligible malaria risk. Of note, the estimated risk of malaria for travelers to Thailand in one study was 1 : 12 254: this may be less than the risk of a serious adverse event secondary to malaria chemoprophylaxis.[9] Such data can help provide an estimate of the risk–benefit ratio for the use of various chemoprophylactic drugs in different geographic areas. Updated malaria information and country-specific risks are available online from several sources, including the Centers for Disease Control and Prevention (CDC), the World Health Organization (WHO), and Health Canada.

Preventing Mosquito Bites (Personal Protection Measures)

All travelers to malaria-endemic areas need to be instructed how best to avoid bites from *Anopheles* mosquitoes, which transmit malaria. Any measure that reduces exposure to the evening and night-time feeding female *Anopheles* mosquito will reduce the risk of acquiring malaria. The travel health advisor should spend time explaining the use of personal protective measures against mosquito bites and encouraging adherence with these measures. Studies have demonstrated that *N,N*-diethyl-3methylbenzamide (DEET)-based repellents provide adequate protection against mosquito bites, and preparations containing approximately 20% DEET can be recommended for adults and children over 2 months.[2,10,11] Controlled trials have also shown that DEET-based insect repellents are effective at preventing vector-borne

©2012 Elsevier Inc
DOI: 10.1016/B978-1-4557-1076-8.00015-6

diseases such as malaria.[12] A randomized placebo-controlled trial examined the use of DEET-based repellents (20% DEET) during the second and third trimesters of pregnancy. No adverse effects were identified in mother or fetus, providing reassurance regarding the use of DEET-based repellents by pregnant women.[13] Another widely used repellent is picaridin (KBR 3023, Bayrepel [RS]-sec-butyl2-[2-hydroxyethyl]piperidine-1-carboxylate). This repellent appears to be less irritating than DEET products and has good cosmetic properties. One controlled field study showed that 19% picaridin was effective and offered a protection equivalent to that of a long-acting DEET formulation.[14] Insecticide-impregnated bed-nets (permethrin or similarly treated) are safe for children and pregnant women and are an effective prevention strategy[15] that is often underused by travelers.

Use of Chemoprophylactic Drugs Where Appropriate

The use of antimalarial drugs and their potential real or perceived adverse effects must be weighed against the risk of acquiring malaria (as described above). The following questions should be addressed before prescribing any antimalarial:

- Will the traveler be exposed to malaria? The risk of malaria exists in urban and rural areas of sub-Saharan Africa and the Indian subcontinent, whereas most urban areas, beach and tourist resort areas of SE Asia, Central and South America do not have sufficient risk of malaria to warrant routine use of chemoprophylaxis
- What type of malaria predominates at the destination, *P. falciparum* or *P. vivax*?
- Will the traveler be in a drug-resistant *P. falciparum* zone?
- Will the traveler have prompt access to medical care (including blood smears prepared with sterile equipment and then properly interpreted) if symptoms of malaria were to occur?
- Are there any contraindications to the use of a particular antimalarial drug? Several issues, including underlying health conditions, drug interactions, pregnancy, and breastfeeding, must be considered. It is also important to determine whether a woman is planning to become pregnant while traveling
- Adherence issues are important. All chemoprophylactic medications need to be started before travel – mefloquine (1–3 weeks), doxycycline, and atovaquone-proguanil (1 day) – taken regularly during travel and continued after leaving the malaria-endemic area (a 4-week, post-travel drug intake is required for all regimens except atovaquone-proguanil and primaquine, where only a week post-travel intake is required).

It is important to note that a number of travelers to low-risk areas, such as urban areas and tourist resorts in SE Asia, continue to be inappropriately prescribed antimalarial drugs that result in unnecessary adverse events but little protection. Improved traveler adherence with antimalarials will likely result when travel medicine practitioners make a concerted effort to identify and carefully counsel the high-risk traveler and avoid unnecessary drugs in the low-risk individual.

Seeking Early Diagnosis and Treatment If Fever Develops During or After Travel

Travelers should be informed that although personal protection measures and the use of chemoprophylaxis can markedly reduce the risk of contracting malaria, these interventions do not guarantee complete protection. Symptoms of malaria may occur as early as 1 week after the first exposure, and as late as several years after leaving a malaria zone whether or not chemosuppression has been used. Approximately

90% of malaria-infected travelers do not become symptomatic until they return home.[16–18] Most travelers who acquire falciparum malaria will develop symptoms within 3 months of exposure.[16–18] Falciparum malaria can be effectively treated early in its course, but delays in therapy may result in serious and even fatal outcomes. The most important factors that determine outcome are early diagnosis and appropriate therapy. Travelers and healthcare providers alike must consider and urgently rule out malaria in any febrile illness that occurs during or after travel to a malaria-endemic area.

Chemoprophylaxis According to Drug Resistance Patterns

Antimalarial drugs are selected based on individual risk assessment (as discussed above) and drug-resistance patterns (Fig. 15.1, Table 15.1). Chloroquine-resistant *P. falciparum* (CRPf) is now widespread in all malaria-endemic areas of the world, except for Mexico, the Caribbean, Central America, Argentina, and parts of the Middle-East and China. *P. falciparum* malaria resistant to chloroquine and mefloquine is still rare except on the borders of Thailand with Cambodia and Myanmar (Burma). Resistance to sulfadoxine-pyrimethamine is now common in the Amazon basin, SE Asia, and in many regions of Africa.

Table 15.1 Malaria Chemoprophylactic Regimens for Persons at Risk by Zone[a]

Zone	Drug(s) of choice[b]	Alternatives
No chloroquine resistance	Chloroquine	Mefloquine, doxycycline or atovaquone/proguanil
Chloroquine resistance	Mefloquine or atovaquone/proguanil or doxycycline	1st choice: primaquine[c]; 2nd choice: chloroquine plus proguanil[d]
Chloroquine and Mefloquine resistance	Doxycycline or atovaquone/proguanil	
Adult Doses		
Chloroquine phosphate	300 mg (base) weekly	
Mefloquine	250 mg (salt in USA; base elsewhere) weekly	
Atovaquone/proguanil	One tablet daily (250 mg/100 mg)	
Doxycycline	100 mg daily	
Primaquine	30 mg (base) daily[c]	
Proguanil	200 mg daily*	

[a]*IMPORTANT NOTE*: Protection from mosquito bites (insecticide-treated bed-nets, DEET-based insect repellents, etc.) is the first line of defense against malaria for all travelers. In the Americas and SE Asia, chemoprophylaxis is recommended only for travelers who will be exposed outdoors during evening or night time in rural areas.
[b]Chloroquine and mefloquine are to be taken once weekly, beginning 1 week before entering the malarial area, during the stay and for 4 weeks after leaving. Doxycycline and proguanil are taken daily, starting 1 day before entering malarial areas, during the stay and for 4 weeks after departure. Atovaquone/proguanil and primaquine are taken once daily, starting 1 day before entering the malarial area, during the stay and may be discontinued 7 days after leaving the endemic area.
[c]Contraindicated in G6PD (glucose-6-phosphate dehydrogenase) deficiency and during pregnancy. Not presently licensed for this use. A G6PD level must be performed before prescribing.
[d]Chloroquine plus proguanil is less efficacious than mefloquine, doxycycline or AP in these areas.
*Should only be used in combination with chloroquine.

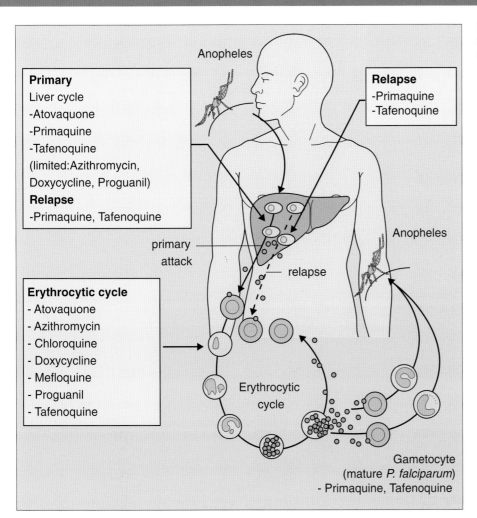

Figure 15.1 The life-cycle of malaria parasites in the human host, showing sites of action of antimalarial drugs.

Chloroquine-resistant *Plasmodium vivax* is also becoming an important problem, particularly in Papua New Guinea, West Papua (formerly Irian Jaya), Vanuatu, Myanmar, and Guyana.

Chloroquine-Sensitive Zones

Chloroquine is the drug of choice for travel to the limited geographic areas where chloroquine resistance has not been described.

Chloroquine-Resistant Zones

For most at-risk travelers to these areas a choice between mefloquine, atovaquone-proguanil, and doxycycline will have to be made. In those with contraindications to or intolerance of these drugs, primaquine or chloroquine plus proguanil may occasionally be used. Deciding which agent is best requires an individual assessment of malaria risk and the specific advantages and disadvantages of each regimen (Tables 15.1–15.6). For drugs such as mefloquine, doxycycline, and chloroquine/proguanil to be optimally effective, they need to be taken for 4 weeks after leaving a malaria-endemic area, although traveler adherence with this component has traditionally been poor.[16–18] Agents such as atovaquone-proguanil and primaquine are called causal prophylactics since they act on malaria parasites early in the life-cycle in the liver, and therefore may be discontinued 1 week after leaving an endemic area. This advantage makes these agents attractive for high-risk but short-duration travel. It is important to note that none of these agents is ideal, and all carry a risk of adverse events that are distressing enough

Table 15.2 Incidence of Any Adverse Event During Malaria Chemoprophylaxis in Non-Immune Travelers

Study	Population	MQ	C+P	DX	A+P
Steffen 1993[8]	Travelers	24	35	–	–
Boudreau 1993[82]	US Marines	43	46	–	–
Barrett 1996[63]	Travelers	41	41	–	–
Nasveld 2000[97]	Austral. Defense	–	–	58	38
Hogh 2000[a34]	Travelers	–	28	–	22
Overbosch 2001[62]	Travelers	68	–	–	71
Schlagenhauf 2003[19]	Travelers	88	86	84	82

MQ, mefloquine; C+P, chloroquine/proguanil; DX, doxycycline; A+P, atovaquone/proguanil.
[a]Drug associated.

to travelers for 1–7% to discontinue their prescribed chemoprophylactic regimen.[2–4,16–18,19]

Chloroquine- and Mefloquine-Resistant Zones

In these regions along the Thai–Myanmar and Thai–Cambodian borders, doxycycline or atovaquone-proguanil are the drugs of choice if chemoprophylaxis is needed in these areas.[2–4]

Table 15.3 Incidence of Severe[a] Events During Malaria Chemoprophylaxis in Travelers

Study	Population	MQ	C+P	DX	A+P
Phillips 1996[64]	Australian	11.2	–	6.5	–
Schlagenhauf 1996[66]	Swiss	11.2	–	–	–
Barrett 1996[63]	UK	17	16	–	–
Steffen 1993[8]	European	13	16	–	–
Hogh[b] 2000[34]	International	–	2	–	0.2
Overbosch[b] 2001[62]	International	5	–	–	1
Schlagenhauf 2003[c][19]	International	10.5	12.4	5.9	6.7

MQ, mefloquine; C+P, chloroquine/proguanil; DX, doxycycline; A+P, atovaquone/proguanil.
[a]Interferes with daily activity.
[b]Stopped taking antimalarials.
[c]Sought medical attention in context of the study.

Table 15.4 Incidence of Serious[a] Adverse Events During Malaria Chemoprophylaxis

Report	Population	MQ	C+P	DX	A+P
MacPherson 1992[68]	Canadian	1/20 000		?	?
Steffen 1993[8]	European	1/10 000	1/13 600		
Croft 1996[70]	UK soldiers	1/6 000			
Barrett 1996[63]	UK	1/600	1/1 200		
Roche Drug Safety 1997	Worldwide	1/20 000			

MQ, mefloquine; C+P, chloroquine/proguanil; DX, doxycycline; A+P, atovaquone/proguanil
[a]Hospitalization.

Table 15.5 Antimalarial Drugs, Doses, and Adverse Effects (Listed Alphabetically) (See Text for Contraindications)

Generic Name	Trade Name	Packaging	Adult Dose	Pediatric Dose	Adverse Effects
Atovaquone/proguanil	Malarone	250 mg atovaquone and 100 mg proguanil (adult tablet)	1 tablet daily (see text)[a]	See text[b] 5–8 kg: ½ pediatric tablet 8–10 kg: ¾ pediatric tablet 10–20 kg: 1 pediatric tablet 20–30 kg: 2 pediatric tablets 30–40 kg: 3 pediatric tablets >40 kg: 1 adult tablet	Nausea, vomiting, abdominal pain, diarrhea, increased transaminases, seizures, rash
Chloroquine[c] phosphate or sulfate	Aralen Avochlot Nivaquine Resochia	150 mg base	300 mg base once weekly[a]	5 mg base once weekly 5–6 kg: 25 mg base 7–10 kg: 50 mg base 11–14 kg: 75 mg base 15–18 kg: 100 mg base 19–24 kg: 125 mg base 25–35 kg: 200 mg base 36–50 kg: 250 mg base >50 kg or if ≥14 years: 300 mg base	Pruritus in black-skinned individuals, nausea, headache, skin eruptions, reversible corneal opacity, nail and mucous membrane discoloration, nerve deafness, photophobia, myopathy, retinopathy with daily use, blood dyscrasias, psychosis, seizures, alopecia
Doxycycline	Vibramycin Vibra-Tabs Doryx	100 mg	100 mg once daily[a]	1.5 mg/kg once daily (max 100 mg daily) <25 kg or if <8 years: contraindicated 25–35 kg: 50 mg 36–50 kg: 75 mg >50 kg or if ≥14 years: 100 mg	GI upset, vaginal candidiasis, photosensitivity, allergic reactions, blood dyscrasias, azotemia in renal diseases, hepatitis
Mefloquine	Lariam Mephaquin	250 mg base (salt in USA)	250 mg base once weekly[a]	<5 kg: no data 5–15 kg: 5 mg/kg once weekly 15–19 kg: 1/4 tablet 20–30 kg: 1/2 tablet 31–45 kg: 3/4 tablet >45 kg: 1 tablet once weekly	Dizziness, diarrhea, nausea, vivid dreams, nightmares, irritability, mood alterations, headache, insomnia, anxiety, seizures, psychosis

Table 15.5 Antimalarial Drugs, Doses, and Adverse Effects (Listed Alphabetically) (See Text for Contraindications)—cont'd

Generic Name	Trade Name	Packaging	Adult Dose	Pediatric Dose	Adverse Effects
Primaquine		15 mg base	30 mg base/day Terminal prophylaxis or radical cure: 15 mg base/day for 14 days[d]	0.5 mg base/day to max of 30 mg base/day Terminal prophylaxis or radical cure: 0.3 mg base/kg per day for 14 days[e]	GI upset, hemolysis in G6PD deficiency, methemoglobinemia
Proguanil	Paludrine	100 mg	200 mg daily: *Note:* Not recommended as a single agent for prophylaxis	5–8 kg: 25 mg (1/4 tablet) 9–16 kg: 50 mg (1/2 tablet) 7–24 kg: 75 mg (3/4 tablet) 25–35 kg: 100 mg (1 tablet) 36–50 kg: 150 mg (1 1/2 tablets) >50 kg or if ≥14 years: 200 mg (2 tablets)	Anorexia, nausea, mouth ulcers

[a]Dose for chemoprophylaxis.
[b]In the USA and EU, a pediatric formulation is available (quarter strength = 62.5 mg atovaquone and 25 mg proguanil). CDC sanctions atovaquone/proguanil for infants >5 kg. WHO allows it for infants weighing over 11 kg.
[c]Chloroquine sulfate (Nivaquine) is not available in USA and Canada, but is available in most malaria-endemic countries in both tablet and syrup form.
[d]Doses are increased to 30 mg base/day for primaquine-resistant *P. vivax*.
[e]Doses are increased to 0.5 mg base/kg per day for primaquine-resistant or tolerant *P vivax*.

Table 15.6 Clinical Utility Score for Current Malaria Chemoprophylactic Regimens

Drug	Efficacy[a]	Tolerability[b]	Convenience[c]	Causal[d]	Cost[e]	Total
Mefloquine	3	1	3	0	3	10
Doxycycline	3	3	2	0	3	11
Chloroquine/proguanil	1	1	1	0	2	5
Primaquine	2	2	1[f]	2	3	10
Atovaquone/proguanil	3	3	2	2	1	11

NOTE: Scores and weighting are arbitrary and can be modified/individualized to specific travelers and itineraries.
[a]Efficacy: 1, <75%; 2, 75–89%; 3, ≥90%.
[b]Tolerability: 1, occasional disabling side-effects; 2, rare disabling side-effects; 3, rare minor side-effects.
[c]Convenience: 1, daily and weekly dosing required; 2, daily dosing required; 3, weekly dosing required.
[d]Causal: 0, no causal activity; 2, causal prophylactic (may be discontinued within 1 week of leaving risk area).
[e]Cost: 1, >US$100 for 1 month of travel; 2, US$50–100; 3, <US$50.
[f]Requires a pre-travel G6PD level resulting in a lower convenience score.

Current Chemoprophylactic Drug Regimens

This section will review currently recommended chemoprophylactic drug regimens, including indications, adverse effects, precautions, and contraindications. The reader is referred elsewhere for other important details of management of malaria-infected patients.[2–4,20]

Chloroquine, Chloroquine/Proguanil

Description, Pharmacology and Mode Of Action

Chloroquine was initially developed in Germany in the 1930s and further evaluated by the Allied powers in the 1940s. It was found to be an outstanding antimalarial drug and has been in continuous use for over 50 years. Although still widely consumed in endemic areas, widespread resistance limits the use of chloroquine and its combinations by travelers. This 4-aminoquinoline drug is chemically a racemate, and both enantiomers have equivalent antimalarial activity. Preparations are available as phosphate, sulfate, and hydrochloride salts, under a wide variety of trade names. The combination of proguanil 200 mg (usually as Paludrine) daily and chloroquine base

300 mg weekly has been used extensively. In some countries, a combined tablet is available that contains chloroquine 100 mg base and proguanil hydrochloride 200 mg (Savarine).

Chloroquine is a potent blood schizonticide, active against the erythrocytic forms of sensitive strains of all four species of malaria, and is also gametocidal against *P. vivax*, *P. malariae* and *P. ovale*.[20] The site of action of chloroquine is within the lysosome of the blood-stage parasite,[21] where it complexes with hemin and prevents its conversion to the non-toxic hemozoin.[22] Proguanil is converted to the active cycloguanil, which is a dihydrofolate reductase inhibitor that acts by interfering with folic–folinic acid systems. Proguanil is effective against the primary exoerythrocytic hepatic forms and is therefore a causal prophylactic. It is also a slow-acting blood schizonticide and has sporonticidal effects against *P. falciparum*.

Efficacy and Drug Resistance

Chloroquine-resistant malaria began to appear in SE Asia and South America in 1960 and reached East Africa in 1978 and West Africa in 1985.[23] Proguanil-resistant *P. falciparum* is widespread and this agent is not recommended as a monoprophylaxis. Chloroquine-resistant *P.*

falciparum (CRPf) is now widespread in many malaria-endemic areas. It is believed that resistance prevents access of chloroquine to the digestive process in the parasite's lysosome, and this process is modulated primarily by mutations in the gene PfCRT, which encodes a transmembrane digestive vacuole protein. Mutations in PfCRT permit the parasite to persist in chloroquine concentrations that kill sensitive parasites.[24–27] Chloroquine-resistant *P. vivax* was been reported in 1989 in New Guinea and later elsewhere in Oceania, India, Asia and parts of South America, and because of the widespread distribution of *P. vivax* (estimated exposure of 2.85 billion people) increasing chloroquine resistance will have far-reaching public health implications.[28] Resistance in this species does not appear to be mediated through mutations in PvCRT.[24]

Only one published randomized controlled trial (RCT) examining the efficacy of chloroquine as malaria chemoprophylaxis for travelers is available. This compared chloroquine with the combination sulfadoxine/pyrimethamine in Austrian workers based in Nigeria[29] and found no significant difference in malaria incidence between medication groups. In the years 1990–1992 Peace Corps volunteers stationed in West Africa had a monthly malaria incidence of 3.8 cases/100 volunteers when they used chloroquine alone. Chloroquine/proguanil users had a monthly incidence of 1.7 cases and mefloquine 0.2 cases/100 volunteers.[30] Croft and Geary[31] reviewed studies of chloroquine plus proguanil and found two published RCTs on the use of chloroquine plus proguanil in non-immune general travelers, where the chloroquine/proguanil combination was not significantly more effective than proguanil alone[32] or a combination of chloroquine with sulfadoxine/pyrimethamine.[33] A more recent study[34] found superior efficacy for atovaquone/proguanil (1 *P. ovale* case in 511 travelers) compared with three *P. falciparum* cases in 511 travelers using chloroquine/proguanil. Using the combination tablet Savarine, French soldiers in Central Africa had a 4.8% incidence of *P. falciparum* malaria compared to 0.6% of doxycycline users.[35]

Tolerability

Croft and Geary have summarized the tolerability evidence of the chloroquine/proguanil combination based on five studies[36–40] conducted in the late 1990s. They found a 1–5% incidence of mild adverse effects (AE) such as depression, dizziness, headache, mouth ulcers, sleeping difficulties, vivid dreams, visual difficulties, vomiting; a 6–10% incidence of mainly gastrointestinal AE; and a high incidence >10% of anorexia. One RCT has shown that atovaquone/proguanil is significantly better tolerated than chloroquine/proguanil,[37] and the most recent RCT[19] has shown poor tolerability of chloroquine/proguanil (as Savarine) compared to doxycycline, mefloquine or atovaquone/proguanil. Serious AE, such as psychotic episodes,[8] have been reported in <1/13 600 users of the chloroquine/proguanil regimen. Keratopathy and retinopathy have been reported in chloroquine users, particularly during long-term use of the drug. Six-monthly ophthalmologic checks are recommended, particularly when the cumulative dose exceeds 100 g.

Contraindications, Precautions, and Drug Interactions[41]

According to the manufacturer, chloroquine is contraindicated in persons hypersensitive to the 4-aminoquinoline compounds and in G6PD-deficient individuals (although significant hemolysis is rare when given at prophylactic and therapeutic doses). Other contraindications are: pre-existing retinopathy, diseases of the central nervous system, myasthenia gravis, disorders of the blood-producing organs, and a history of epilepsy or psychosis. Dosage reduction may be required in patients with hepatic function impairments. Chloroquine and chloroquine/proguanil may be used in pregnancy.

During lactation the drug is present in breast milk, but not in sufficient quantities to either harm or protect the infant. There is no known absolute contraindication for proguanil. Concomitant use of chloroquine and proguanil has been shown to increase the incidence of mouth ulcers. Administration of the oral live typhoid vaccine and live cholera vaccine should be completed 3 days before chloroquine use, and chloroquine may suppress the antibody response to intradermal primary pre-exposure rabies vaccine. Other possible interactions can occur with gold salts, MAO inhibitors, digoxin, and corticosteroids. The activity of methotrexate and other folic acid antagonists is increased by chloroquine use.

Indications and Administration

Chloroquine is the drug of choice in the few malaria-endemic areas free of CRPf. Combining chloroquine and proguanil is an option for CRPf when other first-line antimalarials are contraindicated. Dosage should be calculated in terms of the base. The adult chloroquine dose is 300 mg base weekly (or in some countries 100 mg base daily). Pediatric preparations are available. The recommended children's dosage is 1.5 mg/kg body weight daily. The adult dose of proguanil is 200 mg daily when combined with chloroquine (or 100 mg daily when combined with atovaquone). For children the WHO recommended dosage is 3 mg/kg daily. The combination Savarine is now registered in several European countries and each tablet contains 100 mg chloroquine base and 200 mg proguanil.

Mefloquine

Description, Pharmacology, and Mode of Action

Mefloquine was selected in the 1960s by the Walter Reed Army Institute of Research from nearly 300 quinoline methanol compounds for further investigation because of its high antimalarial activity in animal models.[42] Today, mefloquine is used clinically as a 50:50 racemic mixture of the erythro isomers, and all clinical studies with the drug have used this mixture. The commercial form is available as tablets containing 250 mg mefloquine base. The mefloquine formulation available in the USA contains 250 mg mefloquine hydrochloride (equivalent to 228 mg mefloquine base). Mefloquine has been available for malaria chemoprophylaxis in non-immunes since 1985 in Europe, and since 1990 in the USA, and has been used by >35 million travelers for this indication.

Mefloquine is a potent, long-acting blood schizontocide and is effective against all malarial species, including *P. falciparum* resistant to chloroquine and pyrimethamine-sulfonamide combinations, and the recently recognized fifth species,[43] *Plasmodium knowlesi*. The exact mechanism of activity is unclear, but mefloquine is thought to compete with the complexing protein for heme binding and the resulting drug–heme complex is toxic to the parasite.[44]

Efficacy and Drug Resistance

Mefloquine is recognized as a highly effective malaria chemoprophylaxis for non-immune travelers to high-risk CRPf areas. The first report of mefloquine resistance came from Thailand in 1982, and this region remains a focus of resistance, particularly on the Thai–Cambodian and Thai–Burmese borders, where prophylaxis breakdown has been observed. As reviewed by Mockenhaupt,[45] reports of mefloquine treatment or prophylactic failures have been reported from distinct foci in Asia and, to a lesser extent, from Africa and the Amazon Basin in South America. Studies in 1993 showed high efficacy of mefloquine in travelers. The protective effectiveness of mefloquine in a large cohort of travelers to East Africa was 91%, which was significantly higher than other regimens used at that time: chloroquine/

proguanil (72%), and chloroquine monoprophylaxis at various doses (10–42%).[8] Long-term prophylaxis with mefloquine proved highly effective in Peace Corps volunteers stationed in sub-Saharan Africa, with an incidence of 0.2 infections/month in 100 volunteers. Weekly mefloquine was considered 94% more effective than prophylaxis with chloroquine and 86% more effective than prophylaxis with the chloroquine/proguanil combination.[46] Mefloquine was shown to be highly efficacious (100%) in the prevention of malaria in Indonesian soldiers in Papua,[6] and Rieckmann[47] found mefloquine to be 100% effective against *P. falciparum* in Australian soldiers deployed in Papua New Guinea (PNG). Pergallo[48] reported on the effective use of mefloquine by Italian troops in Mozambique in 1992–1994. When chloroquine/proguanil was the recommended regimen, an attack rate of 17 cases/1000 soldiers per month was noted. The rate dropped significantly to 1.8 cases/1000 per month when chloroquine/proguanil was replaced by mefloquine. The effectiveness of long-term mefloquine in the United Nations Peace Keeping Forces in Cambodia in 1993 was 91.4%.[49] Conversely, mefloquine was found to be incompletely effective in the prevention of malaria in Dutch Marines in Western Cambodia during the period 1992–1993. The attack rate in Marines varied significantly according to the geographical location of the battalions. Of 260 persons assigned to the area Sok San, 43 developed malaria (16%, 6.4/1000 person-weeks) compared to 21 of 2029 stationed elsewhere (1%, 0.5/1000 person-weeks). Mefloquine-resistant parasites were isolated from Dutch and Khmer patients.[50] The use of antimalarials by American troops during Operation Restore Hope in Somalia in 1992–1993 showed high prophylactic efficacy in mefloquine users. Sanchez et al.[51] reported the prophylactic efficacy in an uncontrolled cross-sectional survey of troops at one location (Bale Dogle). Mefloquine users had a malaria rate of 1.15 cases/10 000 person-weeks, compared to 5.49 cases/10 000 person-weeks in doxycycline users. From this and other reports,[52] mefloquine was shown to be more effective than doxycycline in US troops deployed in Somalia. The lower efficacy of doxycycline was attributed to poorer compliance. Mefloquine was shown to provide a high degree of protection in Dutch servicemen (n=125) deployed as part of a disaster relief operation to Goma, Zaire (1994). Despite evidence of exposure to *P. falciparum* as shown by the presence of circumsporozoite antibodies in 11.2% of the group, none developed overt malaria that was attributed to their use of mefloquine prophylaxis.[53] In a German population-based case–control study, mefloquine was considered to be 94.5% effective in preventing malaria in tourists to Kenya.[54]

Prophylactic Failures and Resistance

In many geographic regions, mapping of prophylactic failures, mainly in non-immune individuals, has been used to detect early resistance development, although it should be emphasized that prophylactic failures do not prove resistance. Mefloquine blood concentrations of 620 ng/mL are generally considered necessary to achieve 95% prophylactic efficacy. As defined by Lobel, a prophylactic failure is a confirmed *P. falciparum* infection in persons with mefloquine blood levels in excess of this protective level.[55] Using this definition, an analysis of 44 confirmed *P. falciparum* cases acquired in sub-Saharan Africa[55] showed five volunteers with mefloquine-resistant *P. falciparum* malaria. Other confirmed cases were attributed to poor compliance, and the authors concluded that prevalence of mefloquine-resistant malaria in sub-Saharan Africa is still low. With regard to cross-resistance, there is recent evidence that exposure of parasite populations to antimalarial drug pressure may select for resistance not only to the drug providing the pressure, but also to other novel drugs. This was clearly illustrated in the northern part of Cameroon, West Africa, where the detection of a high level of resistance to mefloquine was

attributed to cross-resistance with quinine,[56] a drug that had been widely deployed for therapy in the area. Resistance to mefloquine appears to be distinct from chloroquine resistance, as shown by the activity of mefloquine against CRPf and by the inefficacy of verapamil to reverse mefloquine resistance, although it does modulate chloroquine resistance. Moreover, in vitro studies have documented an inverse relationship between chloroquine and mefloquine resistance. Mefloquine resistance is, however, associated with halofantrine resistance[57] and quinine resistance.[56,57] Innate resistance, i.e., the existence of small subpopulations of intrinsically resistant malarial parasites within any infecting parasite biomass, is still controversial and may to some extent be explained by cross-resistance to other drugs.[45] The molecular basis of mefloquine resistance is currently unknown, but may be the result of mutation or amplification of certain gene products such as Pgh1, an energy-dependent transporter encoded by the mdr (multidrug resistant) homolog Pfmdr1. Recent transfection studies demonstrate that mutations in pfmdr1 may confer mefloquine resistance to sensitive parasites.[58] Penfluridol, a psychotropic drug, has been reported to reverse mefloquine resistance in *P. falciparum* in vitro.[59]

Tolerability

There is considerable controversy among international experts regarding the tolerability of mefloquine prophylaxis versus alternative regimens such as doxycycline, chloroquine/proguanil, and the combination atovaquone/proguanil. The position of mefloquine as a 21st-century malaria chemoprophylaxis has been reviewed recently,[60] and mefloquine remains an important first-line antimalarial drug; however, tolerability is a key issue with this medication and prescribers need to screen carefully for contraindications and inform mefloquine users of possible adverse events. Regarding tolerability, an overview of the studies and databases comparing the use of malaria chemoprophylactic agents in travelers (Tables 15.2–15.4) shows largely disparate results owing to differing designs, definitions, and methodologies and differing study populations. Regarding the reporting of any AE, the incidence during the use of mefloquine lies in the range 24–88%, and when there is a comparator, is usually equivalent to the incidence reported for almost all chemoprophylactic regimens. A double-blind study comparing all regimens showed that the tolerability of atovaquone/proguanil and doxycycline is superior to that of mefloquine, and women in particular were significantly more likely to experience neuropsychiatric-type adverse events.[19]

Meta-Analysis

A meta-analysis evaluating the efficacy and tolerability of malaria prophylaxis included eight trials in which 4240 non-immune adult participants were randomized to mefloquine or doxycycline or atovaquone/proguanil or chloroquine/proguanil chemoprophylaxis.[61] No 'serious' events occurred in any of the studies, but both atovaquone/proguanil and doxycycline users reported fewer adverse events than mefloquine users.

Moderate/Severe Adverse Events

Although often a subjective report by the traveler, when some measure of severity is applied to AE reporting it appears that 11–17%[8,19,62–67] of travelers using mefloquine are, to some extent, incapacitated by adverse events. The extent of this incapacitation is often difficult to quantify, and a good measure of the impact of adverse events is the extent of chemoprophylaxis curtailment. In a study of 5120 Italian soldiers using either chloroquine/proguanil (C+P) or mefloquine, deployed in Somalia and Mozambique in 1992–1994, the rate of prophylaxis discontinuation in the C+P users was 1.5%, compared to a significantly lower rate of discontinuation in mefloquine users (0.9%).[48] This contrasts with a recent study comparing mefloquine and atovaquone/proguanil (A+P), where subjects receiving the A+P combination regimen had a significantly lower rate of drug-related AE that caused discontinuation of prophylaxis (5% versus 1%).[62] A recent controlled tolerability study showed intermediate withdrawal rates for mefloquine (3.9%) and doxycycline (3.9%) versus chloroquine/proguanil (5.2%) compared with atovaquone/proguanil, which had the lowest withdrawal rate (1.8%).[19]

Serious Adverse Events

These are adverse events that constitute an apparent threat to life, which require or prolong hospitalization, or which result in severe disability.[62] With mefloquine the incidence range is estimated between 1/6000 and 1/10 600,[8,67–69] compared to a rate in chloroquine users of 1/13 600. In a retrospective cohort analysis, serious neuropsychiatric AE were noted for 1/607 mefloquine users versus 1/1181 chloroquine/proguanil users.[63]

Neuropsychiatric Adverse Events

This is the main area of controversy in the tolerability of mefloquine. Neuropsychiatric disorders include two broad categories of symptoms, namely central and peripheral nervous system disorders (including headache, dizziness, vertigo, seizures) and psychiatric disorders (including major psychiatric disorders, affective disorders, anxiety and sleep disturbances). Lobel et al.[46] found an incidence of strange dreams (25%), insomnia (9%), and dizziness (8.4%) in Peace Corps volunteers using long-term mefloquine prophylaxis similar to that reported by users of chloroquine (corresponding incidence 26%, 6.5%, 10%). No severe neuropsychiatric reactions were causally associated with mefloquine use in this study. Steffen et al.[8] reported similar findings in an analysis of tourists (n = 139 164) returning from East Africa. Headache was observed in 6.2% of mefloquine users versus 7.6% of chloroquine/proguanil users, and dizziness, depression and insomnia by 7.6%, 1.8%, and 4.2% of mefloquine users versus 5.5%, 1.7%, and 6.3% of the chloroquine/proguanil group. In this same large cohort study, serious neuropsychiatric AE were observed at a rate of 1/10 600. A total of five probably associated hospitalizations were reported: two cases of seizures, two psychotic episodes and one case of vertigo. The rate of such events in chloroquine users was 1/13 600, with three associated hospitalizations for neuropsychiatric events (one seizure and two psychotic episodes). Croft[70] reported on the experience of the British army with mefloquine, which indicated that the incidence of severe neuropsychiatric reactions arising during a period of prophylaxis lasting 3 months was not higher than 1/6000. In a randomized, double-blind, placebo-controlled ongoing monitoring of AE in Canadian travelers using mefloquine (n = 251) or placebo (n = 238), there was no significant difference in the number or severity of AE reported by either the mefloquine or the placebo users. One clinically significant neuropsychiatric AE, a moderate to severe anxiety attack, occurred in one of the 251 mefloquine users.[68] In a UK retrospective survey with telephone interviews,[63] significantly more neuropsychiatric AE were reported by mefloquine users than by travelers taking the chloroquine/proguanil combination. Neuropsychiatric events classified as disabling were reported by 0.7% of mefloquine and 0.09% of chloroquine/proguanil users, respectively (p = 0.021). Two travelers taking mefloquine (1/607) and one traveler using chloroquine/proguanil (1/1181) were hospitalized for such events. A retrospective survey of returned travelers suggested a causal relationship between neuropsychiatric events during travel and the use of mefloquine prophylaxis.[71] Two controlled studies have shown a significant excess of neuropsychiatric events in mefloquine users versus comparators.[19,62]

The precise role of antimalarial drugs in neuropsychiatric adverse events is difficult to define, and the role of travel as a catalyst for such events should be considered together with other confounding factors such as gender predisposition and the use of recreational drugs and alcohol.[72] The WHO recommends that mefloquine be contraindicated for persons with a personal or family history of psychiatric disorders. In terms of all AE, studies have shown that women are significantly more likely to experience AE.[19,63–65,73] This might be due to dose-related toxicity, and one study has shown an association between low body weight and a relatively high risk of developing AE during malaria prophylaxis.[65] It might be due to reporting bias, greater compliance with prescription,[74] or to gender-related differences in drug absorption, metabolism[64] or CNS distribution. Computer simulations suggest that reduced dosage in women would be effective and might result in improved tolerability.[64,75] An earlier tolerability study aimed to correlate non-serious AE occurring during routine chemoprophylaxis with concentrations of racemic mefloquine, its enantiomers, or the carboxylic acid metabolite.[65] The disposition of mefloquine was found to be highly selective, but neither the concentrations of enantiomers, nor total mefloquine nor metabolite were found to be significantly related to the occurrence of non-serious AE.[72] A role has been suggested for the concomitant use of mefloquine and recreational drugs[64,71] or an interaction between mefloquine and large quantities of alcohol,[75] although concomitant use of small quantities of alcohol does not appear to adversely affect tolerability.[76] Children tolerate mefloquine well,[76a] as do elderly travelers, who report significantly fewer AE than younger counterparts.[77] One report suggests that subjects with AE have slower elimination of mefloquine than the population in general.[78] Some researchers have used animal models to propose mechanisms that may explain the neuropsychiatric profile of adverse events associated with mefloquine. The phenomenon of 'connexin blockade' by mefloquine has been proposed as a possible explanation for some mefloquine-associated adverse events.[79] Careful screening of travelers, with particular attention to contraindications such as personal or family history of epilepsy/seizures or psychiatric disorders, should minimize the occurrence of serious AE. Some travel health advisors recommend starting mefloquine 3 weeks before travel to allow for adverse event screening. Some recommend using a split dose (a half tablet twice weekly) for women with low body weight. Anecdotal reports suggest positive experience with this approach, but no published pharmacokinetic data are available.

Contraindications, Precautions and Drug Interactions

Mefloquine is contraindicated in persons with a history of hypersensitivity to mefloquine or related substances such as quinine. Persons with a history of epilepsy or psychiatric disorders, including active depression, should not use the drug, and concomitant treatment with halofantrine is contraindicated.[2–4,80]

Use of mefloquine in the second and third trimesters for pregnant women who cannot defer travel to high-risk areas has been sanctioned by the manufacturer, WHO, and CDC, and most authorities now allow the use of mefloquine in the first trimester if the expected benefit outweighs the risk.[2–4] It has been suggested by some authorities that pregnancy should be avoided for 3 months after completing prophylaxis because of mefloquine's long half-life, although inadvertent pregnancy while using mefloquine is not considered grounds for pregnancy termination. Mefloquine is secreted into breast milk in small quantities. The effect, if any, on breastfed infants is unknown, but the amount of drug secreted in the breast milk is inadequate to protect the infant from malaria.

A retrospective analysis of a database of antimalarial tolerability data showed that co-medications commonly used by travelers have had no significant clinical impact on the safety of prophylaxis with mefloquine.[81] The co-administration of mefloquine with cardioactive drugs might contribute to the prolongation of QTc intervals, although, in the light of the information currently available, co-administration of mefloquine with such drugs is not contraindicated but should be monitored. Vaccination with oral live typhoid or cholera vaccines should be completed at least 3 days before the first dose of mefloquine. Caution is indicated in persons performing tasks requiring fine coordination,[2–4,80] but a review of performance impact of mefloquine[81–83] suggests that if mefloquine is tolerated by an individual then his or her performance is not undermined by use of the drug.

Indications and Administration

Mefloquine is effective in the prevention of CRPf malaria, except in clearly defined Thai border regions of multidrug resistance. It is a priority antimalarial for travelers to high-risk malaria-endemic areas. The recommended adult dose for chemoprophylaxis is 250 mg base weekly as a single dose (US 228 mg base). Adults weighing <45 kg and children >5 kg require a weekly dose of 5 mg base/kg.

In order to reach steady-state levels of mefloquine in a reduced time-frame (4 days rather than 7–9 weeks with the regular 250 mg/ week regimen) some studies[68,76,82,83] have used a loading dose strategy of 250 mg mefloquine daily for 3 days, followed thereafter by weekly mefloquine dosage. This strategy has also been suggested for last-minute travelers to high-risk areas with chloroquine-resistant CRPf. The advantage is rapid attainment of mefloquine protective levels (620 ng/mL) within 4 days, but this is offset to some extent by a higher proportion of individuals with AE using the loading dose strategy.[82]

Mefloquine and its metabolite are not appreciably removed by hemodialysis.[84] No special dosage adjustments are indicated for dialysis patients to achieve concentrations in plasma similar to those in healthy volunteers.

Doxycycline

Description

The tetracyclines form a class of broad-spectrum antimicrobial agents with activity against Gram-positive and Gram-negative aerobic and anaerobic bacteria, mycoplasma, rickettsia, chlamydiae, and protozoa, including those that cause malaria. Doxycycline and minocycline were derived semi-synthetically in 1967 and 1972, respectively. The only FDA-approved indication for this class of agents is the use of doxycycline for the prophylaxis of *P. falciparum* in short-term travelers (<4 months) to drug-resistant areas.[85,86]

Pharmacology and Mode of Action

Tetracyclines, including doxycycline, are relatively slow-acting schizonticidal agents and are therefore not used alone for treatment. However, numerous studies have established the efficacy of doxycycline as a solo chemoprophylactic agent against *P. vivax* and *P. falciparum* malaria. In addition to its activity against the erythrocytic stage of the parasite, doxycycline is thought to possess some pre-erythrocytic (causal) activity. However, studies examining its efficacy as a causal agent had unacceptably high failure rates, and to be optimally effective doxycycline needs to be taken as a chemosuppressant for 4 weeks after leaving a malaria-endemic area.[2,3,86,,87]

The mechanism of action of tetracyclines in bacteria has been examined in detail and is presumed to be similar in protozoa. Tetracyclines reversibly bind primarily to the 30S ribosomal subunit, thereby inhibiting protein synthesis by preventing the incorporation of new amino acids into the growing peptide chain.[85] In addition, in *P. falciparum* malaria, doxycycline has been shown to impair expression of apicoplast genes required for parasite survival.[88] Doxycycline has several advantages over first-generation tetracyclines, including improved absorption, a broader spectrum, a longer half-life, and an improved safety profile. Doxycycline is well absorbed from the proximal small bowel (>90% oral absorption), and in contrast to other tetracyclines, its uptake does not change significantly with food intake. Doxycycline may be taken with food, and this approach reduces the gastrointestinal irritation occasionally associated with this drug. Doxycycline is highly protein bound (93%), has a small volume of distribution (0.7 L/kg), and is lipid soluble. These features may explain its high blood levels and prolonged half-life, permitting a once-daily dosing regimen. Doxycycline has a half-life of approximately 15–22 h that is unaffected by renal impairment. Doxycycline is eliminated in the urine unchanged by glomerular filtration, and largely unchanged in the feces by biliary and gastrointestinal (GI) secretion. About 40% of the dose is eliminated in the urine in individuals with normal kidney function, whereas those with renal dysfunction are able to eliminate it via the liver–biliary–GI route. Therefore, unlike other tetracyclines, doxycycline may be used in renal failure, and the dose does not need to be adjusted in cases of renal impairment. The drug is not effectively removed by peritoneal dialysis or hemodialysis.[85,86]

Efficacy and Drug Resistance

A number of randomized trials have examined the efficacy of doxycycline as a chemoprophylactic against *Plasmodium* sp.[6,89–98] Four of these studies were randomized, double-blind, and placebo controlled. Two of these trials evaluated semi-immune children or adults in Kenya, and three trials examined non-immune populations in Oceania. The reported protective efficacy in these trials was excellent, ranging from 92% to 99% against *P. falciparum* and 98% for primary *P. vivax* malaria. Doxycycline does not kill *P. vivax* hypnozoites and does not prevent relapses of *P. vivax* and *P. ovale* malaria. In comparative trials in areas with chloroquine-resistant *P. falciparum* malaria, doxycycline has been shown to be equivalent to mefloquine and atovaquone-proguanil and superior to azithromycin and chloroquine/proguanil.[6,93–97] Parasite resistance to doxycycline has not been reported to be an operational problem in any malaria-endemic areas thus far, but prophylactic failures are reported in association with poor adherence, missed and inadequate doses.[99]

Tolerability

The most commonly reported adverse events related to doxycycline use are GI effects (4–33%), including nausea, vomiting, abdominal pain, and diarrhea. These adverse effects are less frequent with doxycycline than with other tetracyclines. Esophageal ulceration is a rare but well-described adverse event associated with doxycycline use that generally presents with retrosternal burning and odynophagia 1–7 days after therapy is initiated.[52,100] In a study of US troops deployed in Somalia, esophageal ulceration due to doxycycline was the most frequent cause of hospitalization attributed to the use of malaria chemoprophylaxis.[52] Taking doxycycline with food and plentiful fluids, in an upright position, can reduce GI adverse effects. Limited data suggest that doxycycline monohydrate and enteric-coated hyclate formulations may have fewer GI adverse effects than regular hyclate formulations.[99]

Dermatologic reactions are also a frequent adverse event associated with doxycycline use. These reactions range from mild paresthesias or exaggerated sunburn in exposed skin to photo-onycholysis (sun-induced separation of nails), severe erythema, bulla formation, and (rarely) Stevens–Johnson syndrome.[85] The reported rate of photosensitivity varies from <7% to 21% or more of users, and the reaction is mild in the majority of cases.[97,101] The risk of photosensitivity may be reduced by the use of appropriate sunscreens (>SPF 15 and protective against both ultraviolet A [UVA] and ultraviolet B [UVB] radiation).[97,102]

Although doxycycline has a lesser effect on normal bacterial flora than other tetracyclines, it still increases the risk of oral and vaginal candidiasis in predisposed individuals. Travelers with a history of these problems who are prescribed doxycycline should be advised to carry an appropriate treatment course of antifungal therapy.

Other uncommon adverse events occasionally attributed to doxy-cycline include dizziness, lightheadedness, darkening or discoloration of the tongue, and (rarely) hepatotoxicity, pancreatitis, or benign intracranial hypertension.[101]

Overall, a number of comparative studies have shown that doxy-cycline used as a chemoprophylactic agent is generally well tolerated and has relatively few reported side-effects.[6,52,90,91,94–98] In clinical trials, doxycycline was tolerated as well as or better than placebo or the comparator drug, with few serious adverse events reported. Randomized controlled trials comparing the tolerability of mefloquine and doxycycline in soldiers deployed in Thailand, and primaquine, doxy-cycline, proguanil/chloroquine, and mefloquine compared with placebo in semi-immune children in Kenya, found no significant differences in tolerability between these agents.[94,103] Ohrt and colleagues compared mefloquine and doxycycline in a randomized placebo-controlled field trial in non-immune soldiers in Papua (Irian Jaya). In this trial both drugs were well tolerated, but doxycycline was better tolerated than mefloquine or placebo with respect to the frequency of reported symptoms.[6] The authors attributed this to the potential of doxycycline to prevent other infectious processes. Anderson and colleagues compared doxycycline and azithromycin in a field trial in semi-immune adults in western Kenya.[94] Both drugs were well tolerated compared with placebo, but there was one case of doxycycline withdrawal due to recurrent vaginitis. There were no significant differences observed in adverse event profiles between the treatment arms, except that azithromycin was protective against dysentery. A randomized comparative trial of antimalarial tolerability reported that doxycycline monohydrate was the best tolerated of the four regimens, mefloquine, atovaquone/proguanil and chloroquine/proguanil.[19]

Adherence with doxycycline, despite its daily dosing schedule, has been reported to be relatively good in studies examining short-term use.[6,91,92,94] Estimating adherence rates in travelers is difficult because such studies require close daily monitoring. Ohrt and colleagues extended their initial comparative study of doxycycline and meflo-quine but did not enforce adherence as they did in the first phase of the study.[6] This resulted in a drop in the protective efficacy of doxy-cycline from 99% (95% CI 94–100%) to 89% (95% CI 78–96%) against all malaria, suggesting a decrease in drug adherence if close monitoring is not done. Similar experience of declining effectiveness over time due to adherence issues has been reported by the US military deployed in Somalia and in Dutch troops deployed in Cambodia.[50–52] US troops in Somalia using doxycycline had fivefold higher attack rates by *P. falciparum* than did mefloquine users. These differences were attributed to poor adherence with daily use rather than to doxy-cycline resistance.[52] Collectively, these studies suggest that adherence with daily doxycycline may be challenging, especially for long-term travelers.

Contraindications, Precautions, and Drug Interactions

Doxycycline administration is not recommended in the following situations:[2–4,85,86]

- Allergy or hypersensitivity to doxycycline or any member of the tetracycline class

- Infants and children under 8 years of age. Tetracyclines bind calcium and may cause permanent yellow-brown discoloration of teeth, damage to tooth enamel, and impairment of skeletal growth in this population. Doxycycline binds calcium less than other tetracyclines, and short courses of doxycycline (such as in the treatment of Rocky Mountain spotted fever) have not been reported to cause clinically significant staining of teeth[104]

- Pregnancy. Doxycycline crosses the placenta and therefore may cause permanent discoloration of teeth, damage to tooth enamel, and impairment of skeletal growth in the fetus (category D drug)

- Breastfeeding. Doxycycline is excreted in breast milk and therefore may cause permanent discoloration of teeth, damage to tooth enamel, impairment of skeletal growth, and photosensitivity in breastfed infants.

Precautions should be taken when using doxycycline in individuals who are susceptible to photosensitivity reactions or who have vaginal yeast infections or thrush. In addition, certain susceptible individuals with asthma may experience an allergic-type reaction to sulfite, which is formed with the oxidation of doxycycline calcium oral suspension. Doxycycline is partially metabolized by the liver; in individuals with significant hepatic dysfunction there may be a prolonged half-life, and a dose adjustment may be required.[85,86]

The safety of long-term doxycycline use (>3 months) has not been adequately studied.[102] Because lower doses of doxycycline and mino-cycline (a related tetracycline) are frequently used for extended periods to treat acne, it has been presumed that long-term use of doxycycline at an adult dose of 100 mg/day is safe. However, serious adverse events, including autoimmune hepatitis, fulminant hepatic failure, a serum-sickness-like illness, and drug-induced lupus erythematosus, have recently been reported with the use of minocycline for acne.[105] It is not known whether doxycycline causes similar adverse events, but doxycycline was not associated with an increased risk of hepatotoxicity in a single reported case–control study.[106] A number of potentially important drug interactions have been associated with doxycycline use,[85,86] including those involving the following drugs and substances:

- Antacids containing divalent or trivalent cations (calcium, aluminum, and magnesium). Doxycycline binds cations, and concomitant administration of antacids will reduce serum levels of doxycycline

- Oral iron, bismuth salts, calcium, cholestyramine or colestipol, and laxatives that contain magnesium. Concomitant ingestion of these compounds may reduce doxycycline absorption. The above agents should not be taken within 1–3 h of doxycycline ingestion

- Barbiturates, phenytoin, and carbamazepine. These drugs induce hepatic microsomal enzyme activity and, if used concurrently with doxycycline, may reduce doxycycline serum levels and half-life and may necessitate a dosage adjustment

- Oral contraceptives. Older literature reported that concurrent use of doxycycline with estrogen-containing birth control pills might result in decreased contraceptive efficacy and recommended an additional method of birth control. However, there are few examples of oral contraceptive failure attributable to doxycycline use, and serum hormone levels in patients taking oral contraceptives have been reported to be unaffected by co-administration of doxycycline. Current evidence suggests that doxycycline can be used concurrently with oral contraceptives without leading to a higher rate of contraceptive failure[99,107]

- Anticoagulants. The anticoagulant activity of oral anticoagulants may be enhanced with concurrent use of doxycycline. Close monitoring of prothrombin time is advised if these drugs are used together

- Vitamin A. The use of tetracyclines with vitamin A has been reported to be associated with benign intracranial hypertension.[86]

Indications and Administration

Doxycycline is currently indicated as an agent of choice for prevention of mefloquine-resistant *P. falciparum* malaria (evening or overnight exposure in rural border areas of Thailand with Myanmar [Burma] or Cambodia), or as an alternative to mefloquine or atovaquone/proguanil for the prevention of CRPf malaria.[2–4] Doxycycline has a long half-life that permits once-daily dosing. The dosage of doxycycline recommended for chemoprophylaxis against drug-sensitive and drug-resistant malaria is 2 mg base/kg of body weight, up to 100 mg base daily. Studies have examined lower-dose regimens, but such regimens have provided inadequate protection.[91,92] Doxycycline should be taken once daily, beginning 1–2 days before entering a malarial area, and should be continued daily while there. Because of its poor causal effect, it must be continued for 4 weeks after leaving the risk area. To reduce the occurrence of GI adverse events, it should be taken in an upright position with food and at least 100 mL of fluid. Doxycycline should not be taken within 3 h of administering an oral antacid or iron.

Atovaquone/Proguanil

Atovaquone/proguanil (AP), a fixed drug combination, is the newest antimalarial to become available, although its individual components have been used for years. AP was first approved in Switzerland in August 1997 and is now approved in many countries for the treatment and prophylaxis of *P. falciparum* malaria.[108]

Description

AP is effective for both the prevention and treatment of malaria. Atovaquone is a hydroxynaphthoquinone compound and, combined with proguanil, an antifolate drug, works synergistically against the erythrocytic stages of all the *Plasmodia* parasites and the liver-stage (causal prophylaxis) of *P. falciparum*.[108a–110] AP is not active against hypnozoites in *P. vivax* and *P. ovale* and does not prevent relapse infections.

Pharmacology and Mode of Action

Atovaquone acts by inhibiting parasite mitochondrial electron transport at the level of the cytochrome bc1 complex, and collapses mitochondrial membrane potential.[111] The plasmodial electron transport system is 1000 times more sensitive to atovaquone than the mammalian electron transport system, which likely explains the selective action and limited side-effects of this drug. Proguanil, as described above, is metabolized to cycloguanil, which acts by inhibiting dihydrofolate reductase (DHFR). The inhibition of DHFR impedes the synthesis of folate cofactors required for parasite DNA synthesis. However, it appears that the mechanism of synergy of proguanil with atovaquone is not mediated through its cycloguanil metabolite. In studies, proguanil alone had no effect on mitochondrial membrane potential or electron transport, but significantly enhanced the ability of atovaquone to collapse mitochondrial membrane potential when used in combination. This might explain why proguanil displays synergistic activity with atovaquone even in the presence of documented proguanil resistance, or in patient populations who are deficient in cytochrome P450 enzymes required for the conversion of proguanil to cycloguanil.[111]

Atovaquone is a highly lipophilic compound with poor bioavailability. Taking atovaquone with dietary fat increases its absorption, and therefore tablets should be taken with a meal or a milky beverage.

Atovaquone is >99% protein bound and is eliminated almost exclusively by biliary excretion. More than 94% can be recovered unchanged in the feces over 21 days and <0.6% in the urine. The elimination half-life is about 2–3 days in adults and 1–2 days in children.[112,113] Pharmacokinetic studies in elderly patients and those with renal and hepatic impairment indicate that no dosage adjustment is required for the elderly, or those with moderate hepatic or mild to moderate renal impairment. However, those with severe renal insufficiency (creatinine clearance <30 mL/min) should not use atovaquone/proguanil because of potential elevated cycloguanil levels and decreased atovaquone levels.

Efficacy and Drug Resistance

Atovaquone/proguanil (AP) is effective against malaria isolates resistant to a variety of other antimalarial drugs. Resistance to atovaquone develops rapidly if this drug is used alone.[114] Resistance to the combination of atovaquone plus proguanil, although uncommon, has been documented in a small number of cases following treatment courses of AP (~25 reported cases).[115–120] Most documented failures have occurred in patients whose malaria was acquired in Africa. In the majority of these cases, the malaria isolates had genetically confirmed markers of resistance, notably mutations in the cytochrome b gene at position 268. Treatment failure not associated with cytochrome b mutations has also been reported in a small number of patients with low plasma drug levels, and rarely in the presence of adequate drug levels.[121] There have been no published reports of documented failure associated with cytochrome b mutations in persons using AP as a chemoprophylactic agent.

Volunteer challenge studies have confirmed that atovaquone, proguanil and the combination have causal activity (they kill parasites as they develop in the liver).[108a,110] In these studies, none of 18 participants randomized to receive atovaquone or atovaquone/ proguanil developed *P. falciparum* malaria following infected mosquito challenge, compared to eight of eight placebo recipients.

In randomized controlled trials, daily atovaquone/proguanil at recommended dosing was highly efficacious in preventing *P. falciparum* malaria in both adults and children. Four published trials have examined the protective efficacy of AP in 534 semi-immune adults and children living in malaria-endemic areas.[122–126] The overall efficacy of AP in the prevention of *P. falciparum* malaria in these trials was 98% (95% CI 91.9–99.9%). The most common reported adverse events attributed to the study drug were headache, abdominal pain, dyspepsia, and diarrhea. However, of note, all adverse events occurred with similar frequency in subjects treated with placebo or AP, and there were no serious adverse events.

The protective efficacy of AP for prevention of *P. falciparum* malaria in non-immune adults and children has been examined in five clinical trials, four of which were randomized and three blinded.[43,62,124] Collectively, the protective efficacy of AP (evaluable in 1361 non-immune individuals, of whom 126 were children under the age of 12) was 96–100% (95% CI 48–100%). However, the determination of protective efficacy in these trials was limited by their small sample size, lack of a placebo control, and, as evidenced by the wide confidence intervals, these studies were inadequately powered for the determination of protective efficacy.

In two of the larger randomized, double-blind clinical trials, <2000 non-immune subjects traveling to a malaria-endemic area received either AP, daily for 1–2 days before travel until 7 days after travel, mefloquine or chloroquine/proguanil, from 1–3 weeks before travel until 4 weeks after travel.[43,62]

All drugs were well tolerated, but AP was significantly better tolerated than either mefloquine or chloroquine/proguanil in these studies.

Drug-related discontinuation rates for AP versus mefloquine were 1.2% versus 5% (p = 0.001) and for AP versus chloroquine/proguanil were 0.2% versus 2% (p = 0.015).[43,62] In a comparative trial of AP versus doxycycline in 175 Australian military participants, there were no prophylactic failures in either arm, but AP was better tolerated, with a significantly lower rate of GI (29% versus 53%) adverse events.[97]

Only one randomized, double-blind, placebo-controlled trial has evaluated the protective efficacy of AP against *P. vivax*. The protective efficacy of AP was 84% (95% CI 45–95%) for *P. vivax* and 96% (95% CI 71–99%) for *P. falciparum*.[125] As AP does not appear to eradicate *P. vivax* hypnozoites it is suggested that travelers to areas where the transmission rates of *P. vivax* are high should be considered for presumptive anti-relapse therapy with primaquine.

Taken together, these studies indicate that AP is an efficacious chemoprophylactic regimen for *P. falciparum*. Additional data are required to establish the efficacy against non-falciparum malaria.

Tolerability

Collectively, the controlled trials indicate that AP at prophylactic doses is well tolerated by both adults and children, with drug discontinuation rates of 0–2%. The most commonly reported adverse events are gastrointestinal, which can often be reduced by taking AP with food. According to the product monograph, when used for malaria prevention the most commonly reported adverse events possibly attributed to AP were headache and abdominal pain; however, in placebo-controlled trials these occurred at similar rates in placebo recipients. In the non-immune traveler studies described above, participants receiving AP reported significantly lower rates of neuropsychiatric adverse events (14% versus 29%) and lower drug discontinuation rates (1.2% versus 5%) than with mefloquine.[62] Compared with CP, AP users reported significantly fewer GI adverse events (12% versus 20%) and lower discontinuation rates (0.2% versus 2%).[34] In a randomized trial in travelers AP was the best-tolerated chemoprophylactic, with discontinuation rates of 1.8% versus 3.9% for mefloquine and doxycycline and 5.2% for chloroquine/proguanil.[19]

Efficacy and tolerability have also been examined in a randomized comparative trial of AP versus CP in pediatric travelers.[126] There were no prophylactic failures, but AP was better tolerated, with no premature discontinuation of AP due to an adverse event compared to 2% of pediatric travelers using CP.

AP treatment and prophylaxis has, rarely, been associated with severe dermatologic adverse events, including erythema mutiforme and Stevens–Johnson syndrome.[127,128] Overall, systematic reviews of the above randomized trials have concluded that AP is a well tolerated and highly efficacious chemoprophylactic agent for the prevention of *P. falciparum* malaria.[129,130]

Contraindications, Precautions, and Drug Interactions

AP is contraindicated in those with severe renal impairment (creatinine clearance <30 mL/min) and those with a history of hypersensitivity to any of the drug components. AP should not be used to treat an individual who has failed AP chemoprophylaxis, or anyone with evidence of severe or complicated malaria.

Recently the CDC have approved AP for chemoprophylaxis in children weighing >5 kg. The WHO and the manufacturer recommend this chemoprophylaxis only for children weighing >11 kg. In December 2003, the US FDA approved its use for the treatment of uncomplicated falciparum malaria in pediatric patients down to 5 kg.

AP is classified as a pregnancy category C drug. Based primarily on lack of data, atovaquone/proguanil is not currently recommended for the prevention of malaria during pregnancy or breastfeeding. However, proguanil is considered safe during pregnancy, and animal studies have revealed no teratogenicity for atovaquone. Three small studies examining AP as treatment in pregnancy suggests that AP is safe and well tolerated, but additional data are needed.[131,132] A recent registry-based cohort study of 570 877 births in Denmark examined whether exposure to AP during the period of maximal susceptibility to teratogenic agents (weeks 3–8) was associated with an increased risk of major birth defects. Although there were a limited number of exposed women, there was no observed increased risk associated with AP exposure during early pregnancy.[133] The USA prescribing information states that atovaquone/proguanil can be used during pregnancy if the potential benefits of therapy outweigh the potential risk to the infant.

AP should not be given with other proguanil-containing medications. Concomitant use with tetracycline has been associated with a 40% decrease in plasma concentrations of atovaquone. Similarly, rifampin, rifabutin, and metoclopramide significantly reduce the level of atovaquone and should not be used concurrently.[132]

Atovaquone appears to lower the steady-state values of azithromycin and also increases plasma concentrations of zidovudine by inhibiting its glucuronidation; however, the clinical implications of the above two interactions are not yet known.[132]

Indications and Administration

AP is currently indicated for the prophylaxis and treatment of *P. falciparum* malaria, including areas where chloroquine and/or mefloquine resistance has been reported. Travelers who have experienced intense exposure to *P. vivax* and *P. ovale* should be considered for radical treatment with primaquine upon leaving the malaria-endemic area. Because of its causal activity, AP is taken 1 day prior to travel in a malarial zone, daily while exposed, and for 7 days upon leaving.

Several European countries initially imposed limited duration of use restrictions on AP use. A randomized double-blind study in Papua demonstrated efficacy and tolerability over a 5-month period, and a 6-month open-label study reported good tolerability.[134,135] Most countries now impose no time limits on the use of AP as a prophylactic agent.

Primaquine

Introduction and Description

Primaquine is an 8-aminoquinoline that has been used for over 50 years for the terminal prophylaxis or radical cure of relapsing forms of malaria (*P. vivax* and *P. ovale*), owing to its ability to eradicate liver hypnozoite stages. Primaquine was rediscovered as a malaria chemoprophylactic agent in the 1990s, based on its ability to eliminate developing liver stages of *P. falciparum* and *P. vivax* (causal prophylaxis).[136,137] Primaquine also has gametocidal activity against and has been used to reduce the transmission of *P. falciparum* in malaria-endemic areas (Fig. 15.1).[138]

Pharmacology and Mode of Action

The precise mechanisms of action of 8-aminoquinoline drugs are unknown. Primaquine localizes within the plasmodial mitochondria, suggesting drug-induced mitochondrial dysfunction as one potential mechanism of action. It is rapidly absorbed from the gastrointestinal tract and rapidly excreted. Peak plasma levels occur within 2–3 h and the mean half-life is approximately 4–5 h. Primaquine is metabolized to a carboxylic acid derivative of unknown antimalarial activity that has a half-life of 24–30 h.[139,140]

Efficacy and Drug Resistance

There have been several randomized controlled field trials: two in Indonesia, two in Colombia, and one in Africa have convincingly demonstrated the prophylactic potential of primaquine. In four studies, adults with little previous experience of malaria were given 30 mg base of daily primaquine for 12–52 weeks. Non-immune immigrants to Papua are intensively exposed to both *P. falciparum* and *P. vivax* malaria. In 1995, a randomized placebo-controlled trial indicated that daily primaquine for up to 1 year had a protective efficacy of 95% (95% CI 57–99%) against *P. falciparum* malaria and 90% (95% CI 58–98%) against *P. vivax* malaria.[141] A subsequent trial in the same region in 1999/2000 over 20 weeks showed a protective efficacy of 88% (48–97%) for *P. falciparum* and >92% (95% CI >37–99%) for *P. vivax*.[142] In placebo-controlled field studies in Colombian soldiers, primaquine was 94% efficacious (95% CI 78–99%) against *P. falciparum* and 85% (95% CI 57–95%) against *P. vivax*.[143] In an attempt to improve the efficacy rate against *P. vivax* malaria, weekly chloroquine was added to the daily primaquine in a subsequent field trial; however, the results were similar to those of primaquine alone.[144]

Relapses of *P. vivax* malaria following standard courses of primaquine (15 mg base/day for 14 days) are commonly reported from Papua New Guinea, Papua, Thailand, and other parts of Southeast Asia and Oceania (failure rates <35%), and less commonly from India and Colombia. Smoak et al.[145] reported high relapse rates in American soldiers deployed to Somalia. Of 60 *P. vivax*-infected soldiers treated with standard doses of chloroquine and primaquine (15 mg base/day for 14 days), 26 relapsed, a failure rate of 43%. Eight soldiers had a second relapse following another course of chloroquine plus primaquine therapy, including several who completed a higher-dose primaquine regimen (30 mg base/day × 14 days).

Tolerability

Randomized controlled trials have shown that daily primaquine is well tolerated, with reported discontinuation rates generally ≤2%. The most commonly identified adverse event has been minor gastrointestinal disturbances, which are minimized by taking the drug with food. In a study by Baird and colleagues primaquine was as well tolerated as placebo.[142]

Contraindications and Precautions

The adverse events of greatest concern with primaquine are methemoglobinemia and hemolysis in glucose-6-phosphate-dehydrogenase (G6PD)-deficient persons. Primaquine-induced hemolysis can be life-threatening in a severely deficient person. Methemoglobinemia is generally not a serious concern when <20% hemoglobin is in the methemoglobin form; only rarely will testing for methemoglobinemia be indicated on clinical grounds, such as with cyanosis, dizziness or dyspnea. Controlled trials have demonstrated that methemoglobinemia levels after 20 or 52 weeks of 30 mg base of primaquine daily were no higher than those following standard 15 mg base daily for 14 days.[141,146] Methemoglobin levels have remained <8.5% in recent trials, well below the 20–30% associated with symptoms.

Primaquine is contraindicated in G6PD deficiency and during pregnancy because of the risk of hemolysis in the fetus. There is limited experience with the prophylactic use of primaquine in children. Prior to receiving primaquine individuals should be confirmed to have a normal G6PD status by laboratory testing.

Primaquine should also not be used in individuals with NADH methemoglobin reductase deficiency or those receiving potentially hemolytic drugs.

Indications and Administration

Randomized controlled trials in Indonesia, South America, and Africa have demonstrated that primaquine is an efficacious and well tolerated chemoprophylactic agent (0.5 mg/kg base per day; adult dose 30 mg base/day) against *P. vivax* and *P. falciparum*. Because of its causal activity, it may be discontinued 1 week after leaving an endemic area. However, primaquine is not currently licensed for this indication. Current pivotal trials may be sufficient to meet regulatory requirements for this indication.

For individuals not taking primaquine as a chemoprophylactic agent, and in whom exposure to *P. vivax* or *P. ovale* malaria is thought to have been particularly high (e.g., long-term expatriates, soldiers, etc.), consideration may be given to the use of primaquine to eliminate latent hepatic parasites by administering a 2-week course (0.5 mg/kg base per day; adult dose 30 mg base/day) after return to a non-endemic area in individuals known to be G6PD normal.[138]

Future Directions

Tafenoquine

Introduction and Description

Tafenoquine is a primaquine analog with a long elimination half-life (14–28 days versus 4–6 h for primaquine). It has activity against liver, blood, and transmission stages of malaria. The long half-life of tafenoquine allows infrequent dosing regimens. When the drug is taken with food, absorption is increased by approximately 50% and the severity of gastrointestinal adverse effects is diminished.[148,149] In vitro and in vivo animal studies indicate that tafenoquine is more potent and less toxic than primaquine (Fig. 15.2).[150]

Efficacy and Drug Resistance

To date, trials have assessed the prophylactic efficacy of tafenoquine in malaria-endemic areas.[151–156] A randomized dose-ranging study of tafenoquine was performed in Gabon in older children and young adults. A loading dose strategy using 25 mg base to 200 mg base of tafenoquine once daily for 3 days was evaluated. Doses of 50 mg, 100 mg, and 200 mg daily for 3 days all showed substantial protective efficacy through 10 weeks of follow-up. Compared to placebo, tafenoquine 200 mg base daily for 3 days provided 100% protection out to week 11.[153] This suggested that a 'fire-and-forget' strategy of 3 daily doses of tafenoquine might be sufficient to protect exposed short-term travelers.

In a randomized placebo-controlled trial in semi-immune adults in western Kenya, 200 mg base daily for 3 days followed by 200 mg weekly for 13 weeks resulted in a protective efficacy of 87% (95% CI 73–93%); 400 mg daily for 3 days followed by 400 mg weekly had a protective efficacy of 89% (95% CI 77–95%). One group received only 400 mg for 3 days at the beginning of the study followed by placebo. The protective efficacy at week 15 in this group was 68% (95% CI 53–79%); however, there were equivalent malaria rates to the weekly-treated groups out to study week 7, again supporting a fire-and-forget dosing strategy.[151]

A randomized trial examined tafenoquine's prophylactic efficacy against *P. falciparum* in semi-immune adults in Ghana.[152] Volunteers received a loading dose of study drug on each of three consecutive days, then a single weekly dose for 12 weeks. Doses of tafenoquine 200 mg base afforded a protective efficacy of approximately 86%, similar to protection afforded by 250 mg mefloquine weekly.

The prophylactic efficacy against *P. vivax* was evaluated in a placebo-controlled trial in 205 non-immune soldiers in the northeastern border regions of Thailand. Using 400 mg base of tafenoquine daily for 3 consecutive days followed by a single monthly dose of 400 mg resulted in a 95% protective efficacy against *P. vivax*.[155] More recently, monthly doses of tafenoquine (400 mg) were assessed in a randomized

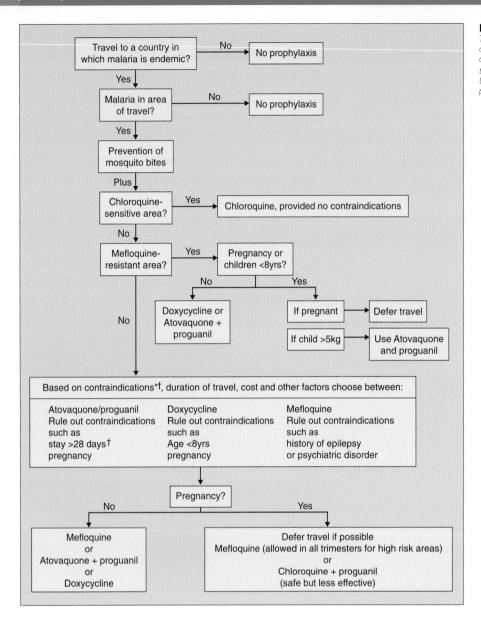

Figure 15.2 Malaria prophylaxis algorithm. [a]*Note: This figure is intended as a visual aid only. Please refer to text and product/package insert monograph for other important details regarding contraindications, precautions, and drug tolerability.* [b]*At present in some countries in Europe (except the UK, Austria, Czech Republic, and France), atovaquone/proguanil is only registered for a maximum period of 28 days.*

double-blind placebo-controlled field trial in 205 Thai soldiers. Protective efficacy against *P. vivax* was 96% (95% CI 76–99%) and against *P. falciparum* was 100% (95% CI 60–100%).[156] Nasveld and colleagues reported the first phase 3 trial of the safety, tolerability, and effectiveness of tafenoquine for malaria prophylaxis. Soldiers received weekly malaria prophylaxis with 200 mg tafenoquine (492 subjects) or 250 mg mefloquine (162 subjects) for 6 months' deployment to Indonesia. No cases of malaria were reported in either group during deployment. Three participants on tafenoquine (0.6%) and none on mefloquine discontinued prophylaxis because of possible drug-related adverse events. Mild vortex keratopathy was detected in 93% of tafenoquine users but none of the mefloquine subjects. The vortex keratopathy was not associated with changes in visual acuity and was fully resolved by 1 year.[157]

Tolerability

The most commonly reported adverse event noted during tafenoquine prevention trials has been mild gastrointestinal upset that was not statistically different from the placebo groups. Other adverse effects have included dermatologic problems, headaches, and mild transient elevations in serum liver transaminases. Initial clinical trials also suggested that longer-term use of tafenoquine might be associated with corneal deposits and increases in serum creatinine. A recent randomized trial of 120 volunteers taking 200 mg of tafenoquine for 6 months showed no clinically significant effects of tafenoquine on ophthalmic or renal function.[158]

Contraindications, Precautions, and Drug Interactions

The potential toxicities of concern with tafenoquine are the same as for primaquine: methemoglobinemia or hemolysis in G6PD-deficient persons. During the Kenyan field trial, two G6PD-deficient individuals were inadvertently given tafenoquine, which resulted in significant intravascular hemolysis requiring blood transfusion in one case. Hemolysis resolved and no renal compromise was observed in spite of hemoglobinuria ('blackwater').[151]

Although methemoglobinemia has been documented in persons receiving tafenoquine, it has not resulted in levels sufficient to induce symptoms or require treatment.[151]

Indications and Administration

The indications for the use of tafenoquine in the treatment or prevention of malaria have yet to be established. Most recent field trials are exploring a weekly dosing schedule, but of particular interest for short-term travelers (<1 month) is a fire-and-forget approach with a 3-day loading dose (three doses over 3 days). Tafenoquine may also be an alternative for terminal prophylaxis and a substitute for primaquine in the therapy of vivax malaria.[149] Tafenoquine's ability to kill sexual stages suggests it might also have an important public health application in transmission blocking.[159]

Drugs Not Recommended for Chemoprophylaxis

A number of agents, not mentioned above, are occasionally used or recommended to travelers to prevent malaria. Although some of these are effective drugs for malaria treatment, their pharmacokinetics, adverse events or toxicities make them inappropriate to prevent malaria.[2–4] Below is a list of drugs that are not recommended for chemoprophylaxis.

Amodiaquine is a 4-aminoquinalone drug that has been available since the 1940s and is structurally similar to chloroquine. It is currently still used for therapy in some sub-Saharan African countries; however, its potential adverse effects include agranulocytosis and hepatitis, and it is not recommended as a chemoprophylactic agent.[140,150]

Pyrimethamine/sulfadoxine (Fansidar) is widely used for the treatment of falciparum malaria in sub-Saharan Africa and occasionally as standby treatment of malaria in travelers. It is not used in a prophylactic setting owing to the risk of severe cutaneous adverse reactions, including Stevens–Johnson syndrome and toxic epidermal necrolysis.[140,150] Other forms of pyrimethamine alone (e.g., Daraprim) are also not recommended due to widespread resistance.

Quinine remains a first-line therapeutic agent for chloroquine-resistant malaria. It is not used as a prophylactic drug because of its short half-life and its frequent treatment-associated adverse effects, including nausea, vomiting, headache, tinnitus, cardiovascular toxicity, and risk of blackwater fever with prolonged use.

Azithromycin is an azalide antimicrobial agent that has been evaluated as a chemosuppressant agent. Although protective against *P. vivax* (>90%), protective efficacy against *P. falciparum* (70–83%) is generally considered to be too low to rely on azithromycin as a single agent to prevent falciparum malaria.[2–4,94,96]

Artemisinin or Qinghaosu derivatives, including Artesunate, are a class of extremely effective therapeutic agents; however, there is currently no role for these drugs as chemoprophylactics.[150,156,160]

Halofantrine is a 9-phenanthrene-methanol drug that continues to be used in some countries as a therapeutic agent for malaria. It is not recommended for the prevention or treatment of malaria owing to its potential to cause potentially fatal cardiac arrhythmias and prolongation of the QTc intervals. These cardiac changes can be especially accentuated when used in combination with other cardiac-altering antimalarials such as mefloquine.[80,161]

Chemoprophylaxis in Special Populations

Pregnancy, Lactation, and Conception

Falciparum malaria in a pregnant woman poses significant risks for the mother, fetus and neonate. Falciparum malaria is associated with an increased risk of spontaneous abortion and stillbirth, intrauterine growth retardation, premature delivery, and maternal mortality. Travel by pregnant women, or women who might become pregnant, to destinations where CRPf malaria is transmitted should be avoided or deferred when possible. This advice is based on the fact that most effective antimalarial regimens against CRPf are neither recommended nor adequately studied during pregnancy, especially in the first trimester.

If a pregnant woman must travel to a CRPf malaria-endemic area, the use of insect repellents and insecticide-treated bed-nets should be strongly encouraged[2–4] and chemoprophylaxis should be used. Chloroquine alone or in combination with proguanil is safe in pregnancy and lactation; however, these agents only offer partial protection in areas with transmission of CRPf. If the travel is to an area where there is intense transmission of CRPf with high-grade chloroquine resistance and travel cannot be deferred, mefloquine may be considered for chemoprophylaxis, A recent evaluation of the use of mefloquine chemoprophylaxis by non-immune pregnant women suggests that it is reasonable to recommend mefloquine prophylaxis in all trimesters when travel cannot be deferred and when the woman is at a high risk of CRPf malaria.[162] For areas with less intense transmission, chloroquine and proguanil chemoprophylaxis can be considered. Some sources recommend supplementation with folic acid for pregnant women taking proguanil.

When possible, conception should be delayed for 3 months from the time of completion of mefloquine; however, inadvertent conception while on mefloquine is not an indication for termination of pregnancy.[3]

At present there are insufficient data on the use of AP in pregnancy or breastfeeding, and therefore it is not recommended unless the potential benefit outweighs the potential risk to the fetus.[2,132] AP is currently licensed for use in children >11 kg; however, it is now recommended by some authorities for children weighing >5 kg.

Doxycycline is contraindicated in pregnancy and breastfeeding. Conception should be delayed until 1 week after completion of doxycycline. Primaquine is contraindicated in pregnancy, although it is considered safe in breastfeeding provided that the infant and mother are both screened for G6PD deficiency.[2] There is currently no safe and effective chemoprophylaxis regimen for pregnant women at risk of mefloquine-resistant *P. falciparum* malaria.

Infants and Children

Young children are at special risk for malaria because of their inability to protect themselves from mosquitoes, the difficulty in administering antimalarial drugs, and the rapidity with which they become severely ill. Parents and guardians must pay particular attention to insect protection measures, including repellents and treated bed-nets.

Malaria chemoprophylaxis in the very young infant is difficult to achieve. Although most antimalarials taken by the mother will be present in breast milk, the drug concentrations are not considered high enough to provide an adequate protective dose to the nursing infant. Thus, malaria prevention in the nursing infant must be addressed separately from what is recommended to the mother.

For pediatric travelers to malarial areas where chloroquine is still effective, the chloroquine dose can be adjusted based on weight (Table 15.6). Chloroquine phosphate pediatric suspension is available in some destination countries, but not in the USA or Canada. If the suspension is not available, chloroquine phosphate tablets (250 mg salt = 150 mg chloroquine base) can be ground up by the pharmacist, and the weight-adjusted dose plus a filler can be put into capsules. Once a week, the capsule can be opened and the chloroquine powder mixed into a syrup to be given to a child. Chocolate syrup is recommended over fruit syrups and jams, as chocolate can effectively mask the bitter taste of the chloroquine and make the mixture palatable to a child. Tablets should also be kept out of sunlight and humidity once removed from the protective packaging. All medication should be kept out of reach of children to avoid overdoses, which may be fatal.

The dosage of proguanil can also be adjusted based on weight. AP (available in a one-quarter strength pediatric tablet) and mefloquine dosage for children can be adjusted based on weight. Mefloquine can be used by children weighing > 5 kg and is well tolerated.[163] Once-weekly mefloquine dosing is convenient for children but the bitter taste of the drug needs to be disguised with chocolate or jam. No data are available on the stability of cut or broken tablets. Doxycycline is contraindicated in children <8 years of age.

In general, children should not rely on standby treatment for malaria; rather, they should be prescribed appropriate chemoprophylaxis and seek medical attention if any febrile illness occurs when traveling.

In immunocompromised travelers *P. falciparum* malaria has been shown to increase HIV-1 replication, and proviral loads and may cause faster progression of HIV-1 disease. HIV-1 infection also appears to make malaria worse, and is associated with higher parasitemia infections and an increase in clinical malaria.[164] Therefore, malaria prevention is particularly important in this population.

The special concern is the possible interaction between antimalarial drugs and anti-retroviral agents. Both mefloquine and protease inhibitors are metabolized by cytochrome P450. Inducers or inhibitors of cytochrome P450 might be expected to alter drug levels of these agents. Mefloquine has been shown to reduce the drug levels of ritonavir, but ritonavir had little effect on mefloquine.[165] There is reported to be less interaction between mefloquine and other protease inhibitors such as nelfinavir or indinavir.[146] Evafirenz is an anti-retroviral with potential neuropsychiatric adverse events, including dizziness, altered concentration, insomnia, abnormal dreaming, sleepiness, confusion, abnormal thinking, memory loss and hallucinations. Although unknown, it is possible that agents such as mefloquine might potentiate these effects. There are few available data on the interaction of other anti-retrovirals with mefloquine.[146,165,166]

Atovaquone increases the level of some nucleoside reverse transcriptase inhibitors (NRTIs) such as stavudine as well as the level of zidovudine plus AZT. Whether this increases the risk of adverse drug events is unknown. There are also few data available regarding the potential interaction of proguanil and anti-retroviral agents.[167]

Doxycycline may cause photosensitivity, similar to anti-retrovirals such as abacavir, and predispose to candidiasis, potential problems for HIV-infected individuals.

Because of potential or unknown interactions between anti-retroviral and antimalarial drugs, it may be advantageous to start an antimalarial drug in advance of the recommended start date in order to monitor for any adverse effects.

Long-Term Travelers

Few data are available on efficacy and tolerability of long-term malaria chemoprophylaxis. Adherence issues are paramount, and the long-term traveler requires expert advice on malaria risk at the destination, possible seasonality, and practical guidance regarding long-term use of medications.[30] Mefloquine has been used successfully for periods up to 2.5 years by Peace Corps volunteers in Africa[30] and was shown to be well tolerated and effective in preventing falciparum malaria. A pharmacokinetic study has shown that toxic accumulation does not occur during long-term intake.[168] Atovaquone/proguanil can be used

for long-term travelers,[169] and in the USA and Canada there is no limit on the period of prophylaxis. In some countries there is a 28-day limit restricting the use of this combination to short-term travel. There are few data on the long-term use of doxycycline malaria chemoprophylaxis for periods longer than 6 months. Insect protection measures such as insecticide-treated bed-nets and effective insect repellents are an essential component of malaria protection for long-term travelers.

Illustrative Cases

Case 1

A 23-year-old woman is about to travel to sub-Saharan Africa for a 2-month safari. She is concerned that she might develop adverse events related to mefloquine while away. She is wondering if there is a way to reassure her that she will be able to tolerate mefloquine before leaving.

Approach

This is a common and appropriate concern voiced by many potential travelers. No-one wants to experience adverse drug events, particularly when they are far from home. This concern most commonly arises with mefloquine use, and a useful approach is to start early with chemoprophylaxis: begin mefloquine prophylaxis 2.5–3 weeks before departure. Since the majority of side-effects occur within the first three doses, this will allow an opportunity to assess adverse events before departure. However, if the individual tolerates three doses of mefloquine, they may be reassured that they will likely tolerate this drug.

Case 2

A business executive in Bangkok is required to take several short (3–5-day) trips to rural Cambodia and rural Laos over the course of the next 3 months. Because standard chemoprophylactic drugs such as doxycycline and mefloquine require use for 4 weeks after malaria exposure, he notes that he will constantly be on antimalarials for many months. He is wondering if there is another option.

Approach

Short and repeated trips to malaria-endemic areas are ideal situations to consider the use of causal antimalarials such as AP and primaquine. Since these drugs only need to be taken for a short time (1 week) after leaving the malaria-endemic area, they are more user-friendly for this type of travel. A similar situation exists in Nairobi, Kenya (one of the few malaria-free areas in East Africa), where travel outside of the city places individuals at risk of chloroquine-resistant *P. falciparum* malaria. European experts recommend the standby treatment approach for many destinations in Southeast Asia.

Case 3

A microbiologist brings her 6-year-old daughter to the travel clinic for advice regarding antimalarial prophylaxis and immunizations for travel to sub-Saharan Africa. The mother elects to use AP for malaria and also requests oral typhoid vaccine. She asks whether the AP will inhibit the immune response to the live oral vaccine.

Approach

Antimicrobial agents can theoretically affect a host immune response to live vaccines. Data in Gabonese children showed that AP did not affect the seroconversion rates to live oral typhoid and cholera vaccines.

Case 4

A 36-year-old client e-mails from Cambodia saying he is having difficulty tolerating doxycycline. He has been able to acquire AP and wants to switch. He wishes to know whether he can discontinue AP 1 week after leaving Cambodia.

Approach

As a causal prophylactic agent, AP is normally discontinued 1 week after leaving a malaria-endemic area. However, all studies have examined the use of AP prior to malaria exposure. It is unknown whether it will work as a causal agent when started after exposure. For this reason, people switching to AP should use the drug as a suppressive rather than a causal agent, and therefore continue it for 4 weeks after leaving the endemic area.

Case 5

A 39-year-old woman visits Papua and uses AP as a chemoprophylactic agent. Some 3 months after returning home she develops *P. vivax* malaria. She asks why she has developed malaria despite using an antimalarial prophylactic agent.

Approach

AP is an efficacious drug to prevent *P. falciparum* and *P. vivax* malaria. However, AP has no activity against liver-stage hypnozoites and therefore cannot prevent relapses of *P. vivax* and *P. ovale* malaria. For individuals who have had extensive exposure to relapsing forms of malaria, consideration should be given to the use of terminal prophylaxis with primaquine upon leaving the malaria-endemic area.

Conclusion

In summary, the use of antimalarial drug regimens should be carefully directed at high-risk travelers, where their benefit most clearly outweighs the risk of adverse events. None of the available regimens are ideal for all travelers, and the travel medicine practitioner should attempt to match the individual's risk of exposure to malaria to the appropriate regimen based on drug efficacy, tolerance, safety, and cost. One strategy to facilitate clinical decision-making is the use of a Clinical Utility Score,[170] in which different attributes of each drug regimen, such as efficacy, tolerance, convenience, cost, etc., are weighted based on clinical trials and experience with these drugs (Table 15.6). The pros and cons are discussed with the client in reaching a suitable choice. This may help provide an objective approach in identifying the 'best choice' drug for an individual traveler. The scores assigned are arbitrary, and users may weigh each variable somewhat differently depending on the specific needs and risk of drug-resistant malaria.

References

1. Hay SI, Cox J, Rogers DJ, et al. Climate change and the resurgence of malaria in the East African highlands. Nature 2002;415:905–9.
2. Centers for Disease Control and Prevention. Health Information for international travel: 2012.
3. Canadian recommendations for the prevention and treatment of malaria among international travelers. Committee to Advise on Tropical Medicine and Travel (CATMAT), Laboratory for Disease Control. Can Commun Dis Rep 2009; Volume 35-S1.
4. World Health Organization (WHO). International travel and health. Geneva: WHO; 2012.
5. Schlagenhauf P, Funk-Baumann M. Malaria maps: PDQ. Travelers' malaria. Hamilton: BC Decker; 2005. p. 81–199.
6. Ohrt C, Ritchie Tl, Widjaja H, et al. Mefloquine compared with doxy cycline for the prophylaxis of malaria in Indonesian soldiers. Ann Intern Med 1997;126:963–72.
7. Leder K, Black J, O'Brien D, et al. Malaria in travelers: a review of the GeoSentinel surveillance network. Clin Infect Dis 2004;29: 1104–12.
8. Steffen R, Fuchs E, Schildknecht J, et al. Mefloquine compared with other malaria chemoprophylactic regimens in tourists visiting East Africa. Lancet 1993;341:1299–303.
9. Hill DR, Behrens RH, Bradley DJ. The risk of malaria in travelers to Thailand. Trans Roy Soc Trop Med Hyg 1996;90:680–1.
10. Fradin MS, Day JF. Comparative efficacy of insect repellents against mosquito bites. N Engl J Med 2002;347:13–8.
11. Anon. Insect repellents. The Medical Letter on Drugs and Therapeutics 2003;43:41–2.
12. Soto J, Medina F, Dember N, et al. Efficacy of permethrin-impregnated uniforms in the prevention of malaria and leishmaniasis in Colombian soldiers. Clin Infect Dis 1995;21:599–602.
13. McGready R. Safety of the insect repellent N, N-diethyl-m-toluamide (DEET) in pregnancy. Am J Trop Med Hyg 2001;65:285–9.
14. Frances SP, Van Dung N, Beebe NW, et al. Field evaluation of repellent formulations against daytime and night-time biting mosquitoes in a tropical rainforest in northern Australia. J Med Entomol 2002;39: 541–4.
15 Lengeler. Cochrane Database Syst Rev 2005. Online. Available: www.thecochranelibrary.com (doi: 10.1002/14651858.CD000363).
16. Kain KC, Keystone JS. Malaria in travelers. Epidemiology, disease and prevention. Infect Dis Clin North Am 1998;12:267–84.
17. Baird JK, Hoffman SL. Prevention of malaria in travelers. Med Clin North Am 1999;83:923–44.
18. Mali S, Kachur SP, Arguin PM. Malaria surveillance–United States, 2010. MMWR Surveill Summ 2012 Mar 2;61:(2):1–17.
19. Schlagenhauf P, Tschopp A, Johnson R, et al. Tolerability of malaria chemoprophylaxis in non-immune travelers to sub-Saharan Africa: multicentre, randomized, double blind, four arm study. BMJ 2003;32:1078–81.
20. World Health Organization. Severe falciparum malaria. Trans R Soc Trop Med Hyg 2000;94: S1–S90.
21. Warhurst DC, Hockley DJ. Mode of action of chloroquine on Plasmodium berghei and P. cynomolgi. Nature 1967;214:935–6.
22. Slater AF, Cerami A. Inhibition by chloroquine of a novel haem polymerase enzyme activity in malaria trophozoites. Nature 1992;355:167–9.
23. Croft Am, Schlagenhauf-Lawlor P. Malaria drug resistance. In: Schlagenhauf-Lawlor P, editor. Travelers' Malaria. 2nd ed. London, Hamilton: BC Decker; 2008. p. 81–8.
24. Rieckmann KH, Davis DR, Hutton DC. Plasmodium vivax resistance to chloroquine? Lancet 1989;2:1183–4.
25. Fidock DA, Nomura T, Talley A, et al. Mutations in the P. falciparum lysosome trans-membrane protein PfCRT and evidence for their role in chloroquine resistance. Mol Cell 2000;6:861–71.
26. Djimde A, Doumbo OK, Cortese JF, et al. A molecular marker for chloroquine-resistant falciparum malaria. N Engl J Med 2001;344: 257–63.
27. Warhurst DC. A molecular marker for chloroquine-resistant malaria. N Engl J Med 2000;344:299–302.
28. Guerra CA, Howes RE, Patil AP, et al. The international limits and population at risk of Plasmodium vivax in 2009. PloS Negl Trop Dis 2010;4(8):e774. Doi: 10.1371)
29. Stemberger H, Leimer R, Widermann G. Tolerability of long-term prophylaxis with Fansidar: a randomized double-blind study in Nigeria. Acta Trop 1984;41:391–9.
30. Chen L, Wilson M, Schlagenhauf P. Prevention of malaria in long-term travelers. JAMA 2006;296:2234 –43.
31. Croft AM, Geary KG. Chloroquine and combinations. In: Schlagenhauf-Lawlor P, editor. Travelers' Malaria. 2nd ed. Hamilton: Decker; 2008. p. 81–8.
32. Wetsteyn JCFM, de Geus A. Comparison of three regimens for malaria prophylaxis in travelers to east, central and southern Africa. BMJ 1993;307:1041–3.

33. Fogh S, Schapira A, Bygbjerg IC, et al. Malaria chemoprophylaxis in travelers to east Africa: a comparative, prospective study of chloroquine plus proguanil with chloroquine plus sulfadoxine-pyrimethamine. BMJ 1988;296:820–2.

34. Hogh B, Clarke P, Camus D, et al. Atovaquone/proguanil versus chloroquine/proguanil for malaria prophylaxis in non-immune travelers: Results from a randomized, double-blind study. Lancet 2000;356:1888–94.

35. Baudon D, Martet G, Pascal B, et al. Efficacy of daily antimalarial chemoprophylaxis in tropical Africa using either doxycycline or chloroquine-proguanil; a study conducted in 1996 in the French Army. Trans R Soc Trop Med Hyg 1999;93:302–3.

36. Huzly D, Schönfeld C, Beurle W, et al. Malaria chemoprophylaxis in German tourists: a prospective study on compliance and adverse reactions. J Travel Med 1996;3:148–55.

37. Chen LH, Wilson ME, Schlagenhauf P. Controversies and misconceptions in malaria chemoprophylaxis for travelers. JAMA 2007;297:2251–63.

38. Durrheim DN, Gammon S, Waner S, et al. Antimalarial prophylaxis-use and adverse events in visitors to the Kruger National Park. S Afr Med J 1999;89:170–5.

39. Peterson E, Ronne T, Ronn A, et al. Reported side-effects to chloroquine, chloroquine plus proguanil, and mefloquine as chemoprophylaxis against malaria in Danish travelers. J Travel Med 2000;7:79–84.

40. Carme B, Péguet C, Nevez G. Chimioprophylaxie du paludisme: tolerance et observance de la mefloquine et de l'association proguanil/chloroquine chez des touristes francais. Bull Soc Pathol Exot 1997;90:273–6.

41. Steffen R, DuPont H.L, editors. Manual of Travel Medicine and Health. Hamilton: Decker; 1999.

42. Schmidt LH, Crosby R, Rasco J, et al. Antimalarial activities of various 4-quinolinemethanols with special attention to WR-142,490 (mefloquine). Antimicrob Agents Chemother 1978;13:1011–30.

43. Bonner U, Divis PC, Färnert A, Singh B. Swedish traveler with Plasmodium knowlesi after visiting Malaysian Borneo. Malaria J 2009; 8:15.

44. Warhurst DC. Antimalarial interaction with ferriprotoporphyrin IX monomer and its relationship to the activity of the blood schizonticides. Ann Trop Med Parasitol 1987;81:65–7.

45. Mockenhaupt FP. Mefloquine resistance in Plasmodium falciparum. Parasitol Today 1995;11:248–53.

46. Lobel HO, Miani M, Eng T, et al. Long term malaria prophylaxis with weekly mefloquine. Lancet 1993;341:848–51.

47. Rieckmann KH, Yeo AE, Davis DR, et al. Recent military experience with malaria chemoprophylaxis. Med J Aust 1993;158:446–9.

48. Pergallo MS, Sabatinelli G, Majori G, et al. Prevention and morbidity in non-immune subjects; a case-control study among Italian troops in Somalia and Mozambique, 1992–1994. Trans R Soc Trop Med Hyg 1997;91:343–6.

49. Axmann A, Félegyhazi CS, Huszar A, et al. Long term malaria prophylaxis with Lariam in Cambodia, 1993. Travel Med Int 1994;12:13–8.

50. Hopperus Buma AP, van Thiel PP, Lobel HO, et al. Long-term prophylaxis with mefloquine in Dutch marines in Cambodia. J Infect Dis 1996;173:1506–9.

51. Sanchez JL, DeFraites RF, Sharp TW, et al. Mefloquine or doxycycline prophylaxis in US troops in Somalia. Lancet 1993;341:1021–2.

52. Wallace MR, Sharp TW, Smoak B, et al. Malaria among United States troops in Somalia. Am J Med 1996;100:49–55.

53. Bwire R, Slootman EJH, Verhave JP, et al. Malaria anticircumsporozoite antibodies in Dutch soldiers returning from sub-Saharan Africa. Trop Med Int Health 1998;3:66–9.

54. Muehlberger N, Jelinek T, Schlipkoeter U, et al. Effectiveness of chemoprophylaxis and other determinants of malaria in travelers to Kenya. Trop Med Int Health 1998;3:357–63.

55. Lobel HO, Varma JK, Miani N, et al. Monitoring for mefloquine-resistant Plasmodium falciparum in Africa: implications for travelers' health. Am J Trop Med Hyg 1998;59:129–32.

56. Brasseur P, Kouamouo J, Moyou-Somo R, et al. Multi-drug resistant falciparum malaria in Cameroon in 1987–1988. II Mefloquine resistance confirmed in vivo and in vitro and its correlation with quinine resistance. Am J Trop Med Hyg 1992;46:8–14.

57. Cowman AF, Galatis D, Thompson JK. Selection for mefloquine resistance in Plasmodium falciparum is linked to amplification of the pfmdr1 gene

and cross resistance to halofantrine and quinine. Proc Nat Acad Sci USA 1994;91:1143–7.

58. Reed MB, Saliba KJ, Caruana SR, et al. Pgh1 modulates sensitivity and resistance to multiple antimalarials in Plasmodium falciparum. Nature 2000;403:906–9.

59. Oduola AMJ, Omitowoju GO, Gerena L, et al. Reversal of mefloquine resistance with penfluridol in isolates of Plasmodium falciparum from south-west Nigeria. Trans R Soc Trop Med Hyg 1993;87:81–3.

60. Schlagenhauf P, Adamcova M, Regep L, et al. The position of mefloquine as a 21st century malaria chemoprophylaxis. Malaria J 2010;9:357.

61. Jacquerioz FA, Croft AM. Drugs for preventing malaria in travellers. Cochrane Database Syst Rev 2009:CD006491.

62. Overbosch D, Schilthuis HS, Bienzle U, et al. Atovaquone/proguanil versus mefloquine for malaria prophylaxis in non-immune travelers: results from a randomized, double-blind study. Clin Infect Dis 2001;33:1015–21.

63. Barrett PJ, Emmins PD, Clarke PD, et al. Comparison of adverse events associated with the use of mefloquine and combination of chloroquine and proguanil as antimalarial prophylaxis: postal and telephone survey of travelers. BMJ 1996;313:525–8.

64. Phillips MA, Kass RB. User acceptability patterns for mefloquine and doxycycline malaria chemoprophylaxis. J Travel Med 1996;3:40–5.

65. Ollivier L, Tifratene K, Josse R, et al. The relationship between body weight and tolerance to mefloquine prophylaxis in non-immune adults; results of a questionnaire-based study. Ann Trop Med Parasitol 2004;6:639–41.

66. Schlagenhauf P, Steffen R, Lobel H, et al. Mefloquine tolerability during chemoprophylaxis: focus on adverse event assessments, stereochemistry and compliance. Trop Med Int Health 1996;1:485–94.

67. CIOMS Working Group. International reporting of adverse drug reactions. CIOMS Working Group Report. Geneva: World Health Organization; 1987.

68. MacPherson D, Gamble K, Tessier D, et al. Mefloquine tolerance-randomized, double-blinded, placebo-controlled study using a loading dose of mefloquine in pre-exposed travelers. Program and Abstracts of the Fifth International Conference on Travel Medicine, Geneva: Switzerland; March 24–7, 1997.

69. Jaspers CA, Hopperus Buma AP, van Thiel PP, et al. Tolerance of mefloquine prophylaxis in Dutch military personnel. Am J Trop Med Hyg 1996;55:230–4.

70. Croft AJM, World MJ. Neuropsychiatric reactions with mefloquine chemoprophylaxis. Lancet 1996;347:326.

71. Potasman I, Beny A, Seligmann H. Neuropsychiatric problems in 2,500 long-term travelers to the tropics. J Travel Med 1999;6:122–33.

72. Schlagenhauf P, Steffen R. Neuropsychiatric events and travel: do anti-malarials play a role? J Travel Med 2000;7:225–6.

73. Schwartz E, Potasman I, Rotenberg M, et al. Serious adverse events of mefloquine in relation to blood level and gender. Am J Trop Med Hyg 2001;65:189–92.

74. Howard PA, Kuile ter FO. CNS adverse events associated with antimalarial agents. Fact or fiction? Drug Safety 1995;12:370–83.

75. Wittes RC, Sagmur R. Adverse reactions to mefloquine associated with ethanol ingestion. Can Med Assoc J 1995;152:515–7.

76. Vuurman EFPM, Muntjewerff ND, Uiterwijk MMC, et al. Effects of mefloquine alone and with alcohol on psychomotor and driving performance. Eur J Clin Pharm 1996;50:475–82.

76a. Schlagenhauf P, Adamcova M, Regep L, et al. Use of mefloquine in children – a review of dosage, pharmacokinetics and tolerability data. Malar J 2011,10:292.

77. Mittelholzer ML, Wall M, Steffen R, et al. Malaria prophylaxis in different age groups. J Travel Med 1996;4:219–23.

78. Jerling M, Rombo L, Hellgren U, et al. Evaluation of mefloquine adverse effects in relation to the plasma concentration. Fourth International Conference on Travel Medicine, Acapulco. Mexico: 23–7 April 1995.

79. Cruikshank SJ, Hopperstad M, Younger M, et al. Potent block of Cx36 and Cx 50 gap junction channels by mefloquine. Proc Natl Acad Sci USA 2004;101:12364–9.

80. CDC. Sudden death in a traveler following halofantrine administration – Togo, 2000. MMWR 2001;50:169–70, 179.

81. Handschin JC, Wall M, Steffen R, et al. Tolerability and effectiveness of malaria chemoprophylaxis with mefloquine or chloroquine with or without co-medication. J Travel Med 1997;4:121–7.

82. Boudreau E, Schuster B, Sanchez J, et al. Tolerability of prophylactic Lariam regimens. Trop Med Parasit 1993;44:257–65.

83. Schlagenhauf P, Lobel HO, Steffen R, et al. Tolerability of mefloquine in Swissair trainee pilots. Am J Trop Med Hyg 1997;56:235–40.

84. Crevoisier C, Joseph I, Fischer M, et al. Influence of hemodialysis on plasma concentration-time profiles of mefloquine in two patients with end-stage renal disease: a prophylactic drug monitoring study. Antimicrob Agents Chemother 1995;39:1892–5.

85. Joshi N, Miller DQ. Doxycycline revisited. Arch Intern Med 1997;157:1421–6.

86. USP DI. Drug Information for the Health Professional, vol.1, 1st ed. Englewood: Micromedex; 2001. p. 2801–12.

87. Shmuklarsky MJ, Boudreau EF, Pang LW, et al. Failure of doxycycline as a causal prophylactic against Plasmodium falciparum malaria in healthy nonimmune volunteers. Ann Intern Med 1994;120:294–9.

88. Dahl EL, Shock JL, Shenai BR, et al. Tetracyclines specifically target the apicoplast of the malaria parasite P. falciparum. Antimicrob Agents Chemother 2006;50:3124–31.

89. Shanks DG, Barnett A, Edstein MD, et al. Effectiveness of doxycycline combined with primaquine for malaria prophylaxis. Med J Aust 1995;162:306–10.

90. Pang LW, Limsomwong N, Boudreau EF, et al. Doxycycline prophylaxis for falciparum malaria. Lancet 1987;1:1161–4.

91. Pang LW, Limsomwong N, Singharaj P. Prophylactic treatment of vivax and falciparum malaria with low-dose doxycycline. J Infect Dis 1988;158:1124–7.

92. Watanasook C, Singharaj P, Suriyamongkol V, et al. Malaria prophylaxis with doxycycline in soldiers deployed to the Thai-Kampuchean border. Southeast Asian J Trop Med Public Health 1989;20:61–4.

93. Baudon D, Martet G, Pascal B, et al. Efficacy of daily antimalarial chemo-prophylaxis in tropical Africa using either doxycycline or chloroquine-proguanil; a study conducted in 1996 in the French Army. Trans R Soc Trop Med Hyg 1999;93:302–3.

94. Weiss WR, Oloo AJ, Johnson A, et al. Daily primaquine is effective for prophylaxis against falciparum malaria in Kenya: comparison with mefloquine, doxycycline, and chloroquine/proguanil. J Infect Dis 1995;171:1569–75.

95. Anderson SL, Oloo AJ, Gordon DM, et al. Successful double-blinded, randomized, placebo-controlled field trial of azithromycin and doxycycline as prophylaxis for malaria in western Kenya. Clin Infect Dis 1998;26:146–50.

96. Taylor WRJ, Richie TL, Fryauff DJ, et al. Malaria prophylaxis using azithromycin: a double-blind, placebo controlled trial in Irian Jaya, Indonesia. Clin Infect Dis 1999;28:74–81.

97. Nasveld PE, Edstein MD, Kitchener SJ, et al. Comparison of the effectiveness of atovaquone/proguanil combination and doxycycline in the chemoprophylaxis of malaria in Australian Defense Force personnel. Program and Abstracts of the 49th Annual Meeting of the American Society of Tropical Medicine and Hygiene; Houston, TX 2000;62:139.

98. Kitchener SJ, Nasveld PE, Gregory RM, et al. Mefloquine and doxycycline malaria prophylaxis in Australian soldiers in East Timor. Med J Aust 2005;182:168–71.

99. Tan KR, Magill AJ, Parise ME, et al. Doxycycline for malaria chemoprophylaxis and treatment: report from the CDC expert meeting on malaria chemoprophylaxis. Am J Trop Med Hyg 2011;84:517–31.

100. Adverse Drug Reactions Advisory Committee. Doxycycline-induced esophageal ulceration. Med J Aust 1994;161:490.

101. Westermann GW, Bohm M, Bonsmann G, et al. Chronic intoxication by doxycycline use for more than 12 years. J Intern Med 1999;246:591–2.

102. Schuhwerk M, Behrens RH. Doxycycline as first line malarial prophylaxis: how safe is it? J Travel Med 1998;5:102.

103. Arthur JD, Echeverria P, Shanks GD, et al. A comparative study of gastrointestinal infections in United States soldiers receiving doxycycline or mefloquine for malaria prophylaxis. Am J Trop Med Hyg 1990;43:606–18.

104. Lochary ME, Lockhart PB, Williams WT. Doxycycline and staining of permanent teeth. Pediatr Infect Dis J 1998;17:429–31.

105. Gottlieb A. Safety of minocycline for acne. Lancet 1997;349:374.

106. Heaton P, Fenwick S, Brewer D. Association between tetracycline or doxycycline and hepatotoxicity: a population based case-control study. L Clin Pharm Ther 2007;32:483–7.

107. Neeley JL, Abate M, Swinker M, et al. The effect of doxycycline on serum levels of ethinyl estradiol, norethindrone, and endogenous progesterone. Obstet Gynecol 1991;77:416–20.

108. Boggild A, Parise M, Lewis L, et al. Atovaquone-Proguanil; Report from CDC Expert Meeting on Malaria Chemoprophylaxis. Amer J Trop Med Hyg 2007;76:208–23.

108a. Shapiro TA, Ranasinha CD, Kumar N, et al. Prophylactic activity of atovaquone against Plasmodium falciparum in humans. Am J Trop Med Hyg 1999;60:831–6.

109. Radloff PD, Philipps J, Hutchinson D, et al. Atovaquone proguanil is an effective treatment for P. ovale and P. malariae malaria. Trans R Soc Trop Med Hyg 1996;90:682.

110. Berman JD, Chulay JD, Dowler M, et al. Causal prophylactic efficacy of Malarone in a human challenge model. Trans R Soc Trop Med Hyg 2001;95:429–32.

111. Srivastava IK, Vaidya AB. A mechanism for the synergistic antimalarial action of atovaquone and proguanil. Antimicrob Agents Chemother 1999;43:1334–9.

112. Beerahee M. Clinical pharmacology of atovaquone and proguanil hydrochloride. J Travel Med 1999;6:S13–7.

113. Pudney M, Gutterage W, Zeman A, et al. Atovaquone and proguanil hydrochloride: a review of nonclinical studies. J Travel Med 1999;6: S8–S12.

114. Looareesuwan S, Viravan C, Webster HK, et al. Clinical studies of atovaquone, alone or in combination with other antimalarial drugs, for treatment of acute uncomplicated malaria in Thailand. Am J Trop Med Hyg 1996;54:62–6.

115. Fivelman QL, Butcher GA, Adagu IS, et al. Malarone treatment failure and in vitro confirmation of resistance of Plasmodium falciparum isolate from Lagos, Nigeria. Malaria J 2002;1:1–4.

116. Schwartz E, Bujanover S, Kain KC. Genetic confirmation of atovaquone-proguanil resistant Plasmodium falciparum malaria acquired by a nonimmune traveler to East Africa. Clin Infect Dis 2003;37:450–1.

117. Schwobel B, Alifrangis M, Salanti A, et al. Different mutation patterns of atovaquone resistance to Plasmodium falciparum in vitro and in vivo: rapid detection of codon 268 polymorphisms in the cytochrome b as a potential in vivo resistance marker. Malaria J 2003;2:5–11.

118. David KP, Alifrangis M, Salanti A, et al. Atovaquone/proguanil resistance in Africa: a case report. Scand J Infect Dis 2003;35:897–8.

119. Farnert A, Lindberg J, Gil P, et al. Evidence of Plasmodium falciparum malaria resistant to atovaquone and proguanil hydrochloride: case reports. BMJ 2003;326:628–9.

120. Kuhn S, Gill MJ, Kain KC. Emergence of atovaquone-proguanil resistance during treatment of Plasmodium falciparum malaria acquired by a non-immune North American traveler to West Africa. Am J Trop Med Hyg 2005;72:407–9.

121. Durand R, Prendki V, Cailhol J, et al. P. falciparum malaria and atovaquone proguanil treatment failure. Emerg Infect Dis 2008;14: 320322.

122. Shanks GD, Gordon DM, Klotz FW, et al. Efficacy and safety of atovaquone/proguanil as suppressive prophylaxis for Plasmodium falciparum malaria. Clin Infect Dis 1998;27:494–9.

123. Lell B, Luckner D, Ndjave M, et al. Randomized placebo-controlled study of atovaquone plus proguanil for malaria prophylaxis in children. Lancet 1998;351:709–13.

124. Sukwa TY, Mulenga M, Chisdaka N, et al. A randomized, double-blind, placebo-controlled field trial to determine the efficacy and safety of Malarone (atovaquone/proguanil) for the prophylaxis of malaria in Zambia. Am J Trop Med Hyg 1999;60:521–5.

125. Ling J, Baird JD, Fryauff DJ, et al. Randomized, placebo-controlled trial of atovaquone/proguanil for the prevention of Plasmodium falciparum or Plasmodium vivax malaria among migrants to Papua, Indonesia. Clin Infect Dis 2002;35:825–33.

126. Camus D, Djossou F, Schilthuis HJ, et al. Atovaquone-proguanil versus chloroquine-proguanil for malaria prophylaxis in nonimmune pediatric travelers: results of an international, randomized, open-label study. Clin Infect Dis 2004;38:1716–23.

127. Emberger M, Lechner A, Zelger B. Stevens-Johnson syndrome associated with Malarone antimalarial prophylaxis. Clin Infect Dis 2003;37:e5–7.

128. Remich S, Otieno W, Polhemus M, et al. Bullous erythema multiforme after treatment with Malarone. Trop Doc 2008;38:190–1.

129. Nakato H, Vivaancos R, Hunter P. A systematic review and meta-analysis of the effectiveness and safety of atovaquone proguanil (Malarone) for chemoprophylaxis against malaria. J Antimicrob Chemother 2007;60:929–36.

130. McGready R, Ashley EA, Moo E, et al. A randomized comparison of artesunate-atovaquone-proguanil versus quinine in treatment for uncomplicated falciparum malaria during pregnancy. J Infect Dis 2005;192:846–53.

131. Pasternak B, Hviid A. Atovaquone proguanil use in early pregnancy and the risk of birth defects. Arch Intern Med 2011;171:259–60.

132. GlaxoSmithKline. Malarone product monograph; 2004;1–36.

133. Jacquerioz F, Croft A. Drugs for preventing malaria in travelers. Cochrane Database Syst Rev 2009; CD006491).

134. Peterson E. The safety of atovaquone proguanil in the long term prophylaxis of nonimmune adults. J Travel Med 2003;10(Suppl. 1):S13–15.

135. Ling J, Baird JK, Fryauff D, et al. Randomized placebo-controlled trial of atovaquone proguanil for the prevention of *P. falciparum* or *P. vivax* malaria among migrants to Papua, Indonesia. Clin Infect Dis 2002;35:825–33.

136. Arnold JAA, Hockwald RS. The effect of continuous and intermittent primaquine therapy on the relapse rate of Chesson strain vivax malaria. J Lab Clin Med 1954;44:429–38.

137. Arnold JAA, Hockwald RS. The antimalarial action of primaquine against the blood and tissue stages of falciparum malaria (Panama, P-F-6 strain). J Lab Clin Med 1955;46:391–7.

138. Hill D, Baird JK, Parise M, et al. Primaquine: report from CDC expert meeting on malaria chemoprophylaxis I. Am J Trop Med Hyg. 2006 Sep;75(3):402–15.

139. Ward SA, Mihaly GW, Edwards G, et al. Pharmacokinetics of Primaquine in man. Comparison of acute versus chronic dosage in Thai subjects. Br J Clin Pharm 1985;19:751–5.

140. Taylor T, Strickland T. Malaria. In: Strickland T, editor. Hunter's Tropical Medicine and Emerging Infectious Diseases. 8th ed. Philadelphia: WB Saunders; 2000.

141. Fryauff DJBJ, Basri H, Sumawinata I, et al. Randomized placebo-controlled trial of primaquine for prophylaxis of falciparum and vivax malaria. Lancet 1995;346:1190–3.

142. Baird KLM, Sismadi P, Gramzinski R, et al. Randomized pivotal trial of primaquine for prophylaxis against malaria in Javanese adults in Papua, Indonesia. Clin Infect Dis 2001;33:1990–7.

143. Soto JTJ, Rodriquez M, Sanchez J, et al. Primaquine prophylaxis against malaria in nonimmune Colombian soldiers: efficacy and toxicity. A randomized, double-blind, placebo-controlled trial. Ann Intern Med 1998;129:241–4.

144. Soto JTJ, Rodriquez M, Sanchez J, et al. Double-blind, randomized, placebo-controlled assessment of chloroquine/primaquine prophylaxis for malaria in nonimmune Colombian soldiers. Clin Infect Dis 1999;29:199–201.

145. Smoak BL, DeFraites RF, Magill AJ, et al. Plasmodium vivax infections in U.S. Army troops: failure of primaquine to prevent relapse in studies from Somalia. Am J Trop Med Hyg 1997;56:231–4.

146. Schippers EF, Hugen PW, den Hartigh J, et al. No drug-drug interaction between nelfinavir or indinavir and mefloquine in HIV-1-infected patients. AIDS 2000;14:2794–5.

147. Kredo T, Mauff K, Van der Walt JS, et al. Interaction between artemether-lumefantrine and nevirapine-based antiretroviral therapy in HIV-1-infected patients. Antimicrob Agents Chemother 2011;55(12):5616–23. Epub 2011 Sep 26.

148. Brueckner RPLK, Lin ET, Schuster BG. First-time-in-humans safety and pharmacokinetics of WR 238605, a new antimalarial. Am J Trop Med Hyg 1998;58:645–9.

149. Walsh DS, Loodreesuwan S, Wilairatana P, et al. Randomized dose-ranging study of the safety and efficacy of WR 238605 (Tafenoquine) in the prevention of relapse of Plasmodium vivax malaria in Thailand. J Infect Dis 1999;180:1282–7.

150. Shanks GD, Kain KC, Keystone JS. Malaria chemoprophylaxis in an age of drug resistance II. Drugs that may be available in the future. Clin Infect Dis 2001;33:381–5.

151. Shanks GD, Klotz FW, Aleman GM, et al. A new primaquine analogue, Tafenoquine (WR238605), for prophylaxis against Plasmodium falciparum malaria. Clin Infect Dis 2001;33:1968–74.

152. Hale BR, Koram KA, Adjuik M, et al. A randomized, double-blinded, placebo-controlled trial of Tafenoquine for prophylaxis against Plasmodium falciparum in Ghana [abstract]. Am J Trop Med Hyg 2000;62:139–40.

153. Hale BR, Owusu-Agyei S, Fryauff DJ, et al. A randomized, double-blind, placebo-controlled, dose-ranging trial of tafenoquine for weekly prophylaxis against Plasmodium falciparum. Clin Infect Dis 2003;36:541–9.

154. Lell BFJ, Missinou MA, Borrmann S, et al. Malaria chemoprophylaxis with Tafenoquine: a randomized study. Lancet 2000;355:2041–5.

155. Walsh DSEC, Sangkharomya S. Randomized, double-blind, placebo controlled evaluation of monthly WR 238605 (Tafenoquine) for prophylaxis of Plasmodium falciparum and P. vivax in Royal Thai Army soldiers. Am J Trop Med Hyg 1999;61:502.

156. Walsh DS, Eamsila C, Sasiprapha T, et al. Efficacy of monthly tafenoquine for prophylaxis of Plasmodium vivax and multidrug-resistant P. falciparum malaria. J Infect Dis 2004;190:1456–63.

157. Nasveld PE, Edstein MD, Reid M, et al; Tafenoquine Study Team. Randomized, double-blind study of the safety, tolerability, and efficacy of tafenoquine versus mefloquine for malaria prophylaxis in nonimmune subjects. Antimicrob Agents Chemother 2010 Feb;54(2):792–8. Epub 2009 Dec 7.

158. Leary K, Riel M, Cantilena L, et al. A randomized, double-blind, safety and tolerability study to assess the ophthalmic and renal effects of tafenoquine 200 mg weekly versus placebo for 6 months in healthy volunteers. Am J Trop Med Hyg 2009 Aug;81(2):356–62.

159. Coleman RECA, Milhous WK. Gametocytocidal and sporontocidal activity of antimalarials against Plasmodium berghei ANKA in ICR Mice and Anopheles stephensi mosquitoes. Am J Trop Med Hyg 1992;46:169–82.

160. Brewer TG, Grate SJ, Peggins JO, et al. Fatal neurotoxicity of arteether and artemether. Am J Trop Med Hyg 1994;51:251–9.

161. World Health Organization. Drug Alert: Halofantrine. Wkly Epidemiol Rec 1993;68:268–70.

162. Schlagenhauf P, Suarez Boutros M, et al. Use of mefloquine chemoprophylaxis by non-immune travelers before and during pregnancy. A critical evaluation of the evidence from 1985–2005. Abstract NECTM, Edinburgh, June, 2006.

163. Schlagenhauf P, et al. Use of mefloquine in children – a review of dosage, pharmacokinetics and tolerability data. Malaria Journal 2011;10:292.

164. Kublin JG, Steketee RW. HIV infection and malaria – understanding the interactions. J Infect Dis 2006;193:1–3.

165. Khaliq Y, Gallicano K, Tisdale C, et al. Pharmacokinetic interaction between mefloquine and ritonavir in healthy volunteers. Br J Clin Pharm 2001;51:591–600.

166. Colebunders R, Nachega J, Van Gompel A. Anti-retroviral treatment and travel to developing countries. J Trav Med 1999;6:27–31.

167. Tessier D. Immunocompromised travelers. In: Schlagenhauf P, editor. Travelers' Malaria. Hamilton: Decker; 2001. p. 324–35.

168. Pennie R.A, Koren G, Crevoisier C. Steady state pharmacokinetics of mefloquine in long-term travelers. Trans Roy Soc Trop Med Hyg 1993:459–62.

169. Petersen E. The safety of atovaquone/proguanil in long-term malaria prophylaxis of non-immune adults. J Travel Med 2003;(Suppl.):S13–5.

170. Kain KC, Shanks GD, Keystone JS. Malaria chemoprophylaxis in an age of drug resistance I. Currently recommended drug regimens. Clin Infect Dis 2001;33:226–34.

16

Self-Diagnosis and Self-Treatment of Malaria by the Traveler

Martin P. Grobusch

Key points

- The concept of standby emergency treatment (SBET) was introduced in the late 1980s
- The principle of SBET: early empiric treatment of suspected malaria is life-saving if there is lack of access to medical care
- Rapid diagnostic tests are not fully reliable as decision-making tools for SBET in the hands of travelers
- The choice of drugs for SBET is dependent on drug resistance and tolerability

Introduction

The global malaria burden is in decline;[1] however, and despite the availability of prophylactic measures,[2–5] a considerable number of travelers contract malaria every year.[6,7]

At present, a comprehensive, single, safe and highly effective method to prevent malaria in travelers to endemic areas is neither available nor in sight, despite considerable recent progress towards an at least partially protective malaria vaccine.[8] Recommendations for the prevention of malaria in travelers are therefore based predominantly on the combination of avoiding mosquito bites ('exposure prophylaxis') and an appropriate chemoprophylactic regimen. Even a combination, however, does not provide 100% protection. More importantly, only a minority of travelers make use of available protective measures. For example, in a cohort of 1659 malaria patients observed in Europe, 60.4% of the European travelers and 72.4% of VFRs had traveled without using chemoprophylaxis,[9] and only a small number of individuals tried to adhere fully to the prevention of insect bites.

Among those individuals who chose to use appropriate chemoprophylaxis, the protection rate varied from 70% to 95% in various prospective and case–control studies.[10,11] This applied not only to established drugs, but also to recently introduced compounds such as atovaquone/proguanil.[12] There are many reasons for chemoprophylaxis failure. Apart from a reduced sensitivity of *Plasmodium* spp. to the antimalarials used, the main reasons for failure are a lack of adherence to the recommended regimen (particularly early cessation of prophylaxis), drug resorption problems (e.g., due to vomiting or diarrhea) and prolonged exoerythrocytic phase times of malaria (i.e., exceeding the period of drug intake).[13]

Each chemoprophylactic agent is linked to a risk of adverse events, with frequencies ranging from 10% to 30%.[11] Apart from taking individual contraindications and intolerances into account, the general risk of adverse events should be weighed against the risk of infection at the destination. This applies particularly to certain groups of travelers and occupational groups, such as airline crews who make frequent short visits to endemic areas over prolonged periods of time, as well as to a larger group of travelers with prolonged duration of travel. It also applies to those with a low to moderate risk of contracting malaria (Figure 16.1).

Regardless of the prophylactic used, one has to keep in mind that infection with *P. falciparum* may lead to very severe disease within a short period of time. This is particularly true for non-immune individuals, such as children in endemic areas and travelers who live in malaria-free regions.

Complications and deaths are predominantly the result of a delay in the initiation of treatment or in the provision of inappropriate therapy. The early diagnosis and treatment of malaria are critical in reducing malaria-related morbidity and mortality.[14]

In developing countries where malaria is endemic, healthcare facilities may be readily available for the management of severe illness. In fact, most febrile illnesses are treated as malaria regardless of the blood film results (which are not infrequently falsely positive). However, in many remote areas optimal medical care is not readily accessible within a reasonable period of time.

For this reason, the concept of standby emergency treatment (SBET) was introduced in the late 1980s[15] and later updated.[16] Travelers are provided with a treatment dose of an appropriate antimalarial drug to be carried and taken in case of a febrile illness, when medical care cannot be reached promptly.

Current guidelines such as the German consensus recommendations[17] embrace the option to abandon chemoprophylaxis in favor of SBET for particular situations, assuming that the traveler will maintain rigorous protection measures against mosquito bites.[18] In Europe, SBET is often recommended in low malaria risk situations such as travel to Thailand and to Central and South America. The CDC recommends that in those rare instances when access to medical care is not available and the traveler develops a febrile illness consistent with malaria, a suitable supply of medication could be self-administered presumptively, but that prompt medical evaluation is imperative.[5] A major problem with SBET is the difficulty that travelers have in making a self-diagnosis of malaria on the basis of clinical symptoms. Since the introduction of new, rapid immunochromatographic tests to detect plasmodial antigens, the question now arises as to whether these tests are suitable for self-diagnosis.

DOI: 10.1016/B978-1-4557-1076-8.00016-8

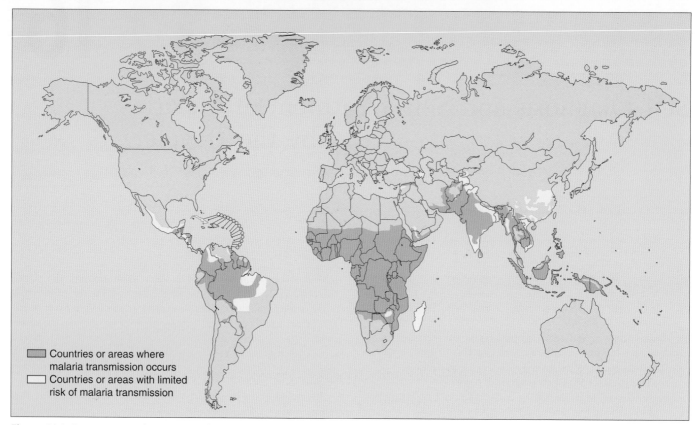

Figure 16.1 Overview on malarious areas of the world and approximate risk of malaria transmission. *(Adapted with kind permission from WHO, Geneva, 2002.)*

Rapid Diagnostic Tests for Malaria

Rationale

Expert examination of thick and thin Giemsa-stained blood smears still remains the diagnostic standard for malaria in both malaria-endemic and non-endemic countries in settings where microscopy expertise and resources to sustain a microscopy unit are readily available. This is not the case, however, in most scenarios, and various authors[19–22] have reviewed new diagnostic approaches for malaria in detail. Microscopy with fluorescent stains,[23] polymerase chain reaction assays[24] and some automated blood cell analyzers[25] offer, to a varying extent, alternatives for laboratory-based diagnostic, epidemiologic and research applications for detection of *Plasmodium* spp. Recently, in the quest for malaria eradication, a research agenda for future improvement of diagnoses and diagnostics has been postulated.[26] However, the most successful alternatives to microscopy are without doubt the rapid immunochromatographic, test-strip-based antigen detection techniques. With the introduction of artemisinin combination therapies (ACTs) for falciparum malaria across most areas of endemicity, rapid diagnostic tests (RDTs) to base rational treatment decisions on now form the backbone of current global malaria control strategies.[27–30] In theory, RDTs might be recommended for use by laypersons for self-diagnosis of malaria, as they do not require a laboratory or much medical expertise to use them.

Principle and Availability of Test Kits

The so-called rapid diagnostic tests (RDTs) for malaria are based on the immunochromatographic detection of plasmodial proteins, namely histidine-rich protein II (HRP-2), and in some tests in combination with parasite-specific aldolase, or parasite-specific lactate dehydrogenase (pLDH).

Test principles and procedures vary depending on the manufacturer. The ready-to-use test kits contain nitrocellulose test strips onto which monoclonal antibodies against HRP-2 or pLDH are immobilized. A small amount of whole blood is applied to the test strip, together with a diluent which hemolyzes the red cells. A detecting antibody attached to colloidal gold or an enzyme against HRP-2, parasite-specific aldolase or pLDH is applied later, or is already integrated into the test strip. After the addition of a buffer solution, the reagents migrate along the test strip.

In a positive case, the complex of parasite protein and detecting antibody is bound to an immobilizing antibody. The colloidal gold, or substrate-enzyme, produces a visible line which can be read with the naked eye. A control line with the antibody against the detecting antibody indicates whether the test was performed correctly. All tests can be performed within 5–15 min. Figure 16.2 illustrates the test principle, Figures 16.3 and 16.4 demonstrate test results, and Table 16.1[21,31–38] details the variety of test formats that have been, or are currently, available. In an attempt to keep abreast with the rapidly growing and constantly changing list of manufacturers, WHO has issued information on available test kits and their evaluation.[39]

Performance of RDTs for Laboratory Diagnosis of Malaria

Several hundred studies that evaluate the different RDTs in various populations have been published and reviewed to date. In comparison to microscopic diagnosis the sensitivity for detecting symptomatic *P. falciparum* infections was high with all rapid tests, having a sensitivity of 85–100% in the majority of studies. In a few cases with proven falciparum malaria rapid tests were already positive at a time when it was impossible to detect parasites microscopically. With low parasitemias, predominantly occurring in semi-immunes, the sensitivity of

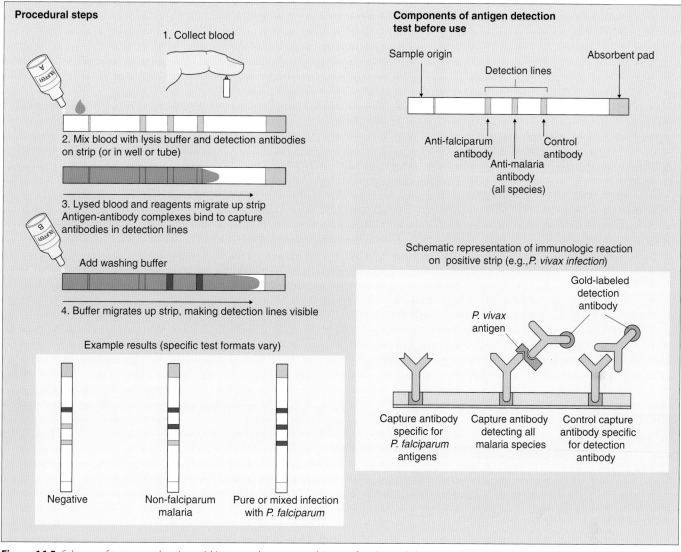

Figure 16.2 Scheme of test procedure in rapid immunochromatographic tests for plasmodial antigen detection. *(Adapted from WHO, Geneva, 2000.)*

Table 16.1 Dipstick Tests for Malaria Diagnosis

Antigen(s)	Species	Brand Name*
HRP-2	P.f.	ParaSight-F[31]
HRP-2	P.f.	Binax Malaria P.f. alias MalaQuick[32]
HRP-2	P.f.	PATH falciparum malaria[33]
HRP-2	P.f.	Paracheck-P.f.[34]
HRP-2	P.f.	Determine Malaria P.f.[35]
HRP-2	P.f.	Quorum RTM[36]
HRP-2 + PMA	P.f. + P.v.	Binax Malaria P.f./P.v.[37]
pLDH isoforms	P.f. + P.v./ non-falciparum spp.	OptiMal[21]
HRP-2 + pLDH isoforms	P.f. + P.v/ non-falciparum spp.	First Response[38]

P.f., *P. falciparum*; P.v., *P. vivax*.

*Brand names are serving only as examples here as there is a multitude of products available, and some older products are becoming unavailable. See WHO 2010 Information[39] for up-to-date information on manufacturers of RDTs.

all tests was significantly lower and reached only 50–70% with parasitemias <100/μL.[40,41] However, false-negative results have also been occasionally recorded with higher parasitemias (>500–1000/μL).[42–45] A false-negative MalaQuick test, in which the *P. falciparum* parasitemia was 30%, became positive after a 1:10 dilution of the patient's blood; a prozone phenomenon with high antigen concentrations was postulated.[44] More importantly, it is estimated that 2–3% of all isolates might lack the HRP-2 gene, thereby making these infections undetectable when using this antigen.[46–48] Also, since mature gametocytes do not produce HRP-2, cases with gametocytes alone will be missed.[49,50] This finding, as well as the fact that HRP-2 antigenemia persists for up to 4 weeks following clinical and parasitologic cure,[22,51] is of relevance when considering test methods for follow-up after therapy.

The specificity in most investigations was in the range of 90–100% in the majority of studies. False-positive results are possible with all tests. They were observed in patients with rheumatoid factor,[52–54] particularly with the ParaSight-F test.

For the detection of *P. vivax* infections, pLDH detection with the OptiMal yielded a high sensitivity and specificity of >90%.[55–57] The ICT Malaria P.F./P.v. test (or RIDA MalaQuick Kombi) yields a similarly high specificity of >90% with *P. vivax* infections, but the overall sensitivity lies between 72% and 75% in most studies,[37] with some studies yielding detection rates even lower than 50%.[58] At low

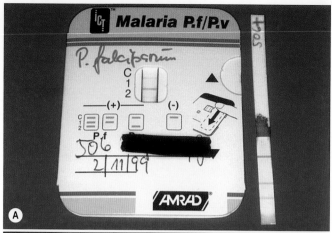

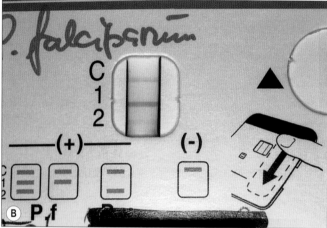

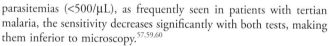

Figure 16.3 (A) RDTs for combined detection of *P. falciparum* and *P. vivax* displaying test results positive for *P. falciparum*. Left side, test format for the detection of histidine-rich protein-2 (HRP-2) in combination with plasmodial aldolase (ICT Malaria P.f./P.v.); right side, test format for the detection of parasite-specific lactate dehydrogenase (pLDH) (OptiMal). **(B)** Close-up view of 'A' to illustrate test result as seen by the examiner.

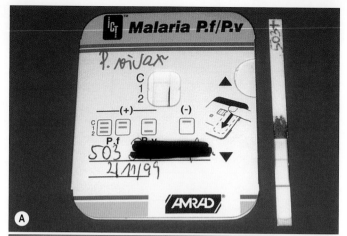

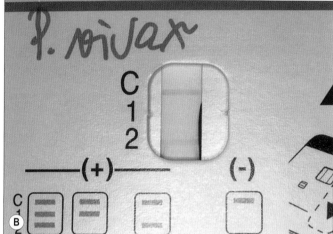

Figure 16.4 (A) RDTs for combined detection of *P. falciparum* and *P. vivax* displaying test results positive for *P. vivax*. Left side, test format for the detection of histidine-rich protein-2 (HRP-2) in combination with plasmodial aldolase (ICT Malaria P.f./P.v.); right side, test format for the detection of parasite-specific lactate dehydrogenase (pLDH) (OptiMal). **(B)** Close-up view of 'A' to illustrate test result as seen by the examiner.

parasitemias (<500/μL), as frequently seen in patients with tertian malaria, the sensitivity decreases significantly with both tests, making them inferior to microscopy.[57,59,60]

For the diagnosis of *P. ovale* and *P. malariae*, comprehensive studies with both antigens (aldolase and pLDH) are lacking. For both tests false-negative results have been reported in patients with established *P. ovale* or *P. malariae* infections,[56,61–63] and in conclusion, none of the available test systems is reliable for the diagnosis of infections with both species.[55] Table 16.2 summarizes characteristic findings for the various test systems.

Performance of RDTs for Self-Use by Travelers

After the introduction of rapid tests, which can be performed without additional technical devices and under field conditions, the question arises whether the self-use of these tests would be a feasible option for travelers to help them decide whether or not to embark on SBET.

In an open, comparative trial to determine whether travelers can successfully use and interpret the ParaSight-F test, 160 visitors to a large travel clinic in Zurich, Switzerland, were asked to test their own blood and to interpret five pre-prepared test strips of the ParaSight-F test: 75% succeeded with self-testing after receiving written instructions only, whereas 90% managed to handle the test correctly after

having received combined written and oral instructions.[64] However, the interpretation of pre-prepared tests was not satisfactory (only 70.6% correct interpretations) and yielded a high rate of false-negative results (14.1%). A comparative study between ParaSight-F and Mala-Quick with 164 participants yielded no significant difference regarding self-testing with both systems, but the MalaQuick test with its cardboard format was considered easier to perform by the laypersons than the test strip format of the ParaSight-F.[65] Reliable results were obtained with both test strips from specimens with parasitemias between 0.1% and 2.0%. Interestingly, in low parasitemias, ParaSight-F test strips were correctly read by 52.1% versus 10.8% with Mala-Quick, but in high parasitemias ParaSight-F test strips were correctly read by only 33.8% versus 96.8% with MalaQuick. Overall, both test systems were associated with unacceptably high levels of false-negative interpretations. The authors concluded that major improvements to assist lay individuals in test performance would be necessary to justify its use by travelers. When asking volunteers for a judgment on the technique, about 67.5% considered self-testing a helpful concept, 31.9% found it indispensable, and only 0.6% judged it superfluous.

In an investigation of 98 European tourists with febrile disease in Kenya under 'field conditions,' only 68% of patients were able to complete the MalaQuick correctly. Most importantly, 10 out of 11 patients with microscopically confirmed falciparum malaria were

Table 16.2 Quality of Malaria Dipstick Tests

Species to be Detected	P. falciparum	P. vivax (Combined With P.f.)	P. ovale + malariae (Combined With P.f. and P.v.)
Antigen(s)	HRP-2, pLDH	PMA, pLDH	PMA, pLDH
Product(s)	Binax Malaria P.f. alias Malaquick[a], ParaSight-F[a] and others; OptiMal[b]	Binax Malaria P.f./P.v. Malaquick[c]; OptiMal[b]	Alias Binax Malaria P.f./P.v. alias Malaquick[c]; OptiMal[b]
Size of database	Large	Intermediate	Small
Study area(s)	Endemic/non-endemic areas	Endemic/non-endemic areas	Endemic/non-endemic areas
Sensitivity versus GS	85–100% in majority of studies	80–95% in majority of studies	All tests unreliable
Specificity versus GS	90–100% in majority of studies	90–100% in majority of studies	All tests unreliable
Tests in direct comparison	No significant differences	pLDH detection superior	All tests unreliable
State-of-the-art	Established knowledge, 'me-too' products work probably equally well	Established knowledge	Established knowledge

GS, gold standard.
[a]Using HRP-2 plasmodial antigen.
[b]Using pLDH plasmodial antigen.
[c]Using plasmodium-specific aldolase and HRP-2 plasmodial antigen.

Table 16.3 Self-Use of Rapid Diagnostic Tests by Travelers

Setting	Test Used	Main Findings
Healthy Swiss travelers: dry run before travel[64] (n = 160)	ParaSight-F	75% success after oral instruction; 90% success after additional oral/written instruction; 14% false-negative interpretation of pre-prepared test; Major technical modifications recommended
Healthy Swiss travelers: dry run prior to travel[65] (n = 164)	ParaSight-F, ICT P.f.	Interpretation problems at low parasitemias (<0.1%); High level of false-negative interpretations; Technical improvement and instruction required
Febrile travelers (Kenya)[66] (n = 98)	ICT P.f.	68% success with manufacturer's instructions only; Only 1 out of 11 patients with confirmed falciparum malaria tested successfully; Intensive training/instruction required
Febrile returning travelers (London)[67] (n = 153)	ICT P.f.	91% success after intensive instruction and assistance obtaining sample; In 22 patients with confirmed falciparum malaria: 100% success, sensitivity 95%, specificity 97%
Expat oilfield workers, self-testing (different countries)[69] (n = 575)	Para-Check Pfor Core malaria Pf	85/575 (15%) of self-test users encountered technical difficulties. Respondents who received poor/no instructions were two times more likely to have difficulties.

Data reproduced from Nothdurft and Jelinek.[64]

unable to self-diagnose their condition by rapid testing (Table 16.3). On the other hand, when these tests were performed by medical personnel, sensitivity and specificity reached 100%. The authors concluded that a considerable proportion of patients might be too sick to correctly diagnose malaria by RDTs and subsequently to start treatment by themselves.[66]

In a prospective study carried out in the UK with 153 returning travelers with an acute febrile illness, only 14 (9%) failed to carry out a MalaQuick test correctly on presentation, using an improved test instruction leaflet. All 22 patients with microscopically confirmed falciparum malaria completed self-testing successfully, and the overall sensitivity reached 95%, with 97% specificity.[67,68] The authors argued that differences in the various studies were possibly due to the poor quality of the manufacturer's instruction sheet, and the customized test procedure. If appropriately validated, a more user-friendly kit could be implemented for travelers without additional instruction and training.

Roukens and colleagues[69] carried out a web-based, cross-sectional study to evaluate self-diagnosis and standby treatment in 2350 non-immune international oilfield employees partaking in a malaria risk reduction programme. Adherence to the programme improved malaria awareness, attitude, and adherence to chemoprophylaxis. Self-testing, however, was difficult and proved to be unsatisfactory regarding the usefulness of this strategy. However, the RDT technology has improved since these early studies in travelers and it may be time to reassess the use of RDTs by travelers.

Table 16.4[66] summarizes the studies dealing with this subject so far. Table 16.5 gives the pros and cons of self-diagnosis.

Standby Emergency Self-Treatment for Malaria

Principle and Rationale for Use

SBET is the self-administration of antimalarial drugs when malaria is suspected, and when prompt medical attention is unavailable within

Table 16.4 Reasons for Failure of Tourists to Obtain Valid Results With Rapid Test for Falciparum Malaria

Reasons for Failure	Number of Patients[a]	
	n	(%)
Unable to draw blood (finger prick)	22	71
Unable to place the blood drop appropriately on the test kit	8	26
Did not wait for the recommended period (8 min)	12	39
Unable to identify the bands indicating the test result	18	58
Unable to interpret the result	27	87

[a]Of a total of 31 patients; some patients failed on more than one point.
Data reproduced from Jelinek et al.[62]

Table 16.5 Pros and Cons of Self-Diagnosis

Pros	Cons
Diagnosis following immediately after onset of symptoms is possible	Test performance and interpretation of results possibly impaired in those already compromised by illness, and in the poorly trained
Relatively inexpensive procedure	Depending on travel conditions, quality of test can be impaired by high humidity and temperature
No loss of transfer time to doctor/waiting time	Risk of 'false security' feeling following false-positive or false-negative test

SBET can be initiated on the grounds of a (preliminary) diagnosis rather than 'blind' treatment based solely on clinical suspicion.

Table 16.6 Possible Indications for Standby Emergency Treatment (SBET)[a]

Stay in areas with low risk of malaria (e.g., beach holiday in Mexico)

No, or suboptimal use of chemoprophylaxis and visit of a remote malaria endemic area without healthcare facilities within reach (e.g., adventure trekking in Sumatra)

Changing itineraries, perhaps with visits to foci with multi-drug resistance not, or inadequately covered by the chosen prophylactic regimen (e.g., traveling in Cambodia using mefloquine prophylaxis or no prophylaxis

Sojourn in malaria-free areas, therefore no continuous chemoprophylaxis, with brief occasional visit(s) to malaria-endemic area(s) (e.g., touring South Africa for 3 weeks including 2 nights in Kruger Park)

Frequent stays in malarious areas for short periods (e.g., air crew weekly 1 overnight stay in New Delhi)

Contraindications, or known intolerance towards recommended chemoprophylactics, therefore no/only 'suboptimal' chemoprophylaxis

Travel for a prolonged period (exceeding 3 months) or residency in malarious areas

Poor motivation towards any chemoprophylaxis

Use of adequate chemoprophylaxis, but feared risk of breakthrough malaria, e.g., on the grounds of low drug levels due to reduced absorption (e.g., because of diarrhea, vomiting) and absence of health service facilities in reach within 24 h

[a]Modified from Schlagenhauf.[65]

Table 16.7 Guidelines for Starting Standby Emergency Treatment (SBET)

Onset of acute febrile disease suggestive for malaria

Sojourn in malaria-endemic area for more than 6 days

Qualified medical care probably not available within next 24 h

Table 16.8 Points to be Discussed or Trained When Counseling Travelers Considering Standby Emergency Treatment (SBET; With or Without Chemoprophylaxis)

SBET is a measure for emergency situations only

Recognition of malaria-suggesting symptoms, stress unspecific character

Indications to self-initiated treatment (see Table 16.7)

Necessity to take a full therapeutic dose

Possibility of adverse events following SBET

Possibility of SBET failure

Necessity to seek medical advice despite initiation of SBET

Necessity to carry on SBET for approximately 4 weeks after the end of exposure

24 h following the onset of symptoms. In her comprehensive review of SBET by travelers, Schlagenhauf[70] points out that presumptive self-treatment is indicated only in emergency situations, and that it must be followed by medical consultation as soon as possible. This implies that a careful risk–benefit analysis, based on an individual's travel, should be carried out before departure. SBET is not indicated for sojourns in areas where travelers have access to good medical care. An indication for SBET may be independent of whether or not a chemoprophylactic agent is being used, since chemoprophylaxis failures are possible with any of the currently available drugs, particularly in areas with high transmission rates and known resistance.

There is a large heterogeneity in expert opinion on whether, and if so, when, to recommend SBET, and to whom. A recent Delphi method analysis of malaria chemoprophylaxis recommendations across Europe highlights this fact, and although SBET was not the focus of this study, it became clear that some experts would prefer SBET over chemoprophylaxis across a range of possible scenarios.[71]

Various national expert committees take slightly different approaches with regard to the estimated real risk of contracting malaria in defined areas. The Swiss recommendation, for example, was to carry SBET rather than to use chemoprophylaxis in areas with a low risk of malaria, since the adverse effects of the drug may far outweigh the risk of malaria. Since malaria symptoms are not specific at the onset of illness, every acute febrile episode occurring after the seventh day in an endemic area must be considered as possible malaria.

The traveler should be informed that malaria can occur in spite of strict adherence to a recommended prophylactic regimen. The traveler must know that SBET is not an alternative to early medical treatment. Still, if a decision for the administration of SBET is made, regardless of the reason, medical help should be sought as soon as possible under all circumstances, to confirm – or rule out – suspected malaria, control the success of therapy and, if necessary, to search for other illnesses.

When counseling the traveler, healthcare providers should keep in mind that SBET should be considered for about 4–8 weeks after the end of the exposure period, to ensure swift intervention in case of a delayed *P. falciparum* infection.

Possible indications for considering SBET are given in Table 16.6;[70] guidelines for use of SBET are given in Table 16.7. Table 16.8 summarizes the essentials to be discussed when counseling travelers with regard to SBET.

Table 16.9 Available Options for Standby Emergency Treatment (SBET)

Generic Name	Trade Name(s)	Amount Per Dosage	SBET[a] Dosage (Adult)
Chloroquine	Aralen, Avlochlor, Nivaquine, Resochin	Tablet: 100 or 150 mg (base); syrups available	600 mg on days 1 and 2, followed by 300 mg on day 3
Sulfadoxine/pyrimethamine	Fansidar	Tablet: 500 mg/25 mg	3 tablets in a single dose
Sulfadoxine/pyrimethamine/mefloquine	Fansimef	Tablet: 500 mg/25 mg/250 mg	3 tablets in a single dose
Sulfalene/pyrimethamine	Metakelfin	Tablet: 500 mg/25 mg	3 tablets in a single dose
Mefloquine	Lariam, Mephaquin	Tablet: 250 mg (US, 228 mg)	5–6 tablets in divided doses[b], depending on body weight
Quinine (sulfate, bisulfate, dihydrochloride, hydrochl.)	Tablet: 300 mg (salt)	600 mg (2 tablets) t.i.d.[c] for 7 days (total of 42 tablets)	
Atovaquone/proguanil	Malarone	Tablet: 250 mg/100 mg	4 tablets daily as a single dose on 3 consecutive days (total of 12 tablets)
Artemether/lumefantrine[d]	Riamet	Tablet: 20 mg/120 mg	4 tablets initially on day 1, followed by a further 4 tablets 8 h later; 4 tablets twice daily on days 2 and 3 (total of 24 tablets)

Note: halofantrine is no longer on the WHO-recommended list; for use under medical supervision only.
[a]SBET, standby emergency treatment;
[b]Manufacturer's recommendation: 25 mg/kg for non-immunes, WHO recommendation: 15 mg/kg (25 mg/kg for certain areas on Thailand border);
[c]t.i.d., three times daily;
[d]There is a paucity of data regarding the efficacy and tolerability of these newer combinations in non-immune travelers.
Data reproduced from Schlagenhauf.[70]

Recommendations for Choice of Drugs

Table 16.9[70] provides a list of drugs suitable for SBET, depending on whether or not drugs are used for chemoprophylaxis. Some drugs listed are not, or are no longer, available or registered in all countries, such as sulfadoxine/pyrimethamine combinations (e.g., Fansidar) or those which are less suitable for SBET owing to their dosage scheme and side-effects profile (e.g., quinine or quinine/tetracycline). Novel drugs – atovaquone/proguanil (Malarone), artemether/lumefantrine (Riamet) – which are only registered and marketed in a limited number of countries, are listed. Halofantrine (Halfan) is not listed, as it is no longer recommended for use because of reports that predisposed patients with QTc interval prolongation and ventricular dysrhythmias can have a life-threatening outcome.[72,73]

The recommendations of the various national expert groups are guided by the report of WHO (Fig. 16.1) in which SBET with chloroquine (Nivaquine, Resochin and other trademarks) is only recommended in zones of limited risk. In those zones of considerable malaria risk, particularly mefloquine (Lariam, Mephaquine), atovaquone/proguanil (Malarone) and artemether/lumefantrine (Riamet) ought to be considered as suitable compounds. Due to increasing mefloquine resistance in the West of Cambodia and along the borders of Thailand with Cambodia, Laos, and Myanmar, for those and adjacent areas atovaquone/proguanil and artemether/lumefantrine are preferred.

For specific contraindications and adverse events profiles of particular drugs, see Chapters 15 and 17 and Table 16.10 for factors influencing SBET.

SBET Recommendations for Pregnant Women, Children, and Chronically Ill Patients

Pregnant women and non-immune children are at particular risk of severe malaria. Therefore, if possible, sojourns in areas with high malaria risk should be avoided. In case of a febrile episode, all efforts should be made to seek medical attention as soon as possible. In

Table 16.10 Factors Influencing Choice of Standby Emergency Treatment (SBET)

The intake of chemoprophylaxis and the drugs used therefore
The expected local plasmodial resistance pattern
Simplicity/complexity of application (tolerability, handling)
Individual contraindications and expected/previously experienced intolerances

pregnant women, quinine is the drug of choice for SBET. Mefloquine should only be used after careful risk–benefit analysis, but not in the first trimester. Sufficient experience with atovaquone/proguanil and artemether/lumefantrine is not yet available. For children heavier than 5 kg, atovaquone/proguanil (>10 kg) and artemether/lumefantrine are suitable for SBET. For newborns lighter than 5 kg quinine is the drug of choice. Table 16.11[70] details drug regimens for SBET suitable for use in children.

For travelers with chronic illnesses who are on medication, a suitable regimen for both chemoprophylaxis and/or SBET has to be tailored carefully to their individual needs. The profile of contraindications, expected drug interactions, and adverse events must be taken into consideration on the background of their underlying illness. For example, mefloquine should be strictly avoided for both prophylaxis and SBET in individuals with a past medical history of neuropsychiatric disorders of any kind.[70]

Balancing of Recommendations

The diagnosis of malaria solely on clinical grounds is unreliable and difficult even for trained medical staff. Fever is the most common and reliable symptom. Even on short trips to developing countries, it is observed with a frequency of 3.8–10%.[14,74]

Travelers appear to have difficulty implementing SBET appropriately. It is particularly feared that the frequency of febrile diseases of

Table 16.11 Drug Regimens for Standby Emergency Treatment (SBET): Children's Dosages[a]

Mefloquine[b]			Sulfadoxine/Pyrimethamine (500 mg/25 mg)		Chloroquine[c] (100 mg base)				Artemether/Lumefantrine[d,e] (20 mg/120 mg)				Atovaquone/Proguanil[d] (250 mg/100 mg)			
Weight (kg)	h 1	h[e], 6–24	Weight (kg)	Single dose	Weight (kg)	Day 1	Day 2	Day 3	Weight (kg)	Day 1	Day 2	Day 3	Weight (kg)	Day 1	Day 2	Day 3
5–6	1/4	1/4	5–6	1/4	5–6	1/2	1/2	1/2	–	–	–	–	–	–	–	–
7–8	1/2	1/4	7–10	1/2	7–10	1	1	1/2	–	–	–	–	–	–	–	–
9–12	3/4	1/2	11–14	3/4	11–14	$1^{1/2}$	$1^{1/2}$	1/2	10–15	2 × 1	2 × 1	2 × 1	11–20	1	1	1
13–16	1	1/2	15–18	1	15–18	2	2	1/2	–	–	–	–	–	–	–	–
17–24	$1^{1/2}$	1	19–29	$1^{1/2}$	19–24	$2^{1/2}$	$2^{1/2}$	1	15–25	2 × 2	2 × 2	2 × 2	21–30	2	2	2
25–35	2	$1^{1/2}$	30–39	$2^{1/2}$	25–35	$3^{1/2}$	$3^{1/2}$	2	25–34	2 × 3	2 × 3	2 × 3	–	–	–	–
36–50	3	2	40–49	$2^{1/2}$	36–50	5	5	$2^{1/2}$	–	–	–	–	31–40	3	3	3

Note: the doses referred to in the table are adult tablets (not pediatric tablets).
[a]Given as tablet fractions.
[b]The total dosage (25 mg [base]/kg) is divided into two doses: 15 mg (base)/kg, followed by 10 mg (base)/kg 6–24 h later.
[c]The total dosage is 25 mg (base)/kg divided over 3 days (tablets usually contain either 100 mg or 150 mg chloroquine base).
[d]There is a paucity of data on efficacy and tolerability of this drug combination in non-immune travelers.
[e]On day 1, the tablets should be taken at 8-h intervals; on days 2 and 3, at 12-h intervals.
[f]h, hour(s).
Data reproduced from Schlagenhauf.[70]

varying origin leads to an uncontrolled over-treatment of malaria, with the combined risk of delayed diagnosis of another illness and antimalarial adverse events.[69] Finally, it has been speculated that SBET recommendations might encourage travelers to abandon chemoprophylaxis altogether.[75–77]

Two large prospective studies have investigated the practical aspects of implementing SBET recommendations. A Swiss study[78] investigated 1187 travelers who received only SBET recommendations without simultaneous chemoprophylaxis (predominantly for journeys to Asia and Latin America). In another study of 2867 German travelers to highly malaria-endemic areas in sub-Saharan Africa chemoprophylaxis and SBET were recommended.[76] Both studies confirmed the high incidence of febrile illness among travelers (8.1% versus 10.4%, respectively) even for short trips to malarial regions (average duration of stay 4 weeks). However, only a small proportion of travelers took SBET in both studies (0.5%, or 1.4% respectively, of all travelers; 4.9%, or 17% respectively, of febrile travelers). In only 10.8%, or 16.7%, respectively, of the latter group, was malaria confirmed retrospectively. A total of 100 (57%) patients sought medical advice after SBET. Out of 30 (15%) of all patients, but predominantly those who took mefloquine or mefloquine-sulfadoxin/pyrimethamine as SBET, one required hospitalization for adverse events, in conjunction with SBET. For travelers who adhered both to advice for chemoprophylaxis and SBET, adherence to chemoprophylaxis was not worse than in comparable studies of chemoprophylaxis alone.[10,11] Both studies pointed out the importance of counseling during which detailed advice in both written and oral form is necessary to ensure a responsible and adequate handling of SBET recommendations by travelers.

In their questionnaire analysis, Roukens et al.[69] found that 44/49 (90%) of self-testing individuals with a positive test result and 115/508 with a negative test result did take SBET, thus highlighting the limitations of the approach. Table 16.12[70] summarizes studies on travelers' use of malaria SBET.

As concluded by Schlagenhauf,[70] the knowledge and behavior of travelers are difficult to predict. In the Swiss study, despite awareness of the need for rapid diagnosis and treatment of malaria, approximately 66% of travelers with a febrile illness failed to seek prompt

Table 16.12 Traveler's Use of Malaria Standby Emergency Treatment (SBET)

Year	Agent	Traveler's Origin	Destination	Use (%)
1987/1988	SDX/PYR	Swiss	Africa	5.4
1989	MQ	Swiss	Africa	3.6
1991	MQ/SDX/PYR	French	Africa	2.1
1992	MQ/SDX/PYR	Swiss	Asia, Americas	0.5
1992/1993	H, MQ, CL SDX/PYR	German	Asia	0.3
			Africa	1.0
1994	H, MQ, SDX/PYR	German	Asia	1.0
			Africa	5.0

CL, chloroquine; H, halofantrine; MQ, mefloquine; MQ/SDX/PYR, mefloquine/sulfadoxine/pyrimethamine (Fansimef); SDX/PYR, sulfadoxine/pyrimethamine (Fansidar).
Data reproduced with kind permission from Schlagenhauf.[70]

medical advice.[78] In a UK survey almost 25% of participants would have acted inappropriately while having malaria-like symptoms, predominantly by resting at home and waiting for resolution of symptoms.[79] On the other hand, the difficulty in deciding correctly – in the absence of diagnostic tools and medical information – that an acute febrile illness is malaria, is highlighted by a German study in which only four (10.4%) of 37 SBET treatment users were found to have significant antibody levels against *P. falciparum*.[77]

Airline crews may be an ideal group to assess the efficacy and safety of SBET alone. After abandoning mefloquine chemoprophylaxis for SBET among Swissair crews traveling to destinations in highly malaria-endemic areas, there was no significant increase in malaria cases observed, although only approximately 1% of crew members took SBET per year.[70,80] Table 16.13 gives the pros and cons of self-treatment.

The current trend in malaria guidelines is to recommend simple, well tolerated regimens as SBET. Drugs of choice are as it stands atovaquone/proguanil and artemether/lumefantrine.

Table 16.13 Pros and Cons of Self-Treatment

Pros	Cons
Swift initiation of therapy, possibly avoiding progression to more severe disease	False treatment based on misdiagnosis, with possible risk of missing underlying, severe, non-malarious condition
Of use if prophylaxis fails	Risk of inappropriate dosages (both too low or too high) or inappropriate drug used
Of use for travelers for whom prophylaxis is inappropriate	Medical advice following initiation of standby emergency treatment (SBET) still ought to be sought

Summary and Outlook

For rational use of SBET, a reliable tool is crucial for rapid self-diagnosis – or exclusion – of malaria in travelers. If performed in the laboratory, the sensitivity and specificity of rapid immunochromatographic 'dipstick' tests almost equal the quality of microscopy results obtained by trained staff. In the only cohort of travelers for which field study data are available, however, serious problems with test performance and interpretation arose, particularly in those individuals who were seriously ill. Although it has been demonstrated that test performance can be considerably improved by adequate information and training, inherent problems of immunochromatographic antigen detection such as false-negative results even with high parasitemias, cannot easily be ignored or overcome.

Conclusion

While earlier experience with the use of RDTs by travelers has proven disappointing, it may be time to reassess this potentially very valuable tool for travelers. As it stands, it remains mandatory that travelers with acute febrile illness should seek medical help as soon as possible in any case. If this is not feasible within a day, the indication for SBET should be independent of a malaria dipstick test result.

The concept of SBET has proved to be a valuable additional tool for reducing malaria illness among travelers. The indication for SBET should be clearly and unambiguously stated by the travel medicine advisor, and the traveler should be informed meticulously. When adequate oral and written instructions, along with comprehensive practical advice, have been provided, it appears that most travelers can make responsible use of the recommendations.

New drugs with better tolerability and efficacy in multidrug resistance areas will ensure that SBET is a useful additional tool for the safety of travelers to malarious areas.

References

1. O'Meara WP, Mangeni JN, Steketee R, et al. Changes in the burden of malaria in sub–Saharan Africa. Lancet Infect Dis 2010;10:545–55.
2. Freedman DO. Clinical practice. Malaria prevention in short-term travelers. N Engl J Med 2008;359:603–12.
3. Schlagenhauf P, Petersen E. Malaria chemoprophylaxis: strategies for risk groups. Clin Microbiol Rev 2008;21:466–72.
4. Uzzan B, Konate L, Diop A, et al. Efficacy of four insect repellents against mosquito bites: a double-blind randomized placebo-controlled field study in Senegal. Fundam Clin Pharmacol 2009;23:589–94.
5. Centers for Disease Control and Prevention. CDC Health Information for International Travel 2012. Atlanta: US Department of Health and Human Services, Public Health Service; 2012.
6. Mali S, Tan KR, Arquin PM. Malaria surveillance – United States, 2009. MMWR Surveill Summ 2011;60:1–15.
7. Odolini S, Parola P, Gkrania-Klotsas E, et al. Travel-related imported infections in Europe, EuroTravNet 2009. Clin Microbiol Infect 2011;doi:10.1111/j.1469–0691.2011.03596.x [Epub ahead of print].
8. The RTS, S Clinical Trials Partnership. First results of phase 3 trial of RTS,S/AS01 malaria vaccine in African children. N Engl J Med 2011;Oct 18 [epub ahead of print].
9. Jelinek T, Schulte C, Behrens R, et al. Imported falciparum malaria in Europe: Sentinel surveillance data from the European network on surveillance of imported disease. Clin Inf Dis 2002;34:572–6.
10. Mühlberger N, Jelinek T, Schlipkoeter U, et al. Effectiveness of chemoprophylaxis and other determinants of malaria in travellers to Kenya. Trop Med Int Health 1998;3:357–63.
11. Steffen R, Fuchs E, Schildknecht J, et al. Mefloquine compared with other chemoprophylactic regimens in tourists visiting East Africa. Lancet 1993;341:1299–303.
12. Lell B, Luckner D, Ndjave M, et al. Randomized placebo-controlled study of atovaquone plus proguanil for malaria prophylaxis in children. Lancet 1998;351:709–13.
13. Grobusch MP, Gobels K, Teichmann D. Is quartan malaria safely prevented by mefloquine prophylaxis? J Travel Med 2004;190:1541–6.
14. Grobusch MP, Kremsner PG. Uncomplicated malaria. Curr Top Microbiol Immunol 2005;295:83–104.
15. World Health Organization. Development of recommendations for the protection of short-stay travellers to malaria-endemic areas: Memorandum from two WHO Meetings. Bull WHO 1988;66:177–96.
16. World Health Organization. Malaria. In: WHO. International travel and health: situation as on 1 January 2002. Geneva: World Health Organization; 2002. p. 130–48.
17. Nothdurft HD, Bialek R, Burchard GD, et al. Consensus recommendations for malaria prophylaxis. Dtsch Med Wochenschr 2005;130:1392–6.
18. Connor BA. Expert recommendations for antimalarial prophylaxis. J Travel Med 2001;8(Suppl. 3):S57–64.
19. Marx A, Pewsner D, Egger M, et al. Meta-analysis: accuracy of rapid tests for malaria in travelers returning from endemic areas. Ann Intern Med 2005;142:836–46.
20. Hänscheid T. Diagnosis of malaria: a review of alternatives to conventional microscopy. Clin Lab Haematol 1999;21:235–45.
21. Makler MT, Palmer CJ, Ager AL. A review of practical techniques for the diagnosis of malaria. Ann Trop Med Parasitol 1998;92:419–33.
22. Moody A. Rapid diagnostic tests for malaria parasites. Clin Microbiol Rev 2002;15:66–78.
23. Lowe BS, Jfa NK, Pederson C, et al. Acridine orange fluorescence techniques as alternatives to traditional Giemsa staining for the diagnosis of malaria in developing countries. Trans R Soc Trop Med Hyg 1996;90:34–6.
24. Snounou G, Viriyakosol S, Jarra W, et al. Identification of the four human malaria parasite species in field samples by the polymerase-chain-reaction and detection of a high prevalence of mixed infections. Molecular Biochem Parasitol 1993;58:283–92.
25. Campuzano-Zuluaga G, Hänscheid T, Grobusch MP. Automated haematology analysis to diagnose malaria. Malar J 2010;9:346.
26. The maERA Consultative Group on Diagnoses and Diagnostics. A research agenda for malaria eradication: Diagnoses and diagnostics. PLoS Medicine 2011;8:e1000396.
27. Wongsrichanalai C, Barcus MJ, Muth S, et al. A review of malaria diagnostic tools: microscopy and rapid diagnostic test (RDT). Am J Trop Med Hyg 2007;77:119–27.
28. Murray CK, Bennett JW. Rapid diagnosis of malaria. Interdiscipl Persp Infect Dis 2009;doi:10.1155/2009/415953.
29. WHO. World Malaria Report:2010. Geneva: World Health Organization; 2010.
30. Abba K, Deeks JJ, Olliaro PL, et al. Rapid diagnostic tests for diagnosing uncomplicated P. falciparum malaria in endemic countries. Cochrane Database of Systematic Reviews 2011; Issue 7. Art. No.: CD008122. DOI:10.1002/14651858.CD008122.pub2.
31. Shiff CJ, Minjas JN, Premji Z. The ParaSight-F(r) test: a simple rapid manual dipstick test to detect Plasmodium falciparum infection. Parasitol Today 1994; 10:494–495.

32. Garcia M, Kirimoama S, Marlborough D, et al. Immunochromatographic test for malaria diagnosis. Lancet 1996; 347:1549.

33. Gaye O, Diouf M, Diallo S. A comparison of thick smears, QBC malaria, PCR and PATH falciparum malaria test strip in Plasmodium falciparum diagnosis. Parasite 1999; 6:273–275.

34. Proux S, Hkirijareon L, Ngamngonkiri C, et al. Paracheck-Pf: a new, inexpensive and reliable rapid test for diagnosis of falciparum malaria. Trop Med Int Health 2001; 6:99–101.

35. Singh N, Valecha N. Evaluation of a rapid diagnostic test, 'Determine malaria pf', in epidemic-prone, forest villages of central India (Madhya Pradesh). Ann Trop Med Parasitol 2000;94:421–427.

36. Wolday D, Balcha F, Fessehaye G, et al. Field trial of the RTM dipstick method for the rapid diagnosis of malaria based on the detection of Plasmodium HRP2 antigen in whole blood. Trop Doct 2001; 31:19–21.

37. Tjitra E, Suprianto S, Dyer M, et al. Field evaluation of the ICT malaria P.f./P.v. immunochromatographic test for detection of Plasmodium falciparum and Plasmodium vivax in patients with a presumptive clinical diagnosis of malaria in Eastern Indonesia. J Clin Microbiol 1999;37:2412–2417.

38. Bharti PK, Silawat N, Singh PP, et al. The usefulness of a new rapid diagnostic test, the First Response Malaria Combo (pLDH/HRP2) Card Test, for malaria diagnosis in the forested Belt of central India. Malar J 2008;11(7):126.

39. WHO. Global Malaria Programme: Information note on recommended selection criteria for procurement of malaria rapid diagnostic tests. World Helath Organization, Geneva 2010.

40. Burchard GD. Malariaschnelltests. Bundesgesundheitsbl Gesundheitsforsch Gesundheitsschutz 1999;42:643–9.

41. Ricci L, Viani I, Piccolo G, et al. Evaluation of OptiMal assay to detect imported malaria in Italy. New Microbiol 2000;23:391–8.

42. Beadle C, Long GW, Weiss WR, et al. Diagnosis of malaria by detection of Plasmodium falciparum HRP-2 antigen with a rapid dipstick antigencapture assay. Lancet 1994;343:564–8.

43. Kodisinghe HM, Perera KLRL, Premawansa S, et al. The ParaSight-F® dipstick test as a routine diagnostic tool for malaria in Sri Lanka. Trans R Soc Trop Med Hyg 1997;91:398–402.

44. Risch L, Bader M, Huber AR. Self-use of rapid tests for malaria diagnosis. Lancet 2000;335:237.

45. Stow NW, Torrens JK, Walker J. An assessment of the accuracy of clinical diagnosis, local microscopy and a rapid immunochromatographic card test in comparison with expert microscopy in the diagnosis of malaria in rural Kenya. Trans R Soc Trop Med Hyg 1999;93:519–20.

46. Pieroni P, Mills CD, Ohrt C, et al. Comparison of the Parasight-F® test and the ICT Malaria P.f.® test with the polymerase chain reaction for the diagnosis of Plasmodium falciparum in travelers. Trans R Soc Trop Med Hyg 1998;92:166–9.

47. Trarore I, Koita O, Doumbo O. Field studies of the ParaSight-F® test in a malaria-endemic area: cost, feasibility, sensitivity, specificity, predictive value and the deletion of the HRP-2 gene among wild type Plasmodium falciparum in Mali [Poster SO2]. Am J Trop Med Hyg 1997;57:272.

48. Uguen C, Rabodonirina M, De Pina JJ, et al. ParaSight-F rapid manual diagnostic test of Plasmodium falciparum infections. Bull World Health Organization 1995;73:643–9.

49. Banchongaksorn T, Yomokgul P, Panyim S, et al. A field trial of the ParaSight-F® test for the diagnosis of Plasmodium falciparum infection Trans R Soc Trop Med Hyg 1996;90:244–5.

50. Craig MH, Sharp BL. Comparative evaluation of four techniques for the diagnosis of Plasmodium falciparum infections. Trans R Soc Trop Med Hyg 1997;91:279–82.

51. Humar A, Ohrt C, Harrington MA, et al. ParaSight-F® test compared with the polymerase chain reaction and microscopy for the diagnosis of Plasmodium falciparum malaria in travelers. Am J Trop Med Hyg 1997;56:44–8.

52. Grobusch MP, Alpermann U, Schwenke S, et al. False-positive rapid tests for malaria in patients with rheumatoid factor. Lancet 1999;353:297.

53. Iqbal J, Sher A, Rub A. Plasmodium falciparum histidine-rich protein 2-based immunocapture diagnostic assay for malaria: cross-reactivity with rheumatoid factors. J Clin Microbiol 2000;38:1184–6.

54. Laferl H, Kandel K, Pichler H. False-positive dipstick test for malaria. N Engl J Med 1997;337:1635–6.

55. Lee MA, Aw LT, Singh M. A comparison of antigen dipstick assays with polymerase chain reaction (PCR) technique and blood film examination in the rapid diagnosis of malaria. Ann Acad Med Singapore 1999;28:498–501.

56. Moody A, Hunt-Cooke A, Gabbett E, et al. Performance of the OptiMal(r) malaria antigen capture dipstick for malaria diagnosis and treatment monitoring at the Hospital for Tropical Diseases, London. Br J Haematol 2000;109:891–4.

57. Palmer CJ, Lindo JF, Klaskala WI, et al. Evaluation of the OptiMal test for rapid diagnosis of Plasmodium vivax and Plasmodium falciparum malaria. J Clin Microbiol 1998;36:203–6.

58. Grobusch MP, Hanscheid T, Gobels K, et al. Sensitivity of P. vivax rapid antigen detection tests and possible implications for self-diagnostic use. Travel Med Infect Dis 2003;1:119–22.

59. Iqbal J, Sher A, Hira PR, et al. Comparison of the OptiMal test with PCR for diagnosis of malaria in immigrants. J Clin Microbiol 1999;37:3644–6.

60. Jelinek T, Grobusch MP, Schwenke S, et al. Sensitivity and specificity of dipstick tests for rapid diagnosis of malaria in nonimmune travelers. J Clin Microbiol 1999;37:721–3.

61. Grobusch MP, Hanscheid T, Zoller T, et al. Rapid immunochromatographic malarial antigen detection unreliable for detecting Plasmodium malariae and Plasmodium ovale. Eur J Clin Microbiol Infect Dis 2002;21:818–20.

62. Hunt-Cooke A, Chiodini PL, Doherty T, et al. Comparison of a parasite lactate dehydrogenase-based immunochromatographic antigen detection assay (OptiMal) with microscopy for the detection of malaria parasites in human blood samples. Am J Trop Med Hyg 1999;60:173–6.

63. John SM, Sudarsanam A, Sitaram U, et al. Evaluation of OptiMal, a dipstick test for the diagnosis of malaria. Ann Trop Med Parasitol 1998;92:621–2.

64. Trachsler M, Schlagenhauf P, Steffen R. Feasibility of a rapid dipstick antigen-capture assay for self-testing of traveller's malaria. Trop Med Int Health 1999;4:442–7.

65. Funk M, Schlagenhauf P, Tschopp A, et al. MalaQuick versus ParaSight F as a diagnostic aid in traveller's malaria. Trans R Soc Trop Med Hyg 1999;93:268–72.

66. Jelinek T, Amsler L, Grobusch MP, et al. Self-use of rapid tests for malaria diagnosis by tourists. Lancet 1999;354:1609.

67. Behrens RH, Whitty CJ Self-use of rapid tests for malaria diagnosis. Lancet 2000;355:237.

68. Nothdurft HD, Jelinek T. Use of rapid tests for and by travelers. In: Schlagenhauf P, editor. Travelers' Malaria. London: BC Decker; 2001. p. 423–30.

69. Roukens AH, Berg J, Barbey A, Visser LG. Performance of self–diagnosis and standby treatment of malaria in international oilfield service employees in the field. Malar J 2008;7:128.

70. Schlagenhauf P. Stand-by emergency self-treatment of malaria by travelers, pp. 316–322. In: Schlagenhauf P, (ed.) Travelers' Malaria. (2nd edition), Hamilton, London, BC Decker 2008.

71. Calleri G, Behrens R, Bisoffi Z, et al. Variability in malaria prophylaxis prescribing across Europe: A Delphi method analysis. J Travel Med 2008;15:294–301.

72. Matson PA, Luby SP, Redd SC, et al. Cardiac effects of standard-dose halofantrine therapy. Am J Trop Med Hyg 1996;54:229–31.

73. World Health Organization 1993. Drug alert: Halofantrine. Wkly Epidemiol Rec 1993;68:268–70.

74. Steffen R, Lobel HO. Epidemiologic basis for the practice of travel medicine. J Wilderness Med 1994;5:56–66.

75. Schlagenhauf P, Steffen R. Stand-by treatment of malaria in travellers: a review. J Trop Med Hyg 1994;97:151–60.

76. Löscher T, Nothdurft HD. Malaria – rapid diagnostic tests and emergency self-treatment. Ther Umsch 2001;58:352–61.

77. Nothdurft HD, Jelinek T, Pechel SM, et al. Stand-by treatment of suspected malaria in travellers. Trop Med Parasitol 1995;46:161–3.

78. Schlagenhauf P, Steffen R, Tschopp A, et al. Behavioural aspects of travellers in their use of malaria presumptive treatment. Bull World Health Organization 1995;73:215–21.

79. Behrens RH, Phillips-Howard PA. What do travellers know about malaria? Lancet 1989;ii:1395–6.

80. Steffen R, Holdener F, Wyss R, et al. Malaria prophylaxis and self-therapy in airline crews. Aviat Space Environ Med 1990;61:942–5.

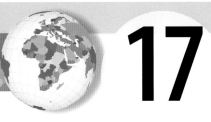

Approach to the Patient with Malaria

Marc Mendelson

Key points

- Malaria constitutes a medical emergency
- Travelers returning from a malaria-endemic area with any fever pattern should be regarded as having malaria until proved otherwise
- Symptoms of malaria are dependent on the plasmodium species, the immune status and the age of the patient, but are not specific to malaria
- As a rule non-immune adults or children suffer from more severe clinical symptoms than semi-immune adults
- Immediate diagnosis and treatment are the key factors in reducing fatalities from malaria
- Malaria treatment options are determined by the species involved, the severity of disease and the expected resistance pattern

Introduction

Malaria remains a significant health problem in travelers to endemic areas. Each year, at least 10 000 travelers fall ill.[1] In falciparum malaria, the dominant cause of malaria in travelers,[2] the mortality rate among imported cases (mostly non-immune adults) is as high as 1.5–7%,[3] compared to ~1% in persons from the endemic area.

Mortality correlates with diagnostic and therapeutic delay, making falciparum malaria a medical emergency. The other four malaria species pathogenic to humans, *Plasmodium vivax*, *Plasmodium ovale* *Plasmodium malariae* and *Plasmodium knowlesi*, are rarely lethal.

Development of Malaria Immunity

Immunity to malaria is not an absolute, protective, sterilizing immunity, but rather a more suppressive type. Persons from malaria-endemic areas, repeatedly exposed to the parasite, develop a relative immunity that inhibits parasite multiplication, rendering the individual an asymptomatic carrier with very low densities of parasites in the blood, which do not cause any harm. Time to develop such immunity depends on the level of transmission and the exposure to malaria infection. In highly endemic (holoendemic) areas, children >5 years

of age rarely suffer acute malaria, whereas in areas with less endemicity, acute malaria is common also in older children. In areas of low endemicity or epidemic outbreaks, immunity may never develop. Expatriates who do not necessarily share the same degree of exposure as indigenous populations should be considered as non-immune. Similarly, persons who have grown up in endemic areas but who have lived for long periods in non-endemic countries lose this type of immunity. When they return to their countries of origin, often to visit friends and relatives (VFR), they form a high-risk group for developing malaria.[4] Chemoprophylaxis is often neglected.

Symptomatology of *P. falciparum* Infections in Non-Immune Individuals

The incubation period for *P. falciparum* is between 1 week and 3 months, or even later in rare cases. A total of 65–95% of non-immune travelers develop symptoms of falciparum malaria within 1 month after leaving an endemic area.[5] The early symptoms of malaria, as with many infectious diseases, are non-specific, highlighting the absolute requirement for a good travel history to be an integral part of all clinical evaluations. Although fever is present in the vast majority (95%) of patients and often accompanied by rigors, the textbook tertian or quartan (*P. malariae*) fever pattern is commonly absent during the first few days of symptoms and may never become apparent, particularly if a timely diagnosis is made and treatment started. Headache, sweating and myalgia occur in about two-thirds of patients, with dry cough in the absence of other respiratory symptoms, diarrhea and other GI symptoms occurring in around one-third. Physical examination in uncomplicated malaria is often unremarkable; splenomegaly may be apparent, as may tender hepatomegaly with or without jaundice and/or pallor. Meningism is rare and should alert the clinician to the possibility of superadded bacterial meningitis.

Severe Falciparum Malaria in Adults

Severe falciparum malaria as defined by WHO (Table 17.1) may develop after 3–7 days of symptoms, although reports exist of non-immune patients dying within 24 h.[6] Prognosis is determined by the number and extent of vital organ systems involved. Splenectomy, pregnancy, corticosteroids, cytotoxic drugs or other immunosuppression, including HIV infection, increase the risk of developing severe malaria.

DOI: 10.1016/B978-1-4557-1076-8.00017-X

Table 17.1 Severe Manifestations of P. Falciparum Malaria in Adults[4]

Clinical Manifestation	Frequency	Prognostic Value
Impaired consciousness or unrousable coma	++	+
Prostration i.e., generalized weakness so that the patient is unable to walk or sit up unaided	+++	?
Failure to feed	+	++
Multiple convulsions – > 2 episodes in 24 hours	+	+++
Deep breathing, respiratory distress (acidotic breathing)	+	+++
Circulatory collapse or shock, systolic BP <70 mmHg in adults and <50 mmHg in children	+++	+
Clinical jaundice plus evidence of vital organ dysfunction	+	+
Hemoglobinuria	+	++
Abnormal spontaneous bleeding	+	+++
Pulmonary edema (radiological)		
Laboratory Findings		
Hypoglycemia (blood glucose <2.2 mmol/L or <40mg/dL)	++	+++
Metabolic acidosis (plasma bicarbonate <15mmol/L)	++	+++
Severe normocytic anemia (Hb <5g/dL, HCT <15%)	+	+
Hemoglobinuria	+	+
Hyperparasitemia (>2% or 100 000/μL in low intensity transmission areas or >5% or 250 000/μL in areas of high stable malaria transmission intensity)	+	++
Hyperlactatemia (lactate > 5mmol/L)	++	+++
Renal impairment (serum creatinine >26.5 μmol/L)	+++	++

Modified from WHO.[6]

The pathogenesis of severe falciparum malaria centers on sequestration of parasitized erythrocytes in the capillaries and venules of vital organs such as the brain. Expression of *P. falciparum* erythrocyte membrane protein 1 (PfEMP1) on the surface of the parasitized erythrocyte leads to binding to endothelial cell receptors such as ICAM-1, E-selectin and, in the placenta, chondroitin sulfate. 'Rosetting' of unparasitized erythrocytes around the sequestered parasitized cells on the endothelium further limits blood flow, and reduced shearing forces in the erythrocyte membrane of unparasitized cells compounds the situation by limiting the ability of cells to negotiate microvascular blood flow obstructions. Sequestration thus leads to local hypoxia. Cytokine production and possibly nitric oxide also play a role in the severe manifestations of malaria.

Cerebral malaria is the most common cause of death in adults with severe malaria, manifesting from mild confusion, to generalized convulsions, to unrousable coma.[6] Other infectious etiologies such as meningitis or encephalitis should be excluded, particularly if meningism is present. Mortality from cerebral malaria is ~20%, but permanent neurological sequelae are rare in survivors.

Occurrence of severe anemia correlates with percentage parasitemia. Parasitemias >2% should be treated as severe malaria in nonimmune subjects.[3] Hemoglobinuria due to hyperparasitemia-related hemolysis may occur, and immune-mediated lysis of quinine-sensitized erythrocytes as a result of previous inadequate treatment may play a role. Jaundice in isolation is common in adults with severe malaria. Mild jaundice may be caused by hemolysis alone, but a very high predominantly unconjugated bilirubin level indicates hepatic dysfunction.

Acute renal failure is often seen as part of multiorgan failure and may still develop with treatment. Prognosis is good with early dialysis.

Pulmonary edema mimicking adult respiratory distress syndrome (ARDS) as a result of increased pulmonary capillary permeability, sometimes compounded by fluid overload, may be a fatal manifestation of severe malaria. Onset is sudden and may occur after several days of therapy when parasites are cleared from blood.

Hypoglycemia related to the malaria infection itself, or as a consequence of insulin release due to quinine treatment, is common. All patients with cerebral malaria or on quinine treatment should have blood glucose monitoring. Despite the very common finding of low platelets and indices of activated intravascular coagulation, clinically evident bleeding is rare in severe malaria.

Recurrence of falciparum malaria per se does not occur, unlike *P. vivax* and *P. ovale* infections, although return of symptoms after treatment is usually due to a low-grade resistance with failure to eradicate parasites. The time to recurrence depends on the initial parasite density, the degree of resistance, and the half-life of the antimalarial drug used; it occurs most frequently within 2–4 weeks after initial treatment. Other mechanisms for treatment failure include poor adherence to antimalarial therapy, or reduced bioavailability of the antimalarial.

Falciparum Malaria in the Indigenous Population in Endemic Areas

Approximately 90% of the malaria occurs in sub-Saharan Africa, where ~1 million children <5 years die from malaria each year. Malaria-related mortality constitutes nearly one-quarter of the total childhood mortality in Africa. Cerebral malaria and severe malaria anemia are the major causes of death.[3]

Owing to the lack of specific diagnostic facilities and the fact that malaria is a common, severe disease, empiric or 'presumptive' therapy for chloroquine-resistant *P. falciparum* is often prescribed, leading to overtreatment for malaria in many endemic countries, particularly in children.[3]

Clinical features of severe falciparum malaria in endemic settings vary according to intensity of transmission. In highly endemic areas, severe anemia predominates in 1–3-year-old children. In areas with lower transmission, cerebral malaria in children between 3 and 7 years of age is a major manifestation, whereas older children and adults are rarely symptomatic, despite low numbers of malaria parasites in the blood. Pregnant women experience a partial loss of malaria immunity resulting in maternal anemia and low-birthweight infants.[7]

Clinical Presentation of Non-Falciparum Malaria

The mean incubation period of *P. vivax* and *P. ovale* malaria after inoculation is 13–14 days. However, some strains of *P. vivax* can remain in the liver for 9–12 months or even longer (*P. vivax hibernans*) before release and subsequent multiplication in the blood will cause symptoms. With the exception of vivax malaria from North India, these strains, previously present in temperate climates, are now nearly extinct.

After the first symptomatic infection, relapse of *P. vivax* and *P. ovale* caused by release of liver forms can occur on several occasions but eventually, after 3–4 years, the infection usually dies out. A relapse is noted in approximately half of those infected with *P. vivax*. The onset is usually within the first 2–3 months.[8] In *P. malariae* infection, relapse has been reported 30–40 years after the original infection.[9] The mechanism for this phenomenon is still not established.

Whereas the fever pattern in first infection with *P. vivax* or *P. ovale* tends to only show a tertian (every 48 hours) pattern after the first few days of fever, the 50% of patients who relapse if primaquine is not used to eradicate liver hypnozoites usually experience a tertian fever from the start of symptoms. Body temperature rises to high levels within a few hours, accompanied by a rigor, i.e., intense shivering and chills, together with headache and myalgia. Profuse sweating starts with defervescence of fever, and gradually the patient recovers over 6–12 hours. In between paroxysms the patient may feel well. Splenomegaly and anemia may develop with time. Eventually, after a few weeks without treatment, the infection gradually resolves. *P. vivax* and *P. ovale* only invade young erythrocytes and therefore do not cause high parasitemias.[10] Complications such as pulmonary edema are rare in vivax malaria.

Microscopic Diagnosis

Microscopic examination remains the gold standard for detecting and identifying malaria parasites with high sensitivity.[11] By carefully examining the thick film a parasite density as low as 5–10 parasites/μL blood can be detected. Contrary to rapid diagnostic tests based on antigen detection, a microscopic examination enables the quantification of the parasitemia necessary for classification of disease severity and parasite response to treatment.

Microscopic examination begins with the collection of a finger-prick or venepuncture blood sample. Both thick and thin blood films are prepared on standard microscopic slides. The thin film, but not the thick film, is fixed with methanol. The slides are then stained, usually with 3–4% Giemsa, rinsed and dried before examination. Preferably, a ×100 oil-immersion lens is used together with a ×10 eyepiece, giving a total magnification of ×1000. The thick film is examined for detection of malaria parasites. Before a thick film is considered negative, at least 100 fields should be examined. This takes an experienced microscopist 7–10 min. The sensitivity is 10–20 times higher examining the thick film. If it is negative, the thin film can be discarded.

In the thin film, the erythrocytes are preserved and the size, shape, and appearance of the parasitized red blood cells can be studied and the percentage of erythrocytes that contain one or more malaria parasites calculated (% parasitemia). This is usually necessary for correct species determination and as part of the assessment of severity. The total time required from finger-prick to the result of the microscopic examination is in the order of not more than 30 min.

Non-immune patients with malaria can sometimes have symptoms before the number of parasites is above the level of detection by microscopic examination. If there is a clinical suspicion of malaria and the examination of a thick film is negative, a microscopic examination should be repeated twice at 6–12-h intervals to rule out malaria. Some laboratories now screen for malaria with rapid antigen detection assays, since microscopic examination requires a high degree of expertise, often lacking in many clinical laboratories.[1] However, the sensitivity of rapid detection assays for malaria is also reduced in low-level parasitemias, and the same need for repeated tests to confidently rule out malaria applies.

Laboratory Parameters in Non-Immunes with Acute Malaria

All travelers with fever returning from a malaria-endemic area must be examined for malaria parasites. Thrombocytopenia (80%)[12] and eosinopenia are common findings. Profound thrombocytopenia is more common in severe malaria with intercurrent sepsis, where a low platelet count also is a negative prognostic factor. Anemia, contrary to expectations, is not a hallmark in uncomplicated malaria. In one study, 32% of adult men and 44% of adult women with malaria had low hemoglobin.[12] There was no difference between falciparum and nonfalciparum (mostly vivax) malaria in the frequency of acute anemia.

C-reactive protein (CRP) is almost always elevated in malaria, and one study has reported a correlation with high parasitemia.[13] However, raised CRP is non-specific. Very high levels (>200 mg/L) are rarely seen and should alert the physician to an intercurrent or superadded bacterial infection (lobar pneumonia, pyelonephritis, or septicemia) as a more probable explanation. Similarly, moderate leukopenia is a common finding in malaria, whereas leukocytosis is rare and again should alert the physician to the possibility of superadded bacterial infection. Increased translocation of Gram-negative bacteria across the gut occurs in patients with falciparum malaria, and if leukocytosis is present a blood culture should be performed and a broad-spectrum antibiotic to cover Gram-negative bacteria should be started empirically. A slight increase in liver enzyme levels is often present. Owing to hemolysis, both bilirubin and lactate dehydrogenase levels are frequently elevated.

Important Differential Diagnosis

As clinical features alone are not specific for malaria, a number of important differential diagnoses should be considered. The list will depend on the travel history and endemic diseases that the traveler will have been exposed to. Furthermore, if there are any localizing clinical features such as rash, which is rare in patients with malaria, or specific abnormal laboratory tests such as the white blood cell differential (Table 17.2), this may help in refining the possibilities.

Common differential diagnoses include influenza and other upper respiratory tract infections, particularly in the winter months, during a country's flu season. Dengue fever is a frequent illness in many

Table 17.2 Differential Diagnoses of Fever in a Returning Traveler Depending on White Blood Count

Leukopenia	Leukocytosis	Eosinophilia
Malaria*	Amebiasis	Schistosomiasis
Enteric Fever	Pyogenic infections	Hydatid disease
Arboviruses e.g., Dengue	Leptospirosis	Filariasis
Rickettsioses	Borreliosis	Strongyloidiasis
Brucellosis		Trichinosis

*Leukocytosis in a patient with malaria is indicative of superadded bacterial infection.

Table 17.3 Advantages and Disadvantages of Antimalarials Commonly Used for Treatment of *P. falciparum* infections

Compound	Advantages	Disadvantages
Chloroquine	Parenteral preparations Inexpensive	Resistance in all malarious areas except north of the Panama channel and Caribbean islands
Sulfadoxine/ pyrimethamine	Single dose, usually well tolerated	Increasing resistance in most malarious areas Slow acting No parenteral preparation
Mefloquine	Effective in Africa and most other malarious areas[a]	No parenteral preparation Side-effects (not lethal)
Quinine	Effective in Africa and most other malarious areas[a] Parenteral preparations	Concentration-dependent side-effects (cinchonism) Long treatment duration (7days)
Atovaquone/ proguanil	Probably effective in most malarious areas Probably well tolerated	Limited experience No parenteral preparation Expensive
Artemisinin[b] derivatives	Effective in all areas[c] Rapid action Parenteral preparations	Long treatment duration (7 days) if not combined as recommended
Artemether/ lumefantrine	Probably effective in most malarious areas Well tolerated	Limited experience No parenteral preparation Expensive Must be taken with lipid meal

[a]Not in areas of Thailand near the borders with Cambodia and Myanmar as well as in western Cambodia.
[b]Artemether, arteether, artesunate, artemisinin and dihydroartemisin.
[c]Reduced in vivo susceptibility of artesunate in western Cambodia.

malaria-endemic areas. Patients with dengue usually complain of severe myalgia and arthralgia (breakbone fever), and headache. Unlike malaria, there is often a macular skin eruption, which classically manifests 'islands of sparing,' although this is by no means universal. Conjunctivitis may also be present. The laboratory findings are similar to those of malaria, with thrombocytopenia and leukopenia characteristic. Septicemia due to *Salmonella typhi or paratyphi* may also mimic malaria early on. Gastrointestinal symptoms are often lacking, but the onset is usually more gradual than in malaria.

If leukocytosis is present, pneumococcal pneumonia should be considered, as patients may present with acute-onset high-grade fever without respiratory symptoms during the first days. Similarly, elderly patients with febrile upper urinary tract infections may present without urinary complaints or low back pain and may be difficult to differentiate from malaria in the first few days of symptoms.

Avoiding 'Doctors Delay'

In all persons who have visited a malaria-endemic area and present with fever or compatible symptoms starting between 1 week after the first possible exposure and 3 months (or even later in rare cases) after the last possible exposure, a diagnosis of falciparum malaria must be excluded.[1] Rare cases of 'airport malaria' exist following importation of plasmodium-carrying anopheline mosquitos from endemic areas.[14] Similarly, malaria from blood products has been described.[15] Hence any patient presenting with fever and rigors should alert the physician to the possibility of malaria. It is recommended that travelers should be urged to demand malaria be excluded if they experience a febrile illness after their return and directly seek medical care at an institution where a good-quality microscopic examination can be performed. As part of the pre-travel counseling, every traveler should be given written information about the symptoms of malaria and what to do if the diagnosis is suspected.

Some Aspects of Chemotherapy in Non-Immune Patients

The treatment of malaria varies depending on the malaria species and the degree of parasitemia, the patient's ability to tolerate oral medication and the drug susceptibility pattern. Chloroquine is still the drug of choice for *P. ovale* and *P. malariae* infections. In many parts of the world (Papua New Guinea and Indonesia, Brazil, Colombia, Ethiopia, Guatemala, Guyana, India, Myanmar, Peru, the Republic of Korea, Solomon Islands, Thailand, and Turkey), *P. vivax* has developed resistance to chloroquine. In these areas, mefloquine or quinine has become the treatment of choice for the blood stages,[1] although

artemesinin derivatives may also be employed. Eradication of liver hypnozoites in *P. vivax* or *P. ovale* infection requires primaquine. This drug will cause hemolysis in persons with G6PD deficiency, which should be checked for before prescribing. In non-falciparum malaria severe disease is rare and oral treatment is usually possible.

Global resistance of *P. falciparum* to chloroquine and antifolates such as sulfadoxine/pyrimethamine makes their use obsolete for this infection. Mefloquine and quinine resistance is also evident in some parts of SE Asia, such as the Trat and Tak provinces of Thailand and adjacent areas in Myanmar and Cambodia. Characteristics of antimalarials used in treatment of *P. falciparum* infections are detailed in Table 17.3.

Artemisinin derivatives (dihydroartemesinin, artesunate, arthemether, arteether) originate from the herb 'quinghao' (*Artemisia annua*) and have been used in traditional Chinese medicine for over 2000 years to control fever. Their advantage over quinine lies in their ability to target malaria parasites in the early blood stages, clearing these from the blood before they can sequester on endothelial surfaces, a characteristic of more mature infected erythrocytes. Their short half-life and the need to prevent the development of resistance necessitate their use as part of combination therapy (artemesinin-combination therapy, ACT) with another effective antimalarial drug.[16] A number of fixed-dose combinations are now available, the most commonly used being Coartem, containing artemether and lumefantrine. If monotherapy is unavoidable the duration of treatment should be lengthened to 7 days. However, a recent report of reduced in vivo susceptibility to artesunate in western Cambodia,[17] characterized by slow parasite clearance, sounds a warning of the potential for *P. falciparum* to become resistant to the artemesin, and it is noteworthy that this area has seen a number of patients treated with artesunate monotherapy.

Intravenous artesunate is now the drug of choice for treatment of severe falciparum malaria in both adults and children.[18,19] The SEQUAMAT study comparing IV artesunate with IV quinine in adults with severe falciparum malaria demonstrated a 34.7% reduction in mortality in the artesunate group,[18] and more recently, the AQUAMAT study in African children showed a reduction of 22.5% mortality in children treated with artesunate.[19] Where artesunate is not available, parenteral quinine with a 20 mg/kg loading dose should be used in conjunction with careful blood glucose monitoring. Once able to take oral medication, the patient should complete treatment with a second antimalarial drug or drug combination. For example, following IV artesunate patients can complete treatment with oral Coartem, or patients on quinine may have doxycycline or clindamycin added to complete therapy.

In the present situation, with varying resistance to most commonly used antimalarials and insufficient data about the performance of new drugs in non-immune populations, it is advised to monitor the parasite response after treatment. The most crucial time for a repeat parasite count is 48 h after initiation of treatment. If the number of parasites at this time is >25% of the initial number, high-grade resistance should be suspected and treatment immediately switched to another drug.

Conclusion

Acute malaria is a medical emergency and must be suspected in all travelers who complain of fever after a stay in an endemic area. Severe *P. falciparum* malaria can develop within a few days after onset of symptoms. Early diagnosis and prompt treatment are of the utmost importance to reduce morbidity and mortality from this preventable infection.

References

1. International Travel and Health. Geneva: WHO; 2010.
2. Freedman DO, Weld, L, Kozarsky PE, et al. Spectrum of disease and relation to place of exposure among ill returned travelers. N Engl J Med 2006;354:119–30.
3. Expert Committee on Malaria. Technical Report Series No. 892. Geneva: WHO; 2000.
4. Leder K, Tong S, Weld L, et al. Illness in travelers visiting friends and relatives: A review of the GeoSentinel Surveillance Network. Clin Infect Dis 2006;43:1185–93.
5. Genton B, D'Acremont V. Clinical features of malaria in returning travelers and migrants. In: Schlagenhauf-Lawlor P, editor. Travellers' Malaria. Hamilton: Decker; 2001. p. 371–92.
6. WHO. Guidelines for the Treatment of Malaria. 2nd ed. Geneva, Switzerland.
7. Marsh K. Clinical features of malaria. In: Wahlgren M, Perlman P, editors. Malaria – Molecular and Clinical Aspects. Amsterdam: Harwood; 1999. p. 87–117.
8. White NJ. Malaria. In: Cook GC, Zumla A, editors. Manson's Tropical Diseases. 22nd ed. London: WB Saunders; 2009. p. 1205–95.
9. WHO. Chemotherapy of Malaria. Revised 2nd ed. Monograph Series No. 27. Geneva: WHO; 1986.
10. WHO. The biology of malaria parasites. Technical Report Series No. 743. Geneva: WHO; 1987.
11. WHO/USAID. Malaria diagnosis. Report of a joint WHO/USAID informal consultation October 25–27, 1999. Geneva: WHO; 2000.
12. Eriksson B, Hellgren U, Rombo L. Changes in erythrocyte sedimentation rate, C-reactive protein and hematological parameters in patients with acute malaria. Scand J Infect Dis 1989;21:435–41.
13. Naik P, Voller A. Serum C-reactive protein levels and falciparum malaria. Trans Roy Soc Trop Med Hyg 1984;78:812–3.
14. Lusina D, Legros F, Esteve V, et al. Airport malaria: Four cases in suburban Paris during summer 1999. Eurosurveillance 2000;5(7):76–80.
15. Kitchen AD, Chiodini PL. Malaria and blood transfusion. Vox Sang 2006;90(2):77–84.
16. WHO. The use of antimalarial drugs. Report of a WHO informal consultation. Geneva: WHO; 2001. p. 13–7 November.
17. Dondorp A, Nosten F, Yi P, et al. Artemesinin resistance in *Plasmodium falciparum* malaria. N Engl J Med 2009;361:455–67.
18. Dondorp A, Nosten F, Stepniewska K, et al. Artesunate versus quinine for treatment of severe falciparum malaria: a randomised trial. Lancet 2005;366:717–25.
19. Dondorp A, Fanello C, Hendriksen I, et al. Artesunate versus quinine in the treatment of severe falciparum malaria in African children (AQUAMAT): an open-label, randomized trial. Lancet 2010;376:1647–57.

18

Epidemiology of Travelers' Diarrhea

John W. Sanders, Mark S. Riddle, and David N. Taylor

Key points

- Travelers' diarrhea (TD) is the most common travel-related health problem
- A major leap in our understanding of travelers' diarrhea occurred when enterotoxigenic *E. coli* (ETEC) was discovered to be a cause of the illness
- Bacteria are the most common cause of TD and ETEC is the most common bacterial pathogen
- Host factors such as age, pre-existing immunity, underlying medical conditions and genetic factors play a role in susceptibility to TD
- Avoidance of high-risk foods, although advisable, is not enough to completely eliminate the risk of acquiring TD

Introduction

Over 100 million travelers from industrialized nations visit tropical and developing areas of the world each year, and there are about 40 million associated cases of diarrhea.[1] One-quarter to more than one-half of these international travelers are afflicted with diarrhea during their trips abroad,[2–8] making this illness the most common travel-related health problem[9,10] (Table 18.1). Diarrheal illness has long been a problem for military forces as well, accounting for more lost man-days during wartime than any other illness.[11–13] Travelers' diarrhea (TD) usually presents as an acute illness, resolving completely in less than a week. About 10% of cases may last up to 2 weeks.[6] Travelers' diarrhea is, for the most part, a mild, self-limited illness; however, even a day of relative incapacitation can disrupt a carefully planned vacation. A 1999 study estimated the average cost for medication, treatment, and missed activities to be US$116.50 per patient with diarrhea on a vacation in Jamaica.[14] Tourists are not the only ones who feel the economic burden of this illness. In addition to the morbidity and mortality of diarrhea, developing nations suffer losses in tourism revenue. Diarrhea-wary travelers often remove high-risk countries from their itineraries.[15] TD is caused by myriad food and water-borne organisms that include bacteria, viruses and parasites. Clarifying the epidemiology and etiology of travelers' diarrhea has the potential to reduce risk in the traveler and lower the endemicity of disease in developing nations.

History

Diarrhea has been a problem for travelers throughout recorded history.[16] There have been many theories as to the causes of diarrhea during travel, including changes in environment, time zone, diet, and exposure to microbial pathogens. Dr Ben Kean was one of the first researchers to conclude that 'turista' or travelers' diarrhea was 'possibly related to shifts in the bacterial population or introduction of "foreign" bacterial strains into the intestinal tract'.[17] He defined travelers' diarrhea as a clinical syndrome. His vivid description of the sudden onset of profuse watery diarrhea remains one of the classic descriptions of an illness. For most of his career, the exact cause of travelers' diarrhea eluded him, but he ruled out all of the known causes and correctly surmised that the primary cause was bacterial, because pre-exposure antibiotic use prevented many of the illnesses. In 1970, Rowe et al. isolated a new serotype of *E. coli*, O148: H28, from a majority of soldiers with diarrhea in Aden, Yemen. A technician working with their organisms in a London laboratory later developed a severe attack of diarrhea, from which *E. coli* 0148: H28 was subsequently recovered in pure culture.[18] Gorbach, Sack and others first associated *E. coli* with an enterotoxin in patients with acute undifferentiated diarrhea in the Indian subcontinent, where it was found to be the most common cause of non-vibrio cholera (profuse watery diarrhea).[19,20] DuPont et al. were able to isolate this enterotoxigenic *E. coli* (ETEC) from US soldiers who became ill in Vietnam.[21] Gorbach, in collaboration with Kean, repeated the studies in Mexico and found that ETEC was the major cause of travelers' diarrhea in that country.[22] Studies performed since then have confirmed that ETEC remains the single most important diarrheal pathogen worldwide. Studies of Peace Corps volunteers have also shown altered bowel flora within days after arriving in a new environment.[23] These westerners were originally colonized with *E. coli* that were susceptible to antibiotics, but a few days after arriving in Thailand these *E. coli* were gradually replaced with indigenous, resistant strains. This rapid change in bowel flora reflects how quickly and easily travelers can acquire diarrhea-producing flora such as ETEC.

Clinical Characteristics

A case of travelers' diarrhea is described as the sudden onset of loose, watery stools associated with abdominal pain, fever, or tenesmus.

Table 18.1 Incidence of Various Health Problems Among European Travelers During a Short Stay in Various Climatic Zones[a]

New or Worsened Disease	% Incidence of Health Problems During Travel		
	Tropics (n = 10 555)	USA/Canada (n = 1300)	Significance, USA, and Canada used as Control Group
Diarrhea	33.9	5.8	p < 0.001
Respiratory infections	13.3	8.5	p < 0.001
Insomnia	10.6	7.0	p < 0.001
Headache	7.8	7.6	ns
Dermatosis	5.7	3.4	p < 0.001
Fever of any origin	3.8	1.2	p < 0.001
Cardiovascular disease	1.6	1.2	ns
Accidents	0.3	0.1	ns

[a]Steffen 1983.[7] ns, not significant.

Table 18.2 Clinical Aspects of Diarrhea Among Americans Traveling to Developing Countries[a]

	Travelers' Diarrhea[b]	All Episodes
Number of travelers	270	358
Travel day of onset	10.6 ± 9.2	9.8 ± 8.5
Stools/day (%)	4.4 ± 2.6	3.7 ± 2.5
1–2	17.4	37.4
3–5	63.0	47.8
>6	19.6	14.9
Duration in days (%)	3.9 ± 5.7	3.7 ± 5.6
1–3	72.1	74.1
4–7	18-9	17
8–14	4.5	4.3
>14	4.5	4.6
Symptoms (%)		
Watery stools	66.3	58.4
Cramping	44.4	33.5
Vomiting	24.4	18-4
Fever	22.2	16.8
Blood	1.5	1.1
Modification of activity (%)	35.2	28.8

[a]Hill 2000.[5]

[b]Travelers' diarrhea defined as ≥3 unformed stools/24 h ± cramping, vomiting, fever or blood or <3 stools/24 h with one or more of the above symptoms. All episodes column includes simple loose motions and travelers' diarrhea.

Rigid criteria for frequency, duration and severity are academic. The sense of urgency can be profound and there may be a few prodromal symptoms, such as stomach gurgling or queasiness. Fever occurs commonly and blood is noted in stools rarely. Nausea and vomiting are also common in the first few hours, adding to the discomfort and water loss (Table 18.2). Dehydration in adults is rarely life-threatening but it is a greater concern for young travelers. Mild dehydration

Table 18.3 Distribution of Enteropathogens Among Patients With TD, 1973–2009[a]

Pathogen	Estimated Distribution of Pathogens by Region (%)		
	Latin America	Africa	South Asia (Indian Subcontinent)
ETEC[b]	34	31	31
EAEC[c]	24	2	16
Shigella	7	9	8
Salmonella	4	6	7
Campylobacter	3	5	8
Aeromonas	1	3	3
Plesiomonas	1	3	5
Norovirus	17	13	unknown
Protozoa	3	3	9
No pathogen identified	49	45	39

[a]Modified from Shah, et al. Am J Trop Med Hyg. 2009. and Bauche, et al. Gastro and Hepatol. 2011.[143]

[b]ETEC, enterotoxigenic Escherichia coli.

[c]EAEC, enteroaggregative Escherichia coli

contributes to a general malaise and other generalized symptoms such as headache and myalgias.[24]

Like most clinical syndromes, there is a spectrum of illness both in severity and type of clinical symptoms. Clinical features and laboratory parameters have proved either too insensitive or too non-specific to be of use in differentiating between pathologic organisms.[25,26] In general, ETEC has tended to cause a milder form of diarrhea than other bacterial agents such as Campylobacter.[24,27] Those who have a mild clinical presentation usually recover more quickly, regardless of the etiology. Depending on the type and location of travel, the onset of diarrhea usually occurs within the first 2 weeks and symptoms usually resolve within 3–4 days.[5,27] Approximately one-quarter of travelers with diarrhea will have to alter their activities, but the majority of these will be incapacitated for <24 h.

Etiology

Isolation rates for pathologic agents among travelers' diarrhea studies have varied from roughly 30% to 60%.[14,28–32] In 1974, Merson et al. identified a pathogen in 63% of travelers who developed TD while traveling in Mexico.[6] Some 20 years later, Jiang et al. conducted a longitudinal study in travelers to Guadalajara, Mexico, that isolated an organism in only 44% of diarrheal cases.[30] Despite advances in laboratory methods and improvements in the handling of stool specimens, isolation rates have not significantly improved. There are a number of variables that might explain why an organism is not isolated from the stool, or why rates vary for specific agents. Antibiotics and bismuth compounds may have been used prior to stool collection; the illness may have waned to the point where few organisms were shed; the stool specimen may have been inadequate to detect the organism; or the appropriate diagnostic test may not have even been used to identify the pathogen. Further complicating the search for infectious etiology, asymptomatic travelers often shed pathogenic organisms in their stool and about 15% of ill travelers have multiple enteric pathogens.[32]

Nonetheless, one consistency remains throughout these studies: enterotoxigenic *E. coli* (ETEC) is the most commonly isolated pathogen (Table 18.3). Future studies are likely to uncover new etiologic agents. The fact that travelers usually respond to antibiotics even if a bacterial pathogen is not isolated suggests that most undiagnosed cases of travelers' diarrhea are bacterial in origin.

Bacteria

Enterotoxigenic *E. coli* (ETEC)

Bacteria are the most common causes of travelers' diarrhea and ETEC is the most common bacterial cause. *Salmonella, Shigella* and *Campylobacter* make up the majority of remaining bacterial pathogens (Table 18.3). All of these are important causes of diarrheal disease in the USA, except ETEC. There is no routine method available to microbiology laboratories for the diagnosis of ETEC. In order to identify an *E. coli* as enterotoxigenic, one must identify the toxin as it is released from bacterial culture, or one must identify the genes for the heat-labile (LT) or heat-stable (ST) toxin produced by strains of ETEC. Neither test is commercially available.

A high number of ETEC organisms are necessary to induce diarrhea.[21] In contrast to an infectious dose of <200 cells for *Shigella*, DuPont et al. demonstrated that 10^8 organisms are required for ETEC to cause diarrhea. These high inocula suggest that a marked breakdown in sanitation, as often happens in developing nations, must occur in order for such high bacterial loads to be ingested. An occasional outbreak of ETEC has occurred in the USA. In 1975, a large water-borne outbreak presented at Crater Lake National Park, when raw sewage entered park water, affecting more than 2000 people.[33] DuPont's study also showed that ETEC pathogenic for animals did not cause disease in humans.[21] This, coupled with ETEC's inability to easily colonize livestock, further supports the suspicion that humans are the main reservoir for ETEC.

In addition to ETEC, there are at least four other groups of *E. coli* that distinctly cause diarrheal illness.[34,35] The role of these groups in travelers' diarrhea is less clear, though future research may provide clarification. Enteroinvasive *E. coli* (EIEC) is closely related to *Shigella* sp. and causes a similar clinical picture of dysentery, but is not a significant cause of TD. Enterohemorrhagic *E. coli* (EHEC) causes hemorrhagic colitis and hemolytic uremic syndrome via shiga-like toxin (SLT). Although EHEC is a significant cause of illness in the USA, Europe, and Japan, it has rarely been acquired in tropical destinations. This is significant because antibiotics are contraindicated for EHEC infections but are commonly used to treat travelers' diarrhea.[36] Enteropathogenic *E. coli* (EPEC) is an important cause of infant diarrhea through an 'attaching and effacing' adherence,[37] but it does not appear to affect travelers to a significant degree. Finally, there is enteroaggregative *E. coli* (EAEC), a recently recognized pathogen that is likely to be a major etiologic agent in travelers' diarrhea. At present, there is no clear understanding of the pathogenesis of diarrhea caused by EAEC. However, in a recent study, EAEC was isolated in 26% of cases of travelers' diarrhea and was second only to ETEC as the most common enteropathogen.[38] It is interesting that this organism explained 26% of cases with unknown etiology, illustrating the importance of bacteria as prominent etiologies of travelers' diarrhea and the need for further study in this area.

Campylobacter spp.

Although *Campylobacter* infections are common in the USA and other developed nations, the incidence of disease is many times higher in developing nations.[39] In such countries, constant, heavy exposure eventually induces an immunity that becomes apparent after the first year of life. Travelers have a high risk of acquiring *Campylobacter* that may reach 10% of total cases on a 2-week trip. Resistance to fluoroquinolones is >70% in Spain and Thailand.[28,40] Azithromycin has become the drug of choice for treating TD in these regions.[41]

Salmonella spp.

Non-*typhi Salmonella* infections have been increasingly common in the USA and other developed countries but are a relatively infrequent cause of TD in developing countries.

Shigella spp.

Shigella becomes more prevalent as sanitary conditions decline. It has been a problem for the US military during deployments in Iraq, Saudi Arabia, and Somalia.[12,42,43] As the duration of deployment increases, *Shigella* becomes a more important cause of diarrhea and dysentery. The low infectious dose increases the incidence of person-to-person transmission and fly-borne disease. Because *Shigella* is a fastidious organism, the true incidence of this organism may be underestimated in conditions where prompt processing of fresh fecal material is not always possible.[44] Recently, a study of diarrhea in Vietnamese children found that 36% of non-dysentery, culture-negative specimens were PCR positive for *Shigella*.[45] As this technology is utilized more frequently, it will not be surprising to find that *Shigella* accounts for more cases of TD than previously recognized.

Vibrio spp.

Vibrio parahaemolyticus and non-O1 *Vibrio cholerae* have been associated with seafood and have been a problem in hotels that offer seafood buffets.[46] *Vibrio cholerae* O1 is a rare cause of TD, but reports from Americans working in Lima, Peru, and Japanese returning from Bali, Indonesia, suggest that westerners can get cholera in endemic areas.[47] The symptoms are the same as those of other causes of TD, and the pathogens cannot be differentiated without culture.

Viruses

Viruses such as norovirus, adenovirus, astrovirus, and rotavirus have been documented as etiologic agents for TD.[12,14,26,32] Most studies have not looked specifically for viral causes of TD. In those that have, many have used electron microscopy or enzyme immunoassay (EIA), which are insensitive, labor-intensive and operator dependent.[48] Newer studies are incorporating polymerase chain reaction (PCR) and reverse-transcriptase PCR to look for viruses and the specific strains responsible for TD.[49–51] The calicivirus family, which includes noroviruses and Sapporo virus, are increasingly recognized as etiologic agents for food-borne, water-borne and person-to-person diarrheal outbreaks that present with nausea, vomiting, and diarrhea. Well-documented outbreaks have occurred aboard cruise ships and in hotels.[52–56] Recently, it was shown that noroviruses were the second most common cause of TD in students from the USA visiting Mexico, accounting for 17% of cases.[57] These viruses are transmitted by the fecal–oral and aerosol routes and are believed to be the most common cause of non-bacterial TD. During the Gulf War, Norwalk virus was a significant cause of diarrhea during the winter months. Once this virus was introduced, person-to-person transmission was believed to have been an important mode of spread, causing substantial morbidity among deployed service members.[58]

Parasites

The most common agents for protracted diarrhea in returning travelers are parasitic infections. The likelihood of parasitic etiology rises commensurately with the duration of diarrheal symptoms. Among travelers in Nepal with diarrhea >14 days, 27% were diagnosed with *Giardia*, in contrast to only 10% who had diarrhea <14 days.[32] The differential for parasitic diarrhea is most likely to include *Giardia lamblia*, *Entamoeba histolytica*, *Cryptosporidium parvum*, and *Cyclospora cayetanensis*. Microsporidia and *Dientamoeba fragilis* are rare causes of persistent low-grade gastrointestinal symptoms.[59–62] Although the risk factors for intestinal parasites are not well defined, it appears that duration of stay is a major factor in acquiring a parasitic pathogen[63] and that this risk is associated with a traveler's continual exposure to human fecal material in drinking water and food.[64]

Giardia Lamblia

The most common protozoal infection in returning travelers is *Giardia lamblia*.[65,66] This organism causes a clinical picture that ranges from an acute self-limited illness to the asymptomatic illness. If untreated, chronic intermittent diarrhea characterized by flatulence, fatigue and weight loss can persist for months.[67,68] Chlorination is ineffective in preventing water-borne infection. In 1997 reliance upon this method of water treatment at a Greek resort hotel resulted in a large *Giardia* outbreak among UK tourists.[69] Filtration or boiling of drinking water will help to prevent infections in such cases, though other possible water-borne sources include recreational water sources. Diagnosis is usually made by stool examination, but multiple careful examinations may be necessary to demonstrate the organism. Stool antigen test kits for *G. lamblia* are available.[70] A duodenal string test has fallen out of favor in recent years.[71]

Entamoeba spp.

In recent years some of the issues in diagnosing and treating *Entamoeba histolytica* infections have been clarified. It is now clear that there are two distinct, but morphologically identical strains of amebae.[72] *E. histololytica* is a pathogen, whose symptoms can range from a self-limited acute illness to severe and even fatal colitis; *E. dispar* is a non-pathogen that often presents in patients who are 'asymptomatic cyst passers'.[73] The organisms cannot be distinguished microscopically, but can be by EIA or PCR.[74,75]

Cyclospora

Cyclospora cayetanensis, along with *Isospora belli*, is a coccidian in the *Eimeria* family of protozoa. Seasonal *Cyclospora* outbreaks have caused up to a third of diarrheal illness in Nepal during the pre-monsoon spring and summer months.[64,76] Imported Guatemalan raspberries have carried *Cyclospora* into the USA, causing outbreaks in summer months.[77] Fatigue and anorexia are extremely prominent, and help distinguish *Cyclospora* infection from other pathogens. Untreated, the illness lasts for an average of 6 weeks.

Isospora Belli

Isospora belli is endemic in tropical and subtropical countries. Healthy travelers to the Caribbean, India, and Africa have returned to the USA with *Isospora* infection. After traveling extensively in West Africa, an American developed chronic diarrhea and cramping abdominal pain.[78] Multiple stool examinations over a 5-week period finally revealed *Isospora belli* in this patient.

Cryptosporidium Parvum

Cryptosporidium is now recognized as a common cause of childhood diarrhea in developing countries[79] and is being increasingly recognized as a cause of diarrhea in travelers to those areas.[80] For example, *Cryptosporidium* was the third most common cause of travelers' diarrhea in military personnel deployed to an area known to have high rates of *Cryptosporidium* in the local children.[79,80] Its resistance to chlorine has led to numerous water-borne outbreaks in US cities, most notably a huge outbreak in Milwaukee, Wisconsin, in 1993.[81] In 34 Finnish students who made a weekend trip to Leningrad, seven returned with symptomatic *Cryptosporidium*, four with *Giardia*, and two with both.[82] In contrast to a mean incubation period of 16 days for *Giardia*, *Cryptosporidium* had a mean incubation of 6 days, and symptoms that lasted 9–23 days. Immunocompromised HIV-infected travelers are particularly susceptible to *Cryptosporidiosis* and should be cautious while traveling abroad.[68]

Blastocystis Hominis

There has long been debate whether this organism causes diarrhea, though the consensus appears to be that it is not a pathogen. A careful case–control study in Kathmandu in 1995 showed that *B. hominis* was found equally often in the stools of diarrhea patients as in control patients with no diarrheal symptoms.[89] It is sensible to continue to look for a recognized pathogen in symptomatic returned travelers who have *B. hominis* in the stool.[83]

Host Factors

People from Europe, the USA, Australia, and Japan comprise the majority of individuals who travel from a developed to a less developed country. They consist of vacationers, business employees, the military, and aid workers. From the developing world, refugees and other displaced persons make up another important at-risk group. Groups and individuals have different demographic and behavioral characteristics that play a role in determining their risk of developing diarrhea.

Age/Gender

Numerous studies have shown that among adults increasing age is significantly protective.[5,7,9,17,29,84] This association persisted even after controlling for preference of adventurous travel, duration of stay, and travel experience. One study found that each additional year of age reduced the incidence of diarrhea by 1%.[4] Younger adult travelers may be at increased risk for a number of reasons. They eat a larger amount of food, and hence pathogens, and they tend to be less selective in the source and type of their food. Additionally, their immune responses to pathogens may differ from those of older travelers. Gender has consistently been shown not to be a factor in developing diarrhea.[14,17,27]

Travelers' Diarrhea in Children

Travelers' diarrhea in children is a relatively neglected area, but it is clear that more adults are now traveling with children and infants. Pitzinger conducted a retrospective study in Zurich to assess the incidence of diarrhea in children.[85] She found that adolescents had a 38% rate of TD, which was as high as in young adults 20–29 years old. Rates declined to 20% in children 7–14 years old and were lowest (8%) in children 3–6 years old. Most notably, children 0–2 years old had the highest diarrhea rates, at 40%[85] (Figure 18.1). In

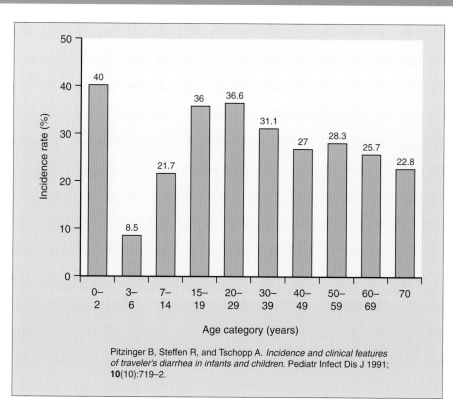

Figure 18.1 Age-specific incidence rates of diarrhea among travelers to the tropics.[91]

Pitzinger B, Steffen R, and Tschopp A. *Incidence and clinical features of traveler's diarrhea in infants and children.* Pediatr Infect Dis J 1991; **10**(10):719–2.

small children, the clinical course tended to be severe and prolonged. In these children, 40% of parents reported that they had consistently practiced dietary preventive measures. More recently, a study reported from the GeoSentinel travel network found that among children reporting for care upon return from travel that diarrhea (28%) was most common, followed by dermatologic disorders (25%), systemic febrile illnesses (23%), and respiratory disorders (11%).[86] Furthermore, diarrhea was classified as acute (80%) or chronic (duration of >2 weeks) (20%), and among acute diarrhea cases no identified pathogen was found in 28%, bacterial diarrhea in 29%, and parasitic etiology in 25%.

Infants still breastfeeding may be an exception. Breastfeeding is the safest nourishment in the absence of other diseases and has saved the lives of millions of children in less developed countries. Infant formula and baby food is available in most urban areas and can be prepared safely. Families moving to a developing country should quickly find a place to live that has a kitchen. The best way to reduce the risk of diarrhea is to have control of how the food is prepared. It is difficult to provide safe foods when trekking with infants. Parents may be able to carry toddlers while trekking, but they must remember that the risk of diarrhea is high. Children's hands will become contaminated, and the dose of organisms necessary to cause disease may be significantly lower in children. Parents who must travel with children merit detailed education regarding dietary prevention, self-treatment, and oral rehydration.

There are few direct data comparing the etiology of TD among children and adults. There are some data describing causes of diarrhea among children returning to developing countries. Available data suggest that the etiology in traveling children is very similar to that in traveling adults. This is understandable, since causes of diarrhea in children living in less-developed countries are the same as those that afflict traveling adults from developed countries.

Country of Origin

A traveler's country of origin appears to be a risk factor for diarrheal illness. While traveling in less-developed regions, residents from more developed countries have the highest attack rates,[9] whereas travelers from lesser developing nations have lower or similar rates than found in the host population.[87] When traveling to developing nations, persons residing in northern countries show significantly higher TD attack rates than those from more southern countries.[14,88] These observations support the theory that attack rates correlate directly with socioeconomic status, as was noted when a diverse group of Panamanians visited Mexico.[89]

Immunity

Protective immunity develops after natural infection with ETEC. The role of specific antigens, such as colonization factors or toxins, or of specific components of the immune system, such as gut IgA or serum IgG, in protective immunity is not well defined. Humans who have recovered from natural infection are protected from challenge with the homologous strain,[21,90,91] so immunity clearly occurs. The decreasing rate of infection associated with increasing age and length of stay in a host nation supports these findings.[92,93] However, the duration of protection stemming from induced immunity is not known. Little protective benefit is derived from having previously visited a specific high-risk country or having traveled in another developing nation.[9,94] Several case series studies have demonstrated that the risk for diarrheal illness in developing nations remains for years after arrival, though there is a demonstrable decrease over time[29,32,92,93] (Figure 18.2). In particularly high endemic environments this risk may be more persistent. A prospective study in Nepal demonstrated no diminution in diarrhea risk within the first year of residence and a high monthly incidence that persisted up to 2 years after arrival.[64]

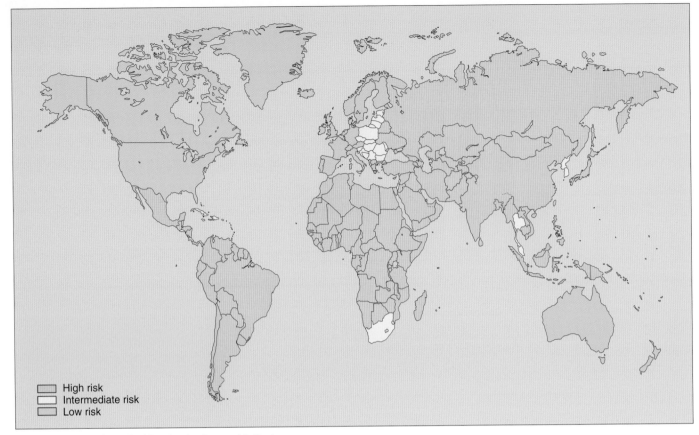

Figure 18.2 Risk of Travelers' Diarrhea by Geographic Region.

Underlying Medical Conditions

Low gastric acidity is thought to be a risk factor for TD.[21] Individuals who are post gastrectomy and those using antacids such as proton pump inhibitors are thought to be at increased risk. Other chronic gastrointestinal problems may worsen during travel and contribute to increased diarrheal symptoms.[94] Underlying medical conditions do not otherwise appear to affect the risk of acquiring diarrhea.[5] The exception to this may be in immunocompromised travelers. Patients with HIV/AIDS are prone to infection from myriad travel-related organisms, ranging from parasites such as *Cryptosporidium*, *Microsporidium* and *Isospora belli* to bacteria such as *Salmonella* and *Campylobacter*.[95]

Specific Host Factors

There are apparently other host factors that make individuals more susceptible to certain infections. For instance, for many years clinicians have observed that some individuals appear to be more resistant to infection with noroviruses than others. Recently it has been learned that noroviruses can only infect individuals who express specific, genetically determined carbohydrate receptors on intestinal cell surfaces. Specifically, noroviruses appear to bind to the H, Lewis, and A histo-blood group antigens expressed in the highest concentrations on enterocytes at villi tips.[96,97] Individuals who are 'non-secretors,' meaning that they do not make H type 1 or Lewis (B), appear to be immune from infection with norovirus.[98] Individuals who are ABO blood group B appear to be more resistant to infection or more likely to have an asymptomatic infection.[98] Persons possessing polymorphism in the promoter (−251 region of the IL-8 gene appear to be more susceptible to diarrhea due to EAEC.[99] A single-nucleotide

polymorphism (SNP) in the human lactoferrin gene (t/t genotype in position codon 632) appears to predispose individuals to TD and to presentation with more markers of intestinal inflammation (blood, mucus, or fecal leukocytes).[100]

Environmental Factors

While traveling in developing nations the environmental risks for TD are omnipresent and often unavoidable. For example, various foods and drinks in less-developed countries have been associated with diarrheal illness. Data also indicate that eating at smaller restaurants or street vendors might put a person at increased risk for TD.[91,101] This suggests that travelers would benefit from avoiding certain foods and eating venues. In Somalia, the US military limited its service members to prepackaged meals from the USA and to water from strictly monitored sources. Vectors for pathogens such as flies were aggressively controlled, and field sanitation facilities were constructed. These tremendous efforts led to a low diarrheal incidence of 4.5% over an 8-week period in a highly endemic region.[42] Most travelers do not find themselves in a position to benefit from such prevention measures, nor would they necessarily want to. However, well-advised travelers may be able to modify their behavior to the extent that risk is significantly reduced.

Pre-Travel Advice

Typically, travelers are urged to follow precautionary recommendations such as 'boil it, cook it, peel it, or forget it.'[102] The benefits of following this sensible advice have been difficult to demonstrate.[6,7,14,88] In a study from 1991, Hill personally provided 784 travelers with detailed counseling and written instructions on the prevention of travelers' diarrhea and the use of empiric therapy according to accepted guidelines. Despite this aggressive education, 34% of the travelers reported significant clinical diarrhea during their trip, and nearly a quarter of these experienced fever and vomiting. Of these, 35% had to alter their travel plans.[5] One prospective study has illustrated some benefit to pre-travel dietary advice.[102] The degree to which patients adhere to this advice and whether it is effective are still matters of debate. It does appear that pre-travel counseling reduces the need for medical assistance while abroad and reduces physician workload in terms of post-travel health visits with returning travelers by 50%.[103]

Travel Packages and Meals

Travelers who choose to travel under an 'all-inclusive package' or with partial board are at higher risk for developing TD than those who choose their own meals.[14,104] A protective effect is seen when people are able to cook their own meals, or eat at the homes of friends or family.[29,101,105] Food appears to be the primary mode of transmission for *E. coli*, *Shigella* and *Salmonella* and norovirus, whereas water seems to be the primary vehicle through which rotavirus is transmitted.[106,107] Tjoa et al. conducted a study in Mexico in 1975 that recovered *E. coli* from food prepared by 39% of restaurants, 55% of street vendors and 40% of small grocery stores. The highest counts of *E. coli* were found in dairy products. The potential perils in dining are further illustrated in the fact that four *Shigella* carriers were found among kitchen personnel in this study.[101]

In a case–control study among expatriate residents of Katmandu in 1992–1993, foods that required reheating and blended drinks held the highest risk of diarrhea.[29] There are conflicting data as to the benefits of bottled water or the risks associated with eating raw vegetables, salads, fresh fruit or ice served in restaurants.[6,29,88] The present data support cooking one's own meals whenever possible, and choosing reputable, safe restaurants able to serve hot, steaming meals if one eats out. Bottled, carbonated beverages should be chosen over juices and fountain drinks. One should also avoid eating salads or other cold dishes that have a higher risk of containing enteric pathogens.

Cruise ships have the task of preparing food for large numbers of travelers, but have limited space for food storage and preparation. Buffet lines are a common means of serving meals aboard ships, and often food is left at room temperature for hours before serving, allowing time for pathogen propagation. ETEC, *Salmonella*, and noroviruses are among those agents found to be causes of food-borne outbreaks aboard ships. As previously noted, norovirus has increasingly been implicated in the literature. Suspect transmission vehicles include shellfish, ice, salads, cake icing and even bottled water. Time reveals the insidious means by which travelers acquire diarrhea. Ill food-handlers and inappropriate handling, hygiene and storage have been at the root of viral outbreaks. Many of these cases can be averted aboard ships if travelers choose a line that cooks food thoroughly, uses pasteurized eggs, and avoids onshore caterers for off-ship excursions.[54]

Person-to-person transmission has also come to light as a probable means of acquiring illness. In a study of diarrhea aboard a cruise ship in which norovirus was implicated, passengers who had shared toilet facilities were twice as likely to acquire gastroenteritis as those who had a private bathroom.[108] Kean found an association between developing diarrhea and having a room-mate with similar symptoms.[17] Once an outbreak has begun, it is difficult to interrupt the cycle of transmission. Classic preventive measures, such as hand-washing, chlorinated water, and flush toilets, are less than effective in preventing norovirus illness in such cases.[48] Among soldiers deployed to Operation Desert Storm, norovirus was a significant cause of diarrheal illness. In this study, canteen use was strongly associated with developing diarrhea. The military typically uses chlorine to treat water, and the CDC has recommended high-level chlorination (10 ppm or 10 mg/L for 30 min or more) as a protective measure, although it acknowledges that even this may be inadequate.[43,109]

Lodging

Guests in luxury four- or five-star hotels often assume that they are protected from developing TD if they eat their meals in the hotel restaurant or from the room service menu. Steffen found that four-star hotels did not offer protection from TD over lesser-rated establishments.[7,94] Travelers should not assume guaranteed protection based on the rating of any establishment. Nonetheless, those undertaking adventurous travel (backpacking, camping, or trekking through rural areas) should be especially cautious, as their risk is higher than that of travelers staying in hotels.[83,85]

Risk by Geographic Region

There are regional differences in the risk and etiology of diarrhea. Black reviewed 34 studies among travelers to Latin America, Asia, and Africa. He found attack rates (median values) for travelers in these three regions to be remarkably similar: Latin America 53% (range 21–100%); Asia 54% (range 21–57%); and Africa 54% (range 36–62%).[15] DuPont has distinguished three grades of risk (high, moderate and low) for travelers' diarrhea.[106] He classifies the above three regions as 'high risk'. Low-risk countries include the USA, Canada, north and central Europe, Australia, and New Zealand. In these countries, the risk does not usually rise above 8%.[9,94] Intermediate risk makes up the remaining regions to include the Caribbean (except Haiti), and the major resorts in the Pacific and northern Mediterranean. Presumably, countries of the former Soviet Union would be included in this category, though data for this region are lacking (Figure 18.2).

If we consider specific etiologies within some of these regions, ETEC is the predominant cause of diarrheal illness in Latin America, Africa, and South Asia,[8,110] but appears to be less common in SE Asia.[111] From a series of studies in Latin America and Africa, Black concluded that these two regions show remarkable similarity in the prevalence of differing etiologic agents.[110] In order of lessening prevalence after ETEC, he noted that rotavirus, norovirus, *Shigella*, *Salmonella*, *G. lambia* and *E. histolytica* were identified most frequently. *Campylobacter* has been noted to be the predominant pathogen among US troops on military exercises in Thailand.[112] It was also the most common pathogen in Morocco during the winter.[113]

In more temperate regions there may be seasonal variation of diarrheal etiology. In Nepal, for example, the greatest number of diarrheal cases occurs during the hot months just before and during the monsoon season, when TD rates typically double. This is the time of year when the fly population is greatest and when indigenous food-borne cases of diarrhea peak among Nepalese.[29] Seasonality is further demonstrated by *Cyclospora* infection rates in Nepal, which consistently peak during the monsoon season and drop to negligible levels throughout the rest of the year, suggesting a water-borne transmission.[64,76] Rotavirus and norovirus infections have typically displayed higher infection rates during the cooler months.[32,114] Other large retrospective studies have failed to demonstrate a seasonal influence on the overall incidence of diarrhea.[7]

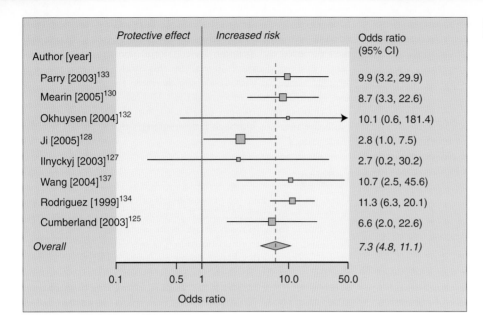

Figure 18.3 Risk of post-infectious irritable bowel syndrome.[134]

Onsequences of Travelers' Diarrhea

Antibiotic-associated diarrhea may affect 2-5% of those treated with fluoroquinolones or macrolides.[115] This clinical diagnosis should be considered in the differential among TD patients who are treated with antibiotics yet who have persistent or worsening symptoms. Other notable complications of TD include reactive arthritis and Campylobacter jejuni-associated Guillain-Barré syndrome.

Chronic diarrhea has been estimated to affect 1% of all travelers.[113] Steffen's study among Swiss travelers in the 1980s showed that 11% of travelers who developed acute diarrhea went on to experience chronic diarrhea.[7] A total of 20 of the 73 cases of chronic diarrhea were associated with protozoa, such as amoeba or Giardia; the rest were undiagnosed. The highest rate of chronic diarrhea was noted after travel in West Africa and East Asia. One-third of the patients became symptomatic only after returning home; some after more than a 1-month delay. Chronic diarrhea ranked second of all travel related illness in days of inability to work. Furthermore, a recent study reported out of the GeoSentinel network found that among long term travelers (trip duration >6 months) compared to short term travelers (<1 month) more often experienced chronic diarrhea, giardiasis, or irritable bowel syndrome (postinfectious), suggesting unique exposures to this traveler sub-population.[116]

Post-Infectious Irritable Bowel Syndrome

Association with Travelers' Diarrhea

A growing recognition of irritable bowel syndrome (PI-IBS) linked to travelers' diarrhea and other acute intestinal infection has come to light. Irritable bowel syndrome (IBS) is a heterogeneous disorder affecting 12% of the population worldwide.[117] Some 40 years ago, and Truelove described IBS symptoms following infective dysentery.[118] Subsequent studies confirmed post-infectious irritable bowel syndrome (PI-IBS) as a sequela of acute gastroenteritis (GE) with reported prevalence ranging from 4% to 31% and relative risk from 2.5 to 11.9.[119,120] Most recently a meta-analysis was conducted to explore differences between reported rates and provide pooled estimates of prevalence and risk and found 14 studies that were eligible for review and inclusion.[118,121-134] Prevalence ranged from 2.6% to 31.6% (see

Figure 18.3). The odds of developing IBS following infective gastroenteritis are 7.3 times greater than the average population, with 12% of GE patients subsequently developing PI-IBS. The risk of PI-IBS specifically associated with TD has been examined in four studies. Most recently a study was reported among 121 US military travelers returning from routine deployment (>6 month follow-up) to the Middle East where a 5-fold increase in incident IBS among those who experienced an episode of TD during travel compared to those that did not was found (17.2% versus 3.7%, p = 0.12).[135] An Israeli traveler sutdy reported that significantly more people (14%) who had TD developed IBS after 6 to 7 months compared with only 2% of those who did not experience travelers' diarrhea.[136] A third study reported an incidence of PI-IBS of 10% in patients who had acquired TD in Mexico.[128] The fourth study reported only a 4% incidence of PI-IBS after TD which was not statistically different compared with those who developed IBS who did not have diarrhea (2%).[123] Taken together, the increased risk for the development of IBS following gastrointestinal infections, including those associated with travelers' diarrhea, reaffirms the need for prevention strategies to reduce the incidence of travelers' diarrhea.

Military Epidemiology

Deployed military personnel are a unique population of travelers that have a long history of being affected by acute infectious diarrhea.[11,137] Although not likely to be fatal, the short-term morbidity associated with diarrhea increases healthcare service use, loss of man-hours, and transient shortages in the deployed force. Although the military has developed extensive capabilities for the provision of clean food and water, diarrhea has continued to be a problem for deployed personnel. A series of studies assessing the health of US troops deployed to Iraq and Afghanistan have found that despite the use of current preventive medicine practices, diarrhea incidence and morbidity remain high, with a monthly attack rate of >30% resulting in over three-quarters of troops reporting at least one episode.[138,139] Nearly half of the troops who developed diarrhea stated that it was severe enough for them to seek medical care at least once, translating to a monthly estimated incidence of six clinic visits per 100 person-months for treatment of diarrhea. Combining results from Iraq and Afghanistan, 46% of the episodes of diarrhea were reported to reduce job performance for an average of 2 days. Extrapolated to the entire population, it was estimated that 13 days of job performance per 100 person-months were lost due to diarrhea. In 14% of the cases diarrhea resulted in the troops being confined to bed for a median of 2 days, and 2% were hospitalized, resulting in an estimated 3.7 days of complete work loss per 100 person-months.[140] During the initial invasion of Iraq, the incidence of diarrhea doubled from the pre-combat to the combat phase, and the perceived impact of these illnesses on the unit increased significantly during the combat phase, resulting in 40% of those ill seeking care from a medical provider, and of these 14% were removed from duty for >24 h.[140]

The pathogens associated with diarrhea in military personnel are typically the same as those that affect civilian travelers.[11] Enterotoxigenic *E. coli* (ETEC) and enteroaggregative *E. coli* (EAEC) were the two most common pathogens isolated from troops deployed in Iraq and Afghanistan.[140] The main risk factor for acquiring diarrhea in military personnel, as with civilian travelers, is the consumption of local food,[13] which was true for two-thirds of troops deployed to Iraq.[141] Most often, personnel choose to eat local food simply to experience the local cuisine, but during the initial 'combat phase' in Iraq, one-third of soldiers reported they were unable to access clean food or water, which probably contributed to the high rates of diarrhea.[140] Furthermore, because military deployments are often associated with overcrowding and poor hygiene, organisms transmitted person-to-person or requiring small inocula for infection may occur in outbreaks. Multiple outbreaks of nausea and vomiting due to noroviruses and severe diarrhea due to *Shigella* species have been reported.[43]

A distinction is sometimes made between travelers' diarrhea and diarrhea among populations living overseas for extended periods, such as military personnel on long deployments. Since the increasingly

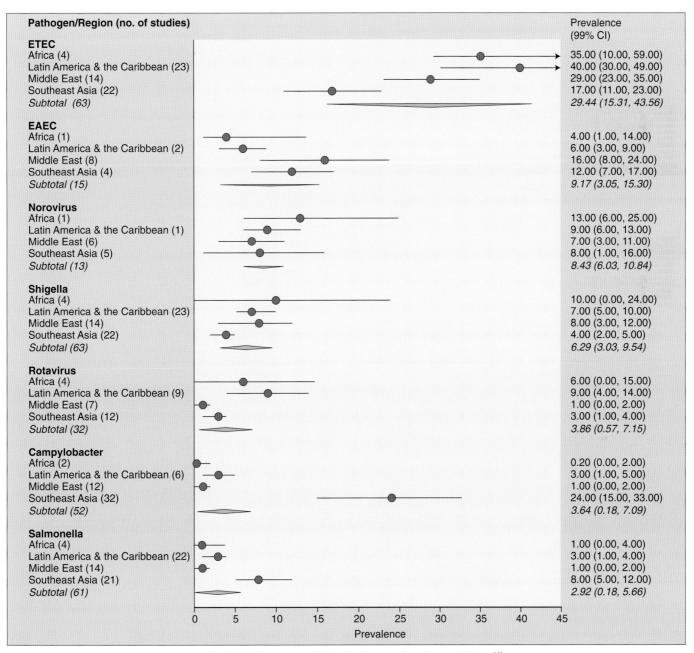

Pathogen/Region (no. of studies)	Prevalence (99% CI)
ETEC	
Africa (4)	35.00 (10.00, 59.00)
Latin America & the Caribbean (23)	40.00 (30.00, 49.00)
Middle East (14)	29.00 (23.00, 35.00)
Southeast Asia (22)	17.00 (11.00, 23.00)
Subtotal (63)	*29.44 (15.31, 43.56)*
EAEC	
Africa (1)	4.00 (1.00, 14.00)
Latin America & the Caribbean (2)	6.00 (3.00, 9.00)
Middle East (8)	16.00 (8.00, 24.00)
Southeast Asia (4)	12.00 (7.00, 17.00)
Subtotal (15)	*9.17 (3.05, 15.30)*
Norovirus	
Africa (1)	13.00 (6.00, 25.00)
Latin America & the Caribbean (1)	9.00 (6.00, 13.00)
Middle East (6)	7.00 (3.00, 11.00)
Southeast Asia (5)	8.00 (1.00, 16.00)
Subtotal (13)	*8.43 (6.03, 10.84)*
Shigella	
Africa (4)	10.00 (0.00, 24.00)
Latin America & the Caribbean (23)	7.00 (5.00, 10.00)
Middle East (14)	8.00 (3.00, 12.00)
Southeast Asia (22)	4.00 (2.00, 5.00)
Subtotal (63)	*6.29 (3.03, 9.54)*
Rotavirus	
Africa (4)	6.00 (0.00, 15.00)
Latin America & the Caribbean (9)	9.00 (4.00, 14.00)
Middle East (7)	1.00 (0.00, 2.00)
Southeast Asia (12)	3.00 (1.00, 4.00)
Subtotal (32)	*3.86 (0.57, 7.15)*
Campylobacter	
Africa (2)	0.20 (0.00, 2.00)
Latin America & the Caribbean (6)	3.00 (1.00, 5.00)
Middle East (12)	1.00 (0.00, 2.00)
Southeast Asia (32)	24.00 (15.00, 33.00)
Subtotal (52)	*3.64 (0.18, 7.09)*
Salmonella	
Africa (4)	1.00 (0.00, 4.00)
Latin America & the Caribbean (22)	3.00 (1.00, 4.00)
Middle East (14)	1.00 (0.00, 2.00)
Southeast Asia (21)	8.00 (5.00, 12.00)
Subtotal (61)	*2.92 (0.18, 5.66)*

Prevalence

Figure 18.4 Pathogen prevalence associated with diarrhea among deployed military and similar populations.[142]

global economy has led to both an increase in short-term travelers and an increase in populations from developed countries moving to and residing for lengthier periods in developing countries, it is important to look for differences in the epidemiology of diarrhea in these groups. A recent systematic review of the literature determined regional estimates of pathogen-specific prevalence and incidence associated with diarrhea among deployed US military and similar populations living for longer periods overseas.[142] A total of 52 studies conducted between January 1990 and June 2005 fulfilled inclusion criteria. A majority of the studies were conducted among US military populations (63%) with foreign military, expatriate (including NGOs and embassy populations) and student populations, each consisting of about 12%. Overall, 37% were from the Middle East, 31% from SE Asia, 24% from Latin America/Caribbean, and 6% from sub-Saharan Africa. Median duration of travel was 1.5 months. Similar to short-term traveler studies, ETEC, *Campylobacter* and *Shigella* were identified as causing 38–45% of diarrhea, with regional and population differences (Figure 18.4). Incidence based on self-report was higher than studies using passive surveillance or clinical-based methods (29 versus 7 versus 6 episodes per 100 person-months, respectively) without regional differences.

Conclusion

TD is a common illness that affects up to half of travelers during their first 2 weeks abroad. Symptoms are for the most part short-lived, but may incapacitate and lay ruin to a carefully planned vacation or business trip. Effective pre-travel counseling may motivate some travelers to avoid risky food and drink, which may in turn reduce diarrheal incidence. Since most TD is bacterial in origin, traveling with appropriate antibiotics for both treatment and prevention is also important.

References

1. Greenwood Z, Black J, Weld L, et al. Gastrointestinal infection among international travelers globally. J Travel Med 2008;15(4):221–8.
2. Ryan ET, Kain KC. Health advice and immunizations for travelers. N Engl J Med 2000;342(23):1716–25.
3. Echeverria P, Blacklow NR, Sanford LB, et al. Travelers' diarrhea among American Peace Corps volunteers in rural Thailand. J Infect Dis 1981;143(6):767–71.
4. Guerrant RL, Rouse JD, Hughes JM, et al. Turista among members of the Yale Glee Club in Latin America. Am J Trop Med Hyg 1980;29(5):895–900.
5. Hill DR. Occurrence and self-treatment of diarrhea in a large cohort of Americans traveling to developing countries. Am J Trop Med Hyg 2000;62(5):585–9.
6. Merson MH, Morris GK, Sack DA, et al. Travelers' diarrhea in Mexico. A prospective study of physicians and family members attending a congress. N Engl J Med 1976;294(24):1299–305.
7. Steffen R, van der Linde F, Gyr K, et al. Epidemiology of diarrhea in travelers. JAMA 1983;249(9):1176–80.
8. von Sonnenburg F, Tornieporth N, Waiyaki P, et al. Risk and aetiology of diarrhoea at various tourist destinations. Lancet 2000;356(9224):133–4.
9. Steffen R. Epidemiology of travellers' diarrhoea. Scand J Gastroenterol Suppl 1983;84:5–17.
10. Steffen R, Rickenbach M, Wilhelm U, et al. Health problems after travel to developing countries. J Infect Dis 1987;156(1):84–91.
11. Connor P, Farthing MJ. Travellers' diarrhoea: a military problem? J R Army Med Corps 1999;145(2):95–101.
12. Hyams KC, Bourgeois AL, Merrell BR, et al. Diarrheal disease during Operation Desert Shield. N Engl J Med 1991;325(20):1423–8.
13. Sanchez JL, Gelnett J, Petruccelli BP, et al. Diarrheal disease incidence and morbidity among United States military personnel during short-term missions overseas. Am J Trop Med Hyg 1998;58(3):299–304.
14. Steffen R, Collard F, Tornieporth N, et al. Epidemiology, etiology, and impact of traveler's diarrhea in Jamaica. JAMA 1999;281(9):811–7.
15. Black RE. Epidemiology of travelers' diarrhea and relative importance of various pathogens. Rev Infect Dis 1990;12(Suppl. 1):S73–9.
16. Lim ML, Wallace MR. Infectious diarrhea in history. Infect Dis Clin North Am 2004;18(2):261–74.
17. Kean BH. The Diarrhea of Travelers to Mexico. Summary of Five-Year Study. Ann Intern Med 1963;59:605–14.
18. Rowe B, Taylor J, Bettelheim KA. An investigation of traveller's diarrhoea. Lancet 1970;1(7636):1–5.
19. Gorbach SL, Banwell JG, Chatterjee BD, et al. Acute undifferentiated human diarrhea in the tropics. I. Alterations in intestinal micrflora. J Clin Invest 1971;50(4):881–9.
20. Sack RB, Gorbach SL, Banwell JG. Enterotoxigenic Escherichia coli isolated from patients with severe cholera-like disease. J Infect Dis 1971;123:378–85.
21. DuPont HL, Formal SB, Hornick RB, et al. Pathogenesis of Escherichia coli diarrhea. N Engl J Med 1971;285(1):1–9.
22. Gorbach SL, Kean BH, Evans DG. Travelers' diarrhea and toxigenic Escherichia coli diarrhea. N Engl J Med 1975;292:933–6.
23. Echeverria P, Sack RB, Blacklow NR, et al. Prophylactic doxycycline for travelers' diarrhea in Thailand. Further supportive evidence of Aeromonas hydrophila as an enteric pathogen. Am J Epidemiol 1984;120(6):912–21.
24. Sanders JW, Isenbarger DW, Walz SE, et al. An observational clinic-based study of diarrheal illness in deployed United States military personnel in Thailand: presentation and outcome of Campylobacter infection. Am J Trop Med Hyg 2002;67(5):533–8.
25. Ericsson CD, Patterson TF, Dupont HL. Clinical presentation as a guide to therapy for travelers' diarrhea. Am J Med Sci 1987;294(2):91–6.
26. Svenungsson B, Lagergren A, Ekwall E, et al. Enteropathogens in adult patients with diarrhea and healthy control subjects: a 1-year prospective study in a Swedish clinic for infectious diseases. Clin Infect Dis 2000;30(5):770–8.
27. Mattila L. Clinical features and duration of traveler's diarrhea in relation to its etiology. Clin Infect Dis 1994;19(4):728–34.
28. Hoge CW, Gambel JM, Srijan A, et al. Trends in antibiotic resistance among diarrheal pathogens isolated in Thailand over 15 years. Clin Infect Dis 1998;26(2):341–5.
29. Hoge CW, Shlim DR, Echeverria P, et al. Epidemiology of diarrhea among expatriate residents living in a highly endemic environment. JAMA 1996;275(7):533–8.
30. Jiang ZD, Mathewson JJ, Ericsson CD, et al. Characterization of enterotoxigenic Escherichia coli strains in patients with travelers' diarrhea acquired in Guadalajara, Mexico, 1992–1997. J Infect Dis 2000;181(2):779–82.
31. Keskimaki M, Mattila L, Peltola H, et al. Prevalence of diarrheagenic Escherichia coli in Finns with or without diarrhea during a round-the-world trip. J Clin Microbiol 2000;38(12):4425–9.
32. Taylor DN, Houston R, Shlim DR, et al. Etiology of diarrhea among travelers and foreign residents in Nepal. JAMA 1988;260(9):1245–8.
33. Rosenberg ML, Koplan JP, Wachsmuth IK, et al. Epidemic diarrhea at Crater Lake from enterotoxigenic Escherichia coli. A large waterborne outbreak. Ann Intern Med 1977;86(6):714–8.
34. Levine MM. Escherichia coli that cause diarrhea: enterotoxigenic, enteropathogenic, enteroinvasive, enterohemorrhagic, and enteroadherent. J Infect Dis 1987;155(3):377–89.
35. Wanke CA. To know Escherichia coli is to know bacterial diarrheal disease. Clin Infect Dis 2001;32(12):1710–2.
36. Wong CS, Jelacic S, Habeeb RL, et al. The risk of the hemolytic-uremic syndrome after antibiotic treatment of Escherichia coli O157: H7 infections. N Engl J Med 2000;342(26):1930–6.
37. Knutton S, Baldwin T, Williams PH, et al. Actin accumulation at sites of bacterial adhesion to tissue culture cells: basis of a new diagnostic test for enteropathogenic and enterohemorrhagic Escherichia coli. Infect Immun 1989;57(4):1290–8.
38. Adachi JA, Jiang ZD, Mathewson JJ, et al. Enteroaggregative Escherichia coli as a major etiologic agent in traveler's diarrhea in 3 regions of the world. Clin Infect Dis 2001;32(12):1706–9.
39. Taylor D. Campylobacter Infections in Developing Countries. In: Nachamkin I, Blaser M, Tompkins L, editors. Campylobacter jejuni:

current status and future trends. Washington, DC: American Society for Microbiology; 1992. p. 20–30.

40. Allos BM. Campylobacter jejuni infections: update on emerging issues and trends. Clin Infect Dis 2001;32(8):1201–6.

41. Kuschner RA, Trofa AF, Thomas RJ, et al. Use of azithromycin for the treatment of Campylobacter enteritis in travelers to Thailand, an area where ciprofloxacin resistance is prevalent. Clin Infect Dis 1995;21(3):536–41.

42. Sharp TW, Thornton SA, Wallace MR, et al. Diarrheal disease among military personnel during Operation Restore Hope, Somalia, 1992–1993. Am J Trop Med Hyg 1995;52(2):188–93.

43. Thornton SA, Sherman SS, Farkas T, et al. Gastroenteritis in US Marines during Operation Iraqi Freedom. Clin Infect Dis 2005;40(4):519–25.

44. Kotloff KL, Winickoff JP, Ivanoff B, et al. Global burden of Shigella infections: implications for vaccine development and implementation of control strategies. Bull World Health Organ 1999;77(8):651–66.

45. Vu DT, Sethabutr O, Von Seidlein L, et al. Detection of Shigella by a PCR assay targeting the ipaH gene suggests increased prevalence of shigellosis in Nha Trang, Vietnam. J Clin Microbiol 2004;42(5):2031–5.

46. Sriratanaban A, Reinprayoon S. Vibrio parahaemolyticus: a major cause of travelers' diarrhea in Bangkok. Am J Trop Med Hyg 1982;31(1):128–30.

47. Taylor DN, Rizzo J, Meza R, et al. Cholera among Americans living in Peru. Clin Infect Dis 1996;22(6):1108–9.

48. Greenberg HB, Matsui SM. Astroviruses and caliciviruses: emerging enteric pathogens. Infect Agents Dis 1992;1(2):71–91.

49. Deneen VC, Hunt JM, Paule CR, et al. The impact of foodborne calicivirus disease: the Minnesota experience. J Infect Dis 2000;181(Suppl 2):S281–3.

50. Moe CL, Gentsch J, Ando T, et al. Application of PCR to detect Norwalk virus in fecal specimens from outbreaks of gastroenteritis. J Clin Microbiol 1994;32(3):642–8.

51. Schwab KJ, Neill FH, Fankhauser RL, et al. Development of methods to detect 'Norwalk-like viruses' (NLVs) and hepatitis A virus in delicatessen foods: application to a food-borne NLV outbreak. Appl Environ Microbiol 2000;66(1):213–8.

52. Herwaldt BL, Lew JF, Moe CL, et al. Characterization of a variant strain of Norwalk virus from a food-borne outbreak of gastroenteritis on a cruise ship in Hawaii. J Clin Microbiol 1994;32(4):861–6.

53. Khan AS, Moe CL, Glass RI, et al. Norwalk virus-associated gastroenteritis traced to ice consumption aboard a cruise ship in Hawaii: comparison and application of molecular method-based assays. J Clin Microbiol 1994;32(2):318–22.

54. Koo D, Maloney K, Tauxe R. Epidemiology of diarrheal disease outbreaks on cruise ships, 1986 through 1993. JAMA 1996;275(7):545–7.

55. McEvoy M, Blake W, Brown D, et al. An outbreak of viral gastroenteritis on a cruise ship. Commun Dis Rep CDR Rev 1996;6(13):R188–92.

56. Sekla L, Stackiw W, Dzogan S, et al. Foodborne gastroenteritis due to Norwalk virus in a Winnipeg hotel. CMAJ 1989;140(12):1461–4.

57. Ko G, Garcia C, Jiang ZD, et al. Noroviruses as a cause of traveler's diarrhea among students from the United States visiting Mexico. J Clin Microbiol 2005;43(12):6126–9.

58. Hyams KC, Malone JD, Kapikian AZ, et al. Norwalk virus infection among Desert Storm troops. J Infect Dis 1993;167:986–7.

59. Cuffari C, Oligny L, Seidman EG. Dientamoeba fragilis masquerading as allergic colitis. J Pediatr Gastroenterol Nutr 1998;26(1):16–20.

60. Raynaud L, Delbac F, Broussolle V et al. Identification of Encephalitozoon intestinalis in travelers with chronic diarrhea by specific PCR amplification. J Clin Microbiol 1998;36(1):37–40.

61. Thielman NM, Guerrant RL. Persistent diarrhea in the returned traveler. Infect Dis Clin North Am 1998;12(2):489–501.

62. Wanke CA, DeGirolami P, Federman M. Enterocytozoon bieneusi infection and diarrheal disease in patients who were not infected with human immunodeficiency virus: case report and review. Clin Infect Dis 1996;23(4):816–8.

63. Herwaldt BL, de Arroyave KR, Wahlquist SP, et al. Multiyear prospective study of intestinal parasitism in a cohort of Peace Corps volunteers in Guatemala. J Clin Microbiol 2001;39(1):34–42.

64. Shlim DR, Hoge CW, Rajah R, et al. Persistent high risk of diarrhea among foreigners in Nepal during the first 2 years of residence. Clin Infect Dis 1999;29(3):613–6.

65. Tomkins AM, James WP, Drasar BS. Proceedings: A malabsorption syndrome in overland travellers to India: mucosal colonization by bacteria. Gut 1974;15(4):340.

66. Wright SG, Tomkins AM, Ridley DS. Giardiasis: clinical and therapeutic aspects. Gut 1977;18(5):343–50.

67. Nash TE, Herrington DA, Losonsky GA, et al. Experimental human infections with Giardia lamblia. J Infect Dis 1987;156(6):974–84.

68. Okhuysen PC. Traveler's diarrhea due to intestinal protozoa. Clin Infect Dis 2001;33(1):110–4.

69. Hardie RM, Wall PG, Gott P, et al. Infectious diarrhea in tourists staying in a resort hotel. Emerg Infect Dis 1999;5(1):168–71.

70. Johnston SP, Ballard MM, Beach MJ, et al. Evaluation of three commercial assays for detection of Giardia and Cryptosporidium organisms in fecal specimens. J Clin Microbiol 2003;41(2):623–6.

71. Goka AK, Rolston DD, Mathan VI, et al. The relative merits of faecal and duodenal juice microscopy in the diagnosis of giardiasis. Trans R Soc Trop Med Hyg 1990;84(1):66–7.

72. Jackson TF. Entamoeba histolytica and Entamoeba dispar are distinct species; clinical, epidemiological and serological evidence. Int J Parasitol 1998;28(1):181–6.

73. Nanda R, Baveja U, Anand BS. Entamoeba histolytica cyst passers: clinical features and outcome in untreated subjects. Lancet 1984;2(8398):301–3.

74. Evangelopoulos A, Legakis N, Vakalis N. Microscopy, PCR and ELISA applied to the epidemiology of amoebiasis in Greece. Parasitol Int 2001;50(3):185–9.

75. Qvarnstrom Y, James C, Xayavong M, et al. Comparison of real-time PCR protocols for differential laboratory diagnosis of amebiasis. J Clin Microbiol 2005;43(11):5491–7.

76. Hoge CW, Shlim DR, Rajah R, et al. Epidemiology of diarrhoeal illness associated with coccidian-like organism among travellers and foreign residents in Nepal. Lancet 1993;341(8854):1175–9.

77. Herwaldt BL, Ackers ML. An outbreak in 1996 of cyclosporiasis associated with imported raspberries. The Cyclospora Working Group. N Engl J Med 1997;336(22):1548–56.

78. Shaffer N, Moore L. Chronic travelers' diarrhea in a normal host due to Isospora belli. J Infect Dis 1989;159(3):596–7.

79. Abdel-Messih IA, Wierzba TF, Abu-Elyazeed R, et al. Diarrhea associated with Cryptosporidium parvum among young children of the Nile River Delta in Egypt. J Trop Pediatr 2005;51(3):154–9.

80. Sanders JW, Putnam SD, Gould P, et al. Diarrheal illness among deployed U.S. military personnel during Operation Bright Star 2001–Egypt. Diagn Microbiol Infect Dis 2005;52(2):85–90.

81. MacKenzie WR, Schell WL, Blair KA, et al. Massive outbreak of waterborne cryptosporidium infection in Milwaukee, Wisconsin: recurrence of illness and risk of secondary transmission. Clin Infect Dis 1995;21(1):57–62.

82. Jokipii AM, Hemila M, Jokipii L. Prospective study of acquisition of Cryptosporidium, Giardia lamblia, and gastrointestinal illness. Lancet 1985;2(8453):487–9.

83. Shlim DR, Hoge CW, Rajah R, et al. Is Blastocystis hominis a cause of diarrhea in travelers? A prospective controlled study in Nepal. Clin Infect Dis 1995;21(1):97–101.

84. Black RE, Merson MH, Rowe B, et al. Enterotoxigenic Escherichia coli diarrhoea: acquired immunity and transmission in an endemic area. Bull World Health Organ 1981;59(2):263–8.

85. Pitzinger B, Steffen R, Tschopp A. Incidence and clinical features of traveler's diarrhea in infants and children. Pediatr Infect Dis J 1991;10(10):719–23.

86. Hagmann S, Neugebauer R, Schwartz E, et al. Illness in children after international travel: analysis from the GeoSentinel Surveillance Network. Pediatrics 2010;125(5):e1072–80.

87. Ryder RW, Wells JG, Gangarosa EJ. A study of travelers' diarrhea in foreign visitors to the United States. J Infect Dis 1977;136:605–7.

88. Loewenstein MS, Balows A, Gangarosa EJ. Turista at an international congress in Mexico. Lancet 1973;1(7802):529–31.

89. Ryder RW, Oquist CA, Greenberg H, et al. Travelers' diarrhea in Panamanian tourists in Mexico. J Infect Dis 1981;144(5):442–8.

90. Levine MM, Nalin DR, Hoover DL, et al. Immunity to enterotoxigenic Escherichia coli. Infect Immun 1979;23(3):729–36.

91. Levine MM, Rennels MB, Cisneros L, et al. Lack of person-to-person transmission of enterotoxigenic Escherichia coli despite close contact. Am J Epidemiol 1980;111(3):347–55.

92. Dupont HL, Haynes GA, Pickering LK, et al. Diarrhea of travelers to Mexico. Relative susceptibility of United States and Latin American students attending a Mexican University. Am J Epidemiol 1977;105(1):37–41.

93. Herwaldt BL, de Arroyave KR, Roberts JM, et al. A multiyear prospective study of the risk factors for and incidence of diarrheal illness in a cohort of Peace Corps volunteers in Guatemala. Ann Intern Med 2000;132(12):982–8.

94. Steffen R. Epidemiologic studies of travelers' diarrhea, severe gastrointestinal infections, and cholera. Rev Infect Dis 1986;8(Suppl 2):S122–30.

95. Guerrant RL, Hughes JM, Lima NL, et al. Diarrhea in developed and developing countries: magnitude, special settings, and etiologies. Rev Infect Dis 1990;12(Suppl 1):S41–50.

96. Marionneau S, Ruvoen N, Le Moullac-Vaidye B, et al. Norwalk virus binds to histo-blood group antigens present on gastroduodenal epithelial cells of secretor individuals. Gastroenterology 2002;122(7):1967–77.

97. Huang P, Farkas T, Marionneau S, et al. Noroviruses bind to human ABO, Lewis, and secretor histo-blood group antigens: identification of 4 distinct strain-specific patterns. J Infect Dis 2003;188(1):19–31.

98. Hutson AM, Atmar RL, Estes MK. Norovirus disease: changing epidemiology and host susceptibility factors. Trends Microbiol 2004;12(6):279–87.

99. Jiang ZD, Okhuysen PC, Guo DC, et al. Genetic susceptibility to enteroaggregative Escherichia coli diarrhea: polymorphism in the interleukin-8 promotor region. J Infect Dis 2003;188(4):506–11.

100. Mohamed JA, DuPont HL, Jiang ZD, et al. A novel single-nucleotide polymorphism in the lactoferrin gene is associated with susceptibility to diarrhea in North American travelers to Mexico. Clin Infect Dis 2007;44(7):945–52.

101. Tjoa WS, DuPont HL, Sullivan P, et al. Location of food consumption and travelers' diarrhea. Am J Epidemiol 1977;106(1):61–6.

102. Kozicki M, Steffen R, Schar M. 'Boil it, cook it, peel it or forget it': does this rule prevent travellers' diarrhoea? Int J Epidemiol 1985;14(1):169–72.

103. McIntosh IB, Reed JM, Power KG. Travellers' diarrhoea and the effect of pre-travel health advice in general practice. Br J Gen Pract 1997;47(415):71–5.

104. Yazdanpanah Y, Beaugerie L, Boelle PY, et al. Risk factors of acute diarrhoea in summer–a nation-wide French case-control study. Epidemiol Infect 2000;124(3):409–16.

105. Ericsson CD, Pickering LK, Sullivan P, et al. The role of location of food consumption in the prevention of travelers' diarrhea in Mexico. Gastroenterology 1980;79(5,Pt 1):812–6.

106. DuPont H. Travellers' diarrhoea. Clin Res Rev 1981;1:225–34.

107. Glass RI, Noel J, Ando T, et al. The epidemiology of enteric caliciviruses from humans: a reassessment using new diagnostics. J Infect Dis 2000;181(Suppl 2):S254–61.

108. Ho MS, Glass RI, Monroe SS, et al. Viral gastroenteritis aboard a cruise ship. Lancet 1989;2(8669):961–5.

109. Parashar U, Quiroz ES, Mounts AW, et al. 'Norwalk-like viruses'. Public health consequences and outbreak management. MMWR Recomm Rep 2001;50(RR-9):1–17.

110. Black RE. Pathogens that cause travelers' diarrhea in Latin America and Africa. Rev Infect Dis 1986;8(Suppl 2):S131–5.

111. Taylor DN, Echeverria P. Etiology and epidemiology of travelers' diarrhea in Asia. Rev Infect Dis 1986;8(Suppl 2):S136–41.

112. Echeverria P, Jackson LR, Hoge CW, et al. Diarrhea in U.S. troops deployed to Thailand. J Clin Microbiol 1993;31(12):3351–2.

113. Mattila L, Siitonen A, Kyronseppa H, et al. Seasonal variation in etiology of travelers' diarrhea. Finnish-Moroccan Study Group. J Infect Dis 1992;165(2):385–8.

114. Bouckenooghe AR, Jiang ZD, De La Cabada FJ, et al. Enterotoxigenic Escherichia coli as cause of diarrhea among Mexican adults and US travelers in Mexico. J Travel Med 2002;9(3):137–40.

124. Ji S, Park H, Lee D, et al. Post-infectious irritable bowel syndrome in patients with Shigella infection. J Gastroenterol Hepatol 2005;20(3):381–6.

125. McKendrick MW, Read NW. Irritable bowel syndrome–post salmonella infection. J Infect 1994;29(1):1–3.

126. Mearin F, Perez-Oliveras M, Perello A, et al. Dyspepsia and irritable bowel syndrome after a Salmonella gastroenteritis outbreak: one-year follow-up cohort study. Gastroenterology 2005;129(1):98–104.

127. Neal KR, Hebden J, Spiller R. Prevalence of gastrointestinal symptoms six months after bacterial gastroenteritis and risk factors for development of the irritable bowel syndrome: postal survey of patients. BMJ 1997;314(7083):779–82.

128. Okhuysen PC, Jiang ZD, Carlin L, et al. Post-diarrhea chronic intestinal symptoms and irritable bowel syndrome in North American travelers to Mexico. Am J Gastroenterol 2004;99(9):1774–8.

129. Parry SD, Stansfield R, Jelley D, et al. Does bacterial gastroenteritis predispose people to functional gastrointestinal disorders? A prospective, community-based, case-control study. Am J Gastroenterol 2003;98(9):1970–5.

130. Rodriguez LA, Ruigomez A. Increased risk of irritable bowel syndrome after bacterial gastroenteritis: cohort study. BMJ 1999;318(7183):565–6.

131. Spiller RC, Jenkins D, Thornley JP, et al. Increased rectal mucosal enteroendocrine cells, T lymphocytes, and increased gut permeability following acute Campylobacter enteritis and in post-dysenteric irritable bowel syndrome. Gut 2000;47(6):804–11.

132. Thornley JP, Jenkins D, Neal K, et al. Relationship of Campylobacter toxigenicity in vitro to the development of postinfectious irritable bowel syndrome. J Infect Dis 2001;184(5):606–9.

133. Wang LH, Fang XC, Pan GZ. Bacillary dysentery as a causative factor of irritable bowel syndrome and its pathogenesis. Gut 2004;53(8):1096–101.

134. Halvorson HA, Schlett CD, Riddle MS. Postinfectious irritable bowel syndrome–a meta-analysis. Am J Gastroenterol 2006;101(8):1894–9; quiz 1942.

135. Trivedi KH, Schlett CD, Tribble DR, et al. The impact of post-infectious functional gastrointestinal disorders and symptoms on the health-related quality of life of US military personnel returning from deployment to the Middle East. Digestive Disease Sciences 2011;in press.

136. Stermer E, Lubezky A, Potasman I, et al. Is traveler's diarrhea a significant risk factor for the development of irritable bowel syndrome? A prospective study. Clin Infect Dis 2006;43(7):898–901.

137. Cook GC. Influence of diarrhoeal disease on military and naval campaigns. J R Soc Med 2001;94(2):95–7.

138. Sanders JW, Putnam SD, Riddle MS, et al. Military importance of diarrhea: Lessons from The Middle East. Curr Opin Gastroenterol 2005;21(1):9–14.

139. Sanders JW, Putnam SD, Riddle MS, et al. The epidemiology of self-reported diarrhea in Operations Iraqi Freedom and Enduring Freedom. Diagn Microbiol Infect Dis 2004;50(2):89–93.

140. Sanders JW, Putnam SD, Frankart C, et al. Impact of illness and non-combat injury during Operations Iraqi Freedom and Enduring Freedom (Afghanistan). Am J Trop Med Hyg 2005;73(4):713–9.

141. Putnam SD, Sanders JW, Frenck RW, et al. Self-reported description of diarrhea among military populations in operations Iraqi Freedom and Enduring Freedom. J Travel Med 2006;13(2):92–9.

142. Riddle MS, Sanders JW, Putnam SD, et al. Incidence, etiology, and impact of diarrhea among long-term travelers (US military and similar populations): a systematic review. Am J Trop Med Hyg 2006;74(5):891–900.

143. Shah N, DuPont HL, Ramsey DJ. Global etiology of travelers' diarrhea: systematic review from 1973 to the present. Am J Trop Med Hyg 2009;80(4):609–14.

144. de la Cabada Bauche J, Dupont HL. New Developments in Traveler's Diarrhea. Gastroenterol Hepatol (N Y) 2011;7(2):88–95.

19

Prevention of Travelers' Diarrhea

Charles D. Ericsson

Key points

- Controlling food and beverage risks for travelers' diarrhea by dietary behavior modification is largely unsuccessful
- Currently available vaccines can protect against only a small proportion of travelers' diarrhea
- Agents such as bismuth subsalicylate and selected antimicrobials effectively prevent a substantial proportion of travelers' diarrhea
- Benefits of prevention include less loss of productivity and vacation and decreased risk of post-infectious irritable bowel syndrome
- The alternative to prophylaxis has been early self-treatment, but the availability now of a safe and effective preventive agent may shift the travelers' diarrhea management paradigm toward more liberal use of prophylaxis

Introduction

Given the incidence and morbidity of travelers' diarrhea, a logical question is: can the syndrome be prevented? After all, preventive measures are generally more cost-effective and practical than treating a disease and its complications. In travelers' diarrhea, preventive modalities need to be compared with the benefits of early self-treatment with the highly efficacious combination of a single dose of antibiotic and an agent such as loperamide.[1–7]

The two major approaches to prevention have been risk avoidance via educational interventions and chemoprophylaxis with antimicrobial and other agents. These prevention strategies are summarized in Table 19.1. Vaccination as a prevention strategy is discussed in more detail in Section 3. Suffice it to say, vaccine protection against typhoid and cholera is not particularly relevant in a discussion of preventing travelers' diarrhea. Both typhoid and cholera are uncommon among travelers and any cross-protection of cholera vaccines against LT toxin-producing E. coli will only afford a small degree of protection against the syndrome in general.

The Impact of Prevention

Any measure that can prevent a substantial percentage of millions of cases of diarrhea should be seriously considered. In 1985, a consensus development conference at the National Institutes of Health concluded, however, that the risk of adverse events associated with millions of people taking antibiotics or bismuth subsalicylate simply exceeded the potential benefits of preventing a relatively trivial, self-limiting syndrome.[8] These experts also expressed concern for such antimicrobial use contributing to the burden of resistance development; however, over the ensuing years many experts have felt that antibiotic use that might contribute to resistance development in a developing nation is very small among travelers compared with injudicious use among the indigenous population. Apparently not considered was the opinion of travelers, who are likely to consider travelers' diarrhea an important syndrome because of its high incidence and considerable potential for vexatious morbidity.

Travelers' diarrhea can potentially affect up to 60–70% of the 80+ million persons traveling from developed to developing countries each year.[9] Although it is rarely lethal, and hospitalization is uncommon, travelers' diarrhea may put a person to bed for a day or ruin a trip. Since the consensus development conference, another important variable has emerged. In one study among many that exemplify the problem, about 18% of those developing travelers' diarrhea had persisting gastrointestinal disturbance 6 months later, compared to a much lower incidence of symptoms among those who did not develop travelers' diarrhea. Over half of the 18% with persisting symptoms met Rome II criteria for irritable bowel syndrome.[10]

The predominant cause of the travelers' diarrhea syndrome was determined to be bacterial enteropathogens, and prophylaxis studies focused on antimicrobial agents. When local strains were susceptible to the antimicrobial agent studied, 80–90% protection against diarrhea could be realized.[1–7]

Bismuth subsalicylate (BSS) afforded 40–65% protection depending on the dose.[11] Other interventions have shown variable but generally disappointing results (e.g., probiotics), or simply have not been adequately studied (e.g., behavior modification). The availability of a safe and effective non-absorbable antimicrobial agent, rifaximin, which is effective in the treatment and prevention of travelers' diarrhea, has re-kindled interest in chemoprophylaxis.

Prevention Strategies

Identifying Hosts at Risk

Classically, chemoprophylaxis was considered based on the riskiness of the traveler's itinerary, the criticality of remaining well during the

Table 19.1 Current Strategies for the Prevention of Travelers' Diarrhea

Strategy	Protection Rates	Comments
Risk behavior modification	Generally low	Considered the cornerstone of prevention; however, advice is often ignored or hard to follow owing to ubiquitous exposure. Must be simple and practical.
Chemoprophylaxis with:		
Bismuth subsalicylate	≤65%	Inconvenient dosing regimen: 2 tablets chewed 4 times a day. May cause black stools and tongue. Salicylate is absorbed, so it should not be used with warfarin and NSAIDs. Not available in all countries.
Absorbable antimicrobial agents Fluoroquinolones (Azithromycin)	50–80%	Once-daily dosing is convenient. Effective when regional microbiology and susceptibilities are considered. May cause side-effects and induce resistance. Less effective in areas with higher resistance. Resistance is high enough worldwide that TMP/SMX can no longer be recommended. Azithromycin has not been studied so efficacy and optimal dose are not known.
Non-absorbed antimicrobial agent, Rifaximin	60–70%	Once-daily dosing is convenient. Very safe. Resistance development not likely a problem. No regional constraints due to resistance. Not available in all countries.
Probiotics	Variable	Clinical trial evidence is conflicting. Relatively safe.

trip, and host risk factors. Known epidemiologic risk factors that do not necessarily argue for chemoprophylaxis are: resident of a developed country traveling to a developing country, no travel to a tropical area in the past 6 months, and higher socioeconomic status.

Chemoprophylaxis might be considered for adventure or 'extreme' travel when travelers will be obliged to consume food and drink under unsanitary conditions, and particularly when they are far removed from medical care and cannot afford even a day's inconvenience, while self-therapy brings the disease under control. Arguably such travelers may also be less likely to respond to attempts at behavior modification. Travelers to developing countries who admit they will disregard safe food and water recommendations might also be candidates for chemoprophylaxis regardless of their itinerary; however, they must be cautioned not to become complacent about their risks, since viral and most parasitic causes of travelers' diarrhea will not be prevented by agents such as azithromycin, fluoroquinolones, or rifaximin.

Criticality of travel is a subjective issue, which ideally should be decided by the traveler after discussion between the practitioner and the client about the risks and benefits of chemoprophylaxis. Business persons who are treated to risky local cuisine and do not wish to offend their hosts by refusing items from the planned menu might be candidates for chemoprophylaxis. Likewise, governmental officials on critical missions might be included. However, does a honeymooning couple critically need chemoprophylaxis? Perhaps the couple should decide after being educated about their risks of travelers' diarrhea and the risks and benefits of chemoprophylaxis. At-risk hosts include those for whom the incidence of diarrhea can be predicted to be higher, or those with higher risks of complications. Although young age (<6 years) is a relative risk factor for travelers' diarrhea, it is generally not considered sufficient to argue for chemoprophylaxis. On the other hand, adolescents and young adults are also relatively at risk and might be candidates, especially if they intend to be adventurous eaters. Conditions that warrant strong consideration of chemoprophylaxis are reduced gastric acidity and diminished host defenses (e.g., immunodeficiency associated with malignancy and its therapy, transplantation, and HIV infection). Some hosts face a potentially worse course of diarrhea (e.g., chronic gastrointestinal disease), a concern for the fetus (e.g., pregnancy), and the possibility that they might not treat themselves adequately (e.g., the elderly).[12] At-risk hosts are summarized in Table 19.2.

Table 19.2 Travelers at Risk of Travelers' Diarrhea

Hosts with increased risk of disease	Hosts with increased risk of complications
Immunocompromised hosts[a]	The elderly[a]
Low gastric acidity[a]	Chronic gastrointestinal disease[a]
Young adults and adventurers or 'extreme' travel[a]	Pregnancy
Higher socioeconomic status	
No travel to tropical areas in the past 6 months	
Travel from developed to underdeveloped countries	
<6 years old	

[a]Classic candidates for chemoprophylaxis. Whereas pregnancy might also benefit from chemoprophylaxis, the limiting factor is safety of an antimicrobial agent.

Education and Behavior Modification

Education and risk behavior modification have always been regarded as one of the pillars in the prevention of travelers' diarrhea. While 'Boil it, cook it, peel it or forget it!' is popular, simple, and generally does make sense, several studies have shown that few travelers actually comply with these kinds of directives. Furthermore, studies have shown conflicting results in the value of following such strict advice. Food and drink can be placed into three categories: safe, probably safe, and unsafe, although hard data for these designations are lacking. Examples are shown in Table 19.3. Travelers probably should be made aware of how food choices affect their likelihood of experiencing diarrhea, but such education is still no guarantee that the traveler will comply with prudent culinary advice.

'Water paranoia' is common among travelers; however, beverage choices, albeit important, probably contribute to travelers' diarrhea less than contaminated foods. Carbonated beverages can be considered safe. Bottled natural water is generally safe, especially if a seal must be broken before consumption. Water supplied in large containers cannot be considered automatically safe: sometimes it is no more than bottled

Table 19.3 Food and Beverage Recommendations for Travelers

Category	Safe	Probably Safe	Unsafe
Beverages	Carbonated soft drinks Carbonated water Boiled water Purified water (iodine or chlorine)	Fresh citric juices Bottled water Packaged (machine-made) ice	Tap water Chipped ice Unpasteurized milk
Food	Hot, thoroughly grilled, boiled Processed and packaged Cooked vegetables and peeled fruits	Dry items Hyperosmolar items (such as jam and syrup) Washed vegetables and fruits	Salads Sauces and 'salsas' Uncooked seafood Raw or poorly cooked meats Unpeeled fruits Unpasteurized dairy products Cold desserts
Setting	Recommended restaurants	Local homes	Street vendors

local water from the regular municipal source. Cans and bottles should be cleaned and dried before consuming their contents. Although boiling water is a very effective way to ensure water safety, this is highly impractical for the short-term traveler. Chemical disinfection with iodine is a practical way to purify water, but the ensuing chemical taste may discourage its use, and iodine should not be used by pregnant travelers and those with thyroid disease. Also, care must be taken to clarify water before iodine disinfection, and close attention must be paid to the amount of iodine to use, the ambient temperature and the duration of disinfection. Chlorine disinfection is less reliable than iodine, since cysts of parasites such as *Giardia* might survive the chlorination process; however, even iodine is not adequately effective against *Cryptosporidium* oocysts or against *Giardia* cysts in heavily contaminated settings.[13]

Commercially available filters exist to supply both large and small supplies of water. Filters are adequate to remove bacteria and parasitic cysts, but viruses will pass through the filter. The combination of a filter with an iodine resin not only removes bacteria and cysts but probably removes many viruses as well.

Water must be kept pure after it has been disinfected. Container handling is of paramount importance, since a contaminated container may defeat the purpose of disinfection, and put the traveler at increased risk (see Ch. 6).

Contaminated food is more of a problem than water. Food may be contaminated at its source (such as with the use of fecal fertilizers on crops), or during preparation due to poor personal hygiene of the cook or food preparer, or inadequate food handling and storage practices. The best advice is to eat food that has been thoroughly and recently cooked and served piping hot. Temperatures in the range of 160°F are necessary, and such food is too hot to eat. Cold foods such as salads, and raw vegetables and fruits, should be avoided. Fresh sauces and condiments (such as 'salsa') that sit on restaurant counters for long periods of time are ideal culture media, and likewise should be avoided. A study of salsas from popular restaurants in Guadalajara, Mexico, showed a high rate of *E. coli* contamination.[14] Unpasteurized milk products, as well as uncooked seafood, are high-risk foods that should not be consumed.

Choice of where food is obtained and consumed also makes a difference. Although not a guarantee, eating meals at a private residence is generally safer than eating out. Eating at a luxury hotel may not be safer than eating at an economy or standard hotel, because many fancy foods are hand-prepared, uncooked, and intentionally served cold. The highest risk comes from food purchased from street vendors. Such food may not be well prepared to start with. The personal hygiene of the vendor is critical, as are food storage practices and the cleanliness of the plates and utensils.

Behavior modification through food and water advice should be as dynamic and candid as possible. Dogmatic advice and long lists of 'bad' foods are likely to be unsuccessful. Drink carbonated beverages or bottled water from a container with a sealed cap; avoid ice. Eat hot, dry or peeled food; avoid salsas, salads, and cold, raw, undercooked or unpasteurized food. However, the impact of even such simple education appears to be minimal. Especially if one identifies a high-risk traveler with a poor attitude toward behavioral modification, the focus should probably be less on education and more on chemoprophylaxis or empiric treatment strategies.[11]

Probiotics and Other Non-Antibiotic Forms of Prophylaxis

Use of probiotics for protection against travelers' diarrhea has long been an attractive idea. The premise behind probiotics is that colonization of the gastrointestinal tract by non-pathogenic microorganisms might displace or prevent infection by pathogenic organisms. Claims of local immunomodulatory effects have also been made. Other authors postulate a change in the intestinal pH, which in turn inhibits growth of enteropathogens. Early studies of probiotics were significantly limited by the lack of standardized organisms, delivery vehicles, and solid clinical trial designs. Later clinical trials with standardized organisms (genetically engineered strains such as *Lactobacillus* GG) have added to the confusion by showing conflicting results. Some trials have shown modest positive effects;[15–18] however, in general, studies have shown modest benefits at best and curious geographic differences that are difficult to understand.[18] At present, probiotic therapy cannot be recommended for the routine prevention of travelers' diarrhea. However, because probiotics are safe, there is no objection if travelers wish to use the products while still exercising careful choices of foods and beverages.

While bulk forming (polycarbophil) or adsorption agents (activated charcoal) have other GI indications, their use for the prevention of travelers' diarrhea cannot be recommended since they lack effectiveness and might interfere with the absorption of drugs. The use of antimotility agents such as loperamide or diphenoxylate/atropine, anticholinergic agents, and calmodulin inhibitors for the prevention of travelers' diarrhea should be discouraged, as they may cause constipation or even ileus, and in the case of diphenoxylate, dependence.

Vaccines

Vaccine development for the agents of travelers' diarrhea has been slow since there are multiple organisms that cause the syndrome. Experimental vaccines include those against *Shigella* spp, *Salmonella typhi*, *Vibrio cholerae* and enterotoxigenic *E. coli*.[19] Available vaccines against *S. typhi* are moderately effective but have little impact on travelers' diarrhea in general, since the incidence of *S. typhi* disease among travelers is low. An oral cholera whole-cell recombinant B-subunit vaccine with cross-protection against heat-labile (LT) toxin-producing *E. coli* disease is available in some parts of the world.[20] If one assumes that LT-only toxin-producing *E. coli* are not important pathogens, then this vaccine might prevent at most 5% of travelers' diarrhea. Vaccinated travelers would still need to be armed with therapeutic drugs and even consider antibiotic chemoprophylaxis. Of course, the latter approach would make the use of vaccine moot, as *E. coli* disease would be prevented by antibiotic prophylaxis. Rotavirus vaccine is currently given to children but probably will not have a major role in preventing rotavirus in adult travelers as many adults have already experienced rotavirus disease.[21]

Antimicrobial Agents

The primary mode of action of bismuth subsalicylate, the active ingredient of Pepto-Bismol, is as an antimicrobial agent. Bismuth subsalicylate disassociates in gastric acid to form bismuth salts, such as bismuth oxychloride. In addition to antimicrobial properties bismuth subsalicylate has anti-secretory properties and a potential for toxin adsorption. Salicylic acid is released as a byproduct of the reaction and is nearly completely absorbed. Chewing a total of eight Pepto-Bismol tablets/day is equivalent to taking 3–4 adult aspirin tablets. Although salicylic acid does not have the same anticoagulant properties as acetylsalicylic acid, travelers taking warfarin or non-steroidal anti-inflammatory agents should avoid bismuth subsalicylate.

Bismuth subsalicylate is an effective and safe agent for the prevention and treatment of travelers' diarrhea.[22] Protection ranges from 40% to 65%, according to the amount and frequency of the dose. For best protection it should be taken as two tablets chewed four times a day.[6,11] The formation of black bismuth salts can discolor the tongue and the resultant blackened stools can mimic melena. Travelers should be advised to rinse their mouths thoroughly after each dose, and especially after the bedtime dose. Gently brushing the tongue at bedtime is recommended to help avoid the otherwise purely esthetic problem of black tongue. Theoretically, the absorbed salicylate may cause tinnitus, but in studies this occurred no more frequently in bismuth subsalicylate-treated patients than in placebo-treated patients. Care should be exercised when using bismuth subsalicylate in patients with impaired renal function. Bismuth subsalicylate can contribute to salicylate intoxication, so it should not be taken with aspirin. Encephalopathy has been anecdotally reported, but the bismuth in bismuth subsalicylate is essentially not absorbed compared to other bismuth compounds, so such reports are exceedingly rare. If doxycycline is used for malaria prevention, travelers should be cautioned not to use concurrent bismuth subsalicylate. The bivalent cations in bismuth subsalicylate preparations can lower the bioavailability of doxycycline.

Much of the early work on travelers' diarrhea prevention focused on the use of prophylactic antimicrobials. Table 19.4 shows currently recommended[6] antimicrobials with the suggested dosing regimens. Although antimicrobials have demonstrated clear efficacy in the prevention of travelers' diarrhea, concerns include side-effects, promoting resistance development, and the use of antimicrobial agents for chemoprophylaxis of a self-limiting syndrome when those agents have more critical other uses.

Table 19.4 Currently Recommended Antimicrobials for the Prevention of Travelers' Diarrhea

Antimicrobial	Daily Oral Dose	Adverse Effects/Comments
Bismuth subsalicylate	8 tabs chewed, in 4 divided doses	Black tongue and stools. Potential for tinnitus and salicylate overdose. Do not use with Coumadin or non-steroidal anti-inflammatory agents
Fluoroquinolones		
Ofloxacin	300 mg	GI upset, rash, dizziness, insomnia, and anxiety
Norfloxacin	400 mg	
Ciprofloxacin	500 mg	Cannot be recommended in SE Asia
Levofloxacin	500 mg	
Rifaximin	200 mg	No different from placebo. Dosage in SE Asia, where relatively resistant Campylobacter is prevalent, is uncertain; some recommend 200 mg BID or 400 mg daily.

Classic studies by Ben Kean noted the utility of the antibiotic neomycin in the prevention of travelers' diarrhea. Then studies with doxycycline dosed at 100 mg/day showed it to be a highly protective agent. Increasing resistance to tetracyclines in developing regions of the world has rendered the use of tetracyclines obsolete.

Trimethoprim and the combination of trimethoprim and sulfamethoxazole (TMP/SMX) were historically the next generation of antimicrobials studied for prevention of diarrhea. These agents provided 71–95% protection in areas where resistance was low; however, rising resistance around the world has compromised the usefulness of these antimicrobials as well. Furthermore, TMP/SMX is ineffective against *Campylobacter jejuni*, an important cause of travelers' diarrhea, particularly in SE Asia, where use of TMP/SMX cannot be recommended for prophylaxis or treatment. While TMP/SMX is relatively inexpensive, easy to administer, and can be used in children, its major disadvantages include rashes, hypersensitivity reactions (including Stevens–Johnson syndrome), bone marrow depression, and gastrointestinal disturbances. Serious side-effects are rare, but need to be considered when prescribing this drug for purposes of prophylaxis.

Until recently, fluoroquinolones were the drugs of choice as effective and relatively safe agents for the prevention of travelers' diarrhea. A study reported in 1994 showed 84% protection.[23] Unfortunately, fluoroquinolone resistance, particularly among *C. jejuni*, is increasingly being reported. In SE Asia, fluoroquinolones can no longer be recommended for prevention of travelers' diarrhea. Adverse reactions to fluoroquinolones include rash, GI intolerance, and central nervous system stimulation manifested as insomnia, nervousness or dizziness. Fluoroquinolones should not be used in pregnant women. For this class of drugs the development of resistance in the community is important, since their broad spectrum of activity, including respiratory tract pathogens, has given them a wide range of clinical applications.

Azithromycin is an antibiotic with efficacy in the treatment of travelers' diarrhea.[24] This agent is attractive for its broad spectrum of activity against enteropathogens including *C. jejuni*, and its availability for use in children and pregnant women. In SE Asia, azithromycin is probably the current drug of choice for treatment of travelers' diarrhea. Although azithromycin should work in prophylaxis, there are no data to guide dosing amounts or frequency of administration.

An ideal antimicrobial agent for the prevention of travelers' diarrhea would be one that has excellent activity against enteric pathogens, is not absorbed (helping to guarantee an excellent safety profile), is safe, has little potential for promoting antibiotic resistance, and has no other uses than in enteric diseases.[1] Rifaximin is just such an agent, which has now been approved for treatment of travelers' diarrhea when invasive pathogens are not suspected.[25–27] It has exclusively intraluminal action with <0.4% gastrointestinal absorption, documented low potential for generating cross-resistance, and a profile of clinical use that is limited to GI syndromes and preventing hepatic encephalopathy. Rifaximin has also been shown to be effective in prevention of travelers' diarrhea and affords 60–70% protection with a single daily 200 mg dose.[28] Fecal levels are about 8000 µg/g of stool after 3 days of therapy, which far exceeds the average MIC (32–50 µg/mL) of enteric pathogens.[25] The availability of such an agent permits consideration of a change in paradigm. The objections of the consensus development conference appear to be largely moot with the availability of rifaximin, although disagreement in general with the concept of chemoprophylaxis will likely continue to exist among some experts.[29] Arguably, chemoprophylaxis with an agent such as rifaximin might now be offered to many short-term travelers rather than only those with special risks.

Prophylaxis Versus Early Treatment

A cogent argument against chemoprophylaxis of travelers' diarrhea is that effective treatment now exists that limits an average case to a matter of hours once therapy with the combination of loperamide and an effective antimicrobial agent is begun.[30] Prior to the availability of rifaximin, chemoprophylaxis required the administration of systemically absorbed antimicrobial agents or bismuth subsalicylate to a large number of patients to prevent about 60–80% of cases. Although chemoprophylaxis with systemically absorbed agents was cost-effective compared to empiric therapy with an antimicrobial agent in terms of saving lost time during trips in a population where the disease prevalence was high, it carried definable potentials for toxicities and drug interactions. Chemoprophylaxis might encourage engagement in risky behavior, and this remains a fair criticism of chemoprophylaxis as an approach because the available systemically absorbed antibiotics do not prevent viral and parasitic disease. Finally, the consensus development conference admitted the efficacy of agents in prophylaxis but could not recommend them, largely owing to known and unknown side-effects.[8] This conclusion was reached despite Pepto-Bismol having been marketed since the turn of the 20th century and unknown side-effects being highly unlikely.

This negative approach failed to deal effectively with high-risk hosts who can easily understand the pros and cons of chemoprophylaxis and the subsequent use of empiric therapy when necessary. Furthermore, while combination therapy limits disease to an average of hours, some travelers will still experience many hours of illness and inconvenience that could have been avoided. Most importantly, aggressive empiric self-treatment still fails to prevent late complications of irritable bowel

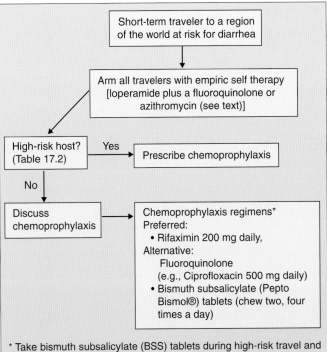

Figure 19.1 Algorithm for the prevention of travelers' diarrhea.

syndrome, a factor that was never considered in the consensus development conference. Finally, since effective treatment can now be realized with a single dose of antibiotic, the cost of medication to prevent disease will likely be more than the cost to treat. However, the cost of lost time and inconvenience likely still would favor the cost-effectiveness of prophylaxis over empiric treatment.

Figure 19.1 offers an approach to chemoprophylaxis[31] that differs from classic approaches that favor self-treatment. Note that in the current algorithm TMP/SMX is no longer featured owing to high resistance worldwide. Fluoroquinolones and azithromycin are reserved for self-treatment. Rifaximin and bismuth subsalicylate are not available in many countries.

Conclusion

Whereas behavior modification is not reliably effective, prophylactic agents such as bismuth subsalicylate and antimicrobials are effective in the prevention of travelers' diarrhea, and presumably in the prevention of post-infectious irritable bowel syndrome.

Chemoprophylaxis has classically been an attractive and effective strategy to prevent travelers' diarrhea, but realistic objections to the approach include the risk of side-effects and complacency about wise food and beverage selection.

With the availability of a safe, non-absorbed agent such as rifaximin, which is effective in prevention and unlikely to promote antimicrobial resistance, prophylaxis should be considered for short-term travelers who are high-risk hosts or taking critical trips, and might be discussed as an option with all travelers.

References

1. DuPont HL, Ericsson CD. Prevention and treatment of travelers' diarrhea. N Engl J Med 1993;328:1821–7.

2. Ericsson CD, DuPont HL. Travelers' diarrhea: approaches to prevention and treatment. Clin Infect Dis 1993;16:616–24.

3. Ansdell VE, Ericsson CD. Prevention and empiric treatment of travelers' diarrhea. Med Clin North Am 1999;83:945–73.

4. Ericsson CD. Travelers' diarrhea. Epidemiology, prevention, and self-treatment. Infect Dis Clin North Am 1998;12:285–303.

5. Ericsson CD. Travelers' diarrhea. Int J Antimicrob Agents 2003;21:116–24.

6. Ericsson CD, DuPont HL, Steffen R, editors. Travelers' Diarrhea. Hamilton: Decker; 2003.

7. Hill DR, Ericsson CD, Pearson RD, et al. The practice of travel medicine: guidelines by the Infectious Diseases Society of America. Clin Infect Dis 2006;43:1499–539.

8. Gorbach SL, Edelman R. Travelers' diarrhea. National Institutes of Health Consensus Development Conference. Bethesda, MD; January 28–30, 1985. Rev Infect Dis 1986;8(Suppl. 2):S109–233.

9. Steffen R, Tornieporth N, Clemens SA, et al. Epidemiology of travelers' diarrhea: details of a global survey. J Travel Med 2004;11:231–7.

10. Okhuysen PC, Jiang ZD, Carlin L, et al. Post diarrhea chronic intestinal symptoms and irritable bowel syndrome in North American travelers to Mexico. Am J Gastroenterol 2004;99:1774–8.

11. DuPont HL. Bismuth subsalicylate in the treatment and prevention of diarrheal disease. Drug Intell Clin Pharm 1987;21:687–93.

12. Ericsson CD. Travelers with pre-existing medical conditions. International J Antimicrob Agents 2003;21:181–8.

13. Gerba CP, Johnson DC, Hasan MN. Efficacy of iodine water purification tablets against Cryptosporidium oocysts and Giardia cysts. Wilderness Environ Med 1997;96:96–100.

14. Adachi JA, Mathewson JJ, Jiang ZD, et al. Enteric pathogens in Mexican sauces of popular restaurants in Guadalajara, Mexico, and Houston, Texas. Ann Intern Med 2002;136:884–7.

15. Hilton E, Kolakowski P, Singer C, et al. Efficacy of Lactobacillus GG as a diarrheal preventative in travelers. J Travel Med 1997;4:41–3.

16. Katelaris PH, Salam I, Farthing MJ. Lactobacilli to prevent travelers' diarrhea? N Engl J Med 1995;333:1360–1.

17. Gorbach SL. Probiotics and gastrointestinal health. Am J Gastroenterol 2000;95: S2–4.

18. Ericsson CD. Nonantimicrobial agents in the prevention and treatment of travelers' diarrhea. Clin Infect Dis 2005;41(Suppl. 8):S557–563.

19. Nataro JP. Vaccines against diarrheal disease. Semin Pediatr Infect Dis 2004;15:272–9.

20. Ryan ET, Calderwood SB. Cholera vaccines. Clin Infect Dis 2000;31:561–5.

21. Dennehy PH. Rotavirus vaccines: an update. Curr Opin Pediatr 2005;17:88–92.

22. Steffen R, DuPont HL, Heusser R, et al. Prevention of travelers' diarrhea by the tablet form of bismuth subsalicylate. Antimicrob Agents Chemother 1986;29:625–7.

23. Heck JE, Staneck JL, Cohen MB, et al. Prevention of travelers' diarrhea: ciprofloxacin versus trimethoprim/sulfamethoxazole in adult volunteers working in Latin America and the Caribbean. J Travel Med 1994;1: 136–42.

24. Adachi JA, Ericsson CD, Jiang Z-D, et al. Azithromycin found to be comparable to levofloxacin in the treatment of US travelers with acute diarrhea acquired in Mexico. Clin Infect Dis 2003;37:1165–71.

25. Ericsson CD, DuPont HL. Rifaximin in the treatment of infectious diarrhea. Chemother 2005;51(Suppl. 1):73–80.

26. DuPont HL, Jiang Z-D, Ericsson CD, et al. Rifaximin versus ciprofloxacin for the treatment of travelers' diarrhea: a randomized, double-blind clinical trial. Clin Infect Dis 2001;33:1807–15.

27. Steffen R, Sack DA, Riopel L, et al. Therapy of travelers' diarrhea with rifaximin on various continents. Am J Gastroenterol 2003;98: 1073–8.

28. DuPont HL, Jiang Z-D, Okhuysen PC, et al. Prevention of travelers' diarrhea with rifaximin, a non-absorbed antibiotic. Annals Intern Med 2005;142:805–12.

29. Gorbach SL. How to hit the runs for fifty million travelers at risk. Ann Intern Med 2005;142:861–2.

30. Adachi JA, Ostrosky-Zeichner L, DuPont HL, et al. Empirical antimicrobial therapy for travelers' diarrhea. Clin Infect Dis 2000;31:1079–83.

31. DuPont HL, Jiang ZD, Okhuysen PC, et al. Antibacterial chemoprophylaxis in the prevention of travelers' diarrhea. Clin Infect Dis 2005;41(Suppl. 8):S571–576.

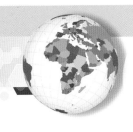

20

Clinical Presentation and Management of Travelers' Diarrhea

Thomas Löscher and Martin Alberer

Key points

- The clinical course and severity of travelers' diarrhea (TD) may be varied, and precise definitions based on number or frequency of bowel movements in a 24 h period are arbitrary
- The mean duration of untreated TD is 3–5 days, but in 8–15% a prolonged course (>1 week) occurs and in 1–3% chronic diarrhea (>4 weeks) will develop
- 50% of patients with TD will be incapacitated for at least 1 day, 20% are confined to bed for 1–2 days, and 5–15% seek professional medical help
- Risk groups prone to more severe and complicated illness are the very young, the old, the immunocompromised, and those suffering from underlying chronic medical conditions
- Diarrhea in travelers might be the initial presentation of other potentially dangerous diseases, such as falciparum malaria

Definition and Spectrum

Most studies define travelers' diarrhea (TD) as the passing of three or more loose stools in a 24 h period, in association with at least one symptom of enteric disease[1,2] such as nausea, vomiting, cramps, fever, fecal urgency, tenesmus, or the passage of bloody, mucoid stools (Table 20.1). However, TD is not a distinct disease but a polyetiological syndrome covering a broad spectrum of mainly infectious enteric diseases caused by a considerable number of various pathogens (see Ch. 18).[3] Therefore, in everyday practice the limits of TD definition are not absolutely precise. Even bowel disturbances that do not fulfill the definition of classic TD (Table 20.1) may be of relevance to the health of the traveler (mild and moderate TD), and can disrupt a business commitment or other travel plans significantly.[4] On the other hand, diarrhea in travelers may be a symptom of severe or systemic disease (Table 20.2), which can be difficult to distinguish clinically from TD, at least in the beginning.[5] In particular, it is important to remember that diarrhea may be a symptom of falciparum malaria, and that TD may be a fatal misdiagnosis in these patients.[6]

Signs and Symptoms

The clinical course and severity of TD vary considerably between studies, depending on geographical differences and variation of the microbial spectrum. TD usually does not start immediately upon arrival, but typically after 3–4 days. Most cases, in some studies up to 90%, manifest during the first 2 weeks.[7] Depending on the duration, purpose, and destination of travel, two or more separate episodes of TD were reported in 5–30% of travelers,[4,7] representing new infections or relapses.

The typical attack begins abruptly. However, in some patients, gastrointestinal symptoms start insidiously (seen more often in TD of protozoal origin). The majority of patients have 3–5 diarrheal stools per day. At least 20% of cases have more frequent bowel movements, with ≥20 stools/24 h.[1,2,7] In most patients the stool is watery. Visible blood in the stool or the presence of bloody, mucoid stools (Fig. 20.2) has been reported in 3–15% of classic TD.[1,4] Concomitant symptoms are frequent and often more disturbing than diarrhea itself. Fecal urgency, nausea, abdominal pain or tenesmus are experienced by almost all patients (Table 20.1). Urgency can be so strong that fecal incontinence occurs. Vomiting does occur, most often within the first hours of disease. Frequent vomiting may be very debilitating and can contribute to significant electrolyte imbalance and fluid loss, especially in infants.

Initial fever lasting for 1–2 days is common (Table 20.1) and has been found at some destinations in up to 40% of patients with classic TD.[1,2] High-grade fever (sometimes with chills) or fever lasting longer than 2 days is more common in classic TD and in cases with an identified pathogen.[1,2] In addition to gastrointestinal symptoms and fever, a variety of general symptoms may occur (i.e., myalgia, arthralgia, cephalgia).

The majority of cases have a self-limited and uncomplicated course. More severe and complicated disease requiring fluid or electrolyte substitution and/or dysentery has been observed in 3–15% in different studies.[4,7] Fatalities from TD are exceedingly rare, and are seen almost only in high-risk groups (see complications) or in severe or enteroinvasive diseases that are beyond the definition of TD (e.g., cholera, shigella, or amebic dysentery).

Mild and moderate TD often last for 1–2 days only.[7] Untreated, the mean duration of classic TD in various studies has been 3–5 days. However, in 8–15% a prolonged course (>1 week) is observed, and in 1–3% chronic diarrhea (>4 weeks) will develop (see Ch. 21).[4,7]

Some patients develop irritable bowel syndrome after an episode of TD, and this has been observed in up to 15% in travelers with more severe TD.[8]

Almost half the patients with classic TD are incapacitated (defined as inability to pursue planned activities) for a mean duration of 1 day.[2]

DOI: 10.1016/B978-1-4557-1076-8.00020-X

Table 20.1 Definition of Travelers' Diarrhea (TD)

Mild TD	One or two unformed stools per 24 h, no additional symptoms	
Moderate TD	One or two unformed stools per 24 h plus at least one of the following symptoms	
Classic TD	≥3 unformed stools per 24 h plus at least one of the following symptoms	
	Symptom	Frequency in various studies (%)
	Nausea	10–70
	Vomiting	4–36
	Cramps	60
	Fever	10–30
	Urgency	>90
	Abdominal pain or tenesmus	80
	Blood in stool	5–15

Table 20.2 Diarrhea as a Symptom of Systemic Infections

Acute Infections	Chronic Infections
Avian influenza	African trypanosomiasis
Brucellosis	Chagas' disease (chronic stage)
Dengue fever	Cytomegaly[b]
Ebola HF	Intestinal tuberculosis
Ehrlichiosis	Histoplasmosis
Hantavirus infection	HIV infection
Influenza A (children)	Lymphogranuloma venereum
Katayama syndrome[a]	*Mycobacterium avium-*
Legionellosis	*intracellulare* infection[b]
Leptospirosis	Schistosomiasis (intestinal)
Listeriosis	Visceral leishmaniasis
Malaria	Whipple's disease
Marburg HF	
Measles	
Ornithosis	
Plague	
Rickettsiosis	
SARS	
Sepsis	
Tick-borne relapsing fever	
Toxic shock syndrome	
Trichinellosis	
Tularemia	
Typhoid/paratyphoid fever	
Viral hepatitis (esp. A and E)	

[a]Acute schistosomiasis.
[b]Usually only in immunocompromised patients.

Approximately 20% of patients are confined to bed for 1–2 days, and 5–15% seek professional medical help.[4] The hospitalization rate is low and usually <2%, but it may increase up to ≥10% depending on the medical circumstances and the microbial spectrum at the destination.[1,4]

Complications

Risk groups, prone to more severe and complicated illness, are the very young, the old, the immunocompromised, and patients suffering from

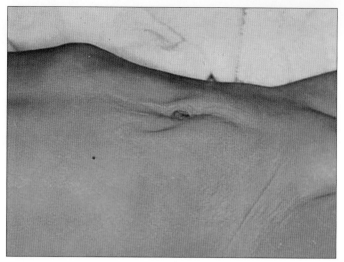

Figure 20.1 'Standing skin folds' as a clinical sign of dehydration in a 7-year-old child with acute watery diarrhea.

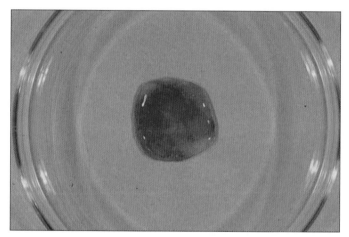

Figure 20.2 Bloody, mucoid diarrhea in a patient with shigellosis.

underlying conditions with special sensitivity to fluid loss or electrolyte imbalance (i.e., diabetes, cardiac, or renal insufficiency).

In patients with profuse watery diarrhea and/or severe and frequent vomiting, the pronounced loss of fluids and electrolytes may cause dehydration, and if not treated adequately, hypotonia, muscle cramps, oliguria, cardiac arrhythmias, coma, and shock may develop. Infants, especially, can develop severe dehydration rapidly (Fig. 20.1), and the same pathogens found in TD are leading causes of mortality in under-5s in developing countries.[9,10]

Enteroinvasive and/or cytotoxin-producing pathogens (Table 20.3)[1,11] may cause significant mucosal injury presenting as dysentery (Fig. 20.2), mucosal inflammation, and ulceration (Fig. 20.3), which can be associated with the risks of severe bleeding or perforation. In addition, invasive pathogens and some absorbable cytotoxins may cause sepsis syndromes and various extraintestinal manifestations such as hemolytic uremic syndrome (enterohemorrhagic *Escherichia coli*, *Shigella dysenteriae*), arthritis, and organ abscesses (e.g., amebic liver abscess, extraintestinal salmonella infection).

Some bacterial pathogens (i.e., *Shigella* spp., *Salmonella* spp., *Yersinia* spp., *Campylobacter* spp.) are associated with the development of reactive arthritis (Reiter's syndrome) up to several weeks after acute

Table 20.3 Pathogenic Mechanisms of Diarrhea

Pathogenesis	Mode of Action	Clinical Presentation	Pathogens (Examples)
Mucosal adherence, superficial invasion	Attachment, colonization and effacement of mucosa	Watery diarrhea, malabsorption	EPEC, EAEC, DAEC, rotavirus, norovirus, *Giardia lamblia*
Toxin production			
Neurotoxin	Action on the autonomous system	Enteric symptoms	*Staphylococcal enterotoxin* B, *Clostridium botulinum*, *Bacillus cereus*
Enterotoxin	Fluid secretion without damage to the mucosa	Watery diarrhea (secretory diarrhea)	*Vibrio cholerae*, ETEC, *Salmonella* spp., *Campylobacter* spp., *Clostridium difficile* toxin A, *Clostridium perfringens* type A
Cytotoxin	Damage to the mucosa	Inflammatory colitis, dysentery	*Shigella dysenteriae* serotype 1, EHEC, *C. difficile* toxin B, *Salmonella* spp., *Campylobacter* spp.
Mucosal invasiveness	Penetration into the mucosa and destruction of epithelial cells	Dysenteric syndrome	*Shigella* spp., EIEC, *Campylobacter* spp., *Yersinia* spp., *Entamoeba histolytica*

EPEC, enteropathogenic *Escherichia coli (E. coli)*; EAEC, enteroaggregative *E. coli*; DAEC, diffusely adhering *E. coli*; ETEC, enterotoxigenic *E. coli*; EHEC, enterohemorrhagic *E. coli*; EIEC, enteroinvasive *E. coli*.

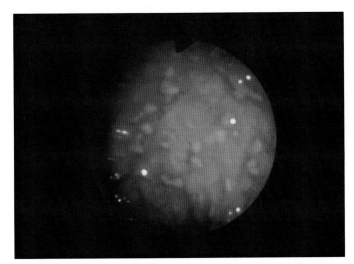

Figure 20.3 Amebic colitis with multiple small (3–5 mm) ulcers of the colon with yellowish exudate and hyperemic borders, and almost normal mucosa between ulcers.

diarrheal disease. Reiter's syndrome is seen predominantly in patients with the HLA-B27 haplotype and can also manifest as urethritis, conjunctivitis, uveitis, and various skin and mucocutaneous lesions. Guillain–Barré syndrome is a rare but important complication of *Campylobacter jejuni* infection.[12]

In patients with AIDS and other immunocompromised people, more severe and chronic courses of TD have been observed.[13,14] In addition, there is an extended spectrum of potential pathogens, and various opportunistic pathogens have to be considered (e.g., CMV, mycobacteria, *Cryptosporidium* spp., microsporidia, *Isospora*, *Cyclospora cayetanensis*).

Differential Diagnosis

Significant information concerning the probable etiological spectrum, severity, and appropriate management can be concluded from the clinical presentation and anamnestic data (Table 20.4). However, it is not possible to predict the etiological agent from the clinical

presentation because the clinical spectrum of the various pathogens causing TD overlaps considerably:

- Bloody, mucoid stools (Fig. 20.2), abdominal cramps, tenesmus and fever are typical for shigellosis. However, full blown dysentery may also occur in infections with *Campylobacter jejuni*, enteroinvasive and enterohemorrhagic *E. coli*, *Salmonella*, *Yersinia* or *Clostridium difficile*. In amebic dysentery, diarrhea often is mucoid and bloodstained, but high fever and abdominal cramps are less common
- Profuse watery diarrhea might suggest cholera, which is rarely a cause of TD. However, enterotoxic *E. coli* and many other pathogens can cause a cholera-like syndrome
- Malabsorptive diarrhea with hyperperistaltic, meteorism, flatulence and urgent, often postprandial bowel movements of voluminous liquid stools without blood or mucus is typical for giardiasis, but can be observed in infections due to enteropathogenic and enteroaggregative *E. coli*, *Cryptosporidium*, *Isospora*, or *Cyclospora*.

Protozoa at most destinations are less frequent causes of TD. However, in persisting gastrointestinal disorders in returning travelers they play a more important role (see Ch. 21). Diarrhea caused by helminth infections (strongyloidiasis, trichuriasis, fasciolopsiasis, schistosomiasis and others) is common in children in developing countries but rare in travelers.

Diarrhea after previous treatment with antibiotics (including chemotherapy of TD) may be caused by toxinogenic *Clostridium difficile*.

Clinical and Diagnostic Features of Specific Agents

Detection of specific enteropathogens in TD patients may have to be interpreted with some caution. Several agents, such as intestinal pathogenic *E. coli*, *Giardia* or *Blastocystis*, can be found commonly also in travelers returning from the tropics without an episode of TD,[15] especially when sensitive methods such as PCR are applied (Table 20.5). In addition, two or more enteropathogens are frequently detected in patients with TD. Therefore, an enteropathogen detected in stool

Table 20.4 Clinical Presentation and Specific Enteropathogens

Symptoms	Fever	Incubation Period	Fecal Leukocytes and Erythrocytes	Enteropathogens
Nausea, vomiting, watery diarrhea	Ø	1–18 h	Negative	ETEC, *Staphylococcus (Staph.) aureus* (toxin), *Bacillus cereus* (toxin), *Clostridium perfringens*
Profuse watery diarrhea, atonic vomiting	Ø	5 h–3 days	Negative	*Vibrio cholerae*, ETEC
Nausea, vomiting, diarrhea, myalgias, cephalgia	Ø/+	12 h–3 days	Negative	Rotavirus, norovirus, and other viruses
Dysentery (bloody, mucoid stools), abdominal cramps	+	1–3 days	Positive	*Shigella* spp., *Campylobacter jejuni*, *Salmonella* spp. *Yersinia* spp., *Clostridium difficile*
Dysentery	Ø/+	Variable	Positive	*Entamoeba histolytica*
Gastrointestinal bleeding	Ø/+	1–3 days	Blood	EHEC, cytomegalovirus[a]
Malabsorptive diarrhea, meteorism, flatulence	Ø	1–2 weeks	Negative	*Giardia lamblia*, *Cryptosporidium* spp., *Cyclospora cayetanensis*, microsporidia[a]

ETEC, enterotoxic *Escherichia coli*; EHEC, enterohemorrhagic *Escherichia coli*.
[a]Almost only in immunocompromised.

Table 20.5 Frequency of Detection (in %) of Various Enteropathogens in a Study on Travelers Returning from the Tropics with and without Diarrhea[15]

Enteropathogen	Travelers with TD	Travelers without TD
Enteroaggregative *E. coli* (EAEC)	45	16.4
Enterotoxigenic *E. coli* (ETEC)	36.2	25.4
Campylobacter spp.	12.3	0
Shigella spp.	6.1	0
Salmonella spp.	2.6	5.4
Norovirus	10.5	3.6
Giardia lamblia	6.1	5.4
Cryptosporidium spp.	2.6	0
Cyclospora cayetanensis	2.6	0
Blastocystis hominis	14.9	3.6
Any enteropathogen detected	95.6	44.6
More than one enteropathogen detected	60.5	12.5

samples may not always be causally related to a concurrent episode of TD.[1,4,15] Nevertheless, specific pathogens are often associated with typical epidemiological, clinical, and diagnostic features.[3]

Bacteria

Enterotoxigenic and Other Escherichia Coli

Enterotoxigenic *E. coli* (ETEC) are a major cause of childhood diarrhea in developing countries as well as in travelers visiting these destinations.[3,16] Infection is acquired through heavily contaminated food or water. ETEC strains may express either or both of two plasmid-encoded toxins causing secretory diarrhea, the heat-labile (LT) and the heat-stable (ST) enterotoxins. LT is closely related to cholera toxin. The clinical spectrum ranges from asymptomatic carriage to profuse watery diarrhea. TD caused by ETEC starts after a short incubation period of a few hours to 2 days with acute-onset diarrhea that may be accompanied by nausea, cramps, and low-grade fever. Vomiting, tenesmus, and high fever are not typical and the stool does not contain blood or leukocytes. However, in some cases a cholera-like illness with

severe dehydration may develop. The symptoms usually subside spontaneously within 3–5 days. A definite diagnosis is possible by detection of the genes encoding LT and ST using PCR or DNA probes, or by assays for the biologic LT/ST activity. However, these laborious procedures are not routinely used in this self-limiting condition, except for studies or in cases that are very severe or of epidemiological importance.

In addition to ETEC, there are at least five other groups of *E. coli* that can cause diarrhea (Table 20.6). Enteroaggregative *E. coli* (EAEC) have been recognized as a common cause of acute and persistent diarrhea, mostly in children in developing countries. In recent years EAEC have also been described as a common cause of TD.[17,18] However, EAEC as well as the poorly described pathotype of diffusely adhering *E. coli* (DAEC) can also be found in a significant number of travelers without enteritis.[15,19] This and other evidence indicates that EAEC and DAEC strains are heterogeneous, and some may be more pathogenic than others.

Enteropathogenic *E. coli* (EPEC) and enteroinvasive *E. coli* (EIEC) are less prominent causes of TD. Enterohemorrhagic *E. coli* (EHEC) and other Shiga toxin-producing *E. coli* (STEC) can cause watery and bloody diarrhea that may be complicated by hemolytic uremic syndrome (HUS). EHEC and STEC are emerging pathogens in industrialized countries. However, they are rarely found as pathogens causing diarrhea in travelers.

Campylobacter

Campylobacter spp. have a worldwide zoonotic distribution and are major causes of food-borne infections in humans. *C. jejuni* is among the most common bacterial enteric infections in all parts of the world and is the leading cause of TD in Southeast Asia.[3] In most studies consumption of contaminated chicken meat has been a major risk factor, but transmission is also possible via other contaminated food and water.[20] Diarrhea starts after an incubation period of 2–5 days and may range in severity from loose stools to massive watery diarrhea or dysentery. Crampy abdominal pain is frequent and may be the predominant or only symptom in some patients. Often GI symptoms are preceded or accompanied by fever, headache, myalgia, and malaise. Usually symptoms last for ≤1 week. However, in some patients prolonged, relapsing, or persistent courses can be seen. Bacteremia, extraintestinal complications, and chronic illness are more common in immunocompromised patients. Guillain–Barré syndrome is estimated to occur at a frequency of 1 case per 2000–3000 infections and

Table 20.6 Intestinal Pathogenic Escherichia coli and Travelers' Diarrhea

Pathotype	Epidemiology	Clinical Features	Diagnosis
ETEC	Contaminated water and food; major cause of childhood diarrhea in DC, leading cause of TD	Acute watery diarrhea, sometimes severe (cholera-like)	PCR or DNA probes for enterotoxin genes (ST/LT)
EAEC/ DAEC	Acute and chronic diarrhea in children in DC and IC, emerging cause of TD	Watery and mucoid diarrhea, persistent diarrhea	TC assay for aggregative or diffuse adherence (e.g., HEp-2 cell assay), PCR for aggR gene
EPEC	Person-to-person transmission; acute and persistent diarrhea in children in DC, cause of TD	Watery diarrhea and vomiting, persistent diarrhea	PCR or DNA probes for eae/bfp genes, TC assay for localized adherence
EIEC	Contaminated food; outbreaks in DC, cause of TD	Watery diarrhea or dysentery	PCR or DNA probes for inv genes
EHEC and other STEC	Food, water, person-to-person spread; major cause of bloody diarrhea in IC, rare cause of TD	Watery and bloody diarrhea, hemolytic uremic syndrome	Detection of Shiga toxins, PCR or DNA probes for stx genes

ETEC, enterotoxigenic *Escherichia coli*; EAEC, enteroaggregative *E. coli*; DAEC, diffusely adherent *E. coli*; EPEC, enteropathogenic *Escherichia coli*; EIEC, enteroinvasive *E. coli*; EHEC, enterohemorrhagic *E. coli*; STEC, Shiga toxin-producing *E. coli*. DC, developing countries; IC, industrialized countries; TC, tissue culture.

usually manifests 2–3 weeks after the diarrheal illness.[12] Reactive arthritis may occur up to several weeks later.

Diagnosis relies on cultural isolation using selective media and microanaerobic conditions. Direct microscopy and carbolfuchsin/Gram staining of stool specimens may show erythrocytes, leukocytes, and vibrio-shaped bacteria with characteristic darting motility.

Salmonella

Enteritis caused by non-typhoidal *Salmonella* is common worldwide and mostly associated with contaminated food products. Typically, watery diarrhea begins within 6–48 h after infection and is often associated with fever lasting 1–3 days, nausea, vomiting, and abdominal cramping. Microscopic examination of stools shows neutrophils, and less frequently erythrocytes. The illness is usually self-limited, lasting for 3–7 days. In some cases, dysenteric illness or profuse cholera-like diarrhea with severe dehydration may develop. Severe and fatal cases do occur, predominantly in neonates, the elderly and immunocompromised patients. Bacteremia develops in some patients and may lead to endovascular or localized infections (e.g., osteoarthritis). In patients with AIDS, *Salmonella* can cause chronic or recurrent bacteremia.

Non-typhoidal *Salmonella* is usually diagnosed by standard culture methods.

Shigella

Shigellosis occurs worldwide, with most cases in children in developing countries. Person-to-person transmission is common, but food-borne and water-borne epidemics are also reported. The infective dose is low compared to other bacterial enteropathogens. Symptoms start after an incubation period of 1–3 days with fever and abdominal cramping followed by watery diarrhea that reflects the small bowel site of infection. About 1 or 2 days later the typical illness of bacillary dysentery may develop, with bloody mucoid stools, tenesmus, and fecal urgency reflecting enteroinvasive colitis. Often diarrhea subsides within 1 week, but in untreated patients symptoms can last for several weeks. Fulminant dysentery, severe dehydration, bacteremia, and even fatalities are reported, occurring predominantly in infants and elderly patients. *Shigella dysenteriae* is associated with more severe disease, and strains producing Shiga toxin may cause hemolytic uremic syndrome. Reactive arthritis (Reiter's syndrome) may develop up to several weeks after re-convalescence.

Shigella can be isolated using standard culture methods. However, *Shigella* are fastidious bacteria and rapid processing of stool samples is essential to obtain high diagnostic yields.

Other Bacterial Agents

Cholera is rarely seen in travelers. However, not all infections with toxigenic *Vibrio cholerae* O1 or O139 will cause severe disease, and some cases may present as uncomplicated TD.[21] *Vibrio parahaemolyticus* and other non-cholera vibrios are abundant in many coastal waters and are usually transmitted by ingestion of seawater or of raw and undercooked seafood. Self-limited, watery diarrhea is typical; some strains may also cause dysentery. *Aeromonas* spp. and *Plesiomonas shigelloides*, ubiquitous inhabitants of fresh water, have also been found as a cause of acute diarrhea in travelers.[3] *Yersinia enterocolitica*, a common cause of acute diarrhea in industrialized countries, has rarely been found as a pathogen in TD. However, this may be an underestimation due to suboptimal isolation methods in the past.[2] *Clostridium difficile* can be a rarer but important cause of diarrhea in travelers and may be seen preferably during or after treatment with antibiotics, including malaria prophylaxis with doxycycline.[22]

Recently, *Arcobacter* species and enterotoxinogenic *Bacteroides fragilis* have been identified as etiologic agents of TD. A study in Mexico, Guatemala and India found that *Arcobacter (A.) butzleri* caused 8% of TD cases[23]. Clinical features are similar to those of *Campylobacter* infection, but *A. butzleri* infections are more frequently associated with a persistent and watery diarrhea and less often with bloody diarrhea. *Arcobacter* has been identified in food at tourist restaurants in Thailand, with most isolated strains being resistant to azithromycin but susceptible to ciprofloxacin.[24] With standard culture methods misclassification as *Campylobacter* is common. More specific cultural, biochemical and molecular methods are required for *Arcobacter* identification and species differentiation.[23]

Enterotoxinogenic *Bacteroides fragilis* (ETBF) causes a clinical syndrome with marked abdominal pain and non-febrile inflammatory diarrhea in both children (age >1 year) and adults. ETBF enterotoxin, a zinc-dependent metalloprotease, was identified via PCR in the stool of 4–13% of cases of TD at various destinations.[23,24]

Viruses

Among the viruses causing gastroenteritis (see Ch. 18), norovirus (NoV) is the most common cause of diarrhea in the adult population of industrialized countries, for both epidemic and sporadic cases. In recent years NoV has also been recognized as the most prominent viral agent of TD, with detection rates between 3% and 17%.[15,25,26] Human pathogenic NoV genotypes are highly contagious and may cause significant outbreaks, e.g., on cruise ships or in resorts. Direct fecal–oral transmission from person to person is considered to be more important than infection via fecally contaminated water and food. NoV may also be transmitted by aerosols generated during vomiting.[27] NoV enteritis typically starts after a short incubation period of 12–48 h with nausea, vomiting and abdominal pain, followed by non-bloody diarrhea with low-grade fever in some patients. The symptoms usually subside within 12–60 hours. Occasionally copious diarrhea, which can result in dehydration and even death, is seen in elderly people and patients with underlying conditions. Partial immunity is short-lived and mostly strain specific.

Rotavirus has been found in up to 10% of patients with TD.[3] Rotavirus infection is highly endemic in developing countries, where it mostly affects children under 5 years. The classic presentation of rotaviral infection at all age groups is fever and vomiting for 2–3 days followed by non-bloody diarrhea. There can be up to 10–20 bowel movements a day, which may rapidly lead to severe dehydration, especially in infants. In healthy adults, viral enteritis tends to be milder and usually lasts for a few days only, leaving protective immunity against infecting serotypes. However, in immunocompromised patients rotavirus can cause chronic and recurrent diarrhea.

A specific diagnosis of both norovirus and rotavirus infections is best made by the use of specific PCR methods to detect viral RNA in stool.

Parasites

Giardia

Although *Giardia lamblia* has not been found as a frequent cause of TD in most studies, it is the most important protozoal cause of diarrhea in travelers and by far the most common pathogen in persistent TD (see Ch. 21). The clinical spectrum ranges from asymptomatic carriage to acute diarrhea and chronic or recurrent gastrointestinal symptoms.[28] Acute giardiasis starts 1 week or more after ingestion of cysts, with watery diarrhea, abdominal pain, bloating, nausea, and vomiting. In most patients symptoms subside within 1–3 weeks. Chronic giardiasis may ensue with or without an antecedent acute episode. Diarrhea is not prominent in all patients and symptoms such as meteorismus, bloating, sulfurous burping, foul-smelling stools, and fatigue may predominate.[28] Symptoms may be continual or episodic and can persist for years. In some cases chronic malabsorption develops, with weight loss, chronic fatigue, and growth retardation in children.

Diagnosis is usually made by detection of *Giardia* trophozoites and/or cysts in stool specimens. Trophozoites may also be found in duodenal biopsies and fluid samplings. Coproantigen ELISA tests for the detection of parasitic antigen in stool have shown high sensitivity and specificity. Since all methods may yield false-negative results, multiple examinations are advisable.

Entamoeba

Historically, *Entamoeba histolytica* has probably been overestimated as a cause of TD. Frequently overdiagnosed in destination laboratories, and with the recent discovery of the two morphologically identical but pathogenically disparate species, it has become clear that the risk of *E. histolytica* infections in travelers is not great. *Entamoeba dispar*, the non-pathogenic species, is 10 times more prevalent than the pathogenic *E. histolytica*.[29]

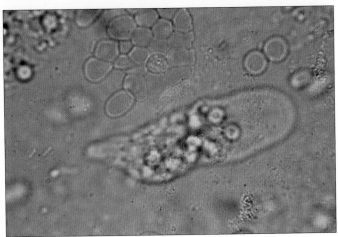

Figure 20.4 Hematophagous trophozoite of *Entamoeba histolytica* in direct microscopy of bloodstained mucus from a fresh fecal sample.

Clinical presentation with intestinal amebiasis usually takes one of three forms. The first is asymptomatic cyst passage detected in screening stool specimens. Non-dysenteric amebiasis, the second form, often presents with cyclical alterations of diarrhea and constipation with fatigue; and the third, amebic colitis is manifested by dysentery, crampy abdominal pain, and tenesmus. Symptomatic colitis usually develops 2–6 weeks after the ingestion of infectious cysts. Extraintestinal manifestations, mostly as amebic liver abscess (see Ch. 53), can evolve with or without preceding colitis, and after variable incubation or latency periods lasting from only a few days up to several years.

In intestinal amebiasis, cysts and trophozoites can be found in fresh or preserved stool specimens. However, it is not possible to distinguish the two morphologically identical species, unless hematophagous trophozoites of *E. histolytica* are detected (Fig. 20.4). Specific coproantigen ELISAs and PCR methods are highly sensitive diagnostic tests and also allow for differentiation between *E. histolytica* and apathogenic *E. dispar*. Serology can be helpful too and shows positive results in cases of amebic colitis or extraintestinal amebiasis, and also in most asymptomatic carriers of *E. histolytica* but not of *E. dispar*.

Cryptosporidium

Cryptosporidium hominis and other *Cryptosporidium* species were first described as opportunistic pathogens causing chronic diarrhea in AIDS patients, sometimes associated with extraintestinal manifestations, including involvement of the biliary and respiratory tract. However, reports of cases in returned travelers and a large water-borne outbreak in Milwaukee, Wisconsin, demonstrated that the immunocompetent were also at risk. Although usually a self-limited diarrheal illness in the immunocompetent, symptoms can still last several weeks.[30] *Cryptosporidium* oocysts in stool samples are not detected by standard parasitological concentration and staining methods. Diagnosis can be made by using modified acid-fast stains (Fig. 20.5) and by coproantigen ELISA or PCR.

Cyclospora

Cyclospora cayetanensis, a coccidian protozoan responsible for syndromes of acute and chronic diarrhea, was first described in outbreaks in Nepal and Peru in the early 1990s. The organism, unrecognized at the time, was probably seen earlier in reports of diarrhea in travelers to Papua New Guinea, Haiti, and Mexico. Reports of cyclosporiasis in returned travelers from many countries worldwide have now been documented. The organism produces a recognizable syndrome of profound fatigue and anorexia in addition to watery diarrhea and other

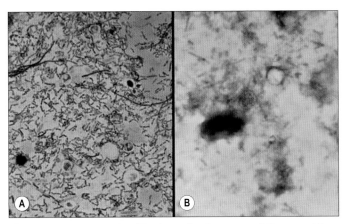

Figure 20.5 Kinjoun stain of fecal samples. **A,** oocysts of *Cryptosporidium* spp. **B,** stained and unstained oocyst of *Cyclospora cayetanensis.*

gastrointestinal symptoms.[31] Untreated cyclosporiasis may last for weeks or longer; may be cyclic or relapsing; and may result in significant dehydration and weight loss. In patients with AIDS, chronic enteritis and biliary tract disease may develop. Similar to cryptosporidiosis, the detection of *Cyclospora* oocysts in stool samples requires specific staining methods (Fig. 20.5).

Other Parasitic Agents

Blastocystis hominis is a protozoon of controversial clinical significance, and probably the most common intestinal parasite of man. In various studies it has been found more frequently in stool samples of patients with TD than in healthy controls. It is hypothesized that the development of diarrhea and other gastrointestinal symptoms is associated with certain subtypes.[32] Diagnosis is usually readily available by microscopy; subtypes can be determined by genotyping.

Microsporidia have occasionally been found as a cause of TD.[33] Even after treatment and resolution of diarrhea, microsporidia may be found in stool. Persistent diarrhea is seen preferably in immunocompromised patients. Diagnosis is made by stool microscopy using specific staining methods or by more sensitive tests, such as PCR.

Helminthic parasites are not a cause of typical TD, but diarrhea may be a symptom of various helminth infections, such as strongyloidiasis, trichuriasis, fasciolopsiasis, intestinal schistosomiasis or trichinellosis. Blood eosinophilia is frequently present. Diagnosis by parasitological stool investigations can be difficult in travelers, as parasite burdens are usually low. Then, serology and new PCR methods may be helpful.

Management of Travelers' Diarrhea

Starting effective treatment for acute TD should help to reduce the immediate and possibly the long-term impact of this condition for travelers. Most cases of travelers' diarrhea are not dehydrating, particularly when effective therapy is begun expeditiously; therefore, the classic role of oral rehydration solutions is much less relevant in the usual management of travelers and will not be dealt with further here. The high prevalence of bacterial microorganisms as the underlying etiological agents of acute TD has made antibiotic therapy the mainstay of treatment. The principles that guide treatment of the returned traveler with acute TD apply also to the informed self-treatment by the traveler acutely ill with TD in the field. The benefits of antibiotic treatment of TD are clear, with treated travelers experiencing both faster resolution and less severe diarrhea. A recent Cochrane analysis demonstrated that travelers receiving antibiotics were almost six times

more likely to have more rapid resolution of diarrhea than untreated travelers.[34] This may also ultimately translate to a lower likelihood of developing chronic diarrhea and irritable bowel syndrome, although clinical trials to confirm this are still lacking.

The earliest antibiotics used to treat travelers' diarrhea were tetracycline and ampicillin. In the early 1980s resistance to these drugs led to the use of trimethoprim/sulfamethoxazole.[35] By the end of that decade, many bacterial enteropathogens had become resistant to this combination, which led to the use of fluoroquinolones, initially nalidixic acid and then norfloxacin and ciprofloxacin. The fluoroquinolones were extremely effective in promptly eradicating the bacterial pathogens and restoring a sense of wellbeing to the traveler, sometimes in a matter of hours. This was true across virtually any destination worldwide until some time in the early 1990s, when the emergence of ciprofloxacin-resistant *Campylobacter* in Thailand led to the empiric use of azithromycin for the treatment of TD in this region.[36] With antimicrobial resistance becoming far more widespread among the common bacterial pathogens associated with TD the choice of currently available antimicrobials will in time become more restricted.

With the growing recognition of resistance patterns the choice of antibiotic for empiric treatment needs to be matched as best as possible to the destination. There is no clear threshold as to when antibiotic resistance mandates a change in empiric treatment. It is known that for certain destinations in Asia, such as Thailand and Nepal, *Campylobacter* isolates comprise approximately 25% of the bacterial pathogens. Considering 70–90% resistance to fluoroquinolones in these regions, one would expect a failure rate of up to 23% in travelers receiving this class of antibiotics for TD.

Azithromycin has been shown to have antibacterial activity that is at least comparable to that of fluoroquinolones but is superior for the treatment of Campylobacter infections.[37] Consequently, azithromycin has become more widely accepted as an effective antibiotic for acute TD, and for several travel destinations this antibiotic is the drug of choice. A newer antibiotic proposed for the treatment of TD is rifaximin. Rifaximin is poorly absorbed and its actions are limited to the lumen of the intestinal tract. Although studies across several countries seemed to indicate that rifaximin was as effective as ciprofloxacin in empiric treatment of TD,[38] the fact that the drug is not absorbed renders it ineffective in treating invasive pathogens such as *Shigella* spp. or *Campylobacter* spp.

So now, instead of a 'one drug fits all' strategy, we are forced to consider factors such as the resistance of specific pathogens, geographic regions, and invasive versus non-invasive organisms. Thus, the empiric treatment of TD is not as simple as it was just a few years ago, requiring a more thoughtful strategy (Fig. 20.6).

Self-Diagnosis and Self-Treatment of Travelers' Diarrhea

Allowing the traveler to recognize acute bacterial diarrhea and be able to distinguish it from less common causes of travelers' diarrhea (e.g., parasitic) made standardization of pre-travel advice possible. Viral gastroenteritis often cannot be distinguished clinically from bacterial diarrhea at the outset, but fortunately for the concept of empiric self therapy, studies have shown that viruses account for only 5–8% of TD. Likewise, toxic gastroenteritis, caused by ingestion of a preformed toxin and not by a bacterial enteric infection, does not appear to be a common cause of travelers' diarrhea. *Giardia* is the most common protozoal pathogen in travelers, accounting for up to 10% of TD at a destination travel medicine clinic in Nepal.[39] With an incubation period of 1–2 weeks, *Giardia* is not usually the cause of TD among short-term travelers. Travelers who prove to have a bacterial pathogen

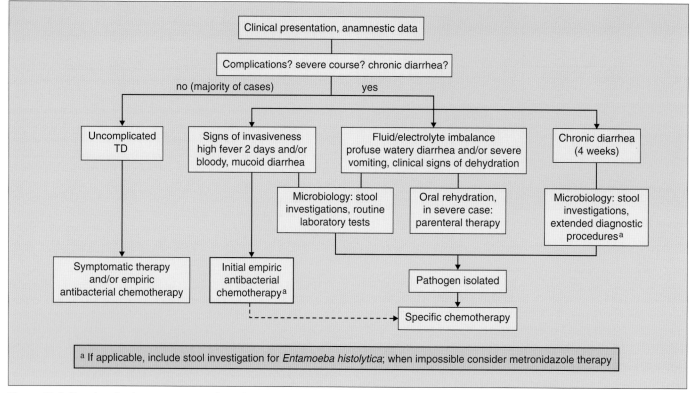

Figure 20.6 Flowchart for the management of travelers' diarrhea (TD).ª (see Chapter 21)

in their stool usually present for evaluation within 3 days of the onset of their illness, whereas those with protozoal pathogens do not present for evaluation until 2 weeks after the onset of their illness.[39] Diarrhea due to *Entamoeba histolytica* is much less common in travelers, accounting for 1–5% of cases in longer-term travelers and expatriates. *Cryptosporidium parvum* is another protozoan that not infrequently causes diarrhea in travelers. The illness is usually self-limiting, with resolution over a week, and in travelers not responding to empiric antibiotic therapy, treatment with nitazoxanide could be considered.[40] *Cyclospora cayetanensis* causes an initial illness indistinguishable from bacterial diarrhea. However, after 2–3 days the severe symptoms subside and a prolonged illness ensues.[41] Whereas TMP/SMX could be given for *Cyclospora* diarrhea, the drug is not effective enough against the majority of much more common bacterial pathogens to be used for initial empiric therapy.

Antibiotics

As bacterial causes of TD far outnumber other microbial etiologies, empiric treatment with an antibiotic directed at enteric bacterial pathogens remains the best and most definitive therapy for TD. However, adjunctive agents such as loperamide used for symptomatic control may also be recommended. The standard treatment regimens consist of 3 days of antibiotic, although when treatment is initiated promptly shorter courses, including single-dose therapy, may reduce the duration of the illness to a few hours (Table 20.7).

The benefit of treating TD with antibiotics has been proven in a number of studies. The effectiveness of a particular antimicrobial agent depends on the etiologic agent and its antibiotic sensitivity. Both as empiric therapy and for treatment of a specific bacterial pathogen, first-line antibiotics include those of the fluoroquinolone class, such as ciprofloxacin or levofloxacin, and the macrolide antibiotic azithromycin.

Table 20.7 Antimicrobial Agents for the Treatment of Acute Travelers' Diarrhea

Antibiotic	Adult dosing regimens
Fluoroquinolone	
Ciprofloxacin	750 mg orally as a single dose, or 500 mg bid for 3* days
Norfloxacin	800 mg single dose, or 400 mg bid for 3* days
Levofloxacin	500 mg single dose, or for 3* days
Azithromycin	1g orally as a single dose or 500 mg daily for 3 days
Rifaximin#	200 mg orally t.i.d. for up to 3 days, or 400 mg bid for 1–3 days or 550 mg once daily

*Preferable in enteroinvasive disease (e.g., dysentery and/or high fever)
#Not in patients with enteroinvasive disease

Fluoroquinolones

Fluoroquinolones have been the mainstay of antimicrobial treatment for TD for the past 2 decades, The combination of fluoroquinolones and loperamide has proved not only to be especially effective in resolving diarrhea but also to be safe, even in patients with *Shigella* dysentery.[42] However, in patients with fever and severe bloody diarrhea it may be prudent to adopt a more cautious approach and initiate treatment with antibiotics alone.

All of the fluoroquinolones are well absorbed and have excellent oral bioavailability, making them suitable for the treatment of enteroinvasive bacteria. They are contraindicated in pregnancy and should be used with caution in young children, although a short course of fluoroquinolones as used for TD is considered safe.[43]

Increasing microbial resistance to the fluoroquinolones, especially among *Campylobacter* isolates, may limit their usefulness in some destinations, such as Thailand and Nepal. However, until good epidemiologic data are available from a larger number of regions throughout Asia, the impact of the growing antimicrobial resistance on the efficacy of fluoroquinolones for TD is uncertain. Despite this gap in our knowledge it appears that fluoroquinolones still work well in most destinations where TD is a risk, and remain first-line agents for most travelers.

Azithromycin

Azithromycin has good activity against a wide range of enteric organisms and appears to be as effective as fluoroquinolones for the treatment of TD acquired in Mexico and Thailand.[44] Azithromycin is active against *Campylobacter* species, providing it with a significant advantage over fluoroquinolones in regions where *Campylobacter* are prevalent. For TD acquired in Thailand and Nepal azithromycin is now the drug of choice.[44]

Rifaximin

Rifaximin is a non-absorbable antibiotic that has recently become more widely available as another option for the treatment of TD, especially diarrhea caused by enterotoxigenic or enteroaggregative *E. coli*. Rifaximin has proved to be less effective than ciprofloxacin for the treatment of invasive enteric bacterial pathogens such as *Shigella* and *Campylobacter*.[45] For travelers who use rifaximin empirically an improvement in symptoms may not be seen if they are infected with an invasive pathogen, and consequently an alternate drug, effective against these pathogens, would need to be taken. Until further information is available about the efficacy of rifaximin for invasive intestinal pathogens it cannot be recommended as an empiric therapeutic option in these patients, or in travelers to regions where invasive pathogens are especially prevalent, such as SE Asia.

If the use of the selected antibiotic fails to result in improvement in 48 hours, this could mean that the diagnosis is wrong (the patient may have a parasitic or viral infection), the bacteria could be resistant to that antibiotic, or (in the case of rifaximin) the patient has an invasive bacterium. In addition co-infection is a possibility. In this circumstance the traveler would need to consider the possibility of an intestinal parasite as the underlying cause for their symptoms.

Antimotility Agents

Anti-motility agents provide symptomatic relief and serve as useful adjuncts to antibiotic therapy in TD.[46] Synthetic opiates, such as loperamide and diphenoxylate, can reduce bowel movement frequency and enable travelers to resume their activities while awaiting the effects of antibiotics. Loperamide also has antisecretory properties and has become the preferred agent of the two because it avoids the anticholinergic side-effects of the atropine contained in diphenoxylate preparations.[47] Although earlier studies suggest these agents should not be used in diarrheal illness associated with high fever or blood in the stool, more recent studies suggest that these medications may be used in such instances as long as antibiotics are administered concurrently. The combination of loperamide with antibiotic results in more rapid relief than either antibiotics or loperamide alone.[48] The recommendations for the use of anti-motility agents in children also vary widely. In the US loperamide and diphenoxylate are not recommended for children <2 years of age, whereas in the UK they are not recommended below 4 years of age and in Australia they are contraindicated in children under the age of 12 years.

Antiemetic Agents

Additional symptomatic treatment may be offered with antiemetics. Most travelers probably do not need antiemetics for empiric therapy in their travel kit, since nausea and vomiting are generally self-limiting in travelers' diarrhea. Antiemetics are available in oral, injectable, or suppository form. Suppositories are a practical way for a traveler to self-treat vomiting, but their usefulness may be limited by the concomitant presence of diarrhea. Orally disintegrating tablets of ondansetron may be effective as they do not require ingestion with fluids. These medications are most effective at the point at which the vomiting is waning and nausea is still prominent. By reducing the nausea and preventing further vomiting, the patient can pursue oral rehydration more vigorously; however, in our experience travelers can also be instructed to continue efforts at rehydration despite occasional vomiting, and they are usually successful in avoiding dehydration and in taking medication between waves of nausea without antiemetics.

Non-Specific Agents

Bismuth subsalicylate (Pepto-Bismol) has been shown in several placebo-controlled studies to reduce stool frequency and shorten the duration of illness.[49] This agent is associated with a 16–18% reduction in unformed stooling compared to over 50% for loperamide. Side-effects include black tongue, black stools, and tinnitus. BSS should be used with caution in travelers on aspirin therapy or anticoagulants, and should be avoided in those who have significant renal insufficiency. In addition, BSS should be avoided in children with viral infections, such as *Varicella* or influenza, because of the risk of Reye syndrome. BSS is not available in many parts of the world, such as Europe, Australia and New Zealand. Other non-specific agents, such as kaolin pectin, activated charcoal, and probiotics such as *Lactobacillus* GG and *Saccharomyces boulardii*, have had a limited role in the treatment of TD.

References

1. Hill DR, Beeching NJ. Travelers' diarrhea. Curr Opin Infect Dis 2010 Oct;23(5):481–7.
2. Al-Abri SS, Beeching NJ, Nye FJ. Travellers' diarrhoea. Lancet Infect Dis 2005;5:349–60.
3. Shah N, DuPont HL, Ramsey DJ. Global etiology of travelers' diarrhea: systematic review from 1973 to the present. Am J Trop Med Hyg 2009;80:609–61.
4. Steffen R, Tornieporth N, Clemens SA, et al. Epidemiology of travelers' diarrhea: details of a global survey. J Travel Med 2004;11:231–7.
5. Reisinger EC, Fritzsche C, Krause R, et al. Diarrhea caused by primarily non-gastrointestinal infections. Nat Clin Pract Gastroenterol Hepatol 2005;2:216–22.
6. Jelinek T, Schulte C, Behrens R, et al. Imported falciparum malaria in Europe: sentinel surveillance data from the European network on surveillance of imported infectious diseases. Clin Infect Dis 2002;34:572–6.
7. Mattila L. Clinical features and duration of travelers' diarrhea in relation to its etiology. Clin Inf Dis 1994;19:728–34.
8. Stermer E, Lubezky A, Potasman I, et al. Is traveler's diarrhea a significant risk factor for the development of irritable bowel syndrome? A prospective study. Clin Inf Dis 2006;43:898–901.
9. Kosek M, Bern C, Guerrant RL. The global burden of diarrheal disease, as estimated from studies published between 1992 and 2000. Bull WHO 2003;81:197–204.
10. World Health Organization. The World Health Report 2010, Geneva: WHO; 2011.
11. Brito GA, Alcantara C, Carneiro-Filho BA, et al. Pathophysiology and impact of enteric bacterial and protozoal infections: new approaches to therapy. Chemotherapy 2005;51:S23–35.
12. McCarthy N, Giesecke J. Incidence of Guillain-Barré syndrome following infection with Campylobacter jejuni. Am J Epidemiol 2001;153:610–4.

13. Baer JT, Vugia DJ, Reingold AL, et al. HIV infection as a risk factor for shigellosis. Emerg Infect Dis 1999;5:820–3.

14. Furrer H, Chan P, Weber R, et al. The Swiss HIV Cohort Study. Increased risk of wasting syndrome in HIV-infected travellers: prospective multicentre study. Trans R Soc Trop Med Hyg 2001;95:484–6.

15. Paschke C, Apelt N, Fleischmann E, et al. Controlled study on enteropathogens in travellers returning from the tropics with and without diarrhoea. Clin Microbiol Infect 2011;17:1194–2000.

16. Vargas M, Gascon J, Gallardo F, et al. Prevalence of diarrheagenic Escherichia coli strains detected by PCR in patients with travelers' diarrhea. Clin Microbiol Infect 1998;4:682–8.

17. Adachi JA, Jiang ZD, Mathewson JJ, et al. Enteroaggregative Escherichia coli as a major etiologic agent in travelers' diarrhea in 3 regions of the world. Clin Infect Dis 2001;32:1706–9.

18. Jiang ZD, Lowe B, Verenkar MP, et al. Prevalence of enteric pathogens among international travelers with diarrhea acquired in Kenya (Mombasa), India (Goa), or Jamaica (Montego Bay). J Infect Dis 2002;185:497–502.

19. Schultsz C, van den Ende J, Cobelens F, et al. Diarrheagenic Escherichia coli and acute and persistent diarrhea in returned travelers. J Clin Microbiol 2000;38:3550–4.

20. Buettner S, Wieland B, Staerk KD, et al. Risk attribution of Campylobacter infection by age group using exposure modelling. Epidemiol Infect 2010;138:1748–61.

21. Zuckerman JN, Rombo L, Fisch A. The true burden and risk of cholera: implications for prevention and control. Lancet Infect Dis 2007;7:521–30.

22. Golledge CL, Riley TV Clostridium difficile-associated diarrhoea after doxycycline malaria prophylaxis. Lancet 1995;345:1377–8.

23. Jiang ZD, Dupont HL, Brown EL, et al. Microbial etiology of travelers' diarrhea in Mexico, Guatemala, and India: importance of enterotoxigenic Bacteroides fragilis and Arcobacter species. J Clin Microbiol 2010;48: 1417–9.

24. de la Cabada Bauche J, Dupont HL. New Developments in Traveler's Diarrhea. Gastroenterol Hepatol 2011;7:88–95.

25. Ajami N, Koo H, Darkoh C, et al. Characterization of norovirus–associated traveler's diarrhea. Clin Infect Dis 2010 Jul 15;51(2):123–30.

26. Apelt N, Hartberger C, Campe H, et al. The Prevalence of Norovirus in returning international travelers with diarrhea. BMC Infect Dis 2010; 10:131.

27. Marks PJ, Vipond IB, Regan FM, et al. A school outbreak of Norwalk-like virus: evidence for airborne transmission. Epidemiol Infect 2003;131: 727–36.

28. Jelinek T, Loscher T. Epidemiology of giardiasis in German travelers. Travel Med 2000;7:70–3.

29. Herbinger KH, Fleischmann E, Weber C, et al. Epidemiological, clinical, and diagnostic data on intestinal infections with Entamoeba histolytica and Entamoeba dispar among returning travelers. Infection 2011 Jun 30. [Epub ahead of print]

30. Okhuysen PC. Travelers' diarrhea due to intestinal protozoa. Clin Infect Dis 2001;33:110–4.

31. Ortega YR, Sanchez R. Update on Cyclospora cayetanensis, a food-borne and waterborne parasite. Clin Microbiol Rev 2010;23:218–34.

32. Stensvold CR, Christiansen DB, Olsen KE, et al. Blastocystis sp. subtype 4 is common in Danish Blastocystis-positive patients presenting with acute diarrhea. Am J Trop Med Hyg 2011;84:883–5.

33. Wichro E, Hoelzl D, Krause R, et al. Microsporidiosis in travel-associated chronic diarrhea in immune-competent patients. Am J Trop Med Hyg 2005;73:285–7.

34. Al-Abri SS, Beeching NJ, Nye FJ. Traveller's diarrhoea. Lancet Infect Dis 2005;5:349–60.

35. Black R. Epidemiology of travelers' diarrhea and relative importance of various pathogens Rev Infect Dis 1990;12(Suppl 1):S73–9.

36. Kuschner RA, Trofa AF, Thomas RJ, et al. Use of azithromycin for the treatment of Campylobacter enteritis in travelers to Thailand, an area where ciprofloxacin resistance is prevalent. Clin Infect Dis 1995;21:536–41.

37. Adachi JA, Ericsson CD, Jiang ZD, et al. Azithromycin found to be comparable to levofloxacin for the treatment of US travelers with acute diarrhea acquired in Mexico. Clin Infect Dis 2003;37:1165–71.

38. Steffen R, Sack DA, Riopel L, et al. Therapy of travelers' diarrhea with rifaximin on various continents. Am J Gastroenterol 2003;98: 1073–8.

39. Shlim DR. Update in Traveler's Diarrhea. Infect Dis Clin North Am 2005;19:137–49.

40. Rossignol JF, Ayoub A, Ayers MS. Treatment of diarrhea caused by C. parvum: a prospective randomized, double-blind, placebo-controlled study of nitazoxanide. J Infect Dis 2001;184:103–6.

41. Shlim DR, Cohen MT, Eaton M, et al. An alga-like organism associated with an outbreak of prolonged diarrhea among foreigners in Nepal. Am J Trop Med Hyg 1991;45:383–9.

42. Steffen R, Jori J, DuPont H, et al. Treatment of travelers diarrhea with fleroxacin: a case study. J Antimicrob Chemother 1993;31:767–76.

43. Adachi J, Ostrosky-Zeichner L, DuPont HL, et al. Empirical antimicrobial therapy for traveler's diarrhea. Clin Infect Dis 2000;31:1079–83.

44. Tribble DR, Sanders JW, Pang LW et al. Traveler's diarrhea in Thailand: Randomized double-blind trial comparing single-dose and 3-day azithromycin-based regimens with a 3-day levofloxacin regimen. Clin Infect Dis 2007;44:338–46.

45. Taylor D, Bourgeois A, Ericsson C, et al. A randomized, double-blind, multicenter study of rifaximin compared with placebo and with ciprofloxacin in the treatment of travelers' diarrhea. Am J Trop Med Hyg 2006;74:1060–6.

46. Schiller LR, Santa Ana CA, Morawski SG, Fordtran JS. Mechanism of the antidiarrheal effects of loperamide. Gastroenterology 1984;86:1475–80.

47. Ericsson CD, Johnson PC. Safety and efficacy of loperamide. Am J Med 1990;88(suppl 6A):10S–4S.

48. Murphy GS, Bedhidatta L, Echeverria P, et al. Ciprofloxacin and loperamide in the treatment of bacillary dysentery. Ann Intern Med 1993;118:582–6.

49. Ericsson CD. Non antimicrobial agents in treatment and prevention of travelers' diarrhea. Clin Infec Dis 2005;41:S557–63.

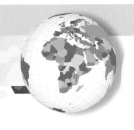

21

Persistent Travelers' Diarrhea

Bradley A. Connor and David R. Shlim

Key points

- Although most cases of travelers' diarrhea are acute and self-limited, it is important for physicians who treat returning travelers to be aware of a significant percentage of patients who develop persistent gastrointestinal symptoms
- The pathogenesis of persistent travelers' diarrhea generally falls into one of three broad categories: persistent infections, post-infectious processes, or chronic gastrointestinal illnesses unmasked by an enteric infection
- Giardiasis is by far the most likely persistent infection to be encountered in these patients, making empiric therapy for it a reasonable option
- Many patients with persistent travelers' diarrhea where no other cause is found suffer from a post-infectious irritable bowel syndrome, although many of these patients have gas bloating and constipation as their predominant symptoms
- Patients with post-infectious irritable bowel syndrome may benefit from antibiotics to eradicate small intestinal bacterial overgrowth

Introduction

Acute and self-limited illnesses comprise the preponderance of cases of travelers' diarrhea. However, an important minority of patients will develop a more protracted course, lasting weeks, months, or even years. Persistent travelers' diarrhea (PTD) is a syndrome frequently encountered by clinicians but poorly studied and characterized. Many of these patients will have long cleared the offending pathogen, and are presenting with post-infectious sequelae: inflammatory, malabsorptive, or functional. Others may be suffering from a chronic noninfectious gastrointestinal disease, such as idiopathic inflammatory bowel disease, colorectal carcinoma, or celiac sprue, which has been unmasked and brought to medical attention by an antecedent enteric infection. When initial stool studies reveal the presence of a persistent pathogen, the management is generally quite straightforward. When this is not the case, however, effective management requires the understanding and application of sound principles of gastroenterology, infectious disease and travel medicine.

Definitions and Epidemiology

Travelers' diarrhea (TD) may be defined as diarrhea which develops while abroad in, or shortly upon return from, a developing country. The dividing line between acute and chronic diarrhea has generally been accepted to occur at a symptom duration of 4 weeks.[1] The term 'persistent diarrhea' (PTD) is often used to describe a syndrome of intermediate duration, lasting >14 days, particularly in children.[2]

In this chapter, the terms chronic and persistent travelers' diarrhea will be used interchangeably to describe a syndrome of at least 3 weeks' duration, although the term persistent is preferred because it is appropriately less precise and implies a process that began acutely but lingered unexpectedly. In addition, in many patients with PTD the diarrhea itself is a relatively minor complaint, overshadowed by associated cramping pain, bloating, excessive flatulence or tenesmus, and even constipation, all of which will be included here under the rubric of PTD.

The incidence of Post-Infectious Irritable Bowel Syndrome (PI-IBS) specifically associated with TD has been examined in four studies. The most recent study was reported among 121 US military travelers returning from routine deployment (>6-month follow-up) to the Middle East, where it was reported that there was an over fivefold increase in incident IBS among those who experienced an episode of TD during travel compared to those that did not (17.2% versus 3.7%, p = 0.12).[3] Another study among travelers from Israel reported that significantly more people (14%) who had TD developed IBS after 6–7 months, compared to only 2% of those who did not have diarrhea.[4] A third study reported an incidence of PI-IBS of 10% in patients who had acquired TD in Mexico.[5] The fourth study reported only a 4% incidence of PI-IBS after TD, which was not statistically different from those who developed IBS who did not have diarrhea (2%).[6] However, this study may have been underpowered and unable to detect a statistical significance for such a small difference in incidence.

In addition to these observational studies, which included a comparison group, a study among healthy young adults living abroad in South America was recently reported where high rates of new-onset dyspepsia appeared to persist upon return from living overseas.[7] The authors did not report an association of functional gastrointestinal disease with acute diarrheal illness during travel, though the risk for these illnesses is known to be high among expatriates. This finding of new-onset dyspepsia among long-term travelers at high risk for acute diarrheal illness is similar to a number of studies documenting higher rates of functional disorders, including dyspepsia and IBS, among US

©2012 Elsevier Inc
DOI: 10.1016/B978-1-4557-1076-8.00021-1

veterans of the first Persian Gulf war.[8,9] Taken together, these studies indicate that the incidence of PI-IBS following TD is a real phenomenon and may range from 4% to 17%.

Pathogenetic Mechanisms

One can broadly subdivide the syndrome of PTD into several pathogenetic subsets: persistent infection, post-infectious processes, and chronic gastrointestinal illnesses unmasked by an infection (Table 21.1).

Persistent Infection or Co-Infection

Infections acquired by travelers often reflect those acquired by the indigenous children of the developing world, the two groups having in common a naïveté to the pathogens of the environment.[10] A more complete list of the relevant pathogens can be found in Table 21.1.

Table 21.1 Differential Diagnosis of Chronic Travelers' Diarrhea

Persistent Infections or Infestations

Protozoans
    Mastigophora: *Giardia lamblia*
    Coccidia: *Cryptosporidium parvum, Isospora belli*
    Ciliophora: *Balantidium coli*
    Microspora: *Enterocytozoon bieneusi, Septata intestinalis*
    Eimeriidae: *Cyclospora cayetanensis*
    Rhizopoda: *Entamoeba histolytica*
    Histomonads and trichomonads: *Dientamoeba fragilis*
Helminths
    Strongyloides stercoralis
    Schistosoma spp.
    Ascaris lumbricoides
    Capillaria philippinensis
Bacteria
    Enterobacteriaceae: *Escherichia coli* (especially enteroadherent), *Shigella* spp., non-typhoidal *Salmonella*
    Campylobacter spp., *Yersinia enterocolitica*
    Vibrionaceae: *Aeromonas* spp., *Plesiomonas* spp.
    Clostridium difficile
Viruses
Unknown pathogen
    Brainerd diarrhea
    Tropical sprue

Post-Infectious Processes

Post-infectious malabsorptive states
    Disaccharide intolerance
    Bacterial overgrowth
Post-infectious irritable bowel syndrome

Chronic Gastrointestinal Diseases Unmasked by an Enteric Infection

Idiopathic inflammatory bowel disease
    Ulcerative colitis
    Crohn's disease
    Microscopic colitis
Celiac sprue
Colorectal adenocarcinoma
Acquired immunodeficiency syndrome (AIDS enteropathy)

Parasites

As a group, parasites are the pathogens most likely to be isolated from patients with PTD, with their probability relative to bacterial infections increasing with increasing duration of symptoms. In a study of travelers to Nepal, protozoans were detected in 10% of travelers with gastrointestinal symptoms lasting <14 days and in 27% of patients with symptoms lasting >14 days.[11,12] Parasites of the proximal small bowel are a particular concern when malabsorption is present in the presenting clinical syndrome. The parasites most likely to be encountered in PTD are discussed in brief below.

Giardia Lamblia

Giardia lamblia is by far the most commonly encountered pathogen in patients with PTD (Fig. 21.1). Suspicion for giardiasis should be particularly high when upper gastrointestinal symptoms predominate (see Clinical approach section).[13] Untreated, symptoms may last for months, even in the immunocompetent host. The diagnosis can often be made through stool microscopy; however, as the parasite infests the very proximal small bowel, it is often too degraded prior to defecation to be recognized at microscopy. It is unclear if specific *Giardia* antigen testing by enzyme-linked immunosorbent assay (ELISA) significantly enhances sensitivity over multiple careful examinations of stool.[14]

Sampling of the duodenum for *Giardia* may be accomplished through several means. A string test, in which a long string is swallowed, carried by peristalsis into the duodenum and extracted per os, has fallen out of favor owing to its unreliability.[15] Upper gastrointestinal endoscopy with aspiration of duodenal fluid and duodenal biopsy is probably the most sensitive means of making the diagnosis. Biopsy specimens generally show the typical trophozoites appearing as small wavy lines inhabiting the intestinal brush border, but not invading the epithelium.

Giardia is usually cured with therapy consisting of metronidazole 250 mg t.i.d. daily for 5 to 7 days or tinidazole as a single 2 g dose. Occasionally, a repeat course may be required. Recently resistance to both metronidazole and tinidazole has been reported. Nitazoxanide 500 mg q 12 hours for 3 days is an alternative. Albendazole 400 mg daily for 5 days, which has cured 100% of children tested, found mixed success in travelers.[16,17] Quinacrine 100 mg t.i.d. and other alternatives are listed in Table 21.2. Given the very high prevalence of *Giardia* in PTD, empiric therapy is reasonable in the appropriate clinical setting, after negative stool microscopy and in lieu of duodenal sampling.

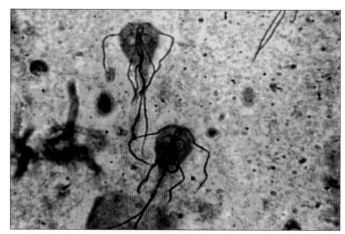

Figure 21.1 *Giardia lamblia* trophozoites, classically described as reminiscent of a face, are seen in this wet prep of stool. *(Courtesy of Murray Wittner, MD, Albert Einstein College of Medicine, Bronx, New York.)*

Table 21.2 Treatment Options for Giardiasis

Drug	Regimen
Metronidazole	250 mg t.i.d. ×5–7 days
Quinacrine	100 mg t.i.d. × 5–7 days
Nitazoxanide	500 mg q 12 hours × 3 days
Paromomycin	25–30 mg/kg per day in 3 doses ×7 days
Albendazole	400 mg q.d. ×5 days
Tinidazole	2 g × 1 day

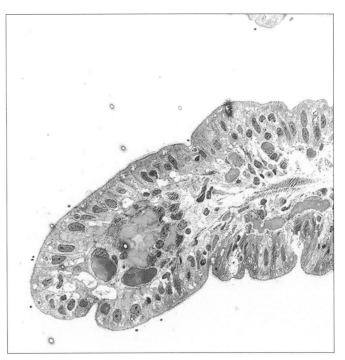

Figure 21.2 Electron microscopy of an endoscopic duodenal biopsy specimen (×1.1K) revealing multiple *Cyclospora cayetanensis* organisms identified with dots around villus.

Entamoeba Histolytica

Entamoeba histolytica has the versatile capacity to produce acute or chronic symptoms, which may vary from mild diarrhea to severe, even fatal, colitis, or dysentery. Its prevalence, however, has probably historically been overestimated as a cause of TD and PTD. Recently we have become aware of *E. dispar*, a morphologically indistinguishable and non-pathogenic protozoan, which seems to vastly outnumber the pathogenic *E. histolytica* in stool isolate prevalence, by a factor of 10 : 1.[18,19] Diagnosis is typically made by finding cysts or trophozoites in stool microscopy specimens or by serology. Illness with amebiasis usually takes one of three forms. The first is asymptomatic cyst passage, detected in screening stool specimens. Non-dysenteric amebiasis, the second form, often presents with cyclical alternations of diarrhea and constipation with fatigue. Amebic colitis, manifested by bloody diarrhea with cramping pain and tenesmus, is the third and most severe form of illness and is relatively uncommon in travelers. Stool specimens from patients falling into the first two categories should be carefully analyzed to ensure that the protozoan found is not *E. dispar*, an isolate which should simply be ignored. Patients in the first category with documented *E. histolytica* should be treated with a luminal cysticidal agent alone, such as paromomycin 500 mg t.i.d. for 10 days, iodoquinol 650 mg t.i.d. for 20 days, or diloxanide furoate.[20–22] For patients in the second and third categories, therapy consists of metronidazole 750 mg t.i.d. for 10 days or tinidazole 2 g daily for 3 days, followed by a luminal cysticidal agent.

Dientamoeba Fragilis

A relatively rare cause of PTD, *Dientamoeba fragilis* is generally diagnosed by stool microscopy and effectively treated by iodoquinol 650 mg t.i.d. for 20 days or tetracycline 500 mg q.i.d. for 10 days.[23]

Microsporidia

Microsporidia including *Enterocytozoon bieneusi* and *Encephalitozoon intestinalis* have been identified in patients with PTD.[24,25]

Cyclospora Cayetanensis

Cyclospora cayetanensis is a coccidian parasite of particular concern in the patient with PTD, as in the untreated state symptoms may be prolonged (Fig. 21.2).[26] In data from Nepal and Peru, before effective therapy was known, cases of diarrhea typically lasted 6 or more weeks.[27,28] Symptoms are usually upper gastrointestinal and associated with profound fatigue, anorexia, weight loss, and malabsorption.[29] Although it is twice as large as *Cryptosporidium*, detection of the 8–10 μm protozoan often requires obtaining a modified acid-fast stain of the stool. Despite often mimicking bacterial gastroenteritis at its onset and giardiasis, unlike the others *Cyclospora* will not respond to either empiric quinolones or metronidazole. The effective therapy, trimethoprim-sulfamethoxazole (given as 1 double-strength tablet b.i.d. for 7–10 days) is now relatively seldom used for treating diarrhea, thus such patients are likely to seek care after having failed multiple empiric therapy regimens.[30]

Cryptosporidium Parvum

Although originally described as an opportunistic pathogen causing diarrhea in AIDS patients, a 1993 water-borne outbreak of *C. parvum* affecting 400 000 Milwaukee residents demonstrated that the immunocompetent were also at significant risk.[31] *C. parvum* has been reported as a cause of PTD in travelers from Egypt, Mauritius, and elsewhere.[32] A large travel-related outbreak occurred when seven out of 34 Finnish students traveling to Leningrad became ill with profuse diarrhea.[33] Like *Cyclospora*, *C. parvum* is more easily found upon acid-fast staining of stool specimens. In the immunocompetent, a self-limited illness usually lasting <1 month is observed. There is evidence of successful treatment of these infections with nitazoxanide, and to a lesser extent paromomycin, in AIDS patients and immunocompetent travelers.[34]

Isospora Belli

Isospora belli has been reported as a cause of diarrhea in travelers returning to the USA from the Caribbean, India, and West Africa.[35] Successful therapy generally includes a 10-day course of trimethoprim-sulfamethoxazole double-strength q.i.d. or pyrimethamine-sulfadiazine.

Bacteria

Enterobacteriaceae

Enterobacteriaceae, such as enterotoxigenic *Escherichia coli* (ETEC), *Campylobacter* and *Salmonella*, which play the major role in acute travelers' diarrhea,[36] are probably a relatively uncommon cause of persistent travelers' diarrhea. Whereas *Salmonella* and *Shigella* have both been reported to result in a carrier state, recrudescence of symptoms is unlikely.

Enteroadherent *E. coli* (EAEC) have been implicated as an important cause of chronic diarrhea in children, AIDS patients, and travelers.[37–39] Fluoroquinolones and rifaximin have been used safely and effectively to treat EAEC in affected travelers.[40,41] *Aeromonas, Plesiomonas* and *Yersinia enterocolitica* are other pathogens to consider for their ability to cause subacute symptoms, and have all been reported in patients with PTD.[42,43]

Clostridium Difficile

C. difficile is an extremely relevant pathogen to consider in the patient with PTD. Its clinical presentation may vary from acute to chronic, and from mildly increased stool frequency to bloody diarrhea to toxic megacolon. Consequently, the initial work-up of PTD should always include a *C. difficile* stool toxin assay. Many PTD patients have taken malaria prophylaxis, including mefloquine, chloroquine or doxycycline, or antibiotics for acute travelers' diarrhea, which place them at risk for this opportunist.[44] It is a special consideration in the patient with continuing PTD which seems refractory to multiple courses of empiric antibiotic therapy. Therapy with metronidazole , oral vancomycin or fidaxomicin is generally successful, although resistance has been reported and recurrence may occur in upwards of 10% of patients.

Unknown Pathogens

There are many patients with a syndrome of PTD which bears the clinical and epidemiological characteristics of a persistent infectious disease, yet in which extensive microbiological analysis has failed to find a responsible pathogen. One has only to look back in recent history to predict that this is a category that will shrink in the future as diagnostic techniques, such as new stains, polymerase chain reaction, and ELISA techniques improve and our knowledge of emerging pathogens increases. Cases of travelers' diarrhea due to *Campylobacter jejuni,* Cryptosporidium parvum, enteroadherent *E. coli* and *Cyclospora cayetanensis* were deemed idiopathic infectious disease until the recent recognition of these organisms as common human pathogens in 1977, 1982, 1985 and 1991, respectively.[45–48]

Tropical Sprue

Tropical sprue identifies a syndrome of persistent travelers' diarrhea associated with malabsorption, steatorrhea, fatigue and deficiencies of vitamins absorbed in both the proximal and distal small bowel (folate and B_{12}, respectively).[49] It most commonly affects longer-term travelers and expatriates in certain areas of endemicity in the tropics, although short-term travelers are still at risk.[50] It occurs more commonly in travelers with close contact with the indigenous population, often follows an acute infectious diarrhea, and is seen in household and seasonal epidemics. It has been included in this section of persistent infections causing PTD as it has long been known to reflect an infectious process. However, although modern microbiology and epidemiology provide evidence to support this statement, the past century has accomplished little in identifying a particular responsible pathogen. Competing theories implicate an overgrowth of mixed bacterial flora versus various protozoan species, including *Cryptosporidium, Isospora* and *Cyclospora*.[51] Endoscopic and histopathological changes resemble those of celiac sprue, including fissuring and scalloping of mucosal folds and villous atrophy with crypt hyperplasia.[49]

The incidence of tropical sprue has declined dramatically over the years. In an active clinic in Nepal geared toward the care of travelers and expatriates, the diagnosis is made only 5–6 times among approximately 1500 patients presenting with diarrhea/year.[52] The reason for this apparent decline in incidence is unknown. Treatment has

generally consisted of tetracycline 250 mg q.i.d. for at least 6 weeks with folate supplements, though shorter courses, b.i.d. dosing and substitution with doxycycline have been tried successfully. Because the diagnosis is currently so rarely made, and the course of treatment is so prolonged, empiric therapy for this should be discouraged.

Brainerd Diarrhea

Brainerd diarrhea was first described in 1983 when an epidemic of chronic diarrhea occurred in Brainerd, Minnesota, in which the unpasteurized milk of a local dairy was epidemiologically identified as the source.[53] Although presumably infectious, extensive microbiological analysis has failed to identify a responsible pathogen and no antimicrobial agents have been found to be effective. At least seven subsequent Brainerd epidemics have been reported since its initial description, including six in the USA, and one on a cruise ship in the Galapagos Islands of Ecuador.[54,55] The watery diarrhea, associated with urgency, frequency (10–20 stools/day), cramping, weight loss, and a waxing and waning pattern, lasts from 2–42 months. At 1 year follow-up of the initial outbreak, 12% of patients were subjectively normal, 40% were improved and 48% had unrelenting diarrhea. Biopsy specimens of the colon revealed a prominence of intraepithelial lymphocytes without markers consistent with microscopic or collagenous colitis. It is unknown whether this entity reflects a frequent cause of sporadic PTD.

Post-infectious Processes

Post-Infectious Malabsorptive States

Malabsorption due to persistent infection or infestation of the proximal small bowel, such as giardiasis or tropical sprue, is readily recognized and understood by most clinicians. Less attention, however, has been paid to the issue of malabsorption that persists after an acute infection, such as a bacterial or viral gastroenteritis, has cleared. Disaccharidases, such as the enzymes used to digest lactose and sucrose, normally reside in the brush border overlying the intestinal epithelium. Any acute inflammatory process will readily disrupt the fragile brush border, leaving the patient with transient lactose and sucrose intolerance, which may take several weeks to resolve.[56,57] In some patients with underlying subclinical disaccharidase deficiency a more permanent lactose intolerance may be seen following gastroenteritis. Exacerbation of symptoms with dairy products and concentrated sweets may not be elicited unless specifically queried, and may not even be apparent to the patient. Malabsorption of xylose, folate and B_{12} has been well documented to occur in the setting of acute gastroenteritis.[58] In most of the patients in this report malabsorption was quite transient; however, a handful showed continued malabsorption lasting weeks to months after the acute gastroenteritis had resolved.

Occasionally, the changes in bowel motility following acute TD can result in stasis and secondary bacterial overgrowth, ultimately leading to a combined osmotic and secretory diarrhea. This diagnosis should be entertained in the setting of positive fecal fat analysis and D-xylose testing in which both non-invasive and endoscopic duodenal sampling have failed to find a persistent pathogen. The diagnosis may be confirmed by lactulose hydrogen breath testing and usually responds to antibiotic therapy, including tetracyclines, amoxicillin-clavulanate, quinolones and rifaximin.[59,60] The prevalence of bacterial overgrowth in the PTD setting is unknown, and many of these patients may be cured by tetracycline empirically administered for tropical sprue. Some authors have suggested that it has been widely underdiagnosed in the setting of chronic gastrointestinal symptoms in general, and there is recent evidence to suggest that in many cases of post-infectious IBS (PI-IBS) (see next section) small intestinal bacterial overgrowth may

Table 21.3 Diagnosis of Post-Infectious IBS

Onset of new IBS symptoms by Rome II criteria:

≥12 weeks (need not be consecutive) in the preceding 6 months of abdominal discomfort or pain with 2 or 3 of the following features:

Relieved by defecation

Onset associated with change in frequency of stool

Onset associated with change in form or appearance of stool

Following an episode of gastroenteritis or travelers' diarrhea

Where work-up for microbial pathogens and underlying gastrointestinal disease is negative

be responsible for many of the hallmark symptoms, including bloating and gas.[61,62]

Post-Infectious Irritable Bowel Syndrome

In the vast majority of patients with PTD, as time passes from the initial bout no specific etiology will be found. Concurrent with the recognition of the importance of PTD as a presenting complaint has been the observation that in a certain number of patients with irritable bowel syndrome the onset of symptoms can be traced to an acute episode of gastroenteritis. Irritable bowel syndrome which develops after acute enteritis has been termed post-infectious irritable bowel syndrome (PI-IBS) (Table 21.3).[63] PI-IBS has recently become a topic of considerable clinical and investigative interest, as evidence validating it as a diagnosis and elucidating its pathophysiology has accumulated. The syndrome of PI-IBS may be the cause of symptoms in the large numbers of patients with persistent travelers' diarrhea in whom no specific etiology is found.

The initial enteric infection is usually characterized by diarrhea and often, but not always, a stool culture positive for bacteria or clinical response to an appropriate antibiotic.[63,64] In most studies, post-infectious IBS has been linked to acute infection with bacterial pathogens, but it may also occur after viral infection[65] or protozoal infection.[66]

Whereas IBS not known to arise from an acute infection is characterized by an insidious onset of symptoms, post-infectious IBS is characterized by the acute or new onset of symptoms in the presence of previously normal bowel function.[63] In post-infectious IBS abnormal bowel habits typically persist continuously from the acute infectious episode, although they may wax and wane. Although symptoms diminish in severity from those of the acute infectious episode, pre-episode bowel function is not regained.

Post-infectious IBS is more often characterized by diarrheal symptoms than by constipation.[67,68] In a sample of 90 patients reporting persistently altered bowel habits after an episode of gastroenteritis, the frequencies of abdominal pain, loose or watery stools, rectal urgency, mucus in the stool, and bloating increased significantly during the 6-month period after the episode of gastroenteritis relative to the 6-month period before.[68] In both IBS and PI-IBS persistent diarrhea may occur; however, constipation-predominant and alternating subtypes also exist in both.[67]

The prognosis of post-infectious IBS has not been systematically assessed, but results of one study suggest that symptoms may persist for years in many patients. In a long-term follow-up of 192 individuals, recovery of normal bowel function was observed 6 years after an episode of gastroenteritis in only 6 of 14 individuals (43%) who developed post-infectious IBS after the episode of gastroenteritis, and

4 of 13 individuals (31%) who had IBS that began before the episode of gastroenteritis.[69]

Although only recently recognized as an important diagnosis in returned travelers, the syndrome was described more than half a century ago. In 1950 Stewart coined the term 'post dysenteric colitis' to describe continued symptoms of diarrhea in British troops after successful treatment of amebic dysentery.[66] Two forms were described, an 'ulcerative' (which in retrospect was probably ulcerative colitis or *Clostridium difficile* colitis), and a functional non-ulcerative form in which continued symptoms predominated but no obvious pathology could be found on sigmoidoscopy. A decade later Chaudhary and Truelove described 130 patients with IBS, 34 of whom dated the onset of their symptoms to an attack of bacterial or amebic dysentery.[70] Since then, others have suggested a high incidence of IBS post-gastrointestinal infection, with estimates ranging from 4% to 31%.[64,68,71–80]

The incidence data should be interpreted with an appreciation of the limitations of the studies. Many of the studies were retrospective and subject to bias. In addition most of the studies did not include a control group to define the incidence of new IBS in the absence of preceding infection.[81] Although most of the studies relied upon the widely accepted Rome I or Rome II criteria for diagnosing IBS, alternative causes of persistent bowel symptoms were often not assessed. This is especially true for patients labeled PI-IBS in the first 3 months after travel, when other causes such as *Clostridium difficile*, protozoan pathogens and temporary post-infective phenomena may be found.

The limitations of these studies notwithstanding, the data suggest that post-infectious IBS may be a relatively common sequela of acute gastroenteritis. The studies that did compare individuals having an acute episode of gastroenteritis with matched control individuals having no gastroenteritis consistently show an elevated incidence of IBS among the individuals with a preceding episode of gastroenteritis.[73,76–79] Across these studies, those with acute gastroenteritis were approximately 2.5–12 times more likely than controls without acute gastroenteritis to develop IBS over follow-up periods of up to 1 year.

Women were significantly more likely than men to develop post-infectious IBS in the Nottingham study,[68] but others observe a male predominance in PI-IBS (author's unpublished data). Age over 60 exerts a protective effect versus ages 19–29 (adjusted relative risk 0.36).

The type of organism responsible for the acute bacterial infection may also influence the risk of developing post-infectious IBS. In studies of community-acquired gastroenteritis, post-infectious IBS was more common after infection with *Campylobacter* and *Shigella* than after infection with *Salmonella*.[63] This difference may be attributed to the more severe mucosal injury and/or the longer duration of initial diarrheal illness caused by *Campylobacter* and *Shigella* compared to *Salmonella*. Consistent with this speculation, in one study bacterial toxicity in vitro was a strong determinant of the probability of developing post-infectious IBS by 3 months after *Campylobacter jejuni* enteritis infection.[74]

Research to date suggests that the duration of acute infectious illness may be the strongest risk factor for post-infectious IBS.[68,78] In a community-based retrospective survey of individuals with culture-positive bacterial gastroenteritis in Nottingham, England, the number of days with acute infectious diarrhea was directly related to the risk of development of post-infectious IBS.[68] Compared with individuals with acute infectious diarrhea lasting 7 days or fewer, those with acute infectious diarrhea lasting 8–14 days, 15–21 days, and ≥22 days were respectively 2.9, 6.5, and 11.4 times more likely to develop post-infectious IBS. The reason why longer duration of illness confers greater risk of developing post-infectious IBS than shorter duration of illness is not known. Insofar as longer duration of illness is a marker for more severe illness, greater illness severity rather than duration of illness per se may confer a risk of developing post-infectious IBS. This would explain the development of PI-IBS following acute TD, which is usually an illness of relatively short (<7 days) duration. This possibility is further supported by the finding that vomiting during acute gastroenteritis appears to protect against the subsequent development of post-infectious IBS, possibly by reducing the amount of inoculum and hence the severity of illness.[68] Some consider this an argument for the early self-treatment or prophylaxis of TD.

Experimental evidence suggests a pathophysiologic role of chronic inflammation following acute bacterial infection in the development of PI-IBS. Those afflicted appear to be unable to downregulate intestinal inflammation. In a recent study of unselected IBS patients there was a decreased prevalence of those with anti-inflammatory cytokines IL-10 and TGF-β, implying more susceptibility to prolonged and severe inflammation. Markers of mucosal inflammation are consistently elevated in patients with post-infectious IBS. The inflammatory cytokine interleukin IL-1β was present at higher levels both during and 3 months after an episode of acute gastroenteritis in the rectal mucosa of eight patients who developed post-infectious IBS, compared to seven patients whose bowel habits returned to normal.[82] Moreover, at the 3-month assessment, IL-1β levels were elevated in the patients with post-infectious IBS, but not in those whose bowel habits normalized after acute gastroenteritis, compared to 18 control individuals who had not had gastroenteritis for at least 2 years before the study. Based on these findings, the authors suggest that inflammation plays a role in causing post-infectious IBS, and that patients who develop post-infectious IBS may be more susceptible than those who do not respond to inflammatory stimuli.[82]

Macroscopic and conventional histologic assessments of the intestinal mucosa of patients with post-infectious IBS generally appear normal within 2 weeks of the acute infectious illness, but chronic inflammation as revealed by quantitative histology persists.[63,83] In a study of 21 patients after a bout of acute *Campylobacter* enteritis and 12 control individuals with no bowel symptoms after *Campylobacter* enteritis, numbers of intraepithelial T lymphocytes and enterochromaffin cells in rectal biopsy specimens were elevated compared to control cell counts 2, 6, and 12 weeks after the episode of enteritis (Fig. 21.1).[83] In a subset of seven patients who remained symptomatic 1 year after the episode of enteritis, counts of both cell types remained significantly higher than those in control subjects. Intraepithelial T lymphocytes and enterochromaffin cells were also increased in a separate group of 10 patients with post-infectious IBS. Cell counts in the latter group were comparable with those in the seven patients who remained symptomatic 1 year after the episode of *Campylobacter* enteritis (Fig. 21.1).[83] These signs of persistent local inflammation were accompanied by increased small-bowel permeability, as reflected by an elevated ratio of urinary excretion of lactulose to mannitol. Together, the increases in T lymphocytes and enterochromaffin cells and in small-bowel permeability reflect persistent mucosal inflammation.

These findings are corroborated by results of a study of 28 patients with newly diagnosed post-infectious IBS after *Campylobacter* infection: 28 age- and sex-matched controls who were asymptomatic after *Campylobacter* infection, and 34 healthy volunteers.[75] Enterochromaffin cell counts and T lymphocytes in rectal biopsy specimens were higher in patients with post-infectious IBS than in either recovered controls or healthy volunteers (Fig. 21.2).[75] For enterochromaffin cells, counts per high-power field were 35.8 in patients with post-infectious IBS compared to 30.6 in recovered controls (p = 0.022 versus IBS) and 29.1 in healthy volunteers (p = 0.006 versus IBS). For T lymphocytes, counts per high-power field were 127.1 in patients with

post-infectious IBS compared to 113.4 in recovered controls (NS versus IBS) and 97.1 in healthy volunteers (p = 0.006 versus IBS).

Enterochromaffin cell hyperplasia, which is thought to be a relatively non-specific response to mucosal injury and inflammation, possibly contributes to the symptoms of post-infectious IBS through serotonin-mediated effects.[63] Enterochromaffin cells are the source of nearly all intestinal mucosal serotonin, which stimulates enteric secretions, activates visceral sensory afferents, and mediates peristalsis.

Chronic Gastrointestinal Diseases Unmasked by an Enteric Infection

Travelers' diarrhea has an important potential to uncover latent non-infectious gastrointestinal disease. In the case of celiac sprue (gluten-sensitive enteropathy) and colonic adenocarcinoma, it seems clear that the acute infection acquired in travel is not causative, but has allowed the underlying pathology to become clinically apparent, bringing the patient to medical attention. In the case of inflammatory bowel disease, it remains somewhat unclear whether the travelers' diarrhea is only unmasking the chronic disease or actually initiating it.

Idiopathic Inflammatory Bowel Disease

Idiopathic inflammatory bowel disease (IBD) was diagnosed in 25% of patients in a retrospective British review of 129 cases of bloody diarrhea acquired during, or within 2 weeks of return from, a tropical sojourn.[84] These patients denied gastrointestinal complaints predating travel, begging the question whether the infection acquired in travel was actually responsible for the initiation of the autoimmune cascade of IBD. As many of the prevailing hypotheses of the pathogenesis of IBD begin with an initiating antigenic pathogen in the setting of an alteration in intestinal permeability and a genetically determined imbalance of pro- and anti-inflammatory responses, such a scenario would seem plausible. The most common form of IBD uncovered in this setting is ulcerative colitis; however, Crohn's disease[85] and microscopic colitis, including collagenous and lymphocytic colitis, have also been seen. The latter group demonstrates a normal gross colonoscopic examination, but random biopsy specimens will demonstrate the underlying inflammatory process.

Celiac Sprue

Celiac sprue is a disease of the small bowel in which genetically susceptible individuals sustain villous atrophy and crypt hyperplasia in response to exposure to antigens found in many grains, leading to malabsorption. From studies of healthy blood donors, we know that clinically apparent disease with malabsorptive diarrhea accounts for only the tip of the celiac sprue iceberg, with the majority of cases being subclinical or presenting with associated symptoms such as osteoporosis or anemia.[86] As 1 in 250 healthy Americans seem to harbor latent celiac disease, based on the screening of blood bank donations, it is important to consider the unmasking of this entity by an enteric superinfection in patients with PTD. The disease is diagnosed by compatible gross and microscopic duodenal examination and by the presence of anti-endomysial, anti-gliadin, anti-tissue transglutaminase antibodies,[87] and is treated by a very effective, if difficult to maintain, gluten-free diet (Fig. 21.3).

Colorectal Cancer

Colorectal cancer must be a consideration in patients with PTD, particularly those passing blood per rectum or found to have fecal occult blood or new iron-deficiency anemia.[88] This is especially true if hematochezia persists after the diarrhea has resolved. In any such patient over the age of 50 a full colonoscopy should be performed, even if the symptoms seem consistent with infectious colitis.

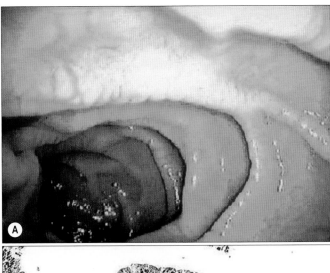

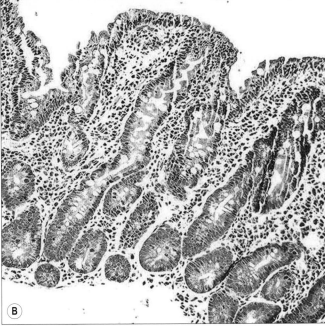

Figure 21.3 (A) Endoscopic photograph of a patient with PTD due to unmasked celiac sprue, showing classic mucosal fissuring and scalloping of folds. **(B)** Low-power light photomicrograph of a duodenal biopsy specimen revealing marked villous blunting and crypt hyperplasia, consistent with sprue. Laboratory values in this patient were notable for iron and folate deficiency, with a normal B_{12} level consistent with a duodenal process and positive antigliadin and anti-tissue transglutaminase antibodies. A gluten-free diet was recommended.

Colorectal cancer is too prevalent, with the average lifetime risk of the individual in Western countries approaching 6%, and the consequences of missing an early diagnosis too great, not to request a complete colonic luminal evaluation in the older patient.

Clinical Approach

History and Physical Examination

It is important to elicit a complete and detailed history of the current illness (Table 21.4). What were the characteristics of the initial illness? Did symptoms start with the abrupt onset of relatively uncomfortable diarrhea suggesting a bacterial pathogen, or were

Table 21.4 Evaluation of the Patient with Persistent Travelers' Diarrhea

Persistent Infection or Co-Infection	
Parasite	Stool O & P × 3, Stool *Giardia* antigen
Clostridium difficile	*C. difficile* toxin assay
	CBC with differential
Tropical sprue	D-xylose test
	Esophagogastroduodenoscopy (EGD) with duodenal aspirate and small bowel biopsy
Post-Infectious Sequelae	
Lactose intolerance	Lactose-restricted diet or lactose tolerance test
	D-Xylose test
PI-IBS	See Table 54.3 (diagnosis of PI-IBS)
Underlying Gastrointestinal Disease	
	Celiac serologies
	IBD serologies
	D-Xylose test
	Gastrointestinal endoscopy
	EGD with duodenal aspirate and small bowel biopsy
	Colonoscopy/sigmoidoscopy with biopsy

initial symptoms more insidious, suggesting protozoan infection? Have the symptoms been consistent throughout? Does the patient truly have persistent diarrhea, or do their persistent symptoms represent separate and distinct episodes of acute diarrhea, the most recent of which brings the patient to the physician? In eliciting the history of current illness it is critical to listen for gaps in wellness: a hiatus of 5–7 days without diarrhea suggests that an infection may have cleared and a new one begun.[89] In addition, vomiting and fever usually occur at the onset of enteric infections, so that if a patient reports weeks of diarrhea followed by the initiation of vomiting and fever, the likelihood is that they are suffering from a new superimposed acute infection, rather than a chronic one. Travelers may develop multiple enteric infections, as suggested in a study of travelers to Nepal, in which 17% were diagnosed with more than one stool pathogen.[90]

The history should be used if possible to localize the pathology anatomically to either small or large bowel. Diarrhea which is large-volume but relatively infrequent should suggest a small bowel process, testament to the bulk of fluid absorption normally occurring in the small bowel, as well as the capacity of the non-inflamed colon as a reservoir for stool. Other symptoms localizing to the upper gastrointestinal tract include nausea, vomiting, eructation, pyrosis, and reflux. Symptoms such as copious flatus or stools that are foul-smelling, floating, or associated with oil droplets suggest a small bowel process associated with malabsorption. The frequent, relatively small-volume diarrhea associated with infraumbilical cramping, implies a colonic process (e.g., Brainerd diarrhea), in which additional symptoms of tenesmus, bloody mucus or frank hematochezia would herald a colitis or dysentery. Fever, sweats or chills would favor the presence of a continued invasive pathogen, but may also be seen in unmasked idiopathic inflammatory bowel disease. Weight loss raises a concern for an ongoing infectious, malabsorptive, inflammatory, or malignant process and should be seen as inconsistent with merely functional syndromes such as PI-IBS.

Another important aspect in the history of current illness is awareness of all preceding diagnostic and therapeutic management. In this regard, it is particularly important to elicit information on medications and/or antibiotics taken, as well as reviewing all pre-, intra- and post-travel care. Many patients will have taken antibacterial agents, malaria prophylaxis etc., predisposing them to antibiotic-associated diarrhea and *C. difficile* in addition to gastrointestinal side-effects of the medications. The particular antibiotics given are important. Did they include broad coverage, as with a fluoroquinolone or macrolide? Did the patient take trimethoprim-sulfamethoxazole, which would have covered *Cyclospora*?

In addition to the careful gastrointestinal history, a detailed travel history is important. In which season did the patient travel (*Cyclospora* being most prevalent in the spring and early summer months in South Asia)? Was the patient in rural or urban areas? Did the symptoms worsen on the flight home? (Air pressure changes in flight may cause inflamed bowel to distend, creating more discomfort.)

Physical examination, though less helpful than history in these patients, remains important. Significant weight loss, abdominal tenderness and the presence of positive fecal occult blood (in the absence of hematochezia) may be useful in directing further evaluation.

Non-Invasive Laboratory Work-Up

Stool Studies

Stool studies should be the first diagnostic step in the evaluation of PTD, after the history and physical examination. These may be very helpful when positive, but are notoriously insensitive. Upper gastrointestinal parasites are often missed and many pathogenic bacteria are not specifically cultured for, and stool cultures may return negative. Initial stool studies should include at least three ova and parasite examinations with wet prep, trichrome stain and modified acid-fast stain, in addition to culture and *C. difficile* toxin assay. A large retrospective review of stool microscopy specimens submitted found that sending three specimens rather than one increased the yield for *E. histolytica*, *G. lamblia*, and *D. fragilis* by 22.7%, 11.3%, and 31.1%, respectively.[91] Acid-fast staining is very helpful in the detection of *Cyclospora*, *Cryptosporidia* and *Isospora* spp., and is not performed unless specifically requested in most laboratories. Concentration of the stool will also increase the yield of finding these protozoans. Antigen assays, such as the one for *G. lamblia*, appear to increase sensitivity only minimally.

The accuracy of fecal light microscopy is exquisitely dependent on the skill, experience and integrity of the technician reading the slides. It is therefore important for clinicians to develop a relationship and a level of confidence with a particular laboratory. Stool microscopy is one area in which laboratories may be insensitive in finding parasites, or overzealous for diagnosing when pathogens are not present.

Another important caveat in obtaining stool microscopy is the potential detection of non-pathogenic protozoans, often identified in avid travelers to developing countries. Many of these are listed in Table 21.5. Unnecessary attention, patient angst and drug therapy have been lavished on these organisms, which are essentially clinically irrelevant and are harmful only in distracting the clinician from further work-up and potential iatrogenic complications of unneeded therapy.

Blood Testing

As in the work-up of any chronic diarrheal illness, reasonable laboratory evaluation for PTD would begin with a complete blood count with differential. Eosinophilia, although suggestive of a parasitic infection, may be seen in cases of invasive helminthic infections but is usually not seen with intestinal protozoan infections. Leukocytosis with neutrophilia favors a bacterial process, and when marked (>20 000 cells/dL) suggests *C. difficile* infection. An elevated

Table 21.5 Non-Pathogenic Protozoans
Entamoeba spp. (non-*histolytica*)
E. hartmanni
E. moshkovskii
E. coli
E. dispar (distinguished from *histolytica* only with specialized analysis)
Blastocystis hominis
Endolimax nana
Iodamoeba butschlii
Chilomastix mesnili
Enteromonas hominis

erythrocyte sedimentation rate or C-reactive protein, although neither sensitive nor specific, may be seen in either an infectious or inflammatory process and should steer the differential diagnosis away from PI-IBS. Abnormalities in albumin or prothrombin time may be seen in malabsorption or malnutrition. Abnormally low values for iron or folate suggest a process in the proximal small bowel, whereas deficiency in vitamin B_{12} generally stems from ileal disease, relating to the area of normal absorption. The presence of both B_{12} and folate deficiency should raise suspicion for tropical sprue in its typical ability to involve wide-reaching segments of the alimentary canal.

D-Xylose testing is indicated as a non-invasive test for small bowel malabsorption. After drinking a 25 g bolus of D-xylose the patient may either submit a 5 h urine collection or have a venous sample drawn. A normal result is excretion of >20% of the xylose load into the urine.

Celiac serologies, including anti-gliadin and tissue transglutaminase antibodies, should be considered and HIV serologies obtained, as enteropathy may be the first clinical marker for HIV infection.

Endoscopic Evaluation

Most patients with PTD who have had non-diagnostic non-invasive evaluation as elaborated above should be considered for an endoscopic evaluation, although empiric therapy is an equally acceptable first-line approach, such as for parasitic illness like *Giardia* or bacterial illness. There are advantages and disadvantages to both strategies. There are no randomized data on the subject of empiric therapy versus endoscopic evaluation for PTD, and generally recommendations have come from infectious disease subspecialists rather than gastroenterologists, the former not having endoscopy as a tool immediately at hand. However, the argument for empiric therapy is the avoidance of procedures that carry some cost and some minimal risk. The use of antimicrobials or antiparasitic agents when no pathogen has been documented may confuse rather than clarify the issue. In addition to the risk of allergic reaction and other side-effects particular to the individual drugs, these medications alter bowel flora and may confuse the picture by introducing antibiotic-associated diarrhea. In addition, a lack of response to an empiric course of therapy may simply reflect antibiotic resistance rather than an incorrect diagnosis. Although empiric therapy remains an important tool in our armamentarium, and an acceptable first-line approach, there are selected groups of patients in whom an endoscopic evaluation should be performed, including (1) patients failing one or two unsuccessful empiric courses, (2) all patients aged >50 with occult or gross fecal blood, and (3) the setting of malabsorptive symptoms or signs. Endoscopy provides a sensitive means of identifying a lingering parasitic infestation or tropical sprue as well as identifying underlying structural gastrointestinal processes, including idiopathic inflammatory bowel disease, celiac sprue, and colorectal carcinoma. It also provides an objective marker to follow in patients with persistent symptoms. From an evidence-based medicine standpoint, it demonstrates a useful diagnostic yield in the work-up of chronic diarrhea in general;[92] however, the yield in PTD remains less well studied.

The choice of upper gastrointestinal endoscopy versus colonoscopy (or sigmoidoscopy) returns us to the importance of the medical history, using the clues as described above for localizing a process to the small or large bowel. Of key importance is that the endoscopist should take biopsies and aspirates of the duodenum at EGD and the colon (and possibly terminal ileum) at lower endoscopy, regardless of the presence of gross mucosal disease, as the changes may be only visible at the microscopic level.

Therapy

Empiric anti-infective therapy is both a useful diagnostic and therapeutic tool. A response to a quinolone or macrolide would simultaneously support the diagnosis of and treat bacterial disease. A response to a nitroimidazole might be similarly useful in clinically suspected giardiasis or amebiasis, as would trimethoprim-sulfamethoxazole for suspected cyclosporiasis. Many authors have recommended empiric courses of therapy for tropical sprue in the patient with PTD and malabsorption.[89] As mentioned previously, this particular approach is no longer recommended for several reasons, including the dramatically diminishing incidence of tropical sprue, the lengthy courses of therapy required, and the increasing awareness of other etiologies, including unmasked celiac disease. In the patient with diarrhea associated with upper gastrointestinal symptoms and without malabsorption, an empiric course of metronidazole to cover giardiasis would be an appropriate intervention.

Symptomatic therapy is another important aspect of the clinical management of PTD and begins with dietary modifications. Owing to the compromise of the brush border with a transient enteric infection, a trial should be undertaken of sequential avoidance of dairy products, sorbitol-containing products, fruit juices, concentrated sweets and high-fat items, in that order. In patients with colitis, a low residue, low-fiber diet should be advised.

Treatment may be empiric, symptomatic, or directed (Table 21.6). Patients with PI-IBS may be helped by a host of empiric treatments such as elimination diets, increasing dietary fiber, digestive enzymes,

probiotics including lactobacillus GG, VSL3, or *Saccharomyces boulardii*.[93] In addition, symptomatic therapies such as antispasmodics (e.g., hyoscyamine), or the judicious use of an antidiarrheal such as loperamide, may reduce symptoms. Low doses of tricyclic antidepressants may help reduce diarrhea by antagonizing the actions of serotonin and acetylcholine. Serotonin 3 (5HT3) antagonists, which increase colonic transit time and improve symptoms in patients with diarrhea-predominant IBS, may be helpful in post-infectious IBS.[94,95] Also, 5HT4 agonists may be helpful in PI-IBS patients with predominance of constipation and bloating.

Insofar as bacteria contribute to the pathophysiology of post-infectious IBS, antibiotics might be useful in its management. Antibiotics could be useful both in treating established PI-IBS and – when they are used either to treat or to prevent acute episodes of bacterial diarrhea – in preventing the development of PI-IBS.

Antibiotics might prove effective in the treatment of established IBS by eradicating bacteria that cause or exacerbate symptoms. Research suggests that small intestinal bacterial overgrowth (SIBO), which is associated with a constellation of symptoms similar to those of IBS, may underlie some of the gastrointestinal symptoms in patients with IBS. In a recent meta-analysis undertaken to assess links between SIBO and IBS, an abnormal lactulose breath test (reflecting the presence of SIBO) was found in 84% of patients with IBS, and eradication of SIBO improved IBS symptoms by 75%, on average.[96]

Antibiotic therapy that reduces SIBO reduces or eliminates IBS symptoms in many patients.[61,62] In a study of 111 patients with IBS meeting Rome I criteria, 84% of whom had an abnormal lactulose breath test at study entry, a course of treatment with the poorly absorbed antibiotic neomycin was associated with a 35% improvement in the Rome composite symptom score, compared to an 11% improvement with placebo. Improvement with neomycin versus placebo on this measure was more marked in the subgroup of patients with an abnormal lactulose breath test at study entry (35% with neomycin versus 4% with placebo). A similar pattern of results was reported for global improvement in IBS. The greatest improvements in IBS symptoms were observed among neomycin-treated patients with normal lactulose breath test results 7 days after completion of treatment.

These data support the potential utility of antibiotics in the treatment of established IBS, particularly those associated with SIBO as reflected in a positive lactulose breath test. As these data were collected from patients with IBS not selected with respect to whether or not they had post-infectious IBS, the findings cannot necessarily be generalized to those with post-infectious IBS. Given the promising results with antibiotics in unselected patients, further study in patients with post-infectious IBS is warranted. Antibiotics with proven efficacy in SIBO are good candidates for additional research. Results of small studies with the poorly absorbed (<0.4%), gut-selective antibiotic rifaximin support its further testing in IBS. In a randomized, double-blind parallel-group study of 21 patients with SIBO, rifaximin given for 7 days at a dose of 1200 mg/day normalized lactulose breath tests in 70% of patients, compared to 27% of patients treated with chlortetracycline.[60] Improvement in functional gastrointestinal symptoms was greater with rifaximin than with chlortetracycline. Likewise, in a randomized, double-blind parallel-group study of 34 patients with functional gastrointestinal symptoms (but not necessarily diagnosed with IBS), rifaximin, but not activated charcoal, improved lactulose breath test results and functional gastrointestinal symptoms.[97,98] In two identically designed, phase 3 double-blind controlled studies in patients with IBS without constipation who were randomized to either rifaximin 550 mg three times daily or placebo for 2 weeks, significantly more patients in the rifaximin group had adequate relief of

Table 21.6 Treatment of PI-IBS
Symptomatic
Elimination diets
Dietary fibre
Digestive enzymes
Probiotics
Antispasmodics
Antidiarrheals
Tricyclic antidepressants
Curative
Treatment course of non-absorbable antibiotic to eradicate associated small intestinal bacterial overgrowth (SIBO) (e.g., rifaximin 550 mg t.i.d. ×14 days)
Followed by low dose pro-kinetic (e.g., erythromycin 50 mg) at bedtime

global IBS symptoms during the first 4 weeks after treatment (primary endpoint) and adequate relief of IBS-related bloating (key secondary endpoint) during the first 4 weeks after treatment.[99]

Some have suggested that the addition of a prokinetic agent such as erythromycin or 5HT4 agonist following an antibiotic treatment course will restore normal gastrointestinal motility, specifically phase III interdigestive waves, and prevent relapse of symptoms.[99]

The increasing recognition that acute bacterial gastroenteritis can frequently cause long-term sequelae, including post-infectious IBS, elevates the importance of effective treatment of the acute bacterial illness as a means of preventing the syndrome. Effective treatment of acute bacterial diarrheal illness with antibiotics might reduce the risk of post-infectious IBS by reducing the duration and severity of acute bacterial diarrheal illness and the associated chronic inflammation that may underlie functional bowel symptoms.

If travelers' diarrhea is a risk factor for the development of PI-IBS, then it stands to reason that early treatment, early self-treatment, or prophylaxis might provide a potential window of opportunity to prevent this complication. Although at present there are no data to support this hypothesis, the potential benefit in preventing this post-infective complication should be considered in addition to the other known benefits from antibiotic therapy of travelers' diarrhea.

Conclusion

This chapter has reviewed the various pathogenetic mechanisms underlying PTD as well as outlining a logical clinical approach to the patient suffering from it. Particularly when initial stool studies fail to reveal a pathogen, considerable clinical acumen is required to appropriately direct diagnostic and therapeutic efforts to pursue diagnoses either not addressed or missed by the initial evaluation. Of course, every effort should be made to identify a persistent infection, and we should remain vigilant for emerging pathogens. It is equally essential, however, for the clinician to develop a level of comfort in the absence of a specific microbiological or histopathologic diagnosis, as the majority of patients with PTD will not have one. In such cases, one must implement the tools of a thorough history and physical examination, blood and stool evaluations, empiric therapy and, on occasion, endoscopy to localize the problem to the small or large bowel, to characterize the problem as a persistent infection, post-infectious syndrome, or the unmasking of a chronic gastrointestinal disease, and to treat the patient accordingly. Many patients with persistent travelers' diarrhea where no other cause is found suffer from post-infectious irritable bowel syndrome (PI-IBS) and may benefit from antibiotics to eradicate small intestinal bacterial overgrowth.

References

1. American Gastroenterological Association Medical Position Statement. Guidelines for the evaluation and management of chronic diarrhea. Gastroenterol 1999;116:1461–3.
2. International Working Group on Persistent Diarrhea. Evaluation of an algorithm for the treatment of persistent diarrhea: A multicenter study. Bull WHO 1996;74:478.
3. Trivedi KH, Schlett CD, Tribble DR, et al. The impact of post-infectious functional gastrointestinal disorders and symptoms on the health-related quality of life of US military personnel returning from deployment to the Middle East. Dig Dis Sci 2011;56:3602–9.
4. Stermer E, Lubezky A, Potasman I, et al. Is traveler's diarrhea a significant risk factor for the development of irritable bowel syndrome? A prospective study. Clin Infect Dis 2006;43:898–901.
5. Okhuysen PC, Jiang ZD, Carlin L, et al. Post-diarrhea chronic intestinal symptoms and irritable bowel syndrome in North American travelers to Mexico. Am J Gastroenterol 2004;99:1774–8.
6. Ilnyckyj A, Balachandra B, Elliott L, et al. Post-traveler's diarrhea irritable bowel syndrome: a prospective study. Am J Gastroenterol 2003;98:596–9.
7. Tuteja AK, Talley NJ, Gelman SS, et al. Development of functional diarrhea, constipation, irritable bowel syndrome, and dyspepsia during and after traveling outside the USA. Dig Dis Sci 2008;53:271–6.
8. Gray GC, Reed RJ, Kaiser KS, et al. Self-reported symptoms and medical conditions among 11,868 Gulf War-era veterans: the Seabee Health Study. Am J Epidemiol 2002;155:1033–44.
9. Sostek MB, Jackson S, Linevsky JK, et al. High prevalence of chronic gastrointestinal symptoms in a National Guard Unit of Persian Gulf veterans. Am J Gastroenterol 1996;91:2494–7.
10. Shlim DR, Hoge CW, Rajah R, et al. Persistent high risk of diarrhea among foreigners in Nepal during the first 2 years of residence. Clin Infect Dis 1999;29:613–6.
11. Hoge CW, Shlim DR, Echevarria P. Epidemiology of diarrhea among expatriate residents living in a highly endemic environment. JAMA 1996;275:533–8.
12. Taylor DN, Houston R, Shlim DR. Etiology of diarrhea among travelers and foreign residents in Nepal. JAMA 1988;260:1245–8.
13. Ortega YR, Adam R. Giardia: overview and update. Clin Infect Dis 1997;25:545–50.
14. Addis DG, Mathews HM, Stewart JM. Evaluation of a commercially available enzyme-linked immunosorbent assay for Giardia lamblia testing in stool. J Clin Microbiol 1991;29:1137.
15. Goka AK, Rolston DD, Mathan VI. The relative merits of faecal and duodenal juice microscopy in the diagnosis of giardiasis. Trans R Soc Trop Med Hyg 1990;84:66.
16. Kollaritsch H, Jeschko E, Wiedermann G. Albendazole is highly effective against cutaneous larva migrans but not against Giardia infection: Results of an open pilot trial in travelers returning from the tropics. Trans R Soc Trop Med Hyg 1993;87:689.
17. Dutta AK, Phadke MA, Bagade AC. A randomized multicentre study to compare the safety and efficacy of albendazole and metronidazole in the treatment of giardiasis in children. Indian J Pediatr 1994;61:689.
18. Jackson TF. Entamoeba histolytica and Entamoeba dispar are distinct species; clinical, epidemiological and serological evidence. Int J Parasitol 1998;28:181.
19. Reed SL. Amebiasis: an update. Clin Infect Dis 1992;14:385–91.
20. Anand AC, Reddy PS, Saiprasad GS, et al. Does non-dysenteric intestinal amoebiasis exist? Lancet 1997;349:89–92.
21. Nanda R, Baveja U, Anand BS. Entamoeba histolytica cyst passers: clinical features and outcome in untreated subjects. Lancet 1984;1:301–3.
22. Petri WA, Singh U. Diagnosis and management of amebiasis. Clin Infect Dis 1999;29:1117–25.
23. Cuffari C, Oligny L, Seidmen EG. Dientamoeba fragilis masquerading as allergic colitis. J Pediatr Gastroenterol Nutr 1998;26:16.
24. Raynaud L, Delbac F, Broussolle V. Identification of Encephalitozoon intestinalis in travelers with chronic diarrhea by specific PCR amplification. J Clin Microbiol 1998;36:37.
25. Wanke CA, DeGirolami P, Federman M. Enterocytozoon bieneusi infection and diarrheal disease in patients who were not infected with human immunodeficiency virus: Case report and review. Clin Infect Dis 1996;23:816.
26. Connor BA, Herwaldt BL. Cyclospora. In: Blaser MJ, Smith PD, Ravdin JI, et al, editors. Infections of the Gastrointestinal Tract. 2nd ed. Maryland: Lippincott, Williams and Wilkins; 2002. p. 1029–38.
27. Herwaldt BL, Ackers ML. An outbreak in 1996 of cyclosporiasis associated with imported raspberries. Cyclospora Work Group. N Engl J Med 1997;336:1548.
28. Hoge CW, Shlim DR, Echeverria P, et al. Epidemiology of diarrhea among expatriate residents living in a highly endemic environment. JAMA 1996;275:533–8.
29. Connor BA, Shlim DR, Scholes JV, et al. Pathologic changes in the small bowel in nine patients with diarrhea associated with a coccidian-like body. Int Med 1993;119:377–82.
30. Hoge CW, Shlim DR, Ghimire M, et al. Placebo-controlled trial of co-trimoxazole for Cyclospora infections among travelers and foreign residents in Nepal. Lancet 1995;345:691–3.

31. MacKenzie WR, Hoxie NJ, Proctor ME, et al. A massive outbreak in Milwaukee of Cryptosporidium infection transmitted through the public water supply. N Engl J Med 1994;331:161.

32. Gatti S, Cevini C, Bruno A, et al. Cryptosporidiosis in tourists returning from Egypt and the island of Mauritius. Clin Infect Dis 1993;16:344–5.

33. Jokipii AMM, Hemila M, Jokipii L. Prospective study of acquisition of Cryptosporidium, Giardia lamblia, and gastrointestinal disease. Lancet 1985;1:487–9.

34. Bissuel F, Cotte L, Rabodonirina M, et al. Paramomycin: an effective treatment for cryptosporidiosis in patients with AIDS. Clin Infect Dis 1994;18:447.

35. Shaffer N, Moore L. Correspondence – chronic travelers' diarrhea in a normal host due to Isospora belli. J Infect Dis 1989;159:596–7.

36. Steffen R, van der Linde F, Gyr K, et al. Epidemiology of diarrhea in travelers. JAMA 1983;249:1176–80.

37. Bhan MK, Raj P, Levine MM. Enteroaggregative Escherichia coli associated with persistent diarrhea in a cohort of rural children in India. J Infect Dis 1989;159:1061–4.

38. Matthewson JJ, Jiang ZD, Zumla A. Hep 2 cell adherent Escherichia coli in patients with human immunodeficiency virus-associated diarrhea. J Infect Dis 1995;171:1636.

39. Gascón J, Vargas M, Quinté L. Enteroaggregative Escherichia coli strains as a cause of travelers' diarrhea: a case control study. J Infect Dis 1998;177:1409–12.

40. Glandt M, Adachi JA, Mathewson JJ, et al. Enteroaggregative Escherichia coli as a cause of travelers' diarrhea: clinical response to ciprofloxacin. Clin Infect Dis 1998;29:335–8.

41. Boockenooghe AR, DuPont HL, Jiang ZD, et al. Markers of enteric inflammation in enteroaggregative Escherichia coli diarrhea in travelers. Am J Trop Med Hyg 2000;62:711–3.

42. Rautelin H, Hanninen ML, Sivonen A. Chronic diarrhea due to a single strain of Aeromonas caviae. Eur J Clin Microbiol Infect Dis 1995;14:51.

43. Rautelin H, Sivonen A, Kuikka A. Enteric Plesiomonas shigelloides infections in Finnish patients. Scand J Infect Dis 1995;27:495.

44. Golledge CL, Riley TV. Clostridium difficile-associated diarrhea after doxycycline malaria prophylaxis. Lancet 1995;345:1377–8.

45. Skirrow MB. Campylobacter enteritis: a 'new' disease. BMJ 1977;2:9–11.

46. Centers for Disease Control. Cryptosporidiosis: an assessment of chemotherapy of males with acquired immunodeficiency syndrome (AIDS). MMWR 1982;31:589–92.

47. Mathewson JJ, Johnson PC, DuPont HL, et al. A newly recognized cause of travelers' diarrhea: Enteroadherent Escherichia coli. J Infect Dis 1985;151:471–5.

48. Hoge CW, Shlim DR, Rajah R, et al. Epidemiology of diarrheal illness associated with coccidian-like organism among travelers and foreign residents in Nepal. Lancet 1993;341:1175–8.

49. Farthing MJG. Tropical malabsorption and tropical diarrhea. In: Feldman M, Scharschmidt BF, Sleisenger MH, editors. Sleisenger & Fordtran's Gastrointestinal and Liver Disease. 6th ed. Philadelphia: WB Saunders; 1998. p. 1574–84.

50. Klipstein FA. Tropical sprue in travelers and expatriates living abroad. Gastroenterology 1981;80:590–600.

51. Cook GC. Aetiology and pathogenesis of postinfective tropical malabsorption (tropical sprue). Lancet 1984;i:721–3.

52. Shlim DR. Response to Letter to the Editor: Tropical sprue as a cause of traveler's diarrhea. Wilderness Environ Med 2000;11:140–1.

53. Osterholm MT, MacDonald KL, White KE. An outbreak of a newly recognized chronic diarrhea syndrome associated with raw milk consumption. JAMA 1986;256:484–90.

54. Mintz ED, Weber JT, Guris D. An outbreak of Brainerd diarrhea among travelers to the Galapagos Islands. J Infect Dis 1998;177:1041.

55. Parsonnet J, Wanke CA, Hack H Idiopathic chronic diarrhea. In: Blaser MJ, Smith PD, Ravidin JI, editors. Infections of the Gastrointestinal Tract. New York, NY: Raven Press; 1995. p. 311–23.

56. Montgomery RD, Beale DJ, Sammons HG, et al. Postinfective malabsorption: a sprue syndrome. BMJ 1973;2:265–8.

57. Greene HL, McCabe DR, Merenstein GB. Protracted diarrhea and malnutrition in infancy: changes in intestinal morphology and disaccharidase activities during treatment with total intravenous nutrition or elemental diets. J Pediatr 1975;87:695.

58. Lindenbaum J. Malabsorption during and after recovery from acute intestinal infection. BMJ 1965;2:326–9.

59. Attar A, Flourie B, Rambaud JC, et al. Antibiotic efficacy in small intestinal bacterial overgrowth-related chronic diarrhea: A crossover, randomized trial. Gastroenterol 1999;117:794–820.

60. Di Stefano M, Malservisi S, Veneto G, et al. Rifaximin versus chlortetracycline in the short term treatment of small intestinal bacterial overgrowth. Aliment Pharmacol Ther 2000;14:551–6.

61. Pimentel M, Chow EJ, Lin HC. Eradication of small intestinal bacterial overgrowth reduces symptoms of irritable bowel syndrome. Am J Gastroenterol 2000;95:3503–6.

62. Pimentel M, Chow EJ, Lin HC. Normalization of lactulose breath testing correlates with symptom improvement in irritable bowel syndrome. A double blind randomized, placebo-controlled study. Am J Gastroenterol 2003;98:412–9.

63. Spiller RC. Post-infectious irritable bowel syndrome. Gastroenterol 2003;124:1662–71.

64. Lee J-S, Jung S-A, Shim K-N, et al. The frequency of post-infectious IBS (PI-IBS) in patients with acute diarrhea and the risk factors for PI-IBS of special reference to the colonoscopic findings (abstract W1686). Program and abstracts of Digestive Disease Week, 105th Annual Meeting of the American Gastroenterological Association, New Orleans, 2004.

65. James C, Thabane M, Borgaonkar MR, et al. Post-infectious irritable bowel syndrome (PI-IBS) is transient following a foodborne outbreak of acute gastroenteritis attributed to a viral pathogen. Gastroenterology 2004;126:S434.

66. Stewart GT. Post-dysenteric colitis. BMJ 1950;1:405–9.

67. Dunlop SP, Jenkins D, Spiller RC. Distinctive clinical, psychological, and histological features of postinfective irritable bowel syndrome. Am J Gastroenterol 2003;98:1578–83.

68. Neal KR, Hebden J, Spiller R. Prevalence of gastrointestinal symptoms six months after bacterial gastroenteritis and risk factors for development of the irritable bowel syndrome: postal survey of patients. BMJ 1997;314:779–82.

69. Neal KR, Barker L, Spiller RC. Prognosis in post-infective irritable bowel syndrome: a six year follow up study. Gut 2002;51:410–3.

70. Chaudhary NA, Truelove SC. The irritable colon syndrome. Quart J Med 1962;123:307–22.

71. McKendrick MW, Read NW. Irritable bowel syndrome – post salmonella infection. J Infect 1994;29:1–3.

72. Gwee KA, Graham JC, McKendrick MW, et al. Psychometric scores and persistence of irritable bowel after infectious diarrhoea. Lancet 1996;347:150–3.

73. Rodriguez LA, Ruigomez A. Increased risk of irritable bowel syndrome after bacterial gastroenteritis: cohort study. BMJ 1999;318:565–6.

74. Thornley JP, Jenkins D, Neal K, et al. Relationship of Campylobacter toxigenicity in vitro to the development of post-infectious irritable bowel syndrome. J Infect Dis 2001;184:606–9.

75. Dunlop SP, Jenkins D, Neal KR, et al. Relative importance of enterochromaffin cell hyperplasia, anxiety, and depression in post-infectious IBS. Gastroenterology 2003;125:1651–9.

76. Ilnyckyj A, Balachandra B, Elliott L, et al. Post-traveler's diarrhea irritable bowel syndrome: a prospective study. Am J Gastroenterol 2003;98:596–9.

77. Parry SD, Stansfield R, Jelley D, et al. Does bacterial gastroenteritis predispose people to functional gastrointestinal disorders? A prospective, community-based, case-control study. Am J Gastroenterol 2003;98:1970–5.

78. Ji SW, Park H, Lee DY, et al. Post-infectious irritable bowel syndrome in patients with Shigella infection: a prospective case-control study. Presented at Digestive Disease Week, May 15–20, 2004; New Orleans.

79. Mearin F, Perez-Oliveras M, Perello A, et al. Irritable bowel syndrome after Salmonella gastroenteritis: one year follow-up prospective cohorts study. Presented at Digestive Disease Week, May 15–20, 2004; New Orleans.

80. Okhuysen PC, Jiang ZD, Carlin L, et al. Post-diarrhea chronic intestinal symptoms and irritable bowel syndrome in North American travelers to Mexico. Am J Gastroenterol 2004;99:1774–8.

81. Barber R, Blakey A. Prevalence of gastrointestinal symptoms after bacterial gastroenteritis. BMJ 1997;314:1903.

82. Gwee KA, Collins SM, Read NW, et al. Increased rectal mucosal expression of interleukin 1beta in recently acquired post-infectious irritable bowel syndrome. Gut 2003;52:523–6.

83. Spiller RC, Jenkins D, Thornley JP, et al. Increased rectal mucosal enteroendocrine cells, T lymphocytes, and increased gut permeability following acute Campylobacter enteritis and in post-dysenteric irritable bowel syndrome. Gut 2000;47:804–11.

84. Harries AD, Myers B, Cook GC. Inflammatory bowel disease: a common cause of bloody diarrhea in visitors to the tropics. BMJ 1985;291:1686–7.

85. Case Records of the Massachusetts General Hospital. Case 29–1992. New Engl J Med 1992;91:182–91.

86. Trevisiol C, Not T, Berti I, et al. Screening for celiac disease in healthy blood donors at two immuno-transfusion centres in northeast Italy. Ital J Gastroenterol Hepatol 1999;31:584–6.

87. Ladinser B, Rossipal E, Pittschieler K. Endomysium antibodies in celiac disease: an improved method. Gut 1994;35:776–8.

88. Case records of the Massachusetts General Hospital. Case 33–1993. N Engl J Med 1993;329:561–8.

89. Taylor DN, Connor BA, Shlim DR. Chronic diarrhea in the returned traveler. Med Clin North Am 1999;83:1033–52.

90. Taylor DN, Houston R, Shlim DR. Etiology of diarrhea among travelers and foreign residents in Nepal. JAMA 1988;260:1245.

91. Hiatt RA, Markell EK, Ng E. How many stool examinations are necessary to detect pathogenic intestinal protozoa? Am J Trop Med Hyg 1995;53:36–9.

92. Shah RJ, Fenoglio-Preiser C, Bleau BL, et al. Usefulness of colonoscopy with biopsy in the evaluation of patients with chronic diarrhea. Am J Gastroenterol 2001;96:1091–5.

93. Kirchhelle A, Fruhwein N, Toburen D. Treatment of persistent diarrhea with S. boulardii in returning travelers: results of a prospective study. Fortschr Med 1996;114:136.

94. Camilleri M, Mayer EA, Drossman DA, et al. Improvement in pain and bowel function in female irritable bowel patients with alosetron, a 5-HT3 receptor antagonist. Aliment Pharmacol Ther 1999;13:1149–59.

95. Houghton LA, Foster JM, Whorwell PJ. Alosetron, a 5HT-3 receptor antagonist, delays colonic transit in patients with irritable bowel syndrome and health volunteers. Aliment Pharmacol Ther 2000;14:775–82.

96. Lin HC Small intestinal bacterial overgrowth: a framework for understanding irritable bowel syndrome. JAMA 2004;292:852–8.

97. Di Stefano M, Strocchi A, Malservisi S, et al. Nonabsorbable antibiotics for managing intestinal gas production and gas-related symptoms. Aliment Pharmacol Ther 2000;15:1001–8.

98. Pimentel M, Park S, Kong Y, et al. Rifaximin, a non-absorbable antibiotic improves the symptoms of irritable bowel syndrome: A double-blind randomized controlled study. Am J Gastroenterol 2005; 100:S321–45.

99. Pimentel M, Lembo A, Chey WD, et al. Rifaximin therapy for patients with irritable bowel syndrome without constipation. N Engl J Med 2011;364:22–32.

22

The Pregnant and Breastfeeding Traveler

Sheila M. Mackell and Susan Anderson

Key points

- Assessment of the pregnant traveler includes a detailed obstetrical history, contraindications to travel, access to medical care abroad, and possible risk activities such as travel modalities, physical recreation and travel at altitude
- With few exceptions, live vaccines are contraindicated during pregnancy. Yellow fever vaccine should be avoided in pregnant and breastfeeding women
- Because malaria poses a considerable hazard to mother and child, prevention measures, including chemoprophylaxis, are paramount
- Food and water precautions are essential in the prevention of pathogens that are of particularly high risk during pregnancy (e.g., hepatitis E, listeriosis, and toxoplasmosis)
- As a general rule, the advantages of breastfeeding outweigh the low risks to the infant that maternal drug therapy might entail

Introduction

The availability of convenient international and domestic travel has opened up possibilities for pregnant women who have any reason to travel. As many working women have chosen to delay childbearing, business travel during pregnancy becomes a reality for many. Long-distance travel has become more common in pregnancy, and pregnant travelers may not be fully informed about the obstetric care and insurance details pertinent to their trip.[1]

Much of the information on the pregnant traveler is based on small studies, anecdotal information, and extrapolation from non-pregnant travelers. Although evidence-based recommendations are ideal, they are lacking for pregnant women. This chapter will summarize available data and experience in this growing field of travelers.

Pre-Travel Preparation

Routine obstetric care begins at approximately 10–12 weeks' gestation, continues monthly until the seventh month, and then every 2 weeks until 36 weeks, when weekly monitoring is standard.[2]

Pre-travel preparation for the pregnant traveler starts with a review of her obstetric and medical history. Any history of pregnancy problems, bleeding, preterm labor, or chronic illness warrants consultation with an obstetrician regarding the advisability of the proposed itinerary. Relative contraindications to travel are listed in Table 22.1.[6]

Counseling on the timing of travel should be done. According to the American Academy of Obstetrics and Gynecology, the safest time for a pregnant woman to travel is the second trimester. The pregnancy is established and the extra weight is not usually a functional limitation for the mother. The risk of miscarriage is highest in all women in the first trimester. Confirming an intrauterine pregnancy prior to travel should be considered a priority. Although first-trimester vaccination is not recommended because of the unknown effects on the developing fetal organs, immunization may be administered after an extensive risk/benefit assessment. In addition, antimalarial chemoprophylaxis carries more uncertainties during the first trimester. Obstetric risks during the third trimester include pregnancy complications such as bleeding, pre-eclampsia, and preterm labor and delivery.

The physiologic changes of pregnancy may affect travel. Reduced exercise and heat tolerance, elevated heart rate due to increased plasma volume, and physiologic anemia may exaggerate travel-related discomforts.

Access to Medical Care Abroad

Awareness of local medical resources and qualified obstetric care at the destination is essential for the pregnant traveler. She should be encouraged to consider in advance how she may feel if pregnancy complications or adverse outcomes occur during or because of her travel. Any sign of an obstetric problem, such as bleeding, abdominal pain, premature rupture of membranes, severe or recurrent headaches, or high blood pressure, should prompt an evaluation by a qualified physician. Investigating the blood supply and screening procedures at the destination (HIV, hepatitis), and knowing her blood type, is wise. While many travel itineraries require a focus on the risk of infectious diseases, maternal trauma remains the leading cause of fetal death. Motor vehicle accidents and falls may cause placental abruption or preterm labor. Extra care needs to be taken later in pregnancy, when balance and position are more difficult to maintain.[7]

Personal health insurance should be checked for limitations to coverage. Unanticipated delivery away from home or approved health-care providers may not be covered by some insurance policies. Evacuation insurance that will specifically cover any pregnancy or delivery

©2012 Elsevier Inc
DOI: 10.1016/B978-1-4557-1076-8.00022-3

Table 22.1 Relative Contraindications for International Travel During Pregnancy[6]

Medical Risk Factors
Valvular heart disease
Chronic organ system dysfunction requiring ongoing assessment and medication
Severe anemia
History of thromboembolic disease

Obstetric Risk Factors
History of miscarriage
Threatened abortion or vaginal bleeding during present pregnancy
Incompetent cervix
Premature labor, premature rupture of membranes, or existing placental abnormalities
History of ectopic pregnancy (should be ruled out prior to travel with ultrasound)
Multiple gestations in present pregnancy
History of toxemia, hypertension, diabetes with any pregnancy
Primigravida >35 or <15 years old

Travel to Destination that May be Hazardous
High altitude
Areas endemic for or where epidemics are occurring of life-threatening food or insect-borne infections
Areas where chloroquine-resistant *Plasmodium falciparum* is endemic
Areas where live vaccines are required and recommended

Adapted from the CDC Health Information for International Travel 2012.[6]

problem is advisable, but may be difficult to obtain. Exclusions to insurance benefits should be carefully scrutinized.

Travel by Air

Flying is not contraindicated in most uncomplicated pregnancies.[8] Airline regulations vary. Most US air carriers require a physician letter beyond the 36th week of gestation for domestic travel and at the 35th week for international travel. The letter should document the status of the pregnancy and the expected delivery date.

Aircraft cabins are routinely pressurized to an altitude of 6500–8000 feet. The corresponding partial pressure of oxygen reduces maternal oxygenation to a far greater extent than that of the fetus. Fetal oxygenation is affected to a much lesser degree owing to the presence of fetal hemoglobin, which binds more tightly to oxygen molecules. The hemoglobin–oxygen dissociation curve permits the fetus to remain oxygenated at a wide fluctuation of maternal oxygen values,[9] hence, the risk of air travel to the fetus is not hypoxia.

Because of the expanded plasma volume and the demands of the developing fetus, mild anemia is common during pregnancy. Iron supplementation is recommended for all pregnant women. If the anemia is more pronounced, and travel is essential, supplemental oxygen can be considered at hemoglobin levels of <8.5 g/dL. Air travel by pregnant women with sickle cell anemia should be considered only after careful review of overall pregnancy status and close consultation with the obstetrician involved.

Cabin humidity aboard the airplane is approximately 8%. In this relatively dry environment, increased fluid intake over normal is recommended to maintain placental blood flow. Six to eight glasses of non-caffeine-containing fluid is the recommended amount for normal daily intake during pregnancy.

During long flights, thrombophlebitis may occur in any traveler due to venous stasis from immobility. A pregnant woman is at increased risk of thrombophlebitis owing to the hormones of pregnancy and the pressure of the uterus on the veins impeding flow.[10] Although no randomized, controlled studies have been done, it is recommended that pregnant women sit in an aisle seat, and stand up and move or walk hourly while on long flights. Support stockings are strongly recommended as they have been shown to reduce the risk of deep-vein thrombosis on long flights.[11] Isometric lower leg exercises may also be done while seated, to promote venous return. Aspirin is not recommended for routine use in pregnancy, particularly during the last 3 months, when increased bleeding and adverse fetal effects may occur. Pregnant women with thrombophilia, a history of thromboembolic events, or genetic predisposition to such problems should consult with their obstetrician for up-to-date antenatal management and prophylaxis during travel.

Radiation exposure during pregnancy should be limited. The 8–14th weeks of gestation are considered the most radiation sensitive for the fetus, as this is when brain and nervous system development occurs. The fetus is exposed to the same amount of radiation as the mother, as the mother's body does not provide an effective shield from radiation. Current Federal Aviation Administration recommendations[12–13] are for a total pregnancy exposure of 1 mS (millisievert), regardless of the number of months flying, or a monthly limit of 0.5 mS. The amount of radiation exposure per flight depends on the aircraft's cruising altitude and the duration of the flight. Further details on these recommendations may be obtained from the US Department of Transportation, Office of Aviation Medicine at: http://www.hf.faa.gov/docs/cami/00_33.pdf. Per-flight dose calculators are available through the FAA for frequent travelers with further interest in their cumulative exposure. Remaining within accepted guidelines on total pregnancy exposure has not been shown to increase fetal malformations, birth defects or miscarriages. There are no data on prenatal radiation exposure and lifetime cancer risk. Prior to its retirement in 2003, it was advised to avoid travel on Concorde, which flew at a higher altitude and involved more radiation exposure. Additionally, limiting flights along polar routes should be considered. Magnetometers at security checkpoints pose no risk of radiation exposure, nor do full body scanners.

Water Sports and Travel by Boat

Pregnant women contemplating a cruise should research the availability of medical care and equipment and trained personnel on board, should pregnancy complications arise. Choices for the treatment of motion sickness are limited by pregnancy (Table 22.2).

The risks of waterskiing during pregnancy are external genital lacerations and forceful water entry into the abdominal cavity via the cervix. Miscarriage or peritonitis may result.

SCUBA diving is generally considered unsafe at any stage of pregnancy. The potential risks to the fetus of decompression sickness, congenital abnormalities, and hyperbaric oxygen exposure, should decompression sickness occur, are unknown.

Exercise

Mild to moderate exercise is not associated with increased pregnancy loss. Running and high-impact aerobics may divert blood from the uterus and thus must be done with care as the pregnancy progresses. The American and British Colleges of Obstetrics and Gynecology recommendations for exercise during pregnancy are as follows:[3,4]

- Maternal heart rate <140 bpm during exercise
- Strenuous activity <15 min
- Avoid core temperature >38°C (100.4°F)
- No exercise in the supine position after the fourth month.

Table 22.2 Medications for Travel Use During Pregnancy and Lactation

Medication	FDA class	Issues during pregnancy	Issues during lactation
Analgesics/antipyretics		Try non-pharmaceutical methods first to treat pain such as rest, heat, massage	
Acetaminophen	B	Safe in low doses short term	Safe
Aspirin	C/D	Avoid last trimester. Has been associated with premature closure of ductus arteriosus in fetus and excessive bleeding Low dose aspirin (60–80 mg) may be used for pre-eclampsia	Unknown
Non-steroidal anti-inflammatory (ibuprofen, naproxen)	B/D (last trimester)	Should not be used in last trimester due to effects on premature closure of ductus arteriosus in fetus and effects on clotting Not teratogenic	Safe
Codeine	B	Use cautiously. May cause respiratory depression and withdrawal symptoms in fetus if used near term	
Hydrocodone	B	Use cautiously. May cause respiratory depression in infant if used near term	
Antibiotics			
Amoxicillin, Amoxicillin/Clavulanic acid (Augmentin) amoxicillin/sulbactam (Unasyn)	B	Safe. Use for treatment of otitis media, sinusitis, strep. throat	Safe
Azithromycin	B	Safe. Use for bronchitis, pneumonia, *Campylobacter*, *Shigella*, *Salmonella*, *E. coli*	Safe
Cephalosporins	B	Safe. Use for otitis, strep., sinusitis, pharyngitis	Safe
Clindamycin oral or vaginal cream	B	Safe, but avoid in first trimester Treat bacterial vaginosis orally or locally in second or third trimester Alternative for malaria treatment when used orally with quinine or quinidine	Safe
Ciprofloxacin, other quinolones	C	Controversial; Can consider for short-term use in severe infections and/or long-term use in life-threatening infections (anthrax) Use if potential benefit justifies risk to fetus	Avoid
Dicloxacillin	B	Safe. Use for skin infections	Safe. Used to treat mastitis
Doxycycline/tetracycline	D	May cause permanent discoloration of the teeth during tooth development, including the last half of pregnancy and children <8 years old May be used in combination with quinine for life-threatening situations such as treatment of malaria	Avoid
Erythromycin (base)	B	Safe	Safe
Nitrofurantoin	B	Drug of choice for UTI. Avoid if G6PD deficient and near term	Safe
Penicillin	B	Safe	Safe
Sulfisoxazole	C/D	Safe Not recommended third trimester due to risk of hyperbilirubinemia	Avoid due to infant risk of kernicterus
Trimethoprim	C	Safe	Safe
Gastrointestinal Antidiarrheal		Replace fluids	
Atropine sulfate diphenoxylate hydrochloride (Lomotil)	C	Avoid during pregnancy	Avoid
Loperamide (Imodium)	C	Use if severe symptoms	Safe
Antiemetics for nausea, heartburn, esophageal reflux		Supportive measures first such as light food (e.g., crackers) upon arising, frequent small meals, protein meal at bedtime, rather than medications	
Antacids	B	May use sparingly for symptoms as needed	Safe
Bismuth subsalicylate (Pepto-Bismol)	D	Avoid Contains salicylate	Avoid

Continued

Table 22.2 Medications for Travel Use During Pregnancy and Lactation—cont'd

Medication	FDA class	Issues during pregnancy	Issues during lactation
Cimetidine, ranitidine, omeprazole	B	Use during the first trimester is not associated with an increase in congenital malformations.	Safe
Metoclopramide (Reglan)	B	Safe in small doses	Safe
Dimenhydrinate (Dramamine)	B	Safe for severe nausea	Safe
Phenothiazines (Compazine)		No longer available in the U.S.	Avoid
		Rare cases of congenital malformations have occurred with use during pregnancy	
Acupressure (Seabands)		Safe	Safe
Emetrol (fluid replacement)	N/A	An oral solution containing balanced amounts of dextrose (glucose) and levulose (fructose) and phosphoric acid with controlled hydrogen ion concentration	Unknown
Ginger	B	Safe	Safe
Meclizine	B	Safe for treatment of severe nausea and vomiting	Safe
Pyridoxine (B6)	A	Safe	Safe
		Used for nausea	
Ondansetron (Zofran)	B	Safe	Safe
Constipation		Increase fiber + fluid in diet first	
Bisacodyl	B	Safe to use occasionally	Safe
Milk of magnesia	B	Safe in small amounts	Safe
Psyllium hydrophilic mucilloid	B	Safe	Safe
Hemorrhoids		Increase fiber + fluid in diet	
Hydrocortisone suppositories	B	Safe occasionally	
URI/congestion/cough		Symptomatic treatment	
Antihistamines			
Chlorpheniramine	B	Use cautiously if severe	Unknown
Cetirizine (Zyrtec)	B	Safe	Unknown
		Non-sedating	
Diphenhydramine (Benadryl)	B	Safe	Avoid
Loratadine (Claritin)	B	Safe	Unknown
		Non-sedating	
Dextromethorphan	C	Probably safe	Safe
		Use in small amounts	
Guaifenesin	C	Probably safe, use only if needed	Unknown
Pseudoephedrine (Sudafed)	C	Avoid first trimester.	Unknown
		Use cautiously	
Saline nasal spray	A	Safe	Safe
Topical nasal decongestants Oxymetazoline (Afrin)	C	Safe	Safe
		Do not use >3 days	
Asthma/allergy			
Inhaled bronchodilators	C	Safe for use if wheezing during pregnancy	Probably safe
Inhaled steroids	C	Use if indicated	Safe
Nasal steroids	C	Use if indicated	Safe
Antimalarials			
Mefloquine	C	Safe for both prophylaxis and treatment	Unknown effect
			Is excreted in breast milk in very small amounts
			Infant also needs prophylaxis
Chloroquine	C	Safe for prophylaxis and treatment	Safe
			Is excreted in small amounts
			Infant needs prophylaxis
Atovaquone/proguanil (Malarone)	C	Avoid in first trimester	No data
		Studies underway to evaluate safety in pregnancy (see text)	
Doxycycline	D	Contraindicated	Avoid
		May be considered for treatment of severe infections	
Halofantrine	C	Embryotoxic	Avoid
		Avoid	

Table 22.2 Medications for Travel Use During Pregnancy and Lactation—cont'd

Medication	FDA class	Issues during pregnancy	Issues during lactation
Primaquine	C	Do not administer during pregnancy because of the possibility that the fetus may be G6PD deficient Continue suppressive treatment until delivery	
Proguanil	C	Not associated with teratogenicity	Unknown
Quinine sulfate	C	Do not use unless life-threatening infection May induce severe hypoglycemia	
Quinidine	C	Relatively safe in pregnancy, but excessive doses may lead to premature labor and overdoses have led to abortions No case reports of teratogenicity to date from quinidine use Has been used in obstetrics since the 1930s.	
Azithromycin	B	Low efficacy Avoid for malaria prophylaxis (see text)	
Insect Repellent			
DEET		Safe Use sparingly as directed	Safe
Antiparasitics			
Albendazole	C	Teratogenic in animal studies Avoid first trimester Treat after delivery if possible May be indicated for serious infections	Excreted in animal milk, unknown in humans Use with caution
Furazolidone	C	Avoid with G6PD deficiency Avoid due to unknown fetal G6PD status	Safety not established
Iodoquinol	C	Use only if indicated for severe infection	Unknown
Metronidazole	B	Avoid first trimester Readily crosses placenta Use only if clearly indicated	Use caution Breast milk concentration similar to plasma. Best to use one dose therapy and delay breastfeeding for 12–24 h
Paromomycin	B	Minimal systemic absorption Recommended for the treatment of severe infections with *Giardia lamblia*, *Entamoeba histolytica* and tapeworm infestations during pregnancy	No information
Praziquantel	B	Used in treatment of severe schistosomiasis Preferable to delay treatment during pregnancy until after delivery, unless absolutely essential	Do not breastfeed on day of treatment and for 72 h following dose
Antivirals			
Aciclovir	B	Use only for severe infections	Safe
Valaciclovir (Valtrex)	B	Limited data show no increase in birth defects, but small studies; use if potential benefit outweighs risk to fetus	Limited data Present in breast milk Use only when indicated and with caution
Altitude sickness			
Acetazolamide (Diamox)	C	Do not use during first trimester Use only if benefit outweighs risk	Discontinue nursing while on drug
Dexamethasone (Decadron)	C	May use if needed for treatment for altitude illness	Avoid breastfeeding during therapy
Calcium channel blockers (Nifedipine)	C	Use only to treat severe symptoms pulmonary edema	Safe
Water purification			
Iodine	D	Avoid, except for short term (2–3 weeks) May lead to goiter and fetal hypothyroidism	Avoid

A total of 30 min of aerobic exercise a day is supported. Hypoglycemia should be avoided. However, some controversy exists concerning these recommendations.[5] Current studies are looking at modification of these recommendations for the woman who was a moderate to competitive athlete before becoming pregnant. Many pregnant women in this group have exceeded the recommendations in the ACOG guidelines without known harm to the fetus. Elite athletes who are pregnant need specific attention to fetal growth assessments and a modification of intense training schedules.

Travel by Automobile

Prudent, but unproven, recommendations regarding automobile travel include limiting prolonged sitting and making frequent stops to permit increased circulation. Care should be taken to position the seatbelt low on the abdomen to prevent fetal compression in a rapid stop. Because lap belts alone are not sufficient restraints, a shoulder–lap belt combination is recommended.

Immunizations

Immunization during pregnancy (Table 22.3) requires a careful evaluation of the potential risk of a vaccine-preventable disease versus the possible risks of vaccination for both the mother and the fetus. Vaccination during pregnancy is indicated in situations where exposure is highly probable and the disease poses a greater risk to the woman or fetus than the vaccination (risk/benefit ratio). Ideally, all women should be vaccinated before pregnancy as part of preconception care. Whenever possible, any pre-travel visit should be used to update the vaccination status of non-pregnant women of reproductive age.

The risks of immunization during pregnancy are largely theoretical. There have been no well-controlled studies of vaccine effects on the fetus. Case reports and post-exposure data comprise the currently available knowledge on vaccinating pregnant women.

In general, vaccinations should be avoided in the first trimester of pregnancy because of the uncertain effect of the vaccine on the developing fetus. Live virus vaccines should be avoided in all trimesters, except in special circumstances. Yellow fever vaccine can be given during pregnancy if travel to a high-risk area is unavoidable.[6] Small numbers of pregnant women inadvertently vaccinated with the yellow fever vaccine have been studied.[14,15] The vaccine did not appear to adversely affect the fetal or maternal outcomes.

The vaccine strain of virus has been documented to be transferred to infants via breast milk. Several case reports have emerged in the past 3 years of infants who have contracted vaccine-strain yellow fever following maternal vaccination.[40] Breastfeeding women should avoid yellow fever vaccine except when exposure cannot be avoided. A letter of waiver may be considered for the pregnant traveler going to a low-risk destination where yellow fever vaccine may be required for entry into the country or for travel between certain countries but the actual risk of acquiring the disease is low.

Malaria and Pregnancy

Malaria affects 300–500 million people a year, resulting in over 800 000 deaths.[16] Morbidity and mortality are the greatest in children and pregnant women. Malaria during pregnancy may have severe consequences. Data indicate that women are more susceptible to malaria during pregnancy and the immediate postpartum period.[17,18] Pregnancy increases the clinical severity of *Plasmodium falciparum* malaria in women both with and without existing immunity.[19] Preferential sequestration of parasitized red blood cells in the placenta may

occur, along with suppression of selected components of the immune system during pregnancy. Intrauterine growth retardation, premature delivery, anemia, fetal loss, maternal death, and/or congenital malaria may result. Maternal and perinatal mortality both increase markedly with infection.

Pregnant travelers need to scrutinize their itinerary and be aware of the increased risk to themselves and their fetus. If a woman is pregnant, or plans to become pregnant and cannot defer travel to a high-risk area, appropriate chemoprophylaxis and maximal personal protective measures are essential. Travel to areas where chloroquine-resistant strains of *Plasmodium falciparum* exist poses increased risk owing to limited data on prophylaxis options. Women who plan to become pregnant while traveling or shortly after also need to be aware of existing information regarding the potential effects of prophylactic or treatment medications on the fetus, and the availability of appropriate medical care should they contract malaria.

Plasmodium vivax malaria occurs more commonly than *P. falciparum* in many parts of the tropics outside Africa.[16] The effects of *P. vivax* infection in pregnancy have not been as well characterized as those of *P. falciparum*, but recent data suggest that *P.vivax* infections may be more serious than previously thought.[17] *P. vivax* malaria during pregnancy is associated with maternal anemia and low birthweight, but does not appear to be associated with miscarriage, stillbirth, or a shortened duration of pregnancy.[20] Though the effects of *P. vivax* infection are less striking than those of *P. falciparum* infection during pregnancy, antimalarial chemoprophylaxis for travel to predominantly *P. vivax*-endemic areas is strongly recommended. Most of the research studies have been conducted on pregnant women living in endemic areas and may not necessarily be extrapolated to non-immune pregnant travelers, who are at higher risk. Terminal prophylaxis with primaquine is not recommended during pregnancy owing to the theoretical risk of having an undiagnosed fetus with G6PD deficiency and the consequent hemolysis that occurs with the use of this drug.

Guidelines for Prevention

Personal Protective Measures

The pregnant traveler should use a combination of physical and chemical barriers to reduce the risk of contracting malaria. Permethrin-treated bed-nets should be recommended. They have been studied in pregnant women in Africa and have not caused any harmful effects on the pregnancy. Prudent application of DEET (diethyl-*m*-toluamide) in a concentration of ≤35%, or picaridin (KBR 3023) may be used safely during pregnancy. The safety of DEET was assessed in a single study of women in the second and third trimester of pregnancy in Thailand.[21] There was no effect on survival, growth, or development at birth or at one year of age in this group of infants. Although DEET was detected in the cord blood of 8% of the infants, there was no effect on survival, development, growth or status at 1 year of age in this group of infants.

Chemoprophylaxis

In recommending pharmacologic prophylaxis to a pregnant woman, the risk of malaria must be weighed with the benefit of the medication (Table 22.4). For travel to chloroquine-sensitive areas, chloroquine may be prescribed safely in the usual adult doses during pregnancy. Chloroquine has been used for decades for both prophylaxis and treatment of malaria during pregnancy without adverse fetal or maternal effects.

If at all possible, travel to areas of chloroquine-resistant *P. falciparum* should be deferred during pregnancy. Mefloquine is currently

Table 22.3 Immunizations During Pregnancy

Immunobiologic agent	Type of vaccine	Issues in pregnancy
Cholera	Inactivated whole cell vaccine	Not recommended for any travelers due to low efficacy
	Killed oral cholera toxin B subunit whole cell killed (Dukoral)	Not available in USA. Available in Canada and Europe
		No live organisms. May be efficacious in high-risk situations but not recommended during pregnancy at this time
	Live attenuated oral cholera vaccine (CVD 103 HgR strain)	Not recommended in pregnancy
		Not available in USA
		Available in Europe
Diphtheria – tetanus – acellular pertussis (Dtap)	Toxoid	None; approved for use in pregnancy and post-partum
ETEC (Dukoral)	Inactivated bacterial ,oral	No safety data in pregnancy
		Vaccination should be weighed against risk of disease
Hepatitis A	Formalin inactivated vaccine	Use only if clearly indicated
	(Combined hepatitis A/Vi capsular polysaccharide)	Data on safety in pregnancy are not available; the theoretical risk of vaccination should be weighed against the risk of disease
Hepatitis B	Recombinant purified hepatitis B surface antigen	Pre-exposure and post-exposure prophylaxis indicated in pregnant women at risk
Hemophilus B conjugate	Polysaccharide	For high-risk persons
Immune globulins (IG) Pooled or hyperimmune	Immune globulins or specific antitoxin serum including antivenin for snakebite, spider-bite, diphtheria antitoxin, HBIG, rabies IG, tetanus IG, RH (D) IG, varicella zoster IG	Give appropriate immunoglobulin or antitoxin as indicated for exposure
Influenza	Inactivated vaccine	Recommended for all pregnant women in their second or third trimester during influenza season
		Indicated for pregnant women in any trimester if history of high-risk medical condition
	Live viral	Not recommended for use in pregnancy
Japanese encephalitis	Vero-cell vaccine	Safety data not available. Risk assessment
Measles Mumps Rubella	Live attenuated	Contraindicated
		Pregnancy should be delayed for 3 months after MMR is given
		Check titer if immunity unknown
		May give immune globulin if exposure
Meningococcal vaccine	Polysaccharide	Administer for high-risk exposure, as per non-pregnant traveler
	Conjugate	Not studied in pregnancy. Theoretical use
Pneumococcus	Polysaccharide	Vaccine used only in high-risk pregnancies
	Conjugate	Post splenectomy
		Not studied in pregnancy. Theoretical use
Polio	Trivalent live attenuated (OPV)	Avoid in previously non-immune individuals due to risk of vaccine-associated paralysis
		ACIP recommends use in outbreak situation
	Killed (IPV)	Preferred over OPV in pregnancy
Rabies	Killed virus	Pre-exposure prophylaxis only when substantial risk for exposure exists
	Human diploid cell rabies vaccine (HDCV) or rabies vaccine adsorbed (RVA)	Post-exposure prophylaxis is indicated during pregnancy
Tick-borne encephalitis	Inactivated	Not recommended in pregnancy
		Practice strict tick-bite precautions
Tetanus – diphtheria	Combined toxoid	Safe in pregnancy
		Use if lack of primary series or no booster within 10 years
Typhoid (Ty21a)	Live-attenuated bacterial, oral	No safety data in pregnancy
		Avoid in pregnancy on theoretical grounds (live vaccine)
Typhoid Vi	Vi capsular polysaccharide	May use for travel to endemic areas
Varicella	Live attenuated	Contraindicated in pregnancy
		Although no teratogenic effects of the vaccine have been documented, pregnancies occurring within 3 months of the vaccine or vaccinations given inadvertently during pregnancy should be reported to the Varivax registry (800–986–8999)
Yellow fever	Live attenuated	Contraindicated except if exposure unavoidable
		Give letter of waiver for travel to low-risk area
		Avoid if breastfeeding

Adapted from CDC Information for International Travel, 2007–2008.[6]

Table 22.4 Malaria Chemoprophylaxis in Pregnant Travelers

Antimalarials	Dose	Comments
Chloroquine-sensitive areas		
Chloroquine (CQ)	300 mg base (equal to 500 mg of phosphate salt) weekly Start 1 week before travel and continue for 4 weeks after travel to malarious zone	Safe Reactions rare
Chloroquine-resistant areas (options for chemoprophylaxis)		
Mefloquine (MQ)	250 mg weekly Start 2–4 weeks before travel and continue for 4 weeks after travel to malarious zone	Considered by FDA to be safe for treatment and prevention in all trimesters. Possible trend in stillbirths noted in some studies Neuropsychiatric reactions
Chemoprophylaxis _not_ recommended in pregnancy		
Atovaquone-proguanil	Atovaquone 250 mg + Proguanil 100 mg 1 tablet daily for 1–2 days before travel and for 1 week after leaving malarious area	Safety of atovaquone in pregnancy _not_ established It is not known whether atovaquone is excreted into human milk Proguanil is excreted into human milk in small quantities Because data are not yet available on safety and efficacy, should not be given to a woman who breastfeeds an infant who weighs <5 kg (11 lbs) unless the potential benefit to the woman outweighs the potential risk to the child (e.g., for a lactating woman who had acquired _P. falciparum_ malaria in an area of multi-drug resistance who could not tolerate other treatment options)
Pyrimethamine		
Azithromycin	250 mg daily	Not recommended for prophylaxis due to limited efficacy. Treatment during pregnancy studies are in progress
Primaquine		Contraindicated in pregnancy due to the possibility of G6PD deficiency in the fetus

the only available recommended antimalarial recommended for use in chloroquine-resistant _P. falciparum_ areas. Until recently mefloquine was considered to be safe primarily during the second and third trimesters. However in 2011 the FDA reclassified mefloquine from category C to category B with respect to its safety in pregnancy, based on their review of the published data on mefloquine use during pregnancy. These data showed that pregnant women who took mefloquine at various doses for both prevention and treatment of malaria did not have an increased risk of teratogenic effects (birth defects) or adverse pregnancy outcomes compared to the background rate in the general population.

Subsequently, the Centers for Disease Control and Prevention (CDC) has recommended mefloquine for pregnant women, both as a malaria treatment option and as an option to prevent malaria infection for _all_ trimesters.[22]

The combination of weekly chloroquine and daily proguanil is safe during pregnancy; however, it is not recommended as a first-line combination owing to its low efficacy in areas of chloroquine resistance. Doxycycline is currently classified as a category C drug in pregnancy. Tetracyclines cross the placenta and can adversely affect fetal skeletal development.[23] The combination of atovaquone plus proguanil (Malarone) is not recommended to date for chemoprophylaxis in pregnancy owing to lack of data on the effects of atovaquone use. It is currently classified as pregnancy category C.

Treatment

There is no convincing evidence that the treatment of malaria during pregnancy adversely affects pregnancy outcome. As noted above, mefloquine has been approved by the FDA for treatment of malaria for all trimesters. Quinine has been used for treatment in the third trimester; however, stillbirths and congenital malformations have been reported. Recurrent hypoglycemia commonly occurs with quinine treatment during pregnancy, and blood glucose should be followed closely to avoid this.

Atovaquone/proguanil has been studied in small numbers of pregnant women for malaria treatment. In two small studies it was well tolerated without adverse effects on the fetus. It is currently considered an option for treatment in multidrug-resistant _P. falciparum_ infections.[23,24] More data are needed to determine whether this combination is safe in pregnancy.

The Qinghaosu derivatives artesunate and artemether have been used to treat malaria in all trimesters of pregnancy. They are well tolerated and no adverse pregnancy outcomes were reported in a study of 441 women treated in Thailand. Further study is needed of the use of these compounds in pregnancy.[25] However, in severe malaria parenteral artemesinin combinations are preferable to quinine in the second and third trimesters because of the problem of quinine-associated hypoglycemia; this occurs less frequently in the first trimester.[26] Although azithromycin alone has not proved reliably efficacious in malaria prophylaxis, studies are under way to evaluate the use of azithromycin in combination with other antimalarials to treat malaria during pregnancy.

Food and Water Precautions

Travelers' Diarrhea

The pregnant traveler needs to make every effort to avoid travelers' diarrhea. This illness is reported in 33–50% of all travelers on a short-term trip to a developing country. All travelers should take meticulous food and water precautions. Food should be thoroughly cooked to avoid the usual bacterial, viral, and protozoal pathogens. Pharmacologic prophylaxis with either antibiotics or bismuth is not recommended routinely for the pregnant traveler. The fever and dehydration that accompany many travelers' diarrhea syndromes may compromise placental blood flow and potentially adversely affect the fetus. Decreased stomach acidity during pregnancy may increase susceptibility to travelers' diarrhea and other enteric pathogens. In addition, some pathogens (*Listeria, Toxoplasma*, hepatitis E) pose an unusually high risk during pregnancy.

Congenital toxoplasmosis may occur if a woman is acutely infected during pregnancy. Approximately 3/1000 infants show evidence of congenital toxoplasmosis; infection is most likely to occur when maternal infection develops in the third trimester. Fewer than half of affected infants are symptomatic at birth. The risk of severe abnormalities may be 5–6%; these include seizures, mental retardation, cerebral palsy, deafness and blindness in the infant. Although the lowest risk of fetal infection is in the first trimester, the majority of those infected have severe disease. Chronic or latent infection almost never causes fetal injury in an otherwise healthy mother.[27] The risk of contracting toxoplasmosis can be diminished by thoroughly cooking meat and wearing gloves for contact with dirt (putting up a tent or other activities that involve contact with dirt). Pregnant women should not change a cat's litter box.

Infection with *Listeria* during pregnancy may cause miscarriage, stillbirth, premature labor, and death of the fetus. *Listeria* is most likely to be found in unpasteurized milk and other soft cheeses. Pregnant women should avoid feta, Brie, Camembert, Mexican-style cheeses, blue-veined cheeses, and deli meats early in pregnancy. Media alerts regarding produce infected with *Listeria* should be adhered so that such foods are avoided while pregnant.

Enterically transmitted hepatitis E infection in pregnancy may cause severe illness in both mother and fetus. It is a major cause of hepatitis outbreaks in India, Nepal, China, Pakistan, Africa, and the former Soviet Union, and has been reported from Central America and SE Asia. Transmission of the virus occurs through the fecal–oral route. Most outbreaks occur as a result of fecal contamination of drinking water. This infection is most common in persons of child-bearing age. Clinical illness can range from mild to severe. Hepatitis E acquired during pregnancy has a particularly high maternal fatality rate (15–30%). In non-pregnant women, severe disease occurs in <1% of individuals. In pregnant women, however, 20–30% may experience fulminant disease.[28] Studies have demonstrated that the maternal fatality rate during pregnancy due to hepatitis E may increase from 2% during the first trimester to 20–30% during the third trimester. The cause of the increased severity during pregnancy is not known. Hepatitis E infection acquired during the third trimester is also associated with fetal morbidity and mortality. A vaccine is in clinical trials but not currently available. If at all possible, pregnant women should avoid travel to areas with a high rate of hepatitis E. Passive immunization with immunoglobulin is not effective in preventing infection. Strict adherence to food and water precautions is critical in the prevention of this infection.

Water Purification

A clean water source should be ensured. Boiling water for 1 min at sea level kills all organisms. As the production of bottled water is not regulated, bottled water should be inspected for a factory-sealed cap. Commercially available ceramic water purifiers remove bacteria and 99–99.9% of viruses. Filters alone do not remove viruses and are not recommended. Heavily contaminated ground water should be pre-treated with chlorine or iodine, and then filtered. Treating water chemically with iodine tablets may be safe for short-term travel (2–3 weeks). Higher, albeit undefined, amounts of iodine ingested during pregnancy may cause fetal goiter and hypothyroidism. The World Health Organization (WHO) recommends 200 μg iodine/day for pregnant women.[29] The pregnant traveler should be familiar with the amount of residual iodine found in iodine tablets.

Treatment

World Health Organization (WHO) oral rehydration solution (ORS) should be used in sufficient quantities to prevent dehydration. Pre-packaged electrolyte or rice-based ORS should be part of the pregnant traveler's medical kit.

Pharmacologic treatment is limited by pregnancy and the potential harm to the fetus. There is no single ideal drug. Ciprofloxacin, the usual drug of choice for non-pregnant adults in Africa, the Middle East and the Western hemisphere, is theoretically contraindicated for use in pregnancy owing to the potential adverse effects on the developing fetal skeleton. However, there have been no reports to date of adverse fetal outcomes in pregnant women who were inadvertently exposed to ciprofloxacin. A recent meta-analysis showed no harmful effects of fluoroquinolones in the first trimester.[30] Until more data are available, ciprofloxacin is not universally recommended unless the possible risk of the infection outweighs the risk of the medication. A single dose of ciprofloxacin may be considered, with informed consent, given the severity of potential infection in pregnancy and the knowledge that a single dose of ciprofloxacin has been shown to be as effective as 3 days of treatment. Of note, ciprofloxacin is recommended in pregnancy if exposure to anthrax is suspected. Azithromycin is a category B (see later, Table 22.5) drug and has good efficacy against *Campylobacter* and ETEC and most other enteric pathogens that cause travelers' diarrhea. Cefixime is an oral third-generation drug that may be used safely in pregnancy. Although it covers *E. coli* and *Salmonella*, it is not an optimal choice for shigellosis or *Campylobacter*.[31] Ampicillin and erythromycin are safe to use in pregnancy, but lack efficacy against common travelers' diarrhea pathogens. Clarithromycin should be avoided. Likewise, furazolidone should be avoided, as it may cause problems in the presence of fetal G6PD-deficiency. Metronidazole may be used when indicated after the first trimester. Paromomycin, a non-absorbed intraluminal amebicide and anti-*Giardia* agent, is safe for use in pregnancy.[32]

Pepto-Bismol is relatively contraindicated owing to data on bismuth toxicity in sheep and the salicylate component, which may cause fetal bleeding. Loperamide may be used in pregnancy, in conjunction with oral rehydration. Medications that may be used safely in pregnancy are listed in Table 22.2.[33]

Table 22.5 Food and Drug Administration Use-in-Pregnancy Ratings

FDA Category/Rating	Description
Category A	Adequate and well-controlled studies in women show no risk to fetus
Category B	No evidence of risk in humans. Either studies in animals show risk, but human findings do not, or, in the absence of human studies, animal findings are negative
Category C	Risk cannot be ruled out. No adequate and well-controlled studies in humans, or animal studies are either positive for fetal risk or lacking as well. Drugs should be given only if the potential benefit justifies the potential risk to the fetus
Category D	There is positive evidence of human fetal risk. Nevertheless, potential benefits may outweigh the potential risks
Category X	Contraindicated in pregnancy. Studies in animals or humans or investigational or post-marketing reports have shown fetal risk that far outweighs any potential benefit to the patient.

Altitude and Pregnancy

Significant issues to consider in contemplating this type of adventure travel during pregnancy include the availability of adequate medical care for the mother or fetus, transport risks and the treatment of enteric infections. Emergency transport may pose risks to the fetus if an unpressurized aircraft is used, or if delivery occurs during transport. Enteric infections should be treated appropriately to avoid maternal dehydration and the possible onset of preterm labor; the limitations of treatment choices have been described above.

Few data have been published on the pregnant woman who travels to altitude (8000 feet, 2400 m) for a short trip. Advice to pregnant women wishing to exercise at altitude is based on isolated observations and a few systematic studies. Few studies have explored the limits of combined exercise and altitude exposure in human pregnancy. Consideration should be given to known physiologic changes of residence at high altitude, the degree of physiologic adaptations to both pregnancy and altitude, and data from the few systematic studies in human pregnancy. Because individual altitude tolerance and exercise capacity cannot be reliably determined at sea level, advice should err on the side of caution and recognize the limitations of the available data.

Short-term travel to moderate altitude does not seem to have negative effects on pregnancy. For women living at altitude, pregnancy-induced hypertension and pre-eclampsia are more common. Infant birthweights are lower at altitude than in infants born at sea level.[34,35] Chronic placental changes occur at altitude, but have not been seen or conclusively studied in the short-term traveler. Low oxygen tension and pressure changes may result in intrauterine growth retardation and an increased risk of premature labor in women who spend most of their pregnancy above 8000 feet.[36]

Studies in pregnant women at altitude show that the human fetus develops normally under low-oxygen conditions. Exposure of a pregnant woman to the hypoxia at high altitude results in acclimatization responses that act to preserve the fetal oxygen supply. The fetus also utilizes several compensatory mechanisms to survive brief periods of hypoxia. While fetal heart rate monitoring data during air travel suggest no compromise of fetal oxygenation, exercise at high altitude may place further stress on oxygen delivery to the fetus. Thus, a pregnant woman who goes to altitude must take time to acclimatize to avoid high-altitude pulmonary edema or additional hypoxic stress.

The risks to the mother and fetus of high-altitude trekking are not well defined physiologically, although fetal bradycardia has been seen with exposure to extreme altitudes.[37] It is reassuring that there have been no reports of injury, pregnancy complications, or losses associated with exercise at altitude (skiing, running, mountain bicycling, trekking, etc.). Studies to date, however, have been conducted at moderate altitudes for short periods and at low intensities. Until more data are available, it is recommended that pregnant women avoid the additional hypoxic stress of extreme altitude.[38]

Pregnancy Planning

Women considering conception should take into account the potential effects of certain vaccinations and medications and plan accordingly, if possible.

Attempts to conceive should be deferred until 1 month after receiving the measles–mumps–rubella (MMR) vaccine. The precaution is based on the theoretical risk of fetal infection with a live viral vaccination. No congenital defects have been reported, and receiving any component of the vaccine singly or in combination is not an indication for pregnancy termination.[39]

Pregnancy should likewise be avoided for 1 month after administration of the varicella vaccine. The VARIVAX pregnancy registry (800-986-8999) is monitoring the maternal and fetal outcomes of women inadvertently vaccinated with varicella vaccine while pregnant or during the 3 months before pregnancy.

Since antimalarial chemoprophylaxis with mefloquine or chloroquine has not been associated with fetal anomalies, it is no longer recommended to wait a specific period of time after exposure to these antimalarials to attempt to conceive.[6] Theoretically, on the basis of drug half-lives, one should wait at least 2 weeks before conceiving when doxycycline, atovaquone/proguanil, or primaquine are used for chemoprophylaxis.

Breastfeeding

Drugs in Breast Milk

Because no randomized controlled trials have been carried out on the safety of medications during lactation, any medication given to a lactating woman should be carefully considered. Most routinely prescribed drugs are safe to use during lactation. Short-acting drugs administered after a feed have the least opportunity to be excreted into milk. Few drugs are absolutely contraindicated while breastfeeding. Quinolones are currently contraindicated for use in children <18 years old. Although ciprofloxacin is excreted into breast milk in small quantities, there have been no adverse reports regarding any effect on breastfed infants.

Malaria Prevention

Mefloquine, chloroquine, tetracyclines and proguanil are excreted into human milk in small amounts. It is not known whether atovaquone or doxycycline is excreted in breast milk. The amount of these drugs is insufficient to protect the nursing infant; therefore, the infant must be adequately protected with an appropriate weight-adjusted dose of antimalarial medication. There is no evidence that amounts excreted in human milk are harmful to a nursing infant.[33]

Immunizations

Lactating mothers may safely receive most vaccinations. Most strains of live viral vaccines are not known to be transmitted in breast milk, with the exception of yellow fever virus and attenuated rubella virus. Infants are usually not infected by the vaccine strain of rubella virus.[39] Transmission of vaccine-strain yellow fever has been documented in nursing mothers, therefore the yellow fever vaccine is strongly discouraged, unless travel is unavoidable.[40] The smallpox vaccine should not be given to nursing mothers, although outbreak situations may lead to a change in this recommendation.[41]

Practicalities

Good breast hygiene should be practiced by the nursing mother while traveling. Human milk protects the infant from many enteric diseases, and breastfeeding should be *strongly* supported for the traveling newborn infant.

For the nursing mother who is traveling without her infant, meticulous attention should be given to maintaining the breast pump. Both manual and electric pumps should be washed with clean water and soap after use and dried in a fly-free environment. Breast milk may be kept at room temperature for 4 h before use, or refrigerated for use within 72 h, though some sources indicate that it may be used for up to 5 days.[42] Frozen breast milk may be stored for up to 4 months.

Women should use the breast pump nearly as frequently as they would nurse the infant to avoid painful breast engorgement or the development of mastitis. If mastitis develops, more frequent pumping, analgesics, and an anti-staphylococcal antibiotic (dicloxacillin or cephalexin) are treatments to consider.

Medications

General principles to consider when prescribing a medication to a pregnant woman include:

- How do the pharmacokinetics of the medication differ during pregnancy?
- Are the adverse reactions or side-effects more common during pregnancy than in the non-pregnant woman?
- What is the potential risk of the medication used to treat or prevent the disease versus the risk of giving the disease to the developing fetus?

The US Food and Drug Administration (FDA) categorizes each medication and immunization used in the USA. As most medications and immunizations have not been tested during pregnancy or lactation, they are categorized as FDA category C (Table 20.5). Other classification systems to estimate fetal risk have been developed in other countries, such as Sweden, Australia, Netherlands, and Denmark. Also, there are a number of website resources with information on the possible teratogenic risk of a particular medication or vaccine.

The American College of Obstetrics and Gynecology has released recommendations regarding the use of antimicrobial therapy during pregnancy. They classify the commonly used antibiotics as:[43]

- Those considered safe (i.e., penicillin and erythromycin base, stearate or ethylsuccinate)
- Those that probably are safe but to be used with caution (i.e., azithromycin, metronidazole, nitrofurantoin)

- Those that are contraindicated (i.e., tetracycline, fluroquinones, and erythromycin estolate).

Other Issues

Medical Kit

The pregnant traveler should carry a medical kit. Aside from the usual first aid, medical and comfort needs, on prolonged trips away from routine OB/GYN care she should consider carrying a sphygmomanometer to monitor blood pressure and urine dipsticks to check for proteinuria. Additional items could include chewable antacids, hydrocortisone cream for hemorrhoids, prenatal vitamins and constipation remedies.

Alternative Medications

The use of herbal remedies has increased over the last several years in all areas of medicine, especially in the area of women's health. Some of these remedies have shown promising application, such as the use of ginger or acupressure for nausea during pregnancy. Women travelers may be tempted to try traditional healing practices or local remedies for symptoms. Pregnant women should be advised that some medicinal herbs may have unknown side-effects, such as inducing uterine contractions or fetal teratogenicity. Until more data are available, all herbal remedies should be used with caution, especially in the first trimester.

References

1. Kingman CE, Economides DL. Travel in pregnancy: pregnant women's experiences and knowledge of health issues. J Travel Med 2003;10:330–3.
2. Gabbe SG. Obstetrics – Normal and Problem Pregnancies. 5th ed. New York: Churchill LivingstoneElsevier; 2007.
3. American College of Obstetricians and Gynecologists; ACOG Committee Opinion, No. 267, January 2002. Exercise during pregnancy and the postpartum period. Obstet Gynecol 2002;99:171–3.
4. Exercise in Pregnancy, RCOG Statement No. 4 –January 2006. Online. Available: http://www.rcog.org.uk/index.asp?PageID=1366
5. Clapp 3rd JF. Exercise during pregnancy. A clinical update. Clin Sports Med 2000;19:273–86.
6. Center for Disease Control. Health Information for International Travel, 2012. US Department of Health and Human Services: Public Health Service; 2012.
7. Rose SR. Pregnancy and travel. Emerg Med Clin N Am 1997;15:95–111.
8. Committee opinion No, 264, December 2001. Air travel during pregnancy. ACOG Committee on Obstetric Practice. Obstet Gynecol 2001;98:1187–8.
9. Huch R, Baumann H, Fallenstein F, et al. Physiologic changes in pregnant women and their fetuses during jet travel. Am J Obstet Gynecol 1986;154:996–1000.
10. Ryan KJ. Kistner's Gynecology and Women's Health. 7th ed. St. Louis: Mosby; 1999.
11. Scurr JH, Machin SJ, Bailey-King S, et al. Frequency and prevention of symptomless deep-vein thrombosis in long-haul flights: a randomised trial. Lancet 2001;357:1485–9.
12. United States Department of Transportation, Office of Aviation Medicine. Online. Available: http://www.hf.faa.gov/docs/cami/00_33.pdf (accessed Feb 25, 2006).
13. Carroll ID. Pregnancy and travel. Clin Fam Pract 2005;7:773–90. Available: http://www.acog.org/from_home/publications/green_journal/2004/v103n6p1326.pdf
14. Robert E, Vial T, Schaefer C, et al. Exposure to yellow fever vaccine in early pregnancy. Vaccine 1999;17:283–5.
16. Suzano CE, Amaral E, Sato HK, et al. The effects of yellow fever immunization (17DD) inadvertently used in early pregnancy during a mass campaign in Brazil. Vaccine 2006;24:1421–6.

16. Kain KC, Keystone JS. Malaria in travelers. Epidemiology, disease, and prevention. Infect Dis Clin North Am 1998;12:267–84.

17. Kochar ,DK Das A, Kochar SK, et al. Severe *Plasmodium vivax* malaria: A report on serial cases from Bikaner in Northwestern India. Am J Trop Med Hyg 2009; 80:194–8. Diagne N. Increased susceptibility to malaria during the early postpartum period. N Engl J Med 2000;343:598–603.

18. Lindsay S, Ansell J, Selman C, et al. Effect of pregnancy on exposure to malaria mosquitoes. Lancet 2000;355:1972.

19. Nathwani D, Currie PF, Douglas JG, et al. *Plasmodium falciparum* malaria in pregnancy: a review. Br J Obstet Gynaecol 1992;99:118–21.

20. Nosten F, McGready R, Simpson JA, et al. Effects of *Plasmodium vivax* malaria in pregnancy. Lancet 1999;354:546–9.

21. McGready R, Hamilton KA, Simpson JA, et al. Safety of the insect repellent N,N-diethyl-M-toluamide (DEET) in pregnancy. Am J Trop Med Hyg 2001;65:285–9.

22. CDC Update: New Recommendations for Mefloquine Use in Pregnancy www.cdc.gov/malaria (accessed 1.1.2012).

23. McGready R, Ashley EA, Moo E, et al. A randomized comparison of artesunate-atovaquone-proguanil versus quinine in treatment for uncomplicated falciparum malaria during pregnancy. J Infect Dis 2005;192:846–53.

24. McGready R, Keo NK, Villegas L, et al. Artesunate-atovaquone-proguanil rescue treatment of multidrug-resistant *Plasmodium falciparum* malaria in pregnancy: a preliminary report. Trans R Soc Trop Med Hyg 2003;97:592–4.

25. McGready R. Artemisinin antimalarials in pregnancy: a prospective treatment study of 539 episodes of multidrug-resistant *Plasmodium falciparum*. Clin Infect Dis 2001;33:2009–16.

26. Guidelines for Treatment of Malaria, second edition 2010 p 47.

27. Gabbe SG, Neibyl JR, Simpson JL, editors. Obstetrics – Normal and Problem Pregnancies. 4th ed. London: Churchill Livingstone; 2002.

28. Aggarwal R, Krawczynski K, Hepatitis E. an overview and recent advances in clinical and laboratory research. J Gastroenterol Hepatol 2000;15:9–20.

29. WHO. Bulletin of the World Health Organization 1996;74:1–3. Reprint 5665. Online. Available: http://whqlibdoc.who.int/hq/1996/WHO_NUT_96.5.pdf

30. Bar-Oz B, Moretti ME, Boskovic R, et al. The safety of quinolones – a meta-analysis of pregnancy outcomes. Eur J Obstet Gynecol Reprod Biol. 2009;143(2):75–8.

31. Salam MA, Seas C, Khan WA, et al. Treatment of shigellosis: IV. Cefixime is ineffective in shigellosis in adults. Ann Intern Med 1995;123:505–8.

32. Rosenblatt JE. Antiparasitic agents. Mayo Clin Proc 1999;74:1161–75.

33. Briggs GG, Freeman RK, Yaffe SJ. Drugs in Pregnancy and Lactation: a Reference Guide to Fetal and Neonatal Risk. 5th ed. Baltimore: Williams & Wilkins; 1998.

34. Niermeyer S. The pregnant altitude visitor. Adv Exp Med Biol 1999;474:65–77.

35. Mortola JP. Birth weight and altitude: a study in Peruvian communities. J Pediatr 2000;136:324–9.

36. Ali KZ, Ali ME, Khalid ME. High altitude and spontaneous preterm birth. Int J Gynaecol Obstet 1996;54:11–5.

37. Hackett PH. High altitude and common medical conditions. In: Hornbein T, Schoene R, editors. High Altitude: an Exploration of Human Adaptation, vol. 161. New York: Dekker; 2001. p. 839–86.

38. Huch R Physical activity at altitude in pregnancy. Sem Perinatol 1996;20:303–14.

39. American Academy of Pediatrics. Rubella. In: Pickering LK, editor. Red Book: Report of the Committee on Infectious Diseases, 2009. 2nd ed. Elk Grove Village: American Academy of Pediatrics; 2003. p. 540.

40. Centers for Disease Control and Prevention. Transmission of yellow fever vaccine virus through breast-feeding: Brazil, 2009. MMWR Morbid Mortal Wkly Rep 2010;59:130–2.

41. Wharton M, Strikas RA, Harpaz R, et al. Recommendations for using smallpox vaccine in a pre-event vaccination program. Supplemental recommendations of the Advisory Committee on Immunization Practices (ACIP) and the Healthcare Infection Control Practices Advisory Committee (HICPAC). MMWR Recomm Rep 2003;52(RR-7):1–16.

42. Academy of Breastfeeding Medicine. Protocol for human milk storage 2010 revision. Online. Available: www.bfmed.org/Resources/Download.aspx?Filename=Protocol_8.pdf (accessed Sept 24,2011).

43. American College of Obstetricians and Gynecologists. Antimicrobial therapy for obstetric patients. ACOG Educational Bulletin No. 245. Washington: ACOG; 1998.

23

The Pediatric and Adolescent Traveler

Andrea P. Summer and Philip R. Fischer

Key points

- With appropriate planning and preparation, frequent rest stops, and liberal food and hydration, travel with children can be very rewarding
- Safety considerations include motor vehicle and aircraft restraints and vigilant supervision during water and land activities
- Sun and insect protection and avoidance of animals are particularly important for children
- When used appropriately, DEET is safe for use in children
- Self-treatment of travelers' diarrhea with antibiotics should be considered, but antimotility agents should be avoided in young children
- It is reasonable to screen long-term travelers upon return from high-risk areas, particularly for exposure to tuberculosis

Introduction

Travel with children offers family fun, cultural broadening, development of world views, and opportunities for service. Despite obvious benefits, though, international travel also opens families to the possibility of inconvenience, injury, and illness. Families, children, and adolescents should all be appropriately prepared[1,2] so that they can maximize the benefits of international travel while avoiding undue risks.

Pre-travel counsel and intervention can help travelers prepare for safe, healthy, and beneficial experiences in a variety of locations.

Pediatric travel medicine is a dynamic process. Supported by four moving 'wheels' (safety and comfort, immunization, avoidance of insect-borne diseases, and diarrhea management), pediatric travelers are carried along on their journeys. The age, health status, and itinerary of the child determine whether all four 'wheels' are powered and how they are used. Health behaviors in each of these four domains are incorporated into the child's trip even as the wheels of the landing gear are raised into an aircraft. The child is then safely propelled on a life-enhancing voyage.

Safety and Comfort

General

Is it Safe for Children to Travel Internationally?

Whether going across a street for minutes or across an ocean for months, all travel carries at least some risk. Those responsible for a child must be convinced that the benefit of the trip outweighs whatever risks the trip might entail. Furthermore, responsible adults should help the traveling child take reasonable precautions to reduce the risks of adverse consequences that might come with the planned travel.

For instance, should a 9-month-old accompany his or her parents on a hike to the summit of Mount Kilimanjaro? One would be hard pressed to identify benefits to the child that would outweigh the risk of mountain sickness that could harm the child and cause the parents to abort their ascent. Should missionary parents take their 2-month-old daughter to their home in rural Kenya? The religious values that the parents perceive in their ministry might prompt them to accept the risk of insect-borne diseases in their baby; at the same time, they should take appropriate precautions. A travel medicine practitioner can help parents wisely choose the timing and destination of proposed trips in light of a risk/benefit balance with the child in mind.

Parents and trip organizers should also be advised to schedule activities with a view to the child's perspective. Running rapidly from museum to museum might not be in a 4-year-old child's best interest, although a visit to a museum between other activities, along with appropriate rest, might give a preschool-aged child a good, age-appropriate view of history and art. Popular books can guide parents in preparing for travel with children.[3,4]

The benefits (indications) of travel must always be balanced with the risks (potential contraindications) for individual children. But, are there absolute contraindications to travel? There probably are no absolute contraindications to travel, but medical conditions can impose relative contraindications that would provide a practitioner with compelling reasons to advise against undertaking certain proposed trips. With adequate planning and with access to appropriate travel health resources and means of transportation, any trip could probably be arranged. Nonetheless, common sense (which is not actually always common) should help guide decisions. Traveling families can also get good advice about local resources and risks by contacting peers who reside in or have traveled to their destinations. Adequately informed, most families will adjust plans and make preparations to avoid undue risks.

©2012 Elsevier Inc
DOI: 10.1016/B978-1-4557-1076-8.00023-5

Schedules

Having carefully considered an itinerary with the children in mind, parents can make sure they have ready access to plenty of food and drink. Adjusting to new climatic areas, children often need to increase their fluid intake. In addition, children should be provided with plenty of rest breaks during their trips.

Air Travel

Is it Safe for Infants to Travel in Commercial Airplanes or Go to High Altitudes?

Data are limited on this and many other aspects of pediatric travel medicine. Nonetheless, available evidence suggests that even though young age has been linked to respiratory and cardiovascular changes in high altitude-like environments, young age is not a contraindication to air travel.

Travel in commercial aircraft includes spending time in a pressurized cabin similar to an environment at ~2700 m above sea level. The oxygen content of the room air at this elevation is similar to that of 15% oxygen at sea level. Would this relative hypoxia be a problem for infants or children? Healthy newborns, infants, and children need not be restricted from air travel based on concerns about alveolar development. Children with pulmonary and cardiac problems and resultant concerns about hypoxia, however, might not tolerate prolonged air travel without supplemental oxygen. Infants less than 1 year of age with a history of neonatal chronic lung disease, even if not requiring oxygen at home, are at risk of hypoxia at altitude and might benefit from in-flight supplemental oxygen.[5]

Might the Relative Hypoxia of Aircraft Cabins Change Normal Breathing Patterns in Infants?

After noting an anecdotal association between air travel and sudden infant death syndrome, researchers studied breathing patterns in babies exposed overnight to 15% oxygen. Babies had lower oxygen saturations in low-oxygen environments and also had more irregular breathing patterns with more respiratory pauses, but no adverse clinical outcomes were noted. It seems that long air flights (or visits/residence at high-elevation locations) might indeed be associated with changes in infant respiratory control. However, it is not clear that these changes are linked to significant health consequences.

What About the Risk of Injury During Air Travel?

There is active debate over the use of restraints for children during routine air travel, but reasonable guidelines have been developed.[6] During automobile travel, safety seats are clearly effective in reducing crash-related injury. Per mile traveled, air crashes are much less frequent than car crashes, and the cost (a ticket for an additional seat) and discomfort (crying with prolonged restraint in a harnessed seat) are not clearly overcome by the benefit (less chance of injury in some sorts of crashes). Thus, it is not clear just what sort of a restraining system might best protect a baby during an air crash. It is clear that sharing an adult's seat belt might cause dangerous abdominal compression in a child who is squeezed between the belt and an adult during sudden deceleration; a child would be safer in an individual belt attached to the adult's seat belt. Since the use of a car safety seat confers at least some theoretical protection, a family might choose to use this seat on a plane even though cost-effectiveness data are not available to support legislation regarding the use of such restraints. Many families reasonably accept the limited benefit data as a reason not to pay the extra expense of a separate seat for an infant. At present there is not widespread agreement to mandate the use of in-flight safety seats for infants.

Assuming that Reasonable Safety Precautions are in Order, What can be Done to Ensure Comfort for a Child and Family Traveling by Air?

Front-row ('bulkhead') seats on most intercontinental flights provide wall-hanging beds that allow horizontal sleep for infants. Aisle access allows an accompanying family member to take 'walks' with a child who tires of prolonged sitting. Parents should help children with seats and trays while food and, especially, hot drinks, are being served so that spills and burns do not occur. Clothing should be comfortable, and fresh clothes should be available when accidental spills and soiling do occur. Fluids should be available to maintain hydration in a fairly dry-air environment. Age-appropriate books, toys, and games can be used to provide entertainment, especially for children who are not able to see a movie screen. Views of specific landmarks from windows, changes of outside lighting, or progress on in-flight maps can be triggers to open surprise packages of new toys to help a child maintain anticipation and enthusiasm for a long voyage. Appropriate scheduling with the child's interests in mind can help maximize the value of airport layovers and breaks in travel during long voyages.

Should Children be Sedated During Long Flights?

Medicines are used to sedate or anesthetize children for painful medical procedures; is a long air trip a 'painful procedure' that should qualify for medical intervention? If so, would this intervention be aimed at helping the child or would it be using pediatric medicine to help the comfort of adult traveling companions? Different families answer these questions differently, and some do choose to sedate their children. Understanding that there are no studies measuring outcomes using pre-flight or in-flight sedation while realizing, nonetheless, that diphenhydramine (1 mg/kg per dose given every 4–6h as needed) is a relatively safe medication, most experts do not advise sedation for traveling children. In fact, pharmacologists have noted a peculiar excitatory response to antihistaminics in children <2 years old. Parents wanting to avoid this paradoxical excitatory response during travel could use a test dose prior to the trip to ensure that the child is not predisposed to an undesired response.

Painful earache bothers some children (and those sitting near them) during the ascent and descent of commercial aircraft, as cabin pressures are adjusted. With ascent, approximately 6% of children experience bothersome pain, and about 10% have pain with descent. Adults who have such pains find preventive efficacy in the use of pseudoephedrine, but a single study of this product in young pediatric travelers showed no decrease in apparent pain. Although untested, physical maneuvers such as sucking, chewing (gum), and swallowing in an effort to open the eustachian tubes may be suggested. Infants should have something to drink readily available during ascent and descent when flight attendants are often not available to bring drinks.

Motor Vehicles

Traumatic injury accounts for more deaths in travelers than do infectious diseases. Motor vehicle accidents are a leading cause of traumatic injury among traveling children. Families should be reminded to supervise their children around streets and roads. Children, like adults, should really 'look both ways' before stepping into streets in countries with driving habits different from their homes.

Families should be particularly careful as they plan road trips: in most developing countries, road travel after dark is dangerous and should be avoided if at all possible. Pre-travel counsel sessions should also include advice about the appropriate restraints for children in cars (Table 23.1). The use of appropriate restraints limits distraction to the driver and thus reduces the risk of collisions. The use of

Table 23.1 General Safety Tips
Always use safety restraint systems when traveling in motor vehicles
Take along car safety seats for children
Inspect lodgings for potential dangers: faulty balconies, exposed wires, uncovered electrical outlets, pest poisons, paint chips
Use sunscreen, SPF30 or higher
Use careful supervision and approved safety devices for water activities
Keep children away from stray or unknown animals, both domestic and wild

restraints also limits the extent of the injuries incurred by children who are in collisions. During the first year of life, children should be restrained in a harness-style safety seat that is strapped securely into the car's backseat. Up to 2 years of age children are at decreased risk of neck injury when they are facing backwards.[6] Children should be restrained in appropriate rear seats until 13 years of age.[6] Families should be reminded that the inconvenience of ensuring the availability of appropriate car seat restraints is less than the 'inconvenience' of life-threatening traumatic injuries. Since child safety seats are often not readily available in foreign sites, families traveling with children should seriously consider taking their own safety seats along. When appropriate restraints are not available, the middle of a rear seat is usually the least dangerous place in a car. A child should not face forward in a car seat that is not attached with a seat belt to the car, but an unrestrained rear-facing safety seat might prevent some crash-related injuries. Unfortunately, seat belts are often not available in many developing countries.

Motion Sickness

Motion sickness can affect children of all ages but most often occurs in children 4–10 years of age. The most common symptom in older children is nausea, whereas ataxia is the predominant symptom in children <5 years of age.[7] Additional symptoms include dizziness, vomiting, sweating and pallor. Non-pharmacologic means are the preferred method of prevention and include avoiding heavy meals before travel, placing children facing forward in the vehicle, and discouraging visual stimuli such as reading or video games. For severe cases, diphenhydramine and dimenhydrinate can be used safely even in young children. Scopolamine is also an option for children ≥13 years. Antidopaminergic medications such as promethazine and prochlorperazine are not recommended for use in children because of the potential for extrapyramidal side-effects.[8] In addition, promethazine carries a warning that includes a contraindication for use in children <2 years and very cautious use in children over 2 years of age owing to the potential for fatal respiratory depression.[9]

Outdoor Activities

Water

In both domestic and foreign destinations, water-related activities are associated with serious injury in travelers.[10] Avoidable risk factors for boating injuries include alcohol use by drivers, and leaving propellers running while people are either swimming near or climbing in or out of the boat. Families planning to use boats during their trips should be counseled about good boating safety practices.

Safety near the water's edge is also important for children. No child should be unsupervised near water, and an adult 'buddy' should always be available in the water near a child playing in the water.

Should children with tympanostomy tubes (ventilation tubes through the eardrums, sometimes referred to as 'pressure equalization' tubes) swim? Surface swimming might moisten the external ear canal but should not push fluid into the middle ear. Thus, splashing and playing at the water's surface is not contraindicated by the presence of tympanostomy tubes. Holding the ears underwater, however, provides enough hydrostatic pressure to force water through the tubes into the middle ears. Therefore, individuals whose eardrums are not intact, whether due to recent perforation or to tympanostomy tube placement, should not dive or hold their ears under water unless they have customized plugs to completely occlude the external ear canals.

Swimmer's ear, or otitis externa, is a superficial infection of the external ear canal that is most common in people who spend significant amounts of time in the water with wet ears. This is not a dangerous condition, and infections can be easily treated (with topical acetic acid or anti-inflammatory drops); concern about swimmer's ear need not limit water activities during travel.

Two medical conditions, long QT syndrome and epilepsy, may increase the risk of drowning in traveling children who choose to play or swim in water. Children with a history of having lost consciousness during water activity should be considered for evaluation for these possible problems prior to international travel. Parents of pediatric travelers known to have either of these conditions should make sure that the underlying condition is adequately treated, and that their child is not more than a couple of arms' lengths from someone who can help should the child lose consciousness in the water.

Skin Protection

Whether vacationing or moving to a new foreign residence, traveling children of all races often have increased outdoor activities with a resultant increase in sun exposure, sometimes at beaches with limited skin coverage and sometimes closer to the equator, where sunlight comes more directly. Sun exposure is clearly linked to acute burns and to subsequent increases in wrinkling, pigmentary changes, and skin cancer. In fact, a blistering sunburn during childhood is a key risk factor predisposing to later malignant melanoma.[11] Sunscreen is both safe and effective at reducing the adverse consequences of sun exposure, but avoidance of both direct and reflective sunlight exposure, especially during the mid-day hours, is important for maximal protection. The potency of sunscreen is measured in terms of sun protection factor (SPF), which is the ratio of the time required to produce minimal erythema on sunscreen-covered skin to the time required to produce the same erythema on uncovered skin under artificial testing conditions. A sunscreen with SPF15 blocks approximately 93% of damaging ultraviolet light, and a sunscreen with SPF30 blocks about 96%. Children should use sunscreen of at least SPF 30. (An inadequately applied 30 will hopefully provide SPF 15.) Sunscreen should be applied 15–30 min before exposure and can be reapplied after washing, swimming, and excessive sweating. Subsequent reapplication after a few hours of ongoing sun exposure is not needed.[12] Sunscreen use is no longer thought to be contraindicated during the first 6 months of life, but young children are better kept in shaded areas or covered than in either reflected or direct sunlight. Clothing provides only partial protection from the penetration of sunlight, and sunscreen can be helpful even for children wearing light clothes in shaded areas.

Altitude

Acute mountain sickness is a potential problem for children as for adults.[13] The exact incidence of acute mountain sickness in children is unknown. Whether headache and malaise are effects of travel or of altitude exposure is not always easily discerned. One study suggested that 28% of school-aged children developed signs of acute mountain sickness when vacationing at 2835 m elevation, but 21% of similar children vacationing at sea level had similar symptoms.[14] In another study of pre-verbal children aged 3–36 months, 22% developed what seemed truly to be acute mountain sickness, suggesting that the risk of children developing symptoms at high altitude is similar to that in adults.[15] Unlike in adults, however, previous experience at altitude by children does not predict the risk of subsequent altitude-related symptoms.[16] Acetazolamide has not been specifically studied as a mountain sickness prophylactic in children, but the medicine is safe in children when used at similar doses for other indications. As for adults, the mainstay of treatment of severe altitude-related illnesses (high-altitude pulmonary edema, high-altitude cerebral edema) is prompt descent. Dexamethasone (for high-altitude cerebral edema, which has not often been reported in children[17,18]) and nifedipine (for high-altitude pulmonary edema) could be helpful adjuncts to treatment of severely affected children.

Staying at high altitude, children undergo physiologic adaptation. Acutely, oxygen saturation drops. Over time, however, oxygen saturation seems to rise as oxygen uptake is enhanced related to increases in ventilation, lung compliance, and pulmonary diffusion. Chest volumes and hemoglobin concentrations also rise. These changes help children grow to tolerate high altitude and to thrive in those environments.

Not all children, however, tolerate continued exposure to high altitude, and some develop life-threatening pulmonary hypertension. Initially, elevated pulmonary artery pressures are provoked by decreased oxygen delivery, but subsequently, pulmonary hypertension can be detrimental. While the incidence of life-threatening pulmonary hypertension in children at high altitude is not known, a study of 15 infant autopsies in Tibet (3600 m elevation) suggested that children of a non-indigenous ethnic group were at a higher risk than were indigenous children, and that most deaths occurred in children who had recently immigrated to the high-altitude setting.[19] The pulmonary hypertension seen in children at high altitude is not completely understood, but seems to be a real occurrence in some children, with newly arrived children of some genetic backgrounds being at greater risk than some other children. Clearly, any child with cardiorespiratory symptoms at high altitude should be carefully evaluated; descent to a lower altitude might be a major part of the treatment plan.

Is sudden infant death syndrome (SIDS, 'crib death,' or 'cot death') more common at high altitude than in children residing at lower elevations? There are no clear data suggesting that sudden infant death is more common at higher elevations, and various studies are not comparable owing to variations in diagnostic criteria. Nonetheless, one study in a relatively low-lying area of the USA suggested that SIDS might occur more commonly in babies residing at higher elevations.[20] At any altitude, the mainstays of SIDS prevention are to have infants sleep in a supine position and to keep infants away from cigarette smoke.

Animal Contact

One of the pleasures of foreign travel is seeing new varieties of animals; however, safety precautions are vitally important around animals.

Obviously, animal bites are to be avoided. Children, especially young children, should not play around unknown animals, and wildlife viewing should always be from a safe distance. Animal bites should prompt a traveling family to visit a physician in view of injury, bacterial contamination, and rabies.

Even without biting, animals can unwittingly transmit illnesses to children. This can vary from family dogs sharing *Toxocara* to raccoons leaving *Baylisascaris*-laden stool in children's play areas to cats carrying plague-infected fleas. Children should be kept safe in areas that are shared with animals, and parents should help traveling children stay clean during and after contact with animals.

As not all animal bites are easily avoided, families should have ready access to cleaning supplies and water to wash and vigorously irrigate any animal bite. Prophylactic antibiotics can be considered for animal bites as well, especially those on the hands or face. Rabies vaccine is sadly neglected by families traveling with children,[21] and pre-exposure rabies vaccination should be considered for all children going to places such as Asia and Africa, where rabies is not uncommon, especially when the trip is of more than 1–2 months' duration. Parents advising children not to pet animals should always remind them that if they disobey and are bitten or scratched, the parents will not be angry as long as the child informs them.

What Precautions Should be Taken for Children With Chronic Medical Conditions?

Pediatric patients with anemia, serious respiratory problems, or congenital heart disease should know how to quickly gain access to oxygen and emergency medications during long trips. Even children with asthma should carry an adequate supply of the medications that they would use for a severe exacerbation. Immunodeficient children should carry appropriate antibiotics with which to begin presumptive therapy while seeking good medical care in inconvenient settings. A specialist's opinion concerning travel would be prudent. Health insurance and evacuation insurance are important considerations for all travelers, but are especially critical for chronically compromised pediatric travelers; unfortunately they are unlikely to be covered if the overseas illness is related to the pre-existing health problem.

Risk-Taking Behaviors

Substance use during travel can represent a significant risk for traveling children, especially adolescents. Traveling teenagers sometimes find themselves with a new sense of freedom. They might be on 'Spring Break' with inexpensive drugs of abuse and partying peers, or they might be imagining that 'When in Rome, do as the Romans' means that they should drink excessively during a European study trip. Pre-travel counsel should remind adolescents and their parents/supervisors to set up careful safety limits to avoid unsafe use of alcohol and other illicit substances during foreign travel (Table 23.2).

Body fluid exposures provide other risks for adolescents[22] and, sometimes, younger children. Children needing injections, such as children with diabetes taking insulin, should carry an adequate supply of sterile equipment and medication. They should also carry adequate documentation about these medical supplies to satisfy curious immigration officials. Travelers should insist that medical testing and treatment involve only sterile supplies. Blood transfusions should only be accepted for life-threatening conditions, and hopefully when safe blood is available. Sexual contact is a significant risk for teenage travelers, whether it occurs with traveling companions or new acquaintances. Abstinence is the safest plan; all teenagers traveling alone should be provided with condoms, as 50% of travelers who had sex with a new partner did not expect this to happen.[23] Body piercing and tattooing, especially when needles are not sterilized between subjects, or when a common tattoo dye source is used for multiple recipients, are well known to transmit hepatitis viruses and human immunodeficiency virus (HIV). Teenage travelers should be advised to avoid any piercing or tattooing.

Table 23.2 Caring for Adolescent Travelers

What to tell them:
    Have a great time!
    Why food and water selection matters
    How insect avoidance prevents sickness
What to give them:
    Update routinely recommended immunizations
    Give appropriate travel vaccines
What they should take along:
    Medical kit (see Table 23.3)
    Water purifier if bottled water not available
What they should do:
    Learn lots
    Use seat belts and helmets appropriately
    Avoid mind-altering substance use
    Avoid potential body fluid contact:
        Tattooing, piercing, non-sterile medical care
        Sexual contact
    Only swim or boat with a friend along
    Use sunscreen
    Avoid stray animals
    Choose food and drink wisely
    Drink lots of pure fluid in case of diarrhea
    Take suggested malaria medicine as directed

Medical Kit for Families With Children

Realizing that proactive safety measures are not always completely successful, responsible adults should carry a medical kit that includes supplies of use to traveling children. A sample of items that might be included is given in Table 23.3. This includes documentation of health situations, first-aid supplies, common medications, and some hygienic supplies. Not only could children with chronic or underlying medical conditions have additional supplies or products included, but also they might wear a medical alert bracelet.

Immunization

Pre-travel consultation provides an opportunity to ensure that the child is current on vaccinations for the home environment. With changing schedules, additional immunizations might be appropriate for some traveling children.[24,25] Various agencies around the world publicize their 'routine' immunization schedules, and the American Academy of Pediatrics updates vaccine recommendations and information regularly.[26] Young travelers might be helped by 'accelerating' the schedule of routine immunizations to provide maximal coverage during their trip (see Ch. 13). Immunization plans should be individualized for special needs children. Prematurely delivered babies are generally immunized according to their chronologic age without changing their immunization schedule in view of their young gestational age. Immunocompromised children should usually avoid live vaccines, but pre-symptomatic children with HIV can still benefit from vaccination against measles, mumps, and rubella. Finally, the selection of specific vaccines for children should be based on careful consideration of the child's activities, age, and medical condition. Children have increased risk for some diseases such as rabies, and young children mount incomplete responses to some vaccines, such as that against meningococcus. (Details about vaccines can be found in Chapters 10, 11, 12 and 13).

Table 23.3 Medical Kit for Traveling Children: Items for Potential Inclusion

Information card noting:
    Name
    Birthdate
    Chronic medical conditions, if any
    Regular medications, if any
    Medical allergies, if any
    Blood type, if known
    Immunization record
    Emergency contact(s)
Supplies:
    Bandages
    Adhesive tape
    Gauze
    Antiseptic cleaning solution
Medications:
    Acetaminophen
    Ibuprofen
    Diphenhydramine
    Topical antibiotic cream or ointment such as mupirocin
    Antibiotic such as azithromycin or ciprofloxacin if risk of
        travelers' diarrhea
    Loperamide if older child
    Regular medications, if any
Products:
    Oral hydration salts
    Sunscreen, SPF15 or 30
    Insect repellent
    Permethrin

Insect-Borne Diseases

More than 1 million children die each year from malaria and other insect-borne diseases. Traveling children should be adequately protected from insect bites, especially in areas where vector-borne diseases are prevalent. Bite avoidance measures include activity scheduling, environmental manipulation, physical barriers, chemical repellents, and insecticides.[27]

Armed with knowledge of insect biting habits, families traveling with children can help schedule activities in such a way that children will reduce their risk of dangerous bites. Tick bites in central Europe, for instance, are more common in the summer than in the winter. Malaria-transmitting mosquitoes bite most in the evening and at night, and can bite either inside or outside. In some areas malaria transmission varies seasonally, with the dry season typically being safer than the rainy season. Some dengue vectors are adapted for urban, indoor, daytime biting; since dengue may be life-threatening in children, families should be careful to avoid even the mosquitoes that are active during the morning and late afternoon hours. Sandflies transmitting leishmaniasis usually bite from dusk to dawn. In areas of leishmaniasis endemicity, children should not camp or play near rodent burrows where sandflies are more active in disease transmission.

Mosquitoes like aquatic environments. They live and breed around water and do not necessarily require much more than a small puddle to support ongoing generations. When possible, children should be kept away from stagnant water, especially during evening and night hours when malaria-carrying mosquitoes are active. Residences, especially when windows are not perfectly screened, should not be surrounded by open water storage containers, puddles, or even plants that can hold water between leaves and stems. Cleaning the environment around dwelling places can markedly reduce the risk of transmission of both malaria and dengue; the latter is transmitted by the *Aedes* mosquito, a small water breeder. Clothes and bed-nets are useful barriers to block many insect bites. During times of insect activity in disease-endemic areas, children are advised to wear long sleeves and long pants or skirts. These clothes should be lightweight for comfort in tropical climates and should be lightly colored to make them less attractive to mosquitoes and other insects.

Bed-nets are highly effective in blocking insects' access to the skin of sleeping children. In areas where mosquitoes and other insects transmit pathogens at night, children should either sleep inside closed, screened, or air-conditioned rooms or else be placed under bed-nets. Bed-nets should be free of tears and should adequately cover the sleeping area so that the child will not sleep with body parts pressed up against the net. Bed-nets are most effective when they are impregnated with an insecticide such as permethrin, a safe chemical derived from the chrysanthemum flower.

The insect repellent DEET (*N,N*,diethyl-*m*-toluamide or *N, N*-diethyl-3-methylbenzamide) has been used safely and effectively in millions of children for more than five decades.[28] Increased concentrations of DEET provide prolonged durations of effective repellent activity, with 5–7% DEET protecting for 1–2 h and 24% DEET protecting for 5 h.[29] Polymerized formulations and near-pure concentrations of DEET seem to provide slightly longer durations of protection from bites, but comparative data are limited. In the past, popular pressure and concern about rare tragic outcomes in association with DEET use stimulated controversy about the use of DEET in children. DEET can cause irritation of the eyes on local contact, and ingested DEET can have systemic complications. There have been serious problems, including neurological events, reported in children who were using DEET inappropriately (more than 10 times a day, licked off the skin) in at least some of the involved children. There have not actually been any good data to support a link between DEET concentration and the risk of adverse outcomes.[30,31] In the USA, both the Environmental Protection Agency[31] and the American Academy of Pediatrics[32] have withdrawn restrictions about DEET concentration for use in children. Children can safely use DEET (Table 23.4) during the entire duration of their exposure to insects. DEET should not, however, be put near the eyes of young children, who might rub it into their eyes, and DEET should not be put on the hands and forearms of children who have the habit of biting or licking those body parts. The newer insect repellent picaridin has comparable efficacy and appears to be less irritating than DEET when used in similar concentrations. Picaridin has low oral, dermal and inhalation toxicity and has been classified by the US Environmental Protection Agency as not likely to be a human carcinogen. It has been used in Europe, Australia, and Latin America for years, but was just recently recommended by

CDC (Centers for Disease Control and Prevention) as a safe and effective alternative to DEET. Picaridin may be used for children of all ages and is considered adequate protection against *Anopheles* mosquitoes when used in concentrations of 20% or higher. 'Natural' botanical repellents containing citronella, eucalyptus, or other products are generally less effective than DEET, as they provide only very short-term (30 min) protection. Perfumed repellents smell nice but might actually attract insects. Environmental insecticides, including those that slowly release insecticide through gradually burning coils, have some (50–75%) protective efficacy.[27] Ultrasonic buzzers and insect electrocuters are not effective in reducing insect bites.

Permethrin and related pyrethroid compounds actually kill a variety of insects on contact. These products are effective against mosquitoes and ticks. They can be sprayed widely in communities, impregnated into bed-nets, or applied to clothes. Bed-nets and clothes lightly moistened with a 0.5% solution or spray of permethrin should be air-dried for about 6 h before coming into contact with children. These nets and clothes are then protective for several weeks, even if laundered. Bed-nets immersed in and impregnated by more concentrated forms of insecticide can maintain their protective role for 6–12 months. The use of impregnated bed-nets reduces bites to children sleeping under the nets as well as to other individuals living in the same area.

Treatment of Bites

Even with good bite avoidance efforts, however, insects do sometimes bite children. Uncomfortable swelling and itching can be relieved with the use of topical or systemic antihistamines, such as diphenhydramine (given at a dose of about 1 mg/kg every 4–6 h, when used orally sedation is not an uncommon side-effect). Bite sites should be kept clean, and scratching should be avoided to prevent the introduction of bacterial pathogens into the inflamed skin. The erythema and induration caused by the bite can increase for 24 h and can persist for ≥48 h. Swelling and redness that are still increasing after 24–48 h could be due to a superimposed secondary bacterial infection. These bacterial infections might be helped by a topical antibiotic such as mupuricin or an oral antibiotic to cover against *Staphylococcus* and *Streptococcus* (such as clindamycin).

For bothersome bites, systemic steroid therapy is reserved for very severe reactions such as those involving anaphylaxis. When a child has a true allergy to bites, with systemic findings such as altered mental status, hypotension, or respiratory obstruction, epinephrine (0.01 mL/kg up to a maximum dose of 0.3–0.5 mL of the 1 : 1000 solution, repeated after 15 min if needed) and, possibly, glucocorticoids can be used.

Additional Preventive Strategies for Specific Insect-Borne Diseases

Malaria

Realizing that malaria may be rapidly life-threatening in children, chemoprophylaxis is usually incorporated into the preventive healthcare plan of children traveling to malaria-endemic areas.[27] The selection of medications depends on the travel itinerary and local resistance patterns, as discussed in Section 4. One of the groups at high risk for malaria during overseas trips includes families who previously came from the destination country and who are returning to visit friends and relatives. Such travelers sometimes bring their children in for pretravel counsel. The child-based visit can serve as a good opportunity to offer necessary intervention to older traveling companions who might otherwise neglect their own care.

Table 23.4 Insect Precautions

Wear light-colored, long-sleeved shirts and long pants

Use bed-nets that have been treated with insecticide

Apply permethrin to clothing

Apply DEET (25–35%) or, for shorter exposures, Picaridin (20%) to exposed skin

Do not apply insect repellent to the face or hands of young children

Children, especially those living in endemic areas, get sicker and get sick more quickly with malaria than their adult counterparts do. Prevention is therefore vitally important. Even though some of a mother's chemoprophylaxis is distributed into breast milk, the dose reaching the child is too low to be effective, and therefore even nursing children need their own chemoprophylaxis.

Mefloquine is safe and effective in children irrespective of age and size.[33] In general, side-effects with mefloquine in prophylactic doses seem to be similar to the effects in adults; however, vomiting, perhaps related to the taste, is frequently reported by people administering mefloquine to children. Mefloquine is given weekly as prophylaxis to children at a dose approximating 5 mg/kg. The weekly dose may be compounded into capsules to open at the time of administration, or the dose may be approximated upward to the nearest one-quarter pill amount. Either way, the tablet may be swallowed quickly by the older child or given crushed to a younger child. The crushed tablet does not taste good and may be mixed with a small volume of an age-appropriate tasty material, such as breast milk, chocolate pudding or syrup, or a cola drink. Emesis within 30 min of administration should prompt the re-administration of a full dose. As in adults, children should be encouraged to drink plenty of fluid as they take mefloquine. Also, as in adults, children with known psychiatric problems, cardiac rhythm disturbances, or an active seizure disorder should take an alternative agent. Children with attention deficit disorders or a remote history of a febrile convulsion should be able to take mefloquine without concern.

The combination of atovaquone and proguanil is, by all available evidence, safe and effective in traveling children. Again, since this product is not available in a liquid formulation, pills can be cut and crushed (and mixed in milk) as needed to provide the appropriate dosing. The smaller 'pediatric' pills provide for ease of dosing in children. Compliance with daily administration and cost are issues for longer-term travelers, but the product seems as valuable in children as in adults. The 5 kg lower weight 'limit' for the use of atovaquone-proguanil is based only on lack of supportive data and is not representative of any particular concern about safety or efficacy. When other chemoprophylactic agents are problematic in small children, the 'off-label' use of atovaquone-proguanil could be considered.

Daily doxycycline is useful in malaria prophylaxis of older children who are unable to take other products, or who are going to areas of mefloquine-resistant malaria. Doxycycline is generally not given to children <8 years of age owing to concerns with the staining of growing teeth. There is also theoretical concern about altering long bone growth, but this does not seem to be a practical problem in children after fetal life. Use of a sunscreen that blocks both UVA and UVB light is advised, especially in those known to have photosensitivity reactions. Adolescent girls using doxycycline might benefit from having antifungal agents available in case vaginal candidiasis becomes symptomatic.

For children traveling to an area where chloroquine-resistant falciparum malaria occurs, prophylaxis is usually with mefloquine, atovaquone-proguanil, or doxycycline except in areas of SE Asia where mefloquine resistance occurs. The choice between these agents depends on health history, age, and personal choice. For children who cannot use any of these options and who have been tested and found to have normal G6PD activity, primaquine could be another option for prophylaxis although this drug is somewhat less effective.

Chloroquine is safe in children of any age and size and can be used when indicated. Liquid formulations of chloroquine sulfate are available in some countries. Otherwise, compounded or crushed chloroquine pills (easiest if not the enteric-coated type) can be used to adjust doses to approximate a 5 mg/kg dose of chloroquine base given orally each week. Despite a very low risk of retinopathy, periodic eye examinations are advisable for children using prophylactic chloroquine for >5 years. (See Section 4 for further details and dosages.) Note: an overdose of chloroquine of 1–2 tablets in an infant may be fatal.

Tick-Borne Diseases

Tick-borne diseases such as Lyme disease, rickettsiosis, encephalitis, and tick paralysis, are problems for children in some areas. Tick bites, like mosquito bites, are successfully prevented by the use of DEET on exposed skin and permethrin impregnation of clothes.

Most tick-borne illnesses do not develop until the ticks have been attached for more than 24 h. Therefore, daily skin examinations while in tick-laden environments are advised. Special attention should be paid to the neck and groin. Ticks may be removed by grasping them at the skin surface and pulling perpendicularly to the skin.

The risk of Lyme disease is possibly reduced by the use of post-bite doxycycline. When particularly large ticks (suggesting a prolonged attachment by the time of discovery) are identified in Lyme-endemic areas, a single 200 mg dose of doxycycline may be given to children ≥8 years of age. Prophylactic antibiotics are not otherwise indicated following tick removal.

Except for tick-borne encephalitis, for which a vaccine is available in Canada and Europe, vaccines are not available for tick-borne diseases.

Yellow Fever and Japanese Encephalitis

Mosquitoes transmit both yellow fever and Japanese encephalitis. Mosquito precautions are effective in preventing many bites. Vaccines, as discussed above and in Section 3, are effective for children at risk of contracting these illnesses during travel.

Diarrhea

Food And Water Hygiene

The principles of preventing fecal–oral transmission of microbes through food and water hygiene are similar for adults and for children. Nonetheless, several pediatric-specific points are important.[34]

Breastfeeding provides good infant nutrition and some anti-infective protection. With exclusive breastfeeding during the first 4–6 months of life, traveling infants will have less exposure to potentially contaminated water/formula. Normal cleaning of the mother's breasts is adequate.

Travelers' diarrhea seems to be more common in infants than in older children. Food and water hygiene should be emphasized to parents of traveling infants (Table 23.5). Many children have a habit of putting their hands in their mouths, either to suck, bite nails, or pick teeth. Parents of such children should be advised to be particularly careful about keeping the hands washed. All children should be reminded to wash their hands before eating. Children in areas of incomplete water purification should be supervised and, as needed, reminded not to use tap water for drinking or for brushing teeth.

Epidemiology of Diarrhea in Pediatric Travelers

The incidence of travelers' diarrhea in one study varied with age.[35] Some 40% of infants 0–2 years of age developed diarrhea during international travel, whereas only 9% of 3–6-year-olds, 22% of 7–14-year-olds and 36% of 15–20-year-olds did so. Infants also seemed to have longer duration and greater severity of travelers' diarrhea than did older children.

Table 23.5 Travelers' Diarrhea

Prevention
  Use purified or bottled water to drink and to brush teeth
  Encourage careful hand washing
  Eat fruits and vegetables that can be washed and/or peeled by consumer
  Consume only foods initially served steaming hot
  Avoid salad bars, cold buffets and street vendors
  Consume pasteurized dairy products only
Management
  Maintain adequate hydration: fluid replacement with oral rehydration solution
  Avoid anti-motility agents (e.g., loperamide) in young children
  Treat presumptively with azithromycin, or ciprofloxacin

The etiologic agents responsible for travelers' diarrhea do not seem to vary between children and adults. Thus, enterotoxigenic and enteroaggregative *Escherichia coli*, *Campylobacter*, *Salmonella*, and *Shigella* are all potential bacterial pathogens in traveling children with diarrhea.

Treatment

Medications to prevent diarrhea are generally not indicated for children. Bismuth subsalicylate has some efficacy, but the link between salicylate use and Reye's syndrome adds a pediatric-specific risk to the use of this product. Prophylactic antibiotics are generally not used, in an effort to avoid the development of resistant bacterial strains among the nasopharyngeal and gastrointestinal flora.

For children with diarrhea, the major risk is dehydration. Therapy should center on oral hydration. When children are not dehydrated, water and routine drinks may be used for hydration. The child should take in a normal 'maintenance' amount of fluid along with enough to fully replace the extra gastrointestinal losses incurred during the illness. When dehydration is present, electrolyte solutions containing ~2% sugar and plenty of salt are best absorbed. To this end, the WHO rehydration solution, commercial products such as Pedialyte or Infalyte, or homemade solutions (2 tablespoons of table sugar and a quarter teaspoon of salt with, if possible, a quarter teaspoon of baking soda mixed in 1 L of pure water) are effective. Fluids may be given via cup, spoon, or syringe. The child can continue with a regular, age-appropriate diet during the diarrheal illness once dehydration is corrected.[36,37]

Antimotility agents are used for adult travelers with bothersome diarrhea. These medications reduce the frequency of stool evacuation, but there is no clear evidence that they actually reduce intestinal fluid loss. Parents of children on antimotility agents should not be fooled into thinking that oral hydration efforts can be relaxed. Some antimotility agents, such as diphenoxylate, are absorbed and can have toxic systemic effects; they are best avoided in young children. Loperamide has minimal systemic effects, though some adverse outcomes have been seen in young children. Loperamide did not reduce the need for rehydration in one infant study, but in another was effective in reducing the severity and duration of diarrhea in children aged 2–11 years. In general, the use of loperamide in infants and young children (<3 years) is not advised owing to the risks of distracting families from needed oral hydration and of slowing the passage of invasive bacteria that might be causing the diarrhea.[36]

Bulking agents such as kaolin change the character of the stool but do not change the net fluid loss. They have not been shown to reduce the severity of diarrhea or the incidence of dehydration. Similarly, binding agents designed to attach to intestinal toxins are of unproven efficacy in children with travelers' diarrhea. Probiotics are being studied and hold some potential for the future in the treatment of children with travelers' diarrhea.

With good oral hydration, travelers' diarrhea is a self-limited illness. Nonetheless, using systemic antibiotics can reduce the duration of symptoms. The agents responsible for travelers' diarrhea in adults and children have become increasingly resistant to sulfa antibiotics. Presumptive antibiotic therapy can shorten the duration of diarrhea in travelers. In areas such as industrialized nations, where *E. coli* O157: H7 is common, the risk of facilitating the development of hemolytic uremic syndrome precludes presumptive antibiotic therapy in children with bloody diarrhea. For the child with typical travelers' diarrhea in a non-industrialized area, the benefit of a shortened illness often outweighs the minimal risks of antibiotic therapy.

Which Antibiotic Should be used in Children?

Azithromycin is effective against the pathogens that cause travelers' diarrhea,[34] is safe in children, and is available in convenient child-friendly dosing formulations. A total of 10 mg/kg per day for up to 3 days as needed is often suggested, but no detailed studies comparing dosing regimens have been done. It is the drug of choice on the Indian subcontinent and in Southeast Asia. Ciprofloxacin (10 mg/kg twice daily for 1–3 days) is often effective against the causes of travelers' diarrhea and, despite early concerns about joint cartilage toxicity, appears to be safe in children.[38] Ciprofloxacin is available in a suspension form that does not need to be refrigerated. Therapy with poorly absorbed antibiotics such as rifaximin has proven efficacy and safety in the treatment of infectious travelers' diarrhea in adults. Even though rifaximin has been shown to be as effective as ciprofloxacin in reducing the duration of travelers' diarrhea, its usefulness in the treatment of travelers' diarrhea caused by invasive organisms is still unclear.[39] Rifaximin is approved for use in children 12 years of age and older but might prove beneficial in younger children as well. Amoxicillin, co-trimoxazole, and erythromycin are much less effective against the causal microorganisms in most traveling children and should be avoided.

Returned/Immigrating Travelers

What Should be Done for Children Returning from International Journeys?

After short trips, an asymptomatic child would not require any specific medical intervention. After longer exposures overseas, even asymptomatic children can benefit from screening for common medical conditions. All returned pediatric travelers and immigrating children should be integrated into ongoing healthcare maintenance and supervision.

After international trips of longer than 3 months' duration, one could consider several screening tests for the returned child.[40] Skin testing for tuberculosis would be useful if the child has been in an area where tuberculosis is common, but an asymptomatic child ideally should wait for 2–3 months after travel to be tested, to avoid a falsely negative result during the 'window' between exposure and skin test positivity. If the child has been in an area of poor hygiene where intestinal parasitoses are common, stool microscopy for ova and parasites is useful. If the child was exposed to fresh water in a schistosomiasis-endemic area, urine and stool tests could be considered, but negative tests do not fully rule out infection; serology is the most sensitive and specific test for this infection. *Strongyloides* serology should always be considered for long-stay travelers.

Table 23.6 Commonly Used Medications in Pediatric Travelers

Medication	Dose	Common Reactions
Malaria Prophylaxis		
Atovaquone-proguanil 250 mg/100 mg adult tab 62.5 mg/25 mg pediatric tab	(5–11 kg) 31.25 mg/12.5 mg (11–20 kg) 62.5 mg/25 mg q. day (21–30 kg) 125 mg/50 mg q. day (31–40 kg) 187.5 mg/75 mg q. day (>40 kg) 250 mg/100 mg q. day	Gastrointestinal symptoms, elevated liver transaminases, dizziness
Chloroquine 300 mg base tab or 150 mg base tab	5 mg/kg base q. week up to a maximum dose of 300 mg base	Gastrointestinal symptoms, blurred vision, rash
Doxycycline 100 mg tab	2 mg/kg daily for children >8 years old (max dose 100 mg)	Gastrointestinal symptoms, rash, photosensitivity, vaginal candidiasis
Mefloquine 250 mg tab	<5 kg, no data (<10 kg) 5 mg/kg q. week (10–19 kg) ¼ tab q. week (20–30 kg) ½ tab q. week (31–45 kg) ¾ tab q. week (>45 kg) 1 tab q. week	Gastrointestinal symptoms, headache, vivid dreams, dizziness, rash
Travelers' Diarrhea – Treatment		
Azithromycin Suspension 100 mg/5 mL or 200 mg/5 mL 250 mg or 500 mg tablet	10 mg/kg once daily up to 3 days	Gastrointestinal symptoms, vaginitis, dizziness, rash
Ciprofloxacin Suspension 250 mg/5 mL or 500 mg/5 mL 100, 250, or 500 mg tablet	10 mg/kg per dose b.i.d., up to 3 days for children >1 year	Gastrointestinal symptoms, headache, dizziness, rash
Anti-motion Sickness		
Dimenhydrinate 12.5 mg/5 mL syrup 50 mg chewable tab	1.25 mg/kg, up to 50 mg. Can be repeated every 6 h; Not for use in children under 2 years	Drowsiness, vertigo, dry mouth, blurred vision
Diphenhydramine 12.5 mg/5 mL syrup 25 mg tab	1 mg/kg, up to 25 mg Can be repeated every 6 h	As with dimenhydrinate
Scopolamine patch	1.5 mg patch. Apply 1 patch q3 days behind ear at least 4 hrs before event.	Dry mouth, drowsiness, dizziness, blurred vision
Altitude Sickness – Prevention		
Acetazolamide 125 mg or 250 mg tab	2.5 mg/kg per dose q. 12 h, up to 250 mg/day	Fatigue, taste changes, gastrointestinal symptoms, electrolyte disorders, tinnitus

An immigrating child who is newly settling in to an industrialized nation may be a candidate for further health screening. A diet history and anthropometric measurements would help guide dietary counsel. Vision and hearing screening may help pick up mild deficits. Dental evaluation is useful to prevent asymptomatic dental caries from progressing to more serious conditions. Depending on the overseas situation from which the child came, there may be value in screening for HIV, hepatitis B antigenemia, hepatitis A and C antibodies, anemia, and lead toxicity in addition to screening for tuberculosis and intestinal and/or urinary parasites. Routine childhood vaccinations should be initiated or updated. Social workers may be able to help with adaptation to a new area. Psychologic referral can help children coming from particularly traumatic situations.

A febrile child who has been in a malaria-endemic area within the preceding 2 months should be immediately evaluated for malaria, even if appropriate prophylactic measures had been used.[41] Blood tests may show evidence of anemia, thrombocytopenia or increased bilirubin.

Thick and thin malaria smears may provide a definitive diagnosis; however, when there is significant concern for the possibility of malaria they should be repeated twice 12–24 h later if initially negative. A child with typhoid fever may present with fever in the absence of localizing physical signs and might have a mild leukopenia; cultures of blood and stool are used for definitive diagnosis. The specific and supportive care measures needed for a febrile returned traveler are similar to those in adults, as long as weight-adjusted medication doses are used. (Details of malaria treatment are discussed in Ch. 17.)

Diarrhea is not uncommon in returned travelers.[42] Diarrhea containing blood and mucus should prompt stool culture for invasive bacterial pathogens (*Campylobacter*, *Escherichia coli* O157: H7, *Shigella*, *Salmonella*, and, sometimes, *Yersinia* and *C. difficile*) as well as stool microscopy for ameba. Except for the very recently returned traveler with acute diarrhea that began in a developing country, antibiotics should be withheld pending culture results (to avoid treatment that is unnecessary or risky for prolonged carriage with *Salmonella* or risky for the development of hemolytic uremic syndrome such as with *E. coli* O157: H7). Hydration and routine feeding should be continued for a returned pediatric traveler with diarrhea. A child with chronic diarrhea should be tested for infectious causes (such as *Giardia* and *Cyclospora*) in addition to being evaluated for inflammatory bowel disease if that seemed likely. However, children may suffer from the same transient post-infectious bowel disorders as adults, namely, lactose intolerance and irritable bowel syndrome.

Dermatologic problems seem more common in returned pediatric travelers than in their adult companions, possibly because of the child's increased skin contact with the environment. Dermatitis from irritation or specific contacts can be treated with humidifying lotions and, when severe, with steroid creams. Infestations such as those caused by penetrating insect larvae or flea eggs can be managed by removing the foreign material, as in adult travelers. Scabies should always be considered when generalized pruritus and a rash are present. Pyogenic bacterial skin infections respond to topical mupirocin (applied 3–4 times daily for 5–10 days); when extensive, oral clindamycin should be used.

Conclusion

Travel offers a wealth of good experiences for children and their families. With careful pre-travel evaluation of the risks and protective interventions, the health risks of travel can be minimized. Medications can be used with attention to the age and size of the traveler (Table 23.6). Managing these risks, healthcare providers and families can ensure that foreign experiences during childhood are memorable and positive.

References

1. Stauffer W, Christenson JC, Fischer PR. Preparing children for international travel. Travel Med Infect Dis 2008;6:101–13.
2. Summer AP, Fischer PR. Travel with infants and children. Clin Fam Pract 2005;7:729–43.
3. Lanigan C, Wheeler M. Lonely Planet Travel with Children. 4th ed. London: Lonely Planet; 2002.
4. Wilson-Howarth J, Ellis M. Your Child's Health Abroad: A Manual for Travelling Parents. Bucks: Bradt Publications; 1998.
5. Udomittipong K, Stick SM, Verheggen M, et al. Pre–flight testing of preterm infants with neonatal lung disease: A retrospective review. Thorax 2006;61:343–7.
6. Durbin DR. Technical Report – child passenger safety. Pediatrics 2011;127:e1050–66.
7. Takahashi M, Ogata M, Miura M. The significance of motion sickness in the vestibular system. J Vestib Res 1997;7:179–87.
8. Lankamp DJ, Willemse J, Pikaar SA, et al. Prochlorperazine in childhood: side-effects. Clin Neurol Neurosurg 1977;80:264–71.
9. Starke, PR, Weaver J, Chowdhury BA. Boxed warning added to promethazine labeling for pediatric use. N Engl J Med 2005; 352(25):2653.
10. Orlowski JP, Szpilman D. Drowning: rescue, resuscitation, and reanimation. Pediatr Clin North Am 2001;48:627–46.
11. Gloster HM, Brodland DG. The epidemiology of skin cancer. Derm Surg 1996;22:217–26.
12. Diffey BL. When should sunscreen be reapplied? J Am Acad Derm 2001;45:882–5.
13. Durmowicz AG. Recognizing high-altitude illnesses in children. J Resp Dis Pediatr 2002;4:34–40.
14. Theis MK, Honigman B, Yip R, et al. Acute mountain sickness in children at 2835 meters. Am J Dis Child 1993;147:143–5.
15. Yaron M, Waldman N, Niermeyer S, et al. The diagnosis of acute mountain sickness in preverbal children. Arch Pediatr Adol Med 1998;152:683–7.
16. Rexhaj E, Garcin S, Rimoldi SF, et al. Reproducibility of acute mountain sickenss in children and adults: a prospective study. Pediatrics 2011;e1445–e1448.
17. Pollard AJ, Niermeyer S, Barry P, et al. Children at high altitude: an inter-national consensus statement by an ad hoc committee of the International Society for Mountain Medicine, 12 March, 2001. High Alt Med Biol 2001;2:389–403.
18. DeMeer K, Heymans HS, Zijlstra WG. Physical adaptation of children to life at high altitude. Eur J Pediatr 1995;154:263–72.
19. Sui GJ, Liu YH, Cheng XS, et al. Subacute infantile mountain sickness. J Pathol 1988;155:161–70.
20. Getts AG, Hill HF. Sudden infant death syndrome: incidence at various altitudes. Dev Med Child Neurol 1982;24:61–8.
21. Arguin PM, Krebs JW, Mandel E, et al. Survey of rabies preexposure and postexposure prophylaxis among missionary personnel stationed outside the United States. J Travel Med 2000;7:10–4.
22. Nield LS. Health implications of a adolescent travel. Pediatr Ann 2011;40:358–61.
23. R. Vivancos I, Abubakar PR. Hunter Foreign travel, casual sex, and sexually transmitted infections: systematic review and meta-analysis. International Journal of Infectious Diseases 2010;14:e842–e851.
24. Greenwood CS, Greenwood NP, Fischer PR. Immunization issues in pediatric travelers. Expert Rev Vaccines 2008;7:651–61.
25. Rongkavilit C. Immunization for pediatric international travelers. Pediatr Ann 2011;40:346–50.
26. American Academy of Pediatrics. Recommended childhood and adolescent immunization schedule – United States. 2011. Pediatrics 2011;127:387–8.
27. Fischer PR, Bialek R. Prevention of malaria in children. Clin Infect Dis 2002;34:493–8.
28. Qui H, Jun HW, McCall JW. Pharmacokinetics, formulation, and safety of insect repellent N,N-diethyl-3-methylbenzamide (DEET): a review. J Am Mosq Control Assoc 1998;14:12–27.
29. Fradin MS, Day JF. Comparative efficacy of insect repellents against mosquito bites. New Engl J Med 2002;347:13–8.
30. Osimitz TG, Murphy JV, Fell LA, et al. Adverse events associated with the use of insect repellents containing N,N-diethyl-m-toluamide (DEET). Regul Toxicol Pharmacol 2010;56(1):93–9.
31. US Environmental Protection Agency. EPA promotes safer use of insect repellent DEET (press release 24 April). Washington, DC: US Environmental Protection Agency; 1998.
32. Weil W.B. New information leads to changes in DEET recommendations. AAP News 2001;Aug:52–3.
33 Use of mefloquine in children – a review of dosage, pharmacokinetics and tolerability data. Malaria J 2011;10:292.
34. Stauffer WM, Konop RJ, Kamat D. Traveling with infants and young children. Part III: travelers' diarrhea. J Travel Med 2002;9:141–50.
35. Pitzinger B, Steffen R, Tschopp A. Incidence and clinical features of travelers' diarrhea in infants and children. Pediatr Infect Dis J 1991;10:719–23.
36. Provisional Committee on Quality Improvement. Practice parameter: the management of acute gastroenteritis in young children. Pediatrics 1996;97:424–33.
37. Duggan C, Nurko S. 'Feeding the gut': the scientific basis for continued enteral nutrition during acute diarrhea. J Pediatr 1997;131:801–8.
38. Grady RW. Systemic quinolone antibiotics in children: a review of the use and safety. Expert Opin Drug Saf 2005;4:623–30.
39. Taylor DN. Poorly absorbed antibiotics for the treatment of travelers' diarrhea. Clin Infect Dis 2005;41:S564–70.
40. Fischer PR, Christenson JC, Pavia AT. Pediatric problems during and after international travel. In: Bia FJ, editor. Travel Medicine Advisor, vol. TC2. Atlanta: American Health Consultants; 1998. p. 9–18.
41. Hickey PW, Cape KE, Masuoka P, et al. A local, regional, and national assessment of pediatric malaria in the United States. J Travel Med 2011;18:153–60.
42. Hagmann S, Neugebauer R, Schwartz E, et al. GeoSentinel Surveillance Network. Illness in children after international travel: analysis from the GeoSentinel Surveillance Network. Pediatrics 2010;125:e1072–80.

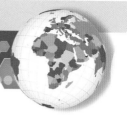

The Older Traveler

Kathryn N. Suh

Key points

- Cardiovascular disease and accidental trauma are the leading causes of death among older travelers
- Older travelers should plan their trip, have their fitness for travel assessed, and seek proper travel health advice well ahead of travel
- All older travelers – regardless of their health – should have adequate health insurance to cover medical and repatriation costs while abroad
- Recommended vaccines may be less immunogenic in the elderly, and the protective efficacy of many travel vaccines is unknown in this population

Introduction

Advancing age is less of a barrier to international travel than at any time in the past. The elderly account for an increasing number of the >940 million travelers who cross international boundaries each year.[1] As the proportion of elderly in the population continues to increase, so too will the number of older travelers – the conveniences of modern-day travel and the increased accessibility of formerly remote or exotic destinations may inspire older travelers to venture farther than they previously thought possible.

Why are Elderly Travelers at Greater Risk?

Older travelers are at increased risk of illness, injury, or death while traveling, even in the absence of pre-existing medical problems. The healthy elderly will often have greater difficulty acclimatizing during travel, take longer to adjust to extremes in temperature or humidity and changes in altitude, and be more prone to motion sickness, jet lag, insomnia, and constipation.

With advancing age comes a greater likelihood of underlying medical conditions, which in turn may make the older traveler more vulnerable to acquiring travel-related infections, and may increase the severity of these illnesses. Specific travel recommendations (e.g., malaria chemoprophylaxis; vaccines) may also be affected by the traveler's medical condition and age (Box 24.1).

While pre-travel assessments tend to focus on the prevention of travel-related infections, it is important to realize that only 1–3% of deaths in travelers are attributable to infectious diseases. The majority are due to natural causes – mostly cardiovascular disease – and trauma.[2–5] Deaths in older travelers are more likely to be due to underlying medical conditions. Older travelers may also be at risk of dying due to injury because they have slowed reaction times, auditory or visual impairment, poor coordination and medication side-effects that may make them more vulnerable to accidents and crime.

General Advice

Choosing a Trip

Planning a trip well ahead of time is especially important for the older traveler. Knowledge of the travel destination(s) and the nature of the trip is key if appropriate advice is to be provided.

For some older travelers, all-inclusive resorts, organized tours, or cruises may be attractive alternatives to individually planned trips. They are usually well organized and feature a predetermined itinerary, choice of activities, leisurely travel with adequate opportunity for rest, reliable accommodations, assistance with luggage, and access (if necessary) to reliable medical care.

Fitness to Travel

An individual's overall fitness for travel should be evaluated by the individual's own physician prior to travel, especially if the agenda includes a marked increase in physical activity. A general check-up is an excellent starting point for the older traveler, but does not replace the need for specific travel advice. A complete medical history and physical examination should be performed. Ideally, this encounter should take place far enough in advance to allow for investigation and treatment of any undiagnosed conditions that might otherwise preclude (or delay) travel.

There are few absolute contraindications to air travel: (1) pneumothorax or pneumomediastinum; (2) acute or unstable coronary syndromes, congestive heart failure, or significant dysrhythmias within 4 weeks of travel; (3) abdominal or intracranial surgery within 1 week, middle ear surgery within 2 weeks, and thoracic or cardiac surgery within 3 weeks; (4) cerebrovascular accidents within 2 weeks; and (5) some infectious diseases during the period of communicability (e.g., chickenpox, measles, tuberculosis).[6] Respiratory tract infections and other pulmonary disorders, anemia, and most communicable diseases are relative contraindications to air travel; with time and appropriate

©2012 Elsevier Inc
DOI: 10.1016/B978-1-4557-1076-8.00024-7

BOX 24.1

General advice for the older traveler

1. Plan your trip well ahead of time to allow for pre-travel health preparation.
2. See your personal physician for a general physical examination prior to travel.
3. If required, consult a travel medicine specialist at least 8 weeks prior to departure (to allow adequate time for immunizations). Be sure that you understand the advice provided, and how to use medications that are prescribed.
4. Start a conditioning program 1–2 months prior to travel, if appropriate.
5. Verify the extent of your current health insurance. Does it cover out-of-country expenses and repatriation costs?
6. When booking travel, make sure that any special requests can be adequately accommodated, and ask about supplemental health insurance (if required) and cancellation insurance. Be certain to clarify limitations and exclusions prior to purchase.
7. Bring a first-aid kit containing commonly used items including medication for self-treatment of diarrhea and constipation.
8. Consider purchasing a medical bracelet if you have underlying medical conditions or medication allergies.
9. Carry any prescription medications with you (do not pack them in checked baggage). Bring extra medications and prescriptions for each.
10. Carry your personal physician's phone number and any relevant medical records with you.
11. If medical services will be required during travel, ask your doctor if these can be arranged ahead of time, before you leave.
12. Bring extra batteries for hearing aids or mechanical devices, and extra eyeglasses. A small repair kit may also come in handy.
13. Acclimatize gradually to heat, cold, and altitude. Drink adequate fluids (add extra salt for hot environments) and drink alcohol and caffeinated beverages judiciously.
14. Seek medical attention if you develop a fever or other health problems during your trip or after your return home. Inform your doctor of your recent travels and the details of your trip.

therapy, most will improve sufficiently to permit travel. It is essential that underlying medical conditions be taken into account prior to recommending *any* pharmacologic agents, including malaria chemoprophylaxis, immunizations, and over-the-counter remedies for common illnesses. Advice for travelers with underlying medical conditions is reviewed elsewhere and will not be discussed in detail here.

If a significant increase in activity is anticipated during travel, a fitness or conditioning program started 1–2 months before can identify potential problems and improve both cardiovascular condition and muscular strength. Exercise stress testing is not routinely recommended during a pre-travel assessment, but may be considered for travelers who will be starting vigorous exercise as part of their trip, or who are anticipating lengthy or remote treks – particularly men over 40 years of age, women over 50, and those with a history of coronary artery disease or two or more risk factors for coronary disease.[7]

Making Travel Arrangements

The specific needs of individual travelers, both during travel and at the destination(s), should be discussed with the travel agent at the time of booking to ensure that they can be accommodated. When making travel reservations, aisle, exit row or bulkhead seats which have increased leg room, may be requested (additional charges may apply); apart from being more comfortable, legs can be stretched without having to stand. On flights where smoking is still permitted, seating in the non-smoking section should be requested if desired. Travelers requiring or preferring special diets for medical or personal reasons should request them 48 h prior to travel; most carriers have a reasonable selection from which to choose, but cannot reliably accommodate last-minute requests.

Travelers should confirm their travel schedules prior to departure. Adequate time should be allowed for travel to the terminal and for check-in. The need for a wheelchair or motorized transportation at the terminal should be arranged with the individual carrier at least 48 h in advance, although in some cases they may be requested from the airline at check-in. While porters are available to assist with luggage in many terminals, this is not always the case; wheeled suitcases with extendable handles may be easier for the older traveler to negotiate through crowded areas.

Health Insurance

More than most other travelers, the older traveler should pay particular attention to ensuring that their health insurance is adequate for their intended travel. Government-funded health insurance plans do not usually cover out-of-country medical expenses; private insurance plans may. If required, supplemental travel insurance can be purchased through several providers, including most insurance and credit card companies and through travel agencies, as well as from travel insurance firms. For any insurance plan, available options, restrictions, and limitations of benefits should be carefully reviewed and clarified with the insurance provider; most carriers will not cover pre-existing health problems if they are responsible for the overseas illness or evacuation ('catch 22'), and will not insure those over 85 years of age. Insurance must be purchased in the country of residence, prior to departure. Some companies will sell travel insurance on a fixed-term basis (e.g., for a 12-month period), suitable for frequent travelers. It may be wise to pay for a few extra days of coverage in case return is delayed. Ensure that the policy will cover repatriation costs, and clarify under what conditions these can be claimed. In foreign countries, payment for medical services may be requested or required 'up front'; an itemized invoice or receipt for medical care or prescription medications will be required for subsequent reimbursement.

Travelers should carry details of any insurance policies with them, including policy numbers. Family or friends at home should also know how to contact the insurance carrier.

Medications and Medical Supplies

Commonly used medications for travel are no different for the older traveler, with the exception of laxatives, as constipation is more common in this age group. Denture adhesive may be difficult to find in some countries: denture wearers should carry a sufficient supply for the entire trip. First-aid medications are not to be used indiscriminately in the elderly, as they can cause uncomfortable and potentially serious side-effects. If possible, older travelers should try to include medications that they have tolerated in the past. Regardless, their use should be reviewed with the traveler prior to departure.

Prescription medications should be carried with the traveler at all times, in carry-on luggage, to minimize the chance of loss or theft. Travelers should bring enough medication to last the duration of the trip, plus an extra several days' worth. A duplicate set of medications, and a prescription for each, should also be carried (in a separate location), in case the first set is lost. Medications should be kept in their original labeled bottles or packs. Some medications and medical supplies – including but not limited to opiate analgesics, narcotics, and needles and syringes – may pose difficulties at border crossings; a legitimate prescription and/or an official (letterhead) letter from a physician can help to overcome this problem. If prescriptions do need to be filled while away from home, it is preferable to obtain the identical medication from the same manufacturer, as differences do exist between different brands of the same medications. The increasing problem of counterfeit medications should be used to dissuade travelers from purchasing cheaper medications while abroad.

Travelers should also carry the name and phone number of their physician and personal contacts in the event of an emergency, as well as a summary of their medical record, a complete list of current medications, and a copy of the most recent electrocardiogram if appropriate.

Medical Services Abroad

Healthcare standards vary greatly throughout the world, and may differ significantly from those in the country of residence. Any acute illness, which alone can be traumatic in the elderly, is made even more stressful by suboptimal care, an unfamiliar environment, and language barriers.

A list of medical services available abroad can be obtained prior to travel through several sources, including the International Association for Medical Assistance to Travelers (IAMAT) (www.iamat.org). Subscribers to Shoreland's Travax EnCompass (www.shoreland.com) or members of International SOS (www.internationalsos.com) can obtain listings of clinics and hospitals in many travel destinations.

Practical Tips during Air Travel

Travelers should wear loose-fitting, comfortable clothing. Intestinal gas expands with altitude and can cause abdominal discomfort, although this is rarely of any medical significance. Furthermore, they should avoid foods that cause bloating (e.g., apple juice, carbonated beverages, sorbitol-containing sugarless gum). Alcohol and caffeinated beverages are both diuretics that should be avoided during flight because dehydration can worsen jet lag and may contribute to the development of deep vein thrombosis.

Medical Conditions Arising during Travel

Motion Sickness

Adults over 50 years of age are less susceptible to motion sickness, possibly due to an age-related decline in vestibular function. See Chapter 43 for tips on how to reduce motion sickness.

Commonly used pharmacologic agents to combat motion sickness, such as dimenhydrinate, diphenhydramine and related antihistamines, and the anticholinergic agent scopolamine (Hyoscine), may cause more adverse effects in the older traveler. Scopolamine can be administered orally, transdermally or intranasally. Although it is one of the most effective oral drugs for motion sickness, the risk of side-effects (drowsiness, dry mouth, blurry vision) is greater than with other agents. Its anticholinergic actions may also precipitate narrow-angle glaucoma, urinary retention (particularly in older men with prostatic hypertrophy) and intestinal ileus. Inhibition of sweating with scopolamine can contribute to heatstroke in warmer climates. Dimenhydrinate and diphenhydramine are generally safer but can also lead to drowsiness, confusion, or ataxia, which may be exaggerated or prolonged in the elderly.

In-Flight Emergencies

In-flight emergencies may be related to the stress of travel, the cabin environment (turbulence, barometric pressure changes), or accident or injury. Unrelated medical emergencies also arise; although less common, they are likely to be the most serious and may necessitate diversion of the flight, which occurs in 4–8% of cases.[8,9] The most commonly reported medical incidents during flight include syncope, trauma, and gastrointestinal, cardiac, or respiratory ailments.[9] Studies have estimated the incidence of in-flight emergencies to be between 22 and 100/million travelers.[8-11] Death during flight is rare, occurring in 0.1–0.8/million travelers.[9,10] Most are sudden cardiac deaths in middle-aged men with no prior history of coronary disease.[12] The increasing use of automated external defibrillators (AEDs) on board may improve survival in some individuals, although commercial airlines are not responsible for delivery of medical care during flight.

Thromboembolic Disease

The exact incidence of venous thromboembolism (VTE) in travelers is unknown; observational studies suggest that VTE occurs in 0–12% of travelers,[13] a risk that appears to be increased two- to fourfold in travelers compared to the population at large.[13-16] Most deep vein thromboses (DVTs) reported in studies have been asymptomatic; their clinical significance and natural history are unclear.[13] Philbrick[13] estimated that 0.05% of travelers will develop a clinically significant DVT, with the risk of a symptomatic pulmonary embolism (PE) being 27 per 1 million flights. Travel-related risk factors for VTE include travel beyond 6–8 hours; other recognized risk factors for VTE include increasing age, a history of prior DVT or PE, thrombophilia, obesity, prolonged immobilization, malignancy, and venous stasis, including varicose veins. A significant proportion of VTE develops after the first week following travel,[15] but often within 96 h of flight.

Recommendations for preventing VTE during travel, including wearing loose clothing, contracting leg muscles frequently while seated, taking frequent short walks when safe to do so, and ensuring adequate hydration with non-alcoholic beverages, have not been proven to reduce VTE risk. Relative immobility, dehydration, lower leg edema, hypoxia, and hypobaric conditions in the cabin may predispose to a thrombophilic state based on measurements of clotting factors, but their role in the development of travel-related VTE is unclear. Compression stockings can reduce the risk of asymptomatic DVT by 90% or more,[17,18] but their effect on clinically apparent VTE is unknown. Compression stockings, aspirin, and subcutaneous heparin are not recommended for VTE prophylaxis in most travelers, but compression stockings or heparin may be indicated for selected (high-risk) patients.

Jet Lag

Jet lag is more common and may be more severe or prolonged in the elderly. Adequate rest prior to, and proper hydration during travel may improve overall wellbeing independent of any effect on jet lag. Dividing long trips into segments (with multiple stopovers) can reduce jet lag, but often with additional inconvenience. Adapting one's daily routine to the current time of day upon reaching the destination can minimize jet lag. Exposure to bright outdoor light may help readjust the circadian rhythm. Other interventions, such as exercise and diet, are unproven in reducing jet lag.

Benzodiazepines provide some relief from sleep disturbances, but can result in daytime sleepiness as well as general drowsiness, impaired memory, and fatigue. These effects may be more pronounced in older travelers, especially those unaccustomed to taking these medications.

Zolpidem, a short-acting imidazopyridine hypnotic that is used for short-term treatment of insomnia, has been shown to be more effective in the treatment of jet lag than melatonin.[19] The elimination half-life and adverse effects of zolpidem, such as confusion, ataxia and falls, and gastrointestinal side-effects (cramps, nausea, vomiting, diarrhea), are increased in the elderly; the initial dosage should be halved (5 mg before bedtime) in the older individual. Clinical trials examining the use of melatonin have reported conflicting results, although a recent meta-analysis[20] and the American Academy of Sleep Medicine[21] support its use. In one dose-finding study, the 5 mg fast-release formulation was most effective in combating jet lag, although lower doses (0.5 mg) were also effective; however, no subjects >65 years of age were included.[22] Melatonin is not currently licensed as a drug but is widely available as a nutritional supplement. The long-term safety of melatonin is unknown. Armodanifil, a racemic isomer of modafenil that is approved for treatment of narcolepsy, increases daytime wakefulness after travel[23] but is not approved for use in jet lag. Limited data suggest that it is well tolerated in older individuals, although a dose reduction may be prudent as systemic drug levels may be increased. The efficacy and safety of armodanifil for jet lag in older travelers have not been assessed.

Hyperthermia and Hypothermia

The elderly are more susceptible to the effects of heat and cold. Proper clothing is essential in both extremes of temperature. Acclimatization to heat or cold may take several days. The older traveler should limit outdoor activity if weather conditions are extreme, or at least gradually adapt to the climate over several days.

Heat

Peripheral vasodilation is impaired with advanced age and perspiration is diminished, reducing the body's cooling mechanisms in hot climates. The thirst response may also be diminished in the elderly, leading to dehydration. The risk of overheating and heatstroke may be further increased by medications that impair thermoregulation, including antihistamines, anticholinergics, β- and calcium channel blockers, diuretics, tricyclic antidepressants, and anti-parkinsonian medications. Older travelers need to use caution in hot weather and drink adequate fluid, avoiding caffeine and alcohol, which will worsen dehydration. Travelers with renal disease and those on diuretics are especially prone to volume and electrolyte abnormalities if they develop dehydration or heatstroke.

Cold

The elderly are also more susceptible to the cold. Heat-generating mechanisms (i.e., shivering) are diminished in older individuals. Appropriate clothing (layered) is essential, and damp clothes should be changed immediately. Alcohol and cigarette smoking can increase the risk of cold-related illnesses (hypothermia and frostbite). Proper hydration is as important in cold climates as it is in the heat.

Altitude Sickness

Altitude sickness refers to several different clinical syndromes, the most common of which is acute mountain sickness (AMS). The effect of age on AMS has been disputed. Some studies have shown advanced age to be protective against AMS, whereas others have found no association between age and AMS. A reasonable level of fitness and adequate acclimatization will minimize the risk of AMS in the elderly. With a 5-day acclimatization period, the healthy older individual can tolerate altitudes of 2500 m well; hypoxemia, sympathetic activation,

pulmonary hypertension, and reduced plasma volume do, however, contribute to reduced exercise capacity.[24] Those with underlying cardiopulmonary disease or anemia may have more severe hypoxemia or cardiac ischemia at higher altitudes. β-blockers can reduce the expected compensatory tachycardia and give rise to dyspnea. Acetazolamide is effective when used for prevention of AMS, although its effects must be carefully considered in the older traveler.

Accidents and Injury

Trauma is a significant cause of morbidity and mortality in the traveler. Between 1975 and 1984 injury accounted for 25% of deaths in US travelers,[2] and 38% of Canadians in 1995.[3] Trauma-related deaths in travelers are more common in males, and in the young and elderly.[2] Motor vehicle accidents and violent deaths are the most common causes of accidental death overall, but causes of death vary by region visited.[25] Other causes include drowning and diving mishaps, falls, and natural disasters. Most (80%) travelers who die from trauma do so before reaching a hospital; even if transport to a hospital occurs, evacuation is often required because of inadequate medical facilities.

Travel-Related Infections in the Elderly

Malaria

Prevention of malaria is essential for any traveler venturing to a malarious area, regardless of age. Adults ≥65 years of age accounted for 5% of all reported cases of malaria in the United States in 2009.[26] Older travelers might be considered less likely to acquire malaria because the activities they pursue may place them at lower risk, but this assumption can lead to fatal outcomes. Illness may be more severe in the elderly, and mortality from malaria increases with age.[27,28] Assessment of malaria risk cannot be ignored in the elderly.

There is no increased toxicity from N,N-diethyl-3-methylbenzamide (DEET) in the elderly. Chemoprophylaxis is always indicated; it can be safely administered in the elderly and may be better tolerated than in younger age groups, but caution must be exercised in certain settings. Chloroquine can rarely cause irreversible retinal damage if used in the presence of known retinal disease, and hearing loss has been reported in those with auditory impairment. Mefloquine should not be used in the presence of cardiac conduction defects or neuropsychiatric disorders, but is otherwise safe to use in the elderly. β-blocker or calcium channel blocker use does not preclude the use of mefloquine. Atovaquone-proguanil is generally well tolerated when used for prophylaxis, but only small numbers of travelers aged ≥65 years have been included in clinical trials.

Travelers' Diarrhea

Young adults are more likely to acquire travelers' diarrhea (TD) than other travelers: they eat more (and more adventurously), and may be less immune to TD pathogens. In theory, older travelers should be more susceptible to TD because decreased gastric acidity – due to achlorhydria, H_2 blocker or proton pump inhibitor use, or prior gastrectomy – lowers the bacterial inoculum required to produce disease, but this has not been proven in epidemiologic studies. Complications of TD, including dehydration and electrolyte imbalance, are more poorly tolerated in the elderly, however, especially in those with underlying cardiac, renal or gastrointestinal disease, diabetes mellitus, the immunosuppressed, and those on diuretics.

Preventive measures emphasizing safe eating and drinking, supportive therapy, and self-treatment should be discussed. Antimicrobial chemoprophylaxis is not recommended for most travelers, but may be considered in the elderly, especially those with underlying health problems such as diabetes or renal insufficiency; however, evidence of benefit is lacking. A daily dose of a fluoroquinolone or azithromycin (depending on the travel itinerary) would be recommended, beginning 1 day prior to departure and continuing until 2 days after the last exposure, for a maximum of 3 weeks. Fluoroquinolones have been associated with Achilles tendinitis, particularly in older adults, and should be used with caution. Azithromycin should be used with caution in those with underlying cardiac disease because of a recent association with sudden cardiac death.[29] Arguments against antimicrobial prophylaxis include the availability of highly effective (even single dose) antimicrobial therapy, adverse effects, development of antimicrobial resistance, and the false sense of security provided. However, the recent introduction of rifaximin, a non-absorbable derivative of rifampin, may change the approach to prophylaxis in the elderly. The drug has few side-effects and has been shown to provide 60–75% protection against non-invasive bacterial causes of travelers' diarrhea.[30,31]

Antimotility agents (loperamide, diphenoxylate hydrochloride-atropine) may be used for symptomatic relief of TD in the absence of bloody diarrhea, but may cause constipation, paralytic ileus, and central nervous system depression (especially with diphenoxylate, which is a narcotic). Anticholinergic side-effects can also contribute to hyperthermia. Older fluoroquinolones (ciprofloxacin, norfloxacin, ofloxacin) remain the antimicrobial agents of choice for treating TD in Africa and the western hemisphere; dose adjustment is required for reduced creatinine clearance. Azithromycin is now the drug of choice in South and Southeast Asia. Rifaximin is also effective for the treatment of TD caused by non-invasive bacterial pathogens.

Sexually Transmitted Infections

Sexually transmitted infections (STIs) are uncommon, accounting for less than 1% of reported illnesses among travelers.[32,33] In contrast, sexual activity is common, with over 20% of travelers engaging in casual sexual activity during travel; over 60% of these encounters occur without use of barrier precautions.[34] While individuals engaging in casual sex during travel are typically young single men,[34] the availability of therapy for erectile dysfunction may influence the risk of acquiring STIs in older travelers, particularly men. Sildenafil (Viagra) use has been associated with an increased risk of unprotected sexual activity and STIs in male travelers having sex with men.[35] Sildenafil is generally well tolerated, but is contraindicated in individuals taking nitrates (who may be overrepresented among older travelers) owing to the risk of severe hypotension, and should be generally avoided in men who have been cautioned against sexual activity because of underlying cardiac disease. Appropriate counseling regarding the risks of sexual activity and the need for barrier precautions is clearly essential, regardless of the age of travelers.

Vaccine-Preventable Infections

Vaccine-induced antibody responses may take longer to develop in the elderly and may be less robust. Therefore, the older traveler should be encouraged to seek travel advice early, preferably at least 8 weeks before travel. Data regarding the immunogenicity and efficacy of many vaccines in the elderly are scarce. Recommendations for travel immunizations are the same as those for younger adults. Only those vaccines for which there are specific issues relevant to the older traveler will be discussed below.

Routine Immunizations

Pneumococcal Vaccine

Travel presents an opportunity to offer pneumococcal polysaccharide (PPV) or conjugate polysaccharide (Pevnar) 23 vaccine to the older adult. Pneumococcal vaccine has become increasingly important for travelers due to widespread antibiotic resistance of *Streptococcus pneumoniae* globally. One dose of PPV is recommended for all adults over 65 years of age. In the elderly, PPV is not associated with a reduction in the incidence of pneumonia, but is effective in reducing invasive pneumococcal disease (i.e., bacteremia).[36] Re-immunization is recommended only for those high-risk individuals immunized before the age of 65; these persons should receive a second dose of PPV once 65, provided at least 5 years have elapsed since the previous dose.

Travel Vaccines

Hepatitis A and B

Hepatitis A is one of the most common vaccine-preventable infections among travelers. Both severity of illness and mortality increase with age. Older travelers who have lived or traveled in endemic regions, or who have a prior history of jaundice, have a higher prevalence of hepatitis A antibody; screening prior to immunization may be cost-effective in this population.

Immunization against hepatitis B should be considered for non-immune travelers to highly endemic regions, and those who are likely to be exposed to blood or sexual contacts. Although seroconversion rates and antibody titers are reduced with advancing age, receipt of hepatitis B vaccine may provide some assurance should unexpected medical care be required in hepatitis B-endemic regions. Injections given with unsterile medical equipment are remarkably frequent in parts of the developing world, particularly North Africa and the Indian subcontinent.[37]

For travelers who are not immune to both hepatitis A and B and for whom vaccination against both is indicated, the combined hepatitis A and B vaccine (Twinrix) is immunogenic in older adults (including those >60 years of age),[38] although antibody titers are again reduced with increasing age and may take longer to develop.

Japanese Encephalitis

Vaccine studies with Japanese encephalitis (JE) vaccine have not been conducted in older, non-immune populations, and the immunogenicity, efficacy, and duration of protection in this age group are unknown.

Travelers' Diarrhea

Travelers' diarrhea (TD) is among the most frequently encountered medical problems among travelers. While vaccination for prevention of TD may not be routinely recommended because of low overall vaccine efficacy (60% against TD due to ETEC, and 25% against TD of all causes), the self-limited nature of most episodes of TD, and the availability of effective agents for treatment of TD, immunization can be considered in individuals who might tolerate TD poorly (see previous section). Efficacy studies of the oral cholera BS-WC vaccine for TD in the elderly are lacking.

Typhoid Fever

Typhoid fever is relatively rare in travelers. Both severity of illness and mortality from typhoid fever increase with age. Vaccine should be offered to older travelers to endemic areas, particularly those visiting friends and relatives ('VFRs') on the Indian subcontinent. No studies using either currently available vaccine preparation (purified Vi polysaccharide vaccine and live attenuated oral vaccine) have specifically examined seroconversion rates or protective efficacy in the elderly, and studies of vaccine efficacy in these travelers are also lacking. A combined hepatitis A/Vi polysaccharide typhoid vaccine is also available in some countries, with the same dosing schedule as that for the individual components. Studies have not been conducted in the elderly.

Varicella

Adult travelers without a history of varicella can be tested for the presence of antibodies and, if seronegative, offered the live attenuated vaccine provided no contraindications exist. Following a single vaccine dose, 75% of adults seroconvert; with a second dose, this rises to >95%. The overall effectiveness of varicella vaccine is approximately 90%, but is lower in adults. There are no immunogenicity or adverse event data for this vaccine when used to prevent primary infection in the elderly. Immunization of the elderly can also provide significant protection against herpes zoster (shingles) and postherpetic neuralgia. It is likely that a single dose of the adult shingles vaccine will be equally as effective as the two-dose varicella vaccine regimen, but data on this approach are lacking.

Yellow Fever

Yellow fever (YF) is rare in travelers. Both the risk of severe disease from YF and the incidence of adverse events from live YF vaccine increase with increasing age, particularly after age 50. Based on passively reported vaccine adverse events, serious side-effects, hospitalization, and death occur in 4.7 per 100 000 vaccinees overall, and in 12.6 per 100 000 in those over 70 years of age.[39] Compared with 19–29-year-olds, serious systemic adverse events are reported 5.9 times as often for those aged 60–69, and 10.7 times more often for those >70.[40] Viscerotropic and neurotropic reactions occur, respectively, in 0.4 and 0.8 per 100 000 vaccine recipients overall, but increase to 1 and 1.6 per 100 000 in persons aged 60 to 69 years, and 2.3 per 100 000 (for both) in those 70 and older.[39] In practical terms, these data suggest that the risks of acquiring YF and of YF vaccine-related adverse events must be carefully considered prior to immunization, and that it would be prudent not to immunize elderly travelers who are at very little risk for YF, even if the vaccine is required by international regulations (e.g., travelers aboard cruise ships stopping at ports along the coast of South America, but not traveling inland where YF is a risk). A medical certificate indicating that the vaccine is 'not indicated or contraindicated for medical reasons' is a reasonable alternative.

Summary

The number of older travelers will only continue to increase in the future. While some limitations and restrictions to travel may be necessary for health reasons, there is little reason why the elderly cannot travel to a broad range of destinations. With adequate preparation and appropriate advice, the elderly traveler can enjoy good health during travel.

Additional Resources

Centers for Disease Control and Prevention. The Yellow Book. CDC Health Information for International Travel 2012. Online. Available: http://wwwnc.cdc.gov/travel/page/yellowbook-2012-home.htm (updated annually).

Committee to Advise on Tropical Medicine and Travel (CATMAT). Statement on older travelers. Can Comm Dis Rep 2011; 37: ACS-2. Online. Available: http://www.phac-aspc.gc.ca/publicat/ccdr-rmtc/11vol37/acs-2/index-eng.php

References

1. World Tourism Organization. Online. Available: http://mkt.unwto.org/sites/all/files/docpdf/unwtohighlights11enhr.pdf. accessed 2011 July 22.
2. Hargarten SW, Baker TD, Guptill K. Overseas fatalities of United States citizen travelers: an analysis of death related to international travel. Ann Emerg Med 1991;20:622–6.
3. MacPherson DW, Guerillot F, Streiner DL, et al. Death and dying abroad: the Canadian experience. J Travel Med 2000;7:227–33.
4. Leggatt PA, Wilks J. Overseas visitor deaths in Australia, 2001 to 2003. J Travel Med 2009;16:243–7.
5. Redman CA, MacLennan A, Walker E. Causes of death abroad: analysis of data on bodies returned for cremation to Scotland. J Travel Med 2011;18:96–101.
6. Aerospace Medical Association. Medical Guidelines for Airline Travel, 2nd ed. Aviat Space Environ Med 2003;74;5 Section II: A1–19.
7. Backer H. Medical limitations to wilderness travel. Emerg Med Clin North Am 1997;15:17–41.
8. Cummins RO, Schubach JA. Frequency and types of medical emergencies among commercial air travelers. JAMA 1989;261:1295–9.
9. Delaune EF 3rd, Lucas RH, Illig P. In-flight medical events and aircraft diversions: one airline's experience. Aviat Space Environ Med 2003;74:62–8.
10. Speizer C, Rennie C, Brenton H. Prevalence of in-flight medical emergencies. Ann Emerg Med 1989;18:26–9.
11. Lyznicki JM, Williams MA, Deitchman SD, et al; Council on Scientific Affairs, American Medical Association. Inflight medical emergencies. Aviat Space Environ Med 2000;71:832–8.
12. Cummins RO, Chapman PJC, Chamberlain DA, et al. In-flight deaths during commercial air travel. How big is the problem? JAMA 1988;259:1983–8.
13. Philbrick JT, Shumate R, Siadaty MS, et al. Air travel and venous thromboembolism: a systematic review. J Gen Intern Med 2007;22:107–14.
14. Kuipers S, Schreijer AJM, Cannegieter SC, et al. Travel and venous thrombosis: a systematic review. J Intern Med 2007;262:615–34.
15. Peerz-Rodriguez E, Jiminez D, Diaz G, et al. Incidence of air travel-related pulmonary embolism at the Madrid-Barajas airport. Arch Intern Med 2003;163:2766–70.
16. Oger E. Incidence of venous thromboembolish: a community-based study in Western France. EPI-GETBP Study Group. Group d'Etude de la Thrombose de Bretagne Occidentale. Thromb Haemost 2000:83;657–66.
17. Clarke MJ, Hopewell S, Juszczak E, et al. Compression stockings for preventing deep vein thrombosis in airline passengers. Cochrane Database Syst Rev 2006;April 19(2):CD004002.
18. Hsieh HF, Lee FP. Graduated compression stockings as prophylaxis for flight-related venous thrombosis: systematic literature review. J Adv Nurs 2005;51:83–98.
19. Suhner A, Schlagenhauf P, Hofer I, et al. Effectiveness and tolerability of melatonin and zolpidem for the alleviation of jet lag. Aviat Space Environ Med 2001;72:638–46.
20. Herxheimer A, Petrie KJ. Melatonin for preventing and treating jet lag. Cochrane Database Syst Rev 2002;(2):CD001520.
21. Morgenthaler TI, Lee-Chiong T, Alessi C, et al. Practice parameters for the clinical evaluation and treatment of circadian rhythm sleep disorders. An American Academy of Sleep Medicine report. Sleep 2007;30:1445–59.
22. Suhner A, Schlagenhauf P, Johnson R, et al. Comparative study to determine the optimal melatonin dosage form for the alleviation of jet lag. Chronobiol Int 1998;15:655–66.
23. Rosenberg RP, Bogan RK, Tiller JM, et al. A phase 3, double-blind, randomized, placebo-controlled study of armodafinil for excessive sleepiness associated with jet lag disorder. Mayo Clin Proc 2010;85:630–8.
24. Levine BD, Zuckerman JH, deFilippi CR. Effect of high-altitude exposure in the elderly. The Tenth Mountain Division study. Circulation 1997;96:1224–32.
25. Tonellato DJ, Guse CE, Hargarten SW. Injury deaths of US citizens abroad: new data source, old travel problem. J Travel Med 2009;16:304–10.

26. Centers for Disease Control and Prevention. Malaria surveillance – United States, 2009. Morb Mort Wkly Rep 2010;60(SS-3):1–15.

27. Greenberg AE, Lobel HO. Mortality from *Plasmodium falciparum* malaria in travelers from the United States, 1959–1987. Ann Intern Med 1990;113:326–7.

28. Legros F, Bouchaud O, Ancelle T, et al. Risk factors for imported fatal *Plasmodium falciparum* malaria, France, 1996–2003. Emerg Infect Dis 2007;13:883–8.

29. Ray WA, Murray KT, Hall K, et al. Azithromycin and the Risk of Cardiovascular Death. N Engl J Med 2012;366:1881–90.

30. DuPont HL, Jiang ZD, Okhuysen PC, et al. A randomized, double-blind, placebo-controlled trial of rifaximin to prevent travelers' diarrhea. Ann Intern Med 2005;142:805–12. Erratum in: Ann Intern Med 2005; 143:239.

31. Martinez-Sandoval F, Ericsson CD, Jiang ZD, et al. Prevention of travelers' diarrhea with rifaximin in US travelers to Mexico. J Travel Med 2010;17:111–7.

32. Field V, Gautret P, Schlagenhauf P, et al. Travel and migration associated infectious diseases morbidity in Europe, 2008. BMC Infect Dis 2010;10:330.

33. Chen LH, Wilson ME, Davis X, et al. Illness in long-term travelers visiting GeoSentinel clinics. Emerg Infect Dis 2009;15:1773–82.

34. Vivancos F, Abubakar I, Hunter PR. Foreign travel, casual sex, and sexually transmitted infections: systematic review and meta-analysisInt J Infect Dis 2010;14:e842–851.

35. Benotsch EG, Seely S, Mikytuck JJ, et al. Substance use, medications for sexual facilitation, and sexual risk behavior among traveling men who have sex with men. Sex Transm Dis 2006;33:706–11.

36. Jackson LA, Neuzil KM, Yu O, et al. Effectiveness of pneumococcal polysaccharide vaccine in older adults. N Engl J Med 2003;348:1747–55.

37. Hutin YJ, Hauri AM, Armstrong GL. Use of injections in healthcare settings worldwide, 2000: literature review and regional estimates. BMJ 2003;327:1075.

38. Wiedermann G. Hepatitis A + B vaccine in elderly persons. J Travel Med 2003;11:130–2.

39. Lindsey NP, Schoreder BA, Miller ER, et al. Adverse event reports following yellow fever vaccination. Vaccine 2008;26:6077–82.

40. Khromava AY, Eidex RB, Weld LH, et al. Yellow fever vaccine: an updated assessment of advanced age as a risk factor for serious adverse events. Vaccine 2005;23:3256–63.

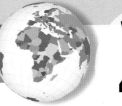

The Physically Challenged Traveler

Kathryn N. Suh

Key points

- The physically challenged have the same rights to travel as the able-bodied, but restrictions or conditions may apply where safety is an issue
- Specific needs and attention that may be required should be arranged ahead of time whenever possible
- A repair kit, extra batteries, and voltage adaptors (if necessary) for medical devices can save time and aggravation while traveling
- Travelers dependent on battery-operated devices should try to use dry-cell batteries, as these are easier and safer to transport
- Service animals should be certified and properly prepared for travel, and any restrictions for their travel clarified prior to departure

Introduction

In the US alone, an estimated 40 million people live with disabilities, over 70% of whom are able to travel. Like advancing age, physical or cognitive disability poses less of a hurdle to international travel today than ever before. Travel companies and carriers have become more aware of the growing number of travelers with disabilities. Furthermore, legislation has been enacted to protect the traveler with special needs against unfair treatment. The Air Carrier Access Act[1] in the US, the Canada Transportation Act[2] in Canada, and the Code of Practice for Access to Air Travel for Disabled People[3] in the UK and Regulation (EC) 1107/2006 of the European Parliament[4] were enacted to allow travelers with disabilities to travel safely and without discrimination on commercial aircraft. Legislation also exists to ensure that travelers with disabilities have improved accessibility to rail and ferry transport. Note that although physically challenged travelers must not be refused transportation because of a disability, some very small commuter aircraft (e.g., those traveling to smaller cities) may be unable to accommodate the traveler with severe physical limitations.

Physical or cognitive limitations should not prevent most affected individuals from traveling. Advanced planning can reduce or eliminate many of the hassles of travel for the individual with a disability and contribute to a positive experience.

General Advice

General advice for the physically challenged traveler is similar to that recommended for other travelers. Issues relevant to specific disabilities will be discussed below. One excellent source of travel information for the disabled is the Society for Accessible Travel and Hospitality website (www.sath.org), which provides an extensive list of resources for the physically challenged traveler. Some additional resources for travelers with disabilities are listed in Box 25-1. An internet search using any widely available search engine can generate many other resources that these travelers may find useful.

An assessment by the traveler's personal physician or physiatrist should precede any trip in order to determine overall fitness to travel, whether the specific disability will impose certain travel restrictions (e.g., on the mode of transportation, or the need for specific accommodations or accompaniment), and to identify other health issues that could pose problems during the trip. Specific recommendations about safe eating and drinking, prevention and self-treatment of travelers' diarrhea and malaria, and immunizations do not differ from those for other travelers, and advice regarding these issues should be sought from a travel medicine specialist.

Careful attention should be paid to health and cancellation insurance: purchase of a supplemental health insurance policy may be prudent. It is important to ensure that the traveler will be covered in spite of his/her disability. Travelers requiring medical equipment, including mobility devices (such as wheelchairs, walkers, prostheses), and hearing and visual aids, should check whether their insurance policy covers theft, loss of, or damage to these devices. Finally, if medical attention will be required while abroad, an appointment(s) arranged prior to departure (with specialists if required) can relieve the stress of finding appropriate medical attention in a foreign country.

Choosing a Trip and Making Travel Arrangements

The nature and severity of disability, and the need for physical assistance, special accommodations, or mobility devices obviously have some bearing on the type of trip that the traveler with a disability can enjoy. Some travel agencies have expertise in arranging trips for the physically challenged, and some organizations specialize in providing group tours or cruises for individuals with particular needs (e.g., dialysis cruises, group travel for the developmentally disabled, or for

DOI: 10.1016/B978-1-4557-1076-8.00025-9

BOX 25.1

Resources for Disabled Travelers

General Information: Organizations

Access-Able Travel Source
www.access-able.com
e-mail: information@access-able.com
PO Box 1796
Wheat Ridge CO 80034 USA
Tel: (303) 232–2979

Disabled Persons Transport Advisory Committee (DPTAC)
www.dptac.independent.gov.uk
e-mail: dptac@dft.gsi.gov.uk
2/23 Great Minster House
76 Marsham Street
London SW1P 4DR United Kingdom
Tel: 020 7944 8011
Textphone: 020 7944 3277

Society for Accessible Travel and Hospitality
www.sath.org
e-mail: sathtravel@aol.com
347 Fifth Avenue
Suite 605
New York NY 10016 USA
Tel: (212) 447–7284

Canadian Transportation Agency
www.cta-otc.gc.ca
e-mail: info@cta-otc.gc.ca
Ottawa, Ontario K1A 0N9 Canada
Tel: (888) 222–2592
TTY: (800) 669–5575

United States Department of Transportation
Federal Aviation Administration
www.faa.gov/passengers/prepare_fly/#disabilities
800 Independence Avenue SW
Washington DC 20591 USA
Tel: (866) 835–5322

General Information: Books

Rosen F. How to Travel: A Guidebook for Persons with a Disability. Chesterfield, MO: Science and Humanities Press, 1997.
http: //sciencehumanitiespress.com/books/preptrav.htm
Science and Humanities Press
PO Box 7151
Chesterfield, MO 63006–7151
Tel: (636) 394–4950
Also available through Amazon (www.amazon.com)

Physically Disabled Travelers

Mobility International USA
www.miusa.org
132 E. Broadway
Suite 343
Eugene OR 97401 USA
Tel: (541) 343–1284
TTY: (541) 343–6812

Royal Association for Disability and Rehabilitation
www.radar.org.uk
e-mail: radar@radar.org.uk
12 City Forum

250 City Road
London EC1V 8AF United Kingdom
Tel: 020 7250 3222
Minicom: 020 7250 4119

Medical Travel, Inc.
www.medicaltravel.org
e-mail: info@medicaltravel.org
16555 White Orchid Lane
Delray Beach FL 33446 USA
Tel: (800) 778–7953 or (407) 438–8010

Accessible Journeys
www.disabilitytravel.com
e-mail: sales@accessiblejourneys.com
35 West Sellers Avenue
Ridley Park PA 19078 USA
Tel: (800) 846–4537 or (610) 521–0339

The Guided Tour Inc.
www.guidedtour.com
e-mail: gtour400@aol.com
7900 Old York Road
Suite 111-B
Elkins Park PA 19027–2310 USA
Tel: (800) 783–5841 or (215) 782–1370
Also arranges tours for developmentally disabled travelers.

Tourism for All
www.tourismforall.org.uk
e-mail: info@tourismforall.org.uk
Tourism for All
c/o Vitalise
Shap Road Industrial Estate
Shap Road
Kendal
Cumbria LA9 6NZ United Kingdom
Tel: 0303 303 0146 or 0044 1539 814 683

Moss Rehab Resource Net Accessible Travel
www.mossresourcenet.org/travel.htm
Information website only

Hearing Impaired Travelers

Canadian Association of the Deaf
www.cad.ca
e-mail: info@cad.ca
203–251 Bank Street
Ottawa ON K2P 1X3 Canada
Tel: (613) 565–2882
TTY/TDD: (613) 565–8882

National Association of the Deaf
www.nad.org
e-mail: available on website
8630 Fenton Street
Suite 820
Silver Spring MD 20910–3819 USA
Tel: (301) 587–1788
TTY/TDD: (301) 587–1789

BOX 25.1

Resources for Disabled Travelers—cont'd

Action on Hearing Loss (formerly the Royal National Institute for Deaf People)
- www.actionhearingloss.org.uk
- e-mail: informationline@hearingloss.org.uk
- 19–23 Featherstone Street
- London EC1Y 8SL United Kingdom
- Tel: 0808 808 0123
- Textphone: 0808 808 9000

World Federation of the Deaf
- www.wfdeaf.org
- e-mail: info@wfdeaf.org
- PO Box 65
- FIN-00401
- Helsinki Finland
- Tel: 358 9 580 3573

Visually Impaired Travelers

American Council of the Blind
- www.acb.org
- e-mail: info@acb.org
- 2200 Wilson Boulevard
- Suite 650
- Arlington VA 22201 USA
- Tel: (800) 424–8666 or (202) 467–5081

Canadian National Institute for the Blind
- www.cnib.ca
- e-mail: info@cnib.ca
- 1929 Bayview Avenue
- Toronto ON M4G 3E8 Canada
- Tel: (800) 563–2642

National Federation of the Blind
- www.nfb.org
- e-mail: available on website

- 200 East Wells Street
- Baltimore, MD 21230 USA
- (410) 659–9314

Royal National Institute for the Blind
- www.rnib.org.uk
- e-mail: available on website
- 105 Judd Street
- London WC1H 9NE United Kingdom
- Tel: 0303 123 9999 (helpline) or 020 7388 1266

Guide Dogs

Guide Dogs for the Blind
- www.guidedogs.com
- e-mail: available on website
- PO Box 151200
- San Rafael CA 94915–1200
- Tel: (800) 295–4050

Guide Dogs for the Blind (Canada)
- www.guidedogs.ca
- e-mail: info@guidedogs.ca
- PO Box 280
- 4120 Rideau Valley Drive North
- Manotick ON K4M 1A3 Canada
- Tel: (613) 692–7777

Developmentally Disabled Travelers

The Guided Tour Inc. (see under Physically Disabled Travelers)

Sprout
- www.gosprout.org
- e-mail: vacations@GoSprout.org
- 893 Amsterdam Avenue
- New York NY 10025 USA
- Tel: (888) 222–9575 or (212) 222–9575
- Specializes in tours for the developmentally disabled.

Author's Note: Reference to or listing of selected organizations does not necessarily signify endorsement by the author. All websites, addresses, and phone numbers were verified at the time of writing.

wheelchair users, etc.). These trips, offered to a variety of destinations, provide the traveler with a predetermined itinerary at a suitable pace, companionship, professional supervision, and medical services where necessary. Some organizations offering these services are listed in Box 25.1.

The specific needs of travelers with disabilities that are likely to arise during travel and at the destination(s) should be discussed with a travel agent, and their availability confirmed prior to booking travel. These arrangements should be verified again at least 48 h prior to departure, and at check-in. Written confirmation of arrangements for special services may also be useful. Because assistance with pre-boarding and disembarking is often required, travelers with disabilities are often the first on and last off the aircraft. This should be taken into account when booking connecting flights, and adequate time should be scheduled between flights. Airlines are responsible for providing help for the traveler with a disability to reach connecting flights. Individuals traveling with a wheelchair, scooter, or other assistive device should inform the carrier and ask how these can be transported. Special seating requests should also be made at the time of booking, e.g., aisle or bulkhead seats may facilitate wheelchair transfers, and seats closer to the washroom may be more convenient for the mobility-impaired. Airlines may not be able to guarantee such requests, but should be able to tell the traveler which seats are most accessible.

When a traveler requests assistance, the airline is obliged to provide access to the aircraft door (preferably by a level entry bridge), an aisle wheelchair, and a seat with removable armrests. Aircraft with <30 seats are generally exempt from these requirements. Airline personnel are not required to transfer passengers from wheelchair to wheelchair, wheelchair to aircraft seat, or wheelchair to lavatory seat. Physically challenged passengers who cannot transfer themselves should travel with a companion or attendant, but carriers may not without reason require a person with a disability to travel with an attendant. Only wide-bodied aircraft with two aisles are required to have fully accessible lavatories, although any aircraft with >60 seats needs to have an on-board wheelchair, and personnel must assist with movement of the wheelchair from the seat to the area outside the lavatory. Airline attendants should assist with managing carry-on baggage, transferring to and from a wheelchair, getting to the washroom (unless lifting or carrying the individual is required), and opening food packages and identifying food. Although they may help with eating, they are not required to do so, nor are they required to help with administering medications or to provide assistance in washrooms. A useful source of information for air travelers with disabilities is a publication entitled *New Horizons*,[5] produced by the US Department of Transportation.

Passenger trains, buses, and ferries in developed countries can usually accommodate the needs of most physically challenged travelers, but these standards are often not the same in the developing world. The transportation company should be notified and any special services requested well in advance. Travelers (or their travel agents) should ensure that hotels, restaurants, and attractions of interest can accommodate their needs. Inquiries about accessible ground transportation to the departure terminal and at the destination(s) (if required) should be made in advance, and reserved well ahead of time if possible. It is best to use a travel agent that is experienced in the unique travel issues of individuals with special needs.

The travel schedule should be confirmed prior to departure. Ample time must be allowed for transportation to the terminal, taking into account the time required for any transfers. Adequate time should also be allowed at the terminal for check-in and for transportation to the departure gate. Any physical assistance, assistive devices required at the terminal (e.g., wheelchairs, or motorized transportation within the terminal), or help with boarding or disembarking should be requested at the time of booking and again at check-in.

Traveling with an Attendant

Some individuals with disabilities may prefer or need to travel with a companion who can assist with their personal needs. The level of assistance required by the traveler should be discussed with the carrier at the time of booking. If the carrier is unable to provide the degree of assistance that it feels the traveler requires, it may request that the individual travel with an attendant. Airlines and other carriers may offer significant discounts for a medically necessary travel companion; proof of disability (medical documents) may be required for this discount to apply.

Circumstances in which the safety of the traveler or fellow passengers can be jeopardized may prevent an individual with a disability from traveling unaccompanied. Examples include cognitive or developmental impairment, severe physical disability impairing mobility, or combined visual and hearing impairments, any of which may prevent the traveler from understanding instructions or taking appropriate action in the event of an emergency. In such cases the carrier may require an attendant (safety assistant) to accompany the traveler, but is not responsible for finding or providing this attendant. Occasionally an off-duty employee traveling on the same flight or a kind-hearted fellow traveler will assume this role. In contrast to a personal travel attendant, the safety assistant is only required to help in the event of an emergency and is not obliged to provide personal assistance to the traveler. If a traveler is denied transportation because a safety assistant is unavailable, compensation should be provided by the carrier.

The Physically Disabled Traveler

Physically challenged travelers may require assistance with boarding and disembarking, and this can be requested at the time of booking and check-in. Most airline carriers will announce pre-boarding and disembarking assistance for those who require it.

BOX 25.2

Practical Tips for the Wheelchair (or Scooter) Traveler

1. Request any special services well in advance, including accessible ground transportation if necessary.
2. Consider insuring the wheelchair or scooter.
3. Have the wheelchair serviced prior to travel.
4. For electric wheelchairs, bring a voltage adapter if necessary; for battery-operated chairs, try to use dry cell batteries (they do not have to be removed).
5. Label the wheelchair and all removable parts with your name and address.
6. Attach instructions for disassembly and reassembly of your chair, and for disconnection and reconnection of batteries if necessary.
7. Arrive early at the terminal.
8. Use your chair within the terminal, then check it at the gate. Remove any removable parts and take them with you before checking it.
9. Make sure the carrier is clear about where the wheelchair is to be returned to you.
10. Bring a repair kit, including tire repair equipment.

Air Travel with a Wheelchair or Scooter

Tips for the wheelchair or scooter traveler are listed in Box 25-2. Wheelchair or scooter rental may be an option for some travelers, particularly short-term travelers or those who depend on these devices only for distance travel. Airlines will transport wheelchairs and scooters at no extra cost to the traveler. Those traveling with a wheelchair or scooter should notify the carrier at the time of making reservations, and should specify whether the device is manual or electric; this should be confirmed with the airline at least 48 h prior to departure. A smaller or lightweight manual wheelchair may be preferable for travel, being easier to transport and less prone to damage. If airport or overnight layovers are scheduled, the traveler can request that the wheelchair or scooter be returned to him or her; this will not only be more convenient for the individual, but will also minimize the risk of loss or damage to the device.

The traveler should verify whether or not the wheelchair or scooter is covered by (or can be added to) an existing insurance policy. Prior to departure, proper functioning of the device should be ensured, and consideration given to having it serviced if this has not been done recently. This might prevent unforeseen mechanical problems that could result in wasted time during the trip. Locating a wheelchair or scooter service agency in the destination may prove useful, just in case. Electric wheelchairs or scooters will require occasional recharging – an appropriate voltage adaptor should be brought along if necessary. The device and any removable parts should be labeled with proper identification prior to travel. Finally, a small repair kit should be carried, including repair equipment for pneumatic tires.

Manual wheelchairs may be stored in the aircraft cabin, depending on their size and the cabin space available. Some smaller aircraft may not allow these items to be stored in the cabin, but the carrier should inform the passenger of this. Newer aircraft (those delivered after 1992 in the US, or after May 2010 for other airlines) must be able to accommodate one folding wheelchair in the cabin, usually on a first-come, first-served basis; if the wheelchair traveler pre-boards, the wheelchair should take priority over carry-on luggage of other passengers boarding at the same terminal. Wheelchairs that are brought on board should not be counted as carry-on baggage. If a wheelchair cannot be brought on board, or if a scooter is used, it can be gate-checked and a baggage claim check obtained for the item; this will allow the traveler to use the device within the terminal and up to the aircraft door. Removable parts (seat cushions, baskets, etc.) should be removed before checking the item. If equipment is battery-powered, dry cell (non-spillable) batteries are preferable; wet cells (spillable), which contain battery acid, must be removed and packed separately in special containers (another item to lose). In some countries, however, removal of dry cell batteries may also be required. Some wheelchairs may need to be disassembled in order to fit into the baggage compartment of certain aircraft, but should be returned to the traveler fully assembled; attaching instructions for disassembly and disconnection of batteries (and reassembly and reconnection) may be helpful for airline personnel. Mobility aids should be returned to the traveler either at (or as close as possible to) the aircraft door or at the baggage claim area, as specified by the traveler.

The carrier is responsible for the intact transportation of any mobility aid to the traveler's destination, including proper disassembly and reassembly. The traveler should not be required to sign any waiver of liability, except when pre-existing damage to the device is present. Damage to (or loss of) wheelchairs, scooters, and batteries does occur during transport, especially in baggage compartments. Damage during flight is the airline's responsibility, and the carrier is obliged to provide a suitable replacement at no cost to the traveler until the damaged item is repaired or replaced. Coverage for loss may vary, depending on the country of travel. For example, during domestic travel, loss (or irreparable damage) of a device by a Canadian carrier requires the carrier to replace it with an identical unit or reimburse the replacement cost, whereas in the US compensation is based on the original purchase price of the device. Liability for loss during international travel is stipulated by the Warsaw Convention,[6] in which assistive devices are not distinguished from other baggage; compensation in these instances may not cover the cost of replacing the device.

The traveler may need to transfer to a wheelchair to board the aircraft. In the US, new wide-bodied aircraft must have one wheelchair on board. Smaller aircraft may require the use of a smaller 'aisle' wheelchair, which the airline should supply. In cases where a ramp to the aircraft door cannot be used, the traveler may need to board the plane by a mechanical lift or use of a 'boarding chair'. Washrooms in older aircraft may be unable to accommodate even aisle wheelchairs, whereas those in newer or remodeled aircraft generally can; new wide-bodied aircraft are required to have a wheelchair-accessible washroom. If an aisle wheelchair will be required on board (e.g., on long flights, where a trip to the washroom may be necessary), it should be requested ahead of time. In addition, travelers should be aware that washrooms are often too small to allow an assistant to accompany them into the washroom. The carrier should provide details about washroom space if this information is requested.

Cruising with a Wheelchair or Scooter

Cruising is an attractive and convenient form of travel for many physically challenged individuals. Newer cruise ships are more user-friendly for the disabled, with features such as wheelchair-accessible washrooms and roll-in showers. In addition, some cruise lines offer cruises specifically for the disabled and are accustomed to the needs of wheelchair travelers.

An appealing feature of most cruises, apart from the all-inclusive nature of travel, is the opportunity to visit many countries by disembarking at several ports of call. Ships can dock if the pier is large enough and in sufficiently deep water to allow this. For wheelchair and scooter travelers, disembarking onto a pier may mean that they and their device have to be carried separately onto the pier; alternatively, the traveler may be seated in the wheelchair or scooter and be 'walked' onto the pier by means of a specialized mechanical contraption which transports both together.

If water is too shallow to permit the ship to dock at shore, the ship will anchor a short distance from land and, weather permitting, passengers must transfer to a smaller ship in order to go ashore, a process known as tendering. Most cruise lines will provide physical assistance to allow the wheelchair traveler to tender.

Ports of call may have many sights to visit in a relatively short period of time. Travelers can usually access these by taxi or other tour company. It may be helpful to inquire about special excursions or services that are available at the different ports when booking the cruise.

Canes, Crutches, Walkers, and Other Medical Devices

Travelers requiring canes, crutches, walkers, and other medical devices can also travel with these at no extra charge. These devices are not included in the carry-on baggage limit, and can generally be stored in the aircraft cabin. The airline's policy regarding replacement of a device in the event of damage or loss should be the same as that for wheelchairs and scooters.

The Hearing-Impaired Traveler

Deaf and hearing-impaired travelers may encounter difficulty with many aspects of travel that others take for granted, such as hearing announcements and using telephones. Hearing impairment may also subject the traveler to potential safety risks, particularly in emergency settings, where verbal or overhead instructions are provided, or where alarms are sounded. If a travel attendant is required, a companion discount may be available. Travelers who use hearing aids should bring extra batteries.

Reservations should be made ahead of time whenever possible; the travel agent, tour company, transportation carriers, and hotels should be informed about hearing difficulties ahead of time. A written confirmation of travel arrangements and a written agenda can help to ensure that travel plans are correct. Travelers should inform the agents at check-in, at the boarding gate, and on the carrier of their impairment. Since information on overhead announcements may go unheard, travelers should request that this information be given to them individually.

Hotel staff must be made aware of a traveler's hearing impairment. Some hotels will provide visual aids for the hearing impaired so that they can be alerted to alarms or phone calls. If these are unavailable, knowledge that a traveler is hearing impaired is essential in the event of an emergency. Teletypewriter (TTY) telephones (synonymous with telecommunications devices for the deaf (TDD), text telephones, and minicoms) allow the hearing impaired (and speech impaired) to use the telephone by typing instead of talking. Such devices may be available at hotels, and should be requested when making reservations.

The Speech-Impaired Traveler

The speech-impaired traveler may also be faced with situations in which an inability to communicate effectively could pose significant problems. As with other disabled travelers, arrangements should be made and confirmed in advance, and travel agents, tour companies, transportation carriers, and hotels notified of the traveler's impairment ahead of time. A written itinerary with details of travel arrangements and addresses of destinations can be helpful if assistance may be required during travel. Flash cards with pictures or written text, a video communicator, or other similar communication devices can also facilitate communication, and may be especially helpful for common inquiries. TTY devices as outlined above should be requested if they are available.

The Visually-Impaired Traveler

Visually-impaired travelers should make advance reservations when possible, arranging any special services ahead of time. They should alert their travel agent, transportation carriers, and hotel staff of their disability. Agents should be informed at the time of making reservations, and again at check-in and at the boarding gate. Written directions and specific addresses are helpful, especially if the traveler will rely on public transportation or taxis. Carrying a white cane will make others aware of the individual's visual impairment.

Some blind travelers may prefer to travel with an escort. Special discounts may be available for travel companions; inquiries about special rates should be made prior to booking travel. Traveling with guide dogs is discussed below.

Service Animals

Service animals are animals that are specifically trained to help an individual with a disability. Dogs are the most common service animals, and as of 15 March 2011 are the only animals that are recognized as such in the United States.[7] Foreign air carriers may not accept animals other than dogs. Although service dogs are most commonly used by the visually impaired, they may also act as guides for the hearing impaired and those with other disabilities. Certification of service dogs is provided by some agencies, but is not necessary in order for them to work as such; however, proof of certification will be required in some circumstances and may be valuable in others. Service dogs are working animals and not pets, and should not be barred entry to areas where pets are disallowed. In the US, the Americans with Disabilities Act stipulates that service animals be permitted to accompany their owners in all areas where the public are allowed, including taxis, public buses, airplanes, restaurants, hotels, and other public facilities.[7] Restrictions may apply, however, where safety concerns take precedence. For example, an individual and his service dog may be prohibited from sitting in an aisle seat or at an emergency exit in an airplane, where the animal may block passage or hinder access to the exit; or a service dog may be barred if its behavior poses a safety risk to others.

Advance preparation can make traveling with a service dog easier (Box 25-3). The dog and its harness may be subjected to detailed inspection for security reasons. The traveler may need to calm the dog or refocus its attention if alarms are set off, or if other dogs (e.g., other guide dogs or security dogs) are present in the terminal. The appropriate individuals and organizations should be aware of the traveler's need for a guide dog, and special arrangements made ahead of time. Some countries may quarantine imported animals; restrictions or requirements for transporting a service dog both into and out of a given country can be clarified by contacting the embassy or consulate of that country. Travelers should also remember to make sure the dog will be allowed to re-enter the home country after travel, and ask what restrictions might apply on return. Prior to travel, a veterinarian should examine the dog and ensure that any required immunizations or routine treatments are up to date. A certificate of health and a record

BOX 25.3

Traveling with a Guide Dog (or Other Service Animal)

1. Contact the embassy or consulate of each country you intend to visit and determine what rules or regulations may apply for entering and leaving the country.
2. Ensure that the animal will be permitted to travel with you, especially for out-of-country travel and if the animal is not a dog.
3. Have your vet examine the dog prior to travel. Make sure immunizations are up to date and obtain a record of the animal's health and immunizations.
4. Have the dog officially certified as a service dog.
5. Consider buying travel health insurance for the dog.
6. Make sure the dog has a sturdy (non-metallic) collar; attach proper identification and date of the most recent rabies immunization to the collar.
7. Bring a harness or vest that will identify your dog as a service dog.
8. Immediately prior to boarding, make sure the dog has exercised and voided.
9. Do not feed or sedate the dog immediately prior to travel.
10. Check with your country of residence to find out what procedures must be followed in order to bring your dog back home after travel.

of immunizations for the dog should be obtained; some countries will require these documents to be certified.

A vest or harness that identifies the dog as a service animal can make others aware that the dog is working and is not a pet. A secure collar with tags identifying the name of the owner, address and phone number, and date of the most recent rabies immunization can be crucial if for some reason animal and owner are separated. A non-metallic collar and harness are preferable, as they will not set off security alarms. The dog should not be fed immediately before travel – a light meal and water 2–4 h previously will satisfy most dogs for up to 12 h of travel. If additional food and/or water will be required en route, folding dog bowls come in handy; the traveler should also carry adequate food for this purpose. The dog should not be sedated before travel, but should be exercised and have voided prior to boarding. If the dog needs to void between connecting flights, it may need to be taken outside of and then brought back into the secure area of the terminal.

Maintenance and feeding of the dog during the trip are the responsibility of the owner. The traveler should remember to pack whatever essentials the dog might need while away from home. Finally, the traveler may consider purchasing health insurance for the dog prior to travel. Some policies will include or offer coverage for veterinary services required during travel, but conditions and limitations should be clarified prior to purchase.

The Developmentally- or Cognitively-Impaired Traveler

Developmental disabilities should not prevent travel. Some organizations specialize in excursions exclusively for developmentally challenged travelers (Box 25.1). General advice given to other travelers also applies to those with developmental or cognitive impairment. These travelers should carry an identification card with the address of their destination, in case they get lost. Any special services required should be arranged when booking travel, and requested again at the time of check-in. Provided that the individual is relatively independent and can understand and follow instructions (e.g., in the event of an emergency), there is no need for accompaniment; if the disability is severe enough to jeopardize the safety of the traveler or fellow travelers, an attendant (safety assistant) may be required.

Summary

Most individuals with disabilities are able to travel. Severe limitations may restrict or even preclude travel, but many physical and cognitive disabilities do not present barriers to traveling. Although some aspects of a trip may be limited, depending on a traveler's specific impairment, proper advanced planning can ensure that physically challenged individuals have a fulfilling, enjoyable, and healthy travel experience.

References

1. United States Department of Transportation. 14CFR Part 382. Nondiscrimination on the basis of disability in air travel (Air Carrier Access Act). July 2003. Online. Available: http://airconsumer.ost.dot.gov/rules/382short.pdf (accessed August 29, 2011); and Rule in effect beginning May 13, 2009. May 2009. Online. Available: http://airconsumer.ost.dot.gov/rules/Part%20382-2008.pdf (accessed September 2, 2011).

2. Canadian Transportation Agency. Summary of regulations covering the accessibility of air travel. November 2010. Online. Available: http://www.otc-cta.gc.ca/eng/publication/summary-regulations-covering-accessibility-air-travel (accessed August 29, 2011).

3. United Kingdom Department for Transport. Access to Air Travel for Disabled Persons and Persons with Reduced Mobility – Code of Practice. July 2008. Online. Available: http://webarchive.nationalarchives.gov.uk/+/http:/www.dft.gov.uk/transportforyou/access/aviationshipping/accesstoairtravelfordisabled.pdf (accessed August 29, 2011).

4. European Commission. Regulation (EC) 1107/2006 of the European Parliament and of the Council of 5 July 2006 concerning the rights of disabled persons and persons with reduced mobility when travelling by air. Online. Available at http://eur-lex.europa.eu/LexUriServ/LexUriServ.do?uri=CELEX:32006R1107:EN:NOT (accessed 29 August 2011).

5. United States Department of Transportation. New horizons: information for the air traveler with a disability. August 2009. Online. Available: http://airconsumer.dot.gov/%5Cpublications%5CHorizons2009Final.pdf (accessed August 29, 2011).

6. Warsaw Convention (amended at the Hague, 1955, and by Protocol No. 4 of Montreal, 1975). Online. Available: http://www.dot.gov/ost/ogc/Warsaw1929.pdf and http://www.dot.gov/ost/ogc/ProtocolNo4.pdf (accessed August 29, 2011).

7. United States Department of Justice Civil Rights Division, Disability Rights Section. ADA 2010 revised requirements: service animals. Online. Available: http://www.ada.gov/service_animals_2010.htm (accessed September 1, 2011).

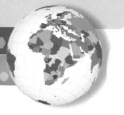

26

The Travelers with Pre-Existing Disease

Anne E. McCarthy and Gerd D. Burchard

Key points

- Prior to travel, early pre-travel health consultation is important, and adequate health insurance, including evacuation insurance, should be arranged
- Copies of prescription medications and medications in original containers should be carried in hand luggage
- When indicated, an assessment of fitness to fly or to travel should be arranged, especially for those with recent surgery or known cardiorespiratory disease
- Patients with diabetes, renal or gastrointestinal disease should maintain adequate hydration and consider antibiotic prophylaxis for the prevention of travelers' diarrhea during short trips
- Individuals with diabetes on insulin therapy should arrange a pre-travel consultation with a diabetes educator

General Principles

Medical advances in the 21st century allow many people with debilitating diseases to live full active lives that include exotic travel. Travel, like life, entails risks that can be minimized with the proper precautions to ensure that the risk does not outweigh the benefits of the travel experience. It is imperative for travelers to understand the risks of their travel, taking into account their particular state of health and their planned itinerary. At times, where choice exists, it may be worthwhile to make a small change in itinerary to minimize health risks without detracting from the benefit of travel.[1,2]

This chapter will address travel medicine considerations for individuals with pre-existing medical conditions, specifically cardiovascular disease, respiratory disease, renal disease, diabetes, gastrointestinal disease (including chronic liver disease), neurological disease, and severe or life-threatening allergies. Considerations for travelers with underlying conditions such as pregnancy (see Ch. 22) and immunodeficiency (see Chs 27 and 28) are presented elsewhere in this text.

Before You Go

Travelers with underlying medical conditions should seek pre-travel care as soon as an international trip is planned, and at a minimum

4–6 weeks before departure. This time is required not only to carry out the pre-travel consultation and administer needed vaccines, but also to provide time to stabilize or optimize underlying disease and to establish a health management plan for the destination country. This health management plan should include prevention strategies and self-treatment instructions for anticipated complications, arrangements for any required routine treatments (such as dialysis), and instructions for where to seek help in the event of particular medical complications. Consideration should be given to the provision of a 24-h medical contact in the event of an unexpected or severe complication (such as an on-call number or e-mail address).

Adequate health insurance is a *must* for travelers with underlying medical conditions. These travelers should ensure that they have a clear understanding of the coverage provided. In particular, they need to know the options for medical evacuation and medical treatment. Many insurance companies will not cover health problems overseas related to pre-existing medical conditions. Read the fine print!

Travelers should carry all medication with them in their hand luggage. This includes medications that are routinely taken and any drugs that are taken on an as-needed basis (such as sublingual nitroglycerine), with enough supply for the duration of the journey plus extra in case of delays. Also, they should carry along with their passport and immunization record an official copy of all prescriptions, with generic names of all medications (most pharmacies are computerized and can provide a printed copy of all medications and instructions for use). It is advisable to have the medication expiry date clearly visible on each prescription label and to carry each medication in its original container (if a smaller container is required, then travelers should visit their pharmacist who can re-package the medication in a smaller container with a new label). Border guards are understandably suspicious about home-packaged medications. Each traveler should be encouraged to discuss with his or her pharmacist the planned journey and ask for storage tips, keeping in mind that 'room temperature' in the planned destination may far exceed temperatures experienced at home. It is prudent to consider providing the traveler with a supply of medications for anticipated complications of their underlying disease (e.g., urinary tract infection) in addition to the routine travel-related medications, with strict instructions as to whether or not medical supervision is required for their use. Drugs used for prevention (e.g., malaria chemoprophylaxis) or treatment (e.g., antibiotics for travelers' diarrhea) of travel-related illness may interfere with the routine medication used to control the underlying disease.

©2012 Elsevier Inc
DOI: 10.1016/B978-1-4557-1076-8.00026-0

Travelers should be warned that, in many countries, many drugs, including antibiotics and oral corticosteroids, are available over the counter but may be inappropriate, dangerous (e.g., a drug no longer licensed at home due to safety concerns), or counterfeit, leading to under- or over-dosing of the medication.

Commercial travel assistance programs are available in some countries. For example, in the US MedicAlert has a program specifically designed for travelers, called the TravelPlus program. More information can be found online at: http://www.medicalert.org/Main/TravelPlusMain.aspx. Travelers should wear a medical alert bracelet or carry medical information on their person (various brands or tags, even electronic, are available) that gives important medical history when the wearer is incapable of providing details. These can save lives, particularly in the event of an acute reversible, but disabling event such as hypoglycemia or allergy. An emergency phone number on the back of each medallion provides healthcare practitioners with details of the medical history.

The International Association for Medical Assistance to Travelers (IAMAT) is a non-profit foundation that provides written information for travelers about health risks, geographical distribution of diseases and immunization requirements for all countries. It also provides a list of western-trained doctors from around the world who speak English in addition to their mother tongue and have agreed to see travelers. (Further information is available at www.iamat.org).

There are many support groups and organizations that work to afford maximum life benefit for those with specific underlying disease, such as the American Diabetes Association (www.diabetes.org). Most of these are easily accessible by phone or on the web. For any traveler with underlying health concerns, the Society for Accessible Travel and Hospitality (www.sath.org) is a valuable resource.

Healthcare providers should supply an official medical letter for any traveler with underlying medical concerns even though it may not be a guarantee for smooth border crossings. The letter, to be carried with the passport, should outline the underlying medical diagnosis, treatment requirements, and the need to carry medications, needles and syringes. Box 26.1 provides a summary of essential health-related items for the traveler with an underlying medical condition.

The Voyage

Air travel, particularly over long distances and multiple time zones, exposes passengers to a number of different conditions that may have adverse effects on those with underlying medical problems.[3]

Airport terminals are often poorly laid out and provide a physical challenge because they require significant commuting between gates.

Wheelchair ground transportation can be arranged through the airlines at the time of the reservation – the traveler must be prepared to supply details of any limitations, since the airline may want to ensure that the individual is fit to fly. In-flight special needs, such as a stretcher, can be arranged through the individual airline. Such special arrangements often require a travel companion or caregiver and may require additional cost.

The cabins of commercial aircraft are pressurized, but only to 6500–8000 ft (2000–2400 m) above sea level; the result is a reduction in available oxygen and expansion of gases within body cavities. The subsequent mild hypoxia in healthy individuals is inconsequential, but may lead to significant compromise in someone with borderline cardiac or respiratory function or with severe anemia. Gas expansion associated with ascent can cause discomfort in some, but lead to significant problems in those who have recently undergone gastrointestinal surgery. Those with ear, nose, dental, and sinus infections should avoid flying because pain or injury may result from the inability to equalize pressure effectively. The need for in-flight supplemental oxygen should be evaluated in those with underlying cardiac or respiratory disease (see below).

Low aircraft cabin humidity (10–20%) may result in mild symptoms, such as dry eyes, nose, and mouth, that can be minimized by maintaining fluids pre-flight and during flight. Occasionally, this dryness may lead to respiratory irritation and an exacerbation of underlying reactive airways diseases.

Prolonged immobilization associated with air travel leads to venous pooling in the lower extremities. Most travelers suffer few consequences other than mild peripheral edema. However, long flights have been causally associated with deep venous thrombosis (DVT) or even pulmonary embolus in some travelers.[4,5] Many airlines promote lower limb exercise in the in-flight magazine and encourage mobility within the cabin. A recent review by Schobersberger et al.[6] categorizes travelers according to their risk of venous thromboembolism:

- Low risk: no personal risk factors (see below). Preventive strategies include regular exercise and maintenance of hydration
- Medium risk: Age >60 years, pregnancy or postpartum period, documented thrombophilia, family history of venous thromboembolism, large varicose veins and/or chronic venous insufficiency, use of oral contraceptive pill or hormone replacement therapy, BMI >30. Preventive strategies include graduated compression stockings
- High-risk: history of venous thromboembolism, active malignancy or other severe illness, immobilization, recent major surgery. Preventive strategies include the use of graduated compression stockings and consideration of low-molecular-weight heparin or fondaparinux.

Health risks associated with air travel may be minimized if the traveler plans carefully and takes some precautions before, during and after the flight (Box 26.2). A simple and useful test to assess whether

---

BOX 26.1

Additional Resources for Information

American Diabetes Association (www.diabetes.org)
American Heart Association (www.heart.org)
American Lung Association (www.lungusa.org)
Anticoagulation Forum (www.acforum.org)
Crohn's and Colitis Foundation of America (www.ccfa.org)
Global Dialysis (www.globaldialysis.com)
International Self-Monitoring Association of Oral Anticoagulated Patients (www.ismaap.org)
US National Home Oxygen Patients Association (www.homeoxygen.org)

BOX 26.2

Essential Items to Be Carried by Travelers with Underlying Medical Conditions

All required medications and print-out of all prescriptions
MedicAlert bracelet
Health insurance
A brief summary of their medical problem including key lab results
Medical contact in destination country
Emergency medical contact at home

Medical Contraindications for Air Flight

Patient sick enough to have a low probability of surviving flight
Any serious and acute contagious disease

Cardiovascular disease:
Unstable angina or chest pain at rest
Recent myocardial infarction – uncomplicated within past 2 weeks; complicated within the past 6 weeks, depending on severity of MI and duration of travel
Coronary artery bypass graft within the past 2 weeks
Compensated heart failure
Uncontrolled arrhythmia
Uncontrolled hypertension with systolic BP >200 mm Hg

Respiratory diseases:
Baseline PaO_2 <70 mm Hg at sea level without supplemental O_2
Pneumothorax within the past 2–3 weeks
Large pleural effusion
Exacerbation or severe chronic obstructive respiratory disease
Breathlessness at rest

Neurologic disease:
Cerebral vascular accident (stroke) within the past 2 weeks
Uncontrolled seizures
Recent surgery or injury where trapped air or gas may be present, such as abdominal trauma, gastrointestinal surgery, craniofacial and ocular surgery

Adapted from International Travel and Health 2002 (WHO), the International Air Transport Association and others.

an individual is fit for air travel is to determine whether he or she can walk 50 m (150 ft) or climb one flight of stairs without severe dyspnea or angina. If there is concern about an individual's fitness to fly the healthcare provider should contact the airline's physician for medical clearance, which is provided on a case-by-case basis. Commercial airlines do have the right to refuse passengers who are medically unfit to travel. Contraindications to flying include those summarized in Box 26.3.

While in the Destination Country

In the destination country, travelers have to adjust to heat, exertion, a novel diet, and possibly altitude. With prior arrangements made through the destination resorts, cruise lines or hotels, special meals can be made available for those with dietary restrictions. It is important for the traveler to realize that available medical resources may be limited; deaths of travelers abroad are mainly due to pre-existing heart disease and accidents. Many of the accidental deaths are preventable. Several studies have determined that 80% of deaths due to injury occurred before the traveler could reach a medical facility, and that infectious diseases (other than pneumonia) accounted for <1% of all overseas deaths.[7–9]

After the Trip

On returning home, ill travelers should seek prompt attention, particularly for any febrile illness, and inform the attending physician about their recent travel history. A differential diagnosis should include possible travel-related illnesses, as these may be life-threatening if not diagnosed and treated appropriately.

Specific Medical Problems

Cardiac Disease

Cardiac events are one of the most common causes of death among adult travelers. Cardiovascular events are also the second most frequent reason for medical evacuation, and cause over 50% of deaths recorded during commercial air travel. Therefore, travelers with underlying cardiac disease should undergo a pre-travel examination to optimize cardiovascular status and define preventive measures, including any in-flight oxygen requirements. Prior to departure, if possible, the traveler should obtain names of specialist physicians in the cities to be visited in case complications arise. The current medication profile and the specific underlying cardiac disease should be reviewed in detail prior to the prescription of any preventive or treatment medication for travel.

In patients with cardiovascular disease, their fitness to fly has to be evaluated. During the flight there are multiple stressors, including altitude-related hypoxia, pressurization, and cramped seating. Hypoxia is reported to have many effects on the circulation, including local vasodilatation of coronary and cerebral vascular beds, increase in heart rate and systemic blood pressure, and increase in pulmonary artery pressure.

Passengers who have suffered an acute coronary syndrome (including STEMI and NSTEMI) can fly 3 days after the event when they are at very low risk (<65 y, first event, successful reperfusion, EF >45%), and after 10 days when they are at medium risk (EF >40%, no symptoms of heart failure, no evidence of inducible ischemia or arrhythmia and no further investigations planned). Patients with hemodynamically significant ventricular arrhythmias should not travel on aircraft. On the other hand, patients with chronic heart failure NYHA III and IV should consider airport assistance between check-in and the aircraft.[10]

Travelers with a history of myocardial infarction or significant heart disease should carry a recent electrocardiogram (EKG) tracing to assist an overseas treating physician in the event that chest pain occurs during the journey. Also, those with pacemakers should carry their pacemaker identification card along with a recent EKG. Although flying is generally safe for those with pacemakers, people with older-style unipolar pacemakers may be susceptible to electronic interference during flight or during security checks. Those with bipolar pacemakers should not be affected. Implantable cardioverter/defibrillators (ICD) may interfere with by handheld security screening devices. Such travelers should carry a physician's letter of explanation with their passport and be sure to inform airport screeners.

Increasing numbers of individuals, including patients with pre-existing cardiac disease, visit high-altitude locations (>2500 m). However, absolute contraindications to high-altitude travel include: unstable angina, uncontrolled arrhythmia, myocardial infarction in the last 3–6 months, decompensated heart failure in the past 3 months, thromboembolic event during the past 3 months, stroke during the past 3–6 months, and poorly controlled hypertension.[11,12]

Concerning vaccinations: Travelers with cardiovascular diseases should get the routine vaccinations as usual. Patients on oral anticoagulants can get all vaccines, as most vaccinations can be given subcutaneously.[13,14]

Concerning malaria prophylaxis: Standby treatment with artemether/lumefantrine is contraindicated in pre-existing cardiac disease. Mefloquine is not recommended for people with cardiac conduction abnormalities, e.g., AV blocks. Co-administration of mefloquine with anti-arrhythmic agents, some β-adrenergic blocking agents, and calcium channel blockers may contribute to prolongation of QTc interval. Drug interactions have to be considered when prescribing mefloquine with warfarin.

Anemia

Anemic patients with unknown underlying disease or unknown source of bleeding should not travel. Also, patients who need regular transfusions should carefully consider their travel route. The minimum hemoglobin for air travel is 9 g/dL (90 g/L).

Air travel with homozygous *sickle cell anemia* is contraindicated, and patients with heterozygous sickle cell anemia can decompensate during air travel. Risk of infection, is elevated.[15]

Patients with functional or anatomic *asplenia* should be vaccinated against meningococcus, pneumococcus and *Hemophilus* (danger of OPSI – overwhelming post-splenectomy syndrome) in addition to routine travel-related vaccines. Malaria risk in these patients can be elevated.

Respiratory Disease

There are many published recommendations for patients with chronic respiratory disease, including air travel.[6–19]

Many patients with chronic lung disease wish to, and do, fly.[20] The most important principle is that patients must be clinically stable at the time they fly. Patients with poor performance status or severe lung disease should not fly, or must fly with oxygen (see below). Pulmonary contraindications to air travel include dyspnea at rest, cyanosis, active bronchospasm and pneumonia. Patients with pulmonary hypertension may suffer clinically significant increases in pulmonary vascular resistance resulting from hypoxic pulmonary constriction; they can only fly when in a stable clinical condition.[21] Reasonable thresholds for lung function are FEV1 <50% for obstructive lung disease and vital capacity <70% for restrictive disease.

In-flight supplemental oxygen is a recognized airline service, but requires planning, a physician's prescription, and possible expense.[22,23] Many types of pulmonary function tests have been used to determine the need for in-flight supplemental oxygen. A simple method recommends the use of in-flight oxygen for all with a PaO_2 of <70 mm Hg at sea level. A more sophisticated test is the hypoxia inhalation test (HIT), which involves a simulation of the hypoxia experienced at altitude to predict an individual's response to air travel.[24] Arrangements for in-flight oxygen can be made through contact with the individual airline at least 48 h prior to departure. A physician's prescription is required for in-flight oxygen and should state flight duration, intermittent or continuous use, and flow rate at 8000 ft (2400 m), with an additional 30–60 min to account for flight delays. In general, a flow rate of 2 L/min is provided to those likely to become hypoxic, with an increase in flow by 1–3 L/min for those on supplemental oxygen at sea level. Travelers are prohibited from using their personal oxygen devices on board an aircraft. In-flight oxygen, when necessary, is always supplied by the airline. It is up to the traveler to arrange any supplemental oxygen requirements for transfer points and layovers, as well as at the final destination. For those routinely on home oxygen, the regular vendor can assist with these arrangements.

Patients with pre-existing lung disease may be at increased risk when they travel to high altitudes, entering an environment of hypobaric hypoxia.[25] Only in some individual cases, such travel may be safely carried out provided a thorough pre-travel evaluation has been conducted and adequate prophylactic measures have been put in place to prevent altitude illness or worsening of the underlying disease.[26–28]

Patients with chronic pulmonary disease may have a tendency for infections in tropical or desert climates. Asthmatic travelers who frequently use inhaled bronchodilators before travel or participate in intensive trekking during travel are at increased risk to develop asthma attacks. Therapy should be intensified to achieve better disease control, with consideration for providing a treatment dose of systemic steroids should they fail to respond to inhalation therapy; intensive trekking should be discouraged.[29]

Concerning vaccinations: In addition to travel-related vaccines, patients with pulmonary diseases should also be vaccinated against influenza and pneumococcal disease.

The British Lung Foundation publishes a free booklet entitled 'Going on holiday with a lung condition', available free of charge from: http://www.lunguk.org/holidays-travel.asp. It contains extensive recommendations for all types of travel for individuals with pulmonary disease.

Renal Disease

Travelers with end-stage renal disease (ESRD) need a prevention and management plan for diarrheal illness; particular emphasis must be placed on fluid management, since dehydration may worsen renal failure. Empiric treatment for travelers' diarrhea, with dosage adjustments based on creatinine clearance, should be provided, along with strict instructions on when to seek medical help. In some cases, antibiotic prophylaxis may be considered. With sufficient notice, dietary restrictions for individuals with renal disease can often be accommodated with the assistance of airlines, hotels and tour operators.

Any arrangements for dialysis should be made well in advance. Peritoneal dialysis is relatively easy to accomplish except for transport of supplies, which are often extremely cumbersome. Also, reliable transport must be organized to ensure that all necessary supplies arrive safely at the destination. Hemodialysis (HD) is available worldwide, but requires several months' notice to implement. Arrangements may be made through the local social worker and/or local branches of the Kidney Foundation (www.kidney.org) or through Global Dialysis (www.globaldialysis.com). The Society for Accessible Travel and Hospitality (www.sath.org) provides information on travel and cruise companies that offer trips specifically tailored for dialysis patients. Arrangements for dialysis must include specific dialysis orders. Some dialysis units require HBV, HCV, and HIV testing, and may refuse anyone who is an HBsAg carrier. Careful scrutiny of any possible hemodialysis (HD) site is essential, owing to the potential for spread of blood-borne pathogens.

Concerning vaccinations: If the dialysis patient is not yet immune to HBV, vaccination using the high-dose series should be carried out prior to travel. Patients with chronic kidney disease may not respond as well to vaccines, but adequate seroresponses have been seen with standard regimens.[30] In addition, patients with chronic renal insufficiency should be vaccinated against influenza and pneumococcal infection. Dukoral® can be considered because fluid loss in case of diarrhea might be harmful.

Concerning malaria prophylaxias: Dialysis does not affect the metabolism of mefloquine and doxycycline. Atovaquone/proguanil (Malarone®) is contraindicated for those with a creatinine clearance <30 L/min. Chloroquine is contraindicated in renal insufficiency.[31]

Diabetes Mellitus

Although those with diabetes may face special challenges during travel, they can usually anticipate or avoid serious problems by meticulous advance planning.[32, 33] However, medication-dependent travelers with diabetes traveling to developing countries do not have symptomatic infectious diseases more often or longer than travelers without diabetes.[34] During the pre-travel evaluation, realistic goals of diabetes control during the voyage should be established; it may be safer to accept higher than normal glucose readings during travel. A physician's letter should be carried with the passport outlining the diagnosis, treatment requirements, and the need to carry medication, needles and syringes.

The American Diabetes Association, ADA (www.diabetes.org) and other groups have valuable resources for travelers with diabetes, including the *Diabetes Monitor*, which contains an edition entitled: 'Traveling with Diabetes' (available online at: www.diabetesmonitor.com). The International Diabetes Federation (www.idf.org) provides a list of regional and country e-mail addresses should one require specialist care abroad.

Adjustment for crossing time zones: All medication should be carried in hand luggage, as insulin may freeze in the aircraft luggage compartment. The traveler with diabetes should anticipate long delays and avoid hypoglycemia by bringing extra food, meals, and glucagon (if appropriate). Frequent monitoring of blood glucose is essential while en route and crossing multiple time zones. Travelers on oral hypoglycemic medication do not require additional dosages and should take their medication according to the local time. For those on insulin therapy, there are many formulae for adjusting insulin dosing during travel (REF).[35] The following is one suggested regimen for insulin adjustment during travel:

- If crossing five or fewer time zones routine insulin dosage should be taken. Frequent blood glucose monitoring should be carried out (every 6 h) and the traveler should anticipate the need for extra insulin and an additional meal or snack.
- Westward travel across six or more time zones leads to a lengthened day. On the day of departure, the routine morning insulin dose is taken and, if appropriate, the evening dose is taken 10–12 h later. Blood sugar should be measured 18 h after the morning dose. If blood sugar is >13 mol/L, the traveler should take one-third of the morning dose and a meal or snack. On the first day at the destination, the usual insulin dose(s) is/are taken according to local time.
- Eastward travel across six or more time zones leads to a shortened day. On the day of departure, the usual insulin dose(s) should be taken, with the evening dose taken 10–12 h after the morning dose. On the day of arrival at the destination, two-thirds of the usual morning dose should be taken with blood sugar determination 10 h later. If routinely on a single-dose schedule and blood sugar is >13 mol/L, then the remaining one-third of the morning dose is required. If routinely on a two-dose schedule and the blood sugar is >13 mol/L, the routine evening dose plus the remaining one-third of the morning dose should be taken. If the blood glucose is <13 mol/L, the routine evening dose alone should be taken. On the second day at the destination, the routine insulin dose(s) is/are taken.

Another approach for insulin adjustment calls for a 2–4% adjustment in insulin dosage for each time zone crossed.[35] For example, a traveler going west over seven time zones would have a lengthened day, necessitating a 20% increase in the long-acting insulin dose.

Carrying insulin: Ideally, insulin should be stored in a refrigerator; however, it is stable at room temperature for up to 1 month. Extremely hot temperatures should be avoided. Those requiring insulin must remember that there is increased insulin absorption in hot climates.

The traveler also should note that altitude may alter glucometer and insulin pump performance.[36]

Complications during travel: A management plan should be in place for any diabetes complications that may arise during the trip (such as a foot ulcer or urinary tract infection). It should include appropriate self-medications and instructions on when to use them, and when to seek medical attention.

Foot injury, with resultant diabetic ulcer and possible secondary infection, is a real concern for the traveler with diabetes. Extensive instructions prior to travel should include the need for frequent sock changes, avoidance of new shoes, diligent foot examinations each night, and careful instructions for foot care and management of ulcers. A prescription should be provided for appropriate antibiotics to be used in event of infection, with strict instructions about when to seek medical attention.

Urinary tract infections are frequent among women with diabetes; due to an increased risk for upper tract involvement, short course antibiotic treatment regimens should be avoided.

Vaccinations: In addition to travel-related vaccines, pneumococcal and influenza vaccines should be up to date. Because of the risks associated with substandard healthcare in developing countries, it would be prudent to vaccinate against hepatitis B.

Travel to high altitude: Beyond 2500 m, freezing, remoteness, hypoxia-induced anorexia, side-effects of medications and the higher incidence of mountain sickness can make diabetes control difficult.[37]

Security measures in different countries: In the US, the Federal Aviation Administration (FAA) has implemented stepped-up security, some of which may affect airline passengers with diabetes. In brief:

- Passengers may board with syringes or insulin delivery systems once it is determined that they have a documented medical need that can be verified by supplying the insulin with a professional, pharmaceutical pre-printed label on the original box
- Passengers who must test their blood glucose levels can board with their lancets as long as the lancets are capped and accompanied by the glucose meter that has the manufacturer's name embossed on it (i.e., One Touch meters say 'One Touch', Accu-Chek meters say 'Accu-Chek')
- Glucagon must be in the pre-printed labeled plastic container or box
- Owing to forgery concerns, prescriptions and letters of medical necessity will not be accepted.

Gastrointestinal Disease

Travelers with decreased gastric acid due to surgery or medications (H_2 blockers and proton pump inhibitors) have lost an important defense against food and water-borne illness. They are more susceptible to illness, since a smaller inoculum of pathogens is more likely to cause disease. For this reason, it is worth considering vaccination with the whole-cell B-subunit cholera vaccine (Dukoral) to protect against ETEC and/or prophylactic antibiotic therapy for travelers' diarrhea (e.g., with ciprofloxacin, azithromycin, rifaximin, according to destination). This should be done with caution as it may predispose to a false sense of security and elicit more risk-taking behavior. For most individuals, it is best to offer antibiotics for self-treatment that should be commenced at the onset of symptoms. Typhoid vaccine should also be considered. In some cases, it may be worthwhile recommending Dukoral that provides some cross-protection against enterotoxigenic *E. coli*. A traveler with a recent ulcer or GI bleed may have problems with intestinal gas expansion at altitude.

Travelers with underlying inflammatory bowel disease (IBD) may experience problems if they acquire food-borne or water-borne infections. Enteric infections may lead to an exacerbation of their underlying disease or cause confusion about the etiology of the symptoms and lead to incorrect management.[38] In those with underlying IBD, it may be worthwhile to consider antibiotic prophylaxis for travelers' diarrhea. Patients with active IBD and complications (such as perianal abscess, severe anemia, fever, extraintestinal manifestations) should not travel. Routine vaccination should be done. However, live vaccines may be contraindicated under immunosuppressive or immunomodulating treatment such as corticosteroids, cyclophosphamide, MTX, leflunomide, AZA, ciclosporin, anti-TNF-α agents and other biologicals[39–41] (see Ch. 27). Prophylaxis of opportunistic infections has to be considered in immunosuppressed IBD patients.[42] Individuals with IBD may benefit from information provided by their national organizations, such as the UK National Association for Colitis and Crohn's Disease (www.nacc.org.uk) or the Australian Crohn's and Colitis Association (www.acca.net.au). Such organizations provide information on many resources for those living with IBD, including lists of international IBD associations.

Individuals with underlying irritable bowel syndrome often experience worsening of their underlying bowel symptoms when they develop travelers' diarrhea. They require particular vigilance in the prevention of travelers' diarrhea and a specific management plan that includes an antibiotic for self-treatment or even antibiotic prophylaxis.

Travelers with colostomies have little problem with air transport but should use a large colostomy bag in case gas expansion leads to increased output. Contraindications to airline travel include any abdominal surgical procedure (including laparoscopy) within 10–14 days and colonoscopy within 24 hours.

Liver Disease

For air travel, it is advisable to carry written confirmation of non-infectivity when jaundiced. Individuals with cirrhosis or chronic alcohol abuse should avoid raw seafood owing to the risk of overwhelming sepsis with *Vibrio vulnificus* and superinfection with hepatitis. Therefore, such travelers should be vaccinated for both hepatitis A and B prior to travel. Also, in this risk group dehydration may lead to severe consequences, such as decompensation of underlying liver disease. Therefore, Dukoral vaccine to protect against ETEC should be considered and empiric antibiotic treatment for travelers' diarrhea should be provided as well as strict instructions for its avoidance and management.

In severe liver disease (Child C) all antimalarial drugs are contraindicated. In moderate impairment atovaquone plus proguanil or mefloquine may be used. In mild impairment: chloroquine, or chloroquine plus proguanil, or atovaquone plus proguanil or mefloquine may be used. Doxycycline should be used only with caution.[43]

Neurologic Disease

Following a stroke or cerebrovascular accident, air travel is possible after 3 days if stable or recovering, though formal medical clearance should be sought if travel is required within 10 days. For those with cerebral artery insufficiency, hypoxia may lead to problems and supplementary oxygen may be advisable. A passenger with epilepsy may be more prone to seizures during a long flight; mild hypoxia and hyperventilation are known precipitating factors, in addition to the aggravation of fatigue, anxiety, and irregular medication. Some airlines instruct intending passengers to increase their regular medication, probably without justification, as in-flight seizures are very infrequent.[44,45]

Some neurological diseases, such as multiple sclerosis and other demyelinating diseases, Guillain-Barré syndrome and myasthenia gravis, can potentially be worsened by infections or vaccinations, and some medications to treat the underlying disease can interact with vaccines:[46]

- Guillain-Barré syndrome (GBS): Refraining from vaccinations should be considered in those fallen ill with GBS following previous immunization, or if the vaccination has exacerbated the symptoms of GBS
- Multiple sclerosis (MS): yellow fever vaccine should be avoided in MS, because it is associated with increased risk of exacerbations of MS.[47,48] The live influenza vaccine should be avoided but the killed vaccine is safe. Individual risk-benefit analysis with yellow fever and other vaccines is important
- Myasthena gravis: Yellow fever vaccination is contraindicated.

Malaria Prophylaxis in Patients with Neurologic Diseases

- Myasthena gravis: Chloroquine and mefloquine are contraindicated. Myasthenic patients always should have a trial of chemoprophylaxis and medical observation before travel[49]
- Convulsive disorders: Mefloquine is contraindicated because of its propensity to worsen seizures; chloroquine has also been associated with seizures. It has been noticed that phenytoin, carbamazepine and barbiturates may shorten the mean half-life of doxycycline, necessitating increased dosage to 100 mg b.i.d. for adults. Malarone seems to be safe in patients with convulsive disorders
- Severe neuropsychiatric disease: mefloquine is contraindicated. Chloroquine should be used with caution because it too has been associated with psychosis (approximately 1 : 13 000 users).

Allergies

Travelers with food allergies may wish to order special meals at the time of airline booking. However, these travelers should keep in mind that such measures are not infallible, and that they should observe the same rigorous precautions that they follow whenever they eat out. Those with life-threatening food allergies should learn how to say, or put in writing in the local language, what they are allergic to in all the countries that they will transit. Also, they should carry pictures of the ingredient or food to be avoided.[50]

Management of allergic symptoms may be different from that at home. It may be worthwhile carrying an emergency anaphylaxis kit (e.g., EpiPen or Anakit). The traveler's medical kit should include antihistamines and possibly a short course of corticosteroids for management of a severe allergic reaction.

Conclusion

Those with underlying health problems should, with appropriate pre-travel planning and behavioral modification, be able to minimize the health risks associated with travel. However, they must have realistic expectations concerning health maintenance and travel restrictions. These individuals at special risk have the option of making use of numerous resources that are now available to make travel an enjoyable and rewarding experience.

References

1. Virk A. Medical advice for international travelers. Mayo Clin Proc 2001;76(8):831–40.

2. Suh KN, Mileno MD. Challenging scenarios in a travel clinic: advising the complex traveler. Infect Dis Clin North Am 2005;19(1):15–47.

3. Davies J. Health risks of air travel. J R Soc Promot Health 1999;119(2):75.

4. Giangrande PL. Thrombosis and air travel. J Travel Med 2000;7(3):149–54.

5. Bartholomew JR, Schaffer JL, McCormick GF. Air travel and venous thromboembolism: minimizing the risk. Cleve Clin J Med 2011;78(2):111–20.

6. Schobersberger W, Schobersberger B, Partsch H. Travel-related thromboembolism: mechanisms and avoidance. Expert Rev Cardiovasc Ther 2009;7:1559–67.

7. MacPherson DW, Gushulak BD, Sandhu J. Death and international travel–the Canadian experience: 1996 to 2004. J Travel Med 2007;14(2):77–84.

8. Leggat PA, Wilks J. Overseas visitor deaths in Australia, 2001 to 2003. J Travel Med 2009;16:243–7.

9. Redman CA, MacLennan A, Walker E. Causes of death abroad: analysis of data on bodies returned for cremation to Scotland. J Travel Med 2011;18:96–101

10. Smith D, Toff W, Joy M, et al. Fitness to fly for passengers with cardiovascular disease. Heart 2010;96(Suppl 2):ii1–16.

11. Dehnert C, Bärtsch P. Can patients with coronary heart disease go to high altitude? High Alt Med Biol 2010 Fall;11(3):183–8.

12. Rimoldi SF, Sartori C, Seiler C, et al. High-altitude exposure in patients with cardiovascular disease: risk assessment and practical recommendations. Prog Cardiovasc Dis 2010;52(6):512–24.

13. Makris M, Conlon CP, Watson HG. Immunization of patients with bleeding disorders. Haemophilia 2003;9(5):541–6.

14. Ringwald J, Strobel J, Eckstein R. Travel and oral anticoagulation. J Travel Med 2009;16(4):276–83.

15. Runel-Belliard C, Lesprit E, Quinet B, et al. Sickle cell children traveling abroad: primary risk is infection. J Travel Med 2009;16(4):253–7.

16. Lien D, Turner M. Recommendations for patients with chronic respiratory disease considering air travel: a statement from the Canadian Thoracic Society. Can Respir J 1998;5(2):95–100.

17. Robson AG, Hartung TK, Innes JA. Laboratory assessment of fitness to fly in patients with lung disease: a practical approach. Eur Respir J 2000;16(2):214–9.

18. Hirche TO, Bradley J, d'Alquen D, et al. European Centres of Reference Network for Cystic Fibrosis (ECORN-CF) Study Group. Travelling with cystic fibrosis: recommendations for patients and care team members. J Cyst Fibros 2010;9(6):385–99.

19. Ahmedzai S, Balfour-Lynn IM, Bewick T, et al. British Thoracic Society Standards of Care Committee. Managing passengers with stable respiratory disease planning air travel: British Thoracic Society recommendations. Thorax. 2011 Sep;66(Suppl 1):i1–30.

20. Edvardsen A, Akerø A, Hardie JA, et al. High prevalence of respiratory symptoms during air travel in patients with COPD. Respir Med 2011;105(1):50–6.

21. Thamm M, Voswinckel R, Tiede H, et al. Air travel can be safe and well tolerated in patients with clinically stable pulmonary hypertension. Pulm Circ 2011;1(2):239–43.

22. Stoller JK, Hoisington E, Auger G. A comparative analysis of arranging in-flight oxygen aboard commercial air carriers. Chest 1999;115(4):991–5.

23. Seccombe LM, Peters MJ. Oxygen supplementation for chronic obstructive pulmonary disease patients during air travel. Curr Opin Pulm Med 2006;12(2):140–4.

24. Kelly PT, Swanney MP, Seccombe LM, et al. Air travel hypoxemia vs. the hypoxia inhalation test in passengers with COPD. Chest 2008;133(4):920–6.

25. Stream JO, Luks AM, Grissom CK. Lung disease at high altitude. Expert Rev Respir Med 2009;3(6):635–50.

26. Luks AM, Swenson ER. Travel to high altitude with pre-existing lung disease. Eur Respir J 2007;29(4):770–92.

27. Brossard L, Brossard C, Jayet PY, et al. Affections pulmonaires et attitude. Rev Med Suisse 2009;5(226):2312–6.

28. Mieske K, Flaherty G, O'Brien T. Journeys to high altitude–risks and recommendations for travelers with preexisting medical conditions. J Travel Med 2010;17(1):48–62.

29. Golan Y, Onn A, Villa Y, et al. Asthma in adventure travelers: a prospective study evaluating the occurrence and risk factors for acute exacerbations. Arch Intern Med 2002;162(21):2421–6.

30. Kausz AT, Gilbertson DT. Overview of vaccination in chronic kidney disease. Adv Chr Kidney Dies 2006;13:209–14

31. Thorogood N, Atwal S, Mills W, et al. The risk of antimalarials in patients with renal failure. Postgrad Med J 2007;83(986):e8.

32. Driessen SO, Cobelens FG, Ligthelm RJ. Travel-related morbidity in travelers with insulin-dependent diabetes mellitus. J Travel Med 1999;6(1):12–5.

33. Burnett JC. Long- and short-haul travel by air: issues for people with diabetes on insulin. J Travel Med 2006;13(5):255–60.

34. Baaten GG, Roukens AH, Geskus RB, et al. Symptoms of infectious diseases in travelers with diabetes mellitus: a prospective study with matched controls. J Travel Med 2010;17(4):256–63.

35. Sane T, Koivisto VA, Nikkanen P, et al. Adjustment of insulin doses of diabetic patients during long distance flights. BMJ 1990;301(6749):421–2.

36. Giordano BP, Thrash W, Hollenbaugh L, et al. Performance of seven blood glucose testing systems at high altitude. Diabetes Educ 1989;15(5):444–8.

37. Thalmann S, Gojanovic B, Jornayvaz FR, et al. Le diabétique en altitude: physiopathologie et consequences pratiques. Rev Med Suisse 2007;3(114):1463–6, 1468.

38. Irving PM, Gibson PR. Infections and IBD. Nat Clin Pract Gastroenterol Hepatol 2008;5(1):18–27.

39. Kotton CN. Vaccines and inflammatory bowel disease. Dig Dis 2010;28(3):525–35.

40. Rahier JF, Moutschen M, Van Gompel A, et al. Vaccinations in patients with immune-mediated inflammatory diseases. Rheumatology (Oxford) 2010;49(10):1815–27.

41. Wasan SK, Baker SE, Skolnik PR, et al. A practical guide to vaccinating the inflammatory bowel disease patient. Am J Gastroenterol 2010;105(6):1231–8.

42. Rahier JF, Moreels T, De Munter P, et al. Prevention of opportunistic infections in patients with inflammatory bowel disease and implications of the ECCO consensus in Belgium. Acta Gastroenterol Belg 2010;73(1): 41–5.

43. Chiodini P, Hill D, Lalloo D, et al. Guidelines for malaria prevention in travellers from the United Kingdom. London: Health Protection Agency; January 2007.

44. Mumford CJ, Warlow CP. Airline policy relating to passengers with epilepsy. Arch Neurol 1995;52(12):1215–8.

45. Schmutzhard E. Flugtauglichkeit bei neurologischen Erkrankungen– Flugreisen und das zentrale Nervensystem. Wien Med Wochenschr 2002;152(17–18):466–8.

46. Giovanetti F. Travel medicine interventions and neurological disease. Travel Med Infect Dis 2007;5(1):7–17.

47. Farez MF, Correale J. Immunizations and risk of multiple sclerosis: systematic review and meta-analysis. J Neurol 2011;258: 1197–206.

48. Farez MF, Correale J. Yellow Fever vaccination and increased relapse rate in travelers with multiple sclerosis. Arch Neurol 2011;68(10):1267–71.

49. Fischer PR, Walker E. Myasthenia and malaria medicines. J Travel Med 2002;9(5):267–8.

50. Kim JS, Sicherer SH. Living with food allergy: allergen avoidance. Pediatr Clin North Am 2011;58(2):459–70.

The Immunocompromised Traveler

Yoram A. Puius, Gerard J. B. Sonder, and Maria D. Mileno

Key points

- Live vaccines should not be given to severely immunocompromised travelers and need to be avoided for at least 3 months after completion of cancer chemotherapy
- Asplenic travelers have increased susceptibility to infection with encapsulated bacteria, *Babesia* species and some enteric bacteria, and respond poorly to polysaccharide vaccines
- After bone marrow transplantation, the highest risk period for acquisition of an infectious disease is in the first 3 months, suggesting that high-risk travel should be avoided during that period

Introduction

The number of people living with immunosuppressive conditions has steadily increased over the past decade, and the complex, unique characteristics of immunocompromised travelers warrant special consideration. As the number of travelers to developing countries has increased tremendously, it is also likely that immunocompromised patients travel more often. Many conditions that had previously been so debilitating as to preclude travel (e.g., rheumatic diseases, inflammatory bowel disease) are now being treated with immunosuppressive medications to make travel for these patients feasible again. All travelers should be advised about the risks of their particular journey. They should be informed on how to avoid risks, how to acquire safe drinking water, and how to seek help should they become ill. There are few absolute contraindications to travel for those who are immunocompromised. Medical providers should carefully review the medical history and needs of their patients prior to travel, and have frank discussions with them regarding the potential risks.

Other chapters in this book are dedicated to the standard approach offered to all travelers, as well as to high-risk groups such as pregnant women, disabled and elderly travelers, or HIV-infected patients. Some individuals may have immune defects, such as common variable immunodeficiency, which make them prone to chronic enteric infections with giardia or campylobacter.[1,2] Other subtle immunodeficiencies caused by interleukin (IL) or interferon (IFN) receptor deficiencies may contribute to increased morbidity from infections, yet there are no data to warrant altering travel advice for these individuals.[3,4] Similarly there are no data to alter travel advice for persons with certain underlying medical conditions considered to predispose to infection (Table 27.1).[5] Here, we address the approach to persons with forms of immunocompromise which can result from use of immunosuppressive medications, solid organ and bone marrow transplantation, cancer chemotherapy, and asplenia. Healthcare workers with these underlying conditions (Table 27.2) are at additional risk. Pretravel discussions should be held regarding avoidance of HIV exposure.[6]

An overview of vaccine recommendations for the immunocompromised traveler is given in Table 27.3. Family members and household contacts of severely immunocompromised persons who may be accompanying the traveler may have previously been vaccinated with live vaccines (such as MMR) to protect the compromised individual, but should not receive the live oral polio vaccine or live intranasal influenza vaccine owing to the risk of transmission. Malaria precautions, including choice of chemoprophylaxis, and prevention of other vector-borne diseases as well as food- and water-borne diseases, generally do not differ from those for immunocompetent travelers.

Corticosteroid and Tumor Necrosis Factor-α Inhibitor Use

Travelers who take high-dose corticosteroids or other agents such as antimetabolites (e.g., methotrexate) and alkylating agents (e.g., cyclophosphamide) for connective tissue diseases and other immune-mediated disorders have an increased risk for a number of travel-related issues. Patients with systemic lupus erythematosus and other autoimmune disorders receiving prednisone doses > 20 mg/day (≈0.3 mg/kg body weight) have an increased risk of serious infections, with up to an eightfold increased risk in persons receiving doses >40 mg/day.[7] Infections with atypical or opportunistic organisms are seen >40 times more often in patients receiving corticosteroids than in those not receiving them. Defects in cell-mediated immunity in these individuals result in weakened responses to immunizations.[8] Live vaccines should be avoided, and a standby course of antibiotics should be given in the event the traveler develops fever (Table 27.3). These patients should receive the influenza vaccine, as corticosteroid therapy does not appear to block the antibody response. Corticosteroid therapy is not a contraindication to receiving live-virus vaccines when the therapy is short-term or low-dose (Table 27.1).[5]

©2012 Elsevier Inc
DOI: 10.1016/B978-1-4557-1076-8.00027-2

Table 27.1 Conditions Which do not Compromise: Prepare as Immunocompetent Travelers[5]

Condition	**Note:** No Immune Compromise if:
Corticosteroid therapy	Short term (<2weeks)
	Low dose (≤20 mg Prednisone/day)
	Alternate day Rx with short-acting preparation over long term
	Replacement Rx (physiologic dose)
	Inhalers
	Topicals
	Injections (intra-articular, bursal, tendon)
	>1 month passed since high doses were used
HIV	>500 CD4 lymphocytes
Leukemia/lymphoma or cancer in remission	>3 months since chemotherapy
Bone marrow transplant	>2 years since transplant
	Patient is not on immunosuppressive agents
	Patient does not have graft-versus-host disease

Autoimmune diseases
  Lupus
  Inflammatory bowel disease
  Rheumatoid arthritis
	Patient is not on immunosuppressive agents
	Note: Data are lacking for persons on immunomodulatory agents

Multiple sclerosis	For MS patients, avoid live virus vaccines if patient is experiencing a current exacerbation and for 6 weeks after the exacerbation resolves
	MS exacerbations may be increased by yellow fever vaccine

Chronic diseases
  Asplenia
  Chronic renal failure
  Cirrhosis/ alcoholism
  Diabetes
  Nutritional deficiencies
	Limited immune deficits exist, yet *no data* exist to suggest decreased vaccine efficacy or increased adverse events with live vaccines

It is also important for these travelers to be aware of the increased risk of acquiring tuberculosis, especially when traveling to developing countries. Several studies have failed to confirm an increased risk of reactivation of tuberculosis in some groups of corticosteroid users. However, conventional wisdom suggests that any patient with a positive tuberculin skin test, a chest radiograph suggestive of tuberculosis, or a history of tuberculosis among close contacts should receive antituberculosis prophylaxis prior to starting corticosteroid therapy.

The use of tumor necrosis factor-α (TNF-α) inhibitors such as infliximab, etanercept, adalimumab, certolizumab, and golimumab for persons with inflammatory rheumatic diseases and Crohn's disease has increased sharply in the past few years. Inhibition of TNF-α predisposes travelers to certain infections that are not common among immunocompetent persons, including reactivation of latent tuberculosis and invasive fungal infections.[9]

Travelers who are recipients of these drugs should be rigorously screened with skin testing, detailed questioning about planned and recent travel, and potential for tuberculosis exposure. As with any patient suspected to have tuberculosis, assessment for symptoms such as cough and weight loss with a chest X-ray is indicated to identify new or reactivating tuberculosis. Induration of 5 mm should be considered a positive PPD reading in this population (as with HIV-infected individuals) instead of the standard 10 mm. Alternatively, the highly specific serum IFN-γ release assays can be considered as an alternative to the PPD.[10]

As use of these agents expands there may be additional infectious risks identified. It is interesting to note that a case–control study of patients on immunosuppressive therapy (including methotrexate, steroids and TNF-α inhibitors) showed no significant increase in travel-associated diarrheal illness, although there was a significant increase in travel-related skin infections;[11] this may merit further study. Little is known about the risks of administering live vaccines to persons taking TNF-α inhibitors, therefore these vaccines should be avoided.

Asplenic Travelers

Once considered a non-essential organ, it is now recognized that the spleen plays a central immunologic role. It actively facilitates phagocytosis, removing blood-borne bacteria, intra-erythrocytic parasites and immune complexes. It also serves as a site for the initiation of both humoral and cellular immunity. Both asplenia (absence of the spleen, mostly postsurgical) and hyposplenism (impairment of splenic function) can result in a higher risk of overwhelming post-splenectomy infection (OPSI). After splenectomy, in addition to the asplenia itself, the underlying reason for splenectomy also plays a role in the subsequent risk of sepsis. Patients who undergo splenectomy for a hematological disease may be at greater risk for infection than those who have splenectomy following trauma. Also, increased mortality due to asplenia occurs in those with underlying reticuloendothelial disease and in patients treated with chemotherapy or radiation. Functional asplenia occurs in all patients with sickle cell disease and after allogeneic hematopoietic stem cell transplantation, and can, in varying degrees of severity, occur in association with a number of other conditions, such as celiac disease, HIV/AIDS, systemic amyloidosis, inflammatory bowel disease and lupus erythematosus.[12]

Most OPSI risk estimates are known from studies in splenectomized patients. Splenectomy is estimated to carry a lifetime risk of overwhelming sepsis of up to 5%, with the highest risk occurring within the first 2 years after splenectomy. The lifetime risk for children who have had a splenectomy reaches 8.1%. The mortality rate of OPSI is 50–70% and most deaths occur within 24 hours after disease onset.[12]

OPSI is mostly caused by encapsulated bacteria and, less frequently, protozoa. Most of the OPSI risk relates to an increased susceptibility to pneumococcal infection. Other important risks include infections due to other encapsulated bacteria such as *Haemophilus influenzae* and *Neisseria meningitides*. Asplenic individuals are also susceptible to overwhelming infection caused by *Babesia* species, a red cell parasite infection transmitted by ticks that largely occurs in temperate and tropical countries, and by *Capnocytophaga canimorsus* following bites from dogs and other animals. Although there are no data to confirm any increased risk of severe malaria in asplenic individuals, it is theoretically possible that the course of malaria in

Table 27.2 Immunization of Healthcare Workers With Underlying Conditions

Vaccine	Severe Immuno-Suppression[a]	Asplenia	Renal Failure	Diabetes	Alcoholism and Alcoholic Cirrhosis
BCG	C	UI	UI	UI	UI
Hepatitis A	UI	UI	UI	UI	R
Hepatitis B	R	R	R	R	R
Influenza	R	R	R	R	R
Measles-mumps-rubella	C	R	R	R	R
Meningococcal	UI	R	UI	UI	UI
Poliovirus vaccine, inactivated (IPV)	UI	UI	UI	UI	UI
Pneumococcal	R	R	R	R	R
Rabies	UI	UI	UI	UI	UI
Tetanus/diphtheria	R	R	R	R	R
Typhoid Vi	UI	UI	UI	UI	UI
Typhoid, Ty21a	C	UI	UI	UI	UI
Varicella	C	R	R	R	R
Vaccinia	C	UI	UI	UI	UI

R, recommended; C, contraindicated; UI, use if indicated.
[a]Severe immunosuppression can be caused by congenital immunodeficiency, leukemia, lymphoma, generalized malignancy or therapy with alkylating agents, antimetabolites, ionizing radiation, or large amounts of corticosteroids.

Table 27.3 Immune Suppression and Immunization

Type of Immune Suppression	Cautions	Suggestions
Travelers with solid organ transplants	Avoid traveling <1 year post-transplant	Pneumococcal, meningococcal, and *H. influenzae* type B vaccines. Hepatitis B and influenza vaccines pre-transplant. Tdap, Td, influenza, IPV as indicated
Travelers status post allogeneic stem cell transplantation	Ideally, defer travel until ≥24 months after transplant	Pneumococcal, meningococcal, and *H. influenzae* type B vaccines. Hepatitis B and influenza vaccines pre-transplant. Tdap, Td, influenza, IPV as indicated
Travelers with hematological malignancies or status post autologous stem cell transplantation	No live virus vaccines <3 months after last therapy	Pneumococcal and *H. influenzae* type B vaccines, ideally 2 weeks before suppressive therapy. Tdap, Td, influenza, IPV as indicated. MMR and varicella if not severely immunosuppressed
Congenital immune disorders	No live vaccines	Intravenous immunoglobulin is used in the management of a number of these disorders but the benefit only lasts for 2–3 weeks
Drug-induced immunosuppression	No live vaccines if taking >20mg/day steroids for >2 weeks	Vaccinate 1 month after last dose of steroid therapy
Other immunosuppressive drugs/therapy[a]	No live vaccines; suppression may last up to 3 months from last dose; can use double dose for hepatitis B vaccine	Vaccinate >1 month after last dose. If vaccinated while receiving immunosuppressive therapy or in the 2 weeks preceding therapy, re-vaccinate >3 months after therapy is discontinued. Immunize as normal

Autoimmune disorders:
  Multiple sclerosis
  Chronic diseases and drugs associated with immune defects
  Hyposplenism
	No live vaccines with significant immunosuppression or during exacerbation of MS	Pneumococcal, influenza, *H. influenzae* type B, hepatitis B vaccines. Pneumococcal, meningococcal, *H. influenzae* type B, and influenza vaccines. Prophylactic Penicillin V
		MS exacerbations may be increased by yellow fever vaccine

Table adapted from Suh and Mileno.[7]
[a]Immunosuppressive agents and procedures: alkylating agents; cyclophosphamide; TNF blocking drugs (infliximab, etanercept, adalimumab, certolizumab, golimumab, etc.); plasma exchange; methotrexate (including low dose), 6-MP + azathioprine; cyclosporine and tacrolimus; total lymphoid irradiation; antilymphocyte globulin.

non-immune asplenic patients is more severe than in patients with a functioning spleen.

The pneumococcal vaccine mostly used for splenectomized and hyposplenic patients is the 23-valent polysaccharide vaccine (PPV-23). Polysaccharide vaccines are only B-cell dependent, induce no T-cell response and therefore no immune memory. Polysaccharide vaccines have low immunogenicity in children and protection is only temporary. Newer conjugate vaccines have been produced by linking polysaccharide to protein carrier molecules, thereby stimulating T and B cells in a concerted fashion. Such conjugation results in increased immunogenicity and the ability to prime for a booster response.

The first conjugated pneumococcal vaccine was a 7-valent vaccine (PCV-7), but later also 9-, 10-, 11- and 13-valent conjugated vaccines became available. Conjugated vaccines are more immunogenic in asplenic patients than polysaccharide vaccines. Often, a conjugate vaccine is given to asplenic patients to obtain long-term protection, followed by the polysaccharide vaccine to obtain protection against more pneumococcal subtypes.

For *H. influenzae* B, a conjugated vaccine is available of which a single vaccination in adults seems sufficient.[13] For *N. meningitides*, a quadrivalent polysaccharide vaccine containing polysaccharides against types A, C, W135 and Y is available, as well as a quadrivalent conjugated vaccine against types ACW135 and Y, and a monovalent conjugated vaccine against type C.[14] Because the risk of OPSI is not necessarily travel related, regardless of travel, asplenic and hyposplenic patients in many countries are advised to undergo vaccination against encapsulated bacteria. The additional risk of OPSI for asplenic patients during travel has not been quantified, and is not necessarily higher than at home. However, healthcare abroad may be of lower quality, or less accessible in the country visited. Also, pneumococcal serotypes may be more resistant to antibiotic treatment. Therefore, the pre-travel consultation should be used to also offer or update the specific vaccinations recommended for asplenic patients. There is no evidence that live vaccines pose any risk to asplenic individuals.

Malaria prevention must include a rigorous discussion of personal protection measures in addition to chemoprophylaxis. Clinicians must emphasize to the asplenic traveler the need for urgent evaluation if fever develops. Other vector-borne diseases may pose a risk and warrant prevention, so tick-bite prevention should be stressed.

Asplenic individuals with fever are advised to seek medical help as soon as possible. Physicians often provide their asplenic travelers with a prescription of amoxicillin/clavulanic acid in the event that they develop illness while abroad, or to start immediately after a cat or dog bite to prevent infection with *Capnocytophaga canimorsus*. Antimicrobial agents that have activity against resistant *Streptococcus pneumoniae, Haemophilus influenzae, and Moraxella catarrhalis* infection, such as extended-spectrum fluoroquinolones, should be provided to asplenic individuals who may not have immediate access to medical care while traveling. Levofloxacin has demonstrated activity against Gram-positive and Gram-negative aerobes implicated in complicated skin infections as well as excellent efficacy for treatment of pneumonia. A higher dose (750 mg, instead of the customary 500 mg dose) ensures high drug concentrations in skin and soft tissue. Alternatively, azithromycin is a well-tolerated broad-spectrum macrolide agent which can be offered for initiation of urgent treatment of suspected upper respiratory infections.

Transplant Recipients

Pre-Travel Counseling for the Transplant Recipient

Transplant recipients are a unique subset of travelers who require additional counseling for a number of reasons. They have increased risk for unusual and opportunistic infections, more severe presentations of typical travel-related infections, and complex medication regimens that may have long-lasting effects on their immune system. However, transplant recipients often do not seek out or receive sufficient pre-travel advice.[15,16]

The most important preventive factor to avoid serious infections while abroad may be to delay travel beyond the period during which these patients are at highest risk. SOT recipients are generally at highest risk of infection in the first month after transplant, and often receive prophylactic anti-infectives for 3–6 months post transplant, but remain at increased risk for invasive pneumococcal disease, community-acquired respiratory pathogens, cytomegalovirus (CMV) reactivation, and invasive fungal infections.[17]

Recipients of allogeneic hematopoietic stem cell transplantation (allo-HSCT) are considered to be functionally asplenic (see the previous section on 'Asplenic travelers'). Infections presenting >100 days post transplant may include invasive pneumococcal disease, *Nocardia*, invasive aspergillosis, HSV, CMV, and respiratory viruses including adenovirus.[18] Patients may be at substantially increased risk if they require high-dose immunosuppressive medications for graft-versus-host disease (GVHD). However, allo-HSCT recipients are presumed immunocompetent at ≥24 months after HSCT if they are not on immunosuppressive therapy and do not have GVHD.

An additional reason to delay travel may be the administration of biologic agents that inhibit or deplete T or B cells, either as part of a peri-transplant immunosuppressive regimen, part of a treatment regimen for an episode of acute rejection, or as part of the treatment for a hematologic malignancy. These agents (such as antithymocyte globulin, muronomab-CD3 , alemtuzumab, basiliximab, daclizumab, or rituximab) may have long-standing effects on immune function for more than a year.

Patients should thoroughly understand food and water safety issues particular to this population, although much of the advice is the same. Guidelines published for safe living after (SOT)[19] and allo-HSCT[20] suggest avoiding the following:

- Raw or undercooked meat, including beef, poultry, pork, lamb, and venison or other wild game, in order to avoid infections caused by Gram-negative enteric organisms (e.g., *E. coli* O157: H7, *Campylobacter*)
- Milk products containing non-pasteurized or raw milk, including soft cheeses, for risk of Gram-negative gastroenteritis
- Cheese containing molds (blue Stilton, Roquefort, gorgonzola) for the theoretical risk of fungal infections
- Unpasteurized fruit or vegetable juices
- Uncooked smoked fish (e.g., salmon, trout) for risk of parasites
- Raw or undercooked eggs, or foods that may contain them (e.g., some preparations of Hollandaise sauce, Caesar and other salad dressings, homemade mayonnaise, and homemade eggnog) owing to risk for infection with *Salmonella enteritidis*
- Combination dishes containing raw or undercooked meats or sweetbreads from these same sources owing to risks of parasitic infection such as toxoplasmosis, trichinellosis, tapeworm and neurocysticercosis
- Unpackaged cold cuts from delicatessens or markets, which may harbor *Listeria*
- Raw or undercooked seafood, such as oysters or clams (viral gastroenteritis, *Vibrio* species, *Cryptosporidium parvum*, hepatitis A).

In situations where the transplant patient or his or her caretaker does not have direct control over food preparation (e.g., in restaurants), they should consume only meat that is cooked until well done.

The environment where the transplant recipient will be traveling should also be reviewed for infectious risks. Of particular concern is minimizing exposure to environmental fungi such as mold or endemic mycoses from soil or caves. Consideration can be made for broader-spectrum prophylaxis (e.g., voriconazole, posaconazole) in selected higher-risk patients who are at risk for exposure to molds[21] or endemic mycoses.[22] Ideally, however, the patient should be counseled to simply avoid high-risk exposures such as spelunking.

Infections from animal bites or scratches or insect stings may be more severe than in the immunocompetent host. Safe sex practices should also be re-emphasized, as some infections which may be sexually transmitted (e.g., HSV, HIV, CMV, viral hepatitis, HPV) may be more severe or complicated in this population. Similar risks may be incurred if the patient receives piercings or tattoos using equipment that may have been suboptimally sterilized; these procedures may also carry the additional risks of infection with non-tuberculous mycobacteria.

Also, transplant recipients have an increased risk for skin cancers, and this risk may be increased by excessive exposure to sunlight. Voriconazole, which is not infrequently prescribed in transplant recipients, is a risk factor for photosensitivity and skin cancer in transplant recipients, particularly among those living in areas with high sun exposure.[23] Specific advice concerning hats and sunblock agents with UVA and UVB protection is warranted.

In the age of global communication – electronic mail, audio/video chatting, international cell phones, faxes – patients who have access to these modes of communication should not hesitate to use them to contact their transplant clinicians for any and all questions.

Medication-Related Issues in the Traveling Transplant Recipient

Immunosuppressive agents for SOT and allo-HSCT are the main cause of increased infection risk, mostly due to suppression of cell-mediated immunity, and sometimes humoral immunity as well. However, recipients need to insure that their immunosuppressive regimens are taken appropriately during their travels to prevent graft rejection, medication toxicity, or over-immunosuppression. These medications may include ciclosporin, tacrolimus, sirolimus, mycophenolate mofetil, azathioprine, and steroids. Also, patients should be counseled to adhere to all prescribed prophylactic antiviral, antibacterial, or antifungal medications.

Patients should travel with an adequate supply of all immunosuppressive and prophylactic medications, with appropriate storage conditions (e.g., a cooler if needed in travel to warm climates). They may consider bringing a written medical history and medication list, and possibly researching ahead of time the closest transplant centers, specialists, pharmacies, dialysis centers, etc.[24]

Calcineurin inhibitors (ciclosporin, tacrolimus, sirolimus) may have significant interactions with travel-related medications,[25] which may include altitude sickness medications (acetazolimide), antimalarials (artemisinins, chloroquine, mefloquine, primaquine, sulfadoxine/pyrimethamine), macrolide antibacterials (azithromycin, clarithromycin), and antifungals (fluconazole). Given the interactions between calcineurin inhibitors and many antimalarial medications, it has been suggested that the patient initiate prophylaxis before travel and have serum levels of the calcineurin inhibitors adjusted before departure.

Travelers should be aware that in other countries interacting agents may be unwittingly prescribed, dispensed by pharmacists, or even available over the counter. All new drugs which are to be taken while abroad should ideally be taken in consultation with a physician or pharmacist, who will be able to take possible interactions into account. Travelers should consider contacting their home transplant clinicians to discuss new medications whenever practical.

Pre-Travel Vaccination of the Transplant Recipient

Recommendations in Tables 27.4 and 27.5 are adapted from guidelines regarding vaccination of SOT recipients[25] and HSCT recipients.[26] In general, live virus vaccines should be avoided, since there is

a risk that disease associated with a vaccine strain might emerge. Inactivated vaccines are safe and important in preventing travel-related infections. However, transplant recipients in general tend to have weaker and less durable antibody responses than normal individuals, and HSCT recipients vaccinated within 6 months of transplant often do not acquire protective immunity.

Hepatitis A vaccine appears to be both safe and immunogenic in liver and renal transplant recipients, and should be given to all transplanted persons. Lifelong once-yearly administration of influenza vaccine should be begun prior to transplant and resume ≥6 months afterwards.

There are also specific recommendations for timing of vaccination following HSCT (Table 27.5). There is no consensus on the precise timing and choice of pneumococcal vaccines in this setting, so the table shows one suggested schedule.[27] MMR vaccine viruses are not transmitted to contacts of vaccine recipients, and varicella vaccine virus transmission is rare. Therefore, family, other close contacts, and healthcare providers of transplant patients should receive the MMR and varicella vaccines if not immune, as well as annual influenza vaccine.

There are reports of successful yellow fever vaccination in allo-HSCT recipients, but the subjects were at least 2 years post transplant and not severely immunosuppressed. (Dr. Bernard Rio, Personal Communication).

Cancer Chemotherapy

Whereas hematological malignancies lead to additional immunosuppression beyond that caused by the chemotherapeutic regimens used to treat them, solid organ tumors may lead to more subtle immune defects. From 1980 to 1997 there was a steady increase in mortality due to aspergillosis associated with malignancy, although mortality rates from endemic mycoses (i.e., histoplasmosis and coccidioidomycosis) remained unchanged. Cryptococcosis is rare in patients with cancer, but it can be confused with lung or brain metastases. Yet, if suspected, serology and CSF culture have good diagnostic yield and therapy usually results in an excellent therapeutic outcome. As with transplant patients, only high-risk exposures may warrant short-term azoles for prophylaxis of endemic mycoses.

Patients receiving immunizations after cancer chemotherapy do not respond as well as normal hosts, with the poorest responses occurring in those with primary hematological malignancies.[28] Persons with chronic lymphocytic leukemia or myeloma are functionally antibody-deficient and will not develop protective responses to most immunizations (Table 27.5). It is better to provide these patients with empiric antibiotics to use if they become febrile while abroad. Live virus vaccines should be avoided until at least 3 months following completion of chemotherapy. It is likely that antibody responses to the other travel immunizations will also be poor.

Post-Exposure Rabies Prophylaxis

The approach to post-exposure prophylaxis for rabies in an immunocompromised patient is often unclear. The Advisory Committee of Immunization Practices (ACIP) guidelines recommend postponing pre-exposure vaccination in immunocompromised patients and refraining from immunosuppressive agents during post-exposure rabies prophylaxis. The authors suggest that post-exposure rabies treatment in immunocompromised individuals may include doubling the dose, monitoring anti-rabies antibody titers daily for at least 1 year,

Table 27.4 Recommendations for Administration of Vaccines Before and after Solid Organ Transplant

Vaccine	Recommended for Use Before Transplantation	Recommended for Use after Transplantation	Re-Immunization Required after Transplantation[a]	Assessment of Immunity Required after Vaccination
Live Attenuated				
Bacille Calmette–Guérin	No	No	No	No
Influenza (intranasal)	Yes	No	No	No
Measles	Yes	No	No	Yes
Mumps	Yes	No	No	No
Oral polio vaccine	Yes	No	No	No
Rotavirus	Yes	No	No	No
Rubella	Yes	No	No	Yes[b]
Salmonella typhi (Vivotif)	Yes	No	No	No
Smallpox (variola)	No	No	No	No
Varicella (Varivax)	Yes	No	No	Yes
Varicella (Zostavax)	Yes	No	No	No
Vibrio cholerae (CVD 103-HgR, Orochol-E)	Yes	No[e]	No	No
Yellow fever	Yes	No	No	No
Inactivated				
Anthrax	No[e]	No[e]	No	No
Diphtheria	Yes	Yes	Yes	No
Hepatitis A	Yes	Yes	Yes[c]	Yes
Hepatitis B	Yes	Yes	Yes[c]	Yes
Human papilloma virus	Yes	Yes	No	No
Inactivated polio vaccine	Yes	Yes	Yes	No
Influenza (intramuscular)	Yes	Yes	Yes	No
Japanese encephalitis	Yes	Yes	Yes	No
Neisseria meningitidis	Yes	Yes[d]	Yes	No
Pertussis (Tdap)	Yes	Yes	Yes	No
Rabies	Yes	Yes[e]	Yes	No
Salmonella typhi (Typhim Vi, intramuscular)	Yes	Yes	Yes	No
Streptococcus pneumoniae	Yes	Yes	Yes	Yes
Tetanus	Yes	Yes	Yes	No
Tetanus	Yes	Yes	Yes	No
Vibrio cholerae (Dukoral)	Yes	Yes[e]	Yes	No

[a]Immunization schedule should be reinstituted once immunosuppression is decreased (typically 6 months to 1 year after transplantation). Once resumed, immunizations should follow the recommended schedule.
[b]Documentation of immunity recommended for women of childbearing age.
[c]Decision to re-immunize should be based on assessment of serological response to the vaccine.
[d]Recommended for college-age students and others at risk.
[e]Recommended for those at risk due to avocation or vocation.

and postponing chemotherapy whenever possible until a protective antibody titer is achieved.[29]

Additional Considerations

Influenza

Most immunosuppressed populations are at higher risk for influenza-associated complications and have a general trend towards impaired humoral vaccine responses. However, these patients can be safely vaccinated with the inactivated seasonal vaccine.[30] If a patient travels to an area with a known high prevalence of influenza, it may be reasonable to send the patient with a supply of appropriate antiviral agents (zanamavir or oseltamivir) to take if an influenza-like illness develops.

Yellow Fever

Travelers with severe immunosuppression should be discouraged from traveling to areas with a high level of yellow fever endemicity. In the event that an immunosuppressed person has not received the yellow fever vaccine and travels to a country requiring it, they should be provided with a waiver letter to the embassy of the country being visited.

Strongyloides

Immunosuppressed travelers are at higher risk of overwhelming strongyloidiasis hyperinfection and septic shock. Walking barefoot, particularly in damp or muddy areas, should be avoided. Closed-toed shoes should be the rule for all immunocompromised travelers. Such exposure may need to be evaluated further with an eosinophil count and

Table 27.5 Recommended Vaccinations for Hematopoietic Stem Cell Transplant (HSCT) Recipients, Including Both Allogeneic and Autologous Recipients

Vaccine or Toxoid	Time after HSCT		
	12 months	14 months	24 months
Inactivated			
Diphtheria, tetanus, acellular pertussis: children aged <7 years	Diphtheria toxoid-tetanus toxoid-acellular pertussis vaccine (DtaP) or diphtheria toxoid (DT)	DtaP or DT	DtaP or DT
Diphtheria, tetanus, acellular pertussis: children aged ≥7 years	Tetanus/diphtheria/acellular pertussis (Tdap)	Tdap	Tdap
Haemophilus influenzae type b (Hib) conjugate	Hib conjugate	Hib conjugate	Hib conjugate
Hepatitis (Hep B)	Hep B	Hep B	Hep B
Pneumococcal[27]	PCV7 (or 10- or 13-valent)	PCV7 (doses at 14 and 18 months)	PPV-23
Hepatitis A	Not routinely; can safely be offered to travelers		
Influenza (intramuscular only)	Lifelong, seasonal administration, beginning before HSCT and resuming at ≥6 months after HSCT		
Meningococcal	Not routinely; can safely be offered to travelers		
Inactivated polio (IPV)	IPV	IPV	IPV
Rabies	Not routinely; can safely be offered to travelers		
Typhoid (intramuscular, Typhim Vi)	Inactivated vaccine can safely be offered to travelers		
Japanese encephalitis	No data on immunogenicity		
Live-Attenuated			
Measles-mumps-rubella (MMR)	–	–	MMR
Varicella vaccine	Contraindicated for HSCT recipients		
Typhoid vaccine (oral, Vivotif)	Avoid, safer alternative available		
Influenza (intranasal)	Avoid, safer alternative available		
Oral polio vaccine	Avoid, safer alternative available		
Yellow fever vaccine	Controversial, few data, avoid		

For these guidelines, HSCT recipients are presumed immunocompetent at ≥24 months after HSCT if they are not on immunosuppressive therapy and do not have graft-versus-host disease (GVHD).

DT, diphtheria toxoid; DtaP, diphtheria toxoid-tetanus toxoid-acellular pertussis; Hib, *Haemophilus influenzae* type b; HSCT, hematopoietic stem cell transplant; IPV, inactivated polio; MMR, measles-mumps-rubella; PCV7, 7-valent conjugated pneumococcal vaccine; PPV-23, 23-valent pneumococcal polysaccharide; Td, tetanus-diphtheria toxoid, Tdap, tetanus-diphtheria-acellular pertussis.

BOX 27.1

General Principles to Consider When Vaccinating Severely Immunocompromised Travelers[5]

- Live viruses are contraindicated
- Additional doses of vaccine may be required for immunocompromised travelers
- There may be decreased protective efficacy due to poor antibody response to vaccines
- If vaccines must be given during immunosuppressive therapy for travel, including the 2 weeks prior to treatment, such persons must be revaccinated >3 months after discontinuing therapy with all indicated vaccines to consider the dose valid
- Household contacts of severely immunocompromised travelers should receive live virus vaccines with the exception of the intransal influenza vaccine or the live oral polio vaccine
- Influenza is the second most frequent vaccine-preventable infection among travelers to tropical and subtropical countries, therefore pre-travel vaccination with inactivated vaccine is extremely important[32]

Strongyloides serology. Infected persons should be treated to avoid severe complications of strongyloidiasis.

Bacterial Gastroenteritis

Antimicrobial prophylaxis for travelers' diarrhea is not routinely recommended for immunosuppressed travelers visiting developing countries; however, in situations where the risk is high, prophylaxis with an antibiotic such as a quinolone or azithromycin may be warranted. Travelers should also be advised regarding how to initiate self-treatment for diarrhea. Recently, rifaximin has been recognized as a safe and effective alternative to ciprofloxacin for the treatment of travelers' diarrhea.[31] This antimicrobial may be especially useful for the immunocompromised traveler, as <1% of the drug is absorbed and there is little potential for drug interactions or adverse events.

References

1. Liesch Z, Hanck C, Werth B, et al. [Diarrhea and weight loss in common variable immunodeficiency]. Z Gastroenterol 2004;42:599–603.
2. Onbasi K, Gunsar F, Sin AZ, et al. Common variable immunodeficiency (CVID) presenting with malabsorption due to giardiasis. Turk J Gastroenterol 2005;16:111–3.

3. de Moraes-Vasconcelos D, Grumach AS, Yamaguti A, et al. Paracoccidioides brasiliensis disseminated disease in a patient with inherited deficiency in the beta1 subunit of the interleukin (IL)-12/IL-23 receptor. Clin Infect Dis 2005;41:e31–7.

4. Zerbe CS, Holland SM. Disseminated histoplasmosis in persons with interferon-gamma receptor 1 deficiency. Clin Infect Dis 2005;41:e38–41.

5. Jong EC, Freedman DO. Immunocompromised travelers. In: Brunette GW, editor. CDC Health Information for International Travel. 2012. Oxford University Press; 2011. p. 522–32.

6. Mileno MD. Occupational HIV exposure. Med Health R I 2000;83:207–10.

7. Suh KN, Mileno MD. Challenging scenarios in a travel clinic: advising the complex traveler. Infect Dis Clin North Am 2005;19:15–47.

8. McDonald E, Jarrett MP, Schiffman G, et al. Persistence of pneumococcal antibodies after immunization in patients with systemic lupus erythematosus. J Rheumatol 1984;11:306–8.

9. Singh JA, Wells GA, Christensen R, et al. Adverse effects of biologics: a network meta-analysis and Cochrane overview. Cochrane Database Syst Rev 2011: CD008794.

10. Mazurek GH, Jereb J, Vernon A, et al. Updated guidelines for using Interferon Gamma Release Assays to detect Mycobacterium tuberculosis infection – United States, 2010. MMWR Recomm Rep 2010;59(RR-05): 1–25.

11. Baaten GG, Geskus RB, Kint JA, et al. A. Symptoms of infectious diseases in immunocompromised travelers: A prospective study with matched controls. J Travel Med 2011;18:318–26.

12. Di Sabatino A, Carsetti R, Corazza GR. Post-splenectomy and hyposplenic states. Lancet 2011;378:86–97.

13. Goldblatt D, Assuri T. The immunological basis for immunization series: Module 9. Haemophilus influenzae type b vaccines. World Health Organization, 2007. (Accessed 27 Sept 2011, at http://www.who.int/immunization/documents/immunological_basis_series/en/index.html.)

14. Borrow R, Balmer P. The immunological basis for immunization series: Module 15: meningococcal disease. World Health Organization, 2010. (Accessed 27 Sept 2011, at http://www.who.int/immunization/documents/immunological_basis_series/en/index.html.)

15. Boggild AK, Sano M, Humar A, et al. Travel patterns and risk behavior in solid organ transplant recipients. J Travel Med 2004;11:37–43.

16. Uslan DZ, Patel R, Virk A. International travel and exposure risks in solid-organ transplant recipients. Transplantation 2008;86:407–12.

17. Fishman JA. Infection in solid-organ transplant recipients. N Engl J Med 2007;357:2601–14.

18. Wingard JR, Hsu J, Hiemenz JW. Hematopoietic stem cell transplantation: an overview of infection risks and epidemiology. Infect Dis Clin North Am 2010;24:257–72.

19. Avery RK, Michaels MG. Strategies for safe living following solid organ transplantation. Am J Transplant 2009;9(Suppl. 4):S252–7.

20. Yokoe D, Casper C, Dubberke E, et al. Safe living after hematopoietic cell transplantation. Bone Marrow Transplant 2009;44:509–19.

21. Marr KA, Bow E, Chiller T, et al. Fungal infection prevention after hematopoietic cell transplantation. Bone Marrow Transplant 2009;44:483–7.

22. Proia L, Miller R. Endemic fungal infections in solid organ transplant recipients. Am J Transplant 2009;9(Suppl. 4):S199–207.

23. Zwald FO, Brown M. Skin cancer in solid organ transplant recipients: advances in therapy and management: part I. Epidemiology of skin cancer in solid organ transplant recipients. J Am Acad Dermatol 2011;65:253–61; quiz 62.

24. Kotton CN, Hibberd PL. Travel medicine and the solid organ transplant recipient. Am J Transplant 2009;9(Suppl 4):S273–81.

25. Kotton CN. Chapter 46: Recommendations for travel-related vaccinations and medications for transplant travelers. In: Kumar D, Humar A, editors. The AST Handbook of Transplant Infections. Hoboken, NJ: Blackwell Publishing; 2011. p. 120–2.

26. Ljungman P, Cordonnier C, Einsele H, et al. Vaccination of hematopoietic cell transplant recipients. Bone Marrow Transplant 2009;44:521–6.

27. Baden L, Wilck M. Chapter 44: Adult vaccination schedule after allogeneic stem cell transplantation. In: Kumar D, Humar A, editors. The AST Handbook of Transplant Infections. Hoboken, NJ: Blackwell Publishing; 2011. p. 113–5.

28. General recommendations on immunization – recommendations of the Advisory Committee on Immunization Practices (ACIP). MMWR Recomm Rep 2011;60:1–64.

29. Rupprecht CE, Briggs D, Brown CM, et al. Use of a Reduced (4-Dose) Vaccine Schedule for Postexposure Prophylaxis to Prevent Human Rabies. 2010 MMWR Recomm Rep 2010:59(RR-2):1–9.

30. Kunisaki KM, Janoff EN. Influenza in immunosuppressed populations: a review of infection frequency, morbidity, mortality, and vaccine responses. Lancet Infect Dis 2009;9:493–504.

31. Koo HL, DuPont HL. Rifaximin: a unique gastrointestinal-selective antibiotic for enteric diseases. Curr Opin Gastroenterol 2010;26:17–25.

32. Mutsch M, Tavernini M, Marx A, et al. Influenza virus infection in travelers to tropical and subtropical countries. Clin Infect Dis 2005;40: 1282–7.

28

The Traveler with HIV

Francesco Castelli, Veronica Del Punta, and Pier Francesco Giorgetti

Key points

- Owing to the availability and effectiveness of anti-HIV drugs, an increasing number of HIV-infected western travelers cross international borders every year
- The HIV-infected traveler may be more prone to travel-related infections, according to his/her immunological status
- Immunizations may be less efficacious and have more adverse effects (live vaccines contraindicated in most cases), depending on the host's immune response
- Drug interactions with antiretroviral agents must be considered
- Behavioral precautions (sexual contacts, food, drink, etc.) need to be carefully addressed during the pre-travel encounter
- Restrictions on international border crossings may be problematic for long-stay travelers

Introduction

As with any sexually transmitted disease, the relationship between human immunodeficiency virus (HIV) infection and travel is complex and multifactorial in nature.

The availability of new potent antiretroviral drugs active against HIV has dramatically improved the natural history of HIV-infected subjects in those countries where HAART (highly active antiretroviral therapy) has become the standard of care. In these countries, mortality and hospitalization rates have decreased steadily and HIV infection has become a chronic condition, manageable on a long-term basis. It is no surprise, therefore, that many HIV-infected persons are willing to travel overseas, including to tropical destinations, as part of their leisure or as an essential component of their professional life.

However, in spite of the common assumption that the availability of HAART would have led to earlier testing, this event has not been observed in practice. Across Europe there is evidence of high rates of late diagnosis – between 15% and 38% of all HIV cases – and that trends are increasing or, at best, unchanged.[1]

Reports indicate that 10–20% of HIV-infected patients with different levels of immunosuppression travel from the United States to foreign destinations,[2] with an increasing trend in recent years.

HIV-infected patients traveled to a considerable extent before the HAART era, and small studies have reported that 30–40% of them became ill abroad or upon return.[3] Therefore, the travel medicine professional is challenged by the reportedly higher infectious disease risk that immunocompromised HIV-infected travelers are likely to face during a stay in developing countries, where circulation of infectious agents is substantially higher than in industrialized countries.

Only very few studies have assessed the incidence of travel-related health problems in HIV-infected subjects. A recent large survey in Canada showed that HIV-infected international travelers were predominantly male (93.2%), with a high educational level (59.4%), a median CD4$^+$ count of 325 cell/µL, taking HAART (89.5%), and less than half were taking prophylactic therapy (42.1%).[4] In the same study about 20% of HIV-infected travelers sought medical care abroad or upon return, a proportion that is similar to that observed in uninfected travelers.

Another study compared fever episodes in HIV-infected and HIV-uninfected travelers, showing that HIV-positive travelers have more respiratory symptoms (61%), enlarged lymph nodes (25%), and abnormal lung auscultation (20%) than the HIV-uninfected travel population. In contrast, fever with no focal symptom was very uncommon (<5%) in HIV-infected travelers. Opportunistic infections (including tuberculosis) and respiratory tract infections were the leading conditions seen in the HIV-infected patients. Both of them represent about 20% of the final diagnoses. Moreover, HIV-positive individuals were more likely to be hospitalized (55%) and to have longer hospital stays (8 days) than HIV-negative ones.[5]

On the other hand, casual sex abroad has been strongly associated with the acquisition of HIV infection. It has been estimated that as many as 35.7% of heterosexually acquired HIV infections reported in The Netherlands in the period 1997–1999 were probably linked to a stay abroad.[6] There has been a recent increase in heterosexually acquired HIV infections among non-Aboriginal men and women in Western Australia, many of whom reported acquiring HIV overseas, mainly via heterosexual intercourse.

This is also true when the migrant population is considered. Difficult socioeconomic conditions, often leading to promiscuous sex, poor access to health services, and low literacy rates, are factors that increase the risk of migrants acquiring sexually transmitted diseases, including HIV.

A Belgian study investigating fever episodes occurring in adult travelers or migrants (>15 years) within 3 months after return/arrival

DOI: 10.1016/B978-1-4557-1076-8.00028-4

showed that HIV testing had been performed in 59% of all patients. Results confirm the different prevalence of HIV infection among three categories: western travelers/expatriates 2%, VFR 11%, foreign visitors/migrants 24%, underlining the major risk of acquiring but also transmitting HIV infection in these particular traveler groups.[5] A study from The Netherlands showed that migrants originating from countries with a high HIV prevalence rank first among heterosexually acquired HIV infections in western European countries, suggesting that heterosexual transmission of HIV occurs mostly within migrant communities.[7]

While recognizing that the disproportionately higher burden of HIV/AIDS is in low-income countries, this chapter will focus mainly on the special precautions that the travel medicine specialist should consider when advising HIV-infected persons traveling from western countries to tropical areas.

Health Risks to the Traveler

Even if the HIV-infected traveler is usually exposed to the same infections as the HIV-negative traveler, traveling to tropical destinations might lead to the acquisition of new opportunistic pathogens, some of which could have a more severe or a chronic course in these patients during or after travel due their immunosuppression.

Travelers' diarrhea may have a more severe and prolonged course. Apart from the usual enteropathogens, less frequent organisms such as *Cryptosporidium parvum*, *Cyclospora cayetanensis* and *Isospora belli* are more likely to produce chronic diarrhea in an HIV-infected individual.

Malaria and HIV infection have a synergistic effect so that co-infection results in higher parasitemia and higher risk of severe malaria; alternatively, recurrent malaria episodes could accelerate HIV progression.

Mycobacterium tuberculosis and HIV co-infection is a major challenge for global health, especially in sub-Saharan Africa, where the prevalence of both infections is high; the risk is particularly high for those with prolonged close contact with the local population.

Sexually transmitted diseases are frequently reported in HIV-infected travelers. It is important to remember that some of them (i.e., syphilis) may present with a more severe course and that co-infection is a risk factor for the transmission of HIV itself to sexual partners.

Toxoplasmosis is distributed worldwide, but travel could be associated with behavioral risk factors for the infection, such as ingestion of poorly cooked meat. The risk of toxoplasma encephalitis in the advanced HIV-infected population is well known.

Leishmaniasis is an important opportunistic infection in patients with AIDS, especially in those with CD4 cell count <200/μL. Visceral leishmaniasis is usually related to the infection by *Leishmania donovani* in Asia and Africa, *L. infantum* in the Mediterranean basin and *L. chagasi* in South America. However, HIV-infected patients can develop the visceral form when infected by non-viscerotropic species, with atypical manifestations.

Chagas' disease is present in Central America and many countries of South America. Patients with HIV infection show a higher parasitemia than HIV-negative subjects, and are at higher risk of reactivation of the disease, mostly in the form of acute meningoencephalitis.[8]

In the field of helminthic infections there is no evidence that trematodes such as schistosomes can cause more severe diseases in HIV-infected patients. Neurocysticercosis in AIDS patients may present with unusual manifestations.[9] *Strongyloides stercoralis* may be an opportunistic agent in AIDS but this theory remains controversial;

however, there is abundant evidence of hyperinfection in those with HTLV-1.

Several mycotic infections are associated with HIV infection. Some of them have a cosmopolitan distribution (*Cryptococcus* spp. and *Histoplasma* spp.), whereas others have a more restricted distribution (*Penicillium marneffei* in Southeast Asia, *Paracoccidioides brasiliensis* in South America and *Sporothrix schenckii* in tropical and subtropical areas of the Americas).[10]

Apart from the infectious risks, the HAART-treated HIV-infected person should be aware of many other potential problems that may arise during travel:

- Antiretroviral drugs should be carried in hand baggage (at least the amount necessary for 10–14 days of treatment), since antiretroviral drugs are not available everywhere in the world
- Since most drug-related adverse events occur within weeks after initiation of therapy, it is preferable to avoid travel within 3 months after antiretroviral therapy has been changed
- Drug-related food and liquid intake may need adjustment in hot climates, where excess fluid loss due to sweating may occur
- Pharmacokinetic interactions with other drugs which may be of potential use during travel should be taken into account
- The cold chain may be necessary for some drugs.

Pre-Travel Advice

Travel-related risks for the HIV-infected traveler depend on the immune status of the subject. As a general rule, travelers with a peripheral CD4+ lymphocytic count >500 cell/μL may travel safely to any destination and may undergo chemoprophylaxis or vaccination as would any immune-competent traveler, with the notable exception of BCG vaccine, which is always contraindicated. On the other hand, special attention and skills are needed to balance infectious risk, medication requirements, and preventive measures in HIV-infected subjects whose CD4+ peripheral count is low. Whenever possible, an expert center in the management of HIV-related complications should be identified in advance in the destination country, and this information should be provided to the traveler. Unfortunately, few HIV-infected international travelers receive authoritative health advice before going abroad. As noted in previous studies, travel medicine physicians were consulted by only 5 to 20% of HIV-positive international travelers.[4]

The most important elements necessary to provide appropriate advice to HIV-infected travelers are reviewed below.

Behavioral Precautions

High priority should be given to the provision of counseling to ensure that the traveler avoids risky sexual practices while abroad, in order to prevent the spread of HIV infection in the host country as well as to prevent the traveler from acquiring other sexually transmitted diseases or additional HIV variants. It has been shown that casual sex is a frequent occurrence in travelers, favored by the lowering of inhibitions by alcohol and recreational drugs.[11] A study on the practices of HIV-positive international travelers revealed that over 20% of travelers reported having had casual sexual activity with new partners while traveling. Of these, fewer than 60% reported condom use during exposure.[4] It has also been proven that other sexually transmitted infections may increase the genital shedding of HIV, which may then facilitate transmission of HIV infection. Furthermore, the possible acquisition of HIV variants other than the original one makes the success of future antiretroviral therapy more difficult to achieve.

Specific and detailed counseling on adequate food and water precautions is mandatory, not only to prevent travelers' diarrhea, which represents the most common medical ailment in the international traveler, but also to avoid the ingestion of possible opportunistic agents that may cause significant illnesses in the subsequent course of their infection. Among those, *Toxoplasma gondii*, *Isospora belli* and *Cryptosporidium parvum* are particularly relevant from a clinical standpoint. Raw vegetables and foods are to be avoided, as well as ice cubes, tap water and fruit juices from street vendors. These simple precautions are clearly underestimated by international travelers, regardless of their HIV status, and particular emphasis needs to be put on them while advising HIV-infected travelers, especially those with low CD4+ cell counts.

It has also been reported that bathing in pools or rivers may increase the risk of skin mycotic, bacterial or helminthic infections. Prolonged sun exposure should be avoided to prevent photosensitivity reactions, which are frequently associated with antiretroviral therapy.

Owing to the possible increased severity of malaria and to the unpredictable pharmacokinetic interactions between antimalarial and antiretroviral drugs (Table 28.1), personal protection measures against mosquito bites (mosquito nets, mosquito repellents, protective clothing, etc.) must be emphasized.

It has also been reported that during travel there is an increased risk of poor adherence to antiretroviral therapy. In a Canadian study, only 44.5% of HIV-infected patients adhered to their therapy while traveling, 26.1% missed only 1–3 doses, and 29.4% either stopped taking their medications altogether or were poorly adherent.[4]

Vaccination

The safety and efficacy of the various vaccinations in HIV-infected persons have been the subject of many debates. Excellent reviews on this topic are available.[12] Four key elements are to be considered in order to make a risk–benefit assessment of a specific vaccine:

1. Risk and Severity of Vaccine-Preventable Disease in the HIV-Infected Traveler

Many infectious diseases are reported to be more frequent and severe in immunocompromised subjects. The incidence of *Salmonella typhi* infection in HIV-infected subjects has been reported to be 25–60 times higher than in the HIV-uninfected population in Peru,[13] and the higher susceptibility of HIV-positive patients to invasive *Salmonella* spp. disease is well described. Typhoid fever may produce life-threatening complications in HIV-infected patients. Although there is no definitive evidence of problems using the live oral vaccine from the Ty21 strain of *Salmonella typhi* in HIV-infected individuals, the typhoid Vi polysaccharide vaccine is preferred regardless of CD4+ level.[14] Non-typhoidal *Salmonellae* (NTS) are increasingly recognized as important pathogens associated with bacteremia, especially in immunosuppressed patients, who experience higher mortality rates.[15]

The yearly incidence of invasive pneumococcal disease may be as high as 1% in the HIV-infected population in the USA, 100 times higher than in the general population.[16] Another reason to consider this vaccine is the increasing resistance of pneumococcal strains globally.

Viral hepatitis is particularly dangerous in HIV-infected patients because hepatitis B and C are more likely to be chronic and to progress more rapidly than in HIV-negative subjects. Hepatitis A infection (HAV), highly prevalent in developing countries, has a more severe course in patients with chronic liver disease, especially hepatitis B and C. HAV excretion has been reported to persist longer in HIV-infected subjects, and the occurrence of hepatitis A, as well as any underlying hepatic disease, may interfere with the regular intake of antiretroviral drugs. On the other hand, the prevalence of HAV immunity in travelers is decreasing, and hepatitis A vaccination should be considered in all previously unexposed HIV-infected individuals. Hepatitis B vaccination should be considered as well for all HIV-infected travelers to high-risk areas.

Apart from the alimentary route, HAV infection may be transmitted sexually in gay men. Epidemics of HAV in men having sex with men (MSM) have been already reported.[17]

There is no evidence that influenza occurs more frequently in HIV-infected individuals, but the incidence of complications has been inconsistently reported to be higher.

Japanese encephalitis (JE) vaccination, indicated for those travelling for 1 month or more in a rural endemic region,[12] is recommended regardless of the immune status of HIV-infected persons.

To date, no information is available on the incidence and/or severity of other vaccine-preventable infections, such as tetanus or diphtheria, in the HIV-infected traveler.

2. Nature of the Vaccine

As for any other clinical situation in which immunosuppression is an issue, live vaccines should be avoided as a general rule, especially when the immune status of the patient is severely compromised (CD4+ peripheral cell count <200 cells/μL). The risk of live vaccines in HAART-treated patients with a satisfactory CD4+ response, but whose CD4+ peripheral count nadir was <200 cells/μL, is still controversial. At least 3–6 months are required after the initiation of HAART therapy before lymphocytes recover full functionality. Current recommendations are that live vaccines may be used safely in HIV-infected patients whose CD4+ peripheral cell count is stable and consistently exceeds 200 cells/μL. A fatal case of measles pneumonia was reported following MMR vaccination in an immunocompromised HIV-infected patient with a CD4+ peripheral count <200 cells/μL. Moreover, the safety of yellow fever vaccination in HIV-infected travelers is still debated, in spite of the absence of adverse events reported in the limited number of HIV-infected vaccinees studied with CD4+ counts >200 cells/μL.[18] These studies did not detect any serious adverse events following immunization among HIV-positive individuals apart from one case of fatal meningo-encephalitis. However, no real evidence about the safety of this vaccine in severely immunocompromised subjects is available.[19] Therefore, yellow fever and measles vaccinations should be limited to situations where a substantial risk of contracting the diseases exists. Inactivated Salk polio vaccine (IPV) should be used instead of the Sabin live polio vaccine (OPV) in HIV travelers. Also, inactivated vaccines should be used instead of live ones against typhoid and cholera, if indicated. BCG vaccine is always to be avoided. However, for those HIV-infected travelers who are likely to be in high-risk situations for tuberculosis (healthcare providers, aid workers in refugee camps, and VFRs) it is advisable to counsel them on how to reduce their exposure to infection, including the possible avoidance of such situations. Polysaccharide vaccines, such as vaccines against *Streptococcus pneumoniae* and *Neisseria meningitidis* appear to elicit a CD4+-independent immune response, as demonstrated by the adequate immune titers obtained in immunocompromised hosts. Despite this consideration, clinical protection against pneumococcal disease is impaired in vaccinees whose CD4+ cell count is <200/μL, regardless of the elicited antibody titer. The protective efficacy of the 23-valent pneumococcal polysaccharide vaccine to prevent invasive pneumococcal disease in HIV-infected persons was not confirmed in a recent trial in Ugandan adults. After 3 years, invasive disease was reported in 15/697 (2.1%) vaccinated subjects and in 10/695 (1.4%) unvaccinated persons, without significant differences.[20] Inactivated,

Table 28.1 Drugs that Should not be Used with Antiretroviral Drugs Because of Pharmacokinetic Interactions (See Table 28.3 for Antimalarial Drugs)

Drug Category	Didanosine	Delaviridine	Efavirenz	Etravirina	Nevirapine	Atazanavir	Darunavir
Analgesics	None	None	None	None	None	None	None
Antiarrhythmics	None	None	Bepridil	None	None	Bepridil, Flecainide, Propafenone, Quinidine	Amiodarone, Bepridil, Lidocaine, Quinidine
Antifungals	None	None	None	None	Itraconazole, Ketoconazole	None	None
Antihistamines	None	Astemizole, Terfenadine	Astemizole, Terfenadine	Astemizole, Terfenadine	None	Astemizole, Terfenadine	Astemizole, Terfenadine
Antimycobacterial	None	Rifabutin, Rifampicin	None	Rifampicin, Rifapentine	Rifampicin	Rifampicin	Rifampicin
Antipsychotics/ Neuroleptics	None	Pimozide	Pimozide	None	None	Pimozide	Pimozide
Anxiolytics/ Hypnotics/ Sedatives	None	Alprazolam, Midazolam (oral), Midazolam (parenteral), Triazolam	Midazolam (oral), Midazolam (parenteral), Triazolam	None	None	Midazolam (oral), Triazolam	Midazolam (oral), Triazolam
β-Blockers	None	None	None	None	None	None	None
Gastrointestinal Agents	None	Cisapride	Cisapride	None	None	Cisapride, Proton pump inhibitors	Cisapride
Lipid-lowering agents	None	Lovastatin, Simvastatin	None	None	None	Lovastatin, Simvastatin	Lovastatin, Simvastatin
Others	Allopurinol					Alfuzosin	Alfuzosin

Drug Category	Fosamprenavir	Indinavir	Lopinavir	Nelfinavir	Ritonavir	Saquinavir	Tripanavir
Analgesics	None	Meperidine, Piroxicam	None	None	Piroxicam	None	None
Antiarrhythmics	Amiodarone, Bepridil, Flecainide, Propafenone, Quinidine	Amiodarone, Bepridil, Flecainide, Propafenone, Quinidine	Amiodarone, Flecainide	Amiodarone, Quinidine	Amiodarone, Bepridil, Flecainide, Propafenone, Quinidine	Amiodarone, Bepridil, Flecainide, Propafenone, Quinidine	Amiodarone, Bepridil, Flecainide, Propafenone, Quinidine
Antifungals	None	None	None	None	Voriconazole	None	None
Antihistamines	Astemizole, Terfenadine	Astemizole, Terfenadine	Astemizole, Terfenadine	Astemizole, Terfenadine	Astemizole, Terfenadine	Astemizole, Terfenadine	Astemizole, Terfenadine
Antimycobacterial	Rifampicin	Rifampicin	Rifampicin	Rifampicin	Rifampicin	Rifampicin	Rifampicin
Antipsychotics/ Neuroleptics	Pimozide	Clozapine, Pimozide	Pimozide	Pimozide	Pimozide	Pimozide	Pimozide
Anxiolytics/ Hypnotics/ Sedatives	Midazolam (oral), Triazolam	Alprazolam, Clorazepate, Diazepam, Estazolam, Flurazepam, Midazolam (oral), Triazolam	Midazolam (oral), Triazolam	Midazolam (oral), Triazolam	Midazolam (oral), Triazolam	Midazolam (oral), Triazolam	Midazolam (oral), Triazolam
β-Blockers	None	None	None	None	None	None	Metoprolol
Gastrointestinal agents	Cisapride	Cisapride	Cisapride	Cisapride, Proton pump inhibitors	Cisapride	Cisapride	Cisapride
Lipid-lowering agents	Lovastatin, Simvastatin	Lovastatin, Simvastatin	Lovastatin, Simvastatin	Lovastatin, Simvastatin	Lovastatin, Simvastatin	Lovastatin, Simvastatin	Lovastatin, Simvastatin
Others	Alfuzosin	Alfuzosin	Alfuzosin	Alfuzosin	Alfuzosin	Alfuzosin	Alfuzosin

Important note: it is advisable to check the package insert before prescribing any medication to HIV-infected persons. Adapted from: www.hiv-druginteractions.org (accessed 15 June 2011). For more and updated details about interactions visit the website.

subunit or polysaccharidic vaccines may be administered safely without risk for the HIV-infected vaccinee, preferably in the early stage of HIV infection to ensure adequate immune response. The 23-valent pneumococcal polysaccharide vaccine (PPV) is not satisfactorily effective in HIV-infected adults and it is not recommended in Africa. In a recent study[21] it was shown that pneumococcal conjugate vaccines (PCV) (7- and 9-valent PCVs) are very effective in preventing invasive pneumococcal disease in HIV-infected children,[22] even if their efficacy and duration are somewhat shorter than in HIV-uninfected children.[23] Although no definitive data are available about the clinical efficacy of PCVs in adult populations, studies in HIV-infected adults show that PCVs are equally immunogenic as PPV.[24] The conjugate vaccine may generate a protective response even at low CD4 counts (<200 cell/ μL), but further studies are needed.

Generally, conjugate vaccines produce higher and longer-lasting serum bactericidal antibody (SBA) titers than polysaccharide ones. The tetravalent conjugate meningococcal vaccine for serogroups A, C, Y and W135 (MCV4) produces protective antibodies to all the involved serogroups both in adults and children >2 years of age. The meningococcal C conjugate vaccine has been proved to be immunogenic in HIV-uninfected children <2 years of age. MCV4 may also be considered for HIV-positive children >2 years of age.[25]

A recent study showed that MCV4 is safe and immunogenic in HIV-infected adolescents, but the immunological response is lower than in uninfected ones, particularly in case of advanced clinical, immunologic or virologic status. A lower antibody response to all four serogroups of the MCV4 vaccine has been shown to be correlated to higher viral load, lower CD4 cell count and more advanced HIV disease stage. Severe immunosuppression (CD4 < 15 cells/ μL) at baseline is associated with the lowest response to the vaccine. Hence, immunization in this group is unlikely to produce protective immunity.[26]

3.   Immune Status of the Traveler

The most reliable and simple marker to quantify the immune status of the HIV-infected traveler, as well as to predict the individual risk to develop clinical opportunistic infections, is the CD4$^+$ lymphocyte count. Also, it may provide important clues to the prediction of the immune response to specific vaccinations, since most vaccines have a CD4-dependent antibody response. The lower the peripheral CD4$^+$ value, the lower the antibody response and the shorter the persistence of antibody titers. These findings have been demonstrated for influenza vaccine, poliomyelitis IPV vaccine, injectable typhoid Vi vaccine, hepatitis A vaccine, and hepatitis B vaccine,[27] but may be true for other vaccines as well. Other studies suggest that there is no correlation between baseline viral load (VL) or CD4 count and response of HIV-infected children to conjugated pneumococcal vaccine.[28] On the contrary, a strong association of baseline VL (but not CD4%) with high-titer antibody response to hepatitis A vaccine has been shown in HIV-infected children.[29]

Vaccination is usually not recommended when the CD4$^+$ peripheral cell count is <200 cells/μL. People with severe immunosuppression should not receive live attenuated viral or bacterial vaccines because they may develop a severe systemic illness due to organism replication. Moreover, their response to inactivated vaccines will be suboptimal. Thus vaccines received by HIV-infected people with CD4 < 200 cells/μL should not be counted; the person should be revaccinated at least 3 months after immune reconstitution with antiretroviral therapy.[30] However, it is interesting to note that children undergoing antiretroviral therapy have been reported to develop a significantly higher anti-measles antibody response than untreated children, regardless of the baseline CD4$^+$ peripheral cell count.

In Thailand, HIV-infected children with satisfactory CD4$^+$ count recovery under HAART showed an effective response after revaccination with childhood vaccines. For this reason, the authors suggest that in endemic areas, HIV-infected children with immune recovery after receiving HAART should be revaccinated.[31]

Most HIV patients under HAART therapy experience a dramatic increase in their absolute peripheral CD4$^+$ cell counts. Nevertheless, since regenerated lymphocytes may recover function only after several months, especially in those patients who experienced a low CD4$^+$ nadir it is safer to consider immunization after at least 3–6 months of the CD4 count > 200 cells/μL in those patients whose CD4$^+$ cell counts had previously fallen below that limit.

4.   Risk of HIV Rebound as a Consequence of Vaccination

The observation that most vaccinations induce a discrete increase in plasma HIV viral load as a result of the activation of the immune system has raised concerns about the appropriateness of vaccination practices among HIV-infected persons. The bulk of the most recent published evidence now shows that the plasma HIV-RNA increase following vaccination is transient, usually returning to pre-vaccination baseline values after 4–6 weeks, and even sooner if the patient is under effective antiretroviral treatment, without any substantial risk of HIV disease progression. On the other hand, it has been suggested that there may be a risk of HIV disease progression following the natural occurrence of many vaccine-preventable diseases.

A summary of current knowledge on vaccination in HIV-infected persons is given in Table 28.2. General principles concerning the immunization of HIV-infected travelers are:

- HIV-infected persons should be vaccinated as early as possible in the course of HIV infection to ensure an adequate immune response to all vaccines
- Inactivated vaccines should be used instead of live vaccines whenever possible
- The CD4$^+$ cell count is a useful marker to predict the response to vaccinations. Vaccinations are less likely to be effective in those with CD4 counts <200 cells/μL
- In patients receiving HAART, at least 3–6 months must elapse before regenerated CD4$^+$ cells may be considered fully functional and predict antibody response. If possible, it is preferable to wait for an effective immune response to develop before vaccination or re-vaccination.

Chemoprophylaxis

Malaria Chemoprophylaxis and Standby Treatment

It is now accepted that HIV infection is a predisposing factor for higher parasitemia and more severe infection, particularly in the HIV-infected pregnant woman, whose immunity to malaria has been reported to be impaired.[32]

Many studies have examined the influence of HIV infection on antimalarial treatment efficacy. Chloroquine treatment for uncomplicated malaria appeared to be less effective in HIV-infected Ugandan children than in HIV-negative controls. Another study evaluated the efficacy of sulfadoxine-pyrimethamine treatment for uncomplicated malaria among adults in Kenya, and showed a higher risk of treatment failure in HIV-1-positive patients than in HIV-1 negative patients.[33]

The correlation between HIV infection and risk of severe malaria is present both in populations living in malaria-endemic areas[34] and in HIV-infected travelers.[35]

On the other hand, acute *Plasmodium falciparum* infection has been demonstrated to induce higher HIV pro-viral loads and to

Table 28.2 Vaccinations in HIV-Infected Travelers

Vaccine	Severity of Vaccine-Preventable Diseases in HIV+ Subjects	Safety and Immunogenicity of Vaccine	Recommendation
Cholera	No data available	Potential risk of vaccine-induced disease for live oral vaccine No data on immune response in HIV+ subjects (effective response to killed whole cell vaccine; after vaccination it may result in a temporary increase in HIV viral load)	Live oral vaccine is contraindicated Use killed (oral or parenteral) vaccine, if substantial risk exists
Diphtheria	No data available	Safe No data on immune response in HIV+ subjects Serologic response found diminished in children with HIV infection but no evidence of increased risk of vaccine adverse effects	Use whenever indicated
Influenza	Possible higher incidence of complication	Safe, but temporary HIV-RNA increase CD4$^+$ dependent immune response Do not vaccinate if CD4$^+$ count is below 100 cells/μL	Recommended in HIV+ subjects
H. influenzae type B	Higher incidence and severity in HIV-infected subjects	Safe, no data on possible HIV-RNA increase Low response if CD4$^+$ count below 100/μL	Early vaccination is recommended in HIV+ subjects
Hepatitis A	Clinical course of hepatitis A is accelerated in patients with chronic hepatitis ART intake may be affected and contagiousness may be prolonged	Safe, but temporary HIV-RNA increase Reduced response if low CD4$^+$ count	Vaccination is recommended for travelers to HAV endemic areas, people at risk (homosexual/bisexual), people with HCV and/or HBV co-infection
Hepatitis B	Progression of hepatitis B is accelerated in HIV+ subjects ART hepatotoxicity may be increased	Safe, but temporary HIV-RNA increase High rate of non-responders. Double-strength dose or additional dose may be required	Early vaccination is recommended in HIV+ subjects. Check antibody titer
Japanese encephalitis	No data available	Safe (Vero-cell vaccine) No data on immune response in HIV+ subjects	Use if substantial risk exists
Measles	Clinical course of measles may be more severe in HIV+ subjects	Vaccination in patients with low CD4$^+$ count may be dangerous Reduced response if low CD4$^+$ count	Avoid vaccination unless high risk of exposure. Avoid vaccination if CD4$^+$ count is below 200/μL
N. meningitidis	Clinical course of meningitis is more severe in HIV+ subjects	Safe Immune response to C serotype may be reduced in HIV+ patients	Use when indicated, particularly in splenectomized subjects traveling to meningitis belt, Umrah, Hadj
Poliomyelitis	No data available	Potential risk of vaccine-induced disease for live oral vaccine (OPV) Reduced response if low CD4$^+$ count	Live oral vaccine (OPV) is contraindicated (also in close contacts). Use killed parenteral (eIPV) vaccine, if substantial risk exists
Str. pneumoniae	Higher incidence and severity in HIV-infected subjects	Safe, but temporary HIV-RNA increase Possible reduced protection if CD4$^+$ count below 200/μL	Usually recommended in HIV+ subjects, but recent reports question its effectiveness (conjugate pneumococcal vaccine led to a better immunological response in immunocompromised host than polysaccharide one)

Table 28.2 Vaccinations in HIV-Infected Travelers—cont'd

Vaccine	Severity of Vaccine-Preventable Diseases in HIV+ Subjects	Safety and Immunogenicity of Vaccine	Recommendation
Rabies	No data available	Safe (inactivated vaccine) The immune response in HIV+ subjects is reduced if CD4< 200cell/μl.	Use if substantial risk exists
Tetanus	No data available	Safe, but temporary HIV-RNA increase Reduced response if low CD4+ count	Use whenever indicated
Tick-borne encephalitis	No data available	Safe (inactivated vaccine) No data on immune response in HIV+ subjects	Use if substantial risk exists
Tuberculosis	Incidence of disease is significantly higher in HIV+ subjects	Live attenuated vaccine (BCG): risk of vaccine-induced diseases	The use of BCG is contraindicated in HIV+ subjects
Typhoid fever	Incidence and severity of salmonellosis are higher in HIV+ subjects	Potential risk of vaccine-induced disease for live oral vaccine No data on immune response in HIV+ subjects	Live oral vaccine is contraindicated. Use Vi parenteral vaccine if exposure is likely
Yellow fever	No data available	Potential risk of vaccine-induced disease in patients with CD4+ below 200/μL No data on immune response in HIV+ subjects (The serological response is significantly decreased in HIV-infected children. Limited experience suggests that it can be given safely and produce protective levels of antibodies in HIV-infected individuals with CD4> 200 cell/μl)	Vaccination may be considered only for HIV+ travelers with CD4 count above 200/μL who are exposed to substantial risk

Modified from Cavassini ML, D'Acremont V, Furrer H, et al. Pharmacotherapy, vaccines and malaria advice for HIV-infected travelers. Expert Opin Pharmacother 2005;6:1–23.

stimulate plasma HIV replication, thus possibly accelerating HIV progression in untreated HIV patients.

As for the non-immune HIV population traveling from industrialized countries to the tropics, the risk of severe malaria is significantly higher in HIV-infected patients with a CD4 cell count <350 cells/μL.[36] The absence of differences in the proportion of severe malaria cases between the HIV-negative population and the HIV-positive population with >350 cells/μL indicates that severe immunosuppression is the major risk factor. The use of personal protection measures such as mosquito repellents, impregnated bed-nets, and protective clothing is to be strongly promoted as first-line protection. As a general rule, chemoprophylaxis in the HIV-infected traveler should follow the same guidelines as for HIV-negative individuals.

Interestingly, in vitro data have demonstrated an antiviral effect of chloroquine[37] and mefloquine.[38] Conversely, some protease inhibitors used to treat HIV infection have been reported in vitro to exert a significant inhibitory effect on *Plasmodium falciparum*: this is demonstrated both for indinavir and nelfinavir associated with artemisinin,[39] and for indinavir in combination with chloroquine.[40]

The consideration that many antimalarial drugs and antiretroviral drugs, particularly the protease inhibitors but also the non-nucleoside reverse transcriptase inhibitors, share a common hepatic metabolic pathway (cytochrome P450) has raised concerns about possible pharmacokinetic interactions. Several studies have evaluated the reciprocal influence of antimalarial and antiretroviral drugs, and these are summarized in Table 28.3.

Chemoprophylaxis and Treatment of Travelers' Diarrhea

In a recent study, 59% of 104 HIV-infected travelers returning from the tropics complained of fever associated with any digestive symptom, and bacterial enteritis was reported in 5%.[5] Some bacterial infections, such as those due to non-typhoidal *Salmonellae* and *Campylobacter* spp, have been reported to be more severe in HIV-positive travelers, with an increased proportion of patients with bacteremia.[41]

For these patients, chemoprophylaxis rather than self-treatment may be considered, depending on the destination and duration of travel, the local antimicrobial resistance spectrum and the severity of immunosuppression. Although most experts do not recommend antibiotic prophylaxis against traveler's diarrhea even in the setting of HIV infection, this approach should be considered in severely immunocompromised individuals.[42]

HIV-infected patients with CD4+ cell counts <200 cells/μL are often administered co-trimoxazole as prophylaxis for *P. jiroveci* pneumonia; this regimen is unlikely to be useful in preventing travelers' diarrhea, as in many areas of the developing world resistant enteropathogens are present. Also, HIV-infected patients are at higher risk of experiencing drug-related hypersensitivity reactions to co-trimoxazole. Fluoroquinolones have proved effective and safe for prevention and treatment of gastrointestinal illness in the HIV-infected population. However, it is important to remember that using this agent for chemoprophylaxis of travelers' diarrhea could promote the selection of resistance in organisms and increase the risk of *Clostridium difficile* infection.

Table 28.3 Effects of HAART on Antimalarial Drugs used for Chemoprophylaxis

Antiretroviral Drugs	Antimalarial Drugs					
	Atovaquone	Chloroquine	Doxycycline	Mefloquine	Primaquine	Proguanil
Nucleoside Reverse Transcriptase Inhibitors (NRTI)						
Abacavir (ABV)	✓	n/a	○	n/a	n/a	n/a
Didanosine (ddI)	✓	n/a	○	n/a	n/a	n/a
Emtricitabine (FTC)	✓	n/a	○	n/a	n/a	n/a
Lamivudine (3TC)	✓	n/a	○	n/a	n/a	n/a
Stavudine (d4T)	✓	n/a	○	n/a	n/a	n/a
Zidovudine (AZT)	✓	n/a	○	n/a	n/a	n/a
Nucleotide Reverse Transcriptase Inhibitors (NRTI)						
Tenofovir (TDF)	✓	n/a	○	n/a	n/a	n/a
Non-Nucleoside Reverse Transcriptase Inhibitors (NNRTI)						
Delavirdine (DLV)	✓	✓	○	✓	○	✓
Efavirenz (EFV)	▲	✓	○	✓	○	▲
Etravirine (TMC 125)	✓	✓	○	✓	○	✓
Nevirapine (NVP)	✓	✓	○	✓	○	✓
Protease Inhibitors (PI)						
Atazanavir (ATV)	▲	✓	○	▲	○	✓
Darunavir (DRV)	▲	✓	○	▲	○	✓
Fosamprenavir (FPV)	✓	✓	○	▲	○	✓
Indinavir (IDV)	▲	✓	○	▲	○	✓
Lopinavir (LPV)	▲	✓	○	▲	○	▲
Nelfinavir (NFV)	✓	✓	○	▲	○	✓
Ritonavir (RTV)	▲	▲	○	▲	○	▲
Saquinavir (SQV)	✓	✓	○	▲	○	✓
Tipranavir (TPV)	▲	✓	○	▲	○	✓
Fusion Inhibitors (FI)						
Enfuvirtide (T20)	n/a	n/a	○	n/a	n/a	n/a
Chemokine Co-Receptor Antagonists						
Maraviroc (MVC)	n/a	n/a	○	n/a	n/a	n/a
Integrase Inhibitors						
Raltegravir (RAL)	n/a	n/a	○	n/a	n/a	n/a

▲, potential interaction; ✓, no clinically significant interaction expected; ○, no clear data available to indicate whether an interaction will occur; n/a, no data available. Adapted from: www.hiv-druginteractions.org updated to June, 15th). For more and updated details about interactions visit the website.

Azithromycin can safely replace fluoroquinolones as early treatment of travelers' diarrhea, especially in those areas of South Asia and Southeast Asia where fluoroquinolone-resistant *Campylobacter* and *Salmonella* strains are highly prevalent. Owing to the higher risk of invasive *Salmonellosis*, 7–14 days of treatment of the diarrheal episode is recommended in the HIV-infected traveler.[27]

Drug interactions

Antiretroviral Drugs

- Nucleoside reverse transcriptase inhibitors (NRTI): abacavir (ABV), didanosine (ddI), emtricitabine (FTC), lamivudine (3TC), stavudine (d4T), zidovudine (AZT)
- Nucleotide reverse transcriptase inhibitors (NtRTI): tenofovir (TDF)
- Non-nucleoside reverse transcriptase inhibitors (NNRTI): delavirdine (DLV), efavirenz (EFV), nevirapine (NVP), etravirina (TMC 125)
- Protease inhibitors (PI): atazanavir (ATV), darunavir (DRV), fosamprenavir (FPV), indinavir (IDV), lopinavir (LPV), nelfinavir (NFV), ritonavir (RTV), saquinavir (SQV), tipranavir (TPV)
- Fusion inhibitors (FI): enfuvirtide (T20)
- Chemokine co-receptor antagonists: maraviroc (MVC)
- Integrase inhibitors: raltegravir (RAL).

As noted above, many of these drugs, especially those belonging to the protease inhibitor class, have a complex metabolic pathway through the hepatic cytochrome P450. The possible interactions between these drugs and other commonly prescribed drugs are numerous and potentially clinically important, resulting in suboptimal or conversely toxic plasma concentrations of the antiretroviral or the companion drug.

Table 28.1 provides a short summary of the potential pharmacokinetic interactions between various commonly used drugs and antiretroviral drugs belonging to the NNRTI and PI classes. Drugs belonging to the NRTI class have less potential for pharmacokinetic interactions. It should be stressed that reliable information is not currently available on the potential interactions of antiretrovirals with most of other pharmacoactive substances, including herbal remedies.

Therefore, the HIV-infected traveler under antiretroviral treatment should avoid taking other non-prescription medications that could lead to potentially serious toxic drug interactions. For more detailed information about interactions visit the website www.hiv-drug-interaction.org.

Healthcare Abroad

Access to specialized healthcare abroad may sometimes be difficult to achieve for HIV-infected travelers. In any case, the HIV-infected traveler should always try to identify in advance a reference center for treatment of HIV/AIDS in the destination country, should the need arise. The Directory of the International Society of Travel Medicine may help the travel medicine professional to identify such expertise abroad before departure. Travelers can visit the website of the National AIDS Manual (NAM), where country-specific information of organizations and services related to the disease can be found (www.aids map. com). HIV-infected travelers should be strongly advised to purchase in advance a health insurance policy covering repatriation costs and flight cancellation insurance, ensuring that HIV infection is covered.

Crossing International Borders

There is no evidence that border restrictions for HIV-infected individuals limit the spread of HIV infection in any given country. WHO has always advised against such restrictions, which are considered to be useless from the perspective of disease transmission. However, in spite of this clear-cut position of the scientific international community, many countries have put in place a variety of entry requirements in an attempt to prevent further spread of the AIDS epidemic locally. Country-specific border requirements change frequently and should be checked by HIV-infected travelers before departure. Possible sources of information include www.hivtravel.org or www.aidsmap.com/countries-and-their-restrictions/page/1504371/

It has long been debated whether migration from HIV-endemic areas in developing countries to western countries is regarded as a risk to the host country. On the other hand, many factors contribute to increase the risk of acquisition of HIV infection in migrants in the host country, mainly via the sexual route: social isolation and single status, poverty and psychological distress may be considered independent risk factors for any sexually transmitted infection, including HIV.[43] A significant epidemiological impact of migration on HIV spread outside migrant communities has never been definitely demonstrated in western countries. From an epidemiological standpoint, the impact of immigration on the HIV epidemic in the host country and on the possible circulation of genetically different strains is still debated. In The Netherlands, a substantial proportion of heterosexually acquired HIV infections has been reported to come from a foreign country.[6] The introduction of non-B subtype HIV strains following migration (migrants, military personnel, tourists, expatriates, etc.) has been demonstrated,[44] with possible implications for therapeutic strategies and the design of preventive vaccines. In Italy, the proportion of notified AIDS cases in migrants has been increasing during recent decades, from 11.0% in 1992 to 32.8% in 2007.[44]

Conclusions

The number of HIV-infected travelers from western countries to the tropics will probably increase in the future as a result of the clinical benefits of HAART, which have dramatically improved the survival rates and quality of life of HIV-infected persons.

Table 28.4 Checklist for HIV-Infected Travelers

Assess CD4 count, viral load and antiretroviral therapy

Consider vaccine efficacy and contraindications, and potential drug interactions

Assess travel risks (especially those with CD4 counts <200 cells/μL) and counsel on infectious disease and risk reduction (consider prophylaxis for travelers' diarrhea for trips <3 weeks)

Encourage traveler to carry current medical history including medications and, if possible, name of an HIV-knowledgeable physician at destination

Advise traveler to determine anonymously any travel restrictions for HIV-infected persons at an intended destination

Adapted from Mileno MD, Bia FJ. The compromised traveler. Infect Dis Clin North Am 1998;12:369–410, with permission.

Most data suggest that HIV patients under HAART with a satisfactory immune status may travel safely to any destination, provided that adequate prophylactic measures are taken (Table 28.4). However, a significant proportion of HIV-infected patients in western countries are unaware of their status, and travel may represent a significant risk.

A particular area of research that needs further investigation concerns the many pharmacokinetic interactions between antiretroviral drugs and antimalarial drugs, since malarial chemoprophylaxis is required for most tropical destinations.

Despite strong advice to the contrary by WHO, many countries still deny entry to HIV-infected travelers requesting long-stay visas.

The impact of migration on the HIV epidemic in the host country has for the most part been reported to be negligible, but the introduction of HIV non-B subtypes may be of concern in some western countries. The provision of adequate access to healthcare is the most potent tool to prevent further spread of HIV infection and other sexually transmitted infections among migrants.

References

1. Adler A, Mounier-Jack S, Coker RJ. Late diagnosis of HIV in Europe: definitional and public health challenges. AIDS Care 2009;21(3):284–93.
2. Franco–Paredes C, Hidron A, Tellez I, et al. HIV infection and travel: pretravel recommendations and health–related risks. Top HIV Med 2009;17(1):2–11.
3. Kemper CA, Linett A, Kane C, et al. Travel with HIV: the compliance and health of HIV-infected adults who travel. Int J STD AIDS 1997;8:44–9.
4. Salit IE, Sano M, Boggild AK, et al. Travel patterns and risk behavior of HIV-positive people traveling internationally. JAMC 2005;172(7):884–8.
5. Bottieau E, Florence E, Clerinx J, et al. Fever after a stay in the tropics: clinical spectrum and outcome in HIV-infected travelers and migrants. J Acquir Immune Defic Syndr 2008;48(5):547–52.
6. Op de Coul EL, Coutinho RA, van der Schoot A, et al. The impact of immigration on env HIV-1 subtype distribution among heterosexuals in the Netherlands: influx of subtype B and non-B strains. AIDS 2001;15(17): 2277–86.
7. Xiridou M, van Venn M, Prins M, et al. How patterns of migration can influence the heterosexual transmission of HIV in The Netherlands. Sex Transm Infect 2011;87(4):289–91.
8. Sartori AM, Ibrahim KY, Nunes Westphalen EV, et al. Manifestations of Chagas disease (American trypanosomiasis) in patients with HIV/AIDS. Ann Trop Med Parasitol 2007;101(1):31–50.
9. Delobel P, Signate A, El Guedj M, et al. Unusual form of neurocysticercosis associated with HIV infection. Eur J Neurol 2004;11:55–8.
10. Karp CL, Auwaerter PG. Coinfection with HIV and tropical infectious diseases. II. Helminthic, fungal, bacterial, and viral pathogens. Clin Infect Dis 2007;45:1214–20.
11. Ward BJ, Plourde P. Travel and sexually transmitted infections. J Travel Med 2006;13(5):300–17.

12. Couzigou C, Voyer C, Shaghaghi CL, et al. Vaccination of HIV-infected traveler. Med Mal Infect 2009;39(1):21–8.

13. Gotuzzo E, Frisancho O, Sanchez J, et al. Association between the acquired immunodeficiency syndrome and infection with *Salmonella typhi* or *Salmonella paratyphi* in an endemic typhoid area. Arch Intern Med 1991;151:381–2.

14. Freedman DO. Advising travelers with specific needs: the immune-compromised traveler. In: Arguin P, Kozarsky PE, Reed C, editors. CDC Health Information for International Travel. Elsevier; 2008. pp. 388–345.

15. Dhanoa A, Fatt QK. Non-typhoidal Salmonella bacteraemia: epidemiology, clinical characteristics and its association with severe immunosuppression. Ann Clin Microbiol Antimicrob 2009;18(8):15.

16. Moore D, Nelson M, Henderson D. Pneumococcal vaccination and HIV infection. Int J STD AIDS 1998;9(1):1–7.

17. Tortajada C, de Olalla PG, Pinto RM, et al. Outbreak of hepatitis among men who have sex with men in Barcelona, Spain, September 2008-March 2009. Eurosurveillance 2009;14:1–3.

18. Goujon C, Tohr M, Feuillie V, et al. Good tolerance and efficacy of yellow fever vaccine among carriers of human immunodeficiency virus. J Travel Med 1995;2:145.

19. WHO. Yellow fever vaccine and HIV infection. Weekly Epidemiological Record Geneva (Switzerland), 28 January 2011;86:37–44

20. French N, Nakiyingi J, Carpenter LM, et al. 23-valent pneumococcal polysaccharide vaccine in HIV-1-infected Ugandan adults: double-blind, randomized and placebo-controlled trial. Lancet 2000;355: 2106–11.

21. French N, Gordon SB, Mwalukomo T, et al. A trial of a 7–valent pneumococcal conjugate vaccine in HIV–infected adults. N Engl J Med 2010;362(9):812–22.

22. Klugman KP, Madhi SA, Huebner RE, et al. A trial of a 9-valent pneumococcal conjugate vaccine in children with and those without HIV infection. N Engl J Med 2003;349:1341–8.

23. Madhi SA, Adrian P, Kuwanda L, et al. Long-term immunogenicity and efficacy of a 9-valent conjugate pneumococcal vaccine in human immune-deficient virus infected and non-infected children in the absence of a booster dose of vaccine. Vaccine 2007;25(13):2451–7.

24. Miiro G, Kayhty H, Watera C, et al. Conjugate pneumococcal vaccine in HIV-infected Ugandans and the effect of past receipt of polysaccharide vaccine. J Infect Dis 2005;192:1801–5.

25. Bortolussi R, Salvadori M. A new meningococcal conjugate vaccine: What should physicians know and do? Paediatr Child Health 2009;14(8): 515–20.

26. Siberry GK, Williams PL, Lujan–Zilbermann J, et al. Phase I/II, open–label trial of safety and immunogenicity of meningococcal (groups A, C, Y, and W–135) polysaccharide diphtheria toxoid conjugate vaccine in human immunodeficiency virus–infected adolescents. Pediatr Infect Dis J 2010;29(5):391–6.

27. Cavassini ML, D'Acremont V, Furrer H, et al. Pharmacotherapy, vaccines and malaria advice for HIV–infected travellers. Expert Opin Pharmacother 2005;6:1–23.

28. Tarragó D, Casal J, Ruiz-Contreras J, et al. Spanish Network Pneumococcus Study Group. Assessment of antibody response elicited by a 7-valent pneumococcal conjugate vaccine in pediatric human immunodeficiency virus infection. Clin Diagn Lab Immunol 2005;12:165–70.

29. Weinberg A, Gona P, Nachman SA, et al. Pediatric AIDS Clinical Trials Group 1008 Team. Antibody responses to hepatitis A virus vaccine in HIV-infected children with evidence of immunologic reconstitution while receiving highly active antiretroviral therapy. J Infect Dis 2006;193: 302–11.

30. CDC Yellow Book. Available online: wwwnc.cdc.gov./travel/ yellowbook/2012.

31. Puthanakit T, Aurpibul L, Yoksan S, et al. A 3-year follow-up of antibody response in HIV-infected children with immune recovery vaccinated with inactivated Japanese encephalitis vaccine. Vaccine 2010;28(36):5900–2.

32. Mount AM, Mwapasa V, Elliott SR, et al. Impairment of humoral immunity to *Plasmodium falciparum* malaria in pregnancy by HIV infection. Lancet 2004;363:1860–7.

33. Shah SN, Smith EE, Obonyo CO, et al. HIV immune-suppression and anti-malarial efficacy: sulfadoxine-pyrimethamine for treatment of uncomplicated malaria in HIV-infected adults in Siaya, Kenya. J Infect Dis 2006;194:1519–28.

34. Chalwe V, Van Geertruyden JP, Mukwamataba D, et al. Increased risk for severe malaria in HIV-1–infected adults, Zambia. Emerg Infect Dis 2009;15(5):749–55.

35. Matteelli A, Casalini C, Bussi G, et al. Imported malaria in an HIV-positive traveller. A case-report with a fatal outcome. J Trav Med 2005;12:222–4.

36. Mouala C, Guiguet M, Houzé S, et al. Impact of HIV infection on severity of imported malaria is restricted to patients with CD4 cell counts < 350 cell/μL. AIDS 2009;23:1997–2004.

37. Savarino A, Gennero L, Chu Hen H, et al. Anti-HIV effects of chloroquine: mechanisms of inhibition and spectrum of activity. AIDS 2001;15: 2221–9.

38. Owen A, Janneh O, Hartkoorn RC, et al. In vitro synergy and enhanced murine brain penetration of saquinavir coadministered with mefloquine. J Pharmacol Exp Ther 2005;314:1039–41.

39. Mishra LC, Bhattacharya A, Sharma M, et al. Short report: HIV protease inhibitors, Indinavir or Nelfinavir, augment antimalarial action of Artemisinin in vitro. Am J Trop Med Hyg 2010;82(1):148–50.

40. Li X, He Z, Chen L, et al. Synergy of the antiretroviral protease inhibitors indinavir and chloroquine against malaria parasites in vitro and in vivo. Parasitol Res 2011 May 3. [Epub ahead of print].

41. Attia A, Huet C, Anglaret X, et al. HIV-1-related morbidity in adults, Abidjan, Cote d'Ivoire: a nidus for bacterial diseases. J Acquir Immune Defic Syndr 2001;28(5):478–86.

42. Bhadelia N, Klotman M, Caplivski D. The HIV-positive traveler. Am J Med 2007;120:574–80.

43. Pezzoli MC, Hamad IE, Scarcella C, et al. HIV infection among illegal migrants, Italy, 2004–2007. Emerg Infect Dis 2009;15(11):1802–04.

44. Thomson MM, Nàjera R. Travel and the introduction of human immune-deficiency virus type 1 non-b subtype genetic forms into western countries. Clin Infect Dis 2001;32:1732–7.

29

The Corporate and Executive Traveler

James Aw and Roger A. Band

Key points

- Corporate traveler risks include those of travel itself as well as corporate-related risks
- The corporate travel medicine consult should include a detailed occupational history, including future anticipated travel to determine occupational-related risks
- 'Fitness to travel' may be part of the corporate travel medicine consult
- Corporate travelers cannot afford to be ill; vaccine schedules may need to be accelerated and updated regularly between trips; cumulative risk must be considered
- A medical threat assessment should be carried out
- A comprehensive travel kit can help mitigate the impact of accidents or illness

Introduction

According to the United Nations World Tourism Organization, 15% of international travel was for business purposes in 2010 – with increasing travel trends in Asia, South America, and Africa. The most significant increase among top international destinations was to China, with an overall increase by 13% to the Asia and Pacific regions. Studies suggest that approximately one-quarter of corporate international travelers make travel plans within 2 weeks of departure, and 19–70% do not seek travel medical advice.[1] The average number of nights in a hotel room for US international business travelers was 8.4 nights.

Several airport survey studies have demonstrated that travelers' knowledge of destination-specific infectious disease risks is poor. European and US travelers (74–83%) seem to recognize the importance of vaccination, but only 15–26% intend to follow preventive food precautions. Studies on business travelers have found that only 16% comply fully with antimalarial chemoprophylaxis, and that they are less likely than tourists to carry antimalarial medication.

Corporate travelers tend to be (a) executives on short trips (<7 days) to multiple urban destinations in five-star hotels; (b) skilled workers sent on specific projects (< 1 month); or (c) expatriate foreign postings (several months to years). A Canadian study classified travel medical risk as (i) high risk: > 4 weeks with ≥ 50% of nights in low-budget hotels; (ii) low risk: < 2 weeks with all nights in a first-class hotel; (iii) intermediate risk: all other types of travel.[2] In rural areas, the level of accommodations may vary from guest houses at established sites to very limited for 'green field' projects. For business travelers, the risk largely depends on the types of activities that will be done at the site during the visit, and the local working environment (infectious disease, public health, occupational health and safety concerns, security). The corporate physician should have a clear understanding of the job requirements and site details of the 'mission'. Access to medical care overseas is an important aspect of corporate travel. Stress associated with work projects, loneliness, and the anonymity of business travel can also lead to unhealthy risky behaviors (i.e., alcohol, decreased exercise, poor eating habits, casual sex, sensation-seeking behavior).

A new field of occupational travel medicine is emerging that will focus on the health characteristics of the business traveler, fitness to travel, and safety risks at the international job sites. Extensive travel has been found to be associated with poorer self-rated health, higher body mass index (BMI) and worse clinical examination results (blood pressure, HDL cholesterol, LDL cholesterol, glucose).[3] In an executive health screened population, poorer health was found in the non-travelers and those with extensive travel (> 14 nights). Health risk appraisal (HRA) surveys by a large multinational corporation found international business travel to be associated with lower risk of self-reported hypertension, higher alcohol consumption, lower confidence in keeping up with the pace of work, and lower perceived flexibility in fulfilling commitments.[4] Frequent flying and longer trips were associated with higher stress-related effects on spouses and children (particularly young children).

The business traveler must quickly adapt into a foreign work environment and successfully complete a work assignment on a tight schedule. Neither employer nor employee can afford to have a mission compromised by travel-related illness. The challenge of corporate travel medicine is providing thorough preventive advice at short notice, and understanding occupational related risks, particularly for non-tourist areas.

Employer Perspective

Fit and Safe for Duty

It is the employer's responsibility to provide a safe workplace for its employees. In developed countries occupational health and safety standards are highly regulated, but less so in developing countries and emerging markets. Business travelers on high-risk trips (longer duration, manual labor, remote areas, industrial hazards) should be in contact with local occupational health and safety officers to ensure

DOI: 10.1016/B978-1-4557-1076-8.00029-6

compliance with local training (environmental risks – chemicals, personal protective equipment, engineering controls in the workplace) and periodic medical monitoring (i.e., mining operations – respiratory, cardiovascular, auditory, etc.). Human rights guidelines also prohibit employers from discrimination based on a medical condition. Corporations may subject employees to foreign posting medical examinations to ensure fitness to travel, and that there are no medical conditions that will prevent the employee performing the essential duties of the job. Employee medical information should always remain confidential from the employer, but an opinion may be rendered by the travel medicine practitioner regarding 'fitness' to travel for the purposes of the assignment. Employees may be reluctant to seek pre-travel advice and health assessments if they are concerned that patient confidentiality on pre-existing medical conditions will not be protected.

Pre- and Post-Travel Health Services

It is in the company's best interests (success of mission, cost of investment) to keep its employees and executives healthy. Often, the most frequent travelers are the key talent and senior leaders in the organization. Larger corporations may retain a corporate medical director and health department that provide in-house pre- and post-travel medical services, executive health and occupational health assessments. Post-travel health assessments for infectious disease, chronic medical conditions (particularly if the destination has limited medical facilities) and psychological screening (stress, culture adaptation for long-term expatriates or frequent travelers) depend on the corporation's willingness to support a program staffed with expertise in the area (i.e., tropical disease experts, psychologists, employee assistance programs). Otherwise, human resource departments (health and safety officers) should have a policy to alert their traveling employees of health risks and direct them to an appropriate healthcare provider (i.e., travel clinic, occupational health consultant). Frequent business travelers may be subject to repetitive job strain, poor sleep patterns, increased alcohol use and family disruptions, which can lead to increased risk of mental health conditions and absenteeism or 'presenteeism' (working while ill with decreased productivity).

Financial Costs of Travel Illness

The financial implications of sick employees related to travel assignments include corporate (i.e., lost productivity, absenteeism and workers compensation) and personal costs (i.e., medical expenses, lost wages). Health insurance claims for World Bank business travelers found an increased number of health claims compared with non-traveling employees for all health conditions considered, including chronic diseases (i.e., asthma, back disorders) – 80% higher for men and 18% higher for women.[5] There are higher claims for infectious diseases and psychological issues. Long-term expatriate travelers are generally considered at higher risk than short-term travelers. It has been estimated that expatriate illness overseas can cost over $500 000, whereas pre-trip vaccination and healthcare screening can cost approximately $500.[6] Expatriates on extended postings tend to have more hospital admissions, infectious diseases, injury, violence, and psychological problems.[7]

Healthy Worker Effect

A study of a US multinational corporation found that employees who engage in low-frequency, short-duration international business travel tended to be healthier than employees who did not travel for business. Comparing 2,962 international travelers and 9,980 non-travelers, international business travel was significantly associated with a lower body mass index, lower blood pressure, excess alcohol consumption, sleep deprivation and diminished confidence to keep up with the pace of work.[4] A Canadian study of middle-aged male executive short-term travelers (<14 days) seen at the Medcan Clinic were found to be a lower risk for cardiovascular disease than patients who did not visit the travel clinic. Selection bias may be a factor when looking at the health characteristics of business travelers. Unhealthy people may not choose to travel; similarly, business managers may not select unhealthy people for assignments requiring travel. The healthy worker effect suggests that employed individuals are healthier than non-working or non-traveling peer groups.

Role of the Corporate Travel Medicine Practitioner

The corporate medical director of a company would be expected to fully understand the job descriptions, nature of assignments and specific regional information for the site visits. This would include knowledge of local infectious disease patterns, security risks and local medical facilities. However, most companies do not have a corporate medical director, so these services are contracted out to local travel clinics. In addition to the usual pre-travel infectious disease counseling and immunization, the consult should include a detailed occupational history (type of job tasks, number of trips over the year, geographical regions of business, established vs. green field sites, urban vs. rural) and review of chronic medical conditions. Pre-trip questionnaires and travel nurse checklists may be helpful. A corporate travel risk assessment should include questioning about all trips anticipated over the coming year, so that vaccination and chemoprophylaxis advice will provide appropriate coverage for anticipated trips. While executive travel may be more confined to office settings and urban settings, other missions may incur increased environmental risks. Pre- and post-travel medical evaluations should have clear clinical protocols, and expectations should be reviewed with the company in advance. Employees should be informed about the confidential nature of the process. Travel practitioners should be familiar with accelerated vaccine schedules (i.e., hepatitis vaccines) and up to date with chemoprophylaxis strategies for both the last-minute traveler (low to intermediate risk) and the long-term expatriate (high risk). The details of immunization and chemoprophylaxis are covered in other chapters. Corporate travel medicine practitioners should also be comfortable with communicating infectious disease risks from an epidemiological perspective (2012 CDC Yellow Book – Travel Epidemiology http://wwwnc.cdc.gov/travel/yellowbook/2012/chapter-1-introduction/travel-epidemiology.htm) and outbreak information (ProMed HealthMap – http://healthmap.org/promed/).

Recommendations to the employer could include mandatory pre-travel consults for high-risk projects, health education bulletins and workshops for staying healthy while traveling (i.e., fitness, nutrition advice). Financial incentives could be used to encourage employees to stay healthy while traveling (i.e., booking at hotels with fitness facilities). Pre- and post-travel medical examinations could be provided. On-site medical services allow for standardization of medical services, improved data tracking, facilitated employee access and potentially improved compliance on follow-up immunization status. Setting up medical facilities overseas for long-term projects requires coordination among several teams (local health, corporate, international network). Human resources and occupational health departments should be prepared for dealing with medical issues overseas, through either local medical networks or medical evacuation companies. To avoid stress, employers may consider creative work scheduling to allow busy corporate travelers 'down time' and rejuvenation after trips. This could allow time to recover from the stressors of long-distance travel.

Employee/Executive Perspective

Medical Threat Assessment

Given the inherent risks of international travel, no-one should be more interested in their health than the travelers themselves. It is therefore imperative that the corporate traveler take a vested interest, ownership of and initiative in their own pre-trip medical planning and medical threat assessment (MTA). An MTA is an all-hazards tool that is used to assess and provides a standardized mechanism for identifying and risk-stratifying potential threats that one may be exposed to during travel, such as violent crime. Anticipating this threat and a multitude of possible scenarios is an easy way to improve personal awareness and safety. Other less common threats that should be considered and planned for include terrorist attacks, epidemics (SARS), environmental stressors (extreme heat or humidity, pollution, sun exposure, altitude, envenomations, and wildlife), the possibility of civil unrest, and more subtle threats such as the reliability of local water or a strategy for water purification.

A preliminary MTA is ideally developed well in advance of an employee's travel. This should include locations of critical facilities (such as hospitals) and a checklist to ensure preventive measures are completed during the planning phase of each trip. This tool is most helpful for companies or employees who make repeated trips to a particular region or destination. When traveling to locations that pose specific medical threats, such as high-altitude regions or areas with dangerous fauna or flora, identifying and obtaining contact information for local experts on the management of associated medical emergencies is advisable. It is useful to have a standardized MTA form that can serve as a checklist during the planning phase of each trip; a detailed example of an MTA can be found in Table 29.1.

VIP vs. Employee – Dignitary Medicine

As the corporate traveler embarks on a company-sponsored journey, either as an individual or as part of a larger contingency, it is profoundly easy to disregard the fact that they are equally at risk for travel-related illness as the average recreational traveler abroad. It is easy to forget that comforts such as higher-end hotels, personal drivers and upscale restaurants do not mitigate the risk of illness, although all of these components of travel can be falsely reassuring.

If you have the misfortune to become ill, it is important that someone (either in person or remotely) is able to make an objective assessment about the safety of having you continue the trip. Specific considerations include: is the medical care superior or equivalent at the next location you are going to?; is the next site further away from a regional medical center or advanced care?; is evacuation more difficult from the next location?; what is the likelihood of progression of disease and/or time course of disease?; and what is the potential impact of an ill person on other members of the traveling party (if not traveling alone)? Decision making must remain objective, even if that means making medically sound recommendations that may curtail or redirect the trip. Whomever you engage to make these complicated decisions must have the appropriate training, practice, and a healthy degree of risk tolerance.

The same overarching principles apply if the traveler is a VIP or dignitary, but the concepts of care differ, with a few very specific caveats. First, security becomes an even higher priority because of targeted violence, which is less of a problem for most employee travelers. That said, the average corporate traveler may be a target simply because of their representation of western wealth. Second, as mentioned above, it is critical that the healthcare provider remain objective: this can be more difficult when caring for a dignitary,

Table 29.1 The medical threat assessment	
Medical Threat Assessment	**Example (Not All-Inclusive)**
Behavioral	Plan for managing travel-related fatigue, alterations in sleep cycle or emotional stress
Emergency contact numbers	Local embassy Hospitals International SOS (http:// www.internationalsos.com/en/) Government liaison offices Trusted transportation sources Trusted local medical provider
Environmental risks	Heat or cold injuries Food-borne illness Sun exposure Altitude Pollution Envenomations and wildlife exposure
Evacuation	Transportation: local transportation assets, company vehicles, options for air travel Locations of critical facilities: Addresses and GPS coordinates of hospitals, intensive care units, and other higher levels of care Transport times Limitations from terrain (e.g., mountains)
Food and water safety	Safety of local water, strategies for water purification, alternative sources of trusted water and food
Infectious disease risk	Prophylaxis requirements (e.g., malaria) Vector-borne disease risk (e.g., dengue, chikungunya ,sand flies, ticks) Respiratory disease Blood-borne disease (e.g., HIV, HCV, HBV) Immunizations (e.g., yellow fever)
Medical Assets	Local hospital capabilities; access to medications, advanced care, safe blood products
Pre-existing medical conditions	Employee's baseline health and underlying medical conditions such as diabetes, hypertension, coronary disease
Trauma/ violence	Road traffic accidents Civil unrest Targeted violence (i.e., assassination) Mass casualty incidents, acts of terrorism, kidnapping

simply because of that person's stature or influence, or because decisions can affect the entire delegation as well as the mission objective and/or agenda. Finally, it must be appreciated that medicine is merely one component of the overall dignitary protection plan. Medical decisions often have consequences for the rest of the team, especially for the logistics, planning, operational, and security personnel. Dignitary Protection Medicine (DPM) physicians must first advocate for the patient but also respect the integrated nature of the environment in which they are working.

Fitness to Travel

The physical and emotional stress of travel, especially international travel, cannot be underestimated. It is imperative that the employee obtain preventative and preparatory health information, either independently or by enlisting the services of an executive medical travel professional. Prevention also includes ensuring that the traveler is able to function in every potential environment, and that he/she does not have pre-existing medical conditions that cannot be cared for under expected circumstances.[3] For example, patients with insulin-dependent diabetes mellitus will need a refrigerator for their insulin. If the medical needs of a certain employee cannot be met, that person should be strongly urged to reconsider their involvement. Special attention should be given to employees who are not accustomed to traveling and foreign-born employees returning to their native country for work-related business. These respective groups of employee travelers may not believe that they are personally at risk, or may not be aware of travel-related risks such as food-borne or vector-borne illnesses, and need additional counseling.

Copies of an employee's medical records should be readily available. Planning for individuals with little or no significant past medical history may only require a basic list, such as allergies, medications (including generic names), blood type, previous medical conditions and surgeries, prior injuries, private physician, and emergency contacts. However, when an employee has a more complex medical history, it is also important to consider having electronic and hard copies of ECGs, radiographs or other imaging studies, as well as reports of invasive diagnostic studies and surgical procedures. This may not always be easy to obtain, especially if confidentiality is a concern, or if a known medical condition can result in denial of entry to a country (e.g., HIV seropositivity). With the development of electronic medical records, health information can be stored securely on the website of the medical provider. This information can then easily be accessed remotely by the traveler. Alternatively, before departure, it may be downloaded onto the smartcard of a hand-held electronic device, into a cell phone's media card or a memory stick, and can even be translated into multiple languages.

Busy travelers not accustomed to taking a medication regularly may need to be reminded to take important chemoprophylaxis, such as antimalarial drugs. Hand-held electronic devices or watches should be programmed to alert the traveler when a medication needs to be taken, regardless of the actual time in the visiting country. Several companies are now in the business of sending regular pre-programmed reminders electronically to cell phones, pagers and hand-held electronic devices concerning medication regimens. Business travelers with chronic conditions should carry medication in sufficient quantity to cover losses and damage or an expected prolongation of the business trip, and should be encouraged to keep these supplies and medications readily accessible, preferably in a carry-on bag. Furthermore, for healthcare workers, a self-treatment kit with 1–4 weeks of post-exposure prophylaxis for HIV might be considered.

Finally, business travelers should be reminded that even in business class, deep-vein thrombosis (DVT) can occur, especially if they lack hydration, indulge in alcohol, and remain immobile. Hypnotics taken during the flight to induce sleep could further increase this risk, as they can act as muscle relaxants and will inevitably reduce movement and hydration. Support stockings may be helpful and usually increase comfort;[8] they can be purchased without a prescription in most pharmacies. To reduce some of the stress associated with frequent travel, it is helpful to learn how to travel light, especially with increased airport security. Carrying heavy luggage, long delays at check-in lines, long waits to retrieve baggage, and arguing about lost, broken or delayed luggage are unnecessary stressors. Small carry-on bags with wheels are ideal.

Dealing with Medical Issues Overseas – Crisis Management, Access to Care

The best approach to dealing with a crisis, especially when out of one's normal comfort zone, is having already established a contingency plan. As previously discussed, the MTA is the perfect tool for this. Access to care, especially in the developing world, where reliable medical care often does not exist, can be very challenging. This becomes even more important for the employee with an existing medical condition or for someone who requires specialty care.

Political unrest (as recently seen in Egypt and other countries in the Middle East), medical illness, emergencies at home and other untoward events may necessitate emergency evacuation from a particular destination. Evacuation planning is an important component of the MTA. The evacuation plan should identify and integrate optimal transport and evacuation routes (such as nearby airports and cities). On an employee-specific basis, certain circumstances may warrant knowing what surgical, diagnostic and higher-level resources are available in the region. This information should be rapidly accessible in order to facilitate real-time decision making in the event of an emergency that may require evacuation.[9]

Medical Travel Kit

Having a personal medical kit is essential. This kit should be very comprehensive and personalized. The complexity of this kit will largely be determined by destination/access to westernized medicine and on the individual employee's risk and comorbidity profile. In addition to antimalarial medication, antibiotics and anti-motility drugs for self-treatment of travelers' diarrhea, the first-aid kit should, at a minimum, include an analgesic and remedies for motion sickness, jet lag, allergic reactions (antihistamines), and constipation.

For the business traveler who makes frequent international trips, it is wise to carry a broad-spectrum antibiotic such as levofloxacin or azithromycin for self-treatment of bowel, skin, and respiratory infections (and with the former, urinary tract infections). Carrying fluconazole for the treatment of yeast infections is more practical than recommending over-the-counter vaginal creams. Alcohol-based hand sanitizer, water purification tablets, insect repellent, and condoms are other essential items. When traveling abroad, medications should be packed in carry-on bags. Since the luggage compartment may freeze during air travel, medication, especially injectable products, inhalers and capsules, could be damaged. Business travelers should be provided with an authorization letter and a full list with generic names of all prescribed medications.

Finally, seemingly trivial medical issues such as skin rashes, thrombosed hemorrhoids, vaginal yeast infections, or panic attacks can have significant consequences for a traveling employee. If a particular employee has a specific recurring issue (UTI, etc.) then prophylaxis for a respective condition should be included in the personal medical kit. The use of a standardized, pre-trip checklist of medications and medical supplies should ensure adequate preparation for these common medical issues (Table 29.2).

In addition to medical supplies, it is important to consider having a supply of non-perishable, high-energy foods (preferably complex carbohydrates). This can be very valuable, especially when the local food source is unsafe (i.e., during a long day in a developing country).

Environmental Risks – Altitude, Remote Areas, Site Surveys, etc.

As alluded to above, aside from vector-borne diseases, there are many diverse environmental risks that should be considered prior to business

Table 29.2 Basic medications and supplies

Medication/Category	Clinical Uses/Drug
Acetazolamide	AMS (acute mountain sickness) prevention or treatment
Analgesics	Pain relief and antipyretics (acetaminophen, ASA, and ibuprofen)
Antidiarrheals	Travelers' diarrhea (loperamide, bismuth)
Antiemetics	Nausea and vomiting (dimenhydrinate, ondansetron)
Antihistamines/allergic reactions	Allergic reaction, anaphylaxis, sleep aid (Diphenhydramine and epinephrine)
Antivirals	Threat-specific post-exposure prophylaxis, (e.g., HIV exposure, influenza exposure or early treatment) (oseltamivir)
Broad-spectrum antibiotics and antimalarials	Malaria prophylaxis (for endemic areas), leptospirosis prophylaxis, bronchitis, pneumonia, anthrax, Chlamydia, skin and soft tissue infections, and topical antifungals (e.g., Atovaquone/proguanil, doxycycline, clindamycin, levofloxacin, amoxicillin/clavulinic acid , azithromycin)
Mosquito repellent	Mitigate vector-borne disease transmission
Personal hygiene	Hand sanitizer, condoms
Sleep aids	Sleep cycle regulation
Sunscreen	Protection against sun exposure
Water and food/snacks	Rehydration, nourishment
Equipment	
Basic first-aid supplies	Bandaids, wound dressings, antibiotic ointment (mupuricin, fucidin), mole skin, safety pins, splints
Tampon	Menses, wound packing, management of epistaxis, ear wick for antibiotics
Tissue adhesives	Wound closure or temporary dental fracture treatment
Trauma equipment and supplies	Tourniquet and hemostatic agent for hemorrhage control, fracture splinting

travel. Other medical threats include: unintentional injuries; extremes of temperature or other weather conditions; difficult terrain, including high altitudes (La Paz, Wenzhuan); contaminated water; improperly prepared food; hazardous materials; infectious diseases; sleep cycle disturbance; harmful wildlife or plants (Black Mamba in Rwanda); and physical or emotional stress. The employee's general physical conditioning and underlying medical conditions are important considerations when assessing these respective external risks. Once potential threats are identified, alternate travel or appropriate contingency plans should be developed.

Special Issues Associated with Business Travel

Stressors and Travel

Sources of stress during travel may be multiple, complex, and vary from person to person. In addition to health concerns related to the destination, the goal of the mission may be difficult to accomplish as a result of these stressors, which include cultural difference, fatigue, sleep deprivation, and health impairment. Additionally, business travel may have a significant and unanticipated impact on the employee and his or her family, which can make the employee traveler less effective at work and less able to manage the other stressors inherent to travel.[10]

Some strategies that may improve the wellbeing of both the traveler and/or his or her family include daily phone or electronic correspondence with loved ones at home (Skype or email), and adding a mid-way stop on long itineraries or those with multiple connections will help to reduce jet lag and provide more preparation time. Personalizing even the most uninviting hotel room and packing comfort items such as preferred music, movies, comfort food, and pictures of family members or pets can help to mitigate stress.

Trauma

A travel medicine consultation cannot be considered complete without addressing the important role of trauma in the deaths of travelers. As mentioned, international business travel may pose health risks well beyond exposure to infectious diseases. Accidental deaths due to motor vehicle accidents and interpersonal violence are an important health risk, and preventive measures should be reviewed prior to travel. According to the World Health Organization, nearly 1.3 million people die annually from motor vehicle crashes, the single greatest cause of death for healthy US citizens traveling abroad, and much of this mortality can be offset by seatbelt and traffic safety compliance; unfortunately, the former are often not available. Furthermore, business travelers must understand that even chauffeured travel by road is risky in rural areas, especially when traveling after dark.

Sexual

About 10% of short-term travelers will have a new sexual partner. Explicit pre-travel counseling is thus recommended for all, without discrimination. Many factors can potentially increase the risk: the exotic new destination, novel sexual practices of potential partners, fatigue, jet lag, insomnia, alcohol intake, difficult business encounters, etc. In some cultures, male business travelers are offered a liaison with a sex worker as part of the process of doing business. For travelers who are likely to be exposed while traveling, a self-treatment kit for post-exposure prophylaxis (PEP) for HIV might be considered. Consideration should be given to local resistance patterns when prescribing a kit for PEP.

Jet Lag

Jet lag is the sleep disorder that results from altering one's innate circadian rhythm in relation to local time.[11] This is the most frequent problem encountered by corporate travelers because the intrinsic circadian rhythm does not take kindly to rapid changes across time zones. Jet lag occurs when several time zones are crossed within a short period. The severity of the jet lag is affected by the length of flight and by the direction of travel.

The dissociation between the body's internal clock and the local time, daylight periods and activities result in symptoms ranging from sleepiness and general malaise to reduced concentration and attention, irritability, and gastrointestinal symptoms. Daytime fatigue is followed by relative insomnia and multiple or early awakening, increasing the discomfort during the following day. The resulting impairment of physical and mental performance may have serious consequences, especially for pilots, business people, athletes, and military personnel. Studies in pilots have shown performance efficiency to decrease by 8.5% after an eastbound flight across eight time zones. Furthermore, there is evidence that chronic jet lag may lead to cognitive deficits, possibly in working memory.[12]

There are several modalities for treating jet lag. Appropriately timed natural light exposure, i.e., getting up early and being exposed to natural sunlight out of doors, will help. This strategy alone or in conjunction with melatonin can be very effective. Another approach is the use of pharmacotherapy to either induce sleep or ward off sleepiness during the waking hours. Finally, maintaining a sleep-wake schedule and optimizing the duration and timing of sleep can help considerably. These strategies can be used independently or as multi-modal therapy.[11]

Selected Infectious Disease Risks

Knowledge of pre-travel advice will be covered in other chapters. Similar principles apply, but corporate travel practitioners should be particularly knowledgeable about vaccination schedules (i.e., accelerated schedules for last-minute travelers), travelers' diarrhea, insect-borne illnesses (dengue fever, malaria, yellow fever) and human-transmitted illnesses (respiratory, sexually transmitted, blood-borne).

Vaccine-Preventable Infections

For the frequent business traveler, there are several important principles to be considered. First, immunizations should be administered not with an individual trip in mind, but rather with the cumulative risk of multiple trips to a particular area. For example, typhoid immunization might not be considered for a 1-week trip to Asia, but the cumulative risk of infection over many trips should make one consider vaccination. Second, business travel is often last-minute, and therefore business travelers should have their travel immunizations updated regularly, even without travel on the immediate horizon, so that they will be protected if international travel is required with little advanced notice. Third, unlike vacationers, business travelers may have considerable financial consequences at stake if they fail to complete work projects or negotiations due to illness. Furthermore, business travelers may be at the whim of foreign colleagues when it comes to their ability to refuse certain foods or activities. Therefore, they must be fully immunized even when risks are considered to be low, especially when the consequence of illness is serious. Finally, there may be financial and/or legal repercussions to a business if appropriate health advice has not been provided to employees who are traveling for the company. Business travelers cannot afford to be sick.

Immunizations recommended for virtually all international business travelers include hepatitis A and B, diphtheria, tetanus, acellular pertussis, polio, influenza, and measles. In addition, vaccines against specific diseases such as typhoid fever, yellow fever, toxigenic *E. coli*, Japanese encephalitis, and rabies should be offered for those at significant risk.

Vector-Borne Diseases and Chemoprophylaxis

Business travelers visiting areas at risk for malaria, dengue fever, yellow fever, Japanese encephalitis and other vector-borne infections should receive proper counseling on personal protection measures to prevent insect bites. With the increase in dengue fever in many major cities in the Caribbean, Central and South America and in Asia, the risk of vector-borne diseases is increasing. Dengue fever is one of the most common mosquito-borne viral diseases in the tropics with no vaccine, so insect protection is the current strategy. Business travelers should be reminded that it is primarily an urban disease transmitted by a day-biting mosquito (*Aedes aegypti*). Re-infection with different serotypes can increase the risk of developing hemorrhagic fever, where the case–fatality ratio approximates 5% worldwide.

Studies have shown that business travelers tend to be well informed of malaria risk, but comply poorly with preventive measures (repellent and medication).[13] Business travelers have been reported to carry self-treatment doses of antimalarials if they anticipate longer periods of exposure or travel frequently to endemic areas. Compliance with anti-malarials in expatriates is particularly poor and decreases over time. Reasons cited include presumed immunity, forgetfulness, conflicting advice, side-effect concerns and daily dosing.[7] Approximately 30% of expatriates develop malaria within 2 years of exposure. Studies in US diplomats found that 83% of malaria cases were *P. falciparum* and 8% *P. vivax*; almost 90% were infected in Africa and 5% in Asia, respectively. The average annual incidence of malaria was highest in West Africa (9 per 1000 personnel), followed by Central and East Africa.

In high-endemic areas for malaria (sub-Saharan Africa, South East Asia, Central America), chemoprophylaxis is usually recommended even for very short stays. Atovaquone-proguanil or primaquine are very good options for this population, as they need to be started the day before exposure and continued for only 7 days after leaving the risk area. When the risk of a 1- or 2- night stay in a low-risk area is carefully reviewed, chemoprophylaxis may not be recommended. In other circumstances where the risk is moderate, the traveler may still decide not to take prophylaxis. However, destinations may change at the last minute. Business travelers should be knowledgeable about the symptoms of malaria, which may appear as early as 7–8 days after exposure, but may be delayed up to 1 year after exposure, for some species. It might be helpful to provide the traveler with a wallet-sized card with a description of malaria symptoms and the recommendation for immediate testing in the case of fever. For travelers to remote areas where proper treatment may not be accessible within 24 h, a self-treatment regimen of atovaquone/proguanil or artemisinin/lumefantrine may be provided.

Conclusion

The travel medical needs of the business traveler are unique. The physician must have an understanding of a broad scope of medical areas to ensure the health and safety of the traveler in addition to a successful mission. Proper planning and customized advice will help corporations protect their employees from the hazards of international travel.

References

1. Hudson TW, Fortuna J. Overview of Selected Infectious Disease risks for the Corporate Traveler. JOEM 2008;50(8):924–34.
2. Duval B, et al. A Population-based comparison between traveler who consulted travel clinics and those who did not. J Travel Med 2003;10: 4–10.
3. Richards C, Rundle AG. Business travel and self-rated health, obesity, and cardiovascular disease risk factors. JOEM 2011;53(4):358–63.
4. Burkholder JD, Joines R, Cunningham-Hill M, Xu B. Health and wellbeing factors associated with international business travel. J Travel Med 2010;17:329–33.
5. Rogers HL, Reilly SM. Health problems associated with international business travel. A critical review of the literature. AAOHN J 2000;48:376–84.
6. Bunn W. Vaccine and international health programs for employees traveling and living abroad. J Travel Med 2001;8(suppl 1):S20–3.
7. Patel D. Occupational travel. Occupational Medicine 2011;61:6–18.
8. Valani R, Cornacchia M, Kube D. Flight diversions due to onboard medical emergencies on an international commercial airline. Aviat Space Environ Med 2010;81:1037–40.

9. Teichman PG, Donchin Y, Kot RJ. International aeromedical evacuation. [Review] [69 refs]. N Engl J Med 2007;356:262–70.

10. Tompkins OS. Business traveler fitness. AAOHN J 2008;56:272.

11. Sack RL. Clinical practice. Jet lag. [Review] [45 refs]. N Engl J Med 2010;362:440–7.

12. Cho K, Ennaceur A, Cole JC, Suh CK. Chronic jet lag produces cognitive deficits. J Neurosci 2000;20:RC66.

13. Farquharson L, Noble LM, Behrens RH. Travel clinic communication and non-adherence to malaria chemoprophylaxis. Travel Medicine & Infectious Disease 2011;9(6):278–83.

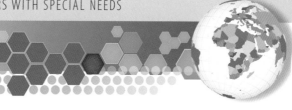

30

International Adoption

Jean-François Chicoine and Dominique Tessier

Key points

- Counseling for international adoption includes: (1) pre-travel health advice for the parents, (2) issues concerning travel with a young child, (3) infectious disease risks from contact between parents and the adoptee, (4) acute and chronic health problems of the adopted child, and (5) parenting counselling and psychosocial support
- Before travel, parents should learn as much as possible about the adoptee's living conditions, culture and health problems, preferably from an international adoption agency or the orphanage; pre-adoption parental preparation courses are recommended for all parents and are mandatory in some host countries
- Pre-travel health advice for adoptive parents includes, in addition to the usual recommendations, greater emphasis on hepatitis B immunization and other infectious diseases
- Adoptees from developing countries, especially those who have been institutionalized or neglected, often suffer from infectious diseases, malnutrition, cognitive and physical developmental delays, attachment issues, and behavioral problems

Introduction

The liberalization of international trade in China, the institutionalization of orphans in Eastern European countries, civil unrest, war, ethnic conflicts, AIDS orphans, natural disasters and the globalization of poverty continue to create a need for a family in more abandoned children. In host countries, the increasing problem of infertility, the regulation of births, family reconstitutions and the recognition of civil rights of illegitimate children are factors that contribute to the need to seek children in other countries. Despite these 'two solitudes', children in need on the one hand, and parents with a desire to have children on the other, the demand for a child exceeds the number of adoptable children in the world, which explains the confusion, in part human, social and moral, related to the topic of international adoption.[1]

Globally, between 30 000 and 40 000 international adoptions take place annually, much fewer than during the previous decade. A decrease of 5–20% was further observed during the past 5 years in all the welcoming countries, except in Italy. Still, every year, approximately 20 000 international adoptions take place in the USA, 4500 in Spain, at the top of European countries for international adoptions, 3300 in France, 1900 in Canada and 900 in Sweden. In North America, most of the adopted children come from China, South Korea, the Russian Federation, India, Haiti, Guatemala, Vietnam, Colombia, Cambodia, Kazakhstan, Ukraine, the Philippines, Madagascar, and Ethiopia. In general, the age at the time of adoption has increased, providing hope for older children looking for a family, but increasing the potential for psychodevelopmental consequences.[2,3]

Ethical Issues

The Hague Convention concerning international adoption stipulates that countries should make it a priority to take measures to ensure that every child be maintained in his/her biological family, or if that is not possible, a proper family should be found for him/her in the country of birth. This statement clearly implies that international adoption should be considered a last resort.[4–6]

Unfortunately, adoption has given rise to the increased trafficking of children, in countries such as in Eastern Europe, Madagascar, Chad, Ethiopia, Ghana, Rwanda, Guatemala, and China, where some children had not really been abandoned, or where their parents entered into direct transactions with the adoptive parties. In the 1990s, the corruption and criminal activities associated with international adoptions drove organizations such as UNICEF to withhold unconditional support for the process. Following discussions with the European Union, and in order to counter the trafficking of children, Romania and eventually Belarus also decided to close its doors to international adoption. International organizations, such as the International Social Service in Geneva, were given the mandate to inform intervening parties worldwide of the evolving terms of adoption in different countries, and to shed light on different problems hindering child protection.

In recent years, a new ethical problem has emerged: the confusion between humanitarian action and international adoption with the pretext of rescuing children. Such conflicts were recently observed in Darfur in 2008 and after the earthquake in Haiti in 2010, at the cost of fraud of both families of origin and at destination, and an assumed loss of cultural identity of targeted children. American legal experts now invoke the fundamental rights of the child in an attempt to

©2012 Elsevier Inc
DOI: 10.1016/B978-1-4557-1076-8.00030-2

violate established adoption conventions by posing the following question: 'Is it moral to buy or adopt a child illegally if, in exchange, it allows him/her to survive poverty or a disaster?'[4–10]

Pre-Adoption Evaluation

Pre-adoption medical consultations are very important. Many parents, blinded by their desire for a child or exhausted by the multiple steps required to adopt one, fail to ask a medical expert to examine the adoption proposal documents. The question of health risks regarding the adoptee is often addressed to the travel health adviser, often at the first immunization consultation. Specific issues of adoption, and support for parents lacking experience, can be very challenging. An evaluation of potential health risks by an expert in international adoption is ideal. To expand access, some multidisciplinary services provide their assessments by electronic means (telephone, e-mail and webcam).[1,10–13]

Additional information on the health of orphans in their countries of origin would go a long way to predict future challenges for adoptive families, i.e., the relative risk of AIDS in Cambodia, fetal alcohol syndrome in the Russian Federation and South Korea, and malnutrition in Ethiopia and Haiti. Unfortunately, the actual medical condition according to written medical documentation, medical imaging, photographs or videos, may turn out to be highly inaccurate.[12] Information on weight, height, cranial circumference, as well as laboratory results for hepatitis B and C, HIV, or syphilis must be evaluated and determined on the basis of all the information provided. The developmental aspects mentioned in the child's file must be measured, especially with low weight or older children, those carrying genetic defects or disabilities, and those adopted after a lengthy hospitalization.[1,11–14]

The work of the medical expert in the pre-adoption process essentially is to try to anticipate the evolution of a child that might have been abandoned, malnourished, or abused. It is also to evaluate whether a child with a disability or illness could receive the appropriate care with the candidate parents.

Although most parents wish to adopt healthy children, an increasing number of parents are now adopting children with HIV or thalassemia major, or correctable deformities such as cleft lip and palate, in order to reduce waiting time. In some countries, parents often have only 72 hours to decide whether or not to adopt the candidate, putting pressure on the professional doing the pre-adoption medical assessment. Such delays and other considerations should not, however, confuse the judgment of the clinician.[1,10–16]

Pre-Adoption Medical Preparation of Caregivers and Families

Before the arrival of the child, all caregivers and family members should be offered immunization against hepatitis B. In China and SE Asia, vertical transmission of hepatitis B is common. The adopted child may thus be a chronic carrier, often HBe antibody positive, and therefore highly infectious. Acute hepatitis B infection among adopting parents is well documented. Fortunately, pre-adoption screening tests for hepatitis B and C and for HIV are now usually performed, reducing the risk of secondary infections. Hepatitis A may represent a significant risk, especially for older parents, caregivers and grandparents. Immunizing the entire family should be considered. If the child is coming from a country highly endemic for tuberculosis, it might be helpful to do a baseline pre-adoption tuberculin skin test (TST) on all potential future household contacts.[1,16–17]

Healthcare professionals should not neglect the risk of infectious diseases, such as measles and mumps, being transmitted by the adopting family to infants and young children adopted from countries with a different epidemiology. It is therefore important to update the immune status for all routine immunizations of all potential close contacts.

The majority of parents will have to travel in order to have their initial encounter with their child, and will thus benefit from a travel medicine consultation. Pre-travel health advice for adoptive parents should include the usual recommendations and a greater emphasis on routine and travel-specific vaccine-preventable diseases.[18]

Travel counseling should address all preventive measures: care related to food and water, vector-borne diseases such as malaria and dengue, and sun and environmental protection. The specific characteristics of the adoption generally confine parents to their hotel rooms in large cities. Therefore, in most areas of the world, malaria chemoprophylaxis is unnecessary. However, in areas highly endemic for malaria, such as Africa, chemoprophylaxis is usually recommended even for very short stays. In considering the choice of chemoprophylaxis for malaria, one must keep in mind the possibility that the mother might become pregnant. There is some evidence that the fertile adopting mother has increased potential for becoming pregnant soon after the adoption. In addition, transmission of cytomegalovirus from the adopted child to the pregnant mother is a consideration. Parents should be advised to wash their hands frequently; carrying an alcohol-based disinfectant may be very useful. A prescription for self-treatment of travelers' diarrhea, such as ciprofloxacin or azithromycin, should not be forgotten.[1,17] Also, institutionalized or previously hospitalized children have a higher incidence of positive MRSA, without consequences for the majority of parents in good health.[19]

The dynamics of group travel can be difficult. International adoption delegations usually have very tight schedules and precise tasks to accomplish in a limited time, often dealing with bureaucratic red tape. Whenever possible, it is preferable to organize a group information session regarding risks and recommended preventive measures. This usually avoids confusion when travelers compare prescriptions or vaccines they received from different healthcare providers, and enables the medical provider to determine whether each traveler should carry his/her own first-aid kit or whether a single group kit would be more appropriate (Table 30.1). If possible, it is advisable to identify within

Table 30.1 Suggestions for First-aid Kit for International Adoption
Milk substitute with or without lactose
Hand cleaner (70% ethyl alcohol)
Hydration cream (glaxal base)
Topical antibiotic (2% mupirocin)
Ophthalmic drops
Topical steroid cream (1% hydrocortisone)
Physiological nasal spray
Clarithromycin or cefixime
Scabicide
Multivitamin
Essential fat supplement (carthamus oil)
Zinc oxide as a diaper rash cream and sunblock
Antipyretic, liquid, pediatric strength
Rehydration preparation
Thermometer

a delegation an individual, preferably someone in the healthcare field, who will be in charge of the first-aid kit, and to ensure that this person understands how to use its contents.[1-20]

Health and repatriation insurance should be purchased before departure. On arrival, adoptive parents should register with their embassy or consulate, especially in a country where the sociopolitical situation is unstable. Keeping a copy of all these documents, including the passport, in a cloud computing system is recommended. Carrying the baby in a front pack during stressful periods, such as check-in at the airport, can help free one's hands while keeping the baby in sight. Security issues need to be reviewed carefully. Most car seats are not approved for use on airplanes but can help maintain children in a more stable and possibly safer position during long flights. Simple measures can be the most useful (see Ch. 23).

As time remains an uncontrollable dimension, jet lag is a common but serious problem for adopting parents. Children tend to adapt faster, but the anxiety of parents and their fear of letting the baby cry, may open the door to unsuitable sleeping patterns and habits. Adults should try to spend time outdoors to be exposed to natural sunlight. If no-one else can take charge of the baby during the night, parents should take turns. Avoidance of caffeine, energy drinks, excessive alcohol, and food too close to bedtime, are commonsense precautions that often need to be reinforced. It is not recommended to co-sleep with the new baby. Laying the child in a crib or on a mattress next to the parent avoids the risk of accidents, including choking or sudden death syndrome.[1]

Adoptee 'Pre-Travel' Consultation

The pre-travel consultation for the adoptee has the very unusual characteristic that it is being done for a traveler about whom there is often little information, except possibly a brief technical report, photograph, or video. Adoptive parents should try to address their questions with other parents (especially those who have successfully completed an international adoption), the adoption agency, associations of adopting parents, and their family doctor or future pediatrician.

Parents should not be too concerned with food allergies and should feed the child as soon as possible. It is essential for parents to be prepared for the fact that in countries such as Haiti, or in Africa, the child might be severely malnourished. Essential nutritional needs must be prioritized and fulfilled. Parents should also know about basic medical care and signs that would warrant a consultation with a healthcare provider. Respiratory infections are common, as are diarrhea and skin problems. A first-aid kit as described in Table 30.1 is well adapted to the specific needs of adoptive parents. Parents should be instructed on the appropriate use of scabicides and carry a topical antibiotic for possible secondary bacterial infection.[1,21-24]

The transition from the orphanage to a loving family is likely to be a tremendous relief for the child, who is used to lying on his/her back under physical constraints, to hunger, to the paucity of human contact, and to the incessant noise of institutional life. Even under these adverse circumstances, an instantaneous attachment between child and parents is more myth than reality. The child will need months or years to deepen the links with the adopting parents. Profoundly deprived children will require a considerable amount of time before being able to find the neurophysiological mechanism that enables bonding to occur. In the weeks following arrival at home, the attachment process will begin. Troubles with sleeping, appetite, and angry outbursts will gradually diminish for most adopted children in the year following their arrival. Children long neglected, abused and adopted at an older age could remain insecure, anxious, aggressive or

avoidant beyond this period. Some may present trauma disorders, development or learning disabilities. Daycare should ideally be delayed for 6–12 months after the adoption. Older children can benefit from a delay in their entry into the school system, to allow optimal recovery with affection, stimulation, and free play.[1,16,25-27]

Health Problems Encountered during Travel

Parents should receive the same advice and medications for themselves as for any other traveler to the country visited. They should be able to properly use rehydration fluids and self-treatment for diarrhea. Personal hygiene measures should be reviewed as well as standard food, water, and insect precautions. They should be informed of signs and symptoms that would require a medical consultation for their child.

The usual items contained in the first-aid kit adapted for international adoption should be sufficient to treat common problems while away. If possible, an overseas doctor should be identified by the embassy, the adoption agency, or an association such as the International Association for Medical Assistance to Travelers (IAMAT), should the need arise for interventions in emergency situations.

Close contact with their new child should not be limited unless there is a very serious risk of infection for the child or the adult. Scabies should not be included in this category, as it is such a common parasite infection in developing countries that parents should be mentally prepared to be confronted by the infection.

Post-Adoption Medical Consultation

Several authors have indicated that the clinical examination after adoption is essential and should include hematologic, biochemical, and serologic screening. A medical evaluation on arrival is important in order to assess nutritional state, identify transmissible infections, evaluate development and possible psychoaffective disturbances, and listen to the concerns of the adopting family. The infectious disease screening should be tailored to the infectious disease epidemiology of the country of origin: malaria in Africa, syphilis in Ethiopia or the Russian Federation, HIV/AIDS in Thailand, Cambodia, and Haiti. The ethnic and geographic origin of the child may mandate other tests, such as hemoglobin electrophoresis, to detect thalassemia or sickle cell disease. Child development should be carefully evaluated. The usual assessment done at Sainte-Justine Hospital in Montreal is given as an example in Table 30.2. Most parents should be supported by a nurse, psychologist, or social worker knowledgeable in adoption.[1,16,21-25]

Nutritional Status

The nutritional status evaluation starts with a thorough clinical examination, followed by an anthropometric evaluation. Weight, height, and cranial parameters are noted and charted on percentile charts to follow the child's progress.[28] The new WHO child growth standards charts are better adapted to the nutrient realities of the world and are now the gold standard.[29] Microcephaly, a common finding among institutionalized children, can be so severe as to alter the interpretation of age.

In Quebec, 808 Chinese girls (average age 11.5 months) were examined consecutively in the month following their arrival.[30] One-quarter of them suffered from wasting and more than half suffered various degrees of stunting. In China, as in Eastern Europe, chronic malnutrition is severe after the age of 1 year.[31] Children adopted from China now arrive better fed than in the previous decade; this is not the case in Haitian children, who are still suffering as much from

Table 30.2 Suggestion for Screening Tests for Newly Arrived International Adoptees

Routine

CBC

Hepatitis B[a] (HbsAg, HbsAb , anti-core antibody)

Hepatitis C[a]

RNA-based anti-HIV-1 and 2 ELISA[a]

Syphilis screening (VDRL or RPR)

Stool O&P (1 to 3)

Strongyloserology

Tuberculin skin test (TST)[a] with or without chest X-ray (at 3 and 12 months post arrival if asymptomatic)

Routine newborns screens: phenylketonuria, thyroid, etc.

Dental evaluation

Hearing screening

Bone age (girls >4 years)

Urinalysis

Optional Depending on Nutritional Status

Serum iron, total iron binding capacity (TIBC), ferritin, albumin, creatinine, transaminases, alkaline phosphatase, calcium, magnesium phosphate, zinc

Serial bone age

Optional, Depending on a Suspected Infection

Chest X-ray

Thick and thin films for malaria

Anti-HCV (RIBA) RNA (PCR)

HIV: HIV viral load, CD4 count

Rubella, varicella, measles, mumps, toxoplasmosis serology, etc.

Optional, Depending on Developmental Assessment

Occupational therapy evaluation or physiotherapist evaluation

Psychological or social worker evaluation

Speech therapist evaluation

Vision screen

Optional, Depending on the Geographic Country of Birth

Hemoglobin electrophoresis, G6PD screening

Lead blood level

[a]Repeat at 6 months–1 year depending on circumstances (American Academy of Pediatrics 2011).

protein–energy malnutrition.[32] Low birthweight, an extended period of malnutrition, and slow cranial growth carry the risk of permanent damage affecting the psychomotor development of the child.[1,3,33] Vitamin and mineral deficiencies are common and are associated with iron deficiency anemia, rickets, and vitamin A visual disturbance.[30] Iron and other mineral supplements should be administered and hematologic follow-up be carried out until the child has fully recovered. Contributing factors such as folic acid deficiency, thalassemia, lead intoxication, and intestinal parasitoses such as hookworm infection, should be evaluated.[1,17]

Growth delay will affect newly adopted children more than any other medical problem.[1,31–34] Height under the third or fifth percentile has been described for nearly one child out of two on his/her first medical evaluation. Genetic, ethnic, environmental, nutritional, psychological, and medical causes should be considered in all cases. More disturbing is the high prevalence of microcephaly in institutionalized children. Improvement may be significant in time, but will not always happen. All of these factors contribute to the great difficulty of evaluating the true age of the child. The possibility of precocious puberty in girls adopted after the age of 4 years should be taken into consideration.[35]

Infectious Disease Issues

Adopted children may be carriers of infections, of which the most serious include HIV, hepatitis B and C, syphilis, and tuberculosis. Some parasitoses may be detrimental to their development and need to be assessed.[17,36–40]

The discovery of infection in the newcomer is rare, thanks in part to the testing of potential candidates in the countries of origin before the decision to adopt is made. Between 2% and 5% of adoptive children may be hepatitis B carriers, having contracted the virus from their biological mother by vertical transmission in China, Vietnam, Thailand, or Cambodia, or by horizontal transmission via syringes or contaminated products in Ukraine or the Russian Federation. Transmission of hepatitis B is well documented to occur between children, especially siblings under the age of 5 years. Hepatitis C-positive serology is reported to occur in <1% of children from China, the Russian Federation, and the Moldavia Republic; this was often due to transplacental transmission of antibodies to children <1 year old. [17]

Adopted children usually come from countries where the prevalence of tuberculosis is 10–20 times higher than in Western Europe or North America. It is not surprising, therefore, to note that the authors found that 2–19% of adopted children had latent tuberculosis on the basis of a positive tuberculin skin test.[17,32] There is no reliable method to distinguish a positive TST caused by BCG vaccination from one caused by infection in spite of the availability of the interferon gamma release assay (IGRA). Because there is some uncertainty about the utility of the IGRA in children <5 years, prior vaccination should not influence the decision of whether or not to treat the individual. Internationally adopted children with positive TST reactions ≥10 mm should undergo chest radiography and careful physical examination in search of clinical evidence of tuberculosis. For immunocompromised children or those with recent known exposure, TST reactions ≥5 mm are considered positive. In the absence of active pulmonary disease or extrapulmonary tuberculosis, children should be offered treatment for latent tuberculosis infection.[41]

Several charts from Eastern Europe mention the possibility of a history of congenital syphilis, and so serological screening is required. The prevalence of parasitic infections is high among adoptive children, except for babies coming from Korea. In several studies, 4–51% of stool samples from adopted children revealed the presence of protozoa, nematodes, and more rarely, cestodes.[17,24,32,38] These infections may contribute to malnutrition, anemia, and psychomotor delays. Hookworm infections and strongyloidiasis are common, the latter frequently reported in children adopted in Haiti.[39]

Immunization Considerations

Both the World Health Organization and the Centers for Disease Control and Prevention consider that immunizations administered to children in developing countries can generally be trusted, and that these adoptees may be considered to be effectively protected provided that there is adequate documentation.[1,3,17,23–24,38] However, other data suggest that this may not be true for children from many orphanages around the world.

In 1998, Hostetter et al. reported this finding for the first time in a study of adopted infants in China and Eastern Europe. Only 35% were immunized against diphtheria, tetanus, and polio, despite vaccination booklets that claimed three vaccine injections after an initial vaccination.[42] The following year, Miller et al. published a new study about children coming mostly from Russia and Eastern Europe with inadequate immunization.[43] In 2002, Strine and colleagues showed that among adopted foreign children aged 19–35 months there was poor vaccination coverage for Haemophilus *influenzae* (type B) and equally poor vaccination coverage for hepatitis B.[44,45] In 2003, Chen published a review of this particular problem and concluded that the results were dependent on the country of origin.[46]

There are many possible explanations for the low levels of protective antibodies noted in some series: breakage of the cold chain, falsification of immunization records, and inappropriate vaccine dosage and use. Almost all children will be appropriately immunized against tuberculosis, diphtheria, tetanus, polio, and pertussis, and, for children >9 months old, against measles. Regarding seroprotection, Cilleruelo et al. found that the best indicator to predict a seroprotective status was the country of origin. The highest rate of protection was found in children from Eastern Europe and, in descending order, India, Latin America, China, and Africa.[47]

It is considered safe to administer most vaccines to a child lacking proof of immunity. Until the availability of more acceptable data in the literature, there is thus a tendency to follow the re-vaccination approach of the USA, as opposed to Europe, where healthcare professionals tend to accept unconfirmed vaccination information instead of repeating immunization. General recommendations for immunization of internationally adopted children are difficult to establish. The American Academy of Pediatrics' position is available in its Red Book.[17]

Child Development

Sensoriperceptive, fine motor and gross motor, cognitive, and language deficiencies are often recorded in children adopted from foreign countries.[1,3,12,14,16,21,25,31,33] Most of these deficiencies are minor and are referred to as 'adoptive normalities. Generally, the post-adoption recovery will be spectacular, supported only by affection and proper feeding.[1,48]

Several series have shown less optimistic developmental evolution among children from Eastern Europe.[48,49] In these circumstances, the interdisciplinary healthcare team should follow closely the development of the child and determine whether it deteriorates into severe developmental disorder.[50]

All adopted children have suffered from abandonment for one reason or another, and others have sustained early, late, or even multiple episodes. Therefore, some families will need professional assistance or coaching in order to better understand the primitive wounds caused by the emotional distress of their child. Socio-affectively, one should remember that an adoption carried out before 8–15 months of age with good conditions at the orphanage or qualified foster home will favor a constructive, loving relationship between parent and child when the adopting parents have the proper tools.

A relational deficiency before and after the adoption can lead to pathologic emotional states in a child. Among them is an emotional insecurity with resistant anxiety that can lead to sleep disorders, lack of self-esteem or academic phobia. Others will be more ambivalent, and will express themselves through angry outbursts and aggression. It is imperative that a social worker, psychologist, educator, or psychiatrist be brought in to assist families who face these challenges and attachment difficulties.[1,14,26,27]

Anxiety in an adopted child is not necessarily related to attachment and can be explained by post-traumatic stress disorder (PTSD).[51,52]

In the months following adoption, the family doctor and pediatrician should be concerned about the emergence of different learning disabilities. Reading, abstraction, or language disorders all are more prevalent in children born with low birthweight or who experienced a deleterious pre-adoption period. Attention deficit disorder (ADD), of which the incidence is up to three times more prevalent, predisposes to abandonment and, since it has a strong genetic component, can explain the child's behavior.[53]

The Social Impact of Adoption

Several Scandinavian, Dutch, and American studies indicate that the majority of overseas adopted children will enjoy a balanced adolescence on a socio-emotional level, both from the familial and an educational point of view. On the other hand, many authors have described an increased number of learning disabilities, behavioral misconducts, and suicide risk in children who have been institutionalized or adopted.[26,27,54–60] Among those most responsible for problems, one finds a diagnosis of attention deficit hyperactivity disorder (ADHD), fetal alcohol syndrome, post-traumatic stress disorder (PTSD) and attachment disorder. Major adoption failures are linked to attachment disorder.[1,16,27,51]

These catastrophic data should, however, be contextualized and interpreted judiciously. An American study compared the evolution of internationally adopted children versus children adopted from the United States and reported that international adoptees evidenced fewer behavioral and emotional problems than domestic adoptees.[59] Central to a successful social adaptation is an identity search. A memory box containing the child's garments at the time of adoption, the plane tickets, and photographs and videos of the trip will facilitate the development of identity. Around the age of 7, children will appreciate scrapbooking activities to make a family tree with roots in their country of origin and branches reaching in out around the world to their new family.[1–61]

From adversity and in abandonment, international adoption brings new challenges and rewards both for the adopted child and the new parents, but most of all, it enables all members to travel a new path towards growth and evolution as a family.[61,62]

References

1. Chicoine JF, Germain P, Lemieux J. L'enfant adopté dans le monde (en quinze chapitres et demi). Éditions de l'hôpital Sainte–Justine, Québec, 2003/ Chicoine, JF, Germain, P., Lemieux J. Genitori adottivi e figli del mondo. Éditions Erickson, Trento, Italy, 2004.
2. Selman P. Données préparées pour Family Helper, site internet www.familyhelper.net/, cité par SSI/CIR 2011.
3. Miller L, Chan W, Comfort K, et al. Health of children adopted from Guatemala: comparison of orphanage and foster care. Pediatrics 2005;115:e710–e717.
4. Conférence de La Haye de droit international privé: http://hcch.e-vision.nl/upload/adostats_us.pdf
5. SSI/CIR no 11–12 2005; no 52 2008; no 3–4 2011.
6. UNICEF. Humanitarian. Action for Children 2011.
7. Ren X. Trafficking in children: China and Asian perspective. International Bureau of Children's Rights, National and International Perspectives, November 20, 2004.
8. Jablonka I. L'arche de Zoé ou le système du déracinement-La vie des idées. www.laviedesidees.fr. 2008.
9. Bartholet E. International Adoption: the human rights position. Global Policy January 2010;1(1).
10. Chicoine JF. Adoption internationale: humanisme et industrie: conférence au Club 44. Suisse: La Chaux-de-Fonds; 2009.
11. Jenista JA. Preadoption review of medical records. Pediatr Ann 2000;29:212–5.
12. Albers LH, Johnson DE, Hostetter MK, et al. Health of children adopted from the former Soviet Union and Eastern Europe: comparison with preadoptive medical records. JAMA 1997;278:922–4.

13. Boone JL, Hostetter MK, Weitzman CC. The predictive accuracy of pre-adoption video review in adoptees from Russian and Eastern European orphanages. Clin Pediatr 2003;42:585–90.

14. Maclean K. The impact of institutionalization on child development. Dev and Psychopathol 2003;15:853–84.

15. Marinopoulos S. et coll. Moïse, Oedipe et Superman: de l'abandon à l'adoption. France: Fayard; 2003.

16. Chicoine JF, Lemieux J. Pratiques en adoption internationale: comment franchir le Rubicon américano-européen. Prisme 2007;46:130–52.

17. American Academy of Pediatrics. Red book 2011 (available online).

18. Wharton M. The epidemiology of varicella-zoster virus infections. Infect Dis Clin North Am 1996;10(3):571–81.

19. Radtke A, & all Internationally adopted children as a source for MRSA. Eurosurveillance 2005;10(42):20.

20. Chicoine JF, Carceller AM, Lebel MH, et al. Détresse psychologique des enfants adoptés après le tremblement de terre survenu à Haïti. Paediatr Child Health 2011;16(50).

21. Mitchell MAS, Jenista JA. Health care of the internationally adopted child. J Pediatr Health Care 1997;11:51–60.

22. Lawson ML, Auger L, Baxter C, et al. A CPSP Survey on Canadian Pediatricians' Experience and Knowledge about the Risks of Infectious Diseases in Children Adopted Internationally. CPS 2006.

23. Aronson J. Medical evaluation and infectious considerations on arrival. Pediatr Ann 2000;29:218–23.

24. Hostetter M. Infectious diseases in internationally adopted children: Findings in children from China, Russia and Eastern Europe. Adv Pediatr Infect Dis 1999;14:147–61.

25. Miller L. Caring for internationally adopted children. N Engl J Med 1999;34:1539–40.

26. Rygaard NP. L'enfant abandonné–Guide de Traitement des Troubles de l'Attachement. 2nd ed. Bruxelles: De boeck; 2007.

27. Schofield G, Beek M. Attachment Handbook for Foster Care and Adoption. Saffron house, London: BAAF; 2006.

28. Miller L. Initial assessment of growth, development and the effects of institutionalization in internationally adopted children. Pediatr Ann 2000;29:224–31.

29. WHO. Growth standards. www.who.int/childgrowth/mgrs/en/

30. Chicoine JF, Blancquaert I, Chicoine L, et al. Bilan de santé de 808 chinoises nouvellement adoptées au Quebec. Tours, France: Résumé XXXIIe congrès de l'association des pédiatres de langue française; 1999.

31. Benoit TC, Jocelyn IJ, Moddemann DE, et al. Romanian adoption: the Manitoba experience. Arch Pediatr Adolesc Med 1996;150:1278–82.

32. Robert M., Carceller AM, Blais D, et al. Health status of adopted children after the Haitian earthquake. Paediatr Child Health 2011;16(52).

33. Johnson D. Long-term medical issues in international adoptees. Pediatr Ann 2000;29:234–41.

34. Proos LA, Hofvander V, Wennquist K, et al. A longitudinal study on anthropometric and clinical development of Indian children adopted in Sweden 1. Clinical and anthropometric condition at arrival. Uppsala J Med Sci 1997;97:79–92.

35. Bourguignon JP, Gerard A, Alvarez-Gonzales ML, et al. Effects of changes in nutritional conditions on timing of puberty: clinical evidence from adopted children and experimental studies in the male rat. Horm Res 1992;38:S97–S105.

36. Davis LC, Weber DJ, Lemon SM. Horizontal transmission of hepatitis B virus. Lancet 1989;1:889–93.

37. Darmany JM. HIV infection and hepatitis B in adopted Romanian children. BMJ 1991;302:1604.

38. Miller LC. International adoption: infectious diseases issues. Clin Infect Dis 2005;40:286–93.

39. Robert M, Carceller AM, Demers AM, et al. Prevalence of strongyloïdes stercoralis in foreign-born children (abstract) ESPID La Haye, 2011.

40. Hersh BS, Popouici F, Jerzek Z, et al. Risk factors for HIV infection among abandoned Romanian children. AIDS 1993;7:1617–24.

41. Trehan I. & coll. Tuberculosis screening in internationally adopted children: the need for initial and repeat testing. Pediatrics 2008;122:e7–e14.

42. Hostetter MK, Johnson DE. Immunization Status of Adoptees from China, Russia, and Eastern Europe. Society for Pediatric Research, 1998 Abstract #851, New Orleans, LA. May 1–4.

43. Miller LC, Comfort K, Kelly N. Immunization status of internationally adopted children [letter]. Pediatrics 1999;13:178.

44. Schulte JM, Maloney S, Aronson J, et al. Evaluating acceptability and completeness of overseas immunization records of internationally adopted children. Pediatrics 2002;109:E22.

45. Strine TW, Barker LE, Mokdad AH, et al. Vaccination coverage of foreign-born children 19 to 35 months of age: findings from the national immunization survey, 1999–2000. Pediatrics 2002;110:e15.

46. Chen LH, Barnett ED, Wilson ME. Preventing infectious diseases during and after international adoption. Ann Intern Med 2003;139:371–8.

47. Cilleruelo MJ. Internationally adopted children: what vaccines should they receive? Vaccine 2008;26:5784–90.

48. Pomerleau A, Malcuit G, Chicoine JF, et al. Health status, cognitive and motor development of young children adopted from China, East Asia and Russia across the first six months after adoption. Int J Behav Dev 2005;29:445–57.

49. Miller L, Chan W, Tirella L, Perrin E. Outcomes of children adopted from Eastern Europe. Int J Behav Dev 2009;33(4):289–98.

50. Lee RM, Seol KO, Sung M, Miller MJ. The behavioral development of Korean children in institutional care and international adoptive families. Minnesota International Adoption Project Team. Developmental Psychology 2010;46(2):468–78.

51. Van der Kolk BA. The neurobiology of childhood trauma and abuse. Adolesc Psychiatric Clin N Am 2003;12:293–317.

52. Cook A, et al. Complex trauma in children and adolescents. Psychiatr Ann 2005;35:390.

53. Lindblad F, Weitoft GR, Hjern A. ADHD in international adoptees: a national cohort study. Eur Child Adolesc Psychiatry 2010;19(1):37–44. Epub 2009 Jun 19.

54. Hodges J, Tizard B. Social and family relationships of ex-institutional adolescents. Child Psychol Psych 1989;30(1):77–97.

55. Faber S. Behavioral sequelae of orphanage life. Pediatr Ann 2000;29:242–8.

56. Verhulst F, Althaus M, Versluis-Den Bieman HJM. Damaging backgrounds: later adjustment of international adoptees. J Am Acad Child Adolesc Psychiatry 1992;29:420–8.

57. Verhulst F, Althaus M, Versluis-Den Bieman HJM, et al. Problem behavior in international adoptees I. An epidemiological study. J Am Acad Child Adolesc Psychiatry 1990;29:94–103. /III. Diagnosis of child psychiatric disorders. J Am Acad Child Adolesc Psychiatry 29:94–103, 1990.

58. Hjern A, Lindblad F, Vinnerljung B. Suicide, psychiatric illness, and social maladjustment in intercountry adoptees in Sweden: a cohort study. The Lancet 2002;360:443–8.

59. Keyes MA, Sharma A, Elkins IJ, et al. The mental health of US adolescents adopted in infancy. Arch Pediatric Adolesc Med 2008;162(5):419–25.

60. Bimmel AL. Problem behavior of internationally adopted adolescents: a review and meta-analysis. Harv Rev Psychiatry 2003 Mar-Apr;11(2):64–77.

61. Grotevant HD. Post-adoption contact, adoption communicative openness, and satisfaction with contact as predictors of externalizing behavior in adolescence and emerging adulthood. Journal of Child Psychology and Psychiatry 2011;52:5.

62. Cyrulnik B. Les vilains petits canards. Éditions Odile Jacob 2001;278.

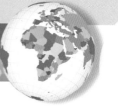

31

Visiting Friends and Relatives

Ronald H. Behrens and Karin Leder

Key points

- VFRs make up a substantial proportion of international travelers
- VFRs traveling to certain countries are at increased risk of typhoid fever, malaria, STIs, and possibly tuberculosis
- Children of VFRs born in industrialized countries, young VFRs, and those from the higher socioeconomic strata of society may be at greater risk of hepatitis A
- VFRs are less likely to seek pre-travel health advice and often travel in high-risk environments that expose them to particular infectious diseases
- Creative strategies are necessary to address the health needs of VFRs, such as community-based education, group sessions for travelers to specific countries, and handouts in multiple languages

Introduction

This chapter focuses on travelers visiting friends and relatives, or VFR travelers. The term VFR refers to travelers who have migrated at some period in the past, but who maintain friends and family links in their country of origin.

Who are VFR Travelers?

Traditionally, VFR travelers have been defined as fulfilling the following criteria: i) travel for which the main intention is to visit friends and relatives; ii) traveling from a higher-income or industrialized country to place of origin in a lower-income or developing country (implying low- to high-risk travel); and iii) ethnicity or cultural background different from those of the host population but similar to the destination population.[1] However, different definitions across studies have been used to describe these travelers, and the appropriateness of this definition given changing travel and global migration patterns has recently been questioned, in particular the need to include the ethnicity and cultural aspects;[2] therefore globally applicable definition of the term is still needed.

VFRs often include immigrants, asylum seekers/refugees, students, economic migrants, and displaced persons. Varied terminology has

been used to reflect citizens of different ethnic and cultural backgrounds from the natives of a country, and encompasses migrants, semi-immune and foreign-born individuals. A number of terms have also been used to describe the natives or majority group of the host country, including "European, non-migrants, nationals and non-immunes", thereby potentially making it difficult to make direct comparisons between population groups referred to in different studies.

Often family members (spouses or children) who were born in the country of residence are also included as VFRs, but better consensus on whether spouses and children should be defined as VFRs would improve uniformity in the use of the term. Ethnic travelers who visit friends and relatives in their country of origin may be three or four generations from the original migrant, but may still have both social and cultural attachments with their country of origin. For example, in some European countries, including the UK, France, and The Netherlands, some cultural and social ideologies and practices are maintained down generations. By contrast, in North American third and fourth generations, these social and cultural factors are often diluted.

We propose that subsequent generations who *maintain cultural identity* with their country of origin, or spouses who adopt this *cultural identity* and who travel to visit friends and relatives, should also be considered VFRs.

Why are VFRs a Risk Group for Travel-Related Illness?

The purpose of travel can influence the pattern of morbidity during and after travel. Both the health of the individual and the public health of the country to which he/she returns may be affected by travel. A number of factors may affect a VFR's risk of illness. Health beliefs held by the traveler will influence the use of pre-travel advice and prophylaxis. Many VFRs believe they will not suffer from infections such as malaria because they consider themselves to be immune, and may feel it unnecessary to seek advice on disease prevention. Many asylum seekers and new immigrants rely on social support but still have problems accessing health services. Pre-travel health advice services are clinic-based and the majority charge for their services. VFR travelers often do not recognize the risks associated with travel, or appreciate the cost/benefit of pre-travel advice and prophylaxis. Also, they may not have confidence in the service and rapport with the health personnel. Language barriers, bureaucracy in the health system, anxiety over immigration status, and ignorance of rights to health services are some of the non-economic

©2012 Elsevier Inc
DOI: 10.1016/B978-1-4557-1076-8.00031-4

reasons why this population may fail to use a travel health service when planning to travel. Most pre-travel health services are accustomed to dealing with the leisure and business traveler, and it is often difficult for those in such practices to adjust for the language and culture of the many diverse and small ethnic groups within a community. Also, this unequal focus of services has led to delays in the treatment of ill returned travelers and can contribute to more severe pathology in this group.

Barriers to Protecting VFR Travelers

- Lack of perception of risk
- Belief that risk of disease is not present
- Lack of awareness of availability of health services
- Language/cultural barriers
- Structural barriers (no travel clinics located nearby)
- Ineffective written materials (not language-appropriate; inappropriate literacy level)
- Financial barriers (including insurance coverage)
- Fear of authorities
- Healthcare professionals' lack of knowledge of VFRs' disease risk and prevention during travel
- Differences in belief systems, including belief in control over one's destiny.

Epidemiology of Travel by VFRs

In the UK, 7.5% of the total population are foreign-born. In 2009, of the 58.6 million visits made by UK citizens abroad, 11.6 million (19.8%) were made by VFRs. Of the 1.1 million visits to sub-Saharan Africa, 36% were undertaken by VFRs, and of 1.4 million visits to the Indian subcontinent 61% were made by VFRs. In the USA in 2009, 49% of the more than 30 million plane trips overseas were made for the purpose of visiting friends and relatives. Overall, VFR travelers now make up nearly half of all visits to disease-endemic areas and have the highest proportion of health problems of all groups of travelers. VFRs stay for longer periods than other groups of visitors, which may be important in their risk exposure to health hazards. Data on the epidemiology of imported hepatitis A, typhoid, malaria, tuberculosis, and HIV help to define important risk factors for different groups of travelers.

Hepatitis A

Hepatitis A virus (HAV) is responsible for roughly 50% of acute hepatitis cases in the USA. Travel is identified as a risk factor in 5–20% of all reported cases in the USA and the UK. Transmission of this RNA picornavirus is by fecal contamination of water or food. In developing countries most children have developed antibodies to HAV by the age of 5 years, although there are high socioeconomic strata of society where children remain susceptible to infection because exposure is limited. Also, as the standard of living improves in developing countries, the age distribution of hepatitis A is shifting to the adult population. A study in New Delhi, India, involving a cross-section of socioeconomic classes, showed that 41% of those between 25 and 35 years of age were still susceptible to hepatitis A.[3] This pattern of reduced transmission is also reflected in the dramatic reduction in hepatitis A risk for travelers, which has fallen nearly 50 fold.[4]

In the developed countries of Europe, parts of North America (except for the Arctic), Japan, and Australia, exposure to HAV is uncommon. The majority of the adult population is antibody negative and therefore susceptible to infection. Those born after 1945 have a HAV-antibody prevalence <20% in many industrialized countries. Adult immigrants born in a developing country are often immune, whereas their children born in a developed country are susceptible to HAV infection. Young children rarely develop clinical symptoms after exposure to HAV, but adults have symptomatic evidence of infection However, in a UK study by Behrens et al.,[5] children under 15 years of age from VFR families traveling to the Indian subcontinent appeared to be twice as likely to develop symptomatic hepatitis A as older travelers. In the same study, ethnic travelers were eight times more likely to develop hepatitis A than tourists or other travelers. This study revealed that the majority of travel-associated cases of hepatitis A (60%) were contracted on the Indian subcontinent. The finding that young VFR travelers developed clinical hepatitis A was unexpected. A recent report from the UK Health Protection Agency stated that VFR travel to Pakistan and other countries in the Indian subcontinent was responsible for the majority of cases of imported hepatitis A.[6]

A review of cases of hepatitis A from The Netherlands revealed a striking seasonal fluctuation in the incidence of HAV over a 5-year period.[7] In the autumn, there was a significant increase in the number of pediatric cases of HAV in Moroccan and Turkish children; these infections were acquired in the summer holiday during visits to relatives in their parents' country of origin. The authors also reported a temporal increase in cases of HAV in adult Dutch citizens in The Netherlands following the seasonal increase in infections in children, and suggested that this was a result of secondary transmission from the imported primary pediatric cases.

A recent review of imported hepatitis A among Swedish travelers between the years 1997 and 2005 found that 55% of all imported cases occurred among VFRs.[8] In the age group 0–14 years, the corresponding figure was 88%. Among Danish travelers, 78% of hepatitis A cases reported between 1980 and 2007 occurred in VFRs, yet only 8% of Danish people are first- or second-generation immigrants.[9] This highlights the disproportionate burden of hepatitis A among VFR travelers, and suggests a rate of infection that is 11 000 times higher in VFRs than native Danes.

Children of immigrant parents are likely to be more vulnerable to hepatitis A for three reasons: the child does not receive pre-travel counseling and immunization; the overseas living conditions are more unhygienic than those encountered by tourists and business travelers; and the contact children make with the local population and environment is more direct and sustained.

Enteric Fever

Most cases of typhoid fever in North America, Europe, and Australia are associated with travel, and it is becoming increasingly clear that VFR travelers are at highest risk. Reports show that 37–91% of travel-associated typhoid fever cases result from travel to the Indian subcontinent (ISC), including Pakistan, India, and Bangladesh.[10] The risk of typhoid among US travelers to the Indian subcontinent is 18 times greater than that to other regions of the world; for foreign-born US citizens the risk is increased by a further 25%.[11] In the UK in 2007, 88% of travel-associated enteric fever cases involved VFR travel[8] (Fig. 31.1). In the USA, VFRs made up a similar high proportion (77%) of reported cases of imported typhoid fever, of which 25% occurred in children.[12] Healthcare presentations with enteric fever have been reported to be seven times more likely among VFRs than in tourist travelers.[13] In contrast to the previous citing of secondary transmission of hepatitis A, there are no reported secondary cases of typhoid.

Malaria

Malaria is one of the most important infectious diseases acquired by travelers to sub-Saharan Africa. This region has the largest global burden of falciparum malaria, and the risk of transmission has been estimated to range from approximately 0.1% per visit to Zimbabwe to as high as 1.7% per visit to Nigeria.[14] Although falciparum malaria from sub-Saharan Africa makes up the largest portion of imported malaria, there is still a small and declining proportion of malaria imported from the Indian subcontinent into the UK.[15]

The surveillance network TropNetEurope reported that 50% of *P. falciparum* cases identified at European sites within this network occurred in VFR travelers.[16] GeoSentinel, the surveillance network of

the International Society of Travel Medicine (ISTM), and Centers for Disease Control and Prevention (CDC), reporting from a wider geographic base, have identified that 35% of malaria cases reported occurred in VFRs.[17] In the US in 2009, 26% of 997 cases of malaria occurred among non-US residents, and of the 701 US civilians with malaria for whom the purpose of travel was known, 63% occurred among those who had traveled for the purpose of visiting friends and relatives.[18] A review of the 39 300 cases of malaria reported to the National Malaria Reference Laboratory surveillance data in the UK between 1987 and 2006 found that 72% of all malaria and 96% of *P. falciparum* infections were acquired in sub-Saharan Africa (mainly Nigeria and Ghana).[19] When cases were stratified by reason for travel, 64.5% malaria occurred among travelers visiting friends and relatives. VFR travelers visiting Africa had a 3.7-fold greater risk of acquiring malaria than other travelers, and for VFR travelers to South Asia there was a 7.7 times greater risk. Recent data from the UK in 2008 (Table 31.1) show that the risk differential of VFRs to West Africa remains the same (3.5 times higher), but the differential for UK VFRs to India has fallen to double that of non-VFRs to India.

Children traveling as VFRs have at least as great a risk of malaria infection as adult ethnic travelers. In a review of pediatric malaria in the UK, 15% of all imported malaria cases between 1990 and 1995 were in children (< 15 years of age).[20] The majority of cases were in VFRs visiting West Africa, and only 50% were taking chemoprophylaxis. A more recent review suggested that 15–85% of pediatric cases of malaria imported into Europe occurred among immigrants, and that VFR was the most common reason for travel.[21]

Another significant contributing factor influencing VFRs' risk of acquiring malaria when traveling to areas of high transmission is their inadequate use of chemoprophylaxis. In a study of malaria among returned travelers, 28% of ethnic travelers used chemoprophylaxis compared with 75% reported usage in tourists with malaria.[22] A similarly low proportion (31%) of Canadian residents of South Indian origin traveling to India intended taking chemoprophylaxis, in spite of the fact that many believed themselves to be at risk.[23] In a study from Brescia,[24] the authors reported that only 11% of migrants started chemoprophylaxis, compared to 55% of non-migrants. The National Analysis of Italian Malaria Cases supports this dismal picture, with 36% of non-migrant and 4% of ethnic travelers using regular prophylaxis during travel to malarious areas.

Even among VFRs who take malaria prophylaxis, there is evidence that their adherence to the prescribed regimen is poorer than for tourist travelers.[25] In a study of malaria risk perception and knowledge among VFR travelers of African ethnicity living in Paris and visiting their country of origin in sub-Saharan Africa, adequate chemoprophylaxis practices (correct drug, dosage, and adherence, including after return) were reported by only 29%.[26] This rate of compliance observed among VFRs is lower than rates observed among European travelers to malaria-endemic countries of 35–63%.[27,28] Three reasons for inadequate chemoprophylaxis were identified: insufficient malaria risk

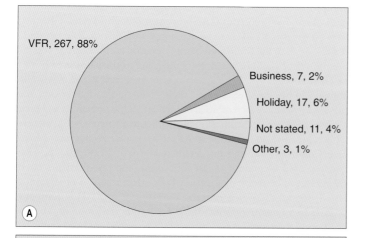

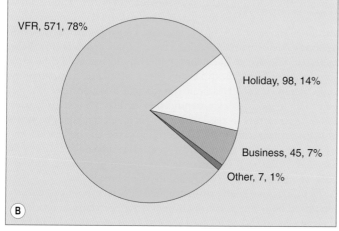

Figure 31.1 Travel-associated cases of enteric fever **(A)** and malaria **(B)** by reason for travel, England, Wales and Northern Ireland, 2007. Taken from Foreign travel-associated illness – a focus on those visiting friends and relatives, 2008 report. Health Protection Agency, UK.

Table 31.1 The Incidence of Malaria in UK Residents Visiting West Africa, India and SE Asia in 2008

	SE Asia	West Africa		India	
	All	All others	VFR	All others	VFR
UK visits	1 512 955	112 952	139 663	517 877	438 93
Malaria case reports	4	115	498	21	39
Incidence cases: 10 000 visits	0.03	10	36	0.41	0.89

(Surveillance data provided courtesy of the Malaria Reference Laboratory, and numbers of travelers provided by the International Passenger Survey, Office for National Statistics, UK. Available online at http://www.statistics.gov.uk/ssd/surveys/international_passenger_survey.asp)

perception; negligence; and absence of the drug after return to France, often because the drugs were left for relatives in Africa. Among reported cases of malaria imported from sub-Saharan Africa to the UK between 1999 and 2006, only 7% of people visiting friends or relatives in their own or their families' country of origin reported having used recommended drugs, compared to 24% of people traveling for other reasons.[19]

The reasons for lack of use of prophylaxis in this high-risk group are likely to be multifactorial. Cost is one issue considered to contribute to the low level of use of malaria chemoprophylaxis by VFRs in the UK.[29] Another contributing factor to low prophylaxis use is lack of knowledge about methods available to prevent malaria. This may relate to lack of awareness of the need to seek health advice before travel, incorrect advice given, or inaccurate beliefs about susceptibility to or risk of malaria in the destination country. Of the ethnic travelers studied on departure from Canada for India, only 54% had sought advice and just one-third planned to use chemoprophylaxis.[23] Only 7% had been prescribed an appropriate regimen, confirming the poor quality of advice being given by some health professionals.

In a population-based study of knowledge, attitudes, and practices of foreign-born Italian citizens, 70% were aware of how malaria was transmitted. Of those who had traveled home to a malarious region, only 18% had sought pre-travel advice; 52% of the total group were unaware of the malaria risk at their destination, and 40% were ignorant of suitable protective measures against infection. The majority of those who had traveled had not taken prophylactic measures on their journey.[24] In a French study of VFRs of African ethnicity visiting their country of origin in sub-Saharan Africa, 26% failed to mention mosquito bites, instead providing incorrect responses such as water transmission, poor personal hygiene, and sun exposure.[26]

Partial immunity to malaria in VFRs and migrant travelers appears to persist for a period after departure from an endemic area, thereby providing some initial protection against severe and fatal disease despite their lack of use of chemoprophylaxis. In two Italian studies, the case-fatality rate for non-immune Italians travelers was 1.6% nationally and 3% in Lombardy, whereas no deaths were reported in the migrant travelers and VFR groups. In the UK, case-fatality rates between 1987 and 2004 were 1.6 deaths/1000 malaria cases in VFRs and 11.7 deaths/1000 malaria cases in tourists; the highest rates were seen in business travelers at 17 deaths/1000 cases (Malaria Reference Laboratory, personal communication). However, the partial protection wanes as time since last exposure to malaria increases. This has been highlighted by a review of malaria cases occurring in African children in Verona, where those who had recently immigrated presented with significantly lower parasitemia, significantly higher platelet counts, shorter parasitemia clearance time and shorter duration of fever than children with malaria who were VFR travelers.[30] In the 2010 annual review of imported malaria in the United States , of patients for whom reason for travel was known, 53% of the severe cases were in VFR travelers.[31] This shows that the threat of severe malaria among VFRs is real, and if a false sense of security among this population has developed it must be dispelled. VFRs must be educated that, as time outside the endemic malaria zone increases, they may become susceptible to severe disease. In practical terms, malaria immunity starts to wane from about 6 months after leaving an endemic zone, and by about 12 months the risk of symptomatic malaria starts to increase.

The imported malaria in many parts of Europe is unlikely to be reduced until the problem of malaria among ethnic travelers is resolved. New and improved chemoprophylaxis regimens are unlikely to have an impact on the pattern of imported malaria, or malaria in individuals who do not have access to sources of these drug regimens. Further research is needed on the behavioral practices of ethnic travel-

ers so that culturally appropriate and practical strategies can be tested and implemented effectively. A community-based intervention program is likely to be the most effective approach to improve knowledge, attitudes, and practices, thereby leading to the enhanced use of pre-travel services.

HIV and Sexually Transmitted Diseases

Although the African ethnic group makes up approximately 0.4% of the total population of the UK,[32] it carries a disproportionate burden of HIV in the country. In the year 2000, 30% of cases were reported to be in black Africans, and 70% of all cases were in one of the many minority ethnic groups.[33] De Cock estimated that the relative risk of acquiring infection during travel in African adults and children was respectively 20 and 355 times higher than in non-African equivalent groups living in the UK. There is evidence of similar high incidence rates of gonorrhea in Afro-Caribbean men living in Leeds, UK: they were 54 times more likely to be diagnosed with this sexually transmitted disease than the white population.[34] Fenton and colleagues[35] examined travel of London-based black Africans to their home countries in Central Africa, and the acquisition of new sexual partners while abroad: 44.5% had returned to their country of origin within the previous 5 years. A total of 40% of men and 21% of women acquired a new sexual partner while abroad. Predictors of new sexual partners while abroad included prior sexual activity with a large number of sexual partners, and previous STDs in the UK. In this group, 42% had not used a condom at last intercourse and one-third perceived themselves to be at risk of acquiring HIV. More than 2% of randomly tested, recently returned travelers were found to be HIV antibody positive in a London hospital, in part reflecting the group of travelers (VFRs and migrants exposed during travel). In this study, a significant risk factor for infection was the patient's place of birth in East, Central, or Southern Africa.[36] The role of travel and risk of HIV is an important one for all travelers: 23% of UK men and 17% of women aged 17–24 have new sexual partners during travel. Ethnic travelers may be at increased risk due to their longer journey, increased likelihood of sexual activity during the trip because of social links to the community, and wider use of local healthcare (for example injections), all of which may lead to potential for transmission of blood-borne pathogens. Recent sero-surveys in the UK have highlighted the high prevalence of heterosexually acquired HIV infections in the UK population who were born abroad, with 63% of new HIV infections in 2009 in England, Wales, and Northern Ireland occurring in black Africans, 68% of whom had acquired their infection abroad.[37]

Hepatitis B infection may be acquired through exposure to infected blood and body fluids. For the reasons described above in relation to transmission of HIV, VFR travelers may be at increased risk of hepatitis B infection. In addition, transmission of hepatitis B within families without a clear documented exposure has been described, and VFRs may have increased exposure to the local population.[38] Hepatitis B transmission in The Netherlands appears to be predominantly heterosexual; however, in 60% of heterosexual cases the source of infection was a partner originating from a hepatitis B-endemic region.

Interventions to address the hazards presented to VFRs by blood-borne pathogens need to be developed and evaluated to ensure effectiveness. They will almost certainly need to be targeted at individual cultural and ethnic groups, rather than consisting of a broad shotgun approach to the problem.

Tuberculosis (TB) in Ethnic Groups

There are considerably more data on the prevalence and risk factors of travel-associated tuberculosis as it relates to immigration. As this is

Table 31.2 Positive Tuberculin Skin Test Correlates in Children Who Travel from the USA to Tuberculosis-Endemic Countries (>100/100 000) or Have Visitors from Endemic Countries

Factor	Odds Ratio (95% Confidence Interval) Multiple Logistic Regression		
	All Children	Born in the US	No BCG
Travel to	3.9 (1.9–7.9)*	4.7 (2.0–11.2)*	5.9 (2.5–13.6)*
Visitor from	2.4 (1.0–5.5)*	3.3 (1.1–10.2)*	2.6 (0.8–8.2)*
Female	1.8 (1.0–3.2)*	2.6 (1.2–6.2)*	3.2 (1.4–7.2)*
BCG	0.8 (0.3–2.2)	12.0 (3.9–36.7)*	NA
Prior TST	0.8 (0.4–1.4)	0.4 (0.2–1.0)	0.7 (0.3–1.5)

*$p < 0.05$.

Lobato & Hopewell. Am J Respiratory and Critical Care Medicine 1998.

a notifiable disease, these data are collected with discipline and detail. In both the USA and Europe there has been an increase in the proportion of cases of tuberculosis in foreign-born individuals. In the US in 2006, 57% of all TB cases and 31% of children and adolescents were in foreign-born populations. Migrants arriving from countries in sub-Saharan Africa have the largest impact on overall TB rates in European countries and in the US,[39,40] and within 2 years of arrival 28% develop a clinical disease. In Europe during 2005, TB in foreign-born individuals from high endemic areas constituted 78%, 73%, and 71% of all cases in Norway, Sweden, and the UK, respectively.

The risk of acquisition of tuberculosis through travel is difficult to assess. Two studies have VFR travel as a risk factor for tuberculosis. In 1984 McCarthy published a retrospective review of tuberculosis in Asians in West Ham, UK. Between 1976 and 1980, 246 cases occurred, of whom 71 (29%) had returned home. When the groups were assessed, almost twice as many cases occurred in those who had returned to visit Asia but had had no TB exposure in the UK as in those who had had exposure to TB in the UK and no history of travel to Asia.[41] Lobato and Hopewell[42] studied children who had traveled from the US to TB-endemic countries using a case–control study and examining tuberculin skin test conversion (Table 31.2). Children who had traveled to TB-endemic regions in the previous 12 months (>100/1 000 000 population rate) were 3.9 times more likely to have a positive skin test than those who had not traveled. In addition, children born in the US who had traveled had a 4.7 odds ratio of a positive skin test. A positive skin test was also found more significantly in children in whose household a visitor had arrived from a country having a high prevalence of TB. No evidence was found of skin conversion in foreign-born children who traveled. There are likely to be many other factors that will affect and influence high rates of tuberculosis in ethnic groups, including the numbers of visits made by relatives from highly endemic countries and the targeted screening of some categories of immigrants on entry to the USA, Australia, and Europe.

Approaches to the VFR Pre-Travel Consultation

Several reviews have addressed travel issues for those returning with families to their countries of origin.[43,44] We will address some of the issues that are important for pre-travel consultation with VFR travelers and their families, and discuss possible approaches to the consultation.

Improving Access to Pre-Travel Services

Opportunities must be sought to engage VFR travelers in pre-travel care. Educating primary care providers about the possibility of travel among their ethnic and foreign-born patients is a first step, so that travel preparation can be viewed as part of routine services for immigrant patients. In this way, the patient can be informed of the need to seek services when travel is planned. Similarly, providers can develop expertise, or a referral network, to provide optimal pre-travel consultation. Community initiatives, such as radio shows in Haitian Creole discussing necessary pre-travel interventions before the holiday travel period (Nicole Prudent, personal communication), providing information regarding the need for pre-travel advice at community-based ethnic events, and other innovative community-based interventions can play an important role in educating travelers. For settings in which there are many immigrant families, a designated health professional in each office might take on the role of local travel medicine 'expert' and gather information for patients, develop personal expertise in travel medicine, and arrange for needed vaccines to be available on site. Primary care sites offering travel medicine services on site, without the need for referral to a separate site or clinic, would increase access to these services. Clinics serving patients who travel frequently to specific parts of the world might consider holding group travel preparation sessions.

Language barriers can impair the ability to provide appropriate pre-travel advice. When healthcare professionals fluent in the patient's language are unavailable, medically trained interpreters are desirable. Ideally, handouts should be provided in the patient's language, and it should be ascertained whether the patient is comfortable reading that language. If the consultation is not in the patient's first language, literacy level should be tactfully assessed before assuming that handouts would be helpful. Ideally, medications should be labeled in the patient's most fluent language. Handouts in multiple languages prepared by William Stauffer and colleagues in Minnesota are available and can be found at http://www.tropical.umn.edu (under travel handouts), or http://www.tropical.umn.edu/TTM/VFR/index.htm.

Routine Immunizations

Updating routine immunizations is an important part of the pre-travel consultation. Although VFR travelers are likely to have received routine immunizations against diseases such as tetanus, measles, and polio in their home countries, they may not have been immunized against varicella, influenza, or pneumococcal disease. Infants traveling to regions with risk of measles transmission can receive a dose of MMR vaccine as early as 6 months of age. If the vaccine is administered before the optimal time, parents must be warned that the routine MMR should be repeated when it is due according to the standard schedule. Hepatitis B vaccine is beginning to be incorporated into routine immunization schedules, but many VFRs may not have benefited from these recent changes. Hepatitis B vaccine is particularly important for VFR children, who are at highest risk for chronic carriage and acquisition from close contact with child carriers in developing countries. Another challenge for VFR travelers may be difficulty in producing documents indicating receipt of routine vaccines. Travel medicine providers can assist in providing durable documents for use in other settings.

Travel-Specific Immunizations

All travelers should be offered vaccines appropriate for their destination according to standard sources of pre-travel advice and information. As discussed earlier in this chapter, VFRs are likely to be at increased risk of some diseases, but may be more likely to be immune to others. An approach to travel medicine counseling that takes into account these differences is likely to be of most benefit to the traveler.

Table 31.3 Travel Vaccines – Special Considerations for VFRs

Vaccine	Considerations in VFRs	Approach to Management
Hepatitis A	Adults more likely to be immune; children may be at increased risk due to increased exposures relative to non-VFR travelers	Consider sero-testing for adults before immunizing; provide documentation of sero-status
Typhoid	Increased risk of disease	Consider immunization even for trips of short duration; counsel about food and water precautions
Yellow fever	May have immunity due to previous disease or immunization; but testing not available routinely	Inquire about availability of prior vaccine records; immunize per current recommendations
Japanese encephalitis	May have immunity due to previous disease or immunization; but testing not available routinely	Immunize per current recommendations
Meningococcal disease	May be at increased risk due to increased contact with the local population; increased risk for travel to the Hajj	Consider immunization with the conjugate polysaccharide quadrivalent vaccine
Rabies	May be at increased risk due to increased exposure to infected animals; children may be at particular risk	Consider pre-exposure prophylaxis; counsel about management of animal bites/exposures
Hepatitis B	May be at increased risk of disease due to increased contact with local population during travel and lower immunization rates against hepatitis B	Offer hepatitis B vaccine to those who are non-immune; screen for hepatitis B infection before immunizing in patients from endemic countries

Table 31.3 lists travel vaccines and special considerations in VFR travelers.

VFRs are more likely to have pre-existing antibody to hepatitis A and are candidates for sero-testing before immunizing with hepatitis A vaccine. This strategy has been examined by several studies and has been found to be cost-effective when prevalence of immunity is above cut-off values that depend on the relative costs of vaccine and sero-testing.[45] Seroprevalence rates of antibody to hepatitis A generally exceed values required for cost-effectiveness in adult VFRs.[46] Logistical and financial challenges may exist that impede efforts to perform the cost-effective strategy of testing before immunizing. For example, the patient's insurance may pay for the vaccine but not sero-testing, or the patient may be unable to return for a second visit to receive vaccine should sero-testing indicate lack of antibody. Still, for VFR travelers, consideration should be given to screening before immunization with hepatitis A vaccine. Providing the traveler with adequate explanation and documentation to indicate presumed lifelong protection against hepatitis A will facilitate subsequent pre-travel consultation.

VFRs are at increased risk of typhoid, especially those traveling to the Indian subcontinent, and provision of typhoid vaccine is sensible for these travelers. For travelers to other destinations, offering typhoid vaccine to those who will be at increased risk by virtue of living circumstances, duration of travel, or exposure to contaminated food and water, is indicated. These factors may be present more commonly for VFR travelers.

Exposure to vector-borne vaccine-preventable diseases such as yellow fever and Japanese encephalitis may be greater for VFR travelers owing to length of stay and living circumstances. VFR travelers may also be at decreased risk for yellow fever if they are protected through prior immunization. In the absence of documentation of previous immunization, VFR travelers should be immunized according to current recommendations.

VFR travelers may be at increased risk of meningococcal disease because of increased exposure to local populations who may be carriers of the bacterium. This risk has been described for visitors to the *Hajj* in Mecca, Saudi Arabia.[47] Still, the risk of meningococcal disease is very low for all travelers, and standard recommendations are appropriate. Children in some countries now receive routine immunization

with meningococcal conjugate vaccines; it must be kept in mind that not all such vaccines include serogroup A, the most common epidemic strain in sub-Saharan Africa.

Risk of exposure to rabies is present in many parts of the world. All travelers should be told of rabies risk and offered pre-exposure prophylaxis if exposure may be long or high risk. This is particularly of concern for children, who are the highest risk for animal bites. Even more important is a discussion of a plan to follow should a rabies exposure occur, including first-aid treatment and the need for both rabies immunoglobulin and vaccination. Owing to the high cost of the vaccine, VFR travelers may be less likely to be vaccinated against rabies or to have evacuation insurance or other means of traveling to sites where appropriate care can be obtained.

Malaria Prevention

Although VFR travelers are clearly at risk of malaria, there may be significant barriers to the use of preventive measures. Travelers may have beliefs about specific antimalarials, or may not feel they are necessary because of faith in their own immunity. Such medications may be prohibitively expensive, or may not be covered by insurance plans. Discussions about malaria prevention need to include information that permits travelers to make informed decisions for themselves and their families. For example, it may be important to discuss the problem of waning immunity after long stays away from the home country, the risk of severe disease in non-foreign-born children, and the reason why antimalarials being prescribed may not be the familiar ones used in a patient's country of origin. Use of personal protective measures to prevent insect bites can be discussed in a way that emphasizes disease prevention as well as prevention of the annoying sound of mosquitoes at night, or the discomfort of multiple bites.

General Travel Advice

Pre-travel advice must be given with sensitivity for VFR travelers. Focusing on behaviors that will promote a healthy or more comfortable trip (bed-nets and repellents, food and water precautions) may be more effective than discussions about increased risks of travel to the destination country. Travelers can be asked about health problems encountered on previous trips: those who have suffered malaria or severe diarrhea are usually highly motivated to seek and follow health advice before travel. Eliciting from the traveler a description of the living circumstances during travel, if known, will help to focus the discussion on specific health promotion behaviors and strategies. One common situation is when a spouse or potential spouse, born and raised in a developed country, is taken to meet family members. They may feel awkward about asking for special measures to be taken, such as the need to boil drinking water. Empowering travelers with specific strategies (invoking 'allergies', doctor's instructions, etc.) to deal with these situations can be extremely helpful. VFR families may be advised about the situation of children brought up in developed countries who have not built up immunity to certain diseases, and therefore need additional protective measures.

Families often appreciate written or pictorial materials. Care should be taken that these are language or literacy level-appropriate. Attention should be paid to the fact that families may be influenced by the opinions of senior members of the family or the community, and care may need to be taken when such opinions include incorrect or unhelpful information. If there are specific foods or cultural practices associated with increased risk of disease, time should be taken to describe means of reducing risk in such circumstances. For example, handshaking is important in many cultures, often in settings where no soap and water are available. Carrying alcohol-based or other antiseptic hand rubs may be a good solution. Another frequent problem is when travelers are offered potentially contaminated food or water; working with travelers to formulate strategies to handle these awkward situations may be extremely useful. In addition, medication for self-treatment of common travel-related problems such as travelers' diarrhea should be supplied to VFRs, and the reasons for not relying on locally manufactured medicines (e.g., counterfeit drugs, antibiotic resistance) should be explained.

Information about general safety, especially with respect to transportation, is appropriate for VFRs. Discussion about seat belt use, helmet use when motorcycles are used for transport of adults and children, and where the safest seats are in public vehicles, may be helpful. Most important of all is the need to discourage VFRs from traveling by road in rural areas after dark because of the potential poor quality of the drivers, vehicles, and roads.

Conclusion

VFRs have the highest morbidity from infectious diseases, including typhoid, hepatitis A, malaria, tuberculosis, and HIV. These increased risks appear to be associated with decreased access to pre-travel healthcare, beliefs about susceptibility to infection, and living circumstances during travel. This pattern of morbidity is being increasingly recognized, but there is still a lack of data on the major contributing factors to the problem. Improvements in travel medicine practice, including the development of new antimalarial drugs and novel vaccines, have been of little benefit to this group of travelers, as can be seen from the increasing trend of morbidity. Efforts to improve access to pre-travel services and adapt information provided to the languages and cultures of ethnic travelers have the potential to yield measurable benefits for VFR travelers.

Acknowledgment

We recognize the contribution made by Elizabeth Barnett to the earlier chapter on VFRs.

References

1. CDC Travelers' Health Yellow Book, 2012. Chapter 8: VFRs: Immigrants returning home to visit friends and relatives. (Accessed at http://wwwnc.cdc.gov/travel/yellowbook/2012/chapter-8-advising-travelers-with-specific-needs/immigrants-returning-home-to-visit-friends-and-relatives-vfrs.htm.)
2. Barnett ED, MacPherson DW, Stauffer WM, et al. The visiting friends or relatives traveler in the 21st century: time for a new definition. J Travel Med 2010;17:163–70.
3. Das K, Jain A, Gupta S, et al. The changing epidemiological pattern of hepatitis A in an urban population of India: Emergence of a trend similar to the European countries. Eur J Epidemiol 2000;16:507–10.
4. Mutsch M, Spicher V, Gut C, et al. Hepatitis A virus infections in travelers, 1988–2004. Clin Infect Dis 2006;42:490–7.
5. Behrens RH, Collins M, Botto B, Heptonstall J. Risk for British travelers of acquiring hepatitis A. BMJ 1995;311:193.
6. Foreign travel-associated illness – a focus on those visiting friends and relatives, 2008 report. Health Protection Agency, UK.
7. Termorshuizen F, Van De Laar MJW. Epidemiology of hepatitis A in the Netherlands, 1957–1998. Nederlands Tijdschrift voor Geneeskunde 1998;142:2364–8.
8. Askling HH, Rombo L, Andersson Y, et al. Hepatitis A risk in travelers. J Travel Med 2009;16:233–8.
9. Nielsen US, Larsen CS, Howitz M, et al. Hepatitis A among Danish travelers 1980–2007. J Infection 2009;58:47–52.
10. Caumes E, Belanger F, Brucker G, et al. Diseases observed after return from travels outside Europe. 109 cases. Presse Medicale 1991;20:1483–6.
11. Mermin JH, Townes JM, Gerber M, et al. Typhoid fever in the United States, 1985–1994: changing risks of international travel and increasing antimicrobial resistance. Arch Intern Med 1998;158:633–8.
12. Steinberg EB, Frisch A, Rossiter S, et al. Typhoid fever in travelers: who should we vaccinate? In: 49th Annual Meeting of the American Society of Tropical Medicine and Hygiene; 2000; 2000. p. 158–9.
13. Leder K, Tong S, Weld L, et al. Illness in travelers visiting friends and relatives: a review of the GeoSentinel Surveillance Network. Clin Infect Dis 2006;43:1185–93.
14. Muentener P, Schlagenhauf P, Steffen R. Imported malaria (1985–95): Trends and perspectives. Bul World Health Org 1999;77:560–6.
15. Behrens RH, Bisoffi Z, Bjorkman A, et al. Malaria prophylaxis policy for travelers from Europe to the Indian Subcontinent. Malar J 2006;5:7.
16. Jelinek T, Schulte C, Behrens R, et al. Imported Falciparum malaria in Europe: sentinel surveillance data from the European network on surveillance of imported infectious diseases. Clin Infect Dis 2002;34: 572–6.
17. Leder K, Black J, O'Brien D, et al. Malaria in travelers: a review of the GeoSentinel surveillance network. Clin Infect Dis 2004;39:1104–12.
18. Centers for Disease Control and Prevention. Malaria Surveillance – United States, 2007. MMWR 2009;58.
19. Smith AD, Bradley DJ, Smith V, et al. Imported malaria and high risk groups: observational study using UK surveillance data 1987–2006. BMJ 2008;337:a120.
20. Brabin BJ, Ganley Y. Imported malaria in children in the UK. Arch Dis Child 1997;77:76–81.
21. Ladhani S, Aibara RJ, Riordan FA, et al. Imported malaria in children: a review of clinical studies. Lancet Infect Dis 2007;7:349–57.
22. Behrens RH, Curtis CF. Malaria in travelers: Epidemiology and prevention. Brit Med Bull 1993;49:363–81.
23. Dos Santos CC, Anvar A, Keystone JS, et al. Survey of use of malaria prevention measures by Canadians visiting India. Can Med Assoc J 1999;160:195–200.
24. Castelli F, Matteelli A, Caligaris S, et al. Malaria in migrants. Parassitologia 1999;41:261–5.
25. Joshi MS, Lalvani A. 'Home from home': Risk perceptions, malaria and the use of chemoprophylaxis among UK South Asians. Ethn Health 2010;15:365–75.
26. Pistone T, Guibert P, Gay F, et al. Malaria risk perception, knowledge and prophylaxis practices among travelers of African ethnicity living in Paris and

visiting their country of origin in sub-Saharan Africa. T Roy Soc Trop Med H 2007;101:990–5.

27. Hamer DH, Connor BA. Travel health knowledge, attitudes and practices among United States travelers. J Travel Med 2004;11:23–6.

28. Malvy D, Pistone T, Rezvani A, et al. Risk of malaria among French adult travelers. Travel Med Infect Dis 2006;4:259–69.

29. Badrinath P, Ejidokun OO, Barnes N, et al. Change in NHS regulations may have caused increase in malaria. BMJ 1998;316:1746–7.

30. Mascarello M, Allegranzi B, Angheben A, et al. Imported malaria in adults and children: Epidemiological and clinical characteristics of 380 consecutive cases observed in Verona, Italy. J Travel Med 2008;15:229–36.

31. CDC Malaria surveillance United States–2010. MMWR 2010;6:1–17.

32. Office of Population Censuses and Surveys. The 1991 census; 1993.

33. Anonymous. AIDS and HIV infection in the United Kingdom: Monthly report. Communicable Diseases Review Weekly 2001;11:11–3.

34. De Cock KM, Low N. HIV and AIDS, other sexually transmitted diseases, and tuberculosis in ethnic minorities in United Kingdom: Is surveillance serving its purpose? BMJ 1997;314:1747–51.

35. Fenton KA, Chinouya M, Davidson O, et al. HIV transmission risk among sub-Saharan Africans in London traveling to their countries of origin. AIDS 2001;15:1442–5.

36. Hawkes S, Malin A, Araru T, et al. HIV infection among heterosexual travelers attending the Hospital for Tropical Diseases, London. Genitourin Med 1992;68:309–11.

37. HIV in the United Kingdom: 2010 Report. Health Protection Agency. (Accessed at http://www.hpa.org.uk/web/HPAwebFile/HPAweb_C/1287145367237.)

38. Vernon TM, Wright RA, Kohler PF, Merrill DA. Hepatitis A and B in the family unit. Nonparenteral transmission by asymptomatic children. JAMA 1976;235:2829–31.

39. Gilbert RL, Antoine D, French CE, et al. The impact of immigration on tuberculosis rates in the United Kingdom compared with other European countries. Int J Tuberc Lung Dis 2009;13:645–51.

40. Cain KP, Benoit SR, Winston CA, et al. Tuberculosis among foreign-born persons in the United States. JAMA 2008;300:405–12.

41. McCarthy OR. Asian immigrant tuberculosis–the effect of visiting Asia. Brit J Dis Chest 1984;78:248–53.

42. Lobato MN, Hopewell PC. Mycobacterium tuberculosis infection after travel to or contact with visitors from countries with a high prevalence of tuberculosis. Am J Resp Crit Care 1998;158:1871–5.

43. Angell SY, Behrens RH. Risk assessment and disease prevention in travelers visiting friends and relatives. Infect Dis Clin N Am 2005;19:49–65.

44. Bacaner N, Stauffer B, Boulware DR, et al. Travel medicine considerations for North American immigrants visiting friends and relatives. JAMA 2004;291:2856–64.

45. Rubio PP. Critical value of prevalence for vaccination programmes. The case of hepatitis A vaccination in Spain. Vaccine 1997;15:1445–50.

46. Fishbain JT, Eckart RE, Harner KC, et al. Empiric immunisation versus serologic screening: developing a cost-effctive strategy for the use of hepatitis A immunisation in travelers. J Travel Med 2002;9:71–5.

47. Wilder-Smith A, Goh KT, Barkham T, et al. Hajj-associated outbreak strain of Neisseria meningitidis serogroup W135: estimates of the attack rate in a defined population and the risk of invasive disease developing in carriers. Clin Infect Dis 2003;36:679–83.

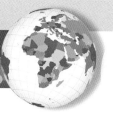

32

Expatriates

Kenneth Gamble, Ted Lankester, Deborah Lovell-Hawker, and Evelyn Sharp

Key points

- During pre-departure appointments, assess current health status, pre-existing health conditions and psychological resilience
- Ensure travelers are fully immunized, and well informed about prevention of malaria and other common conditions in their place of employment
- Cross-cultural training concerning the international assignment and re-entry issues is a priority
- Preparation should include contingency plans for evacuation and repatriation
- Appropriate, well-informed self-care is central to successful health abroad

Expatriate is derived from two Latin words: *ex-* 'out' and *patria* 'native country', and in this chapter it refers to individuals or families who reside in a foreign country for more than 3 months for vocational purposes. In the 29 OECD countries reviewed in a study by the Organization for Economic Cooperation and Development, 36.3 million persons were expatriates from another OECD country.[1] The length of stay necessitates some form of assimilation into the host culture.

There is a large variation in the health support expatriates receive. Many volunteers receive little pre-travel preparation and may have poor access to adequate healthcare abroad. Age, gender, behavior, climate, environmental factors, and exposure to infectious diseases influence risk. Lifestyle, which depends on personality, wealth and available opportunities for risk-taking activities, dramatically influences risk. Occupation location and nationality expose a minority to danger from the violence of extremist groups.[2,3]

Intense, prolonged exposure to physical, environmental, political, and social challenges affects the psychosocial wellbeing of the expatriate. Therefore, screening, preparation, and care before, during, and after the assignment necessitate an integrative model of care.

Understanding the Risks

An understanding of epidemiology helps prioritize preventive measures and affects healthcare strategies.

Morbidity

Surveillance systems designed to monitor health events among expatriates while on assignment have demonstrated similar trends, as shown in Table 32.1.[4,5]

GeoSentinel, a global, provider-based sentinel surveillance system, compiled clinical data from 4039 long-term travelers (trip duration >6 months). Per 1000 travelers, long-term travelers more often experienced chronic diarrhea, giardiasis, *P. falciparum* and *P. vivax* malaria, cutaneous leishmaniasis, schistosomiasis, and *Entamoeba histolytica* diarrhea than their short-term counterparts. Psychological problems, particularly depression and stress, were reported significantly more often, as was the incidence of fatigue lasting >1 month.[6]

Stress

In a survey of 390 missionaries, Parshall[7] found that 97% reported experiencing tension, 88% found anger to be a problem, and 20% had taken tranquilizers.

In another study, 46% of respondents reported that they had experienced a psychological illness of clinical severity either while they were away or on their return home. In 87% of cases the primary diagnosis was depression; 4% of the cases had received a diagnosis of post-traumatic stress disorder.[8]

Premature Attrition

The cost of premature attrition is a major problem. Some 20–40% of all expatriate managers return home early owing to their inability to adjust to the new culture. Moreover, nearly half of those who remain function below their normal level of productivity while working as expatriates.[9]

Mortality Data

Frame[10] and Hargarten[11] observed that vehicle crashes were the leading cause of death among missionaries and Peace Corps Volunteers (PCVs). A recent study of violence among humanitarian workers indicates that attacks against aid workers have increased sharply, and intentional violence was responsible for most of their deaths. The most dangerous location remained the road, and vehicle-based attacks were the most common context for violence.[2]

©2012 Elsevier Inc
DOI: 10.1016/B978-1-4557-1076-8.00032-6

Table 32.1 The Most Commonly Reported Health Problems

Event	Percent Frequency (Per Year)
Diarrheal disease	48
Respiratory illnesses	27
Injuries	20
Skin conditions	19
Psychological	4

Table 32.2 Checklist for Pre-Departure Assessment

Update the immunizations
Evaluate the prophylaxis regimen for persons in malaria endemic regions
   Record adverse reactions if they limit use of specific medications
   Evaluate compliance regimen
   Review personal protection measures
Record relevant history and positive physical findings
Record abnormal laboratory findings
   Provide a management plan for new problems
   Report on long-term problems that were identified
Review health issues that impact placement
   Outline management responsibilities for sending organization

Pre-Departure Assessment

The Purpose of Pre-Departure Assessments

Evidence in the literature on the specifics of pre-travel assessment is sparse. Generally agreed guidelines comprise:

- Risk appraisal
- Counsel regarding appropriate immunization, malaria prophylaxis and minimizing preventable illness
- Third-party health appraisal for sending organizations to circumvent legal liability.

The Sending Organization: Protecting Their Investment

Transition from one country to another interrupts people's connection with their primary care provider, a connection that is fundamental to successful guideline-centered healthcare. Sending organizations have a duty of care toward personnel, since occupational health affects the wellbeing of the taskforce. Thus, shared responsibility for healthcare is essential, and requires cooperation between the expatriate, healthcare professionals and the sending agency.

Candidates may be required to have a 'third-party assessment' by an 'agent'. The sending organization is responsible for defining the purpose of the evaluation; the healthcare provider is responsible for assessing current health, personal, and occupational health risk factors. The employee must grant formal consent before the healthcare provider can release confidential information to the employer. Conclusions and directives should be discussed with the candidate.

When complete, the health assessment should serve to:

- Establish a risk profile for each individual
- Ensure appropriate management of chronic health conditions (e.g., hypertension and diabetes), leading up to the transfer of care when deployed
- Encourage the adoption of appropriate preventive measures related to personal and occupational risk (the individual and healthcare provider's joint responsibility)
- Empower the individual to effect meaningful self-care (Table 32.2).

Pre-Departure Medical Assessment

This assessment is a comprehensive risk appraisal and provides an ideal opportunity to ensure that all candidates receive guideline-centered care.[12] Studies indicate that up to 50% of the general population may not be compliant with national guidelines.[13] Structured health histories and focused physical assessments improve outcomes.[14] Location, duration of stay, and age of the employee determine the content of screening procedures. Management of pre-existing conditions should accord with guidelines in the applicant's country of origin.

Additional testing may be necessary, depending on the nature of the assignment and to ensure compliance with the host government's regulations.

Few conditions absolutely contraindicate cross-cultural assignments. However, many pre-existing ailments – such as cardiac conditions, diabetes mellitus, inflammatory bowel disease, and reactive airway disease – could suddenly change or be exacerbated by environmental conditions or infectious diseases.

Pre-Departure Psychological Assessment

Pre-departure psychological assessments are imperative, given that 20–40% of expatriate managers return home early owing to failure to adjust to the new culture. Similar results have been reported for all overseas employees. Personal and family stress is thought to be the primary cause of early repatriation. Therefore, it is recommended that candidates for cross-cultural assignments have a pre-departure psychological assessment.

A pre-departure psychological assessment will:

- Indicate how the candidate is likely to be affected by living and working in a different culture
- Evaluate the impact of cultural change on the relationship with partner or spouse
- Evaluate the impact of the transition on any children
- Determine any vulnerability to psychological disorders
- Determine coping and resiliency factors
- Foster dialogue
- Guide personnel managers on employee selection and preparations.

Psychological Interview

There should be a reassessment before every new assignment. One study found that approximately 25% of people applying for a new expatriate position were suffering from depression or another psychological condition.[8]

One predictor of an expatriate's adjustment is the spouse's adjustment.[15] If a couple is moving overseas together, it is useful to interview them both separately and together. If the couple has children, assess the whole family. Concern about children is a common cause of early return.

Psychological Interview – When There Is No Time or Expertise

A 'triage' approach could be adopted. Health professionals need to identify and discuss relevant issues and encourage specialist referral if significant issues are present.

Salient issues in an abbreviated psychological interview are:

- Current mental state (e.g., any current symptoms of depression)
- Current stressors, what causes stress and how it is handled (e.g., illness in family, aging parents, recent bereavements/traumas, etc.)
- History of psychiatric or psychological problems (including depression, eating disorders, self-harm, alcohol or drug misuse, psychotic symptoms)
- Symptoms of traumatic stress or other anxiety conditions (obsessive–compulsive tendencies, phobias, panic attacks)
- Any psychological treatment, counseling, antidepressant medication or other psychiatric treatment received
- Family psychiatric history.

Managing The Outcome

Knowledge of vulnerabilities can assist in placement. In some cases it is wise to advise delaying the move until there has been time to engage in cross-cultural training and personal or marital therapy. Moving to a new culture inevitably involves loss; therefore, a delay may also be advisable if the candidate has suffered from a recent bereavement or relationship breakdown. Those who have successfully overcome past difficulties and have developed effective coping strategies may adjust and perform well as expatriates. However, Foyle et al.[16] found that affective disorders among expatriates were associated with a personal history of depressed mood, and a family history of suicide, psychosis, personality disorder, or neuroses. The risk for a relapse is greatest during the first 5 years following a major episode of depression.

When making a psychological referral, clearly identify the issues that are of greatest concern. Is the employee being assigned to a hardship post, a leadership role (e.g., that forced the resignation of the previous leader), or to a politically sensitive region that makes diplomatic skills an essential prerequisite?

The Role of Psychometric Testing

Some psychometric tests might add useful information when used alongside a clinical interview. No one test covers all aspects, and none has yet been reliably validated in cross-cultural settings.

It is essential that these tests are interpreted by someone with expertise, training, and an understanding of the inherent deficiencies.[17]

Pre-Departure: Preparation

Many expatriates report feeling under-prepared for their international assignment,[18] although GeoSentinel found that 70% of long-term travelers had received pre-travel medical advice.[6]

A comprehensive preparation program reduces both psychological and medical problems and reduces attrition. When preparing material on health risks, ask three practical questions:

1. Is it likely to happen?
2. Will your audience recognize the risk when it does happen?
3. Is there a practical solution or management option if it does happen?

Immunizations

Immunization counsel is addressed in Chapters 12 and 13. However, some considerations are particularly relevant for the expatriate community and will be briefly addressed.

Hepatitis A

The hepatitis A vaccine is responsible for a radical reduction in the incidence of hepatitis A among expatriates. Before the widespread availability of this vaccine, the incidence was as high as 17/1000 per month; therefore, a universal immunization program is clearly warranted.

Hepatitis B

Hepatitis B is an established risk for expatriates, with an incidence as high as 1–5% per year. Although largely related to unprotected intercourse in non-monogamous relationships, exposure especially through re-used needles is significant in communities where the prevalence of hepatitis B is high. A prospective study in 124 unvaccinated Dutch missionaries living in Nigeria showed a higher seroconversion rate in children. Attendance at a local school and having a Nigerian child living in the home were cited as risk factors. Given significant risks, the efficacy of the vaccine and the relatively low cost, universal immunization for the expatriate task force and their children is justified.[6]

Japanese Encephalitis

When evaluating the risk of Japanese encephalitis (JE) among travelers, the CDC identified 24 cases, all of whom were expatriates; six died and 50% of the remainder had permanent neurological deficits. Expatriates dwelling in endemic rural areas should be immunized against JE. Residents in urban settings are generally not advised to receive this vaccine. However, consider the cumulative risk of exposure in rural or peri-urban areas.

Rabies

Countries at greatest risk include those in Asia, Africa, and Latin America. Most post-exposure treatment is for dog bites, although the risk should be considered for most mammalian bites. Post-exposure treatment should parallel the risk of exposure, which is approximately 1/1000 volunteers/month among expatriates living in rabies enzootic regions.[19] However, limited data available suggest that in the majority of cases management is suboptimal.

The following should be vaccinated if going to affected regions:

- Families with children
- Families with pets
- Those remote from reliable healthcare
- Personnel in countries where access to human or purified equine rabies immunoglobulin and/or modern tissue culture vaccines is limited
- Personnel who visit or travel into remote regions.

Expatriates should 'streetproof' their children to prevent animal bites.

Malaria

Risk Factors

Malaria (see Chapters 14–17 for details) is the leading cause of death among expatriates who die from infectious diseases, and GeoSentinel found that the risk of malaria was significantly greater in long-term travelers.[6] The infection continues to pose a threat in sub-Saharan Africa, Papua New Guinea and Papua Indonesia (Irian Jaya), where the rate of malaria is at least 10 times greater than in other malarious countries.[20] The incidence of malaria in expatriates ranges from 31/1000 per year in Asia to 209/1000 per year in West Africa.

Myths and Practices Among Expatriates

Seasoned expatriates frequently ignore orthodox medical counsel, instead relying on their own 'experience', untrained advisors, colleagues or anecdotal evidence. Personal protection measures are overlooked and compliance with prophylaxis is poor. Less than 75% of expatriates take the recommended regimen; expatriates frequently change their medication without advice. Among US Army Rangers in Afghanistan, the self-reported compliance rate was 52% for weekly prophylaxis, 41% for terminal chemoprophylaxis, 31% for both weekly and terminal chemoprophylaxis, 82% for treating uniforms with permethrin and 20% for application of insect repellents.[21]

Many judge the value of using prophylaxis on personal experience. Those who have false-positive malaria smears conclude that an appropriate medication is ineffective.

Malaria and Pregnancy

Plasmodium falciparum infection during pregnancy increases the risk of abortion, maternal anemia, intrauterine growth retardation, prematurity, and stillbirth, and is a risk factor for neonatal death. Susceptibility to malaria increases during the second and third trimesters, reaching its peak during the first 60 days postpartum. However, many pregnant expatriates, fearing adverse outcomes, stop their prophylaxis. Risks from mefloquine or other commonly accepted regimens are far less than from malaria. Likewise, mosquito repellents that include DEET are safe during pregnancy.

Malaria Prevention In Children

Children and adolescents are at special risk of malaria, perhaps because of poor compliance or inaccurate calculation of the dose,[22] and may rapidly become seriously ill. Babies, breastfed infants, and children must be protected against mosquito bites (e.g., by sleeping under treated bed-nets) and receive malaria chemoprophylaxis. Children are possibly at greater risk than adults for DEET toxicity, although the complications recorded in the literature, including seizures, are very rare. The American Academy of Pediatrics recommends 30% DEET in children down to 2 months of age.

Self-Diagnosis

Self-diagnostic kits have proved to be accurate and reliable in the hands of laboratory workers but less accurate in the hands of travelers.[23] Motivated expatriates in high-risk settings remote from medical care have a growing comfort with this technology. Self-diagnosis with reliable kits could prove to be a major advance in the management of malaria among expatriates[6] (see Ch. 16).

Tuberculosis

The exponential development of multidrug-resistant tuberculosis is a major concern for expatriates. The incidence of latent mycobacterium tuberculosis is about 3% per year for aid workers and their children, mirroring the infection rate in the host community. The risk for healthcare workers is considerably higher.[24]

The European and North American guidelines are distinctly different. In the UK, BCG vaccination is offered to those without contraindications who are going to a developing country or high-risk location or occupation for >1 month. In North America, BCG is not recommended for adults and is not available through the public health system; however, some advocate the immunization of children under 5.

Diarrheal Diseases

GeoSentinel found that ingestion was the most common attributable route of transmission for diseases in long-term travelers.[6] Expatriates who reside in 'high risk communities' for <2 years are likely to experience attack rates similar to those of short-term travelers.[25] The severity may gradually decrease over time. Variance in the attack rate is related to regional and seasonal deviation and etiologic agents; therefore, expatriate families should be trained to anticipate such and be instructed in self-treatment protocols.

Self-Treatment Regimens for a Range of Infectious Diseases

Provide expatriates with broad-spectrum antibiotics such as levofloxacin or azithromycin, effective against most bacterial infections, if they live in or travel to areas remote from good healthcare. Simplify the regimen to ensure that it will be easy to remember. For example, in adults levofloxacin can be taken as follows:

A. *Above the waist* (respiratory or skin infections): 1 tablet daily for 6 days.

B. *Below the waist* (bowel and bladder infections): 1 tablet, 500 mg, daily for 3 days.

The '6 above and 3 below' rule appears to be easy to follow and gives the expatriate the security of being able to manage most common infections in a reliable manner.

Risk Behavior

Excessive alcohol consumption (see Ch. 47), drug abuse and a high rate of extramarital sexual activity are common amongst expatriates.[26] Peer pressure and expectations, loss of norms, boredom, stress, loneliness, separation from the social support network, spousal separation or avoidance strategies are among reasons cited for these behavioral changes.

Sexually Transmitted Diseases

Sexually transmitted diseases have historically proved to be a major public health challenge. A study of approximately 900 Dutch expatriates living in four different geographic regions showed that 41% of men and 31% of women reported having sex with casual or steady local partners. Of concern is the inconsistent use of condoms, especially among those who had two or more partners.

HIV

HIV transmission is primarily correlated with occupational hazards and sexual activity. Expatriates may need pre-departure HIV testing for visa applications. Consideration should also be given to control programs for blood-borne pathogens, found to be of greater prevalence in long-term travelers.[6]

Infection Control Policies

Guidelines for post-exposure prophylaxis following an occupational health exposure have been carefully crafted and are continually under review. Guidelines on sexual assault have been developed based on similar principles. An increasing number of agencies now provide these kits, but individuals must still take personal responsibility. Aid workers perceived to have a high occupational risk of HIV exposure, including doctors, nurses, and medical students, are encouraged to have access to a 5–7-day starter package, designed for prompt treatment yet providing time to access the complete treatment course. A

28-day supply may be preferable in regions with limited access to antiretroviral agents.

Basic principles include:

- Sending organizations should develop policies regarding all blood-borne pathogens
- Pre-departure training should be provided
- Provisions and protocols should be established for rape and/or sexual exposure, and occupational exposure
- Protocols should be regularly updated in accordance with international guidelines.

Health Briefing: Possible Structure

Most personnel assigned to an international setting will have at least one private consultation with a travel medicine specialist, specifically for vaccines and malaria counsel. Time constraints limit the scope of this encounter. Group sessions are often very manageable and are a more cost-effective approach to the educational component of preparation. However, web-based educational modules and SMS technology may prove to be even more viable and cost-effective medium for education.

The curriculum should include the following topics:

- Vaccine counsel
- Basic hygiene and sanitation: food and water preparation, sewage disposal
- Injury prevention and security
- Self-management of the commonest medical ailments
- Diarrhea
- Respiratory tract infections
- Malaria
- Skin diseases
- Sexual health
- General health: sleep, diet, exercise, rest and relaxation, work–life balance, alcohol and drug abuse
- Personal medical supplies and emergency kits
- Minimizing road crashes, and swimming and domestic accidents
- How to select healthcare providers.

Health Briefing: 'The Extended Family'

Careful food, water, and domestic hygiene can greatly minimize infection in the expatriate family, as can following sensible eating practices when eating out or visiting local households.

Psychological Training and Preparation

Signs of stress and 'culture shock' are normal. Therefore, expatriates should be encouraged to accept as normal mild stress-related symptoms (e.g., sleeping problems, poor concentration, fatigue, tearfulness, irritability, weight changes, indecisiveness), but also to be aware that if these persist or combine they may indicate more significant stress, whose causes must be recognized and addressed.

Information and General Counsel

Expatriates should have information about how to recognize and handle stress and how to access help should any symptoms persist or become more severe. For mild difficulties, self-help books and information (available over the internet) may be sufficient. Professional help is essential in cases of psychoses, severe depression, suicidal ideation, anorexia nervosa, post-traumatic stress disorder, and serious

behavioral difficulties in a child. If appropriate treatment is not available locally, there may be a need for repatriation. A handout for use in such briefings is shown in Table 32.3.

Stress Briefing: Possible Structure

- If expatriates have worked in similar situations before, start by asking what they found most stressful, what their reactions were, and what helped them
- Discuss what they expect this placement will be like. Unrealistic expectations can be a major cause of stress
- What do they think might be stressful or difficult this time? Discuss in detail how they are likely to cope. (Change is itself a cause of stress)
- When they are under stress, how does it generally affect them?
- How have they coped with previous stressful experiences? What have they learned that might be helpful this time?
- What will they do to relax?
- What social support network do they have? (How can they build up a stronger network of friends?) Who will they talk to if they feel low or under stress? Who will they contact if they have significant problems? (Ensure there is a named person)
- Discuss stress management techniques and help them identify strategies that they might find useful (e.g., exercise)
- Encourage sufficient time to rest and relax. Excessive working hours contribute to difficulties, which can cause premature return. It is especially important that they make time to spend with their partner or family
- How do they feel about the organization? What support is available?
- What are their views on security arrangements?
- Thinking ahead, encourage them to have appropriate psychological support when they return 'home' at the end of their placement, and to take sufficient time off before resuming work.

Culture Shock and the U-Curve Hypothesis

Cultural adaption, commonly known as 'culture shock', is a long and varied process. This adjustment depends on factors that correspond both to expatriates' personal values and the new culture.

Cultural adaptation can be divided into psychological adaptation (measured by mood), and sociocultural adaptation (measured by social competence in the new environment). Motives and expectations have an influence on both. For instance, a businessperson who embeds exclusively in the expatriate community may appear to be well adapted psychologically, but may not have adapted socioculturally.

In 1955 Lysgaard[27] described a U-curve model of adjustment, depicted in four chronological steps:

1. The 'honeymoon period': An initial stage of fascination, lasting a few days to many weeks. The expatriate is a detached observer. Everything is new and exciting. Short-term travelers may never leave this stage.
2. Disillusionment: The expatriate, no longer a spectator, becomes disillusioned. The new culture begins to intrude on the expatriate's normal habits, creating practical problems. The expatriate may feel overwhelmed and inadequate, and experience an inability to respond instinctively to linguistic and cultural cues. Feelings of irritability, anxiety, loneliness, frustration, confusion, disorientation, self-blame, depression,

Table 32.3 Health and Stress Management Strategies for Expatriates

1. Remember that it takes time to adjust to a new culture. Do not expect to fit in straight away.

2. We are all more vulnerable when we are tired. Ensure that you get enough rest. Take at least 1 day off work each week, and have regular holidays. People who work 'all the hours' are at risk of burnout. Make sure that you fit leisure time into each week. Leisure is not an optional extra, it is a necessary ingredient for health.

3. Moderate exercise (such as walking) is good for both mental health and physical health. Make time to be active in ways you enjoy (and are possible and safe in your new location).

4. Avoid too much alcohol, caffeine, or nicotine, as these can increase symptoms of stress.

5. Look after your health:
   Eat a balanced diet; drink plenty of water
   Avoid excessive exposure to sun
   Accidents are more likely when you are tired, so:
   Take enough rest
   Take special care when driving
   Do not drive at night
   Do not 'drink and drive'
   Adhere to the malaria prevention guidelines.
   If a change is necessary, seek the wisdom of an expert in that area.

6. If you become ill, take enough time off to recuperate, rather than trying to continue working while unwell.

7. If other people have unrealistic expectations of you, discuss the situation with them. Check out any information that seems ambiguous or unclear. Do not be afraid to ask questions.

8. Relationship problems can be especially stressful when you are cut off from your normal circle of family and friends. If a problem arises, try to speak about it objectively with the person concerned, and see if you can resolve it. Try to give encouragement to others when possible.

9. Maintain regular contact with friends at home. This can make life more pleasant while you are away, and ease the transition when you return home.

10. Some people find it helpful to record their thoughts and feelings in a journal or in letters. Research suggests that this can be good for your physical health as well as your emotional wellbeing. Solutions to problems may emerge as you write.

11. If you are used to being an expert, it can be difficult to suddenly become a newcomer who has to learn new ways of doing things. Acknowledging this frustration and trying to be patient can make it easier to bear.

12. Remember that it is completely normal to experience some signs of stress when living in a different culture. Most expatriates have times when they have problems concentrating or sleeping; become unusually irritable; feel overwhelmed; feel tearful or low; have difficulty making decisions; experience changes in their appetite; etc. If you experience such symptoms, remind yourself that this is a normal part of the adjustment process. Let people know that you are feeling under stress. Recognizing your limitations is a sign of strength, not a sign of weakness. It is best to acknowledge and deal with stress early on, so that it does not escalate.

13. Seek professional help if any symptoms of stress persist for more than a few weeks, or if they start to interfere with your ability to work or to function well. Also, seek help if you find that you are drinking excessive amounts of alcohol as a way of coping.

14. Try to maintain your sense of humor, and have some fun!

and hostility towards the new culture are common during this stage.

3. **Partial adjustment:** The expatriate develops an understanding of the culture and its cues, and functions reasonably well. However, some anxiety about the culture remains.

4. **Adjustment:** Both cultures are re-evaluated. Good and bad elements can be perceived in each. The expatriate feels in control, more relaxed, confident about their ability to live independently, and they are able to react warmly towards local people, and to accept their customs.

This process is not always predictable. Some may bypass or fail to reach certain stages. Only rarely do people fully adapt and become equally comfortable in both new and old cultures. See Table 32.4 for another breakdown of cultural adjustment.

Research has provided some support for the U-curve hypothesis, although there have been very few well-designed longitudinal studies. Despite limitations, the U-curve remains a popular model, and many travelers affirm that it accurately describes their experience.

'Normal' Adjustment Difficulties

The most taxing part of life overseas is often not short-lived traumas but cultural frustrations, relationship problems, and dissatisfaction with work or the organization they work with.[8,28] Mild stress-related symptoms are common during the process of acculturation (Table 32.5). Studies suggest that 15–25% of international students have significant adjustment difficulties regarding homesickness, loneliness or depression, whereas fewer 'home' students suffer from such difficulties.[29] Living and working alongside colleagues who are stressed also takes its toll.

While reluctance to acknowledge emotional difficulties is common, many are willing to consult a health professional about somatic complaints.[6] For example, anxiety over living in the new culture may cause expatriates to over-react to minor physical complaints. A tendency to invalidate one's feelings (i.e., to conclude 'I should not feel this way') is a predictor of the development of psychological disorders among overseas aid workers.[8] 'Normalization' assists in breaking the cycle.

Table 32.4 Cultural Adaptation: Stages of Adjustment

1. Before you go, expect: anticipation and anxiety.
2. When you first arrive, expect: a 'honeymoon' period, when everything is new and interesting – it is an adventure.
3. When the 'honeymoon' comes to an end: you may miss home, and become depressed, irritable, and anxious. Everything may seem too much effort. Remember that these feelings are normal and will pass.
4. Adjustment: The new culture begins to feel like home. You are able to enjoy your experiences again.
5. Leaving: Saying goodbyes can be difficult.
6. Readjustment when you return home: You may experience 'reverse culture shock', feeling that you no longer quite 'fit' back in your own culture. For example, the supermarkets may seem overwhelmingly big; people may appear unfriendly, you may feel isolated or that no-one really understands what your life abroad has been like. You may feel very tired, so try to take sufficient time off work. Feeling low is common and will pass with time – do not tell yourself that you are 'over reacting'.

In each stage you can aim to manage stress through:

S Social support (family and friends)
T Talk, do not bottle-up feelings
R Rest and relax
E Exercise and eat sensibly
S Sleep enough
S Sing, laugh, and do what you enjoy.

Table 32.5 Symptoms of Stress, Which May Occur during Cultural Adaptation

Physical
  Tiredness: difficulty in sleeping or spending a lot of time in bed; nightmares; headaches; back pain; inability to relax; dry mouth and throat; feeling sick or dizzy; pounding heart; sweating and trembling; stomach-ache and diarrhea; loss of appetite, or over-eating; feeling very hot or cold; shortness of breath; shallow, fast breathing; hyper-vigilance; irregular menstruation; frequent need to urinate; increased risk of ulcers; high blood pressure and coronary heart disease

Emotional
  Depression: tearfulness or feeling a desire to cry but being unable to; mood swings; anger (at self or others); agitation; impatience; guilt and shame; shock; feelings of helplessness and inadequacy; feeling different or isolated from others; feeling overwhelmed/unable to cope; feeling rushed all the time; anxiety; panic/phobias; loss of sense of humor; boredom; lowered self-esteem; loss of confidence; unrealistic expectations (of self and others); insecurity; self-centered/inability to think about others; feelings of vulnerability; feeling worthless

Behavioral
  Withdrawal from others or becoming dependent on them; irritability; critical of self and others; relationship problems; lack of self-care; nail biting; picking at skin; speaking in slow monotonous voice, or fast, agitated speech; taking unnecessary risks (e.g., when driving); trying to do several things at once; lack of initiative; working long hours; poor productivity; loss of job satisfaction; carelessness; absenteeism; promiscuity, or loss of interest in sex; increased smoking or use of alcohol or drugs (including prescription drugs); excessive spending or other activities to try to take one's mind off the situation; loss of motivation; self-harm or suicidal behavior

Cognitive
  Concentration and memory difficulties; indecisiveness; procrastination; pessimism; thinking in 'all or nothing' terms; very sensitive to criticism; self-critical thoughts; loss of interest in previously enjoyed activities; imagining the worst will happen; preoccupation with health; expecting to die young; less flexible; confusion and disorientation; excessive fears (e.g., about being attacked); trying to avoid thinking about problems; flashbacks, or intrusive thoughts about difficulties; hindsight thinking ('if only …' 'why didn't I …'); negative thoughts about oneself, one's work, family, the future and the world; time seems to slow down or speed up; suicidal thoughts

Spiritual/philosophical
  Questioning the meaning of life; loss of purpose; loss of hope; changes in beliefs; doubts; giving up faith; legalism; rigidity; cynicism; loss of sense of community with others; sense of being abandoned; submission to excessive control (e.g., may join a religious cult); spiritual dryness; unforgivingness; bitterness; feeling distant from God; difficulty praying; anger at God or at life

Be alert for symptoms that go beyond normal culture shock. Depression remains the most common psychological disorder reported by expatriates. In rare instances expatriates become overwhelmed by unhappiness, refuse to integrate into the new culture, neglect self-care and regular duties. E-mails and phone calls echo their distress. Uncomplicated clinical depression will often go undetected. Those with a family or personal history of psychiatric disorder are at greater risk of developing an affective disorder when overseas, though depression may affect those without a previous history.[8,16] In cases of severe depression, suicide risk should be assessed and appropriate action taken to ensure the safety of the individual.

Anxiety disorders (including post-traumatic stress disorder) are reported among overseas workers, and should be treated with the recognized effective treatments for such disorders. Adjustment difficulties play a part in the development of problems such as eating disorders. A higher than expected proportion of development workers appear to develop chronic fatigue syndrome while working overseas.[6,30,31]

Non-mefloquine psychosis, also reported more commonly among long-term travelers, may be triggered by stress,[6] often where there has been a family history of such problems. When assessing psychiatric symptoms, it is important to ask about the use of any medication (e.g., malaria prophylaxis including mefloquine).

Non-working spouses of overseas workers may experience more adjustment problems than their working partners.[29] Their needs should be taken into account, and they should be encouraged to build up a network of friends and to find their own role.

Most overseas workers who become clinically depressed do not tell their organization. Sometimes relief is sought from excessive alcohol intake, drug abuse, and sexual activity.[32] Many expatriates prefer to complete their assignment and then return home, rather than returning prematurely due to 'psychological difficulties'. Early return is often regarded as failure. Provide emotional support and help them identify the stresses that are contributing to their difficulties.

Children

Cultural adjustment is generally easier if the individual feels it was voluntary, predictable, and they had time to prepare. It is important to realize that expatriate children often do not experience these advantages. It is important to help them feel less powerless and explain why the family is moving, and to seek out their views, and to attempt to prepare them for the move well in advance. Children should be encouraged to ask questions, should be involved choosing which toys and clothes are brought along, and, where old enough, involved in school selection.

On arrival in the new culture, parents need to take plenty of time to listen to and talk with their children, particularly about adjustment difficulties. Otherwise, children may feel that they are less important than their parent's job, which can lead to a loss of their self-esteem and self-confidence. Keeping up routines (such as stories at bedtime) helps children feel secure. For most children, 'home' is wherever their parents are. They can adapt to relocation, especially if they are able to keep in touch with friends. Parents should teach their children about appropriate and inappropriate touching. In certain cultures children are disciplined at school by a teacher touching their (clothed) genitals, and in others, babies are masturbated to send them to sleep. If children are to be looked after by other people, parents should try to ensure that no inappropriate behavior will take place.

Children may become anxious if they perceive that their parents are anxious. Symptoms of stress vary with age, but common symptoms among children include regressing to behaviors that they had grown out of (e.g., clinging, bed-wetting, thumb sucking); appetite loss; abdominal pain or headaches; sleeping problems and nightmares, fears, social withdrawal, and angry outbursts. Most children get over such problems relatively quickly as they feel more familiar with the new environment. Reading about normal child development can help parents determine normal patterns of behavior. If they are unusual, seek professional help.

Often expatriate children have to accept that they live in a highly mobile community, where friends come and go constantly. There may be family separations too, if children are sent to boarding school. Some react to this by becoming self-sufficient and deciding never to form deep relationships, as goodbyes seem too painful. This may reduce the pain of parting, but leaves a sense of constant loneliness.

Others move so often (e.g., in military families) that they conclude that there is no point in planning ahead (as plans have been changed and their hopes disappointed so often). Some decide that it is not worth addressing problems or conflict, because they can move away instead. Consequently, as adults they may decide to move whenever they face problems (e.g., changing college if they decide they do not like their course; seeking divorce rather than attempting to resolve marital conflict, etc.).

It is generally wise to avoid a first cross-cultural experience during the often-turbulent adolescent years. If the move is unavoidable, extra support should be offered.

Pollock and Van Reken[33] have provided excellent accounts of the experience of expatriate children and what are referred to as Third Culture Kids (see later), and offer many useful suggestions.

Factors That Can Facilitate Cultural Adaptation

Good psychological briefing, educational material, and cross-cultural training before departure play an important part in equipping expatriates to adapt well.[34]

Establishing a routine can provide a feeling of security and consistency. During this time, it is helpful to actively seek out positive aspects of the new culture. It is generally useful for expatriates to have a mentor, such as a seasoned expatriate, to guide them through the adjustment process. Local mentors can explain the reasons for customs, and help the newcomer to begin to understand the culture more fully. Friendship with locals and expatriates, and ongoing support from friends and family in the home country play a crucial role in cultural adaptation.

Adjustment takes time. Pressure for productivity adds to the strain felt. Allow time for adjustment without having to meet demanding goals during the initial period. However, setting and achieving a few small, achievable goals can dissipate feelings of inadequacy, helplessness and frustration. Accepting practical help will reduce frustration.

Expatriates are something of a novelty in many areas. Local people may stare, call after them, beg from them, or follow them around. Even local colleagues and friends can seem intrusive. For instance, in many cultures people think nothing of asking questions such as, 'How much do you earn?', 'How old are you?', or 'Why are you not married?' The easiest way to deal with such questions is to think in advance of a suitable response.

Although it is a difficult process for many people, cultural adaption can lead to personal growth and greater self-confidence and self-esteem. Most expatriates rate their overseas experience as positive overall.[8] Children who move to a different culture also tend to rate the experience as a positive one in retrospect.

Security Issues and Evacuation Policies

Traumatic incidents, such as terrorist bombing, war situations, evacuations, hostage taking, rape, robbery, riots, violence, road crashes or natural disasters, are commonly reported. Training in crisis management is relevant, at least for team leaders. The manual *Supporting staff responding to disasters: Recruitment, briefing and on-going care* provides detailed information about the recruitment, briefing and support of expatriates working in disaster zones or other difficult or insecure settings.

Relational Factors

Interpersonal issues are common causes of frustration and attrition. Training in problem-solving skills, negotiation techniques and conflict resolution can be effective in reducing stress and enhancing productivity.

If children are to be included in the move, it is important to help the parents understand how to make the cross-cultural transition successful for their children.

Caring for Expatriates in International Settings

Not all expatriates remain healthy. Approximately 8% of travelers to the developing world will seek medical attention during or after their travel. Cross-cultural challenges may expose some health issues.

Models of Care

- Self-reliant staff that develop their own network of healthcare providers
- Reliance on national healthcare providers who have received international training
- Utilization of international clinics staffed by persons who are also members of the expatriate community, or medical facilities staffed by members of the same organization (e.g., mission hospitals).

Self-Care

Consultants in the USA estimate that 80% of care is 'self-care', defined as diagnosing and managing medical symptoms without a healthcare professional. Although no formal studies have been done to determine how effective expatriates are in this discipline, most pre-travel counsel is accessible for this intelligent and motivated group. It is reasonable to conclude that expatriates can become proficient in key aspects of self-care when safeguarded with appropriate support.

Telemedicine and the Internet

Chat rooms and bulletin boards with health news could improve the depth and quality of self-care. The number of countries with access to web-based products is steadily increasing.

Most seek help from healthcare professionals for more complex medical problems, which can be achieved through telemedicine portals. SMS technology, personal health information on 'smartcards', mobile phone apps and new forms of innovative technology are likely to become major tools in enhancing the care of travelers.

Repatriation and Medical Evacuation

For a minority of problems, medical evacuation may be necessary. An analysis of 504 aeromedical evacuations for one relief organization demonstrated that the majority of adult evacuations were related to trauma (32.7%), followed by general internal medicine (24.4%) and neurology (14.5%). The top three diagnoses in the pediatric population were meningitis (20.9%), cerebrocranial trauma (16.7%), and fractures of the lower leg (8.4%). Middle-aged patients accounted for 75% of the psychiatric cases. The median duration of illness prior to travel was 7 days.[35]

Organizational Support

Organizations should have clear policies on evacuation, abuse, and hostage situations that expatriates are asked to adhere to as a condition of their contract. During periods of political unrest, expatriates may lack the capacity to exercise sound judgment. Appropriate evidence-based forms of debriefing and psychological support should be offered to all who are evacuated in times of crisis.[36] Training in 'psychological first aid' and peer support should be offered to suitable team members working in the same vicinity, especially if in vulnerable or remote situations.

Employers must also ensure their staff have adequate time off, and where appropriate more formal rest and relaxation procedures which they are encouraged to follow. They will need adequate support on their return home, which is often neglected.

Returning Home

Just as there are many reasons for traveling abroad, so there are many reasons for returning home. People may return early for personal, family or agency reasons. Unexpected return may be associated with considerable distress and cost. Even a planned return can be stressful, and may call for psychological care on returning home. 'Reverse culture shock' is the term given to the common reaction that many experience on coming back to their home country. After the initial joy and sometimes relief at being back, there can follow a sense of not belonging and of finding once-familiar things strange and overwhelming.

When people return home after a stressful incident they often perceive themselves to be in some way inadequate, guilty, or aggrieved. Using the model of a normal reaction to an abnormal circumstance can sometimes hasten resolution.

The Value of a Combined Physical and Psychological Approach

Physical and psychological health are often so related in returning expatriates that to look at one without the other offers an incomplete picture.

We must look at the returning traveler from an integrated perspective, using a model that includes both physical and psychosocial

Table 32.6 Examples of Questions in the Medical History Which Include Both Physical and Psychological Components for Loss of Wellbeing

Where has the traveler been? Obtain details on locations, lifestyle, and security risks to inform whether medical investigations or counseling are needed.

What paid or voluntary work has the traveler been doing? Those in the voluntary sector often work long hours with low pay and inadequate time off, leading to cumulative stress.

What occupational health risks has the worker been exposed to? e.g., leptospirosis from flood waters, symptoms of post-traumatic stress from working in war zones?

What types of leisure and recreational interest have been followed? e.g., swimming in African lakes with a risk of schistosomiasis; scuba diving, surfing or white-water rafting where frightening experiences may cause flashbacks or threaten the enjoyment of previously valued leisure pursuits.

Are there medical concerns the traveler wants to discuss, e.g., sexual health risks including HIV? Alternatively, has a romantic bond been fractured on coming home? Is the possibility of pregnancy a worry?

Has the traveler felt he or she has betrayed strongly held religious or moral convictions by a behavior or event? Has this led to guilt or a painful questioning of religious conviction? Is spiritual counseling needed?

Are there significant sleep disturbances? What are the possible causes?

Is the traveler feeling abnormally tired? The problem may have multiple physical and psychological factors.

What has the average weekly consumption of alcohol been? Has the traveler been abusing drugs?

health. This is a valuable approach for the increasing number of long-term travelers in a globalized world returning from anywhere to anywhere, who may have been exposed to diverse and multiple pursuits, experiences and stressors. A classic study by Peppiatt and Byass on the health of 212 returning missionaries illustrates the blurred boundaries between physical and psychological health on those returning from overseas and illustrates the importance of this paradigm of care.[37] On the one hand, they found that full blood counts and stool tests were valuable because of a significant number of abnormal results even in asymptomatic returnees, but they concluded that a careful history and psychological assessment were equally important. Subsequent experience in travel medicine, where physicians often overlook anything but physical symptoms and causes, gives this conclusion ongoing relevance.

The questions in Table 32.6 help to underline how essential this twin approach is for travelers re-entering their home country.

Of course, many returning travelers will not exhibit significant physical or psychological problems. In our enthusiasm to identify problems, we must not assume that a traveler's denial of any health problems means important concerns are necessarily being concealed.

Table 32.7 gives examples of the interplay between physical and psychological causation and health from one travel clinic.

Who Should Be Seen for a Medical Check on Return Home?

From the experience of those seeing returning long-term travelers a consensus is emerging of which are most in need of a medical check

Table 32.7 Some Recent Examples from a Clinic in London of Concerns Expressed by Long-Term Travelers

Effects of living in a war zone for 12 months.

Living and working with a 'difficult colleague' from another nationality or with a different personality type.

Worries about a slipped condom after too many bottles of beer in a bar in southern Africa.

Inability to face friends, climate and supermarkets back at home after 6 months on a year-out in rural Uganda.

The rape of a nun on a hospital compound only verbalized after 3 years of agonizing fear and shame.

Depression and alcohol addiction after 2 bored years as the unfulfilled spouse of an international civil servant.

Returning to live with parents, who fail to understand or sympathize with their children's travels saying only: 'And when are you going to get a proper job?'

Persistent panic attacks. Are they a result of Kalashnikov-wielding boy soldiers, or mefloquine, or a mixture of both?

Concern and anxiety that the employing agency fails to care for its staff after they have completed their contract, with an unwillingness to pay for medical checks and counseling.

Adapted from InterHealth, London.

Table 32.8 Principles of Confidential Review: Face-to-Face, by Telephone, or Video Conferencing

Post assignment or mid assignment as part of routine psychosocial support to provide opportunity to reflect on personal impact of assignment

Provides a relaxed, unhurried setting that fosters confidence in raising sensitive issues

Session not reported to sending organization without proper consent

Review includes:

    Assignment issues

    Personal issues

    Current circumstances

    Looking forward

    Check on psychological health including concerns as below:

        Poor general health

        High stress levels, stress-related illness, burnout, fatigue, chronic fatigue

        Worries about sexual health

        Safety – e.g., ability to observe security protocols, capacity for concern for others, etc.

        High-risk behaviors, including alcohol, drugs, unsafe sex, unsafe driving, breaching security protocols etc.

        Alcohol or any other behaviors deemed to have become problematic

        Post-traumatic stress

        Depression, anxiety, panic disorder or other psychological condition

        Bizarre behavior or possible psychosis

        Unexplained changes and/or other concerns with a psychological impact

Adapted from InterHealth London 2011.
Source: Annie Hargrave, InterHealth London 2011.

on their return home. These have been summarized in a publication by People in Aid, an agency specializing in the care and support of aid workers. They include:

- Those unwell, symptomatic, or abnormally tired
- Those exposed to a potential health risk, which may come to light later, e.g., exposure to HIV, *Chlamydia* or other sexually transmitted infection, or to schistosomiasis through swimming in Lake Malawi
- Those whose style of living or travel have put them at special risk, including the military, aid and relief workers involved in famine, war, relief situations and in providing assistance in natural disasters such as floods and earthquakes
- Those whose colleagues or families have significant, or perceived, concerns about their health
- The worried 'probably well'
- Those feeling unduly stressed or depressed after returning home on account of reverse culture shock, acute, post-traumatic or cumulative stress.

What Should the Physician Be Looking For?

A practitioner working entirely on a biomedical model may fail to identify or offer care to those travelers with the greatest health needs, commonly expressed in paramedical symptoms or body language. As practitioners, we need to develop our skills, both as competent health professionals and as skilled listeners. Here are some examples:

- Health and safety risks
- Psychosocial factors, including failed expectations, causes of sleep disturbance and signs of stress
- Indicators of excess alcohol consumption or drug abuse
- Risks specific to hostile or dangerous environments
- Occupational or lifestyle risks from HIV and other sexually transmitted diseases, including hepatitis B or C.

Table 32.8 outlines an assessment for those returning overseas after home assignment.

At End of the Consultation

Often travelers will feel reassured and encouraged by their appointments with a physician or psychological health practitioner, but often, too, worries and questions may reappear unless an adequate 'sign-off' has been carried out. Before the traveler leaves the practitioner should ask themselves: Have I:

- Addressed the real and perceived concerns of the traveler?
- Drawn-up an action plan?
- Explained how and when any test results will be reported back to the client?
- Arranged for any referrals?
- Agreed whether any further psychological support is needed?
- Sought the client's permission and arranged results to be sent to the normal medical attendant?
- Given contact details in case health concerns persist?

Factors Influencing the Ease of Reintegration

Those who have lived abroad for longer tend to find readjustment harder. In one study of American returnees, 64% reported significant culture shock on repatriation, and in another survey 64% of Dutch and 80% of Japanese expatriates said they found coming home more difficult than adjustment overseas.[38] Often, the greater the integration in the foreign culture, the greater the difficulty of reintegration.

When an assignment has ended badly or abruptly, the reaction is likely to be more complicated and accompanied by anger or anxiety. The reaction will also be affected by other stresses in the person's life.

On returning home, perceptions of what is acceptable in dress, social and business behavior may have altered. A study of returned aid workers found that a high percentage reported feeling predominantly negative emotions on returning home.[8] McNair found that the most common reported difficulties were feeling disorientated, problems finding a job, lack of understanding from family and friends, and financial difficulties.[39]

Coming home is easier if there are supportive family and friends to return to. The ease with which people can now keep in contact with home via e-mail and mobile phone may mean that the transition is easier.

For some, coming home signifies the end of a career, e.g., military service, or the end of paid employment, as in retirement, so there is the challenge of a double adjustment.

Issues for Families

A returning spouse, partner or parent may find that their role in the family has to be re-established or even renegotiated. An independent son or daughter returning to the family home may find they are being treated as a child again. There may be little understanding of the kind of life and experience the family member has been through.

Richardson, in a study of expatriate wives returning to the UK, found that 70% admitted to loneliness, boredom and depression when readapting to life at home.

Younger children may not have formed strong attachments to the country they are leaving, but may react to the upheaval of transition by reverting to earlier stages of childhood, e.g., bed-wetting, thumb sucking, temper tantrums, or physical symptoms such as abdominal pain. They may experience a sense of loss if there has been a relationship with a local nanny or house help.

Older children will have stronger friendships, both in school and in the community. For them, returning may be much harder than for their parents, but this may go unrecognized if parents do not understand about 'Third Culture Kids' (TCKs) and assume that their children are now 'back home'. The term TCKs, first used by Useem and Downie, applies to those who do not fully belong to the culture of their parents or to the culture in which they have grown up, but to a third culture that incorporates aspects of both. Although for many this leads to greater adaptability and a wider view of the world, it makes reintegration harder, especially during the teenage years. They may be drawn to friendships with others who do not fit in and so identify with the marginalized, or with those regarded as 'undesirable' by their parents. They may respond to feelings of alienation by using drugs or excess alcohol, or by dropping out of school or college.

What Can Be Done to Make Return Easier?

Preparation before return is important. Children need some explanation of what is happening in language and terms they can grasp and, like parents, can be helped by good leave-taking. Saying goodbyes, having leaving ceremonies and exchanging gifts can be very helpful in coming to terms with the losses associated with leaving.

A record of memories from overseas may also aid the process of integrating the experience into life at home. Diaries, scrapbooks, photos, e-mails, letters or video clips can help children understand the story of their own life and reduce the sense of dislocation in a new culture.

For many people, talking about their experience abroad with family and friends may be sufficient, but for some the opportunity to reflect on the experience in a structured way is more helpful. Many people returning from working abroad find a confidential review beneficial (Table 32.6). The role of psychological debriefing for expatriates is still under discussion despite the negative findings of a Cochrane review related to critical incident debriefing for people exposed to traumatic incidents.

When coping strategies fail, there is a need for additional help. Counseling may be necessary to look at past experiences and reactions that have contributed to present difficulties. Cognitive behavior therapy (CBT) can be useful in identifying and challenging faulty thought patterns that lead to distressing emotions and unhelpful behaviors. If more severe disorders develop, such as post-traumatic stress disorder or depression, full assessment and appropriate treatment is needed. (Table 32.8)

The opportunity to share experiences through meeting or social networking sites can be very helpful, and children benefit from discovering that there are others like them with a third culture upbringing. There are internet groups available, and some organizations run holidays where returning children can meet up and find common ground.

For people of all ages, the experience of traveling abroad is often both enriching and challenging. Returning is often no less challenging, and requires attention to both physical and psychological health.[40]

Key References

Bernard K, Graitcer P, van der Vlugt T, et al. Epidemiological surveillance in Peace Corps Volunteers: A model for monitoring health in temporary residents of developing countries. International Journal of Epidemiology 1989;18:220–6.

Chen LH. Illness in Long-Term Travelers Visiting GeoSentinel Clinics. Emerging Infectious Diseases 2009.

Dahlgren AL, Deroo L, Avril J, et al. Health risks and risk-taking behaviors among International Committee of the Red Cross (ICRC) expatriates returning from humanitarian missions. Journal of Travel Medicine 2009 Nov-Dec;16(6):382–90.

Hamer DH, Ruffing R, Callahan MV, et al. Knowledge and use of measures to reduce health risks by corporate expatriate employees in western Ghana. Journal of Travel Medicine 2008 Jul-Aug;15(4):237–42.

Lankester T. Health care of the long-term traveller. Travel Medicine And Infectious Disease 2005 Aug;3(3):143–55.

Lovell D. Psychological adjustment among returned overseas aid workers. Bangor: University of Wales; 1997.

Lovell-Hawker D. Supporting staff responding to disasters: Recruitment, briefing and on-going care. 4th ed. London: People In Aid; 2011.

McNair. Room for improvement: the management and support of relief and development workers. London: Overseas Development Institute; 1995.

Peppiatt R, Byass P. A survey of the health of British missionaries. British Journal of General Practice 1991;(41):159–62.

Pollock D, Van Reken R. The Third Culture Kid Experience: growing up among worlds. Yarmouth, Maine: Intercultural Press; 1999.

References

1. Dumont J-C, Lemaître G. Counting Immigrants and Expatriates in OECD Countries: A New Perspective: Organization for Economic Cooperation and Development [OECD]2005 June 22, 2005 Contract No.: JT00187033.
2. Stoddard A, Harmer A, DiDomenico V. Providing aid in insecure environments: Humanitarian Policy Group. April 2009.
3. Dahlgren AL, Deroo L, Avril J, et al. Health risks and risk-taking behaviors among International Committee of the Red Cross (ICRC) expatriates returning from humanitarian missions. J Travel Med 2009 Nov-Dec; 16(6):382–90.

4. Bernard K, Graitcer P, van der Vlugt T, et al. Epidemiological surveillance in Peace Corps Volunteers: A model for monitoring health in temporary residents of developing countries. Int J Epidemiol 1989;18:220–6.

5. WR. L, Frankenfield D, Frame J. Morbidity among refugee relief workers. J Travel Med 1994;1:111–2.

6. Chen LH. Illness in Long-Term Travelers Visiting GeoSentinel Clinics. Emerg Infect Dis 2009.

7. Parshall P. How spiritual are missionaries? In: O'Donnell K, O'Donnell M, editors. Helping Missionaries Grow: Readings in Mental Health and Missions. Pasadena: William Carey Library; 1988. p. 75–82.

8. Lovell D. Psychological adjustment among returned overseas aid workers. Bangor: University of Wales; 1997.

9. Deshpande SP, Viswesvaran C. Is cross-cultural training of expatriate managers effective: A meta analysis. Int J Intercult Rel 1992;16: 295–310.

10. Frame J, Lange W, Frankenfield D. Mortality trends of American missionaries in Africa, 1945–1985. The American Society of Tropical Medicine and Hygiene 1992;46:686–90.

11. Hargarten S, Baker S. Fatalities in the Peace Corps. A retrospective study:1962 through 1983. JAMA 1985;254:1326–9.

12. Atlas SJ, Grant RW, Ferris TG, et al. Patient–physician connectedness and quality of primary care. Ann Intern Med 2 March 2009;150(5): 325–35.

13. Yarnall K, Pollak K, Ostbye T, et al. Primary care: is there enough time for prevention? Am J Public Health 2003;93:635–41.

14. Backman JW. The patient-computer interview: A neglected tool that can aid the clinician. Mayo Clinic Proc 2003;78:67–78.

15. Stroh L, Dennis L, Cramer T. Predictors of expatriate adjustment. Int J Organizational Analysis 1994;2:176–92.

16. Foyle M, Beer M, Watson J. Expatriate mental health. Acta Psychiat Scand 1998;97:278–83.

17. Schnurr P, Friedman M, Rosenberg S. Premilitary MMPI scores as predictors of combat-related PTSD symptoms. Am J Psychiat 1993;150:479–83.

18. Dunbar E, Ehrlich M. Preparation of the international employee: Career and consultation needs. Consult Psychol J 1993;45:18–24.

19. Arguin P, Krebs J, Mandel E, et al. Survey of rabies preexposure and postexposure prophylaxis among missionary personnel stationed outside the United States. J Travel Med 2000;7:10–4.

20. Adera T, Wolfe M, McGuire RK, et al. Risk factors for malaria among expatriates living in Kampala, Uganda: The need for adherence to chemoprophylactic regimens. Am J Trop Med 1995;52:207–12.

21. Kotwal R, Wenzel R, Sterling R, et al. An outbreak of malaria in US Army Rangers returning from Afghanistan. JAMA 2005;293:212–6.

22. Lobel H, Varma J, Miani M, et al. Monitoring for mefloquine-resistant Plasmodium falciparum in Africa: Implications for travelers' health. Am J Trop Med Hyg 1998;59:129–32.

23. Funk M, Schlagenhauf P, Tschopp A, Steffen R. MalaQuick versus ParaSight F as a diagnostic aid in travellers' malaria. Trans R Soc Trop Med Hyg 1999;93:268–72.

24. Cobelens F, Deutekom Hv, Draayer-Jansen I, et al. Association of tuberculin sensitivity in Dutch adults with history of travel to areas with a high incidence of tuberculosis. Clin Infect Dis 2001;33:300–4.

25. Shlim D, Hoge C, Rajah R, et al. Persistent high risk of diarrhea among foreigners in Nepal during the first 2 years of residence. Clin Infect Dis 1999;29:613–6.

26. Hamer DH, Ruffing R, Callahan MV, et al. Knowledge and use of measures to reduce health risks by corporate expatriate employees in western Ghana. J Travel Med 2008 Jul-Aug;15(4):237–42.

27. Lysgaard S. Adjustment in a foreign society: Norwegian Fulbright grantees visiting the United States. Int Soc Sci Bull 1955;7:45–51.

28. Taft R. Coping with unfamiliar cultures. In: Warren N, editor. Studies in Cross-cultural Psychology. London: Academic Press; 1977.

29. Church A. Sojourner adjustmen. Psychol Bull 1982;91:540–72.

30. Lovell D. Chronic fatigue syndrome among overseas development workers: A qualitative study. J Travel Med 1999;6:16–23.

31. Nasser M. Comparative study of the prevalence of abnormal eating attitudes among Arab female students at both London and Cairo universities. Psychol Med 1986;16:621–5.

32. De Graaf R, Van Zessen G, Houweling H. Underlying reasons for sexual conduct and condom use among expatriates posted in AIDS endemic areas. AIDS Care 1998;10(6):651–65.

33. Pollock D, Van Reken R. The Third Culture Kid Experience: growing up among worlds. Yarmouth, Maine: Intercultural Press; 1999.

34. Lovell-Hawker D. Supporting Staff Responding to Disasters: Recruitment, Briefing and On-going Care. 4th ed. London: People In Aid; 2011.

35. Sand M, Bollenbach M, Sand D, et al. Epidemiology of aeromedical evacuation: an analysis of 504 cases. J Travel Med 2010 Nov-Dec; 17(6):405–9.

36. Hawker DM, Durkin J, Hawker DS. To debrief or not to debrief our heroes: that is the question. Clin Psychol Psychother 2011;18:453–63.

37. Peppiatt R, Byass P. A survey of the health of British missionaries. Brit J Gen Pract 1991;(41):159–62.

38. Storti C. The Art of Coming Home. London: Nicholas Brealey; 2001.

39. McNair. Room for Improvement: the Management and Support of Relief and Development Workers. London: Overseas Development Institute; 1995.

40. Lankester T. Health care of the long-term traveller. Travel Med Infect Dis 2005 Aug;3(3):143–55.

33

The Migrant Patient

Elizabeth D. Barnett

Key points

- Knowledge of birth and migration history is critical for providing optimal healthcare to all patients, but especially migrants
- Tuberculosis and hepatitis B screening should be considered for all migrants
- Migrants should receive healthcare and immunizations according to locally accepted clinical guidelines
- Screening for conditions related to birth country and migrant history should be considered for all migrants
- Attention should be paid at all levels to strategies that optimize the healthy migrant advantage

Foreign-born individuals now make up significant and increasing proportions of the population of many countries. It is important now more than ever for all healthcare professionals to be able to provide appropriate healthcare for migrant patients. The purpose of this chapter is to review some fundamental concepts about the care of foreign-born individuals in the context of the epidemiology of some common health problems of immigrants.

In 2010, more than 200 million people, or 3.1% of the earth's population, crossed international borders for the purpose of immigration. Migrants make up more than 40% of the 2010 population of Singapore, Israel, and Jordan, more than 20% of the population of Australia, Canada, and Switzerland, and more than 10% of the population of the United States, Spain, Germany, France, and the United Kingdom.[1] Although no standardized international screening protocols exist for health assessment of new arrivals, several countries have developed screening guidelines, most often designed for specific groups of migrants such as refugees, international adoptees, or those from particular regions of the world. Some of these are designed for all migrants, whereas others were developed to address specific health problems identified in particular groups of migrants. An example of the first are the extensive evidence-based recommendations developed by Pottie et al. in Canada, and an example of the latter is the program to screen South American, primarily Bolivian, migrants in Spain for Chagas' disease.[2,3] Many other countries, including Australia, the United Kingdom, and the United States, provide guidance about screening for immigrants and refugees.[4–6]

Migrant populations differ from the native-born in many ways with respect to health. Some of these are obvious: different language and culture, different experiences of health systems and approaches to curative and preventive healthcare, and different exposures to diseases and other environmental conditions affecting health, such as air pollution and extremes of climate. Others are more subtle, such as varying exposures to infectious diseases of long latency, such as hepatitis B, tuberculosis, and human papillomavirus. Whatever the differences, foreign-born individuals need healthcare according to local standards for diagnosis and management, but also need attention to conditions that may be present or occur in the future due to exposures related to their country of origin and migration route. Thus the first step in the care of migrants from any part of the world must be attention to complete migration history: 'Where were you born and where have you traveled?'

Health Evaluation of Migrants

Migrants should have access to the same standard of healthcare as the native-born population. In addition, migrants will need additional assessment for conditions that may be present as a result of exposures or experiences occurring in the country of birth or during migration. Examples include tuberculosis, hepatitis B, HIV, and parasitic diseases. Some of these health conditions may not be familiar to health professionals in countries in which migrants settle and will therefore provide additional challenges when caring for migrant patients. Migrant populations, especially refugee populations, may change frequently, making it even more difficult to identify health problems specific to migrants from particular geographic regions. Still, there is increasing attention being paid to this challenge, and increasing numbers of sources of information available to aid clinicians in facing this challenge.[1,6]

Specific Conditions Deserving of Health Screening for Migrants (Boxes 33.1 and 33.2)

Tuberculosis

In 2010 there were an estimated 8.8 million new cases and a prevalence of 12 million cases.[7] These numbers do not consider the much larger number of individuals with latent tuberculosis infection (LTBI): those who have been infected and could develop active disease at a later date. Studies of new immigrants in the United States show rates of positive tuberculin skin tests to range from 25% to 70%, suggesting

©2012 Elsevier Inc
DOI: 10.1016/B978-1-4557-1076-8.00033-8

BOX 33.1

Evaluation and Screening of Migrants Appropriate for Most New Arrivals

Medical and migration history

Physical examination, including hearing, vision, and dental examinations

Complete blood count with differential

Tuberculin skin test

Hepatitis B testing

Urinalysis

Syphilis testing

HIV testing (adolescents and adults; consider for children)

Mental health screening

Age-appropriate immunizations

BOX 33.2

Screening of Migrants to be Considered Based on Birth and Migration History, Age, Gender, or Specific Symptoms or Risk Factors

Hepatitis C

Strongyloides

Schistosomiasis

Malaria

Intestinal parasites

Lead level

Diabetes

Hypertension

Pregnancy

Unmet contraceptive needs

Pap smear

---

that the potential burden of disease is substantial.[8] Efforts to address tuberculosis in migrants include identification and treatment of individuals with infectious tuberculosis before migration, and testing and treatment of migrants upon arrival. Although many migrants are tested and treated successfully, there are an even larger number who are not screened upon arrival and may be infected and at risk for the development of tuberculosis later in life. Another group may undergo screening, be diagnosed with LTBI, but decline treatment, leaving them at risk for reactivation disease later in life.

Most experts agree that virtually all new arrivals should be screened for tuberculosis as soon as possible after arrival, and that those who screen positive should be evaluated and treated either for active tuberculosis or for latent tuberculosis infection. Those who decline treatment can be informed of their risk for active tuberculosis, especially if they become immunocompromised at a later date.

Opinion is mixed about which type of screening is most appropriate. The tuberculin skin test, long the standard for tuberculosis screening, has several limitations, including false-positive results in those who have been immunized with BCG vaccine, and the need for two visits. Interferon-γ (IFN-γ) release assays (IGRAs), while not producing false-positive results with BCG, are limited by greater cost and limited availability.[9] The currently available IGRAs also are not recommended for certain groups, including children under 5 years of age, immunocompromised individuals, and those who may have recently

been exposed to tuberculosis. Individual sites or practitioners that evaluate migrants will need to assess which of the screening tests best meets their needs and is available to them.

Migrants who screen positive for tuberculosis will need to receive appropriate evaluation for active disease, including a chest radiograph and evaluation for extrapulmonary tuberculosis. If this evaluation does not reveal disease, the individual will need to be offered treatment for LTBI, taking into consideration the wide range of beliefs about tuberculosis and its treatment held by many immigrant groups. As the treatment lasts for many months and adherence is often challenging, these programs are most successful when treatment can be provided with attention to the language and culture of the migrant populations being served. Shorter-course regimens, such as directly observed isoniazid-rifapentine, may facilitate adherence to LTBI treatment.[10]

Hepatitis B

As many as 350 million individuals worldwide are chronically infected with hepatitis B; 500 000–700 000 deaths annually can be attributed to this infection.[11] Although many countries have initiated immunization programs, these did not come soon enough for many individuals who are already infected. Screening of immigrant groups in the United States reveals rates of infection ranging from 4.3% to 14%.[8] Many migrants come from countries where the prevalence of hepatitis B infection is higher than that of their country of resettlement.

Screening for hepatitis B should be considered for any migrant who may have risk factors for hepatitis B infection, or who comes from a higher-risk area. In the US, screening is recommended specifically for migrants who come from countries with a prevalence of hepatitis B infection ≥2%.[12] The cost-effectiveness of this strategy was demonstrated recently.[13] Healthcare professionals seeing migrant patients for the first time should be especially vigilant to make sure individuals who have been immunized have been tested for hepatitis B infection, as many case reports exist of migrants immunized on arrival without testing who present at a later time with complications of unrecognized hepatitis B infection. Individuals with hepatitis B infection need close monitoring for complications, preferably with attention paid to the health beliefs of the individual, especially those related to testing and treatment of asymptomatic conditions.[14]

Human Immunodeficiency Virus

Human immunodeficiency virus (HIV) screening poses unique challenges for healthcare professionals caring for immigrants. There is still significant stigma associated with an HIV diagnosis and many barriers to testing and access to treatment, including fears about breaches of confidentiality and perceptions of the implications of the diagnosis. Until early 2010, the US required HIV testing for those entering the country as immigrants or wanting to change immigration status when in the US. Today, many new immigrants and healthcare professionals may still believe this testing is being done. At the same time, although the US does not collect data about new HIV diagnoses by country of birth, data from several states suggest that the proportion of individuals living with HIV is greater in the foreign-born in some areas than it is in the US-born.[15] In addition, a study in The Netherlands suggested that immigrants may be at greater risk for HIV in the country of resettlement than in their country of origin, owing to the concentration of social and sexual networks in immigrant communities.[16] Unfortunately, the concept that HIV-infected immigrants pose a risk to the local population persists in both the lay population as well with some healthcare professionals. Focusing on identifying and providing appropriate education, testing, and treatment is more helpful in reducing the burden of disease in immigrant communities in many locations.

Testing for HIV should be considered for all adult and adolescent new immigrants from countries where prevalence is >1%, and also considered for children.[1] Accomplishing this may require special attention to the culture-specific concerns about confidentiality and stigma, and to the concept of testing and treatment for conditions not currently resulting in symptoms of illness.

Parasitic Disease Screening

Newly arrived immigrants may be offered testing for parasites in three ways. The first involves collection of up to three stool samples for testing for gastrointestinal pathogens; the second, serologic testing for specific parasites; and the third, diagnostic testing focused on signs and symptoms identified in patients, such as biopsies of affected tissue. Stool testing is most effective for parasites that remain in the GI tract, such as *Giardia*, *Ascaris*, and other helminths. It may also identify pathogens that are capable of providing systemic illness, such as *Schistosoma* species or *Entamoeba histolytica*. Treatment for specific parasites can be provided once identified.

A recent assessment of the effectiveness of pre-migration treatment of refugees has demonstrated a significant reduction in pathogenic helminths in refugees upon arrival in the United States.[17] Although these results suggest that post-arrival screening for stool ova and parasites could be curtailed in this specific population, this may not be possible for refugee groups resettling in other countries and for non-refugee immigrants.

Eosinophilia may suggest parasitic infection, usually with a parasite that has a tissue phase. If eosinophilia is identified, specific serologic or other diagnostic testing may be required. Depending on the migration route of the individual, some of the specific serologic tests that could be considered include those for *Strongyloides*, schistosomiasis, or filarial diseases, including lymphatic filariasis, onchocerciasis, or loiasis. Additional information about evaluation of eosinophilia can be found in Chapter 55.

Immigrants may present years after migration with signs or symptoms of parasitic diseases. Examples include heart or gastrointestinal disease in Chagas' disease and lymphedema in lymphatic filariasis. One of the most dreaded late presentations of parasitic diseases is *Strongyloides* hyperinfection syndrome, which may occur in an individual who sustains an illness or starts a medication resulting in an immunocompromised status.

Healthcare professionals will need to become familiar with their patient population and provide screening tests appropriately for that population. They may need to identify local expertise in the diagnosis and treatment of parasitic infection, especially those familiar with differences in the presentation of these infections in immigrants who have resided for extensive periods in the endemic area compared with the ways in which these diseases present in travelers. In addition, when immigrants face illnesses or therapies that could result in immunocompromise, health professionals will need to be vigilant to consider screening or empiric treatment for *Strongyloides* as well as tuberculosis.

General Screening Tests

Immigrants should receive standard healthcare screening according to guidelines and protocols in the country of resettlement. Screening tests that are helpful in particular for migrants include complete blood count with differential (to identify anemia, either due to iron deficiency or to hemoglobinopathy; eosinophilia associated with possible parasitic infection; leukopenia, potentially associated with HIV infection; and platelet abnormalities), urinalysis (to identify hematuria, proteinuria, or glucosuria), HIV testing, STD assessment (RPR or other screening test for syphilis, urine for GC and *Chlamydia* if appropriate), lead screening for children, and parasite screening with stool samples. Individuals with eosinophilia will need additional assessment for parasitic infection, including history and physical examination and serologic testing for parasites appropriate to the epidemiology and findings from history and physical examination. A varicella antibody test has been found to be cost-effective in those who have not been immunized, and malaria screening may be appropriate for those coming from areas of high malaria prevalence, especially if they have symptoms (fever) or signs (thrombocytopenia, anemia) associated with malaria. Screening tests that may be done if there are specific indications include hepatitis C and *Helicobacter pylori* screening.

Other screening tests appropriate for migrants include vision, hearing, and dental screening and mental health assessment. Screening for mental health problems is particularly challenging in some immigrant populations, and requires use of appropriate interpreters, patience and careful listening, and willingness to learn about the circumstances leading to the patient's distress.[18]

Immunizations

Immunizations should be provided according to local recommendations. Records of immunizations received in the country of origin or along the migration route may be accepted as valid if the month and year of the vaccine are recorded, and if the vaccine was given according to the accepted schedules in the country of resettlement. For example, many countries give the first measles vaccine before 1 year of age; if the country of resettlement does not accept such a vaccine as valid according to its schedules, the dose will need to be repeated.

Records of individuals who have received hepatitis B vaccine should be reviewed carefully. If from a risk country, attention should be paid to whether the vaccine was given at birth, and whether it was given with hepatitis B immunoglobulin, whether the individual's mother is infected with hepatitis B, and if the individual has ever been tested for hepatitis B. Even if vaccine has been given, if not given at birth to an infant born to a mother who was not infected, it is prudent to consider testing for hepatitis B infection.[12]

Vaccines may be available in the resettlement country that were not available in the country of birth. Examples include tetanus, diphtheria, and acellular pertussis (Tdap), conjugate pneumococcal, human papilloma virus, and zoster vaccines. These should be offered to individuals who are in the appropriate age groups according to locally accepted schedules.

Healthy Migrant Effect

Immigrants may arrive in their country of resettlement healthier in many ways than the local population. Sadly, this 'healthy migrant advantage' may disappear over time. Factors affecting this change include the adoption of less healthy lifestyle choices, lack of ability to exercise as much or to eat as healthy foods, exposure to pollution or violence in some large cities or neighborhoods, and poverty. Healthcare professionals can be influential in helping to maintain this healthy migrant advantage by addressing the challenges of resettlement, providing access to healthcare and information about healthy life style choices, and by advocating for a system that optimizes care given to immigrant groups.

Core Values and Best Practices in the Care of Immigrant Patients

A set of core values can be identified for providers working with migrants which include global health equity, respect, trust, cultural humility and compassion.[19] These core values can equip healthcare professionals with some tools to address health disparities for immigrants and refugees and barriers to their care, including incomplete screening and treatment, inadequate insurance coverage or access to care, lack of cultural and linguistic competence on the part of healthcare professionals, and shortage of bilingual and bicultural providers. In 2004, the Minnesota Immigrant Health Task Force identified action steps to reduce barriers that prevent immigrants from receiving optimal healthcare.[20] These action steps include providing equal access to care to all, providing care in the patient's language of choice using trained interpreters, recognizing the costs of healthcare for immigrants, developing clinical guidelines and best practice models of healthcare, diversifying the healthcare work force, using bilingual and bicultural community health workers, and training healthcare professionals about care of immigrant patients and migrants about the local healthcare system and maintaining health.

Conclusion

Caring for migrant patients and their families is becoming a nearly universal experience for healthcare providers in most countries. There is a specific body of knowledge that can be learned to equip healthcare professionals to provide optimal healthcare for immigrant patients, including providing a standard of care equivalent to that provided to the local population and attending to diseases and conditions related to the country of origin and migration route. Providing this care can reduce health disparities that exist for immigrant and refugee patients.

References

1. United Nations Department of Economic and Social Affairs Population Division. Trends in International Migrant Stock, the 2008 revision. 2009 [accessed 15 June 2012]; Available from: http://esa.un.org/migration.
2. Pottie K, Greenaway C, Feightner J, et al. Evidence-based clinical guidelines for immigrants and refugees. Canadian Medical Association Journal 2011; DOI: 10.1503/cmaj.090313. Available at: http://www.cmaj.ca/content/early/2011/07/25/cmaj.090313 (accessed 15 June 2012).
3. Navarro M, Perez-Ayala A, Gulonnet A, et al. Targeted screening and health education for Chagas disease tailored to at-risk migrants in Spain, 2007–2010. Euro Surveill 16(38):pii=19973, 2011. Available at: http://www.eurosurveillance.org/ViewArticle.aspx?ArticleId=19973 (accessed 15 June 2012).
4. Australian Government Department of Immigration and Citizenship. Fact Sheet 22 – The Health Requirement. [cited 2010 September 29]; Available from: http://www.immi.gov.au/media/fact-sheets/22health.htm#d (accessed 15 June 2012).
5. Health Protection Agency. Assessing Migrant Patients. Available from: http://www.hpa.org.uk/MigrantHealthGuide/AssessingMigrantPatients/.
6. Centers for Disease Control and Prevention. Immigrant and Refugee Health Domestic Guidelines. Available at: http: //www.cdc.gov/immigrantrefugeehealth/guidelines/domestic/checklist.html. (accessed 15 June 2012).
7. Global Tuberculosis Control: WHO report. 2010. Available at: http://www.who.int/tb/publications/global_report/2011/gtbr11_full.pdf (accessed 15 June 2012).
8. Seybolt L, Barnett ED, Stauffer W. US medical screening for immigrants and refugees: Clinical issues. In: Walker PF, Barnett ED, editors. Immigrant Medicine. Philadelphia: Saunders Elsevier; 2007. pp. 135–50.
9. Centers for Disease Control and Prevention. Fact Sheet: Interferon gamma release assays – (IGRAs) – Blood tests for TB infection. Available at: http://www.cdc.gov/tb/publications/factsheets/testing/IGRA.htm (accessed 15 June 2012).
10. Jereb JA, Goldberg SV, Powell K, et al. Recommendations for use of an isoniazid-rifapentine regimen with direct observation to treat latent *Mycobacterium tuberculsis* infection. MMWR 60:1650–3, 2011.
11. Hepatitis. WHO. Available at: http://www.who.int/immunization/topics/hepatitis/en/index.html (accessed 15 June 2012).
12. Weinbaum CM, Williams I, Mast E, et al. Recommendations for identification and public health management of persons with chronic hepatitis B infection. MMWR 57(RR08):1–20, 2008.
13. Eckman Mtt, Kaiser TE, Sherman KE. The cost-effectiveness of screening for chronic hepatitis B infection in the United States. CID 2011. DOI: 10.1093/CID/CIR199.
14. Hassanein T. Screening and diagnosing hepatitis B infection: Immigrant and Special Populations. Adv Stud Med 9:82–8, 2009. Available at: http://www.jhasim.com/files/articlefiles/pdf/ASIM_V9-3_article1.pdf (accessed 15 June 2012).
15. Crosby SS, Piwowarczyk LA, Cooper ER. HIV infection. In: Walker PF, Barnett ED, editors. Immigrant Medicine. Philadelphia: Saunders Elsevier; 2007. p. 361–73.
16. Xiridou M, van Veen M, Coutinho R, et al. Changes in patterns of migration barely influence the heterosexual HIV epidemic in Europe. Eighteenth International AIDS Conference, Vienna, abstract WEAC0104. 2010.
17. Swanson S, Phares C, Mamo B, et al. Albendazole therapy and enteric parasites in United States-bound refugees. NEJM 2012;366: 1498–507.
18. Eisenman DP. Screening for mental health problems and history of torture. In: Walker PF, Barnett ED, editors. Immigrant Medicine. Philadelphia: Saunders Elsevier; 2007. p. 633–38.
19. Walker PF, Barnett ED. An introduction to the field of refugee and immigrant healthcare. In: Walker PF, Barnett ED, editors. Immigrant Medicine. Philadelphia: Saunders Elsevier; 2007. p. 1–9.
20. Ohmans P. Action steps to improve the health of new Americans. In: Walker PF, Barnett ED, editors. Immigrant Medicine. Philadelphia: Saunders Elsevier; 2007. p. 27–35.

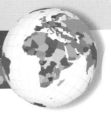

34

Humanitarian Aid Workers

Shiri Tenenboim and Eli Schwartz

Key points

- Humanitarian aid workers (HAWs) typically travel for extended periods, work in close proximity to local populations, and work in high-risk environments in low-resource regions
- Although morbidity might be high, death during volunteer missions is not common and is usually not attributable to infectious diseases. Nor is medical evacuation common
- Owing to the nature of their work, HAWs are often unable to avoid high-risk behavior and frequently encounter stressful conditions, leading to psychological repercussions
- Pre-and post-travel physical and psychological screening evaluations, in addition to routine healthcare, are essential among this population

Introduction

Traveling to extreme environments for the purpose of providing humanitarian aid is becoming a common trend. The number of humanitarian agencies, including both United Nations bodies (UN) and non-governmental organizations (NGOs), involved in complex emergencies and other humanitarian aid missions has increased significantly in the last two decades and has been accompanied by an increase in the number of recruited personnel designated to work in complex environments.[1,2]

The humanitarian aid workers (HAW) community is an extremely diverse group of organizations and individuals, making it difficult to describe holistically. Most HAW originate from North America or West and Central Europe and their popular destinations include Africa (especially the sub-Saharan region) and South East Asia, but the Caribbean, Central and South America, as well as Eastern Europe, are also temporary homes for many aid workers. They may travel for a period ranging from a few days to a few years and practice many different kinds of aid (medical, educational, agriculture, etc.). Most of them are in their 20s or 30s, but some are older or even much older. They may be professional or non-professional, and they may travel in large groups, in families with children, or as individuals.[1–7]

Data about the extent of this phenomenon are still scarce. However, two surveys done in the US in an interval of two decades demonstrated an increase in the percentage of travelers reporting volunteer work as their main travel purpose. Out of 2445 surveyed Americans who traveled to developing countries between 1984 and 1989, 5% did so for the purpose of voluntary/missionary activities.[7] In 2009, the number more than tripled, with 17% reporting traveling as volunteers or medical aid providers.[8]

The Geosentinel Network, which is the largest database of travel-related morbidity around the world, documented that 40% of long-term travelers (>6 months abroad) traveled for volunteer or missionary purposes. Also, 7% of short-term travelers (<1 month) traveled for similar reasons.[9] If this reflects the nature of traveling, aid workers may become – if they are not already – a group of travelers that pose a specific challenge for travel medicine practitioners, as well as for mental health specialists. This group might be different from the typical traveler since they tend to travel for longer periods,[9,10] work in close proximity to local populations, and practice high-risk professions (medical work, peacekeeping missions, security, drivers, etc.) in low-resource environments with poor infrastructures. In addition they tend to practice high-risk behaviors.[2,11]

Despite the fact that there are limited data focusing on this group, Peace Corps volunteers (PCVs), the International Committee of the Red Cross (ICRC), and various UN agency employees can represent a good source of information. These groups however constitute a relatively well-kept aid-workers group, with oiled recruiting, screening and surveillance programs. This contrasts significantly with the many other volunteers sent on behalf of small, sometimes very inexperienced NGOs. Additional data may be extrapolated from publications regarding expatriate populations, long-term travelers, or other data regarding aid workers from different organizations. Therefore, generalization should be applied carefully, and personally tailored recommendations should be favored.

Mortality in Humanitarian Workers

The risk of death among aid workers is influenced dramatically by the nature of their work and the country and situation in which they act. Traveling to areas following natural disasters or to areas with ongoing violent conflict is common, as is engaging in high-risk work such as peacekeeping missions, security or medicine.

©2012 Elsevier Inc
DOI: 10.1016/B978-1-4557-1076-8.00034-X

Nevertheless, published data clearly demonstrate that death during volunteer missions is not common, and neither is medical evacuation. Contrary to the common perception, 'obscure' tropical diseases are rarely the cause of death: most deaths are due to relatively trivial causes.

Between 1961 and 1983, 185 out of 105 539 PCVs died during missions. Almost 70% of these deaths were caused by unintentional injuries (especially motor vehicle accidents). In the following 20 years (1984–2003) an additional 66 deaths occurred during service, out of a total of 71 198 volunteers. Among the 66 deaths, 45 were from unintentional injuries, 11 were due to homicide, seven from chronic illnesses (five people died from heart conditions, two from cancer), and only two were due to infectious diseases (one from malaria and one from sepsis). Almost all the fatal injuries were in volunteers aged 18–34, and deaths from chronic illnesses were more common in the older age group.[5]

Comparing the first two decades and the following two decades of Peace Corps activity has shown a decline in the overall death rate by more than half. This decrease was mainly attributed to the decline in motor vehicle accidents and the decreasing number of deaths from chronic illness. These changes resulted from restriction of motorcycle use by volunteers and better pre-travel screening of applicants with chronic diseases.[5,6]

In another report, which examined the mortality pattern of a more diverse group of volunteers, 382 deaths of humanitarian workers serving during the years 1985–1998 were analyzed. They were employed by different NGOs, in addition to the ICRC and various UN agencies. In this group, intentional violence was the cause of death in 68% of cases, and motor vehicle accidents were responsible for an additional 17% of all deaths.

Again, illnesses were not a common cause of death: only 8% of volunteers died from diseases or natural causes. Interestingly, one-third of deaths in workers from NGOs were due to diseases, compared to only 5% of worker fatalities from the UN. This may be explained by a better pre-travel medical screening and preparedness carried out by the UN, compared to the small NGOs; this emphasizes the importance of recruiting and the pre-travel training process leading to the wellbeing of volunteers.[12]

Morbidity in Humanitarian Workers

Although catastrophic events leading to death during aid missions are uncommon, morbidity is significantly higher than in the home country. This was reflected in a recent survey conducted among ICRC personnel serving an average period of 11 months. Among them, one-third (36.4%) reported a decline in health after returning, and 72.8% reported having at least one medical problem during their mission. The rate of medical problems identified among them varied between regions, while traveling to Africa seemed to pose a greater risk in almost all reported categories of medical issues.[2]

Morbidity during missions comprises a wide range of illnesses. This may include conditions with similar incidence to those reported in routine travelers, as well as conditions which seem to be exceptionally more prevalent among volunteers. As usual, enteric-transmitted diseases are the most common disorder among all groups of travelers, including HAW, as well as febrile diseases. On the other hand, it appears that psychological problems, gynecological complaints, and dental emergencies are reported much more commonly among HAW (Table 34.1).

We highlight some of the conditions we believe require special attention, or those which may influence the health recommendations that should be provided to HAW.

Table 34.1 Medical Problems Reported by ICRC Expatriates on Missions Compared to Those Reported in Ill Returned Travelers

Medical Problem	ICRC[2] n = 1250 %	GeoSentinel[13] n = 17353 %
Diarrhea	44	33
Fever	25.9	22
Fatigue	19.9	NA
Gastrointestinal (not diarrhea)	15.6	8.2
Neuropsychological	14.6	2.7
Dermatological	16.3	17
Dental	12.6	0.1
Gynecological/obstetric	8.5	0.3
Cardiovascular	1.7	0.8
Sexually transmitted diseases	0.3	NA

Malaria

Malaria-endemic countries are common destinations for aid workers. The length of stay in the host country poses a big challenge for the consulting physician recommending the proper chemoprophylaxis in order to minimize side-effects and ensure adherence to treatment (see Ch. 15).

Despite prior knowledge about transmission of the parasite, relief workers fail to continuously incorporate protective measures into their daily life. A comparison of knowledge regarding health risks during travel between humanitarian aid workers and other travelers was done at the Institut Pasteur in France. Although NGO travelers had better knowledge about the transmission route of malaria, no difference was observed regarding practical knowledge about means of prevention or symptoms requiring prompt medical consultation.[10]

Chemoprophylaxis is often neglected during the course of the missions.[3,10,13] In addition, workers were at risk of malaria over-diagnosing and over-treatment practices, while missing the correct diagnoses and treatment.[2]

Tuberculosis

Tuberculosis (TB) is one of the most prevalent infections in the world. The World Health Organization (WHO) estimates that one-third of the world's population is currently infected with the TB bacillus. Scattered data are available regarding infection risk among travelers and aid workers.

Unlike long-term travelers for tourist purposes, aid workers have a higher tendency to work and live in close proximity to local communities. PCVs are typically housed together with local host families, and many other volunteers work in the health and education systems, where they are at higher risk of acquiring a TB infection.

In a Dutch study, 1.8% of Dutch travelers to high TB-endemic regions were identified as newly TB-infected patients. The overall incidence rate was 2.8 per 1000 person-months of travel after the exclusion of healthcare workers. The infection rate is of a similar magnitude to the average risk for the local population. Not surprisingly, working in patient care abroad, a common volunteering target, was an independent risk factor, with an odds ratio of 5.3.[14]

Furthermore, US PCVs have significantly higher rates of TB than the average population in the US, having a PPD conversion rate of 1.283 per 1000 volunteer-months, albeit lower than those reported in the Dutch trial. Despite this rate of newly infected persons, active TB cases are very rare.[4]

Table 34.2 Incidence of PPD Conversion Rate Among PCVs by Region[4]

Region	Total PPD Conversion Rate Per 1000 Volunteer-Months
Africa	1.464
Europe and Central Asia	1.442
South-East Asia	1.364
Central America	1.272
Caribbean	0.994
South America	0.739
Pacific Islands	0.547

Table 34.3 Countries with High Incidence of PPD Conversion Rate among PCVs[4]

Country of Volunteering	PPD Conversion Rate Per 1000 Volunteer-Months
Hungary	5.514
Guinea-Bissau	5.309
Ethiopia	3.384
Côte d'Ivoire	3.161
Cameroon	3.104
Albania	2.799
China	2.788
West Russia	2.632
Kazakhstan	2.426
Turkmenistan	2.421

The average infection rate has a large variation between different regions and countries (Tables 34.2 and 34.3).

HIV/AIDS

Data regarding HIV infection in travelers or humanitarian workers are scarce. The data that do exist suggest a very low rate of transmission,[9,15] although this probably does not reflect true numbers, especially among volunteers who engage in medical work.

The primarily recognized route of HIV transmission is through unprotected sex. Numerous reports suggest that sexual relationships in general, and unprotected contacts in particular, are common among aid workers.[2,11] Those returning from longer missions were more likely to have engaged in sexual risk behavior, as were men and younger volunteers.

Occupational exposure is another possible source of infection. It has long been established that healthcare workers are at increased risk of acquiring HIV through percutaneous or mucosal exposure. Healthcare workers traveling to high-prevalence HIV countries are estimated to be at an even higher risk. A British study found that the risk of healthcare workers in developing areas acquiring HIV infection through work was 1.5% over 5 years, which represented 1 in every 333 workers per year.[16]

Almost a third of British medical students doing an elective period in a hospital in developing countries had experienced at least one exposure to potentially infectious body fluids during their clinical training; 75% of these exposures were unreported;[17] 23% of American medical volunteers reported exposure to blood splash, and 2.3% experienced needle-stick.[18] But the exposure itself does not necessarily differ from the exposure in a western hospital, and the risk of transmission during a single needle-stick exposure is estimated to be only 0.3%. Nonetheless, the risk is probably much higher owing to variables present especially in developing counties settings, such as:

- Lower standards of sanitation of needles and other medical devices, absence of continuous and stable supply of protective measures such as gloves and gowns
- Higher prevalence of patients with high viral load
- Lack of appropriate knowledge or access to post-exposure prophylaxis treatment (PEP).

The latter is crucial, as it may minimize dramatically the risk of infection following a dangerous exposure.

Needle-stick exposure poses a risk to a wide range of diseases other than HIV/AIDS. Among other potential infections are dengue virus and other hemorrhagic fever viruses, syphilis, trypanosomiasis, and others.[19] Hepatitis B and C viruses are of special importance in low- and middle-income countries. Viruses that can easily be transmitted by needle-stick are highly prevalent in most developing countries, thereby posing a potential risk to the HAW.

Rabies

The risk of rabies is considered to increase with longer duration of travel. Because volunteers tend to travel for longer periods, and as they tend to stay in more deserted areas, post-disaster areas, or even to work in farms or directly with animals, one may assume they might even be at greater risk than usual: 7% of Norwegian missionaries and aid workers serving in different regions were exposed to proven or suspected rabies during their mission.[20] PCVs are 10 times more likely to be exposed to rabies risk abroad than in the US,[21] and numbers are as high as 3120 bites per 100 000 volunteers per year.

Dental Care

Oral health is an essential component of wellbeing, and dental emergencies may pose a big challenge to volunteers in developing countries. Dental services are often lacking or inadequate, with most developing countries having extremely low density of dentists per population. It appears that dental problems are a common complaint of long-term travelers, expatriates, and volunteers: 8% of cases that led to business trip cessation were reported to be caused by dental emergencies.[22] Among US Peace Corps volunteers serving 2 years in Madagascar, dental problems were reported as the fourth most common health problem, with 3.7% of volunteers reporting an event during service.[3] Similar numbers were reported by Peace Corps volunteers in Africa, and even higher numbers were noted among ICRC personnel.[2]

Mental Health

Mental health problems are consistently among the most reported by relief workers overseas (Table 34.1). It seems, however, that the extent of the phenomenon is overlooked and that the emotional needs of volunteers are often left unmet.

The anthropologist Kalervo Oberg was the first to apply the term 'cultural shock' to people who travel outside of their familiar culture.[23] The term suggests that travel and the experience of a new culture, considered a positive and exciting experience by most people, may be an unpleasant surprise or even shocking for others. Contact with an unfamiliar culture can lead to anxiety, stress, mental illness, and, in extreme cases, physical illness and suicide.[24–26] Exposure to extreme events with multiple casualties poses an even greater risk of long-term mental consequences.[27–29]

Relief workers are usually younger and motivated individuals, who travel to places that are both geographically and culturally remote from their daily experience, often without their family or familiar companion. They may travel to war zones and disaster areas, where they may be exposed to large-scale death and suffering. They often have great aspirations – sometimes unrealistic – about their future volunteer work and its effect on the community. These may all serve as precipitating factors to the development of emotional distress expressed by a wide range of symptoms, and may even develop into more serious mental conditions.

As many as 2% of PCVs in Madagascar seek mental health counseling outside of the routine support provided by the organization. The rate of reported mental health problems was more than double among other volunteers in the entire African region.[3]

Upon return home 42.6% of ICRC volunteers reported that the mission had been more stressful than they had expected: 30% reported exhaustion for at least 1 week during their mission, and similar numbers reported sleeping problems; 10% used sleeping pills. Other reported behavioral changes may also be contributors to stress: 14% declared increased alcohol consumption, 43% admitted to have been smoking more than usual during missions, and an additional 10% started to smoke for the first time. These behavioral changes were more common among those reporting exhaustion; 3% used drugs, mainly cannabis, during their stay.[2]

Migration itself is known to be a risk factor for suicide.[25] Suicide as a leading cause of death among international volunteers was first noticed in the Peace Corps: 13% of all reported deaths from 1981 to 1983 were due to suicide. These numbers declined drastically after a better screening procedure was instituted, with only one reported suicide in the following 20 years.[6,7] Unfortunately, many organizations do not have a parallel screening process and follow-up capabilities similar to the Peace Corps.

Finally, it should be emphasized that culture shock and emotional distress may also occur upon return home. This readjustment back to their own culture after a period of time abroad has been termed 'reverse culture shock.' In this part of their life, the volunteers might be left alone, without even the support of the organization or the expatriate group they may have had during the mission, leading to the feeling that they are alone in their struggle to readjust to their new circumstances.

Health Recommendations for the Relief Worker Traveling to Challenging Work Zones

Relief workers are a diverse group of organizations and individuals, thus general health recommendations should be tailored according to the age of the volunteer, the duration of travel, destination, nature of work and other variables. Nevertheless, we believe that proper volunteer preparation should include solid screening procedures, personal pre-travel counseling by a physician, and psychological preparedness.

During missions, especially those that are long-term or to crisis areas, volunteers should undergo a refreshment of health guidelines regarding wide-range risk behavior activities, either individually or in a group. In addition, debriefing mechanisms should be implemented, with emphasis on peer support.

Post-travel follow-up is unfortunately a neglected topic. The emotional and physical aspects of the volunteer should be addressed to ensure proper resettlement into his or her culture and community. This recommendation should be executed both by a treating physician and by the recruiting humanitarian organization, and a comprehensive

program, if feasible, is favored. For pre-travel screening see Tables 34.4 to 34.11.

Table 34.4 Physical Screening
Review of medical history, with emphasis on chronic health conditions and psychiatric history
Complete physical examination
High-risk individuals should undergo screening for possible hidden heart conditions: ECG, stress test
Dental examination

Table 34.5 Laboratory and Other Diagnostics
Routine laboratory screening: CBC, fasting glucose, kidney and liver function etc.
Baseline serological tests – HIV, HBV, HCV
TB screening (PPD or IGRT)
Pregnancy test for women of childbearing age
Malignancy screening (colonoscopy, mammography and Pap smears according to national screening recommendations)

Table 34.6 Vaccinations and Medications
Updating routine vaccinations and adding travel vaccines according to destination and duration of travel
Chronic medication supply for a minimum of 3 months and sustained mechanisms for future shipments of drugs. Use of local brands is not highly recommended
Self-treatment medications: diarrheal diseases (fluoroquinolone or substitutes), malaria standby therapy, first-aid kit
Malaria prophylaxis as needed
HIV post-exposure prophylaxis
Malaria rapid test kit (for groups)

Table 34.7 Personal Protection
Mosquito repellent
Male condoms
Personal supply of needles for injection or intravenous treatment
For volunteers in the medical field: protective clothing (gloves, gowns, goggles), face masks

Table 34.8 Psychological, Cultural and Environmental Preparedness
Psychological assessment to evaluate the ability of the volunteer to adjust to the specific mission
Encourage recruiting organizations to develop and implement pre-travel preparedness programs including background regarding host country, work environment, and cross-cultural issues
Promote knowledge regarding risk behaviors with possible health implications. This may include a wide range of topics such as traffic accidents awareness, safe sex, TB or schistosomiasis prevention

Table 34.9 During Mission

Continuous professional accompaniment of the volunteer to minimize insecurity and stress

Periodic oral and/or written refreshment of personal safety and risk behaviors recommendations

Consider group administration of malaria prophylaxis or a reminding mechanism to maximize adherence

Regular debriefing sessions, either in a group or one-on-one, allowing volunteers to express stress and difficulties during mission

If post-traumatic stress disorder (PTSD) signs or symptoms are suspected, prompt professional intervention

During long missions, an annual personal medical consult is advised

Table 34.10 Post-Mission Evaluation

Specific signs and symptoms reported by the volunteer should be addressed according to medical standards. If there are no specific medical complaints:

Anamnesis with emphasis on high-risk exposures to different pathogens, which may be asymptomatic

Routine laboratory tests as during pre-travel session

Repeat pre-travel serology tests (HIV, HBV, HCV)

Repeat TB screening test

Stool examination for ova and parasites

Table 34.11 Psychological Evaluation

Debriefing session(s) upon return

Encouragement of peer support

Monitoring the readjustment of long-term volunteers, as well as their children

Specific evaluation of PTSD signs and symptoms, especially following crisis intervention missions

References

1. UNHCR. The State of the World's Refugees. 2006; Chapter 3. http://www.unhcr.org/4a4dc1a89.html#

2. Dahlgren AL, Deroo L, Avril J, et al. Health risks and risk–taking behaviors among International Committee of the Red Cross (ICRC) expatriates returning from humanitarian missions. J Travel Med 2009 Nov–Dec;16(6):382–90.

3. Leutscher PD, Bagley SW. Health-related challenges in United States Peace Corps Volunteers serving for two years in Madagascar. J Travel Med 2003 Sep–Oct;10(5):263–7.

4. Jung P, Banks RH. Tuberculosis risk in US Peace Corps Volunteers, 1996 to 2005. J Travel Med 2008 Mar–Apr;15(2):87–94.

5. Nurthen NM, Jung P. Fatalities in the Peace Corps: a retrospective study, 1984 to 2003. J Travel Med 2008 Mar–Apr;15(2):95–101.

6. Hargarten SW, Baker SP. Fatalities in the Peace Corps. A retrospective study: 1962 through 1983. JAMA 1985 Sep 13;254(10):1326–9.

7. Hill DR. Pre-travel health, immunization status, and demographics of travel to the developing world for individuals visiting a travel medicine service. Am J Trop Med Hyg 1991 Aug;45(2):263–70.

8. LaRocque RC, Rao SR, Tsibris A, et al. Pre-travel health advice-seeking behavior among US international travelers departing from Boston Logan International Airport. J Travel Med 2010 Nov-Dec;17(6):387–91.

9. Chen LH, Wilson ME, Davis X, et al; GeoSentinel Surveillance Network. Illness in long-term travelers visiting GeoSentinel clinics. Emerg Infect Dis 2009 Nov;15(11):1773–82.

10. Goesch JN, Simons de Fanti A, Bechet S, Consigny PH. Comparison of knowledge on travel related health risks and their prevention among humanitarian aid workers and other travellers consulting at the Institut Pasteur travel clinic in Paris, France. Travel Med Infect Dis 2010 Nov;8(6):364–72. Epub 2010 Oct 27.

11. Moore J, Beeker C, Harrison JS, et al. HIV risk behavior among Peace Corps Volunteers. AIDS 1995 Jul;9(7):795–9.

12. Sheik M, Gutierrez MI, Bolton P, et al. Deaths among humanitarian workers. BMJ 2000 Jul 15;321(7254):166–8.

13. Freedman DO, Weld LH, Kozarsky PE, et al; GeoSentinel Surveillance Network. Spectrum of disease and relation to place of exposure among ill returned travelers. N Engl J Med 2006 Jan 12;354(2):119–30.

14. Cobelens FG, van Deutekom H, Draayer-Jansen IW, et al. Risk of infection with Mycobacterium tuberculosis in travellers to areas of high tuberculosis endemicity. Lancet 2000 Aug 5;356(9228):461–5.

15. Eng TR, O'Brien TR, Bernard KW, et al. HIV-1 and HIV-2 infections among U.S. Peace Corps Volunteers returning from West Africa. J Travel Med 1995 Sep 1;2(3):174–7.

16. Gilks CF, Wilkinson D. Reducing the risk of nosocomial HIV infection in British health workers working overseas: role of post-exposure prophylaxis. BMJ 1998 Apr 11;316(7138):1158–60.

17. Gamester CF, Tilzey AJ, Banatvala JE. Medical students' risk of infection with bloodborne viruses at home and abroad: questionnaire survey. BMJ 1999 Jan 16;318(7177):158–60.

18. Uslan DZ, Virk A. Postexposure chemoprophylaxis for occupational exposure to human immunodeficiency virus in traveling healthcare workers. J Travel Med 2005 Jan–Feb;12(1):14–8.

19. Tarantola A, Abiteboul D, Rachline A. Infection risks following accidental exposure to blood or body fluids in healthcare workers: a review of pathogens transmitted in published cases. Am J Infect Control 2006 Aug;34(6):367–75.

20. Bjorvatn B, Gundersen SG. Rabies exposure among Norwegian missionaries working abroad. Scand J Infect Dis 1980;12(4):257–64.

21. Banta JE, Jungblut E. Health problems encountered by the Peace Corps overseas. Am J Public Health Nations Health 1966 Dec;56(12):2121–5.

22. -0Callahan MV, Hamer DH. On the medical edge: preparation of expatriates, refugee and disaster relief workers, and Peace Corps volunteers. Infect Dis Clin North Am 2005 Mar;19(1):85–101.

23. Oberg K. Culture shock: adjustment to new cultural environments. Practical Anthropol 1960;7:l77–82.

24. Stewart L, Leggat PA. Culture shock and travelers. J Travel Med 1998 Jun;5(2):84–8.

25. Stack S. The effects of interstate migration on suicide. Int J Soc Psychiatry 1980;26(1):17–26.

26. World Health Organization/UN Joint Medical Services. Occupational health of field personnel in complex emergencies: report a pilot study. WHO/EHA 98.4. July 1998.

27. Fullerton CS, Ursano RJ, Wang L. Acute stress disorder, posttraumatic stress disorder, and depression in disaster or rescue workers. Am J Psychiatry 2004;161:1370–6.

28. Ozen S, Aytekin S. Frequency of PTSD in a group of search and rescue workers two months after 2003 Bingol (Turkey) earthquake. J Nerv Ment Dis 2004;192:573–5.

29. Guo U, Chen C, Lu M, et al. Posttraumatic stress disorder among professional and non-professional rescuers involved in an earthquake in Taiwan. Psychiatry Res 2004;127:35–41.

35

Expedition Medicine

Eric L. Weiss and Trish Batchelor

Key points

- The expedition physician must first assess his/her expertise and responsibility to determine whether the role is appropriate
- Pre-travel preparation includes a risk assessment analysis, and risk management strategies, including the development of a first-aid kit
- Potential medical problems are most often determined by the health of the group, the nature of the activities and the environment in which they are carried out
- Meticulous preparation, medical expertise, communication and problem-solving skills, creativity and improvisation are qualities that make for a successful expedition physician

Introduction

In the early 1900s expeditions were the reserve of the privileged few who could devote months or even years of their lives to the pursuit of discovery. The heroic exploits of the early Antarctic explorers such as Scott and Shackleton define our concept of 'expedition'. What, now, a century later, is an expedition? The *Collins English Dictionary* defines an expedition as 'an organized journey or voyage, esp. for exploration or for a scientific or military purpose'.[1] The range of expeditions undertaken today is enormous. In the UK alone, it is estimated that the 'expedition market' involves between 1200 and 1500 travelers annually.[2] At one end of the scale are those whom one would consider the 'purists' – the Scotts and Shackletons of our era. These are the individuals who impose a stratagem of 'arbitrary self-limitation'[3] to overcome the lack of 'blank places' on our earth. These individuals will often travel alone or in very small groups with little or no support, for example Goran Kropp, a Swede who rode his bicycle from Sweden to the base of Mt Everest and then climbed to the summit entirely unsupported. For the majority of people, however, an expedition is a group exercise. This may be a group of friends or colleagues, a university or school group, a commercial climbing trip, an ecological group or perhaps a charity support group. A uniting theme is that expeditions will usually visit areas of climatic extremes (mountains, polar regions, desert, the tropical jungle, or the ocean) and that they will undertake some kind of activity, whether this be scientific research or an adventure activity such as climbing, kayaking, rafting, diving, caving, or sailing.

Expedition doctors are rarely paid to accompany such a group. Often they are invited by friends or have an interest in the particular activity being undertaken. In fact, many expeditions leave with no physician or other medical provider – here is another opportunity for travel medicine outreach and education. The aim of the expedition doctor is to minimize risk by taking sensible precautions – advising on the correct pre-travel preparation, managing potential environmental risks, and being as prepared as possible to manage emergencies that may arise. Risk cannot be eliminated, and neither should it be – part of the appeal of undertaking an expedition is an element of risk. However, as in all aspects of travel medicine, wise pre-planning can only contribute to a successful journey.

Many of the topics relevant to expedition doctors are covered in more detail in other chapters of this book – particularly high-altitude medicine, diving, remote destinations, psychological disorders, diarrhea, and food and water issues. This chapter attempts to give some guidance on deciding whether being an expedition doctor is right for you; how to prepare yourself and your group for the expedition; how to put together an appropriate first-aid kit; an awareness of common problems that may occur in various climatic conditions or undertaking particular activities; and how to deal with some of the more difficult situations you may be faced with on your journey.

To solve a problem which has long resisted the skill and persistence of others is an irresistible magnet in every sphere of human activity.

(Sir John Hunt, expedition leader of the first successful ascent of Everest)

Questions to Ask

The opportunity to be a trip physician may come as an unexpected phone call or e-mail, or at other times the expedition physician may be a founding member of the expeditionary team. Either way, there are important questions to ask, both of yourself and of the organizing group, to ensure a good match of expectation, ability, and responsibility.

Perhaps the overriding consideration for the expedition physician-to-be is a careful evaluation of the expedition team. Strong communication abilities, interpersonal skills, and sensitivity are all vital components for all members of the expedition leadership – physician

©2012 Elsevier Inc
DOI: 10.1016/B978-1-4557-1076-8.00035-1

included. Be honest with yourself regarding your personality, your skills, and your overall suitability for this exciting, but often demanding role. For more challenging expeditions to austere environments, strong interpersonal skills are obviously important for all team members. However, for more commercially organized group expeditions or trips, the expedition physician will likely be a member of the staff; it is essential that he or she be willing and able to work as a team player.

The converse is also true: the organizing group also needs to be willing to grant medical authority to the physician. Everyone's respective roles and responsibilities need to be clearly defined long before the first medical issues arise, far from the peaceful comforts of the meeting room. Even then, medical action (once the patient has been medically stabilized) should take place in a coordinated fashion, with all team members aware of and agreeing on the plan. For all this to work smoothly, there are questions that every potential expedition physician should put on the table. Before, during, and after the trip, what are the physician's responsibilities to the program? Will he or she be responsible for pre-travel medical screening? Will a health questionnaire be administered, and who will write the questions? In borderline cases, who has the final say regarding passenger participation? And who will provide 'pre-travel' education and information to leadership and participants alike? The authors feel strongly that these responsibilities fall clearly in the expedition physician's domain. Since it may be less clear what is the role of the physician regarding non-medical issues, this also should be discussed. Some programs simply want a physician available should a medical situation arise, while others view the physician as an integral member of the leadership team. The more challenging the expedition the more important it is to be a member of the team.

Other issues that need to be considered include the provision or requirement of travel health/repatriation insurance. Many companies allow this to be an optional addition for their participants, setting the stage for difficult situations and/or decision making later on. Be aware that traditional limits on payment (often US$5000 in the USA) or on pre-existing illness with standard policies are insufficient for even the most 'vanilla' of expeditions. The expedition physician is in a position to lobby for appropriate attention to be paid to this often neglected issue.

Responsibility for the expedition medical kit is another very important issue for discussion. Smaller expeditions may expect the physician to be completely responsible for the medical kit, whereas other programs may have an established kit built at the corporate office. The latter may be perfectly acceptable, but it is essential that the trip physician be very familiar with the kit contents, both in name as well as in location. Taking the kit apart and putting it back together several times before departure would be wise, not only to breed familiarity, but also to ensure inventory completeness.

Not to be forgotten in the pre-adventure enthusiasm are the issues of compensation, and, unfortunately, liability. The latter is more an issue for physicians who work where the ratio of legal to medical professionals is higher and will be discussed separately below. The former should simply be put on the table before the significant responsibility of providing on-trip medical care is agreed to and assumed.

Depending on the size, nature, duration, destination(s) of the expedition, being included may be sufficient reward. For more commercially oriented trips, the trip physician is typically not charged the same fee that his or her fellow passengers may have to pay. Some companies may only reduce the fee, rather than eliminate it all together. Perhaps physician family members may participate at a reduced rate. The expectant expedition physician should be wisely counseled that the trip at hand may include a significant amount of

work. Clearly, many factors are at play here. Young, healthy travelers going on a short rafting expedition are less likely to need significant medical intervention than a group of elderly travelers on a 4-week around-the-world trip (see quote by Iain McIntosh, below). For programs where the need for medical care may be expected to be high, it is not unreasonable to ask for payment for services rendered.

One should avoid at all costs accompanying the elderly devotees on tours specially designed for them, with a suicidal urge to embark on a holiday of a lifetime to the end of the earth. These old-timers carry their chronic disorders with them and are always accompanied by suitcases full of medicaments. Grounded by gout and arthritis, deterred by dyspnoea and congestion, few are fit enough to view the sights of global travel and seek recompense by monopolizing the attention of the captive tour-doctor to his/her great discomfort. The holiday spirit, can, however, be experienced to excess in younger groups where over-indulgence in cheap, potent, local libations brings maudlin merriment, self-inflicted injury, drunken coma and resultant inconvenience to the harassed group medic.

It is well to eschew well-publicized jaunts to conquer K4 or climb to some inaccessible summit in Bhutan. The 'tigers' of the high tops frequently peel off the mountain at a moment of maximal discomfort for the expedition doctor and rendering first aid, where exposure is both vertical and climatic, is not without hazard. Simple school trips to Gwent or Tangier must also be viewed with misgiving for youngsters start vomiting the moment the boat leaves the harbour, if not before, and a series of bruises, breaks and blood-letting will exasperate the medical companion.

Better by far to choose a group of the middle-aged in robust health, long separated from the boisterous over activity of youth, devoid of desire to climb impossible peaks and seeking only their creature comforts and a modicum of culture in a distant sunny clime. They never wander very far from life's simpler pleasures such as hot baths, flushing loos and good cuisine.

(Iain McIntosh, 1992)[4]

In sum, there are many issues to be considered before signing up for the exciting, but often challenging, role as expedition physician. Be sure you are comfortable with expected roles and responsibility, do not underestimate the amount of work involved, and be satisfied with the compensation offered, even if it is simply the opportunity to participate in an adventure that will hopefully broaden your horizons forever.

Risk Assessment and Preparation

After positively answering the question: 'Am I right for this expedition' (and 'Is it right for me?'), it is now time to prepare. A risk assessment analysis should be prepared. All the potential aspects of the trip that could cause a problem should be reviewed, and ways to minimize the risks should be thought through. It is prudent to reduce the risk to acceptable levels, as ultimately it is the expedition physician who will have to deal with the medical problems that will arise.

Personal Preparation

The expedition physician will need to learn as much as possible about the group members, the environment it is traveling to, and the activities the group will be undertaking.

A medical questionnaire (Table 35.1) is designed to (a) identify group members who may be unsuitable for the trip and (b) identify members with pre-existing conditions.

Table 35.1 Sample Medical Questionnaire for Group Members

Personal details
  Name
  D.O.B.
  Address
  Phone contacts
  E-mail address
Next of kin to be contacted in an emergency
  Name
  Address
  Phone contacts: Home:
Work:
Mobile:
  E-mail address
Regular doctor
  Name
  Address
  Contact phone numbers: Surgery:
Emergency:
  E-mail address
When did you last see your regular doctor and why?
  Do you have any current medical problems? If so, please provide details.
  Have you ever had any medical or psychological problems in the past? If so, please provide details.
  Have you ever had any surgery?
  Have you been hospitalized in the past 2 years, and if so, why?
  Do you take any prescribed medications?
  Do you take any over-the-counter or herbal medications?
  Do you have any allergies including drugs, foods, stings, Band-Aids etc.?
  What is your blood group?
  Do you drink alcohol? If so how many per day of:
Wine:
Beer:
Spirits:
  Have you traveled to less developed countries before? If so, when, and did you have any problems while you were away?
  Activity, as relevant, e.g., what is the highest altitude you have climbed/trekked to? How deep was your deepest dive? etc.
  Environmentally specific questions as relevant, e.g., have you suffered from altitude sickness before? Have you suffered from the bends before? If so, provide details.
  We have provided a list of recommended immunizations – please mark below the date you received them. List as appropriate.
  What was your most recent blood pressure reading and when was this taken?
  Do you have any particular medical concerns regarding this trip?

Having to say 'no' to a potential participant is one of the more difficult tasks you may be faced with – this is more likely to happen on a commercial expedition. It is possible that the individual concerned will dispute the decision; therefore, it is recommended that one ask for a second opinion from an expert in the relevant field. This may not be necessary if a positive relationship is established with the individual's personal physician. This is a relatively uncommon scenario. More frequently, some trip members will have pre-existing conditions that do not warrant exclusion from the trip, but require

extra preparation. Most pre-existing conditions can be successfully controlled as long as the group member is honest about his/her condition, the appropriate pre-trip preparation has been undertaken, and you as the physician are prepared to manage any exacerbations that may occur as a result of the conditions of the trip. It would be wise to obtain a report from the individual's regular physician including laboratory work, X-ray and EKG interpretation, and contact information (including e-mail and mobile phone).

It is important for the trip physician to be prepared to handle almost any emergency that may occur. A background combining primary care, emergency medicine, and tropical or travel medicine would be ideal. Apart from the management of common travel-related illness, such as diarrhea and problems specific to the environment to be visited, the following are some suggestions of prerequisite skills necessary to ensure that the physician is adequately equipped before the expedition is undertaken:

- Basic resuscitation skills on an emergency life support (ELS), advanced cardiac life support (ACLS) or acute trauma life support (ATLS) course should be renewed or taken up
- Management of chronic disease exacerbation (CHF, CAD, asthma, and diabetes) should be reviewed
- Comfortable with SAM splint (or equivalent) to improvise immobilization for common orthopedic conditions including fractures
- Familiarity with shoulder, ankle, and elbow dislocation management
- Comfortable with the use of sports tape to treat common sprains and strains
- Knowledge of basic dental skills, e.g., using cavit for temporary fillings
- Management of epistaxis
- Proficiency with wound care, including lacerations, burns, and foreign bodies
- Comfortable with dealing with minor ophthalmological problems, such as corneal foreign body, corneal abrasions, etc.
- Knowledge of the use of basic transportation and evacuation systems.

The other major contributors to potential medical problems are the expedition environment and the activities the group is undertaking. Learn as much as possible about the trip environment. Environmental extremes of heat, cold, humidity, altitude, depth, UV exposure, or motion all have their consequent medical problems. Table 35.2 gives some examples to consider. Learn about the endemic diseases of the country – some will be preventable with immunizations or medications, while others will be preventable by behavior modification, such as insect avoidance and personal hygiene. Will you be able to diagnose and manage these conditions without sophisticated laboratory support? There may be concerns about specific forms of wildlife, particularly venomous reptiles. The expedition physician can learn about the environment to be visited by reading (the bibliography at the end of this section is a good starting point), speaking with doctors or group members who have been to similar environments before, or undertaking one of the increasing number of courses available which focus on specific environmental hazards and activities.

You will also need to be prepared for the health risks specific to the activity you are undertaking, e.g., the risk of dislocated shoulders in kayakers, decompression illness in divers, etc. In preparing for a potential 'worst case scenario', an evacuation plan should be in place (Fig. 35.1). You should have made contact with your assistance company and learned as much as possible about any local healthcare facilities

Table 35.2 Risk Assessment – An Example of Some Potential Risks

Aspect of Trip	Potential Risk
The team	
Pre-existing medical conditions	Deterioration in extreme or remote conditions resulting in medical emergency/death
Fitness of members	Lack of fitness leading to increased risk of injury or illness
Adequate pre-travel preparation	Lack of adequate preparation leading to risk of preventable diseases, e.g., Hep A, malaria
Experience and training of members	Less experience and training will lead to increased risk of mishap
Attitudes	Willingness to follow guidelines will reduce risk
Equipment	Poorly maintained equipment adds risk
Team dynamics	A harmonious team is less risky
The environment	
Mountains	Altitude sickness, serious injuries, frostbite, snow blindness, UV damage, hypothermia
Desert	Heat exhaustion, dehydration, UV damage
Tropics/jungle	Heat exhaustion, dehydration, skin infections, wildlife
Ocean	UV damage, sea sickness, decompression illness, CAGE, dehydration, venomous stingers, coral cuts
All less developed countries	Poor food and water hygiene leading to enteric diseases
Specific endemic diseases	Insect-borne diseases, e.g., malaria, dengue, JBE, trypanosomiasis, myiasis, etc.
Wildlife	Bites, envenomation, stings, injuries
Transport/road conditions	Motor vehicle accidents/plane accidents leading to serious injury or death
The activity	
Mountaineering	AMS, serious injuries from falls, hypothermia, frostbite, snow blindness, UV damage
Trekking	AMS, UV damage, minor injuries
Kayaking	Drowning, shoulder dislocations
Diving	Decompression illness, CAGE, coral cuts
Sailing	Drowning, injuries, motion sickness
Caving	Drowning, suffocation
Local population	
Political climate	Risk of kidnapping, terrorist activities, piracy
Attitudes to foreigners	Risk of theft, injury, rape
Hygiene standards	Enteric disease
Medical facilities	Nosocomial infection in local medical facilities (esp. Hep B, HIV)

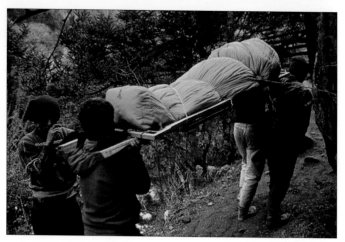

Figure 35.1 Litter evacuation. Nightmare in Nepal – Be Prepared, Do Your Homework, and Do Not Forget Evacuation Insurance. (*Photograph courtesy of Eric Weiss.*)

that may be accessible. In a very few parts of the world there are well-organized rescue facilities in place, e.g., the Himalayan Rescue Association in Nepal; however, in most areas for expedition, there will be a dearth of reliable local medical facilities.

Safety and security issues are paramount. In their study looking at the incidence of health problems on expeditions, the Royal Geographical Society of Britain recorded only two deaths out of 2381 participants in 19 000 expedition days. These were two Indonesian members of a trip to Irian Jaya who were kidnapped by West Papuan independence fighters.[4] In particular, many of the world's highest mountains are in countries with unstable political situations (India, Nepal, Tibet, and Pakistan), and piracy on the ocean is a real threat to long-term ocean-goers. The local Department of Foreign Affairs website provides updated information (Table 35.3).

Preparing your group members is vitally important – you should be the one to provide them with specific pre-travel health recommendations, including appropriate immunizations, malaria prophylaxis (if relevant), and general health advice. If you run a travel medicine clinic this can be a 'marketing' opportunity for you, otherwise you should refer your members to a travel medicine clinic with staff who are knowledgeable about the type of risks associated with the trip. For remote expeditions where the rabies risk is high, you should think about ensuring that all of your members are immunized against rabies, as in many parts of the world obtaining human rabies immunoglobulin is impossible. Travel medicine advice for groups is notoriously inconsistent if supplied by different providers: ensuring consistency also gives a sense of confidence to group members. Although you will be bringing your own extensive medical kit, it is sensible to ensure that each member of the group also carries a basic kit – you do not want to be a 'day and night pharmacy' for basic over-the-counter medications. The only exception to this rule may be travel with a group of students under the age of 18 and on whom you prefer to keep a very close eye. Your group members should receive clear written information about the environmental conditions they are going to face so that they can be mentally and physically prepared. If appropriate, you may even consider giving advice on pre-travel fitness training.

One often-ignored element of group preparation is ensuring that there are other members who can perform first aid in a remote setting. It would be unwise to be the only person in the group capable of managing common medical problems. There are an increasing number of first-aid courses with an emphasis on the wilderness setting being

Table 35-3 Useful Websites

Subject Area	URL
Mountaineering	
International Society of Mountain Medicine	www.ismmed.org
High altitude medicine guide	www.high-altitude-medicine.com
The British Mountaineering Council UIAA Mountain Medicine Centre	www.thebmc.co.uk
The International Porter Protection Group	www.ippg.net
Kayaking and rafting	
America Canoe Association	www.acanet.org
The American White Water Affiliation	www.americanwhitewater.org
Canadian Recreational Canoeing Association	www.paddlingcanada.com
British Canoe Union	www.bcu.org.uk
Scuba diving	
South Pacific Underwater Medical Society	www.spums.org.au
Divers Alert Network	www.diversalertnetwork.org
Undersea and Hyperbaric Medicine Society	www.uhms.org
Safety and security	
US Dept of State	www.state.gov
UK Foreign and Commonwealth Office	www.fco.gov.uk
Canada Dept of Foreign Affairs	www.voyage.gc.ca/dest/sos/warnings-en.asp
Australian Department of Foreign Affairs and Trade	www.smarttraveller.gov.au
New Zealand Dept of Foreign Affairs	www.safetravel.govt.nz
German Foreign Office	www.ayswaertiges-amt.de/diplo/en/Startseite.html

run for lay people. Consider asking other members of the expedition leadership (or other interested parties) to take this or similar courses. Poll the expedition participants for persons with medical training. Retired or off-duty physicians and other healthcare providers can provide useful extra hands and expertise.

A group meeting, if possible, is the ideal environment in which to give a medical briefing to your group – this can be an excellent opportunity to dispel any myths and resolve any conflicting advice that people invariably will have received.

First-Aid Kits

Nowhere does the adage 'the right tool for the job' ring more true than when trying to deal with a brisk nosebleed or case of urinary tract obstruction while away from your local emergency department. The expedition physician must be creative and innovative when it comes to caring for those in his or her charge, and this includes the ability to improvise with materials at hand if the first-aid kit is not. That being said, duct tape or safety pins are usually no substitute for the 'right tool', so careful consideration of your first-aid kit's contents is an essential component of pre-trip planning.

Contents

Expedition participants play several important roles in respect to the trip first-aid kit. Certainly everyone should be advised to travel with his or her own personal kit, including the simple remedies that many use on a regular basis. Having travelers consider any medication or first aid-oriented product that they have used in the past year is a good trigger for what ought to come along. The expedition physician should also carefully review the health status of each participant, and be certain to anticipate potential medical conditions or exacerbations while designing the kit. In addition to being participant specific, the kit should also be itinerary specific: consider the environmental risks as well, such as altitude, cold, or heat illness. It is useful to divide the kit contents into categories (wound care, ears/nose/throat, antibiotics, dental, etc.) while planning the contents (Table 35.4). Pack items that can be used creatively for several purposes – for example, a Foley catheter can also be used to control epistaxis, or as a tourniquet. Lastly, the participants themselves unknowingly may provide some degree of buffer for the physician, since often they may have an item you need in their personal stash. This is obviously more likely to occur in a larger, commercial group.

Design

In addition to its contents, the actual kit design is an important feature. The expedition physician needs to be very familiar with the contents as well as their location. Having to struggle to find the epinephrine or nitroglycerin in an emergency situation is not optimal. To have all of the 'emergency' drugs/interventions in a separate pull-away pouch can be very helpful. For day excursions where the group will be away from packs or baggage, the physician should make up a 'day pack', which includes not only the emergency pouch above, but also the commonly used agents, such as analgesics, antibiotics, loperamide, and bandaging materials.

Supplies

Another consideration is drug and supply availability on the road. If the expedition needs to be truly self-sufficient, careful consideration needs to be paid to both first-aid kit components and amounts. If there is an ability to re-stock while on the road, be certain to have a system of tracking first-aid kit use. For kits that will be re-used, a careful post-trip inventory check is critical.

A final consideration is perhaps the most difficult. Where will you, as expedition physician, draw the line? Will you include intravenous supplies? What about airway equipment, such as laryngoscopes and endotracheal tubes? The size and cost of automatic external defibrillators (AEDs) have come down significantly such that they are now increasingly being included in expedition medical kits. The weight and size of the first-aid kit are obviously important considerations, but so too are issues of 'what then?' If your patient requires respiratory support in the middle of nowhere, how long can you reasonably sustain such efforts? 'Triage' becomes even more important, as well as more difficult, when far from home.

Liability

In the USA, the issue of medical legal exposure quickly arises in any environment where a healthcare provider is involved with caring for patients. Unfortunately, over time this issue is being exported around the world. However, medical legal sensitivity does not mean that fear of lawsuit needs to drive all decision making, or even be a constant concern. Providing quality patient care and documentation that serves

Table 35-4 Example of Physician-Level First-Aid Kit

Emergency
    Epinephrine 1: 1000 (1 mg/mL)
    Nitroglycerin spray, metered dose inhaler
    Oral glucose gel
    Pocket mask (e.g., by Laerdal)
    Diphenhydramine 50 mg/mL injectable vial
    Albuterol metered dose inhaler
    No. 11 scalpel
    No. 10 scalpel
    5.0 endotracheal tube, cuffed
    1 mL pre-packaged syringe (27 gauge needle)
    3 mL pre-packaged syringe (21 gauge needle)
    Oral airways (assorted sizes)
    Laryngoscope with Macintosh 3 blade
    McGill forceps
    Nasal trumpet (30 french)
    Foley catheter (16 french)
    Sawyer snake bite extractor
    Morphine sulfate
    Diazepam
Other injectables
    Promethazine
    Furosemide
    Dexamethasone
Wound care/preparation
    0.25% bupivacaine
    0.25% bupivacaine w/epinephrine
    20 mL irrigating syringe
    Povidone iodine solution
    Povidone iodine swab stick
    Needle driver
    Mosquito clam
    Iris scissors
    Toothed forceps
    3 mL syringe (25 gauge needle)
    5 mL syringe (25 gauge needle)
    Alcohol wipes
Wound closure
    Dermabond tissue glue
    Disposable skin stapler
    6.0 Surgilene suture
    5.0 Surgilene suture
    4.0 Surgilene suture
    4.0 Dexon suture
    Steri-Strips (3 mm, 5 mm)
    Tincture of benzoin swabs
Wound dressings
    Band-Aids (assorted sizes)
    2 × 2 gauze
    4 × 4 gauze
    2-inch Kling gauze
    Polysporin ointment
    One inch cloth tape
    ½ inch pink tape
    Xeroform gauze
    Q-tips
    Mole skin

    Sam splint
    Ace wrap
    Duct tape
Eyes, ears, nose and throat
    Sterile eyewash
    Tetracaine drops
    Mydriacyl drops
    Sulamyd drops
    Ciprofloxacin drops
    Erythromycin ointment
    Fluorescein strips
    Ophthalmoscope/otoscope
    Alligator forceps
    Earwick
    Cortisporin otic suspension
    Rhinoguard epistaxis device
    Lidocaine 2% jelly
    Ear speculum
    Afrin nasal spray
    Sucrets (oral anesthetic)
    Dental
    'Tempadent' (dental filling)
    Oil of clove
Dermatologic
    Topical steroid (sample size)
    Clotrimazole cream (sample size)
    Topical 'sting relief'
    Sunscreen (UVA & UVB blocker)
Oral medications
    Pain/sedation
    Acetaminophen
    Ibuprofen
    Acetaminophen/hydrocodone
    Diazepam
    Haloperidol
Antibiotics
    Ciprofloxacin
    Azithromycin
    Penicillin VK
Gastrointestinal
    Imodium AD
    Docusate sodium (stool softener)
    Oral rehydration salt packets
    Ranitidine
Cough/cold
    Sudafed decongestant
    Echinacea herbal supplement
    Zinc tablets
Altitude
    Acetazolamide 125 mg
    Dexamethasone 4 mg
    Nifedipine 10 mg
Other
    Diphenhydramine
    Prednisone
    Caffeine (nodose)

Table 35.4 Example of Physician-Level First-Aid Kit—cont'd

Miscellaneous	
21 and 25 gauge butterfly needles	Stethoscope
Small ziplock plastic bags w/labels	BP cuff
Small breakout emergency medical bag	Safety pins
One liter normal saline	Lighter
Trauma scissors	Small notepad
Latex gloves	Pen or other writing instrument
Small flashlight	Pregnancy test
Electronic thermometer	Urine dip-stick test
Eye protection	Pocket pharmacopeia reference
	Pocket emergency medicine reference

as a good communication tool should be your guiding principle. That being said, the expedition physician would be wise to consider malpractice insurance because there is, in fact, some liability assumed.

The simplest way to do this, if you are currently covered through your practice, is to approach your insurance provider and ask that a 'rider' be added to the existing policy. Often this can be accomplished at no additional expense, or perhaps a one-time fee will be involved. The other terms of your insurance will remain the same. Detailed discussion of 'occurrence' versus 'claims made' insurance, with a 'tail', is beyond the scope of this discussion, but if these terms are unfamiliar, it would be wise to familiarize yourself with them. Simply stated, occurrence coverage will cover any event that occurs within the timeframe of the policy – if a trip participant chose to bring a lawsuit several years later, you would still be provided for. In contrast, the 'claims made' insurance policy covers you against malpractice claims only during the time you are paying premiums. Legal action years later may find you unprotected, unless a 'tail' to your policy is purchased. The 'tail' extends the policy for a fixed period of time, for a fixed price, naturally.

If you are providing medical services on behalf of a larger travel organization, it is possible to be covered under the auspices of the parent company. This practice, however, is rare – most travel companies looking for a 'trip physician' will require the physician to provide his/her own malpractice insurance. Do not overlook this issue during your discussions with such a company. The expedition physician assumes liability even if not formally paid. Simply receiving a trip discount brings responsibility and potential exposure. So-called 'Good Samaritan' laws do not apply here.

If you currently have no malpractice insurance, and the expedition itself is unable or unwilling to provide this, it is wise to explore insurance options for the duration of the trip. That being said, this sort of coverage is increasingly difficult to obtain. One physician, having exhausted the local options, actually turned to Lloyds of London to craft a customized insurance product.

In summary, medical legal exposure is one of the unfortunate realities of providing medical care in almost any situation. Signing up as the expedition physician will ensure adventure, but also bring added responsibility. Although practicing 'good medicine' is the best advice, having a good malpractice policy will provide an additional layer of comfort.

On the Road

As expedition medical officer, the responsibility will be that of caring for the group members should they become ill or injured, managing medical emergencies that may occur, and organizing evacuations and repatriations should they be necessary. In the field of wilderness medicine, the following attributes have been suggested as desirable for a 'wilderness physician' and they translate well into selection criteria for an expedition doctor: 'forethought, preparation, experience, confidence in your knowledge and abilities, the ability to step into a 'wilderness' mindset, and especially, the ability to take a thorough history, do a meticulous and accurate physical examination, and draw the proper conclusions from your findings'.[5] All this has to be accomplished in potentially hostile environmental conditions, with no back-up and limited communications.

It is important to remember that the group will probably include local staff – their health on the expedition is also the expedition physician's area of responsibility. There is a popular misconception that porters in the developing world are made of 'tougher stuff' than Westerners. Recently, the health of porters, particularly in the Himalayas and the Andes, has been studied, and it has been found that even on commercial high-altitude treks, porters are just as likely as Western trekkers to become ill or injured at altitude.[6] Concerned individuals have established an organization known as the International Porter Protection Group (IPPG) to educate trekking and climbing groups of their responsibilities to their local staff (www.ippg.net).

It is very wise to lay down the ground rules at the beginning of your trip – you should set aside a specific time each day for 'clinic'. All non-urgent problems should be dealt with at this time, including problems of the local staff. Treating the local population is a contentious issue[7] and will be discussed later.

This section will look briefly at the more common types of expedition and the conditions for which the expedition physician should be prepared. Some aspects will be covered in more detail in other chapters, and specific texts should be consulted for more detailed information.

There has been little published research on the actual incidence of medical problems on expeditions. Physicians will have a 'feel' for the emergencies they should be prepared for, but how does this correlate with what actually happens in the field?

The Expedition Advisory Center of the Royal Geographic Society in London has established a 'medical cell' that is studying the incidence of medical problems during expeditions. Data published by them in 2000 examined expeditions that were in the field between 1995 and 1997.[2] These data are based on the voluntary submission of questionnaires from expedition leaders. The study authors recorded information from 36% of the expeditions registered with the Society over this period.

Their data examined 2381 participants in 246 expeditions who visited 105 different countries for a total of 19 000 man-days in the field. Of these expeditions, 41% visited the mountains, 33% the tropics, and the remainder visited variously polar regions, desert, or marine environments. Group sizes ranged from 1 to 90 members, with a mean of nine. The average length of trip was 8 weeks, with a range of 2 weeks to >3 months. The main purposes were scientific study (45%), adventure (39%), community work (2%), and a mix of science and adventure (14%).

Most notably, only 13% of expeditions had a physician accompanying them to provide medical care. Some 65% relied on a trained 'first aider', 6% on a registered nurse, and 4% on a paramedic. Lastly, 13% of the expeditions reviewed had no-one with any medical training accompanying them. This is a marked improvement on data collected in 1983, which showed that 52% of 95 expeditions had no individual with even basic first-aid training accompanying them.[8] Nearly three-quarters of the groups reported medical problems. A total of 181 groups reported a total of 835 incidents, an incident rate of 6.4/1000 person-days in the field. A total of 78% of incidents were classified as mild (the person could return to their activity after treatment); 17% were intermediate (the person was unable to return to activity but did not require evacuation), and 5% were serious (resulting in death, evacuation, or hospitalization). Repatriation back to the UK was required by only 0.3% of expeditioners.

Not surprisingly, the most common problem affecting expedition members was gastrointestinal illness, particularly diarrhea – this accounted for 33% of problems recorded. Similar figures were reported by the British 1992 winter expedition to Mt Everest[9] and reflect the rate of GI illness in travelers to less developed countries in general (Table 35.5). What may be a nuisance for the leisure traveler

Table 35-5 Conditions Treated on British Mt Everest Winter Expedition	
Category	**Number of Cases**
GIT	
Gastroenteritis	43 (30%)
Upper GI bleed	1
Dyspepsia	2
Persistent vomiting	1
Hemorrhoids	3
TRAUMA	
# Tibia	1
STI incl. lacerations	10
RESPIRATORY	
Sore throat	14
High altitude cough	18
Cough induced intercostal myalgia	2
Respiratory tract infection	5
Persistent nasal congestion	2
ENVIRONMENTAL	
Hypothermia	2
Sunburn	5
AMS mild	24
AMS severe	2
Frostbite	6
GENERAL MEDICAL	
Ileofemoral venous thrombosis	1
Insomnia	5
Macular hemorrhage	1
Presumed retinal ischemia	1
DENTAL	
Abscess	2
Lost crown	2

can be a devastating illness that risks the success of an expedition (see Chs 18–21 for more detail.) The expedition physician should ensure that the incidence of any specific pathogens that could be of concern during the trip has been researched, e.g., are you visiting Nepal before the monsoon season, when *Cyclospora* is a problem? Ensure that your method of water purification and armamentarium of antibiotics reflect the pathogens to which your group will be exposed. Anecdotally, it appears that individuals who are suffering from an intercurrent illness such as diarrhea are more susceptible to altitude sickness.[10] In an expedition situation, any illness should be treated at an early stage.

'General medical conditions' accounted for 21% of problems recorded by the RGS expeditioners; these included chest, ear and skin infections, typhoid fever, 23 cases of confirmed or suspected malaria, seven cases of dengue fever, and 16 disabling drug side-effects. Interestingly, mefloquine was felt to be the offending drug in 75% of these cases.

A total of 17% of problems were classified as 'orthopedic'. These were predominantly falls on rough terrain, burns, lacerations, bruises, and concussion. Only 11 people were involved in motor vehicle accidents and one in an avalanche. Of the problems, 14% were 'environmental' – 50% of these were altitude related, with sunstroke and heat exhaustion making up 35%; 8% were unwell as result of arthropod or other wildlife bites – particularly scorpions, snakes, and jellyfish. Surgical disorders were rare and accounted for only 3% of complaints, including two cases of appendicitis, 10 minor dental problems, and 13 cases of minor ophthalmic trauma.

Of the serious disorders, altitude sickness accounted for 27% of cases, 'general medical' (predominantly malaria) for 27%, and serious fractures or dislocations in the mountains for 23%. Two deaths were recorded, both as a result of kidnapping. The authors suggest that 'participation in a well-planned expedition is comparatively safe, with a medical incident rate of 6.4 per 1000 person-days and a death rate of 1 per 12 00 participants'.[2] They compared this with the risk of a medical incident at other events in which young people participate: 10 per 1000 at a scout camp; 17 per 1000 at a rock concert, and 28 per 1000 running a marathon.[11]

There is no doubt that the level of risk varies according to the style of expedition that one is undertaking. As only 13% of the studied expeditions took a medical officer with them, it is tempting to suggest that many of them would be considered relatively low risk by the organizers and participants. High-altitude mountaineering is known to be a very dangerous pastime, with a death rate of 2.9%.[12] An analysis of British mountaineering deaths on peaks of over 7000 m from 1968 to 1987 documented a mortality rate of 4.3/100 mountaineers. A total of 70% of deaths were due to falls, avalanches, or crevasse accidents.[13]

Although acute psychiatric problems appear to be rare on expeditions, they are without doubt one of the more difficult problems to manage in a remote area. Expeditions will invariably involve significant levels of stress, discomfort, and interpersonal conflict. Although most individuals will cope under these circumstances, there is a small chance that an individual may decompensate, resulting in a psychiatric crisis. Pre-travel screening is crucial in trying to avoid such potential problems. There are no hard and fast rules, but some issues to consider include:

- Past behavior. Find out what your team members have done in the past and speak to people who have traveled with them – how have they coped under difficult circumstances previously. Past behavior is a better predictor of future behavior than words and intentions

- Enthusiasm of the individual for not only the trip but also for life in general. What are the person's motivators? Negative reasons for joining a trip (such as getting over a major life crisis) are not necessarily a contraindication to joining the group, but these issues should be explored prior to departure
- Past mental health history. Very serious thought should be given before considering someone with a past history of hospitalization for a psychiatric illness.

A good team leader will be working on keeping open and effective communication throughout the team, and a good team physician should be unobtrusively monitoring the mental health of his or her group.

Acute psychosis is a diagnosis much feared by the team doctor. In the case of travel, most cases of acute psychosis occur in individuals with no past history of mental illness. The exact diagnosis under these circumstances has not been systematically studied; however, it has been suggested that acute situational psychosis is the most common psychiatric diagnosis during travel.[14] The team doctor should have an injectable antipsychotic in the medical kit, and follow-up medication as required. Repatriation is often very difficult in these situations, as patients need to be stabilized before they board a passenger aircraft and will often need a medical (Dr or RN) escort home. A lack of familiar medical facilities and personnel in developing countries can further exacerbate the situation.

Other less dramatic problems include: dealing with 'difficult' patients, such as the hypochondriac, or potentially more dangerously, the stoic. Those who have never traveled to a less developed country before may find the whole experience overwhelming and may develop symptoms such as anxiety, fear, depression, being overanxious about their health, insomnia, and withdrawal. Some doctors have coined the term PUTA – Psychologically Unfit to Travel in Asia – to describe this condition.[15] This can, of course, occur at any destination away from the individual's home.

Post-traumatic stress disorder is a serious consideration in anyone who has been involved in a major trauma while traveling. It is important that the trip physician remains involved with such individuals and ensures appropriate follow-up on their return home.

The most insidious danger on any expedition where men have to rub shoulders for weeks is a mental sickness which might be called 'expedition fever' – a psychological condition which makes even the most peaceful person irritable, angry, furious, absolutely desperate because his perceptive capacity gradually shrinks until he sees only his companions' faults while their good qualities are no longer recorded by his grey matter.[16]

Polar environments

Travel to polar regions has increased enormously over recent years. In 1998, there were 37 winter stations run by 18 nations located south of the 60th parallel, and over 1000 tourists and adventurers visited Antarctica during the summer season.[17] Virtually all published data on polar medicine have studied individuals working in these research stations.[17–19] While these stations do have medical facilities and usually one physician, conditions are extreme and emergencies can be very difficult to manage.[20]

Analysis of problems on Antarctic bases shows that the most common cause of medical consultation is injury or poisoning (42% of cases). Other frequent problems are categorized as respiratory (9.7%), skin and subcutaneous tissue (9.6%), CNS (7.5%), gastrointestinal (7.4%), infections and parasitic diseases (7.3%), musculoskeletal and connective tissue (7.1%), and psychiatric disorders

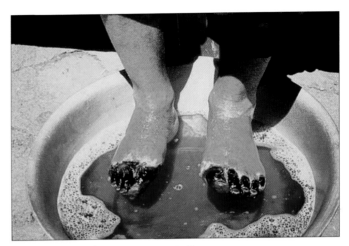

Figure 35.2 Frostbite. *(Courtesy Dr. Jim Duff)*

(2.3%). According to the researchers 'high rates of dental problems and skin diseases contrasted with low rates of disease related to the environment (e.g., cold injury, sunburn, snow blindness) and psychiatric problems'.[18] British investigators have reported similar results. In a retrospective study of medical records compiled by the British Antarctic Survey from 1986 to 1995, only 2.5% of medical consultations were for cold injury. A total of 95% of these cases were frostbite (Fig. 35.2); in three-quarters of cases this was superficial, and most commonly affected the face. Trench foot and hypothermia accounted for only a very small number of cases. The majority of the cases occurred as a result of recreational skiing or snowmobile driving. The most significant factor associated with the development of frostbite was previous cold injury. The authors conclude that 'cold injury is uncommon on Antarctica. In spite of these findings the subject warrants a continued high profile, since under most circumstances frostbite may be regarded as an entirely preventable occurrence.'[19] This pattern of illness and injury is in contrast to what one might expect of small group expeditions to these regions that do not have access to the climate-controlled facilities of a scientific base.

Mountaineering

Increasingly, mountaineering expeditions are becoming high-profile public events. Books such as *Into Thin Air* chronicling the tragic events of 1996 on Mt Everest have highlighted the danger inherent in high-altitude climbing. Those who have survived the 1970s and 1980s climbing scene are the exceptions rather than the norm (Figs 35.3, 35.4). Many classics of mountaineering literature are based on stories of serious falls and miraculous survivals.[21,22] Technical climbing, even at moderate altitudes, has a significant death rate. Analysis of mortality data in the New Zealand Alps (Mt Cook is the highest mountain, at just over 3000 m) showed that the risk of death in the more technically difficult areas of the park was 6.5/1000 days – a similar rate to that reported for high-altitude climbing.[23] The world's two highest mountains, Everest and K2, have significant mortality rates.[24]

Since many of the world's highest and most challenging mountains are located in countries known to have high rates of enteric disease (Nepal, Pakistan, India, Tibet, Peru, Bolivia, Kazakhstan, etc.) it is not surprising that diarrhea ranks highest on the list of likely problems encountered on a mountaineering expedition. Meticulous attention to hygiene standards on arrival in the host country, on the walk in, and at base camp is necessary to try and minimize this risk

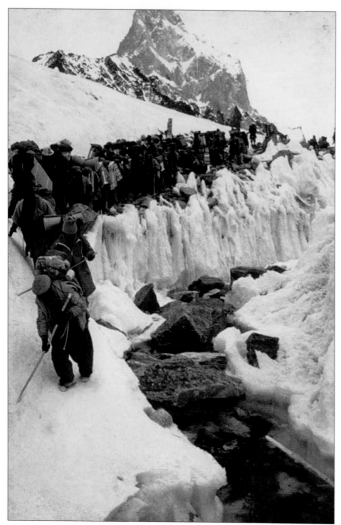

Figure 35.3 Porters approaching K2 in the Karakoram Himalaya. *(Courtesy Dr. Jim Duff)*

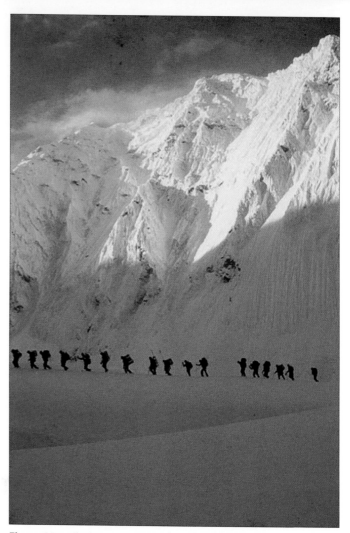

Figure 35.4 Climbers on Mt. Everest. *(Courtesy Dr. Jim Duff)*

– often a huge challenge. Early treatment is recommended to limit the debilitation that can be caused by a bout of bacteria-induced diarrhea.

> The next phase of the expedition is ambitious: climb Rakaposhi, a huge mountain reaching into sky and cloud. But ambition has left, replaced by unshakeable illness in us all. A combination of dysentery and dehydration flattens me, and I end up back in Karambad, in the hospital for a day, and I'm prostrate for a week. It was a small thing that entered our guts, bacterial in dimension, but devastating out of all proportion to its size. Our conversation dwells on it. Bowels and intestines.[25]

Respiratory problems are also frequent – particularly the ubiquitous high-altitude cough, known as the Khumbu cough in the Everest region of Nepal. 'Sore throat, chronic cough, and bronchitis are nearly universal in persons who spend more than two weeks at an extreme altitude (over 5500 m)'.[26] Of note is that these symptoms are not usually accompanied by the traditional signs of infection, such as fever, myalgias or lymphadenopathy. The disorder is considered to be the result of a combination of obligate mouth-breathing due to exertion, the cold dry air, and the addition of vasomotor rhinitis.

Acute mountain sickness, frostbite, hypothermia, UV keratitis, and sunburn are the most common environmental problems to be

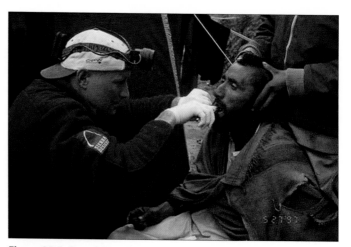

Figure 35.5 Dental Extraction.

prepared for. Dental problems often pose a significant challenge for doctors in remote areas – it would be wise to gain some basic dental skills before going on a major expedition (Fig. 35.5). Replacing lost fillings and managing dental abscesses appear to be the most common issues.

Major trauma is the greatest fear of the mountaineering expedition doctor. Falls are likely to be serious and to result in major injuries. Larger expeditions will carry commercial splinting and traction systems to stabilize such patients.[10] If traveling with a smaller expedition, you should familiarize yourself with possible methods of improvised splinting and traction systems. An excellent review of this topic can be found by Weiss and Donner in *Wilderness Medicine*.[27] Blood and fluid loss can present a potentially life-threatening situation. Intravenous isotonic crystalloids, or perhaps colloids, should be carried. Cross-transfusion between group members is potentially an option. This can be done by creating a donor–recipient chart after checking each group member for blood group, antibodies, and blood-borne infection. There are also commercial cross-matching kits available for use in the field, but these do not provide any information about infectivity. Field blood transfusion would certainly be an enormous medical and logistical challenge. Depending on circumstance, proactive physicians could consider blood bank 'insurance', which provides alarm center-dispatched couriers armed with pints of blood, but even so the logistics here would be challenging.

Many doctors involved in climbing expeditions are experienced climbers themselves. There is also a more formal qualification known as the International Diploma of Mountain Medicine. These European-based courses are intensive, with over 100 h of course-work, and require a certain level of mountaineering skill. There are two parts to the course, the common thread and then a choice of one of the specialty courses studying mountain rescue or expedition and wilderness medicine.[28]

Dr Jim Duff shares his experience as team doctor on a daring, small group climb of the north face of Everest by four Australians in 1988. Two of the team summitted on a route that is still considered one of the most difficult on the mountain:

After several weeks of hard and unsupported effort a team of four climbers set off from their high camp in a bid for the summit. Taking a purist approach, no fixed rope or supplemental oxygen was used on this summit push. The climbers accepted that they were essentially soloing on the mountain as each person had little in reserve to help the others.

On a 100-meter steep mixed section one of the climbers discovered he had a broken crampon. He was in a precarious position and the crampon required repair. In order to achieve this he had to remove all of his gloves apart from the lowest layer, a pair of Thinsulate gloves. The climber's hands became increasingly frostbitten as he continued up to the top of the west ridge and he was within 50 vertical meters of the summit when his friends returned from the summit and he accompanied them back down to their top camp in the dark. On return to top camp radio contact was established. This was our only means of communication for diagnosis and treatment over the next 40 hours, before the climber reached the foot of the mountain face. He was met at the base of the face and treated with oxygen, but no rewarming was attempted until his return to base camp when we could ensure that no refreezing would occur. This climber ultimately lost all of his fingers down to the PIP joint and required ongoing physical and emotional support until surgery was performed some months later, and beyond.

This case demonstrates some of the unique aspects of providing care in such extreme circumstances: equipment failure is a potent source of injury or death; the treating physician may be remote from the victim and may need to treat by proxy; victims of severe injuries such as this one need long-term support. As the initial emotional shock wears off, depression is common.

Useful websites are listed in Table 35.3.

Desert environments

Desert environments are characterized by high daytime temperatures, low night-time temperatures, and potentially huge temperature variations over a single 24-h period – up to 45°F.[29] Additionally, there is little surface water, minimal vegetation, clear sunny skies, potentially strong winds, and sparse human habitation. Planning ahead in such an unforgiving environment is essential – 'in deserts, travelers have the potential to kill themselves quite easily through bad planning, and this is a wasteful way to go'.[30]

Clearly, the major health risks in desert environments result from heat and UV exposure. Humans do have some ability to adapt to heat (as opposed to cold), but this takes at least 7–10 days.[31] There should be adequate time for acclimatization before starting the expedition, and activities should be designed to reduce the risk of heat exhaustion or, more seriously, heat stroke. Activity should be avoided during the hottest part of the day (usually 10 am until 3 pm), and appropriate clothing should be worn. As little skin as possible should be exposed to the sun. Broad-brimmed or legionnaire-style hats are a necessity, as are sunglasses. Shoes should balance the need for protection against the harsh surface and comfort in order to avoid blisters. Awareness of the symptoms of heat exhaustion and dehydration among group members is paramount: they should ensure they are keeping an eye on one another. Important warning signs include headache, nausea, dizziness, vomiting, and anorexia. Recent work on hikers in the Grand Canyon has highlighted the risk of exercise-induced hyponatremia, which can occur as a result of over-hydration in individuals exercising in conditions of extreme heat.[32] The authors note 'heat exhaustion is difficult to distinguish from mild hyponatremia; we did not find statistically significant differences in symptoms or signs until clinically apparent alterations in mental status appeared'. They found that hyponatremia was the most common cause of serious illness related to exercising in the heat, and that altered mental status, convulsions (in the absence of hypoglycemia and extreme hyperpyrexia), and the development or progression of symptoms after the cessation of exercise were suggestive of hyponatremia. The remarkably simple prevention for this serious problem is the regular ingestion of sodium-containing foods.

Heat exhaustion may also progress to heat stroke – a true medical emergency. Before 1950, the mortality rate for heat stroke was between 40% and 75%,[31] and without the benefits of a hospital emergency department, or a knowledgeable trip physician, this statistic is likely to hold true in the field. The obvious answer is to avoid the problem in the first place through behavior modification. However, the expedition physician needs to be familiar with the clinical spectrum of heat illness and its management in the field.

Jungle/tropical environments

Although heat is also the main threat in tropical jungle environments, it is the accompanying humidity that characterizes these areas, and significantly increases the risk of heat-related illness (see quote below by Redmond O'Hanlon).

First-time visitors to such regions may waste an enormous amount of time trying to stay dry, when in reality this is a futile effort. It is, however, worth making an effort to stay dry at night, and to have dry clothes to change into at the end of the day. Skin is particularly vulnerable to the constant wetness of jungle travel, with fungal infections, maceration, cuts that refuse to heal, and prickly heat all potential problems. As with all hot environments, careful attention to fluid and electrolyte replacement is essential to avoid heat exhaustion, hyponatremia, and heat stroke. Water is generally abundant in these environments, but will usually require purification to avoid enteric disease.

Malaria and other vector-borne disease are likely to be a significant risk in most tropical jungle areas. These important topics are covered elsewhere in this book.

Other arthropods such as ants, chiggers, botfly, sandflies, wasps, bees, spiders, and scorpions may also be prevalent in your patch of the jungle. Mammals such as bats are a rabies risk, snakes and fish such as Candiru, piranha, eels, and stingrays have fearsome reputations. Research your destination thoroughly so you are aware of the potential hazards you may encounter.

> The heat seemed insufferable, a very different heat from the dazzling sunlight of the river-side, an all-enclosing airless clamminess that radiated from the damp leaves, the slippery humus, the great boles of the trees. My shirt was as wet as if I had worn it for a swim in the river. With a humidity of 98% there is nowhere for sweat to evaporate, no relief by cooling, just an added body-stocking of salt, slime, smell and moisture.

(Redmond O'Hanlon: *Into the Heart of Borneo*)

Kayaking and Rafting

White-water enthusiasts are now traveling to increasingly remote destinations in their aim to run 'first descents'. The Himalayas – particularly Nepal, Bhutan, and Tibet – are renowned for their difficult rivers.

Rivers are graded from class I to class VI, class VI describing runs that 'exemplify the extremes of difficulty, unpredictability, and danger. The consequences of error are very severe, and rescue may be impossible.'[33] A well-publicized white water kayak trip to the Tsangpo River in Tibet exemplifies the exploratory and dangerous nature of some kayak expeditions.[34]

Health risks of particular relevance to white water kayak and raft trips include:

- Ingestion or immersion in contaminated water. Apart from the obvious risk of contracting enteric disease from swallowing water, diseases such as leptospirosis and schistosomiasis have been contracted by groups undertaking trips on rivers in countries such as Borneo, Costa Rica, Thailand, and Ethiopia[35–37]
- Dehydration – despite proximity to water, heat and strenuous activity may result in inadequate fluid replacement
- Drowning and near-drowning. Almost all fatalities on rivers are the result of submersion.[38] Wearing a PFD (personal flotation device, or life jacket) may reduce the risk of drowning. However, on extreme rivers, entrapment may be inescapable
- Trauma. One of the injuries commonly associated with kayaking is anterior shoulder dislocation. If you are accompanying a kayak trip you should learn to feel comfortable with relocation techniques. One analysis of white-water injuries showed that shoulder dislocation accounted for 16% of injuries. Other common injuries included fractures (17%), leg injuries (13%), near drowning (13%), and lacerations (10%).[38] Ankle injuries commonly occur as a result of portaging (carrying the raft or kayak overland in areas where the river is not navigable), or while scouting ahead. Head injuries in a remote area can be disastrous: participants should always be expected to wear a helmet and a PFD in white water
  - Blisters from paddles, and other abrasions can be slow to heal in the constantly wet environment
  - Burns are a significant risk as a result of campfires lit at evening riverside camps

- UV damage from sun exposure is exacerbated by almost 100% reflection of UV by the water.

Doctors accompanying kayaking or rafting expeditions should be particularly versed in managing trauma.

Useful websites are listed in Table 35.3.

Scuba Diving Expeditions

Scuba diving is covered in detail in Chapter 40. Doctors accompanying dive trips should have undertaken extra training in hyperbaric medicine. Participants should be carefully screened. They should have a recent and thorough diving medical and should be screened for past diving-related problems, particularly DCI (decompression illness). A contingency plan for the management of DCI, including the location of the closest hyperbaric chamber and a plan for how to get there, should be made in advance. An update on basic skills and emergency responses for all members of the group is wise – a common cause of dive accidents is a failure to respond rapidly to an emergency. Equipment failure poses a real risk in scuba diving, so thorough attention to maintenance of equipment is essential.

While some dive expeditions will be undertaken in cold environments (there are many commercial dive trips to the Antarctic), most dive locations are in the warmer tropical areas of the world. In particular, the expedition physician should ensure that the group has appropriate malaria chemoprophylaxis if relevant, e.g., many authorities still recommend avoiding mefloquine in divers. The availability of Malarone (atovaquone/proguanil combination) has made the choice of malaria chemoprophylaxis easier for divers. Other vector-borne diseases are also likely to be prevalent. The expedition physician should ensure that the group is insured specifically for diving – many policies will actively exclude cover for treatment in a recompression chamber, or evacuation to such a facility. Groups such as DAN (Divers Alert Network) offer specialized insurance packages for diving, including phone support with a doctor trained in hyperbaric medicine, and cover for evacuation to the nearest recompression chamber. There are few data on the exact risk of diving expeditions; however, data on recreational divers show that the most common cause of hospitalization is decompression illness. One Australian study looking at hospital admissions in tourists to the state of Queensland found that in a 3-year period there were 296 overseas visitors admitted for water-related injuries. A total of 55% of these were to treat decompression illness, 15% were for fractures or dislocations (predominantly as a result of rafting and kayaking) and 15% for drowning and non-fatal submersion.[39]

Specific problems to try and avoid with pre-planning, while still being prepared to manage, include:

- Coral cuts. These are notorious for developing secondary infection. Divers should wear protective clothing to minimize the risk of coral cuts
- 'Swimmers ear'
- Biting venomous sea creatures, such as sea snakes or blue-ringed octopus. Ensure the area to be visited has been thoroughly researched in order to be aware of specific risks
- Stinging sea creatures, such as the box jellyfish or the Portuguese Man-of-War. Be prepared with acetic acid (vinegar) to inactivate the stinging organelles
- Penetrating injury (sea urchin spines)
- Marine-acquired wound infection (*Vibrio* species)
- Ciguatera poisoning if catching your own fish.[40] Commercial kits are available for detection of this toxin and may be useful
- Decompression illness

- Barotrauma of any gas-filled space
- Arterial gas embolism
- Motion sickness
- Severe sunburn.

Useful websites are listed in Table 35.3.

The Luxury Expedition

Rather than the rigors of the outback or the Spartan existence of base camp, the expedition physician may find him/herself surrounded by relative luxury during the high-end luxury 'expedition'. A variety of factors have contributed to a new breed of upscale adventure travelers. As our population has aged, a lucky few have found themselves with an abundance of time, money, and desire to travel the world. Many travel companies provide 'high-end' adventure travel, from safaris to large private jets. The clientele are often older, and arguably sicker, than the average traveler. They have also paid for a very expensive trip and may have a different set of expectations regarding their medical care. This being said, these travelers are also often sophisticated, fun-loving, well-read, world-traveled, and wonderful expedition companions.

Advice for the physician joining such a group would include extra attention to pre-travel health screening and considerations that the medical kit needs to be able to accommodate for the potentially special needs of the group. Although still rigorous, such an expedition opens the door to a different set of travelers: chronic, stable illness is common. 'Clinic hours' before dinner, or on the jet, provide both a sense of service and help to manage the physician's time. Lastly, having a supply of alternative remedies such as zinc tablets or *Echinacea* will help keep the peace during the invariable outbreak of upper respiratory infections.

Local Healthcare

Although serious emergencies on expedition are rare, they will provide you with the greatest level of stress. You should establish an evacuation plan and find out as much as you can about any local medical facilities that may be available.

The most logical way to prepare for any serious medical situation is to make contact with an evacuation assistance company in the middle to late planning stages of the expedition. In general, insurance companies contract assistance companies to undertake communication with the expedition doctor/local medical facility should an emergency occur, and to organize repatriation to the nearest relevant medical facility. It is also possible to have a corporate subscription directly with an evacuation company. Assistance companies have an extensive network of local care providers, and generally have practical experience of the quality of care that is available in a given location.

Contacting the assistance provider allows them to be aware of your activities and location and therefore be forewarned of any potential problems. It is far better that they are aware that there is a group of 20 paddlers in a remote area of Tibet, rather than being contacted for the first time in the middle of an emergency. If they feel that the risk is warranted, they will set up a contingency network. Making this contact ensures that financial issues are also taken care of, as larger companies will have provisional guarantees pre-organized with local care providers.

Among the countries popular for expeditions, Nepal is unique in that it has a very comprehensive rescue network, with multiple helicopter companies offering their services. In this situation, access to a satellite phone will allow easy access to a helicopter rescue company.

Limitations on rescue are imposed by weather and altitude/location, rather than access to facilities. This is one country where the involvement of an assistance company may not be required until repatriation back to Katmandu. However, one should still be aware of the local facilities with which the assistance company has arrangements – this will facilitate further management, whether it be hospitalization, repatriation to Bangkok or repatriation home. Nepal is also unusual in that there are two well-respected private medical clinics run by Western-trained physicians and usually staffed by a number of Western doctors. In most countries, finding reliable local medical care is far more difficult. Ideas for trying to find local facilities include contacting doctors who have previously visited the area in question, contacting local members of the ISTM, and contacting members of IAMAT. If the expedition physician is able to locate the closest reasonable facility prior to the expedition, it would be valuable to visit the facility and meet the treating physicians there, so that the level of care available can be fully assessed. This will assist enormously when communicating with the assistance company should an evacuation be required. One important challenge is when to decide to turn over the care of your patient to another provider or medical team. Although the expedition physician has an obvious duty to care for his/her patient, he/she also has a duty to be available to care for the other members of the expedition, who may well be pressed, for a variety of reasons, to move on. This highlights the importance of having other members of the group trained in first aid, so that you are not entirely indispensable! An evacuation will be an enormously stressful situation – pre-planning for the eventuality can be enormously helpful.

Difficult Situations

Above and beyond the obvious challenges of group medical care in an austere environment, there are several other situations that may or may not arise to challenge you in your role as expedition physician. Some depend on the nature of your expedition (trekking to Everest base-camp or beyond, versus an organized tour of the Galapagos), some on your destination (Middle East versus Northern Europe), and some simply on circumstance.

Medical Care of Others

It is not uncommon for expeditions, even to relatively remote parts of the globe, to cross paths with other expeditions. This can be an opportunity for cultural exchange, learning from groups who are returning from your destination, and even occasionally shifting the load of food or equipment. There may, however, be an expectation of sharing the expedition physician and medical supplies. This can be acutely problematic in the setting of another group that is not medically prepared and/or is dealing with an acute medical problem. Obviously, for urgent or life-threatening cases medical concerns come first. But non-urgent requests can strain the time and resources of the medical team. Plenty of expedition physicians have awoken to a line outside the tent of porters or climbers seeking medical attention. The expedition physician and other members of the team should be prepared for this eventuality. Again, preparation is key: will there be other groups at your destination? Is it appropriate to contact them in advance of the trip? Should extra medical supplies be packed, and if so, how much? Discussing this situation in advance and deciding on a 'party line' will help when the situation arises.

More difficult is the issue of providing medical care to the local population. This will be less of an issue for the average commercial trip, but can be a challenging situation for expeditions traveling through local villages. Locals may go out of their way to pursue medical assistance or advice from a traveling physician. As with caring for other expeditions, this issue needs to be thought through and prepared for in advance.

Safety and Security

Although technically not the responsibility of the expedition physician, as a member of the expedition team it is not uncommon for the physician to get involved in issues of safety and security for the group. Obviously, if there is a threat of injury or harm, the medical concerns can quickly become paramount. As with many of the other issues touched on in this chapter, preparation is extremely important. The expedition leadership should do their homework on their destination. US State Department, or equivalent, information should be sought out and read. Friends or colleagues who have traveled recently to your destination can provide invaluable inside advice. Be familiar with the local cultural and political situation, and have at hand emergency contact information for local police as well as appropriate embassies or consulates. A substantial supply of local currency can be invaluable. It is important to register your group members with the local embassy if your itinerary permits it, especially if there is a risk of social unrest in the country.

Increasingly available technology allows for excellent communication fixes through international cellular telephones and smartphones. Even satellite-based phones can be taken, with many vendors offering 'emergency only' subscription services which are worth looking into.

Useful websites are listed in Table 35.3.

Repatriation

Despite best efforts at screening trip participants and at keeping them well on the trip, the situation may arise where one of the group becomes sufficiently injured or ill to warrant emergency evacuation to a site where more sophisticated medical care can be provided. When this happens, the expedition physician's role can become quite challenging.

The first issue will be one of communication. Does the group have the means of calling for help? Even an investment in a satellite phone does not ensure success in all parts of the world, and one might need to rely on a porter or other messenger to deliver word on foot. In this case, it will have been extremely important to have set up a plan in advance. For example, in Nepal, a private or even a military helicopter can be requested to evacuate an ill or injured trekker, but only if that trek is registered in advance with the appropriate authorities. More commonly, phone communication is available, but the issue of advanced planning is just as important.

There are many excellent companies dedicated to the medical repatriation of sick or injured travelers. The arrival of a sophisticated medical team, ready to swoop the patient off in a dedicated jet air ambulance, is a relief for both patient and physician alike. But this moment comes at a price, and that price can be steep if the team is unprepared.

Aeromedical evacuation, with a physician-based team, can easily cost over US$10 000. This raises several very important points. It is essential on any international expedition where there is a risk of significant illness or injury, that each participant carry insurance to cover medical repatriation. In addition, pay particular attention to the 'cap' on the policy: less expensive policies may only cover up to US$5000, leaving the patient with significant financial liability. Also, pre-existing illness clauses should be looked for and addressed if appropriate. The notion of paying out of pocket and then submitting receipts to your insurance company once back home is simply not practical for anything but the most minor of medical problems.

Note also that the first stop for such an evacuation may not be 'back home', but rather to a relatively local center where appropriate medical interventions can be provided. This may cause some fear or frustration for the ill passenger. Setting expectations, but also working closely with the medical repatriation company (and at times lobbying on behalf of the patient or family) are important roles for the expedition physician.

Lastly, the expedition physician caring for a patient who needs to be hospitalized or repatriated is faced with a difficult decision. When does he or she leave the patient to rejoin the group for which he or she continues to have overall medical responsibility? This is a complicated question depending on many variables, and should be discussed with expedition leadership as soon as possible.

Death Overseas

There can be no more challenging situation for the expedition physician than to have one of the team die under his or her watch. The circumstances can of course vary, ranging from an accident taking the life of a young and healthy climber to the sad, but not entirely unexpected death of a chronically ill elderly traveler on their last tour of the Caribbean. In any case, the issues for the trip physician are many.

For the patient suffering from a life-threatening illness or injury, there is the issue of coordinating local care and/or repatriation. Transporting an infirm victim from a remote location can be difficult, but even at the local hospital there are a number of obvious challenging issues, such as language, finances, and physician or equipment availability. Less obvious can be issues of gender (male expedition physician and female patient, or vice versa), hours of operation (hospital pharmacy is closed overnight), and medical culture. Western physicians may be surprised to find a system where medications and supplies need to be purchased (cash only) at a pharmacy and then provided to the local doctors for use. Also, friends or family may be expected to provide nursing care, such as bathing the patient, simple wound care, and providing meals. It is important for the expedition physician to be aware of these potential issues when coordinating local medical care for the group.

Emotionally, having one of the team die while under your care is very difficult. The fact that other physicians or health professionals may have been involved may actually make the situation more difficult. It is difficult somewhere where you do not speak the language, do not know the system, and are left with a nagging feeling that you should have done more. Other members of your team will have the same feeling, and a post-incident debriefing session is very important.

Practically, there are a number of issues that need to be handled in the event of a death overseas. Foremost is the need for communication. The victim's next of kin should be advised of injury, illness, or death as soon as possible. Also, communicating with the expedition's parent company or organization is very important. They may be able to coordinate communication and other efforts back home. Local burial or cremation may be available, depending on the desires of the victim's family. Repatriation of remains is usually arranged by the appropriate local embassy or consulate. Regulations may require that the deceased be embalmed prior to transport. Regardless, repatriation of remains can be an expensive proposition, and monies will need to be provided before any action will be taken. Early involvement of the local embassy or consulate is advantageous, but do not overestimate their ability to intervene and problem solve on your behalf.

Back Home

On the return home, the expedition physician's obligations will depend upon the style of trip undertaken.

If you have been employed by a company, you should write a trip report outlining the medical problems you encountered, how they may be better prevented next time, comments on your experience with the evacuation company (if relevant), and any improvements you could recommend to the group and individual medical kits. If the company plans to employ a physician for their next trip, it is wise to make contact so the next trip doctor can be informed of any relevant issues.

If you had any dealings with local caregivers, a letter of thanks and information on the outcome of the patient they cared for will be greatly appreciated, and will undoubtedly pave the way for even better relations should another injured or ill expedition member come their way in the future.

Finally, it is important to remember the health of the group in the post-travel period. It is wise to give them a list of symptoms and signs to be aware of over the ensuing weeks, based on the incubation times of common endemic diseases in the area visited. If there were any exposures that require screening for at a later stage, e.g., for schistosomiasis after 3 months, they should be given an appropriate protocol to follow with their local physician. Additionally, group members should have your contact details so they can get in touch if they are concerned or need their regular physician to discuss any issues with you. You should keep in contact with anyone who has had a significant injury that will require extensive post-travel treatment, e.g., frostbite. And of course, anyone who has been involved in a significant trauma or rescue situation should be counseled regarding post-traumatic stress disorder and advised to seek care should they develop symptoms.

Post-travel illness is covered in detail in Chapters 52–57.

Conclusion

The role of the expedition physician has come a long way in the past century, coinciding in part with the sense of the world becoming ever smaller while our need for exploration and self-discovery grows ever larger. Such a personal expedition is no longer restricted to the extremely wealthy and privileged, although to a lesser degree this continues to be true. More and more, groups of travelers are organizing to explore the vastness of nature, the richness of other cultures, or the depths of their own spirits. The field of travel medicine has matured along with this change in travel patterns, and as such even so-called 'adventure travelers' are paying more attention to their health and more liberally involving physicians and other travel medicine professionals in the medical aspects of their planning.

The expedition physician, whether accompanying the team to the summit or simply advising the group from the office, has an increasingly complex role to play. The job begins long before departure with assessing the health of the party, educating participants, building a quality medical kit, doing destination homework, and working closely with other members of the expedition leadership. Once on the road, the job responsibilities become more obvious, but there are many hidden pitfalls, including difficult patients, challenges to time and resources, and perhaps having to deal with significant injury, illness, or death in an environment that is extremely remote both physically and culturally.

On the other hand, there are numerous rewards, not the least of which is traveling to an interesting or physically challenging corner of the globe. There is satisfaction to be had from providing quality healthcare with little besides a medical kit and personal creativity, improvising solutions while actually finding time to enjoy the expedition itself. It is hoped that, for your next expedition, this chapter will be one of the essential tools in your 'pre-travel' medical kit.

References

1. McLeod WT, editor. The New Collins Concise Dictionary of the English Language. London: Collins; 1986.
2. Anderson SR, Johnson CJ. Expedition health and safety: a risk assessment. J R Soc Med 2000;93:557–62.
3. Roberts D, editor. Points Unknown: A Century of Great Exploration. New York: WW Norton; 2000.
4. Iain McIntosh. Trials and tribulations of an expedition doctor. Trav Med Int 1992;72–7.
5. Bowman WD. Perspectives on being a wilderness physician: is wilderness medicine more than a special body of knowledge? Wild Env Med 2001;12:165–7.
6. Basnyat B, Litch JA. Medical problems of porters and trekkers in the Nepal Himalaya. Wild Env Med 1997;8:78–81.
7. Bishop RA, Litch JA. Medical Tourism can do Harm. London: BMJ Publishing; 2000. p. 320.
8. Johnson CJH. Expedition medicine, a survey of 95 expeditions. Travel Med Int 1984;2:239–42.
9. A'Court CHD, Stables RH, Travis J. How to do it: Doctor on a mountaineering expedition. BMJ 1995;310:1248–52.
10. Prativa Pandey. Personal communication from Dr Prativa Pandey MD. Medical Director, the CIWEC Clinic Kathmandu, Nepal.
11. Hodgetts TJ, Cooke MW. The Largest Mass Gathering. London: BMJ Publishing; 1999. p. 318.
12. Shlim DR, Houston C. Helicopter rescues and deaths among trekkers in Nepal. JAMA 1989;261:1017–9.
13. Pollard A, Clarke C. Deaths during mountaineering at extreme altitudes. Lancet 1988;1:1277.
14. Shlim DR. Psychological aspects of adventure travel. Wild Med Lett 2001;18:1–6.
15. Duff J, Gormly P. First aid and survival in mountain and remote areas. Katmandu: Dr Jim Duff: 158.
16. Taylor A. Antarctic Psychology. Wellington: DSIR Science Information Publishing Centre; 1987.
17. Lugg DJ. Antarctic medicine. JAMA 2000;283:2082–4.
18. Sullivan P, Gormly PJ, Lugg DJ, et al. The Australian Antarctic Research Expeditions Health Register: three years of operation. In: Postl B, Gilbert P, Goodwill J, et al, editors. Circumpolar Health 90. Winnipeg: University of Manitoba Press; 1991.
19. Cattermole TJ. The epidemiology of cold injury in Antarctica. Aviat Space Environ Med 1999;70:135–40.
20. Priddy RE. An 'acute abdomen' in Antarctica. MJA 1985;143:108–11.
21. Plowright RK. Crevasse fall in the Antarctic: a patient's perspective. MJA 2000;173:583–4.
22. Lamberth PG. Death in Antarctica. MJA 2001;175:583–4.
23. Malcolm M. Mountaineering fatalities in Mt Cook National Park. NZ Med J 2001;114:78–80.
24. Huey RB, Eguskitsa X. Supplemental oxygen and mountaineer death rates on K2 and Everest. JAMA 2000;284:181.
25. Child G. Mixed Emotions. Seattle: The Mountaineers; 1997.
26. Hackett PH, Roach RC. High altitude medicine. In: Auerbach PS, editor. Wilderness Medicine, St Louis: Mosby; 2001. p. 2–43.
27. Weiss EA, Donner HJ. Wilderness improvisation. In: Auerbach PS, editor. Wilderness Medicine. St Louis: Mosby; 2001. p. 466–94.
28. Peters P. Practical aspects in mountain medicine education. Wild Environ Med 2000;11:262–8.
29. Otten EJ. Desert survival. Wild Med Lett 2000;17:2.
30. Dryden M. Tropical and desert expeditions. In: Warrell D, Anderson S, editors. The Royal Geographical Society Expedition Medicine. London: Profile Books; 1998.
31. Gaffin SL, Moran DS. Pathophysiology of heat-related illnesses. In: Auerbach PS, editor. Wilderness Medicine. St Louis: Mosby; 2001. p. 240–89.

32. Backer HD, Shopes E, Collins SL, et al. Exertional heat illness and hyponatremia in hikers. Am J Emerg Med 1999;17:532–8.

33. American Whitewater Affiliation. Safety Code of the American Whitewater Affiliation. New York: Phoenicia; 1989.

34. Balf T. The Last River. The Tragic Race for Shangri-la. New York: Crown; 2000.

35. Centres for Disease Control and Prevention. Outbreak of Leptospirosis among white-water rafters – Costa Rica 1996. MMWR 1997;46:577–9.

36. Pinner R. Update on emerging infections: Outbreak of acute febrile illness among athletes participating in eco-challenge – Sabah 2000 – Borneo, Malaysia 2000. Ann Emerg Med 2001;38:83–6.

37. Istre GR, Fontaine RE, Tarr J, et al. Acute Schistosomiasis among Americans rafting the Omo River, Ethiopia. JAMA 1984;251:508–10.

38. Weiss EA. Whitewater medicine and rescue. In: Auerbach PS, editor. Wilderness Medicine. St Louis: Mosby; 2001:729–45.

39. Wilks J, Coory M. Overseas visitors admitted to Queensland hospitals for water-related injuries. MJA 2000;173:244–6.

40. Farstad DJ, Chow T. A brief case report and review of Ciguatera poisoning. Wild Environ Med 2001;12:263–9.

36

Medical Tourism

C. Virginia Lee and Linda R. Taggart

Key points

- Medical tourism describes the phenomenon of people traveling outside their home country for the primary purpose of receiving medical treatment
- The most common categories of procedures sought are cosmetic surgery, dentistry, cardiology (cardiac surgery), and orthopedic surgery
- Common destination in developing countries include Thailand, Mexico, Singapore, India, Malaysia, Cuba, Brazil, Argentina, and Costa Rica
- The risks of postoperative complications can compound the risks of international travel
- Long-term follow-up when the medical tourist returns home may be complicated by lack of documentation provided on the services received at the destination facility

Introduction

Since antiquity, people have traveled in search of healing. There are places throughout the world that have come to be thought of as healing places. These places have aspects in the natural, built, symbolic, and social environment that people associate with healing.[1] Many of these places, such as Lourdes in France, continue to attract pilgrims.

In more modern times, there has been a great deal of interest in creating spaces that are therapeutic. Florence Nightingale introduced early concepts such as healing being facilitated through the provision of fresh air, adequate lighting, and good accommodations for staff.[2] In 1984, *Science* magazine published a study by Roger Ulrich showing that patients in hospital rooms that looked out on the natural world healed faster. Architects have worked with medical researchers to design buildings such as hospitals and wellness spas to facilitate healing.[3] Many of these modern 'healing places' continue to draw travelers.

The travelers to places discussed above would be more accurately considered to be health tourists. Health tourism includes those going to:

- Hospitals for conventional medicine, invasive treatments, and/or state-of-the-art technology

- Wellness centers and spas that offer complementary medicine and traditional natural preventive medicine
- Destination spas offering body and mind treatment backed with medical knowledge and treatments such as hydrotherapy tubs, steam baths, and therapeutic massage.

This chapter will focus on the first group, those individuals traveling internationally for conventional medical treatment in hospitals or clinics.

Medical Tourism

Medical tourism is the term commonly used to describe the phenomenon of people traveling outside their home country primarily for the purpose of seeking medical treatment.[4, 5] Traditionally, international medical travel was done by patients from less developed countries to major medical centers in a developed country for treatment that was not available in their home country. However, the term 'medical tourism' generally refers to people from developed countries traveling to less developed countries for medical care. In a recent Hastings Center Report, Cohen suggested separating medical tourism into three types:

- Services that are illegal in both the patient's home country and the destination country, such as organ sales
- Services that are illegal in the patient's home country but legal in the destination country, such as some stem cell therapies
- Services that are legal in both the patient's home country and the destination country, such as joint replacement.[6]

Each of these types of medical tourism presents different ethical and other issues for clinicians working with patients considering traveling for these services. A list of advantages and disadvantages of medical travel is summarized in Table 36.1.[7]

Medical travel is expected to increase significantly in the next 5–10 years.[5] However, very few reliable epidemiologic data on medical tourism currently exist. Prevalence estimates for medical tourism range from 60 000 to 750 000 medical tourists annually.[5,8] One reason for the differences in estimates is that various groups define medical tourism in different ways, and may include travelers going to spas and for traditional healing. Another is that certain groups, such as McKinley & Company, do not consider Mexico and Canada as destinations for their estimates. However, a report by the Deloitte Center for

©2012 Elsevier Inc

DOI: 10.1016/B978-1-4557-1076-8.00036-3

Table 36.1 Advantages and Disadvantages of Medical Travel

Advantages
Lower healthcare costs
Total overall cost
Co-pays and deductibles
More luxurious accommodations than stateside hospitals, including 'recovery resorts'
Not subject to federal oversight, such as the US Food and Drug Administration*
Possibility of incorporating leisure activities into the trip

Disadvantages
Not for emergent procedures
Not subject to federal oversight, such as the US Food and Drug Administration*
Laws regulating insurance coverage may vary
Limited tort options in event of a bad outcome
Potential language and cultural barriers
Requires travel
Risks of long-distance travel
Same logistical challenges as any out-of-town medical care
Risks of adverse outcomes, especially infection, possibly with drug-resistant organisms
Use of local resources and healthcare personnel that otherwise might be available to the indigenous population of low-income countries

*An advantage for those seeking alternative therapies; a disadvantage if federal oversight is a proxy for effectiveness and safety.

Health Solutions predicted that by 2012 >9 million Americans would travel abroad for medical care. [9]

The most common categories of procedures that people pursue during medical tourism trips include cosmetic surgery, dentistry, cardiology (cardiac surgery), and orthopedic surgery.[4, 10] Other surgeries include bariatric and reproductive procedures. Common destinations include Thailand, Mexico, Singapore, India, Malaysia, Cuba, Brazil, Argentina, and Costa Rica.[4, 11] The type of procedure and the destination need to be considered when reviewing the risk of travel for medical care.

The majority of medical tourists currently rely on private companies or 'medical concierge' services to identify foreign healthcare facilities and pay for their care out of pocket. Some insurers and large employers have been developing alliances with overseas hospitals as a means to control healthcare costs, and several major medical schools in the United States have developed joint initiatives with overseas providers, such as the Harvard Medical School Dubai Center, The Johns Hopkins Singapore International Medical Center, and the Duke-National University of Singapore.[12, 13] At present it is not known whether such joint ventures will serve to increase the number of people who go abroad for healthcare.

General Considerations Related to Medical Treatment Abroad

Patients who do elect to travel should consult a travel healthcare practitioner for advice tailored to individual health needs, preferably at least 4–6 weeks in advance of travel. In addition to the considerations for healthy travelers, medical tourists should consider the risks associated with surgery and travel – either while ill or while recovering

from treatment. The Aerospace Medical Association has published medical guidelines for airline travel that provide useful information on the risks of travel with certain medical conditions.[14] Air pressure within an aircraft is equivalent to the pressure at an altitude of 6000–8000 feet, rather than sea level. Individuals are advised not to travel for 10 days after chest or abdominal surgery to avoid risks associated with this change in barometric pressure.[15] Flying and surgery both increase the risk of deep venous thrombosis and the subsequent formation of pulmonary embolus. Severe headaches have also been reported in individuals who traveled by air within a week of receiving a spinal anesthetic.

When advising travelers considering a trip overseas for medical care, clinicians should consider the guiding principles developed by the American Medical Association (AMA) for employers, insurance companies, and other entities that facilitate or offer incentives for care outside the United States.[16] These guidelines discuss ensuring the voluntary nature of the care, the need to use an accredited facility, legal recourse, and transfer of data between facilities.[16] In addition, patients should be advised that they should arrange for follow-up care in their home country prior to travel.[16]

Healthcare providers can advise prospective medical tourists to determine whether healthcare facilities where they are considering receiving care are accredited by the Joint Commission International (JCI). JCI is the international division of the Joint Commission Resources, a US-based not-for-profit affiliate of the Joint Commission, and provides accreditation to hospitals, ambulatory care facilities, clinical laboratories and other healthcare organizations.[17] Successful accreditation of hospitals requires that two groups of standards are met, patient-centered standards and healthcare organization management standards.[18] Patient-centered standards include maintaining confidentiality, obtaining informed consent for treatments, having qualified individuals to conduct patient assessments, and providing adequate resources, including appropriate laboratory services, medical imaging and medications. Healthcare organization management standards include having a quality improvement and patient safety program, an infection prevention and control program, and a process to verify credentials of their medical staff. As of 2011, JCI has accredited 325 international hospitals.[19] As the credentialing issues become less of a factor, it is anticipated that more insurance providers will offer incentives for their patients to travel overseas for care. Other organizations provide a similar service, including Accreditation Canada International and Quality Healthcare Advice Trent Accreditation, which is based in the United Kingdom.[20]

Numerous ethical concerns have been raised in relation to medical tourism. Concerns for patients undergoing procedures abroad are the lack of data on quality of care and difficulty achieving continuity of care.[21] In addition, there may be broader public health implications. For example, in countries with publicly funded healthcare systems, the general public in the patient's home country may indirectly incur costs for follow-up care and ongoing treatment received after patients return home from procedures carried out elsewhere.[22] There are also unknown implications on the healthcare system of the country providing the procedure. Proponents of medical tourism believe it will improve health for local populations by encouraging technological advancements in the medical field and providing a source of economic growth. However, others are concerned that physicians and other healthcare resources will be diverted from local populations to provide for international patients.[23] Finally, numerous concerns have been raised about exploitation of individuals who sell their organs for transplant or eggs for fertility treatments, or who provide surrogacy services.[24, 25]

Cosmetic Surgery Tourism

The American Society of Plastic Surgeons (ASPS) advises individuals who have had cosmetic procedures of the face, eyelids, and nose, or who have had laser treatments, to wait 7–10 days before flying. Patients are also advised to avoid 'vacation' activities such as sunbathing, drinking alcohol, swimming, taking long tours, and engaging in strenuous activities or exercise after surgery.[26]

For cosmetic surgery, the American Society for Plastic Surgery developed a briefing paper that includes a patient safety checklist for plastic surgery in the United States.[27] This checklist includes questions to be asked and places for information on the procedures. These recommendations include asking the surgeon about their qualifications, their experience with the procedure, the expected recovery period, and how complications will be managed. Some of the recommendations are more difficult for those traveling to other countries, such as having a medical evaluation done prior to the procedure.

The International Society for Aesthetic Plastic Surgeons was organized by the United Nations in 1970. The society represents over 1900 board-certified esthetic plastic surgeons in 91 countries. ISAPS has developed a set of key guidelines for plastic surgery travelers.[28] The guidelines cover such areas as the surgeon training and certification and that of the facility. They also caution travelers to ensure that key personnel speak the traveler's language fluently as a way to avoid complications. Other key issues include aftercare and complications. Travelers should be clear on how these will be handled, and whether additional payment will be required for any necessary revision surgeries.

Dental Tourism

The American Dental Association (ADA) provides informational documents, including *Traveler's Guide to Safe Dental Care* through the Global Dental Safety Organization for Safety and Asepsis Procedures.[29] Although the ADA guidelines were not developed for medical tourists, they provide useful information for travelers to consider when selecting a facility or planning a trip for medical or dental care. A major concern for dental procedures is infectious complications, so travelers planning to go for dental care should inquire about the sterilization and disinfection procedures in the office. Particular caution is required if the traveler is going to an area that has problems with drinking water contamination. In those areas, sterile or boiled water is required for all surgical procedures. The patient should be sure that new needles and gloves are used, and that hands are washed between each procedure.

Transplant Tourism

One form of medical tourism that is very controversial is sometimes called 'transplant tourism': travel for the purpose of receiving an organ purchased from an unrelated donor for transplant.[30] It is estimated that 5–10% of all kidney transplants in 2007 were from commercial living donors or vendors (although most of these were not 'transplant tourism').[31, 32] In 2004, the World Health Assembly Resolution 57.18 encouraged member countries to 'take measures to protect the poorest and vulnerable groups from 'transplant tourism' and the sale of tissues and organs'.[33] A meeting in 2008 in Istanbul, Turkey, addressed the issue of 'transplant tourism' and 'organ trafficking' and resulted in a call for these activities to be prohibited.[34] In view of those events, the World Health Organization (WHO) revised the Guiding Principles on Human Cell, Tissue and Organ Transplantation and released those revised principles in March 2009.[33] A 2007 report on the international organ trade found that China, the Philippines, and Pakistan were the largest organ-exporting countries.[35] Several studies have indicated some potential problems that travelers and healthcare providers should be aware of when considering transplantation overseas: lack of documentation related to the donor and the procedures, patients receiving less immunosuppressive medication than is current practice to use in the United States, and the majority of patients not receiving antibiotic prophylaxis.[19, 36, 37] However, it is not clear whether these issues are representative of the issues faced by all patients who travel for transplants. Data comparing complications rates between transplants performed in a patient's home country with those in lower-income countries are limited, for a variety of reasons. For example, transplant tourists tend to be more ill than other medical tourists, and generally only those transplant patients with complications are seen in their local hospitals upon returning to their home country.

Bariatric Tourism

Apart from following general recommendations for medical tourism, individuals seeking bariatric surgery abroad should be reminded that obesity is often considered a chronic disease, even after bariatric surgery.[38] As a result, some bariatric surgeons have suggested that a multidisciplinary care team skilled in the ongoing management of patients after bariatric surgery should be involved in the follow-up plan.[38] In addition to monitoring for surgical complications, the team can also assist with complications that arise due to rapid weight loss or from ongoing obesity. Patients should be encouraged to liaise with an appropriate center in their home country before undergoing surgery abroad.

Reproductive Tourism

Increasingly, patients are traveling to other countries or different regions within their own country to access fertility treatments that are difficult to obtain locally. This may be due to procedures being illegal in their home country, or unavailable owing to lack of local expertise, cost, or long waiting times.[25] Patients may therefore travel to countries where they are able to access donor eggs or surrogates, or have more embryos implanted than are allowed locally. In some areas reproductive care may exclude certain patient groups, so single women or those in same-sex relationships may travel abroad to seek care. Finally, some may travel for added privacy. Although there are limited data on outcomes, the majority of studies have shown high patient satisfaction. However, language and communication problems were the most common problems experienced by patients.[25]

Medications

Travelers, whether they are seeking health or medical care, need to be aware of the global problem of counterfeit medications. The content of these medications varies widely, from insufficient active ingredients to toxic levels of active ingredients, or the addition of toxic additives. While it is difficult to estimate the extent of the problem, it is more prevalent in low-income countries where regulatory and enforcement systems are weak. WHO estimates that 10–30% of medicines sold in developing countries are counterfeit.[39] CDC recommends that travelers carry a sufficient amount of their routine medications and drugs needed for the trip. Travelers should also be advised to carry copies of their prescriptions and a list of all medications they take, including the brand name, generic name, and the manufacturer.[40] Herbal medicines used in complementary or traditional healing centers also lack standardization and may carry similar risks to counterfeit medications.

Adverse Effects and Complications

Although many medical tourists hope to achieve a similar quality of care to that in their home country at a reduced cost, there are currently few or no outcome data from international centres.[23] In addition to the overall quality of care, one specific potential concern is that infection control practices may not be as rigorous as those in the patient's home country, and rates of various blood-borne infections in the local population may be higher. Contaminated instruments or blood products could therefore lead to acquisition of HIV, or hepatitis B or C. One study comparing patients transplanted abroad to those transplanted in their home country of Saudi Arabia revealed that those traveling abroad were more likely to have hepatitis C seroconversion.[41]

Postoperative wound infections due to non-tuberculous mycobacteria have also been associated with medical tourism. In 1998, nine patients who underwent liposuction or liposculpture procedures in Venezuela were found to have confirmed or probable infection due to rapidly growing mycobacteria.[42] In another report, 20 US residents returning from cosmetic surgery in the Dominican Republic in 2003–2004 developed infection with *Mycobacterium abscessus*.[43] An average of 9 months of antimicrobial therapy was required to achieve cure. These reports also highlight the difficulty of identifying outbreaks related to surgical procedures when follow-up care is not confined to the treating institution. Since these infections developed a median time of 2 weeks or more after the procedure, patients usually presented after arriving in their home country, making it more difficult to identify that an outbreak had occurred.

Even in the absence of infection, foreign travel has also been identified as a risk factor for colonization with resistant organisms. A prospective study from Sweden in 2010 demonstrated that international travel is a major risk factor for colonization with ESBL-producing Enterobacteriaceae.[44] Another concerning organism is the New Delhi metallo-β-lactamase-1 (NDM-1), first described in 2009 in a Swedish man who had been hospitalized in India.[45] Organisms that express NDM-1 have now been reported in Canada, the United States, Turkey, Japan, China, Singapore, Australia, and many European countries, including the United Kingdom.[46]

Patients may also have difficulty finding follow-up care upon their return home. Surgeons may not wish to see patients returning from procedures done internationally if they disapprove of the patient's choice to seek care abroad, or have concerns related to the potential for litigation if the patient has a complicated course following treatment.[23] Therefore, patients should arrange for appropriate follow-up care before traveling. Furthermore, even if clinicians are willing to see patients returning from an international trip for medical procedures, they face many challenges. Documentation on the procedures and treatments performed may be incomplete or unavailable. Aftercare for a patient who received a transplant or has developed a wound infection in the absence of adequate information on the immunosuppressive medications given or the antibiotics provided, can lead to the development of further complications.[47]

Finally, options for legal recourse may be limited by local laws and difficulty navigating a foreign legal system. Even when successful, the amount of compensation may be considerably less than that in the patient's home country.[23]

References

1. Gesler WM. Healing Places. Lanham, Md.; Oxford: Rowman & Littlefield; 2003.
2. Nightingale F. Notes on Hospitals: 2 papers; with evidence given to the royal commissioners on the state of the army in 1857. 3rd , enlarg ed. Lond: 1863.
3. Sternberg EM. Healing Spaces: The Science of Place and Well-being. Cambridge, Mass.: Belknap Press of Harvard University Press; 2009.
4. Reed CM. Medical tourism. Med Clin North Am 2008 Nov;92(6):1433, 46, xi.
5. Ehrbeck T, Guevara C, Mango PD. McKinsey Quarterly. 2008.
6. Cohen IG. Medical tourism: The view from ten thousand feet. Hastings Cent Rep 2010 Mar-Apr;40(2):11–2.
7. Huntington MK. The expanding scope of medical travel. Am Fam Physician 2011 Oct 15;84(8):863–4.
8. US. Department of Commerce. Office of travel and tourism industries survey of international air travelers US to overseas and Mexico by birth and citizenship. 2008 report, 2008 January-December.2009. 2009.
9. Deloitte Center for Health Solutions. Medical Tourism: Customers in Search of Value. 2008.
10. Horowitz MD, Rosensweig JA, Jones CA. Medical tourism: Globalization of the healthcare marketplace. Med Gen Med 2007 Nov 13;9(4):33.
11. Bookman MZ, Bookman KR. Medical Tourism in Developing Countries. Basingstoke: Palgrave; 2007.
12. Einhorn B. Outsourcing the patients. BusinessWeek. March 13, 2008.
13. Galland Z. Medical tourism: The insurance debate. BusinessWeek. November 9, 2008.
14. Aerospace Medical Association. Medical guidelines for airline travel, 2nd edition. Aviat Space Environ Med 2003;74(5):A1–19.
15. Air travel. Updated February 2009. Available from: http://www.merck.com/mmpe/sec22/ch333/ch333b.html#CBBIEDEH.
16. New AMA guidelines on medical tourism [Internet]. Available from: New AMA Guidelines on Medical Tourism.
17. Joint Commission International [Internet]. Available from: www.jointcommissioninternational.org/.
18. Joint Commission International. Joint Commission International accreditation standards for hospitals, 4th edition. Joint Commission International; 2010.
19. Merion RM, Barnes AD, Lin M, et al. Transplants in foreign countries among patients removed from the US transplant waiting list. Am J Transplant 2008 Apr;8(4 Pt 2):988–96.
20. Travelling for treatment [Internet]. Updated Nov 11, 2011. Available from: http://www.nathnac.org/travel/misc/medicaltourism_010911.htm#Introduction, 2011.
21. Snyder J, Crooks VA. Medical tourism and bariatric surgery: More moral challenges. Am J Bioeth 2010 Dec;10(12):28–30.
22. Johnston R, Crooks VA, Adams K, et al. An industry perspective on Canadian patients' involvement in medical tourism: Implications for public health. BMC Public Health 2011 May 31;11:416.
23. Weiss EM, Spataro PF, Kodner IJ, et al. Banding in Bangkok, CABG in Calcutta: The United States physician and the growing field of medical tourism. Surgery 2010 Sep;148(3):597–601.
24. Martin D. Professional and public ethics united in condemnation of transplant tourism. Am J Bioeth 2010 Feb;10(2):18–20.
25. Hudson N, Culley L, Blyth E, et al. Cross-border reproductive care: A review of the literature. Reprod Biomed Online 2011 Jun;22(7):673–85.
26. Doheny K. Sick? don't fly. but if you must, get prepped before takeoff. Los Angeles Times. 2004 Oct 17, 2004; Sect. Travel.
27. Cosmetic surgery tourism briefing paper [Internet]; updated July 2010. Available from: http://www.plasticsurgery.org/Media/Briefing_Papers/Cosmetic_Surgery_Tourism.html.
28. The key guidelines for plastic surgery travelers [Internet]. Available from: http://www.isaps.org/medical-procedures-abroad-the-key-guidelines-for-plastic-surgery-travelers.html.
29. Traveler's guide to safe dental care [Internet]; 2001. Available from: http://www.osap.org/?page=TravelersGuide&hhSearchTerms=traveler's+and+guide.
30. World Health Organization. Human organ and tissue transplantation. March 26, 2009. Report No.: A62/12.

31. US. Health Resources and Services Administration, Healthcare Systems Bureau, Division of Transplantation. 2007 annual report of the US. organ procurement and transplantation network and the scientific registry of transplant recipients: Transplant data 1997–2006. Rockville, MD: 2007.

32. Budiani-Saberi DA, Delmonico FL. Organ trafficking and transplant tourism: A commentary on the global realities. Am J Transplant 2008 May;8(5):925–9.

33. Draft guiding principles on human organ transplantation [Internet]. Available from: http://www.who.int/ethics/topics/transplantation_guiding_principles/en/index2.html.

34. Steering Committee of the Istanbul Summit. Organ trafficking and transplant tourism and commercialism: The declaration of Istanbul. Lancet 2008 Jul 5;372(9632):5–6.

35. Shimazono Y. The state of the international organ trade: A provisional picture based on integration of available information. Bull World Health Organ 2007 Dec;85(12):955–62.

36. Gill J, Madhira BR, Gjertson D, et al. Transplant tourism in the United States: A single-center experience. Clin J Am Soc Nephrol 2008 Nov;3(6):1820–8.

37. Sajjad I, Baines LS, Patel P, et al. Commercialization of kidney transplants: A systematic review of outcomes in recipients and donors. Am J Nephrol 2008;28(5):744–54.

38. Birch DW, Vu L, Karmali S, et al. Medical tourism in bariatric surgery. Am J Surg 2010 May;199(5):604–8.

39. World Health Organization. Medicines: Spurious/falsely-labelled/falsified/counterfeit (SFFC) medicines. 2010 Jan 2010. Report No.: Fact Sheet Number 275.

40. Counterfeit drugs and travel [Internet]; 2008. Available from: http://wwwnc.cdc.gov/travel/page/counterfeit-drugs.htm.

41. Alghamdi SA, Nabi ZG, Alkhafaji DM, et al. Transplant tourism outcome: A single center experience. Transplantation 2010 Jul 27;90(2):184–8.

42. Centers for Disease Control and Prevention (CDC). Rapidly growing mycobacterial infection following liposuction and liposculpture–Caracas, Venezuela, 1996–1998. MMWR Morb Mortal Wkly Rep 1998 Dec 18;47(49):1065–7.

43. Furuya EY, Paez A, Srinivasan A, et al. Outbreak of mycobacterium abscess wound infections among 'lipotourists' from the United States who underwent abdominoplasty in the Dominican Republic. Clin Infect Dis 2008 Apr 15;46(8):1181–8.

44. Tangden T, Cars O, Melhus A, et al. Foreign travel is a major risk factor for colonization with escherichia coli producing CTX-M-type extended-spectrum beta-lactamases: A prospective study with Swedish volunteers. Antimicrob Agents Chemother 2010 Sep;54(9):3564–8.

45. Yong D, Toleman MA, Giske CG, et al. Characterization of a new metallo-beta-lactamase gene, bla(NDM-1), and a novel erythromycin esterase gene carried on a unique genetic structure in klebsiella pneumoniae sequence type 14 from India. Antimicrob Agents Chemother 2009 Dec;53(12):5046–54.

46. Kumarasamy KK, Toleman MA, Walsh TR, et al. Emergence of a new antibiotic resistance mechanism in India, Pakistan, and the UK: A molecular, biological, and epidemiological study. Lancet Infect Dis 2010 Sep;10(9):597–602.

47. Jones JW, McCullough LB. What to do when a patient's international medical care goes south. J Vasc Surg 2007 Nov;46(5):1077–9.

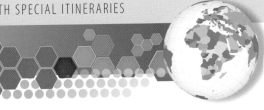

37

Cruise Ship Travel

Carter D. Hill

Key points

- Cruise ships can be amplifiers of infectious diseases due to the close human proximity of semi-closed ship environments
- The most common diagnoses of cruise passengers evaluated in cruise ship infirmaries include upper respiratory infections, injury, seasickness, and gastrointestinal illness
- Cruise ship passengers may experience clusters of brief self-limited diarrheal disease, although this rate is much lower risk than on land
- Ensure the traveler has medical insurance (health and repatriation) that covers conditions in international waters

Introduction

Cruise ship travel has gained tremendous popularity over the last three decades. In 2010, 15 million passengers on 187 ships sailed on North American cruises. Surveys show that three travel categories virtually tie for lead in generating the highest satisfaction levels: cruising, friends/relatives, and resort trips, at 45% each.[1] Cruise destinations such as the Caribbean and Mediterranean have gained popularity due to climate as well as accessibility to many ports. The ever-expanding cruise itineraries, which include diverse ports of call, along with a growth in the number of embarkation ports and onboard amenities, provide travelers with convenient and comfortable means to sample different parts of the world in a short amount of time.[2]

With the growing popularity of recreational cruises, gastrointestinal (GI) and respiratory disease outbreaks may be amplified by the densely populated, semi-closed cruise environment, which compels international passengers and crew to share many activities and resources. Moreover, passengers can acquire a new infectious disease while in port through contaminated food, water, or infected people.[3] Environmental contamination of cruise ships may result in protracted outbreaks due to infected crew and passengers who remain on board during successive voyages. Sanitation and disease surveillance programs developed through the cooperation of the cruise industry and public health agencies have led to improved detection and control of communicable diseases.[4] Understanding the most

frequently reported diseases on cruise ships, their source and mode of transmission, prevention measures, and available ship medical care facilities can lead to better preparedness for a healthy cruise vacation.[5]

The Cruise Industry

The North American Cruise Industry

Ships carrying 13 or more passengers are considered under international law to be passenger ships. They include sailboats, yachts, river cruise ships, and ocean cruise ships. Sailboats and yachts are best known for niche travel, such as 'eco-touring.' River cruises are popular for providing an informal, intimate atmosphere while traveling to places such as the Nile and the Amazon. Ocean cruises make up the greatest portion of ship-based leisure travel, with the North American cruise industry accounting for the major part of the global ocean cruise market. The North American cruise industry consists of cruise lines that market cruises primarily to North Americans but have embarkation ports all over the world. The Caribbean remains the top cruise destination, followed by Alaska, the Mediterranean, and other parts of Europe. Depending on the type of cruise, the duration can range from hours (e.g., gambling cruises) to several months (e.g., round-the-world cruises). The average duration of a cruise is 9 days, and approximately 58% of cruising passengers choose 6–8-day cruises. The typical 7-day cruise allows passengers ample time to visit 3–5 ports and explore different locales and cultures.[1]

The Passengers and Crew

Compared to US residents on non-cruise vacations (defined by those spending 3 nights or more away from home for leisure trips), cruisers tend to be older (49% are over the age of 50), have higher income levels, and are likely to plan a vacation 4–6 months in advance,[1] allowing time for pre-travel health preparation. A typical cruise ship will have a passenger-to-crew ratio of around 3:1. Cruise ships employ crew from around the world: on average, 50 nationalities will be represented in a crew of 1200.[6] The origin of crew will depend on the cruise line and their designated occupation on the ship. Crew members may stay aboard a cruise ship for months on successive voyages, carrying out specialized tasks with the aim of achieving higher-quality service.

©2012 Elsevier Inc
DOI: 10.1016/B978-1-4557-1076-8.00037-5

Cruise Health, Sanitation, and Safety Regulations

International Regulations

In 2005 the World Health Organization (WHO) revised the International Sanitary Regulations (ISR) (in force in 2007) for international regulations and standards binding 194 countries. The overall goal of the revised ISR is to support ship and port sanitation, disease surveillance, and response to infectious diseases (www.who.int/ihr/en). It provides oversight of safe food and water, appropriate waste disposal and vector control, requirements for ship construction and operation, and for sanitary measures on ships.

The safety of cruise ship passengers and crew members is of paramount importance to cruise lines.[7] Safety regulations for international shipping, including cruise ships, are promulgated by the International Maritime Organization (IMO) in its International Convention for Safety of Life at Sea (SOLAS).[8] SOLAS addresses a variety of issues pertaining to passenger and crew safety, including fire protection, lifesaving equipment and procedures, and radio communications. The primary responsibility for implementing the SOLAS standards and other IMO conventions lies with the ship's country of maritime registry or flag state. State maritime agencies at ports of call, such as the United States Coast Guard for ships sailing in US territorial waters, have the legal authority to inspect vessels to ensure compliance with IMO conventions.[8]

US Regulations

The Centers for Disease Control and Prevention (CDC) Vessel Sanitation Program (VSP at http://www.cdc.gov/nceh/vsp/) has responsibility for ensuring appropriate levels of sanitation and health aboard cruise ships arriving at US ports, including facilities that could affect public health, such as food storage, ventilation systems, and pools or spas (www.cdc.gov/quarantine/index.html)/. VSP (Vessel Sanitation Program) develops guidelines and provides consultation to help shipbuilders and renovators meet construction standards. VSP also conducts unannounced, biannual sanitation inspections of US-bound cruise ships that have international itineraries. A score of at least 86 (out of 100) is considered a pass. Up-to-date sanitation inspection scores of cruise ships are available on the VSP website and are published monthly in the 'Summary of Inspections of International Cruise Ships' (http://wwwn.cdc.gov/InspectionQueryTool/InspectionGreenSheetRpt.aspx). Other than acute gastroenteritis (AGE) requirements, all international passenger conveyances bound for the US are legally required to report to US Quarantine, at least 24 hours before arrival, ship cases with certain febrile syndromes suggestive of a communicable disease, as well as any deaths. Diseases on the list are primarily those with pandemic potential (http://www.cdc.gov/ncezid/dgmq/).

Cruise Lines International Association (CLIA) and their member lines participate in domestic and international maritime policy development, and compliance guidelines on behalf of its 25 member cruise lines (which represent the vast majority of the North America cruise industry).[7]

Medical Care Aboard Cruise Ships

CLIA member cruise lines state that they follow the 'Health Care Guidelines for Cruise Ship Medical Facilities'[9] developed by the American College of Emergency Physicians (ACEP) Cruise Ship and Maritime Medicine Section (http://www.acep.org/Content.aspx?id=29980). This ACEP section is composed of physicians actively involved

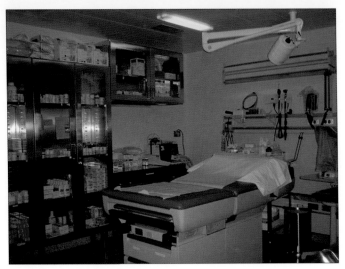

Figure 37.1 Cruise Ship Medical Examination Room. *(Courtesy of Dr R. Wheeler.)*

in cruise ship medicine. Their objective is to advance the capabilities of cruise ship medical facilities and the quality of medical care provided aboard cruise ships. The guidelines address standards for medical facility design, medical staff qualifications, diagnostic equipment, and formulary selection, with a goal of providing general and emergency medical services to passengers and crew.[9]

Medical care aboard cruise ships is designed to provide cruise line passengers and crew members with timely access to comprehensive services for minor to severe illness and injury (Fig. 37.1). Most of the medical conditions that arise aboard ship can be treated as they would be at a doctor's office or ambulatory care center at home. The medical facility is staffed several hours a day for routine medical evaluations. The medical staff is also available 24 hours per day to respond to medical emergencies. More serious problems (such as myocardial infarction, respiratory distress, or cerebrovascular accidents) may require emergency evacuation to an appropriate shore-side hospital after the patient is stabilized in the ship's medical facility.[10]

Most modern cruise ships are equipped to perform a variety of laboratory tests (which may include complete blood count, blood sugar, electrolytes, chemistries, cardiac enzymes, pregnancy testing, and urinalysis), radiography, cardiac monitoring, and advanced life-support procedures.[9] The ship's formulary includes medications for treating common medical problems and a variety of more serious conditions, including infections, injuries, respiratory distress, and cardiac disorders.

Illness on Cruise Ships

The spectrum of illnesses occurring aboard cruise ships generally follows land-based incidences. It can vary depending on the demographics of passengers and crew on board. Two studies involving retrospective reviews of cruise ship medical logs showed that about half of all passengers seeking care aboard cruise ships were older than 64 years. Respiratory tract infection was the most common diagnosis, followed by injuries, nervous system problems (e.g., seasickness), and gastrointestinal illness. About 90% of illnesses on cruise ships were not considered serious or life-threatening, but of those that were, asthma, arrhythmia, angina, and congestive heart failure were among the most common. More than 95% of ill persons seen by the medical clinic were treated on board. The remainder required either temporary or permanent disembarkation for shore-side medical care.[11,12]

Documented outbreaks of infectious diseases aboard cruise ships have been most commonly related to gastrointestinal (norovirus) and respiratory infections (influenza, *Legionella*). Clusters of illnesses related to vaccine-preventable diseases (other than influenza) such as rubella and varicella have also been reported.

Respiratory Infections

Upper respiratory tract infections are the most frequent diagnosis in cruise ship medical facilities, accounting for approximately 29% of passenger visits.[11] The semi-closed and crowded environment of cruise ships may allow for increased person-to-person transmission of respiratory viruses. In addition, ship resources such as contaminated whirlpools or water supply, and even infected crew or passengers remaining on board for multiple voyages, may serve as reservoirs for respiratory pathogens, causing continuous transmission of illness on consecutive cruises. The two most frequently documented etiologic agents of cruise ship-related pneumonia outbreaks are *Legionella* and influenza viruses.

Influenza

Influenza A and B outbreaks among cruise ships crew and passengers can occur throughout the year, even when seasonal influenza activity is absent in the region of the cruise. The convergence and intermingling of international crew and passengers from parts of the world where influenza is in circulation can lead to the introduction and rapid spread of influenza aboard ships. Vaccination of most crew members annually helps with secondary infections. Substantial morbidity may result from cruise influenza outbreaks owing to the presence of a large percentage of elderly and chronically ill passengers, both of whom are at higher risk for complications and death due to influenza infection.

Clinicians can also play an important role in preventing influenza and other respiratory disease outbreaks aboard ships by:

- asking travelers to refrain from traveling while ill, and if illness develops during the trip to practice respiratory hygiene measures and minimize contact with other people, including the cruise staff
- providing vaccination or, if necessary, prophylactic antiviral medication, especially to high-risk populations as well as their close contacts, and those traveling in large tour groups, even if travel occurs during summer.

Legionnaires' Disease

The most commonly established causes of the outbreaks included contamination of ships' water supply, air conditioning systems, or spa pools.[13] The largest documented culture-confirmed cruise ship outbreak of legionnaires' disease occurred in 1994. It involved a total of 50 passengers during nine separate sailings of the same ship.[4] Illness due to infection through bacteria-laden aerosols generated by the spas was associated with immersion in, and spending time around, the whirlpool. This outbreak was detected 3 months after it began, when a New Jersey physician notified the state health department that three hospitalized patients with atypical pneumonia had been on the same cruise ship, which highlights the delay in detection of cruise-associated legionnaires' disease. Symptom onset is typically 2–10 days post exposure without person-to-person spread. Most cruise ships have urinary antigen testing capability.

Clinicians can also play an important role in the control of cruise travel-related legionnaires' infection through rapid case detection among pneumonia patients by:

- inquiring about travel history, including cruise travel
- performing appropriate diagnostic tests (both rapid and culture-based tests)
- promptly reporting cases to state and local health departments. (email: travellegionella@cdc.gov)

Gastrointestinal Illness

The estimated likelihood of contracting gastroenteritis aboard a 7-day cruise is < 1%.[11,14] Acute gastrointestinal disease (AGE) accounts for < 10% of passenger visits to the ship's infirmary.[11] Cruise outbreaks of gastroenteritis due to bacterial and viral pathogens, particularly noroviruses (NoV), are well recognized.[14] The number of outbreaks of gastroenteritis on cruise ships has increased since 2002 owing to the worldwide resurgence of NoV.

Water-Borne Diseases

A review of data from cruise ship water-borne diseases outbreaks during the period 1970–2003 showed that enterotoxigenic *Escherichia coli* (ETEC) is the pathogen most frequently linked to cruise ship water-borne GI outbreaks. Other organisms that may cause water-borne GI outbreaks on cruise ships include *Salmonella* spp, *Shigella* sp, *Cryptosporidium* spp, and *Giardia intestinalis* and NoV. However, in about one-quarter of outbreaks the specific cause cannot be identified.[15]

Cruise ships can prevent water-borne disease outbreaks by ensuring that water is obtained from safe and reliable sources at ports and stored safely; loading water properly at ports to avoid cross-contamination; conducting extra disinfection treatments of water if it is suspected to be contaminated; monitoring residual disinfectants in distribution systems; and ensuring regular inspections and maintenance of the ship's potable water systems.

Food-Borne Diseases

An epidemiologic review of cruise ship food-borne disease outbreaks that occurred from 1970 through 2003 showed that 82% were caused by bacterial pathogens and the rest by viruses, parasites, or unknown sources.

Cruise dining typically offers elaborate meals consisting of a large assortment of foods, which usually involve preparation by multiple food handlers and in many steps, resulting in an increased chance of food mishandling and contamination.[16]

Norovirus

The total number of reported GI outbreaks on cruise ships increased from 4 in 2001 to 11 in 2010. This increase, as well as the frequency of AGE cases on cruise ships, was attributed to noroviruses (NoV).[14]

NoV are the most common cause of viral gastroenteritis and AGE in the United States, with 23 million cases yearly.[5,14] NoV are transmitted via the fecal–oral route, directly person to person, from contaminated food and water, or by contact with contaminated surfaces or objects. Aerosolized vomit has also been suspected as a mode of transmission. During NoV outbreaks on cruises the original source of infection may be an infected person or food. Further spread, resulting in large numbers of illnesses, mainly occurs by person-to-person transmission of the virus.[16] Most NoV outbreaks can be characterized by high attack rates, a high prevalence of vomiting, short duration of illness, and absence of an identifiable pathogen on culture. The key to controlling the spread of NoV on cruise ships is the rapid implementation of infection control measures at the first signs of an AGE outbreak. Typically, the ship gives printed instructions to the passengers about illness prevention and control measures to be followed. During safety orientation at the beginning of most cruises, hand-washing tips are provided, as well as other sanitation measures such as frequent cleaning of common areas, staterooms, elevator buttons, and hand rails, and limiting guest contact with serving utensils in buffet lines during first 2 days of the cruise. Recommend seeking medical care in the ship's infirmary as soon as GI symptoms develop (see Fig. 37.1).[17]

Miscellaneous

Vaccine-Preventable Diseases (VPD)

In addition to influenza, cruise ships have had outbreaks of other routine vaccine-preventable diseases (VPD), such as rubella and varicella. Most often, such illnesses are traced to crew originating from developing countries in which immunity to routine VPD may be low. The densely populated environment of cruise ships and the social interactions between crew and passengers allow for person-to-person spread of VPD among susceptible persons. Pregnant women, along with other potentially susceptible groups of cruise travelers, such as the elderly, the immunosuppressed, and children, need to check their immune status to routine VPD before travel. MMR (measles, mumps, rubella) and varicella vaccines are not ubiquitously provided for all employees on cruise ships, and unvaccinated crew members may serve as a potential reservoir for these diseases to high-risk travelers.

Other Communicable Diseases

The CDC Quarantine Stations receive case reports from US-bound ships of other communicable diseases (mostly among crew) such as measles, mumps, rubella, and varicella, tuberculosis, typhoid, and hepatitis A and B.[18]

Injuries

After respiratory infection, injuries are the second most common reason for passengers to seek medical care aboard cruise ships, accounting for 18% of infirmary visits.[11] The most common injuries seen are sprains, contusions, and superficial wounds. Reported cruise-related injuries most frequently occur on decks and stairs, in passengers' own cabins, or ashore during port calls.[11] Some of the most severe injuries occur during tendering procedures.

Seasickness

Most cruise itineraries tend to sail in the calm waters of the Caribbean or the Mediterranean. Modern cruise ships are also constructed with roll stabilizers, which minimize turbulence. Even so, seasickness is a common concern of many cruise travelers and is among the top four reasons for infirmary visits.[11] Some passengers are sensitive to motion and require pharmacologic prevention and treatment with antihistamines, antimuscarinic, or antidopaminergic agents[6] (see Ch. 43). Alternative medicines may also help some individuals. The association between passenger cabin location and risk of motion sickness is controversial, but common perception persists that central cabins are the least seasickness-inducing. A recent study found that cabin location is only associated with the risk of seasickness when the passenger is seated or standing. Passengers who are able to readily lie down can reduce their risk for motion sickness irrespective of their cabin

location. Additionally, elderly passengers should be cautioned about the overuse of even OTC medications that may affect balance, mental status, or urinary function.

Health Preparation and Prevention Measures for Cruise Travel

Pre-travel health preparation for cruise travel can be challenging because of planned visits to multiple countries and participation in a variety of shipboard and shore-side activities/excursions. In making health risk assessments, healthcare providers should consider a broad range of issues. These include the travelers' health condition and immunity to routine VPD, including influenza, pneumococcus (>65s), MMR (two lifetime vaccinations unless born prior to 1957), the need for special immunizations and chemoprophylaxis based on the cruise ship's itinerary, and health-related risk behaviors during cruise travel[19] (Table 37.1). Cruise ship passengers should be encouraged to consult a travel health advisor for appropriate recommendations. A commonly overlooked risk occurs with the shore excursions off the ships! The International Society of Travel Medicine maintains a list of travel clinics online at www.istm.org.

Pre-Travel

During pre-travel counseling, clinicians should carefully review the traveler's medical conditions to assess whether they can endure the stress of travel and whether they have any special health needs, for example wheelchair access (gangways are often inadequate/unsafe for morbidly obese guests), oxygen (concentrators much preferred), or dialysis.[5,6] Women who will be ≥24 weeks gestation on final day of cruise are not accepted for travel on most cruise lines. Cruise travel can expose travelers to infectious agents, pollutants, changes in diet, physical exertion, extremes of weather, and other conditions that can exacerbate chronic medical conditions. However, cruise tours are available that provide care by onboard specialists, such as pulmonologists and nephrologists, for persons with certain physical impairments, such as chronic obstructive pulmonary disease (COPD) and renal failure requiring hemodialysis. Travelers with medical conditions should be advised to contact and make arrangements with the cruise line/travel agent about their specific medical needs before departure.[6] Cruise ships built during the past 10 years generally have some cabins designed to accommodate wheelchairs. Information regarding wheelchair access can be obtained from the individual cruise lines or the CLIA website.[6] Depending on the medical condition, some cruise lines may require that the traveler have a travel companion. Assisted-living type of care must be provided by passenger. Medical facilities on most modern cruise ships are comparable to those of a community urgent care center, some much better. However, limitations and variability in the level of care available exist between cruise lines and individual ships – and at shore-side hospitals during port stops.[6] For this reason, and to protect the health of others on board, passengers with acute medical complaints or those who acquire an infectious disease before travel should be encouraged to postpone travel and call the cruise lines to discuss alternatives. Cancellation insurance may be purchased from the cruise line.

Regardless of age and underlying medical conditions, all passengers should be up to date with routine age-appropriate vaccinations (see Table 37.1). Given previous cruise ship outbreaks of VPD such as rubella, chickenpox, and influenza, immunity to these diseases should be ensured, especially in high-risk populations (e.g., the elderly, immunosuppressed, or pregnant women). Consideration should be given to influenza vaccination, especially to travelers at high risk for

Table 37.1 Clinicians' Checklist: Pre-Travel Health Preparation of Cruise Ship Travelers[5,6,19,21]

Review
  Presence of acute medical complaints
  Past medical history (presence of chronic illnesses)
  Medication list
  Vaccination history:
    Routine – (see Ch. 10)
    Special travel – (See Ch. 12; typhoid, rabies, yellow fever, Japanese encephalitis, meningococcal
  Travel itinerary and style of travel – countries to be visited during stops and activities
Assess
  Medical feasibility of travel
  Cruise ship facilities: http://www2.cruising.org/CruiseLines/index.cfm
  Cruise ship sanitation score: http://www.cdc.gov/nceh/vsp/desc/about_inspections.htm
  Recent or ongoing GI outbreaks on ship: http://www.cdc.gov/nceh/vsp/surv/gilist.htm
  Health risks and needs based on itinerary: www.who.int; www.cdc.gov/travel/destinat.htm
  Vaccines required (routine and others based on itinerary): Routine: www.who.int; http://www.cdc.gov/vaccines/pubs/ACIP-list.htm; www.cdc.gov/travel/destinat.htm
  Malaria chemoprophylaxis (Ch. 15, based on itinerary) (same resources as above)
Insect repellent (based on itinerary and shore-side activities) (same resources as above)
Provide to/discuss with traveler
  Adequate supply of all medication (ship's formulary is limited and adequate supply for entire cruise is necessary, controlled meds in original Rx bottle). Hand-carry and do not place in checked luggage
  Written personal medical information (include patient demographics, health and travel insurance, contact information of health-care provider and next of kin, medical history, current medications and pertinent lab data (EKG)
  Routine immunizations, if not up to date (Ch.s 10–13, especially for children)
  Other immunizations if indicated (Ch. 12, based on itinerary)
  Malaria prophylaxis if indicated (Ch. 15, based on itinerary)
  Influenza antiviral medication (Ch. 56, based on risk assessment)
  Guidance about mosquito prevention (Ch. 14)
  Guidance about sun protection
Travel advice – pre-travel health preparation, during travel healthy habits, and after travel follow-up (Table 37.2)

complications from influenza and their close contacts, or those who will be traveling with a large group (any time of the year) or visiting the tropics or the southern hemisphere during April to September. Clinicians may consider prescribing a recommended antiviral medication for treatment or prophylaxis of influenza for high-risk patients or travel during summer months.[20]

The traveler's planned itinerary – which countries will be visited, duration of stay, and shore-side excursions and activities – provides crucial insights for determining the need for special immunizations (such as typhoid, rabies, yellow fever, Japanese encephalitis, and meningococcal) and chemoprophylaxis (e.g., for malaria and influenza). If warranted by the location of shore-side stays and outdoor activities, travelers should be advised to include mosquito and sun

protection in their travel kit (for more information on travel kits, see Ch. 8). Travelers, especially those with known health conditions, should carry a written/digital summary of essential health information that could facilitate their care on board or at a shore-side hospital during a medical emergency.[6] This personal medical information sheet (sample available in reference 6) should include information on the traveler's demographics, allergies, chronic conditions, blood type, medication list, contact information of the physician and next of kin, and medical and travel insurance information.[5,6] Important laboratory information, such as an ECG or chest radiograph, if abnormal, should also be attached to the medical information sheet.[6] All prospective cruise travelers should be strongly advised to contact their health insurance carriers in advance of travel and to consider purchasing additional insurance to cover reimbursement for medical evacuation and health services in foreign countries.[5,6] Often, gaps in regular coverage require the additional travel insurance, which can often be found in a travel package offered by cruise lines, usually costing 5–7% of the total package price.[6] However, if only supplemental medical evacuation insurance is needed, the cost can be as low as $70 per person for 1 year of coverage.[6]

During Travel

Clinicians should remind cruise travelers to exercise health-conscious behavior during their journey. Travelers should use caution in selecting the food and water they consume and should practice good hygiene (wash hands, cover coughs and sneezes, etc.) to reduce their risk of getting ill from an infectious disease (Table 37.2).[19] Passengers should ensure that food they consume is thoroughly cooked, inquire whether pasteurized eggs were used for foods requiring a large number of eggs as ingredients (e.g., custards or flan), and evaluate the risks of eating food off the ship at ports. During shore-side excursions pre-packaged foods should not be kept for long hours at unsuitable temperatures, and passengers should drink bottled water. Practicing good hand and respiratory hygiene is important in preventing illnesses that are transmitted from person to person, either by direct contact, by respiratory routes, or through contaminated environments.[21]

After Travel

Passengers should be urged to follow up with their healthcare provider for any fever or flu-like illness that develops up to a year after travel.[21] Clinicians should inquire about cruise travel in all cases of pneumonia, other respiratory illnesses, gastrointestinal illnesses, or suspected communicable disease. Appropriate diagnostic testing, both rapid and culture-based, better enables public health investigations to link an illness to a source. Viral isolation (via nasopharyngeal specimens) is essential to identify new and unusual imported strains of influenza and other respiratory pathogens.[4] Clinicians can help enhance surveillance and characterization of cruise ship-associated illnesses by identifying and reporting notifiable diseases or conditions and possible clusters of diseases to public health agencies (http://www.cdc.gov/quarantine/QuarantineStationContactListFull.html).

Conclusion

Since 1980, the number of cruise passengers on CLIA member lines has grown at an average annual rate of 7.4%. An estimated 16 million passengers are forecast to sail in 2011 (73% from North America).[2] The occurrence of shipboard illnesses and outbreaks related to gastrointestinal, respiratory, and vaccine-preventable diseases has led to

Table 37.2 Travel Health Advice for Cruise Ship Travelers[19,20,21,22]

Before travel

Notify cruise ship of special medical needs (e.g., wheelchair access, bariatric equipment, oxygen concentrators, food allergies/sensitivities, dietary restrictions, injectable meds like insulin/syringes for sharps containers or refrigeration, scooter access/storage/charging). See Ch. 25

Wheelchair assistance for embarking/disembarking is generally available but should be requested in advance. Medical equipment during cruise including wheelchairs, concentrators, CPAP equipment, etc. needs to be requested from an approved vendor well before sailing (e.g., Special Needs at Sea at http://www.specialneedsatsea.com/)

Clients with medical/electronic equipment should insure voltage of the ship is compatible and cabins have enough outlets; extension cords/Surge protectors may need to be packed

Ensure adequate insurance coverage for medical evacuation (N America $25K min, Caribbean $50K min, S America $100K min, Asia/Africa $200K min) and healthcare abroad

Prepare first-aid kit (see Ch. 8)

Infants <6 months cannot travel on most CLIA vessels and some sailings require infant be 1 year old on or before day cruise starts

Postpone travel if illness develops

Obtain mosquito prevention (with DEET) See Ch. 7

Obtain sun protection

During travel (while on cruise and on-shore):

To prevent getting food- and water-borne diseases

Ensure all food consumed is thoroughly cooked

Inquire about use of pasteurized eggs for foods with eggs as main ingredient (e.g., flan, omelets)

Evaluate the risks of eating any food, especially off the ship

Ensure correct temperature of cold and hot foods

Ensure pre-packaged food for shore-side excursions is stored at appropriate temperature

To prevent spread of germs

Follow good hand hygiene:

Wash hands frequently with soap and water

If soap and water not available, alcohol-based disposable wipes or gel sanitizers containing at least 60% alcohol may be used

Follow good respiratory hygiene:

Cover mouth and nose with tissue when coughing or sneezing

If tissue not available, cough or sneeze into upper sleeve, not hands

Put used tissue in waste basket

Avoid close contact with people who are sick

Be sure to report illness to cruise staff if they are unaware

Stay well hydrated by drinking water

Get plenty of rest

Avoid excessive alcohol intake

After travel:

Report to doctor for illnesses especially with fever or respiratory symptoms (Chs. 53 and 56)

improved infectious diseases surveillance and control strategies by the cruise industry and public health agencies.[5] Pre-travel health preparations and knowledge of available medical care aboard cruise ships are important for cruise travelers, especially given that approximately one-third are senior citizens who may have chronic illnesses or who may be at greater risk for some infectious diseases.[6] Because medical facilities aboard cruise ships are designed to provide basic emergency medical care, travelers should be encouraged to consult their health insurance provider regarding extra coverage while away from their home country and for medical evacuation.[6,9] Healthcare providers can contribute to a healthy cruise environment through rapid detection, diagnosis, and public health reporting of cruise-related communicable diseases in returned ill travelers.[5,22]

Acknowledgement

Division of Global Migration and Quarantine, National Center for Preparedness, Detection, and Control of Infectious Disease, Centers for Disease Control and Prevention, Atlanta, Georgia, Robert Wheeler, Kiren Mitruka, Linda Allen, Grant Tarling, Bud Darr, and Eilif Dahl.

References

1. Cruise Lines International Association (CLIA). 2011 Market Profile Study (http://www.cruising.org/).
2. Cruise industry overview: Cruise Lines International Association (US); 2011. Available from: http://www.cruising.org/vacation/pressroom-research.
3. Widdowson MA, Cramer EH, Hadley L, et al. Outbreaks of acute gastroenteritis on cruise ships and on land: identification of a predominant circulating strain of norovirus – United States 2002. J Infect Dis 2004;190:27–36.
4. Jernigan DB, Hofmann J, Cetron MS, et al. Outbreak of Legionnaires' disease among cruise ship passengers exposed to a contaminated whirlpool spa. Lancet 1996 Feb;24;347:494–9.
5. Lawrence DN. Outbreaks of gastrointestinal diseases on cruise ships: lessons from three decades of progress. Curr Infect Dis Rep 2004;6:115–23.
6. Wheeler RE. Travel health at sea: cruise ship medicine. In: Zuckerman JN, editor. Principle and Practices of Travel Medicine. New York: John Wiley and Sons; 2001. p. 275–87.
7. Cruise industry source book – 2007 edition [online]. Arlington (Virginia): Cruise Lines International Association. 2007 Feb [cited 2007 Mar 29]. Available from: www.cruising.org/press/sourcebook2007/index.cfm.
8. International Convention for the Safety of Life at Sea (SOLAS) [online]. London: International Maritime Organization; 1974. [cited 2006 Feb 1]. Available from: www.imo.org./home.asp?flash=false.
9. Health care guidelines for cruise ship medical facilities [online]. Irving (TX): American College of Emergency Physicians, Section on Cruise Ship and Maritime Medicine; April 2011. (www.acep.org/webportal/PracticeResources/issues/cruiseship)
10. Prina LD, Orazi UN, Weber RE. Evaluation of emergency air evacuation of critically ill patients from cruise ships. J Travel Med 2001;8:285–92.
11. Peake DE, Gray CL, Ludwig, et al. Descriptive epidemiology of injury and illness among cruise ship passengers. Ann Emerg Med 1999;33:67–72.
12. Dahl E. Anatomy of a world cruise. J Travel Med 1999;6:168–71.
13. World Health Organization (WHO). Sanitation on Ships: Compendium of Outbreaks of Foodborne and Waterborne Disease and Legionnaire's disease Associated with Ships, 1970–2000. Geneva: WHO; 2001.
14. Cramer EH, Blanton CJ, Blanton LH, et al. Epidemiology of gastroenteritis on cruise ships, 2001–2004. Am J Prevent Med 2006 Mar;30(3):252–7. (http://www.cdc.gov/nceh/vsp/surv/glist.html#years)
15. Rooney RR, Bartram JK, Cramer EH, et al. A review of outbreaks of waterborne disease associated with ships: evidence for risk management. Public Health Rep 2004 Jul/Aug;119(4):435–42.
16. Rooney RR, Cramer EH, Mantha S. A review of outbreaks of foodborne disease associated with passenger ships: evidence for risk management. Public Health Rep 2004 Jul/Aug;119:427–34.

17. Dahl E. Dealing with gastrointestinal illness on a cruise ship. Part 1: description of sanitation measures. Part 2: an isolation study. Int Marit Health 2004;55(1–4):19–29.

18. Quarantine Activity Report System, Version 4.1. Atlanta (GA): Division of Global Migration and Quarantine, National Center for Preparedness, Detection, and Control of Infectious Disease, Centers for Disease Control and Prevention, US Department of Health and Human Services; 2006.

19. Cruising tips. Vessel Sanitation Program, National Center for Environmental Health [online]. Atlanta: Centers for Disease Control and Prevention; 2006. [cited 2006 Jan 29]. Available from: www.cdc.gov/nceh/vsp/pub/ CruisingTips/cruisingtips.htm.

20. Centers for Disease Control and Prevention (CDC). Prevention and Control of Influenza. Recommendations of the Advisory Committee on Immunization Practices. MMWR 2006 July 28;55(RR 10):1–42.

21. Travelers' Health [online]. Atlanta: Centers for Disease Control and Prevention, Department of Health and Human Services. 2005 July 14. [cited 30 Jan 2006]. National Center for Infectious Diseases, Division of Global Migration and Quarantine; [about 2 screens]. Available from: www.cdc.gov/travel/destinat.htm

22. Slaten DD, Mitruka K, Cruise Ship Travel. Chapter 6. Yellow Book; 2012. (http://wwwnc.cdc.gov/travel/yellowbook/2012/chapter-6-conveyance-and-transportation-issues/cruise-ship-travel.htm).

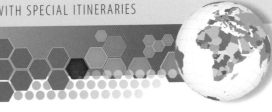

38

Mass Gatherings

Annelies Wilder-Smith and Robert Steffen

Key points

- Mass gatherings are the temporary collection of large numbers of people at one site or location for a common purpose
- Mass gatherings present some of the most complex management challenges faced by governments and organizers
- Mass gatherings may lead to three potential infectious disease public health threats: the risk of importation of infectious diseases usually not seen in the country of the gathering; the amplification of transmission during the event; and lastly the international spread of infectious disease via the visitors and travelers returning to their home countries
- While infectious diseases may be of greater global public health relevance, non-communicable diseases and accidents usually have a higher local impact with respect to morbidity and mortality during mass gatherings

Mass gatherings are the temporary collection of large numbers of people at one site or location for a common purpose. The purpose of the mass gathering can be manifold, such as major sport events, e.g., the Olympic Games, the FIFA World Cup, other spectator events (e.g., air shows, concerts), or pilgrimages (the *Hajj* pilgrimage for example), or religious mass gatherings (such as Papal visits) and political or business (e.g., conferences, trade fairs). Gatherings can be short-term (for a few hours as in a sporting event or concert) or longer (for several days to weeks, as in the Olympic Games or the *Hajj*). A gathering can be held at one location or spread over different sites.

The sizes of mass gatherings vary. For example, there were around 3.2 million spectators during the FIFA World Cup in Germany in 2006; the *Hajj* pilgrimage usually attracts some 2 million Muslims; the Hindu pilgrimage Kumbh Mela in India can attract more than 10 million pilgrims. There is no consensus on a threshold of the number of people that constitute a mass gathering. The number may be as few as 1000 people, although 25 000 is more common. International events draw persons from all over the world, including heads of state

and international dignitaries, as well as masses from the lowest socio-economic strata, thereby presenting problems of security, language, and cultural and dietary specificities.

There is no simple definition of a mass gathering. Large masses of people may be at certain venues, such as international airports, in shopping centers or mass tourism settings, but yet they are not considered a mass gathering. Most mass gatherings are planned, but spontaneous mass gatherings may also occur, such as for a Papal funeral. There can be similar visitor numbers and health risks at organized mass gatherings that attract media attention (such as the Olympics) and those that do not, such as trade fairs, certain religious events, etc.

There is also no specified relation to the potential risks to public health or even public health emergencies of international concern. As far as epidemic potential and public health implications are concerned, mass gatherings need to be differentiated from humanitarian emergencies. Mass gatherings are non-emergency events that have usually been planned ahead, whereas humanitarian emergencies are the result of unplanned occurrences, possibly in association with natural disasters, civil conflict or war. The purpose, location, characteristics and number of participants, and duration of the event will determine the nature of a mass gathering.

The best definition is probably the one by the World Health Organization (WHO), which defines mass gatherings as 'events attended by a sufficient number of people to strain the planning and response resources of a community, state or nation'.

Mass gatherings present some of the most complex management challenges faced by governments and organizers. The influx of large numbers of people, often from different countries and cultures, and the infrastructural changes needed to support them are a formidable challenge for any public health system. Effective management of mass casualty incidents requires coordinated efforts across a wide variety of sectors, some of which may have little experience of working with the health sector. Even if the existing health services and other support services of the host community have adequate capacity to manage the regular disease burden affecting its own population (including occasional outbreaks and large accidents), the influx of large numbers of people, together with the infrastructural changes needed to support the event, can place severe strains on such services, compromising the ability to detect a developing problem and carry out an effective response.

©2012 Elsevier Inc
DOI: 10.1016/B978-1-4557-1076-8.00038-7

Mass gatherings have been a target for terrorist attacks. Mass gatherings may also attract deliberate releases of chemical, biological or radioactive agents, or even bomb attacks.

Following requests for assistance from several WHO member states that were hosting mass gatherings, in 2007 a program on mass gatherings was established by WHO's Department of Global Alert and Response. Its mandate is to provide advice or technical assistance on health protection, disease prevention and planning, and alert and response measures for mass gatherings.

Furthermore, the *Lancet* organized a conference on Mass Gathering Medicine, 23–25 October 2010; and a series on issues of mass gatherings was commissioned for the year 2011.[1]

In this chapter, the focus will be both on communicable and non-communicable disease risks associated with mass gatherings, with a focus on some well-documented mass gatherings such as the *Hajj* and the Olympics.

Communicable Diseases

The high population density at a mass gathering event has the immense potential to amplify infectious diseases. As mass gatherings draw visitors from countries around the world, there are three potential public health problems: the risk of importation of infectious diseases usually not seen in the country of the gathering; the amplification of transmission during the event; and the international spread of infectious disease via the visitors and travelers returning to their home countries. Surveillance and public health response may not be developed for diseases that are usually not endemic in the host country. Furthermore, gatherings with international participants potentially pose specific challenges for implementing control measures, such as contact tracing in case of an outbreak.

Despite the theoretical concerns, however, infectious diseases have historically not been a major issue in association with mass gatherings, except for the *Hajj* pilgrimage. The Hindu pilgrimage Kumbh Mela is likely to be associated with outbreaks of diarrheal diseases, but published reports are lacking.

The close proximity of people during mass gatherings provides ideal grounds for rapid spread of influenza. The decision to proceed with a mass gathering or to restrict, modify, postpone, or cancel the event due to pandemic influenza should be based on a thorough risk assessment. Event planners undertake such an assessment in partnership with local and national public health authorities. The risk assessment may take into account available information at global, national, and local levels, such as severity of illness, and periods of communicability and incubation. If the severity of illness is high and the periods of communicability or incubation are less than the duration of the event, there is a greater risk of overwhelming the local health services; however, if the periods of communicability or incubation are of longer duration, the greater impact may be in the participants' home communities upon their return home. It is recommended that these risk factors be assessed against the social disruption that may be caused by the cancellation of an event.

Hajj Pilgrimage

The potential for spread of infectious diseases associated with the *Hajj* is well recognized. *Hajj*, the unique annual mass gathering of over 2 million Muslims from all over the world, presents enormous challenges to the authorities in Saudi Arabia[2] (Fig. 38.1) . Saudi Arabia has developed a comprehensive program which is updated annually, to ensure that all aspects of *Hajj* rituals are conducted safely and without major incident.[3] The inevitable overcrowding in a confined

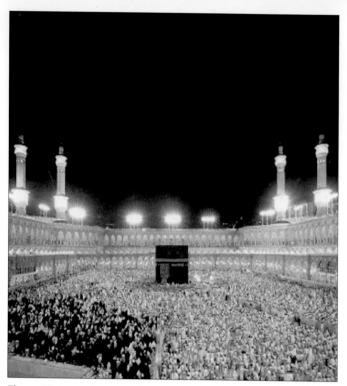

Figure 38.1 Hajj, the unique annual mass gathering of over 2 million Muslims from all over the world.

area of such large numbers increases the risk of respiratory infections. The *Hajj* has historically been associated with outbreaks of meningococcal disease, with a major outbreak of serogroup A occurring in 1998.[4,5] In response to this outbreak, the Ministry of Health in Saudi Arabia introduced vaccination against serogroup A as a *Hajj* visa requirement. In 2000 and 2001 other outbreaks occurred, this time related to serogroup W135.[6] The outbreaks of meningococcal W135 strains in 2000 and 2001 with the associated high mortality showed the potential for international spread at mass gatherings.

Although H1N1 was a concern prior to the *Hajj* 2009, massive amplification of this pandemic through the *Hajj* did not take place, partly because of the preventive measures that were taken, and partly because the *Hajj* in 2009 took place at the tail end of the epidemic.[7]

Olympics

Mass events such as the Olympic Games provide an opportunity to strengthen the health system's capacity to manage health emergencies as well as to promote preventive services and healthy lifestyles.[8] The experience of the Olympics 2008 in Beijing, China, shows that it is possible to advance a public health agenda by capitalizing on the attention generated by the Games among Government agencies and civil society.

Non-Communicable Diseases and Accidents

Whereas infectious diseases may be of greater global public health relevance, non-communicable diseases and accidents usually have a higher local impact with respect to morbidity and mortality during mass gatherings. For example, during the 1996 Olympics in Atlanta, USA, a review of all medical records at the Olympic medical site was undertaken.[9] Spectators and volunteers accounted for most (88.9%, $p<0.001$) of the 1059 visits for heat-related illness. Injuries, accounting for 35% of all medical visits, were more common among athletes (51.9% of their visits, $p<0.001$) than among other groups. Injuries accounted for 31.4% of all other groups combined. Overall physician treatment rate was 4.2 per 10 000 in attendance (range, 1.6–30.1 per 10 000).

A number of risk factors have been identified. With respect to environmental factors, meteorological conditions, both heat and cold, play a leading role. Further, infrastructure and crowd density are decisive for the wellbeing of the attendants at a mass gathering or a disaster. Considering host factors, age is the most important factor, as demonstrated at the *Hajj*, where a large proportion of older adults participate, many with pre-existing illness which may be aggravated by heat or exertion. Gender may be an issue, as young women tend more often to collapse due to hypotension and dehydration; on the other hand, patients with fall injuries tend to be women aged over 40 years. Emotional stress such as at sporting tournaments has been associated with severe acute cardiovascular events. Alcohol and drug consumption may result in aggression, as shown in sports events, or coma, as reported from street parades.

Planning

In order to meet the challenges posed by a mass gathering, countries and organizers must conduct advanced risk assessment, planning and system enhancement. Event planners and other stakeholders are advised to work in close collaboration with local public health officials when planning events, taking into account local factors while conducting a risk assessment of the event. Conducting a risk assessment of a planned event will assist event planners, stakeholders, and local public health officials to determine whether an event should be cancelled, modified, or postponed. Pre-planning includes a multi-sectoral approach (http://www.wpro.who.int/publications/PUB_9789290614593.htm). This includes assessing the local health services, medical emergency services and blood supply, and public health preparation for potential nuclear, biological, chemical and explosive terrorist actions. It also includes ensuring food safety, air quality, and vector control where needed. These are critical to identifying potential public health risks, both natural and manmade, and to preventing, minimizing and responding to public health emergencies.

Surveillance and health response mechanisms should be upgraded to take into account possible importation of diseases not usually seen in the host country. Surveillance should focus on issues identified in a formal risk assessment but should cover all hazards.

Individual Pre-Gathering Advice

The travel health professional advising individuals planning to attend a mass gathering should offer the usual pre-travel advice depending on destination, which should include advice on appropriate immunizations, malaria prophylaxis (if the gathering takes place in a malaria-endemic area), advice on food and water hygiene and avoidance of traffic accidents. With regard to immunizations, particular attention should be given to recommending influenza vaccination. Furthermore, the importance of being immune against measles cannot be over-emphasized, particularly in light of declining vaccine coverage rates in some countries or poor coverage in others, highlighting that routine immunizations should be up to date. If prolonged crowding conditions are to be expected, quadrivalent meningococcal vaccine may be indicated. The quadrivalent meningococcal vaccine is a *Hajj* visa requirement. As much as possible, travelers must be made aware of the risk of stampede, so that they are aware of the danger and can avoid critical situations.

References

1. Mass gatherings medicine. Lancet Infect Dis 2010;10(10):653.
2. Ahmed QA, Arabi YM, Memish ZA. Health risks at the Hajj. Lancet 2006;367(9515):1008–15.
3. Shafi S, Booy R, Haworth E, et al. Hajj: health lessons for mass gatherings. J Infect Public Health 2008;1(1):27–32.
4. Wilder-Smith A. Meningococcal vaccine in travelers. Curr Opin Infect Dis 2007;20(5):454–60.
5. Wilder-Smith A. Meningococcal disease: risk for international travellers and vaccine strategies. Travel Med Infect Dis 2008;6(4):182–6.
6. Wilder-Smith A, Goh KT, Barkham T, Paton NI. Hajj-associated outbreak strain of Neisseria meningitidis serogroup W135: estimates of the attack rate in a defined population and the risk of invasive disease developing in carriers. Clin Infect Dis 2003;36(6):679–83.
7. Memish ZA, McNab SJ, Mahoney F, et al. Establishment of public health security in Saudi Arabia for the 2009 Hajj in response to pandemic influenza A H1N1. Lancet 2009;374(9703):1786–91.
8. Amiri N, Chami G. Medical services at the Olympics: a monumental challenge. CMAJ 2010;182(5):E229–30.
9. Wetterhall SF, Coulombier DM, Herndon JM, et al. Medical care delivery at the 1996 Olympic Games. Centers for Disease Control and Prevention Olympics Surveillance Unit. JAMA 1998;279(18):1463–8.

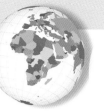

39

High-Altitude Medicine

Thomas E. Dietz and Peter H. Hackett

Key points

- Most individuals, even those with chronic illness, can enjoy traveling to altitude as long as they are properly advised and are careful to acclimatize
- Hypoxia, lower temperature, UV radiation, and dehydration are the challenges one faces at altitude
- Acute mountain sickness is common and affects up to 40% of individuals even at moderate altitudes (2000–3500 m) at popular ski resorts
- Management of acute mountain sickness includes: no further ascent until symptoms resolve, descent to lower altitude if no improvement, and descent if any signs of cerebral or pulmonary edema develop
- A variety of medications are available for both prevention and treatment of high-altitude illness, especially acetazolamide, dexamethasone, nifedipine, and PDE-5 inhibitors

Introduction

The increasing popularity and accessibility of adventure travel trips to high-altitude locations, as well as employment opportunities in these locations, make it more important than ever for travel medicine physicians to understand the medical problems associated with high altitude. This chapter discusses the unique aspects of the high-altitude environment, acclimatization, the high-altitude illnesses, the impact of high altitude on pre-existing medical conditions, and whether a pre-existing condition might adversely affect acclimatization to high altitude. A list of online resources is included in Table 39.1. For more detailed recent reviews, see references[1,2].

The High-Altitude Environment

The high-altitude environment refers to elevations >1500 m (4900 ft). Moderate altitude includes the elevations of most mountain and ski resorts, 2000–3500 m (6600–11 500 ft). Arterial oxygen saturation is well maintained at these altitudes, but mild tissue hypoxia results from low arterial PO$_2$ (PaO$_2$), and altitude illness is common. Very high altitude refers to altitudes of 3500–5500 m (11 500–18 000 ft). In

this range, arterial oxygen saturation is not maintained, and extreme hypoxemia can occur during sleep, exercise, and illness. High-altitude pulmonary and cerebral edema is most common in this range. Extreme altitude is > 5500 m (18 000 ft). Above this altitude, successful long-term acclimatization is impossible and deterioration ensues; no long-term human habitations exist above 5500 m. Individuals must progressively acclimatize to intermediate altitudes to reach extreme altitude.

Hypoxia is the primary physiological insult on ascent to high altitude. The fraction of oxygen in the atmosphere remains constant (0.21), but as barometric pressure decreases on ascent to altitude, so does the partial pressure of oxygen (Fig. 39.1). The inspired partial pressure of oxygen (PiO$_2$) is lower than atmospheric oxygen partial pressure because of water vapor pressure in the airways. At the altitude of Denver, Colorado (1600 m), PiO$_2$ is 18% lower than at sea level (122 versus 149 mmHg); in Breckenridge, Colorado (2860 m) it is 105 mmHg; while at La Paz, Bolivia (4000 m), PiO$_2$ is only 86.4 mmHg, which is equivalent to breathing a gas mixture of 12% oxygen at sea level. Thus, the high-altitude environment produces significant alveolar and consequent arterial hypoxemia.

The high-altitude environment offers a number of stresses in addition to hypoxia. Temperature decreases with ascent to altitude, of the order of 6.5°C per 1000 m; the effects of hypoxia and cold can be additive in terms of predisposing to problems such as frostbite and high-altitude pulmonary edema. Ultraviolet radiation increases by 4% per 300 m gain in altitude, owing to less water vapor and particulate matter in the high-altitude atmosphere; this predisposes to sunburn, UV keratoconjunctivitis, and cataracts. Dehydration is common because of increased insensible water loss from the airways and skin.

Acclimatization

The body's response to altitude depends on both the degree and the rate of onset of hypoxia. Acute hypoxia causes feelings of unreality, dizziness, dim vision, and rapid unconsciousness given sufficient hypoxic stress; for example, sudden exposure to an altitude equivalent to the summit of Mt. Everest (8848 m; PiO$_2$ 43 mmHg) will result in unconsciousness within 2 minutes. However, individuals developing the same degree of hypoxia over days to weeks are able to function relatively well. This process of adjusting to hypoxia, termed acclimatization, is a complex process with great variability involving over 200 genes activated by hypoxia, with a series of compensatory changes in multiple organ systems over differing time courses from days to weeks,

DOI: 10.1016/B978-1-4557-1076-8.00039-9

Table 39.1 Online Information Resources on Altitude Illness

International Society for Mountain Medicine: www.ismmed.org
> Detailed practical information on altitude illness available for both physicians and non-physicians. Includes diagnostic criteria for AMS, HACE, and HAPE, as well as AMS scoring tools for adults and children. An 'ask the experts' section is available for difficult cases.

Institute for Altitude Medicine: http://www.altitudemedicine.org
> A thorough information source for high-altitude travelers, with availability for consultation with experts.

The High Altitude Medicine Guide: www.high-altitude-medicine.com
> Information on altitude illness and other health issues for travelers and their physicians. Has a practical tutorial on field hyperbaric treatment, and comparisons of the various portable hyperbaric bags.

ICAR-MEDCOM: http://www.ikar-cisa.org
> A collection of articles on medical management of mountaineering emergencies, including a suggested alpine medical kit. Presented by the International Commission for Mountain Emergency Medicine. From the home page navigate to Alpine Medicine, then Recommendations; from there you can download each position paper as a pdf file.

Wilderness Medical Society: www.wms.org
> Complete archives of Wilderness and Environmental Medicine and the prior *Journal of Wilderness Medicine*. Archives are open, but the current issue is only accessible to subscribers and WMS members.

Altitude.org: http://www.altitude.org/
> Information on altitude illness prevention and treatment for travelers and physicians, including a barometric pressure calculator.

MEDEX: http://medex.org.uk/
> MEDEX organizes high altitude medical research expeditions. They have an excellent booklet Travel at High Altitude, available in 12 different languages, which can be downloaded for free as a pdf file at http://medex.org.uk//medex_book/about_book.php

and even years. There are limits to the body's ability to adjust to hypoxia; the severity and rate of onset of the hypoxic stress and individual physiology determine whether acclimatization will be successful or fail, resulting in high-altitude illness.

Over the past several years great advances have been made in our knowledge of the molecular basis of human response to hypoxia. Central to this is hypoxia-inducible factor (HIF), an oxygen-sensitive transcription factor that under hypoxic conditions modulates the expression of hundreds of genes involved in angiogenesis, apoptosis, regulation of metabolism, cell proliferation, and many other aspects of basic cell physiology.[3,4]

Although the fundamental process occurs in the metabolic machinery of the cell, which takes time to adjust, acute physiologic responses are essential. The most important and immediate response of the body to hypoxia is an increase in minute ventilation, triggered by oxygen-sensing cells in the carotid body. First with an increase in tidal volume and then respiratory frequency, increased ventilation produces a higher alveolar PO_2, thereby reducing hypoxic stress. Concomitantly, a lower alveolar CO_2 produces a respiratory alkalosis, which acts as a brake on the brain respiratory center and limits the increase in ventilation. Only after renal compensation (excretion of bicarbonate ion) does the blood pH return to near-normal levels and the full increase in ventilation

take place. This process, termed ventilatory acclimatization, requires approximately 4 days at a given altitude, and is greatly enhanced by acetazolamide. Patients with insufficient carotid body response (genetic or acquired) or pulmonary or (rarely) renal disease may have an inadequate ventilatory response and therefore not adapt well to high altitude.

Just as the ventilatory pump increases in order to supply more oxygen to the blood, the circulatory pump increases to provide more circulating oxygen to the tissues. Ascent to high altitude, through sympathetic activation, initially increases resting heart rate and cardiac output, and mildly increases blood pressure. The healthy heart tolerates extreme hypoxia well; even with PaO_2 <30 mmHg, ECG and echocardiogram evaluation in experimental subjects showed no evidence of ischemia, no wall motion abnormalities, and no depressed contractility.[5,6]

The pulmonary circulation reacts to hypoxia with vasoconstriction, owing to smooth muscle activation in the vessel walls. This response is arguably beneficial, somewhat improving ventilation/perfusion matching and gas exchange. The resulting pulmonary hypertension, however, can lead to a number of pathological syndromes at high altitude, including high-altitude pulmonary edema and altitude-related right heart failure.

Cerebral blood flow increases immediately on ascent to high altitude, and then returns toward normal over the first week of acclimatization. This response is variable, but the average increase is 24% at 3810 m, and more at higher altitude. Whether this increased flow relates to the headache of acute mountain sickness is likely but not proven.

Hemoglobin concentration increases on ascent to high altitude, thereby enhancing the oxygen-carrying capacity of the blood. In the first few days it increases secondary to reduction in plasma volume (i.e., hemoconcentration). Over weeks to months, hemoglobin concentration increases due to augmented red cell production stimulated by erythropoietin.

The oxyhemoglobin dissociation curve remains unchanged until the marked alkalosis of extreme altitude shifts it to the left, thereby facilitating loading of the hemoglobin with oxygen in the pulmonary capillary. Reinforcing the notion that a left-shifted hemoglobin is an advantage at high altitude, individuals with a rare naturally occurring left-shifted hemoglobin have exceptional performance at altitude. Whether those with a right-shifted oxyhemoglobin dissociation curve are at a disadvantage at altitude is unknown.

Effects of High Altitude on Exercise

High-altitude hypoxia dramatically affects aerobic but not anaerobic exercise performance. Maximum oxygen consumption (VO_{2max}) decreases approximately 10% for every 1000 m of altitude, starting at 1500 m. As a result, a person exercising at altitude to the same degree as at sea level will be operating at a higher percentage of VO_{2max}, will become more easily fatigued and will reach anaerobic threshold earlier. Also, because of the large increase in exercise ventilation, breathlessness becomes a limiting factor. The result is that persons exercising at high altitude must exercise less intensely to avoid exhaustion, and rest more frequently. Endurance time (minutes to exhaustion at 75% of altitude-specific VO_{2max}) does improve, by as much as 40% after 12 days.[7]

Sleep at High Altitude

Sleep architecture is altered at high altitude, and results in a slight change in sleep stages, frequent arousals, and nearly universal

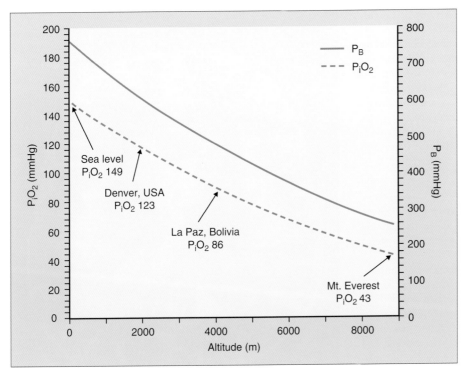

Figure 39.1 Barometric pressure and PiO₂ at altitude. Barometric pressure (P_B) decreases exponentially with increasing altitude; FiO₂ is a constant 21% of P_B, but the partial pressure of oxygen in inspired air (PiO₂) is decreased because of water vapor added as the air is warmed and humidified in the respiratory tree.

subjective reporting of disturbed or unsatisfactory sleep. After 3–4 nights at a given altitude this generally improves, though periodic breathing (Cheyne–Stokes) during sleep is 'normal' at altitudes >2700 m.

High-Altitude Syndromes

Altitude illness refers to the syndromes that result from hypoxia; the target organs are the brain and the lung. High-altitude headache (HAH), acute mountain sickness (AMS) and high-altitude cerebral edema (HACE) reflect the brain pathophysiology; symptomatic pulmonary hypertension and high-altitude pulmonary edema (HAPE) reflect that of the lung. These illnesses generally occur at altitudes above 2500 m, though particularly sensitive individuals can become ill as low as 1800 m. Everyone traveling to altitude is at risk, regardless of the level of physical fitness or previous altitude experience.

High-Altitude Headache

Epidemiology

Headache at altitude is common. In one study, women and persons suffering from headaches at low altitude had more severe headaches, but not more headaches than other trekkers; older persons were less susceptible.[8] Headache may be the harbinger of AMS, but often it is the only symptom. Half of those with headaches did not have AMS by the Lake Louise criteria (defined as headache plus at least one of four other symptoms in the context of a recent altitude gain).

Pathophysiology

The pathophysiology is thought to be multifactorial. Vasodilatation seems to be the primary event, with possible activation of the trigeminovascular system by both mechanical and chemical stimuli. In addition, altered threshold of pain at high altitude may play a role.[9] The

rapid onset and quick relief with oxygen therapy make edema an unlikely cause of HAH, and favor vasodilatation.

Clinical Presentation and Diagnosis

The International Headache Society has defined HAH by the following: headache with at least two of the following characteristics: 1. bilateral; 2. frontal or frontotemporal; 3. dull or pressing quality; 4. mild or moderate intensity; and 5. aggravated by exertion, movement, straining, coughing, or bending. Additionally, the headache must occur with an ascent to altitude > 2500 m, develop within 24 hours after ascent, and resolve within 8 hours after descent.[10]

Treatment

Management of HAH is symptomatic, with analgesics such as non-steroidal anti-inflammatory drugs (NSAIDs) and acetaminophen generally being effective. There have been mixed results using 5-HT1 receptor agonists (sumatriptan). With or without AMS, oxygen is often rapidly effective in treating the headache.

Prevention

Recent studies suggest that ASA or ibuprofen may help prevent high-altitude headache in situations at low-risk for AMS, although they are not as effective as acetazolamide in moderate-to high-risk settings.

Acute Mountain Sickness and High-Altitude Cerebral Edema

Epidemiology

The incidence of AMS varies, depending on the rate of ascent and the highest altitude reached. In moderate altitude (2000–3500 m) ski resorts, the incidence ranges from 10% to 40%. In those who hike above 4000 m, 25–50% will suffer from AMS. Travelers flying to a high-altitude destination such as Lhasa, Tibet (3810 m) or La Paz, Bolivia (4000 m) can expect an incidence of 25–35%.

Susceptibility to AMS demonstrates great individual variability because of genetic differences. Individual susceptibility is reproducible: a past history of AMS is the best predictor. Men, women, and children are at equal risk, although the risk is slightly decreased after age 50. See Pollard et al. for an excellent consensus document on children at altitude,[11] and recent reviews.[12,13] Although physical fitness provides no protection from AMS, obesity seems to increase the odds of developing AMS. Exposure to high altitude within the previous 3 months reduces susceptibility on re-ascent.

Pathophysiology of AMS/HACE

The exact pathophysiology of AMS/HACE is unknown. The current hypothesis is that hypoxia elicits hemodynamic and neurohumoral responses in both the brain and lung that ultimately result in edema from capillary leakage in microvascular beds.[14,15]

Whether mild AMS is actually due to brain edema seems unlikely. Recent magnetic resonance imaging (MRI) studies demonstrated that the brain swells on ascent to altitude in both those with and without AMS, presumably from vasodilatation. True edema, however, was not detected, except with severe AMS and HACE.[9,16] Factors that might contribute to a hydrostatic brain edema (HACE) are multiple and include sustained cerebral vasodilatation, impaired cerebral autoregulation, and elevated cerebral capillary pressure as well as alterations in the permeability of the blood–brain barrier through cytokine activation.[17]

Clinical Presentation and Diagnosis

AMS is a syndrome of non-specific symptoms and a broad spectrum of severity. Diagnostic criteria and scoring tools for altitude illness for both adults and children are available online (Table 39.1). AMS occurs in non-acclimatized persons in the first 48 h after ascent to altitudes >2500 m, especially after rapid ascent (1 day or less). Symptoms usually begin a few hours after arrival at the new altitude, but may arise a day later (often after the first night's sleep). The cardinal symptom is headache, typically bifrontal and throbbing. Gastrointestinal symptoms (anorexia, nausea or vomiting), and constitutional symptoms (weakness, lightheadedness, or lassitude) are common. AMS is thus similar to an alcohol hangover, or to a non-specific viral infection, but without fever and myalgia. Fluid retention is characteristic of AMS, and victims often report reduced urination, in contrast to the spontaneous diuresis observed with successful acclimatization. As AMS progresses the headache worsens, and vomiting, oliguria, and increased lassitude develop. Ataxia and altered level of consciousness herald the onset of clinical HACE (Fig. 39.2).

Patients with AMS appear ill but lack characteristic physical findings. Heart rate and blood pressure are variable and non-diagnostic. Unless HACE is present, neurological examination is normal. Funduscopy may reveal retinal hemorrhages, but these are not specific to AMS. Pulmonary crackles may be present, but oxygen saturation will be normal or at most slightly lower than in acclimatized persons at the same elevation. Peripheral and facial edema may be present, particularly in women.

Most conditions similar to AMS can be excluded by history and physical examination. Onset of symptoms >3 days after ascent, lack of headache, or failure to improve with descent, oxygen, or dexamethasone suggest another diagnosis. Dehydration is commonly confused with AMS, as it can cause headache, weakness, nausea, and decreased urine output.

The natural history of AMS varies with altitude, ascent rate, and other factors. In general, symptoms improve slowly, with complete

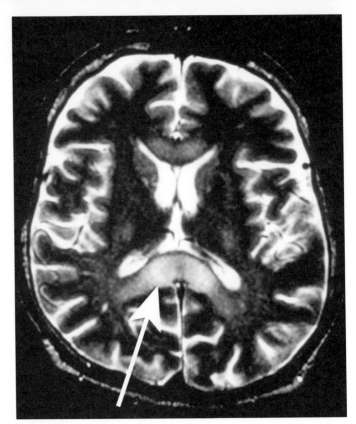

Figure 39.2 Magnetic resonance image (MRI) demonstrating reversible vasogenic edema in the splenium of the corpus callosum (arrow) in a climber with high altitude cerebral edema. *Courtesy of P. Hackett.*

resolution in 1–2 days. A small percentage (<10%) of persons with AMS will go on to develop HACE, especially with continued ascent in the presence of AMS symptoms. Whereas AMS has no characteristic physical findings, HACE is an encephalopathy and is characterized by gait ataxia, severe lassitude, and altered consciousness.

Untreated, HACE may progress to stupor and coma over hours to days, and death is due to brain herniation. Ataxia commonly persists for days to weeks after descent, but persistent mental status changes or the presence of focal neurological deficits should prompt a complete neurological evaluation. Brain tumors that suddenly become symptomatic at altitude,[18] Guillain–Barré syndrome, severe hyponatremia, and cortical blindness have all been misdiagnosed as HACE. The typical MRI finding of increased T_2 signal in the corpus callosum acutely, or evidence of hemosiderin deposits on T_{2^*} or SWI sequences even years later will confirm the diagnosis. Patients who survive typically have full recovery after descending, but reports of persistent neurological sequelae exist.

Treatment

Management of AMS follows three axioms: (1) no further ascent until symptoms resolve; (2) descent to a lower altitude if no improvement with medical therapy; and (3) immediate descent at the first sign of HACE; see Luks et al. for a consensus guideline to prevention and treatment of acute altitude illness.[19] It is not possible to predict the eventual severity from the initial clinical presentation, and patients must be watched closely for progression of illness.

Suggested medications for high-altitude travelers are listed in Table 39.2. Table 39.3 provides a variety of common clinical scenarios and

Table 39.2 Medications for Travelers to High Altitude

Agent	Indication	Dose	Adverse Effects	Comments
Acetazolamide	Prevention of AMS	125–250 mg orally twice a day beginning 24 h before ascent and continuing during ascent and for at least 48 h after arrival at highest altitude	COMMON: Paresthesiae; polyuria; alters taste of carbonated beverages PRECAUTIONS: Sulfonamide reactions possible; avoided in breastfeeding; can decrease therapeutic levels of lithium	Can be taken episodically for symptoms; no rebound effect; pregnancy category C; allergic cross-reactivity with sulfa antibiotics uncommon
	Treatment of AMS	250 mg orally every 12 h		
	Pediatric prevention & treatment of AMS	2.5 mg/kg body weight orally every 12 h		
	Periodic breathing	125 mg orally 1 h before bed		
Dexamethasone	Treatment of AMS	4 mg every 6 h orally, i.m. or i.v. until descent	Mood changes; hyperglycemia; dyspepsia	Rapidly improves AMS symptoms; can be lifesaving in HACE; may improve HACE enough to facilitate descent; no value in treating HAPE; pregnancy category C but preferably avoided by women who are pregnant or breastfeeding. In our opinion, dexamethasone use should be limited to 72 hours
	HACE	8 mg initially, then 4 mg every 6 h orally, i.m. or i.v.		
	Pediatric HACE	0.15 mg/kg every 6 h orally, i.m. or i.v., not to exceed 16 mg/d		
	Prevention of HAPE	8 mg every 12 h orally during ascent		
Ginkgo biloba	Prevention of AMS	80–120 mg orally twice daily starting 5 days before ascent and continuing to highest altitude	Occasional headache; rare reports of bleeding	Requires further study; preparations are not standardized and vary in potency; may be used by women who are pregnant or breastfeeding
Nifedipine	Prevention of HAPE	30 mg SR formulation orally every 12 h	Reflex tachycardia; hypotension (uncommon)	No value in AMS or HACE; not necessary if supplemental oxygen available; pregnancy category C
	Treatment of HAPE	10 mg orally initially, then 30 mg of extended release formulation orally every 12 h		
Salmeterol	Prevention of HAPE	125 mcg inhaled every 12 h, starting the day before ascent and continuing while at altitude	COMMON: Palpitations, tachycardia, tremor, hypokalemia, headache, nausea	May be reasonable to use in treatment of HAPE; not for monotherapy
Sildenafil/ tadalafil	Prevention of HAPE	Sildenafil 50 mg orally every 8 h while ascending and continuing at altitude / Tadalafil 10 mg orally every 12 h while ascending	COMMON: Headache, dyspepsia, flushing	May be reasonable to use in treatment of HAPE
Ondansetron	Symptomatic treatment of nausea and vomiting	4 mg orally disintegrating tablet every 4 h	Usually minimal; may cause dizziness, drowsiness, headache	Pregnancy category B
Hydrocodone	Symptomatic treatment of high altitude cough	5–10 mg orally every 4 h	Causes sedation Contraindicated with HACE	May also be helpful for pain of intercostal muscle strain associated with cough
Zolpidem	Insomnia	5–10 mg orally	Rare, short-acting	Does not depress ventilation at high altitude; pregnancy category B

AMS, acute mountain sickness; HACE, high-altitude cerebral edema; HAPE, high-altitude pulmonary edema; i.v., intravenous; i.m., intramuscular.

Pregnancy category B: No evidence of risk in humans. Adequate, well-controlled studies in pregnant women have not shown increased risk of fetal abnormalities despite adverse findings in animals, or in the absence of adequate human studies, animal studies show no fetal risk. The chance of fetal harm is remote, but remains a possibility.

Pregnancy category C: Risk cannot be ruled out. Adequate, well-controlled human studies are lacking, and animal studies have shown risk or are lacking as well. Use only if potential benefits outweigh the potential risks.

Table 39.3 Options for Management of High-Altitude Illness

Clinical Presentation		Management
Mild acute mountain sickness		
	Mild to moderate headache with nausea, dizziness or fatigue within first 24 h of ascent to high altitude (>2500 m).	Stop ascent, rest, and acclimatize Descend 500 m or more Speed acclimatization with acetazolamide (125–250 mg orally twice daily) Treat symptoms with mild analgesics and antiemetics or use a combination of these approaches
Moderate acute mountain sickness		
	Moderate to severe headache with marked nausea or vomiting, weakness, dizziness, lassitude, and peripheral edema 12–24 h after rapid ascent to high altitude.	Stop ascent, rest, treat medically Descend 500 m or more Give acetazolamide (250 mg orally twice daily), or dexamethasone (4 mg orally or intramuscularly every 6 h), or both Administer low-flow oxygen (1–2 L/min) or use a portable hyperbaric chamber Treat symptoms or use a combination of these approaches
High-altitude cerebral edema		
	Confusion, lassitude, and ataxia 48 h after ascent to high altitude; complained of a headache the day before onset of the confusion.	Start immediate descent or evacuation If descent is delayed or not possible, use a portable hyperbaric chamber and/or administer oxygen (2–4 L/min) Administer dexamethasone 8 mg intramuscularly, intravenously, or orally initially, then 4 mg every 6 h
High-altitude pulmonary edema		
	Cough, weakness, dyspnea, chest congestion 60 h after arrival at a ski resort at 2750 m.	Administer oxygen (2–4 L/min, to keep SaO_2 >90%) If oxygen is not available, use a portable hyperbaric chamber If oxygen and hyperbaric chamber not available, start immediate descent, minimizing exertion and cold stress If descent/oxygen unavailable, administer nifedipine (10 mg orally initially, then 30 mg extended release formulation every 12 h), or sildenafil or tadalafil

suggests management options. Descent to an altitude below that at which symptoms started is always effective treatment, but may not be practical given the topography, or possible given the patient's ultimate trekking or climbing goals or group resources. A descent of 500–1000 m is usually sufficient. Acetazolamide speeds acclimatization and thus hastens resolution of the illness, but this requires 12–24 h. Dexamethasone rapidly reverses symptoms (2–4 h), but does not improve acclimatization. Therefore, it is logical to use both agents if the victim does not descend. Acetazolamide can be taken episodically without fear of rebound symptoms when it is discontinued. Oxygen is extremely effective, but availability may be limited. Dexamethasone should be continued for 1–2 days after descent in persons with uncomplicated HACE, or until the mental status clears in cases of severe HACE.

Portable hyperbaric chambers made of coated fabric (e.g., Gamow Bag, CERTEC, and PAC), are now widely available among adventure travel groups, on expeditions, and in high-altitude clinics (Fig. 39.3). The patient is placed completely within the bag, which is sealed shut and inflated with a manually operated pump, pressurizing the inside to 105–220 mmHg (2–4 psi) above ambient atmospheric pressure. This effects a physiologic descent, and is equivalent to low-flow oxygen.

Coca leaf tea is widely recommended in South America and in the popular press as a cure for altitude illness; however, there are no studies to support this claim. Coca leaf tea may act as a mild stimulant and

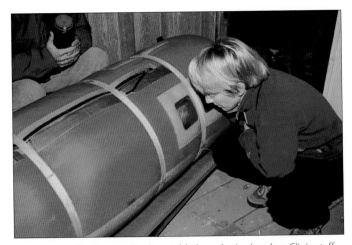

Figure 39.3 The Gamow Bag® portable hyperbaric chamber. Clinic staff talks with a patient undergoing hyperbaric treatment for high-altitude pulmonary edema at 4250 m in Nepal. *Courtesy of T. Dietz.*

improve wellbeing at altitude, which may be its primary effect. Garlic has also been advocated for prophylaxis and treatment of altitude illness. Animal studies show efficacy in preventing hypoxic pulmonary hypertension, but studies in humans are lacking and its use cannot be recommended at present. Treatments shown to have no benefit include

Table 39.4 Practical Advice for Travelers to Altitude
Go slowly
Avoid overexertion
Avoid abrupt ascent to sleeping elevations > 3000 m
Spend one to two nights at an intermediate elevation (2500–3000 m) before further ascent
Above 3000 m, sleeping elevations should not increase by more than 500 m per night
When topography or village locations dictate more rapid ascent, or after every 1000 m gained, spend a second night at the same elevation
Day hikes to higher elevations, with return to lower sleeping elevations help to improve acclimatization
Avoid alcohol consumption in the first 2 days at a new, higher elevation
Memorize the Golden Rules of Altitude
The Golden Rules of Altitude:
If you feel unwell at altitude, it is altitude illness until proven otherwise
If you have symptoms of AMS, go no higher
If your symptoms are worsening (or with HACE or HAPE), you must go down immediately

Note: Thanks to Dr David Shlim, who originally popularized The Golden Rules of Altitude.

naproxen, calcium channel blockers, phenytoin and antacids. Alcohol and other respiratory depressants should be avoided in someone with AMS owing to the risk of exaggerated hypoxemia.

Prevention

Recommendations on staged ascents are generally adequate for the average person, but some persons will still become ill despite a slow, staged ascent. Persons traveling to high altitude should allow adequate time for acclimatization, and pay careful attention to symptoms. Helpful guidelines to avoid altitude illness are included in Table 39.4; see also Luks et al.[19]

Many travelers wonder how long acclimatization lasts after a sojourn to high altitude. Some value in preventing AMS will persist for a month or more, but only a few days at sea level can render one susceptible to HAPE. Improved exercise ability will last for weeks if altitude exposure was for weeks or more.

Acetazolamide (Table 39.2) effectively prevents AMS;[20,21] it accelerates acclimatization by inducing a bicarbonate diuresis, stimulating ventilation and improving sleep breathing patterns. It does not mask symptoms of AMS. Since it is also useful for treatment,[22] acetazolamide should be in the high-altitude traveler's medical kit, along with written instructions. A recent survey concluded that trekkers carrying acetazolamide did not know how to use it properly. Dexamethasone also effectively prevents AMS, but does not improve acclimatization.[21] Owing to concern about rebound symptoms and the side-effect profile, this medication cannot be routinely recommended for prophylaxis.

Several controlled trials have shown that *Ginkgo biloba* extract may be effective in preventing AMS, with both gradual and rapid ascents.[14,23–25] The data on efficacy are not clear, due in part to differing study designs, small study sizes, and the lack of standardization in *Ginkgo biloba* preparations. *Ginkgo biloba* is safe and inexpensive, and may be a reasonable prophylaxis alternative to acetazolamide; however,

preliminary data suggest that acetazolamide is superior for the prevention of AMS.

High-Altitude Pulmonary Edema

Epidemiology

The reported incidence of HAPE varies from 0.01% to 15%, depending on the altitude, ascent rate, and the population at risk.[1] Individual susceptibility based on genetic factors is perhaps the greatest risk factor, with male gender also being suggested as a risk factor. There is no clear association with age. Pre-existing medical conditions associated with PHT or a restricted pulmonary vascular bed will greatly increase susceptibility to HAPE. Exercise increases the risk of HAPE since it increases cardiac output and pulmonary artery pressure at altitude.

Pathophysiology

HAPE is a non-cardiogenic, hydrostatic pulmonary edema, characterized by PHT and increased capillary pressure. Left ventricular function in HAPE is normal. Although increased pulmonary artery pressure due to hypoxic pulmonary vasoconstriction occurs in all who ascend to high altitude, it is exaggerated in those susceptible to HAPE, again primarily a genetically determined susceptibility.[26–30]

Clinical Presentation and Diagnosis

HAPE occurs 2–4 days after ascent to high altitude, often worsening at night. Decreased exercise performance is the earliest symptom, usually associated with a dry cough. The early course is subtle; as the illness progresses, the cough worsens and becomes productive; dyspnea can be severe, tachycardia and tachypnea develop, and drowsiness or other CNS symptoms may develop. Patchy unilateral or bilateral fluffy infiltrates and a normal cardiac silhouette on chest X-ray are characteristic of HAPE (Fig. 39.4). The presence of a fever has led to misdiagnosis (as pneumonia) and to subsequent deaths.

HAPE varies in severity from mild to immediately life-threatening. It can be fatal within a few hours, and is the most common cause of death related to high altitude. Differential diagnosis is sometimes problematic: HAPE improves dramatically with descent or oxygen, whereas other diagnoses do not and should be pursued in patients who do not fit this pattern.

Treatment

The treatment of HAPE depends on the severity of illness and logistics (see Tables 39.2 and 39.3). In remote locations, where oxygen and medical care may be unavailable, persons with HAPE need to be urgently evacuated to a lower altitude. Exertion must be minimized as it augments PHT and worsens hypoxemia. Mild HAPE responds rapidly to a descent of 500–1000 m. If oxygen is available, bed rest with supplemental oxygen may be adequate, but in severe HAPE high-flow oxygen (4 L/min or more) may be required for more than 24 hours. Hyperbaric therapy with a fabric pressure bag is equivalent to low-flow oxygen (2 L/min); treatments can be given in 1-hour increments. If oxygen is not available, immediate descent is life-saving; waiting for a helicopter evacuation has resulted in needless deaths.

If oxygen and descent are not available, drugs that reduce pulmonary artery pressure may be useful but are not as effective. Nifedipine reduces pulmonary vascular resistance and PAP during HAPE, and slightly improves arterial oxygenation, but clinical improvement is not dramatic. Nifedipine is well tolerated and is unlikely to cause

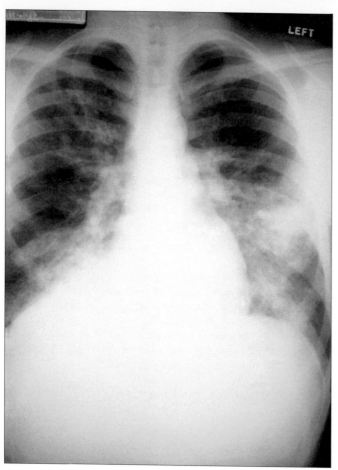

Figure 39.4 Chest radiograph of a patient with high-altitude pulmonary edema. Note the normal heart size and extensive bilateral infiltrates, consistent with high-altitude pulmonary edema. *Courtesy of P. Hackett.*

significant hypotension in healthy persons. Sildenafil and tadalafil effectively reduce pulmonary artery pressure at altitude and have shown value in the prevention of HAPE, but have not yet been studied for treatment. No drugs are as effective as oxygen and descent.

As with HACE, prognosis is excellent for survivors, with rapid clearing of the edema fluid and no long-term sequelae. Patients may need from 2 days to 2 weeks to recover completely; after all symptoms have resolved, cautious re-ascent is acceptable. Patients with mild to moderate HAPE at ski resorts will typically resume skiing after 3 days of oxygen therapy. See also Luks et al.[19]

Prevention

See AMS prevention; the same staged ascent recommendations are useful for HAPE prevention.

The indication for chemoprophylaxis of HAPE is repeated episodes. Whether one previous episode should encourage prophylaxis is arguable, but demonstrated susceptibility certainly requires caution. Often a slower ascent is the only preventive method required. Effective agents for prevention of HAPE include (Table 39.2) nifedipine, salmeterol, the PDE-5 inhibitors sildenafil and tadalafil, and dexamethasone.[19,31–34] Those with a history of HAPE should carry nifedipine to use either prophylactically or with the first signs of HAPE. Salmeterol reduced HAPE by 50% in susceptible persons, appears safe, and should be considered an adjunct for treatment as well, though it has not yet been studied for this indication. Both

dexamethasone and PDE-5 inhibitors have been shown to reduce pulmonary artery pressures at altitude, and also effectively prevent HAPE, although the optimal dose has not been established for these medications.

Other Altitude-Related Conditions

Syncope within the first 24 h at high altitude is a well-recognized entity termed 'high-altitude syncope'. This form of neurocardiogenic syncope[35] does not imply an underlying condition; a complete evaluation is generally unnecessary unless a second episode occurs.

The occurrence of focal neurological deficits, such as transient ischemic attacks in otherwise healthy individuals, has been noted at high altitude.[1] These are not part of the altitude illness spectrum and require further evaluation. Patients with previously undiagnosed arteriovenous malformation (AVM), cerebral aneurysm and brain tumors have all become symptomatic on ascent to high altitude,[18] and both ischemic and hemorrhagic stroke have also been reported.

High-altitude retinal hemorrhage (HARH) is common and usually asymptomatic. The incidence of HARH varies from 4% at 4243 m to >50% at 5360 m in one study.[36] For those who develop visual changes, evacuation to a lower altitude is recommended.[36] No reports claim that such visual changes are progressive in persons who remain at altitude. HARH resolves completely within a few weeks after descent.

Peripheral edema is common at high altitude, especially in women.[1] It is not necessarily associated with altitude illness, but anyone with edema must be evaluated for AMS. Edema will resolve with decent. Diuretics work well; however, one must be cautious to avoid dehydration.

High-altitude cough increases with elevation, and is a significant cause of morbidity among extreme-altitude climbers. The cough is paroxysmal, and sometimes sufficiently forceful to fracture ribs. Sputum is frequently purulent, but fever is absent. Normal exercise performance, lack of dyspnea at rest, and absence of râles or cyanosis help distinguish high-altitude cough from HAPE. A concurrent sore throat is common, without any abnormal findings on examination. The cause of high-altitude cough is unknown but probably multifactorial, including mucosal injury from hyperventilation of cold, dry air, airway inflammation, hypoxic bronchoconstriction, and alteration in the cough threshold. Treatment is symptomatic.

The intense UV light when reflected off snow at high altitude can easily cause damage to the unprotected eye, resulting in UV keratitis, also known as 'snow blindness.' Although it can be intensely painful and debilitating, it is self-limited and without sequelae, resolving in 24–48 h. Treatment consists of antibiotic ointment, analgesics, and perhaps eye patching. This injury is entirely preventable by proper use of sunglasses with good UV-absorbing characteristics. If sunglasses are not available, any material can be placed across the orbits, such as tape or cloth, with horizontal slits to provide essential vision.

Effect of Altitude on Common Medical Conditions

Some pre-existing medical conditions may be exacerbated by high altitude, or may affect the ability to acclimatize or susceptibility to altitude illness. Although data are scant, case reports, and a growing number of controlled studies support some reasonable recommendations.[37] Table 39.5 lists common medical conditions in terms of risk stratification for moderate altitude, up to 3500 m; above this altitude data are very scarce.

Table 39.5 Advisability of Ascent to High Altitude (up to 3000 m)

Minimal Risk	Some Documented Risk – Consider Medical Monitoring, Availability of Oxygen	Substantial Risk – Ascent Not Advised
Children and elderly	Carotid surgery or irradiation	COPD, severe
Physically fit and unfit	Sleep-disordered breathing and apnea	Coronary artery disease, with poorly controlled angina
Obesity	COPD, moderate	
Chronic obstructive pulmonary disease (COPD), mild	Cystic fibrosis	CHF, uncompensated
Asthma	Hypertension, poorly controlled	Congenital heart disease: ASD, PDA, Down's syndrome
Hypertension, controlled	Coronary artery disease, with stable angina	Pulmonary hypertension
Coronary artery bypass grafting, angioplasty, or stenting (without angina)	Arrhythmias, high-grade	Pulmonary vascular abnormalities
Anemia, stable	Congestive heart failure (CHF), compensated	Sickle cell anemia (with history of crises)
Migraine	Sickle cell trait	Pregnancy, high-risk
Seizure disorder, on medication	Cerebrovascular disorders	
Diabetes mellitus	Seizure disorder, not on medication	
LASIK, PRK	Radial keratotomy	
Oral contraceptives	Diabetic retinopathy	
Pregnancy, low-risk		
Psychiatric disorders		
Neoplastic diseases		
Inflammatory conditions		

Table 39.6 Oxygen Resources for Travelers

Access-Able Travel Tips: http://www.access-able.com/tips/oxy.html
  A travel web site oriented toward disabled persons that has a nice page with general tips on traveling with oxygen.
National Home Oxygen Patients Association: http://www.homeoxygen.org/airline-travel-with-oxygen
  The NHOPA has general information about flying with oxygen, a list of oxygen concentrators approved for airline use, and links to the oxygen concentrator makers.
TravelO2: http://www.travelo2.com
  TravelO2.com provides worldwide oxygen services to supplementary-oxygen-dependent travelers. They can arrange for oxygen on airline flights, during connections in airports, and for use while traveling away from home.
Oxygen To Go: http://oxygentogo.com/travelers
  Oxygen To Go provides rental oxygen concentrators for travelers with short to longer-term needs.
OxyTravel: http://www.linde-healthcare.com/en/about_linde_healthcare/Patient-focused_care/oxytravel/index.html
  A service of Linde Healthcare that helps coordinate oxygen for worldwide travelers.
Oxygen Worldwide: http://www.oxygenworldwide.com/
  Oxygen worldwide provides oxygen services for international travelers.

Pulmonary and Cardiac Problems

Because the body increases ventilation in response to altitude exposure, any condition that affects this response might be expected to affect high-altitude tolerance. Persons who have had carotid artery surgery or neck irradiation lose carotid body function and are therefore more hypoxic at high altitude, and perhaps more susceptible to altitude illness.[38]

Patients with sleep-disordered breathing (SDB) are often hypoxemic at low altitude, and might be much more hypoxemic at high altitude. Supplemental nocturnal oxygen may be advisable, at least for those who are hypoxic at low altitude. In addition, patients on Bi-PAP or CPAP need to make sure that their machine has pressure compensating features; machines without this can be off by as much as 10 cmH$_2$O pressure at 2500–3000 m. In general, obstructive sleep apnea improves on ascent to high altitude but converts to a central apnea; thus, acetazolamide may be useful in these patients.

Patients with hypoxemic lung disease are physiologically at a higher altitude (they have a decreased PaO$_2$) than healthy persons. On ascent to altitude, they might develop altitude illness at relatively lower altitudes, and their exaggerated hypoxemia would likely have other consequences as well. Surprisingly, only one field study has addressed the issue of COPD and altitude, and that was at the modest altitude of 1920 m.[39] Minor symptoms occurred, but patients did acclimatize

similarly to healthy persons. Nonetheless, oxygen prescriptions should be provided to these travelers to be used if necessary. Mobile oxygen services (Table 39.6) are widely available in mountain resorts and communities, especially in developed countries. For those with COPD who are on oxygen at low altitude, the FiO$_2$ needs to be increased by the ratio of the old barometric pressure over the new barometric pressure. Some experts have suggested that the PaO$_2$ at high altitude can be predicted from sea-level hypoxic gas breathing, but testing is not generally available in travel clinics, and the correlation between altitude PaO$_2$ and symptoms is weak.

Patients with cystic fibrosis have been reported to do poorly at high altitude. Hypoxic testing has not been useful in predicting the need for supplemental oxygen. These patients should be monitored and might require oxygen therapy. All patients with chronic lung disease can be advised to carry a pulse oximeter when traveling to high altitude; these devices are now easily available and inexpensive, and patients can monitor their own oxygen saturation according to their physician's instructions.

Numerous studies have demonstrated that patients with allergic asthma do better at high altitude because of decreased allergens and pollution, and decreased air density.[40] Exercise-induced bronchospasm (EIB) was not exacerbated at 1500 m,[41] but this needs to be studied at higher altitudes. Anecdotally, patients with EIB do well at high altitude, but, like all asthmatics, they need to be prepared in the event of an asthma attack. These patients should always have their inhalers on their person, not in a bag or pack from which they can be separated, and they should have a course of steroids to use as necessary. Asthma is not a contraindication to high-altitude exposure.

Permanent dwellers at high altitude have lower blood pressure than their low-altitude counterparts.[42] Persons with hypertension who move to high altitude also benefit because of a slowing of progression and even regression of the disease after months to years in residence.[43] In contrast, acute induction to high altitude is associated with a slight increase in blood pressure in normotensives (5–10 mmHg in both systolic and diastolic pressure). In those with hypertension the increase is similar to that in normotensives, but individual variation is great.[44] The first goal with hypertensive patients is to optimize the medical regimen at low altitude. Because certain individuals with hypertension may have a significant increase in blood pressure on ascent to altitude, and since this abnormal response cannot be predicted, hypertensives should monitor their blood pressure and consider taking with them additional medication, particularly if their hypertension is not well controlled at lower altitude. The ideal medication to help control altitude-aggravated hypertension is unknown. Since the increase is transient and resolves with descent, treatment is often unnecessary. For those with symptoms, their regular medication can be increased. Rarely, a new or second medication is added; calcium channel blockers may be superior to α-blockers[45] and ACE inhibitors are of unknown value.[46]

Limited available data do not suggest an increased risk of sudden cardiac death in travelers to high-altitude locations.[47] Most often, individuals doing exercise at high altitude are accustomed to exercise at low altitude and are reasonably fit. However, exercise and hypoxia together seem to be more stressful than either alone (especially in the sedentary), and any male older than 40 contemplating a trip to high altitude involving exercise should be conditioned to exercise prior to departing the lowlands.[48]

The slight increase in heart rate and systolic BP on ascent to altitude causes a small increase in myocardial work. As a result, patients with angina may have onset of ischemia at slightly lower workloads than at low altitude.[49] Patients with angina, then, should stay on their medications, reduce their activities somewhat during the first 3 days at altitude, and perhaps transiently increase their anti-anginal medication if they are more symptomatic than usual.

Patients with previous coronary artery bypass surgery, coronary artery angioplasty or stenting can be stratified into risk categories on the basis of symptoms and exercise treadmill test, as suggested by Hultgren.[50] These patients are considered at high risk for an acute coronary event only if they have a positive exercise treadmill test. Alexander has proposed other criteria for high risk during altitude exposure: ejection fraction <35%, a fall in exercise systolic blood pressure, ST segment depression >2 mm at peak heart rate, and high-grade ventricular ectopy.[51]

Perhaps the most common scenario regarding CAD and altitude exposure in the setting of a travel medicine practice is how to assess risk in a man >50 years old without known CAD but who has risk factors for CAD. The same risk stratification should be done as if the client were starting an exercise program at low altitude. For those with no symptoms, no evidence of CAD on ECG and no risk factors, an exercise treadmill test (ETT) is optional. For those without symptoms or evidence of CAD but one or more risk factors, a negative ETT assigns the person to the low-risk category, and a positive ETT requires further evaluation. For men <50 years with normal ECG and either none or one risk factor, ETT is not indicated.[50]

Limited data and anecdotal observations suggest that patients with active heart failure decompensate at high altitude and should probably avoid altitude, whereas those with CAD without active CHF may tolerate moderate altitudes without difficulty.[52] Supplemental oxygen should be considered.

Children (and adults) with shunts such as atrial septal defect, patent ductus arteriosus, and those with Down's syndrome with various defects have developed severe HAPE at modest altitudes of 2500–3000 m.[53,54] Children with a heart murmur that is not clearly benign should be evaluated prior to altitude exposure of more than 1 day's duration. Those with cyanotic congenital heart disease should avoid high altitude unless using supplemental oxygen.

Pulmonary hypertension (PHT) of any etiology is aggravated by altitude exposure and carries a substantial risk of developing HAPE. Unless PHT is mild, ascent without oxygen should generally be avoided. Persons with other congenital or acquired abnormalities of the pulmonary circulation (e.g., congenital agenesis of a pulmonary artery, thromboembolic pulmonary vascular disease, granulomatous mediastinitis, restrictive lung disease) are also at high risk of HAPE and should not go to high altitude without supplemental oxygen.[53]

Hematologic Disorders

Sickle cell anemia, with a history of crises, is a contraindication to high-altitude travel unless with supplemental oxygen. Even the cabin pressure of commercial jets (1500–2500 m equivalent altitude) will precipitate crises in 20% of those with hemoglobin SS, SC and sickle-thalassemia. Persons with sickle cell trait are at small risk of splenic infarction or vaso-occlusive crisis at high altitude, although the exact risk is difficult to quantitate. Left upper quadrant pain at high altitude should raise the suspicion of splenic infarction because of the sickle cell trait, even in phenotypic Caucasians. Persons with low hemoglobin concentration seem to tolerate high altitude surprisingly well; they are not prone to altitude illness, although greater dyspnea and fatigue may develop.

Neurologic Disorders

Whether ascent to high altitude will increase the frequency or severity of headaches in lowlanders with migraine is not clear, but ascent can certainly trigger migraine in some persons, regardless of a prior history of migraine at sea level. Observations have included new focal defects (visual and other) with migraine at altitude.[55,56] Migraine must be included in the differential diagnosis of AMS at altitude. Triptan medication (sumatriptan), often effective for migraine, has had some success with altitude headache, suggesting an overlap of mechanism between migraine and high-altitude headache.

Military studies have noted an increased incidence of ischemic stroke at high altitude, and similar data need to be collected in tourists. Predisposing factors that may contribute to cerebrovascular thrombosis at high altitude include dehydration and polycythemia. Because of the significant cerebral vasodilatation on ascent to altitude, persons with cerebrovascular structural abnormalities, such as arteriovenous malformation or aneurysm, may be at risk for an untoward event. The experiences of one of the authors (PH) in the field suggest that it is crucial to advise patients with known cerebrovascular disorders to be very cautious at altitude, report any symptoms, and to perhaps avoid sleeping altitudes >3000 m.

Anecdotal reports indicate that ascent to high altitude may lower the seizure threshold. For those with new-onset seizure, subsequent evaluation often reveals a previously unknown seizure focus. Persons with well-controlled seizure disorder at low altitude seem to be at no increased risk at altitude if they continue their medication. Individuals with a previous history of seizure but currently not on medication should consider anticonvulsant medication when traveling to high altitude, especially for extended trips to sleeping altitudes >2500 m.

Diabetes

Some diabetics have more problems at high altitude. First episodes of diabetic ketoacidosis, and death, have been observed in fit trekkers at high altitude (Shlim, personal communication, 2002). None, however, had been monitoring their blood glucose. Expeditions with diabetics have had both positive and negative feedback regarding the health of these individuals.[57,58] Problems encountered have included poorly functioning glucometers, possibly related to the cold, confusion between AMS and hypoglycemia, ketoacidosis secondary to nausea and vomiting of AMS, and remoteness of medical care. Taking extra time to acclimatize, keeping glucometers in special bags next to the skin, and active monitoring of glucose, fluid and carbohydrate intake can make a high-altitude journey successful.

Ophthalmologic Conditions

As the cornea and the retina are the eye structures most affected by altitude, patients with corneal and retinal conditions may be at increased risk on ascent to high altitude.[59] Persons who have had radial keratotomy no longer have structurally normal corneas, and on ascent to altitude the typical altitude-related swelling of the cornea is not uniform. Central flattening and peripheral expansion can result in a significant hyperopic shift, up to three diopters. The problem is also likely to become worse with decreasing accommodation as one ages. In contrast, photorefractive keratotomy (PRK) is a laser technique that shaves the anterior cornea uniformly, without incisions, and does not produce significant visual change at altitude. There are no definitive data regarding altitude responses to laser in situ keratomileusis (LASIK) surgery. Those with a history of RK can correct their vision by bringing with them glasses of increasing plus power. No information exists as to whether high altitude may contribute to or aggravate the retinal microangiopathy of hypertension, diabetes, or other diseases. Patients with retinopathy should probably avoid very high sleeping altitudes, >3500 m.

Contact lenses are used successfully at high altitude, though a few precautions are worth mentioning. Lenses in a case with liquid should not be allowed to freeze. Good hygiene can be difficult and requires forethought. The contact wearer should bring backup glasses. Rewetting solution and fluoroquinolone drops should be in the person's kit, and should also be kept from freezing.

Obstetrics/Gynecology

There are no data to suggest that women on oral contraceptives at altitude have a greater risk of thrombosis than at sea level. Anecdotal evidence shared by those working at the high-altitude clinics in Nepal has substantiated this. Nonetheless, women on mountaineering expeditions might constitute a special case because of prolonged exposure to extreme altitude and the attendant problems of dehydration, polycythemia, and immobility. Many expedition doctors recommend an aspirin a day for extreme altitude climbers, and especially for women using oral contraceptives.[60]

There are no data to suggest an increase in pregnancy complications in lowland women who travel transiently to high altitude. Pregnancy in high-altitude dwellers is associated with complications such as pregnancy-associated hypertension, pre-eclampsia, and infants small for gestational age, and it is reasonable to wonder whether this fact has any relevance for altitude sojourners. So far, for altitudes up to 2500 m, study results are reassuring. In addition, laboratory data in humans and animals have shown that fetuses with normal circulation tolerate levels of acute hypoxia far exceeding moderate altitude exposure. However, these studies also concluded that a compromised placental–fetal circulation could be unmasked at high altitude. Therefore, when advising a pregnant woman contemplating travel to altitude, it seems prudent to make sure the pregnancy is normal. Remoteness from medical care, the quality of available medical care, the risks of trauma and other issues related to wilderness or developing world travel are probably more important than the issue of moderate hypoxia.

Psychiatric Conditions

There are no data to help the physician advise persons with psychiatric illness about the risks of altitude exposure. Studies demonstrating effects of hypoxia on mood and personality in normal subjects suggest that some changes take place starting at about 4000 m. An interview might help determine whether the individual has realistic expectations of the trip, and whether the particular trip is suitable for them. A frequent question is whether common psychiatric medications, such as lithium and selective serotonin reuptake inhibitors (SSRIs), are a problem at high altitude. Lithium excretion has been studied and is normal at high altitude, but little else is known. This is an important area for further study. We advise patients on psychotropic medications to stay on them, to be careful to avoid altitude illness, and to descend if problematic symptoms develop. Again, what may be of greater concern than the risk of altitude-related problems may be the remoteness of the environment for those who may suffer from anxiety or depression.

References

1. Hackett PH, Roach RC. High altitude medicine and physiology. In: Auerbach PA, editor. Wilderness Medicine. 6th ed. Elsevier; 2012.
2. Barry PW, Pollard AJ. Altitude illness. BMJ 2003;326(7395):915–9.
3. Rey S, Semenza GL. Hypoxia-inducible factor-1-dependent mechanisms of vascularization and vascular remodeling. Cardiovasc Res 2010.
4. Smith TG, Robbins PA, Ratcliffe PJ. The human side of hypoxia-inducible factor. Br J Haematol 2008;141:325–34.
5. Suarez J, Alexander JK, Houston CS. Enhanced left ventricular systolic performance at high altitude during Operation Everest II. Am J Cardiol 1987;60:137–42.
6. Reeves JT, Groves BM, Sutton JR, et al. Operation Everest II: Preservation of cardiac function at extreme altitude. J Appl Physiol 1987;63:531–9.
7. Maher JT, Jones LG, Hartley LH. Effects of high altitude exposure on submaximal endurance capacity of men. J Appl Physiol 1974;37:895–8.
8. Silber E, Sonnenberg P, Collier DJ, et al. Clinical features of headache at altitude: a prospective study. Neurology 2003;60:1167–71.
9. Sanchez del Rio M, Moskowitz MA. High altitude headache. In: Roach RC, Wagner PD, Hackett PH, editors. Hypoxia: Into the Next Millennium. New York: Plenum/Kluwer Academic Publishing; 1999. p. 145–53.
10. The International Classification of Headache Disorders: 2nd edition. Cephalalgia 2004;24(Suppl 1):9–160.
11. Pollard AJ, Niermeyer S. Children at high altitude: an international consensus statement by an ad hoc committee of the International Society for Mountain Medicine, March 12, 2001. High Alt Med Biol 2001;2:389–403.
12. Niermeyer S, Andrade Mollinedo P, Huicho L. Child health and living at high altitude. Arch Dis Child 2009;94:806–11.
13. Yaron M, Niermeyer S. Travel to high altitude with young children: An approach for clinicians. High Alt Med Biol 2008;9:265–9.
14. Hackett P, Roach RC. High-altitude illness. N Eng J Med 2001;345:107–14.
15. Wilson MH, Newman S, Imray CH. The cerebral effects of ascent to high altitudes. Lancet Neurol 2009;8:175–91.
16. Hackett PH, Yarnell PR, Hill R, et al. High-altitude cerebral edema evaluated with magnetic resonance imaging: clinical correlation and pathophysiology. JAMA 1998;280(22):1920–5.
17. Hackett PH, Roach RC. High altitude cerebral edema. High Alt Med Biol 2004;5:136–46.
18. Shlim DR, Meijer HJ. Suddenly symptomatic brain tumors at altitude. Ann Emerg Med 1991;20:315–6.
19. Luks AM, McIntosh SE, Grissom CK, et al. Wilderness Medical Society consensus guidelines for the prevention and treatment of acute altitude illness. Wilderness Environ Med 2010;21:146–55. Epub 2010 Mar 10.
20. Basnyat B, Gertsch JH, Johnson EW, et al. Efficacy of low-dose acetazolamide (125 mg BID) for the prophylaxis of acute mountain sickness: a prospective, double-blind, randomized, placebo-controlled trial. High Alt Med Biol 2003;4:45–52.

21. Reid LD, Carter KA, Ellsworth A. Acetazolamide or dexamethasone for prevention of acute mountain sickness: a meta-analysis. J Wild Med 1994;5(1):34–48.

22. Grissom CK, Roach RC, Sarnquist FH, et al. Acetazolamide in the treatment of acute mountain sickness: clinical efficacy and effect on gas exchange. Ann Intern Med 1992;116(6):461–5.

23. Gertsch JH, Basnyat B, Johnson EW, et al. Randomised, double blind, placebo controlled comparison of ginkgo biloba and acetazolamide for prevention of acute mountain sickness among Himalayan trekkers. BMJ 2004;328:797.

24. Maakestad K, Leadbetter G, Olson S, et al. Ginkgo biloba reduces incidence and severity of acute mountain sickness. Wilderness Environ Med 2001;12(1):51.

25. Roncin JP, Schwartz F. P DA. EGb 761 in control of acute mountain sickness and vascular reactivity to cold exposure. Aviat Space Environ Med 1996;67(5):445–52.

26. Bärtsch P, Mairbaurl H, Maggiorini M, et al. Physiological aspects of high-altitude pulmonary edema. J Appl Physiol 2005;98:1101–10.

27. Dehnert C, Berger M, Mairbaurl H, et al. High altitude pulmonary edema: a pressure-induced leak. Respir Physiol Neurobiol 2007;158:266–73.

28. Luks AM. Do we have a 'best practice' for treating high altitude pulmonary edema? High Alt Med Biol 2008;9:111–4.

29. Maggiorini M. High altitude-induced pulmonary oedema. Cardiovasc Res 2006;72:41–50.

30. Scherrer U, Rexhaj E, Jayet PY, et al. New insights in the pathogenesis of high-altitude pulmonary edema. Prog Cardiovasc Dis 2010;52:485–92.

31. Ghofrani HA, Reichenberger F, Kohstall MG, et al. Sildenafil increased exercise capacity during hypoxia at low altitudes and at Mount Everest base camp: a randomized, double-blind, placebo-controlled crossover trial. Ann Int Med 2004;141(3):169–77.

32. Maggiorini M, Brunner-La Rocca H-P, Peth S, et al. Both tadalafil and dexamethasone may reduce the incidence of high-altitude pulmonary edema; a randomized trial. Ann Intern Med 2006;145:497–506.

33. Richalet JP, Gratadour P, Robach P, et al. Sildenafil inhibits altitude-induced hypoxemia and pulmonary hypertension. Am J Resp Crit Care 2005;171:275–81.

34. Sartori C, Allemann Y, Duplain H, et al. Salmeterol for the prevention of high-altitude pulmonary edema. NEJM 2002;346(21):1631–6.

35. Freitas J, Costa O, Carvalho MJ, et al. High altitude-related neurocardiogenic syncope. Am J Cardiol 1996;77:1021.

36. Butler FK, Harris DJ, Reynold RD. Altitude retinopathy on Mount Everest, 1989. Ophthalmology 1992;99(5):739–46.

37. Hackett P. High altitude and common medical conditions. In: Hornbein T, Schoene R, editors. High Altitude: An Exploration of Human Adaptation. NY, NY: Dekker; 2001. p. 839–86.

38. Basnyat B, Litch J. Another patient with neck irradiation and increased susceptibility to acute mountain sickness [Letter]. Wilderness Environ Med 1997;8:176.

39. Graham WG, Houston CS. Short-term adaptation to moderate altitude. Patients with chronic obstructive pulmonary disease. JAMA 1978;240:1491–4.

40. Boner A, Comis A, Schiassi M, et al. Bronchial reactivity in asthmatic children at high and low altitude. Effect of budesonide. Amer J Resp Crit Care 1995;151:1194–200.

41. Matsuda S, Onda T, Iikura Y. Bronchial responses of asthmatic patients in an atmosphere-changing chamber. Inter Arch Allergy Immunol 1995;107:402–5.

42. Hultgren HN. Reduction of systemic arterial blood pressure at high altitude. Adv Cardiology 1979;5:49–55.

43. Mirrakhimov M, Winslow R. The cardiovascular system at high altitude. In: Fregly M, Blatteis C, editors. Section 4: Environmental Physiology. Oxford: Oxford University Press (American Physiological Society); 1996. p. 1241–57.

44. Savonitto S, Giovanni C, Doveri G, et al. Effects of acute exposure to altitude (3,460 m) on blood pressure response to dynamic and isometric exercise in men with systemic hypertension. Am J Cardiol 1992;70:1493–7.

45. Deuber HJ. Treatment of hypertension and coronary heart disease during stays at high altitude (Abstract). Aviat Space Environ Med 1989;60:119.

46. Hultgren HN. Effects of altitude upon cardiovascular diseases. J Wild Med 1992;3:301–8.

47. Shlim DR, Gallie J. The causes of death among trekkers in Nepal. Int J Sports Med 1992;13(1):S74–6.

48. Burtscher M, Philadelphy M, Likar R. Sudden cardiac death during mountain hiking and downhill skiing. N Engl J Med 1993;329:1738–9.

49. Levine BD, Zuckerman JH, deFilippi CR. Effect of high-altitude exposure in the elderly: the Tenth Mountain Division study. Circulation 1997;96(4):1224–32.

50. Hultgren H. Coronary heart disease and trekking. J Wild Med 1990;1:154–61.

51. Alexander JK. Coronary heart disease at altitude. Tex Heart Inst J 1994;21:261–6.

52. Erdmann J, Sun KT, Masar P, et al. Effects of exposure to altitude on men with coronary artery disease and impaired left ventricular function. Am J Cardiology 1998;81:266–70.

53. Das BB, Wolfe RR, Chan KC, et al. High-altitude pulmonary edema in children with underlying cardiopulmonary disorders and pulmonary hypertension living at altitude. Arch Ped Adolescent Med 2004;158:1170–6.

54. Durmowicz A. Pulmonary edema in 6 children with Down syndrome during travel to moderate altitude. Pediatrics 2001;108(2):443–7.

55. Dietz TE, McKiel VH. Transient high altitude expressive aphasia. High Alt Med Biol 2000;1:207–11.

56. Murdoch DR. Focal neurological deficits and migraine at high altitude (Letter). J Neurol Neurosurg Psychiatr 1995;58:637.

57. Moore K, Thompson C, Hayes R. Diabetes and extreme altitude mountaineering. Brit J Sport Med 2001;35:83.

58. Admetlla J, Leal C, Ricart A. Management of diabetes at high altitude. Brit J Sport Med 2001;35:282–3.

59. Butler FK. The eye at altitude. Int Ophthalmol Clin 1999;39:59–78.

60. Jean D, Leal C, Kriemler S, et al. Medical recommendations for women going to altitude, A Medical Commission UIAA consensus paper. High Alt Med Biol 2005;6:22–31.

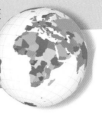
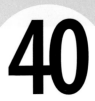

40

Diving Medicine

Karen J. Marienau and Paul M. Arguin

Key points

- Drowning is the most common cause of death in divers; however, a few antecedent triggers and events account for the majority of the deaths due to drowning, most of which are preventable
- Disorders from the altered pressure during diving can be broadly characterized as barotrauma, due to overexpansion of gas within body compartments, and decompression sickness, due to too rapid a return to atmospheric pressure
- Decompression illness includes decompression sickness and arterial gas embolism; they have different causes, but treatment is the same
- Many people with underlying chronic illnesses or disabilities may dive as long as their medical problems are stable prior to diving and they have taken appropriate measures to ensure their safety
- Many excellent sources of diving safety and preventive guidelines are available for physicians and travelers to learn about diving and associated risks, and the management of complications

Introduction

Recreational scuba diving has become increasingly popular.[1] There are an estimated 1–3 million certified US sport divers.[2] Because many diving destinations are in tropical or remote locations, travel medicine practitioners may be in a unique position to provide diving-related assessments and advice to individuals who seek a pre-travel medicine consult.

Diving is a high-risk sport, but with proper training and adherence to safe diving practices, most people will have enjoyable, uneventful dives. The incidence of decompression illness is an estimated 5–80 per 100 000 dives.[3] Among American and European Divers Alert Network (DAN) members the risk of death is 1/6000 dives per year. In comparison, the risk of jogging-related death is 1/7700 joggers per year.[4] Although drowning is the official cause of death for 70% of dive-related fatalities, the most common triggers leading to death are air supply problems, emergency ascent, cardiac health issues, entrapment/entanglement, and buoyancy issues.[4,5] Because physiological changes

due to exposure to ambient pressure during and after dives can result in dive-related disorders, physicians practicing travel, primary care, or emergency medicine need to be familiar with the unique characteristics of the underwater environment, understand diving-related disorders, know how to recognize and diagnose them, be familiar with treatments for those disorders, and know the recommendations for determining fitness to dive.[1,6–8]

Fitness to Dive

Medical Evaluation for Diving

Certain levels of physical and psychological fitness are necessary for safe diving.[9] Anyone who desires to learn to scuba dive should have an initial medical evaluation that focuses on the heart, lung, ears, sinuses, and psychological status, and identifies chronic conditions. Divers should have periodic re-evaluations to determine continued fitness with advancing age, and regarding existing or new medical conditions. The World Recreational Scuba Training Council (RSTC) (www.wrstc.com) provides physical examination guidelines for determining fitness to dive, including a comprehensive discussion of conditions that are relative or absolute contraindications. These guidelines are endorsed by the Divers Alert Network (DAN) (www.diversalertnetwork.org) and the Undersea and Hyperbaric Medicine Society (UMHS) (www.membership.uhms.org).[10]

Age

Because of the physiological changes that tend to occur with advancing age, older divers need to have a realistic appraisal of their abilities and not exceed them. The RSTC, UHMS, and DAN recommend that persons >40 years of age undergo risk assessment for coronary artery disease as an essential part of their fitness to dive evaluation.[1,10]

The minimum age normally permitted for diving certification is 12 years, although there are no formal age restrictions. Considerations for children include physical and emotional maturity, eustachian tube function, strength, and equipment fit.[11,12]

Women and Diving

Other than pregnancy, there are no contraindications to diving that are specific to women. If menses is a known trigger for migraine headaches, it may be advisable to avoid diving during menstruation.[13–15]

©2012 Elsevier Inc
DOI: 10.1016/B978-1-4557-1076-8.00040-5

Common Medical Disorders and Diving

Although several conditions may be relative or absolute contraindications, many divers with medical conditions may safely dive provided recommendations are followed.[10,16,17] Some medications may be contraindicated for diving,[18] but many are relatively safe (Table 40.1). Divers are advised against starting a new medicine before or during a trip: they should take the medication for a sufficient time before

Table 40.1 Medications and Diving	
Medication or Medication Class	**Comments**
Sedatives/ analgesics	Narcotics contraindicated
	Non-steroidal anti-inflammatory drugs safe
	Acetaminophen safe
Cardiovascular agents	Some anti-hypertensive drugs may impair exercise tolerance[1]
Insulin	Insulin requirements may change[2]
	Lower levels of glucose/glucagon measured in some diabetics while diving
Antipsychotics	Contraindicated
Anticonvulsants	Contraindicated[3]
Antimicrobial agents	Appear safe, unless underlying acute illness for which there is a contraindication
Antimalarials	Mefloquine may induce adverse events confused with decompression sickness. Test doses may be taken prior to diving to make sure tolerated. Atovaquone-proguanil or doxycycline may be better choices depending upon the circumstances[4–6]
Antihistamines	Depends on medication and underlying cause for its administration[7]
Decongestants	Pseudoephedrine may decrease risk and severity of otic barotraumas[8]
Anti-motion sickness agents	Some may cause sedation; scopolamine has been used safely[9]
Antidepressants	Some may cause sedation, affect concentration, decrease alertness or impair decision-making[10]

[1]Caruso JL. Cardiovascular fitness and diving. Alert Diver Jul/Aug 1999. Available at: http://www.diversalertnetwork.org/medical/articles/article.asp?articleid=11 (accessed 10/13/11).

[2]Bonomo M, Cairoli R, Verde G, et al. Safety of recreational scuba diving in type 1 diabetic patients: the Deep Monitoring programme. Diabetes Metab 2009;35(2):101–7.

[3]Howard GM. Radloff M, Sevier TL. Epilepsy and sports participation. Current Sports Med Reports 2004;3(1):15–9.

[4]Mefloquine and scuba diving. N Z Med J 1995;108:514.

[5]Goodyer L, Rice L, Martin A.Wright D. Choice of and adherence to prophylactic antimalarials. J Trav Med 2011;18(4):245–9.

[6]Riemsdijk MM, Ditter JM, Sturkenboom MCJM, et al. Neuropsychiatric events during prophylactic use of mefloquine before travel. Eur J Clin Pharmacol 2010;58:441–5.

[7]Taylor DM, O'Toole KS, Auble TE, et al. The psychometric and cardiac effects of dimenhydrinate in the hyperbaric environment. Pharmacotherapy 2000;20(9):1051–4.

[8]Brown M, Jones J, Krohmer J. Pseudoephedrine for the prevention of barotitis media: a controlled clinical trial in underwater divers. Ann Emerg Med 1992;21(7):849–52.

[9]Williams TH, Wilkinson AR, Davis FM, et al. Effects of transcutaneous scopolamine and depth on diver performance. Undersea Biomed Res 1988;15:89–98.

[10]McGown L. Medications for depression and fitness to dive. Alert Diver May/June 2005. Available at: http://www.diversalertnetwork.org/medical/articles/article.asp?articleid=72 (accessed 10/13/11).

traveling in case adverse effects occur, and if so, change to a different medication if possible. Antimalarial drugs are an exception to this general advice, as they are started before entering a malaria-endemic area. Most antimalarial drugs are considered to be safe for diving, with the exception of mefloquine because of its higher incidence of side-effects.[19–22]

Coronary Artery Disease

DAN surveillance data indicate that cardiac conditions are the number two cause of diving-related deaths, second only to drowning.[5] In addition to the increased myocardial oxygen demands from swimming and carrying diving tanks, preload is increased due to immersion-induced increase in central venous return, and afterload is increased due to cold-induced vasoconstriction.[1,16,23] Fitness to dive is optimal when a diver can reach a maximum capacity of 13 metabolic equivalents, as this allows a diver to exercise comfortably at 8–9 metabolic equivalents, and provides leeway for responding to unexpected physical demands.[1,17]

Patent Foramen Ovale

PFO-associated DCS risk has long been a source of controversy.[1,17] Evidence suggests that screening the average diver for PFO is not indicated. Although known PFO is not an absolute contraindication to diving, these divers should consider avoiding decompression dives, limiting bottom time, and using oxygen-enriched breathing mixes to maximize safety.[1,3]

Asthma

Evidence for an increased relative risk of barotrauma or DCS among divers with well-controlled asthma is equivocal.[1,17] The RSTC and UHMS recommend that people with mild to moderate well-controlled asthma with normal spirometry can be permitted to dive.[17–24]

Diabetes Mellitus

Fitness to dive criteria for physically fit people with well-controlled diabetes mellitus were first established in 1994.[25] Guidelines developed in 2005 recommend that adults with diabetes mellitus may dive provided they have been on a stable dose of insulin for 1 year or oral hypoglycemic agents for at least 3 months; have a glycosylated hemoglobin level of ≤9%; have had no significant episodes of hypo- or hyperglycemia for 1 year; have no secondary complications of diabetes; and have hypoglycemia awareness.[26]

Previous Spontaneous Pneumothorax

A history of spontaneous pneumothorax is considered a contraindication to diving because of the increased risk of pulmonary barotrauma.[1]

Diving Physics and Physiologic Changes Related to Diving

Atmospheric pressure – the amount of pressure exerted by the air above the earth's surface – at sea level is equal to 14.7 pounds per square inch or 1 absolute atmosphere (ATA) when standardized.[27,28] Underwater pressure is the weight of the water at a given depth plus atmospheric pressure, and increases linearly with depth by 1 ATA for every 33 feet of seawater (fsw) or every 34 feet of fresh water. The pressure at a depth of 33 fsw is 2 ATA, at 66 fsw it is 3 ATA, etc.[8,27] Air is the breathing gas used for scuba diving. Breathing air under pressure and the changes in pressure during and after a dive cause physiologic changes, some of which can result in injuries, and even death.

Two gas laws are key to understanding the physiological changes associated with diving and how injuries can occur. Boyle's Law describes how the volume of gas in an enclosed space changes with changes in pressure. As ambient pressure increases, the volume of gas decreases, and vice versa. Barotrauma, or tissue damage resulting from the inability to equalize pressure in a gas-filled space with ambient pressure, occurs when a diver fails to equalize those pressures with the pressure of the surrounding water during descent (compression) or ascent (decompression). The risk of barotrauma is greatest at depths of 33 fsw or less, and can occur at depths of as little as 4 fsw.[1,8,27]

Henry's Law describes how the partial pressure of inspired gases changes with changes in ambient pressure. During an air dive, inspired nitrogen (inert) is dissolved into the blood and tissues, the degree to which depends both on depth and duration at depth. As ambient pressure decreases during ascent, nitrogen is gradually eliminated from the body.[8,27] If a diver ascends too rapidly, or ascends to altitudes above sea level too soon after a dive, the dissolved nitrogen comes out of solution too quickly and forms bubbles in extravascular and intravascular tissues, resulting in decompression sickness.

Diving Disorders

Barotrauma (non-pulmonary)

Middle-Ear Barotrauma

Middle-ear barotrauma ('middle-ear squeeze') is the most common diving injury, occurring in 30% of first-time divers and 10% of experienced divers.[1,29] Although usually mild, it may have serious consequences. Pressure in the middle ear is equalized with the surrounding water pressure via the eustachian tube and nasopharynx. Middle-ear squeeze most often occurs during descent (usually in the first 33 fsw). Pressure is equalized by opening the eustachian tubes via Valsalva maneuvers or by swallowing or moving the jaw, which allow pressurized air from the scuba tank to enter the middle-ear space via the regulator in the mouth.[6,28,30,31] Pain during descent is the hallmark of middle-ear squeeze; the diver should ascend to a depth where equalization does occur, then re-descend slowly. If unable to equalize, the dive should be aborted.

If descent continues without pressure equalization, vascular congestion, hemorrhage, tympanic membrane deformation and rupture may follow, along with hearing loss and tinnitus.[29,30] If rupture occurs and cold water rushes into the middle ear, vertigo secondary to caloric stimulation may occur, as well as nausea, vomiting, and disorientation. Common causes of eustachian tube dysfunction are descending faster than equalization can occur; acute or chronic inflammation; nasal congestion or obstruction; anatomical deformities; tympanic membrane scarring; prolonged use of nasal decongestants; and excessive smoking.[31]

Although most common during descent, middle-ear barotrauma may also occur during ascent ('reverse squeeze') if the eustachian tube becomes blocked.[1,6,31] It can be caused by cerumen in the external canal, stenosis, atresia, a tight-fitting hood, or from rebound edema if the effects of decongestants taken before a dive wear off before ascending to the surface.

Alternobaric vertigo is a fairly common occurrence in divers, but the risk of life-threatening situations is low.[30,32] It develops because of asymmetric pressure changes in the middle ear that are transmitted via the oval and round window membranes to the vestibular system, resulting in a sensation of spinning and disorientation, and possibly nausea or vomiting (rare).[32] It is usually associated with middle-ear equalization difficulties and occurs primarily during ascent. Vertigo

may be stopped by halting the ascent, or by descending and then slowing continuing ascent. Repeated occurrences may warrant evaluation by an otorhinolaryngologist knowledgeable about diving disorders.[30,32]

Inner-Ear Barotrauma

Inner-ear barotrauma results from difficulty equalizing middle-ear pressure, but unlike middle-ear barotrauma, is relatively rare.[33] Consequences can be severe, from round or oval window rupture with possible perilymph fistulae, to cochlear hemorrhage with sensorineural hearing loss and vestibular dysfunction. Round window rupture is more likely with overly forceful Valsalva maneuvers that raise cerebrospinal fluid and inner-ear pressures, and leads to tinnitus and hearing loss. Since manifestations of inner-ear barotrauma can mimic those of inner-ear decompression sickness (DCS), it is important to determine which is the most likely cause because the treatments are markedly different. When in doubt, recompression for suspected inner-ear DCS should be the priority. Recompression has not been shown to cause further damage if inner ear barotrauma has occurred.[6] Divers with inner-ear barotrauma should be referred to an otorhinolaryngologist.

Sinus Barotrauma

The paranasal sinuses are the second most common sites of barotrauma, usually due to transient nasal pathology or chronic sinusitis. The ostia draining mucus from the sinuses can easily become blocked with minimal inflammation. If the pressures between the sinuses and the surrounding water are not equalized, barotrauma results. It most often occurs during descent, when the relative negative pressure in the sinus cavity causes edema of the mucous membranes or pulls them away from the sinus walls, resulting in severe pain over the affected sinus and bleeding into the cavity.[1,6,28,31] Unless damage has already occurred, ascent to a lower depth brings immediate relief. Sinus barotrauma may also occur during ascent (reverse sinus squeeze). Descending to a depth of relief and slow ascent usually resolves the problem.[28] If sinus barotrauma has occurred during a dive, epistaxis may be noticed on reaching the surface. Palliative treatment is usually sufficient.

Preventing Ear and Sinus Barotrauma

Most common barotraumas can be prevented by paying careful attention to pressure equalization during descent, descending slowly in a feet-first position, and avoiding diving with significant nasal, otic, or sinus congestion. Taking systemic or nasal decongestants before a dive can be helpful, but must be used with caution because of the potential for a rebound effect and reverse squeeze during ascent.[1]

Pulmonary Barotrauma

During ascent compressed air inside a diver's lungs expands. If not allowed to escape by exhaling, or if air is trapped in a lung segment by local obstruction, the expanding gas may lead to pulmonary over-inflation and alveolar tissue rupture.[1,6,34] The resultant interstitial emphysema causes no symptoms unless further distribution of the air occurs. Four important pulmonary over-inflation syndromes may result as air migrates into the surrounding tissues or arterial circulation: subcutaneous emphysema, pneumomediastinum, pneumothorax, and arterial gas embolism.

Arterial Gas Embolism (AGE)

Arterial gas embolism (AGE), the most serious of the pulmonary over-inflation syndromes, is potentially life-threatening and requires immediate treatment. It occurs when air bubbles enter the arterial circulation via the pulmonary veins and left heart, and lodge in arterioles and capillaries. Although the brain is especially susceptible to AGE, it may occur in the heart and other organs. Almost all cases present within 5–10 minutes of surfacing and manifest as gross neurological deficits, including unconsciousness, confusion, motor or sensory deficits, visual disturbances, seizures, personality changes, and headache. Paralysis and numbness may develop with spinal cord involvement. If emboli occlude coronary arteries, chest pain, myocardial infarction, and cardiovascular collapse may occur.[1,6,31,34] AGE may occur from very shallow or very brief dives if a diver breath-holds with the lungs maximally expanded.

The major risk factor for AGE or one of the other pulmonary overinflation syndromes in divers with healthy lungs is breath-holding during ascent, or shooting to the surface too rapidly for exhalation to compensate for the degree of gas expansion. These situations often result from panic associated with running out of air, equipment dysfunction, or loss of buoyancy control. Chronic or acute lung conditions predispose a diver to pulmonary barotrauma from local obstruction, including chronic obstructive pulmonary disease, acute and chronic bronchitis, severe asthma, pulmonary blebs, pulmonary abscesses, and restrictive lung diseases.

Decompression Sickness (DCS)

Decompression sickness (DCS) or 'the bends' is a continuum of injury due to the formation of bubbles in blood and tissues. Incidence among recreational divers is approximately 2–3 cases per 10 000 dives.[35] The pathophysiology is very complicated; important factors include the rates of gas absorption by tissues (saturation), gas elimination (desaturation), and other poorly predictable factors that contribute to bubble formation.[36] The inert nitrogen in air is absorbed into blood and tissues during the dive because of its increased partial pressure at depth (Henry's Law). The degree and rate of tissue saturation that occurs depends primarily on the lipid versus aqueous content of the tissues, their blood supply, the depth of the dive, and time at depth.[6,37,38]

During ascent nitrogen is eliminated through the lungs; however, complete equilibrium is not reached until several hours after a dive. Unlike AGE, DCS does not occur in shallow water, and bubbles are primarily venous. If a diver ascends too fast or has dived outside no-decompression limits without making required decompression stops, the dissolved nitrogen will become supersaturated and form bubbles. These primarily venous bubbles can cause tissue injury through mechanical and biochemical effects, with manifestations ranging from trivial to fatal.[1,6,37,38]

Several dive tables provide guidelines for safe depth and time exposures to minimize the risk of DCS. Dive computers address the same issues but perform continuous calculations of the partial pressure of inert gases in the body based on the actual depth and time profile of the diver. One can dive within the limits of the accepted dive tables or dive computers and still develop DCS.[6,8] Clinical manifestations of DCS can be caused by the direct effect of bubbles in the tissues (autochthonous bubbles) or in the bloodstream (circulating bubbles), as well as by indirect effects resulting from endothelial damage by intravascular bubbles and interactions with formed elements of the blood and plasma proteins.[31,36] Autochthonous bubbles can exert pressure on nerves, stretch and tear tissue leading to hemorrhage, and exert pressure in the tissue causing restriction or obstruction of blood flow. Arterial bubbles can act as emboli, blocking the blood supply of almost any tissue and leading to hypoxia, cell injury, and death. Venous bubbles can cause venous obstruction leading to tissue hypoxia, cell injury, and death. Venous bubbles carried to the lung as emboli can partially block pulmonary blood flow and cause pulmonary DCS, resulting in pulmonary edema, hypoxia and hypercarbia.[6]

DCS Type I and Type II

Signs and symptoms of DCS occur relatively soon after a dive: 42% occur within 1 hour of surfacing; 60% within 3 hours; and 98% within 24 hours.[36,39] DCS is categorized into type I and type II; however, they may occur simultaneously. DCS type I (non-systemic or musculoskeletal) is most common, is not life-threatening, and may involve the skin, lymphatic system, or muscles and joints (musculoskeletal pain-only). Musculoskeletal pain-only is the most common manifestation of DCS type I, most often involving the shoulder, elbow, wrist, hand, knee, or ankle joints, tends to be asymmetrical, and may shift in character and temporal pattern. The pain may be mild or excruciating; is often described as a deep, dull ache; may be difficult to localize initially; is present at rest; and is usually not affected by movement. Any pain occurring in the abdominal and thoracic areas or the hips should be considered as symptoms of spinal cord involvement and treated as DCS type II.[39]

Pruritus, with or without a faint rash, the most common skin manifestation, tends to be associated with wearing a dry suit, is generally transient, and does not require recompression treatment. Another skin manifestation, cutis marmorata, is more serious and should be treated as DCS type II. It may begin with pruritus and erythema, and progresses to distinctive bluish-red patches with adjacent areas of pallor producing the mottled appearance. Lymphatic obstruction creates pain in the involved lymph nodes and swelling of tissues drained by the nodes. Recompression usually provide prompt pain relief, but the swelling may persist for a while.[6,39]

Any neurologic, cardiopulmonary, or vestibular manifestation is categorized as DCS type II and requires urgent recompression.[1,6,31,38] Generally, the sooner the onset of symptoms after a dive, the more severe the case and the more rapid the progression. Neurologic involvement is the most common type II DCS and may be caused by spinal cord or cerebral involvement; spinal DCS is most frequent.[31] Presenting manifestations include numbness, weakness, gait abnormality, paresthesias, loss of bladder and bowel control, paralysis, visual deficits, personality changes, impaired consciousness, seizures, or coma. Low back or abdominal pain may indicate spinal DCS. Signs and symptoms may wax and wane.

Pulmonary DCS, or 'the chokes,' is a rare condition caused by massive venous bubbling in the pulmonary vasculature. Chest pain aggravated by inspiration may be the first symptom; cough and increased respiratory rate often occur. Without immediate recompression increased pulmonary congestion, respiratory failure, shock, and death may rapidly ensue. Victims usually recover with prompt treatment.[1,38,39]

Inner-ear or vestibular DCS (the 'staggers') presents with tinnitus, hearing loss, vertigo, dizziness, and nausea or vomiting. The dive profile and timing of symptom onset should help differentiate this condition from inner-ear barotrauma. If in doubt, treat as for DCS.[1,38,39]

Unusual fatigue or exhaustion after a dive is probably due to bubbles in unusual locations and the associated biochemical changes. Unusual fatigue should be considered a symptom of DCS.[39]

Decompression Illness

Decompression illness (DCI) is a term that combines DCS types I and II and AGE. Although treatment is the same, it is important to distinguish between DCS type II and AGE because of potential implications for future diving. The dive history and profile will usually distinguish between the two.[1,38,39]

DCI Treatment

Primary first aid for DCI is 100% oxygen and medical stabilization, followed by recompression in a hyperbaric chamber. Recompression in a chamber while breathing 100% oxygen is usually advised even if manifestations resolve with oxygen alone, because DCI can recur after initial onset. Hyperbaric treatment reduces bubble volume and increases the pressure gradient between alveolar and tissue nitrogen, which quickly resolve bubbles, relieving mechanical pressure on tissues and promoting the redistribution of bubbles lodged in the microcirculation. Hyperbaric oxygen also oxygenates compromised tissues and ameliorates inflammatory responses that contribute to tissue injury.[38,39] The US Navy Treatment Table 6, or an equivalent, is the most common recompression schedule used for treating DCI; Treatment Table 5 may be used for pain-only DCS type I. Treatment is usually successful if it has not been excessively delayed, although some patients may require repeat treatments over a course of days to weeks, and a smaller percentage may have permanent, residual deficits.[38–40]

Preventing DCI

Proper training, properly functioning diving equipment, and knowing and diving within one's limitations are critical to safe diving. Most cases of AGE are due to rapid or uncontrolled ascent accompanied by breath-holding, or are associated with underlying pulmonary conditions that cause local obstruction.[38] A case review found that 3/4 of AGE fatalities were triggered when divers exhausted their breathing gas, panicked, or developed equipment problems, and 96% were associated with emergency ascent.[5]

Ascending too fast, deep, long dives, and approaching or diving beyond the limits of no-decompression are the primary factors leading to DCS, hence strict adherence to dive table or dive computer recommendations is paramount to minimizing DCS risk. Following recommendations for repetitive dives and for flying after diving, or ascending to altitude after diving, is also important in reducing risk.[6,31,38]

Since diving in cold water and hard exercise at depth increase the risk of DCS, following a more conservative dive plan is recommended when diving under those conditions. Other possible risk factors, but for which evidence is inconclusive, include dehydration, obesity, poor physical condition, hard exercise after surfacing, and alcohol use before or after diving, as well as individual risk factors that have not been identified.[31,38,41,42] Being well hydrated, diving within one's physical limitations, seeking periodic re-evaluation of fitness for diving, cancelling a dive if feeling unwell, and avoiding certain behaviors can help minimize the risk of DCS.

Awareness of signs and symptoms of DCS, understanding that DCS can occur even when staying within safe diving limits, AND seeking evaluation promptly if symptoms develop will help ensure full recovery should DCS occur. DCS that manifests subtly may be attributed to other causes, such as overexertion, heavy lifting or a tight wetsuit, resulting in a delay in treatment. Denial has actually been noted as the first symptom of DCS.[45] Other reasons for delay in seeking treatment include rationalization, embarrassment, or cost.[31]

Flying after Diving

Modern aircraft cabins are pressurized from approximately 2400 to 8000 feet. Flying too soon after diving increases the risk for DCS because of the decrease in atmospheric pressure. Consensus guidelines, updated in 2002, apply to recreational air dives followed by flights at cabin altitudes of 2000–8000 feet for divers *without* symptoms of DCS.[43] For a single no-decompression dive, one should wait at least 12 hours before flying; for multiple dives per day or multiple days of diving, waiting 18 hours is recommended; and for dives requiring decompression stops (decompression dives) waiting 'substantially longer than 18 hours appears prudent.' Guidelines as for flying after diving should be followed for other modes of ascending to higher altitudes after diving, such as driving or hiking.[44]

Diving at Altitude

Diving at an elevation >1000 feet is considered altitude diving. Certification is highly recommended because of the increased risk of DCS and other hazards. Different tables and algorithms from those used at sea level are required owing to the reduction in surface pressure at altitude.[44–47] Recommendations when diving at altitude include: an ascent rate of 0.5 ft/s; mandatory safety stops; avoiding repetitive dives, or at a maximum, no more than two dives per day; and waiting 24 hours between a dive and increasing altitude by more than 2000 feet.[45]

Returning to Diving Following Diving Trauma or Illness

Diving-related conditions should have resolved before persons attempt to dive again. For a safe return to diving, there should be no increased risk of recurrence or worsening of tissue damage (Table 40.2).

Table 40.2 Recommendations for Returning to Diving Following Barotrauma and Decompression Sickness

Condition	Recommendations (Minimum)	Comments
Middle-ear barotrauma	When hearing is normal, tympanic membrane is intact, eustachian tubes can function[30,31]	
Inner-ear barotrauma	Evaluation and clearance by otorhinolaryngologist[33]	Should have knowledge of diving-related injuries
Pulmonary barotrauma (AGE[a])	4 weeks if complete resolution of signs/symptoms[31,42,43]	Evaluation for possible underlying pulmonary pathology
DCS[b] type I (pain-only)	2 weeks[31,42,43]	
DCS[b] type II (minor neurological involvement)	4–6 weeks after complete resolution of signs/symptoms[31,42,43]	
DCS[b] type II (severe neurological manifestations or residual signs or symptoms)	No further diving[31,42,43]	
DCS[b] type II, multiple bouts	Refer to diving medical specialist owing to possible increased susceptibility to DCS[45]	Even if DCS is relatively minor and completely resolves, and especially if other divers following same dive profile are DCS-free

[a]Arterial gas embolism.
[b]Decompression sickness.

Other Diving Hazards

Nitrogen Narcosis

Also known as the 'rapture of the deep,' nitrogen narcosis is a state of altered mental status, most notably euphoria, and confusion caused by intoxication with dissolved nitrogen due to its narcotic effects under pressure. Its effect is related to depth and rapidity of descent. During air dives, narcosis usually appears at approximately 130 fsw, and intensifies with deeper depths. Susceptibility to the effects of nitrogen varies among divers and some may experience narcosis at shallower depths. Disregard for personal safety, such as removing the regulator mouthpiece or swimming to unsafe depths, is the greatest hazard of nitrogen narcosis.[6,31]

Diving Resources

Professional and recreational international diving organizations are valuable resources. Many, such as DAN (http://www.diversalertnetwork.org), have websites with diving safety tips and articles for divers and health practitioners; http://en.wikipedia.org/wiki has a comprehensive list of international diving organizations. Dive accident insurance is highly recommended and can be purchased through DAN or other diving organizations. Costs of treatment and emergency transport to a hyperbaric chamber can be in the thousands of dollars, and should not be a deterrent to treatment.

References

1. Lynch JH, Bove AA. Diving medicine: A review of current evidence. J Am Board Fam Med 2009;22:399–407.
2. How many people scuba dive? It's not an easy answer to find. In: http://www.scuba-diving-smiles.com/how-many-people-scuba-dive.html (accessed 9/19/2011).
3. Bove AA, Moon RE. Patent foramen ovale – is it important to divers? In: Alert Diver, Sept/Oct 2004. Available at: http://www.diversalertnetwork.org/medical/articles/article.asp?articleid=70 (accessed 9/5/2011).
4. Vann RD, Lang MA, editors. Recreational Diving Fatalities. Proceedings of the Dives Alert Network 2010 April 8–10 Workshop. Durham, NC. Available at: https://d35gjurzz1vdcl.cloudfront.net/ftw-files/Fatalities_Proceedings.pdf (Accessed 9/15/11).
5. Denoble PJ, Caruso JL, Dear Gde L, et al. Common causes of open-circuit recreational diving fatalities. Undersea Hyperb Med 2008;35(6):393–406.
6. Underwater physiology and diving disorders. In: U.S. Navy Diving Manual, volume 1, revision 6. Available at: http://www.supsalv.org/00c3_publications.asp (last accessed 09/30/11): 3–22-3-55.
7. Taylor L. Diving physics. In: Bove AA, Davis JC, editors. Diving Medicine. 4th ed. Philadelphia, PA: Saunders; 2004. p. 11–35.
8. Spira A. Diving and marine medicine review part I: Diving physics and physiology. J Travel Med 1999;6:32–44.
9. Bove AA. Medical evaluation in sport diving. In: Bove AA, Davis JC, editors. Diving Medicine. 4th ed. Philadelphia, PA: Saunders; 2004. p. 519–33.
10. Medical guidelines. Recreational Scuba Training Council. Available at: http://www.wrstc.com/downloads/10%20-%20Medical%20Guidelines.pdf (accessed 9/20/11).
11. Bove AA. Diving in the elderly and the young. In: Bove AA, Davis JC, editors. Diving Medicine. 4th ed. Philadelphia, PA: Saunders; 2004. p. 411–20.
12. Dembert ML, Keith JF. Evaluating the potential pediatric scuba diver. Am J Dis Child 1986;140:1135–41.
13. Taylor MB. Women in diving. In: Bove AA, Davis JC, editors. Diving Medicine. 4th ed. Philadelphia, PA: Saunders; 2004. p. 381–409.
14. Uguccini DM, Moon RE, Taylor MB. Fitness and diving issues for women. Alert Diver Jan/Feb 1999. Available at: http://www.diversalertnetwork.org/medical/articles/article.asp?articleid=9. (Accessed 9/26/11).
15. Held HE, Pollock NW. The risks of pregnancy and diving. Available at: http://www.diversalertnetwork.org/medical/articles/article.asp?articleid=86 (accessed 9/13/11).
16. Strauss MB, Borer RC. Diving medicine: contemporary topics and their controversies. Am J Emerg Med 2001;19:232–8.
17. Harrison D, Lloyd-Smith R, Khazei A, et al. Controversies in the medical clearance of recreational scuba divers: updates on asthma, diabetes mellitus, coronary artery disease, and patent foramen ovale. Curr Sports Med Rep 2005;4:275–81.
18. Dowse MS, Cridge C, Smerdon G. The use of drugs by UK recreational divers: prescribed and over-the-counter medications. Diving Hyperb Med 2011;41(1):16–21.
19. Leigh D. DAN discusses malaria and antimalarial drugs. Alert Diver Sept 2002. Available at: http://www.diversalertnetwork.org/medical/articles/article.asp?articleid=80 (accessed 10/13/11).
20. Wright D. Mefloquine and scuba diving. N Z Med J 1995;108:514.
21. Goodyer L, Rice L, Martin A. Choice of and adherence to prophylactic antimalarials. J Trav Med 2011;18(4):245–9.
22. Riemsdijk MM, Ditter JM, Sturkenboom MCJM, et al. Neuropsychiatric events during prophylactic use of mefloquine before travel. Eur J Clin Pharmacol 2010;58:441–5.
23. Bove AA. Cardiovascular disorders and diving. In: Bove AA, Davis JC, editors. Diving Medicine. 4th ed. Philadelphia, PA: Saunders; 2004. p. 485–506.
24. Godden D, Currie G, Denison D, et al. British Thoracic Society guidelines on respiratory aspects of fitness for diving. Thorax 2003; 58:3–13.
25. Scott DK, Marks AD. Diabetes and diving. In: Bove AA, Davis JC, editors. Diving Medicine. 4th ed. Philadelphia, PA: Saunders; 2004. p. 507–18.
26. Pollock NW, Uguccioni DM, Dear Gde L, editors. Diabetes and recreational diving: guidelines for the future. Proceedings of the UHMS/DAN 2005 June 19 Workshop. Durham, NC: Divers Alert Network; 2005. Guidelines available at: http://www.diversalertnetwork.org/news/download/SummaryGuidelines.pdf (accessed 8/29/11).
27. Underwater physics. In: U.S. Navy Diving Manual, volume 1, revision 6. Available at: http://www.supsalv.org/00c3_publications.asp (last accessed 09/30/11): 2–1-2-29.
28. Brandt MT. Oral and maxillofacial aspects of diving medicine. Military Medicine 2004;169:137–41.
29. Hunter SE, Farmer JC. Ear and sinus problems in diving. In: Bove AA, Davis JC, editors. Diving Medicine. 4th ed. Philadelphia, PA: Saunders; 2004. p. 431–59.
30. Uzun C. Evaluation of predive parameters related to Eustacian tube dysfunction for symptomatic middle ear barotraumas in divers. Otol Neurotol 2005;26:59–64.
31. Spira A. Diving and marine medicine review part II: Diving diseases. J Travel Med 1999;6:180–98.
32. Klingmann C, Knauth M, Praetorius M, et al. Alternobaric vertigo – really a hazard? Otol Neruol 2006;27:1120–5.
33. Shupak A. Recurrent diving-related inner ear barotrauma. Otol Neurotol 2006;27:1193–6.
34. Neuman TS. Pulmonary barotrauma. In: Bove AA, Davis JC, editors. Diving Medicine. 4th ed. Philadelphia, PA: Saunders; 2004. p. 185–94.
35. Pollock NW, editor. Divers Alert Network Annual Diving Report 2008. Durham, NC: Divers Alert Network; 2008.
36. Francis JT, Mitchell SJ. Pathophysiology of decompression sickness. In: Bove AA, Davis JC, editors. Diving Medicine. 4th ed. Philadelphia, PA: Saunders; 2004. p. 165–83.
37. Vann RD. Mechanisms and risks of decompression. In: Bove AA, Davis JC, editors. Diving Medicine. 4th ed. Philadelphia, PA: Saunders; 2004. p. 127–64.
38. Vann RD, Butler FK, Mitchell SJ, et al. Decompression illness. Lancet 2010;377:153–64.
39. Diagnosis and treatment of DCS and AGE. In: U.S. Navy Diving Manual, volume 5, revision 6. Available at: http://www.supsalv.org/00c3_publications.asp (last accessed 09/30/11): 20–1-20-36.
40. Moon RE. Treatment of decompression illness. In: Bove AA, Davis JC, editors. Diving Medicine. 4th ed. Philadelphia, PA: Saunders; 2004. p. 195–217.

41. Thalmann ED. Decompression illness: what is it and what is the treatment? Alert Diver Mar/Apr 2004. Available at: http://www.diversalertnetwork.org/medical/articles/article.asp?articleid=65 (accessed 9/30/11).

42. Dovenbarger J. Obesity and Diving. Available at: http://www.diversalertnetwork.org/medical/faq/faq.aspx?faqid=144 (Accessed 8/30/11).

43. Sheffiel Paul, Vann Richard, editors. Flying After Diving Workshop Proceedings. Durham, N.C. Divers Alert Network, 2004. Available at: http://www.diversalertnetwork.org/research/projects/fad/workshop/FADWorkshopProceedings.pdf (accessed 8/3/11).

44. Air decompression. In: U.S. Navy Diving Manual, volume 5, revision 6. Available at: http://www.supsalv.org/00c3_publications.asp (last accessed 09/30/11): 9–46–9-86.

45. Ware J. Diving at Altitude. Available at: http://www.scuba-doc.com/divealt.html (accessed 8/31/11).

46. Egi SM, Brubank AO. Diving at altitude: a review of decompression strategies. Undersea Hyperb Med 1995;22(3):281–300.

47. Paulev P-E, Zubieta-Calleja G. High altitude diving depth. Res Sports Med 2007;15(3):213–23.

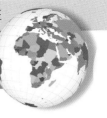

41

Extremes of Temperature and Hydration

Yoram Epstein and Daniel S. Moran

Key points

- Prevention of exertional heatstroke requires following a variety of guidelines: matching activity levels to fitness; acclimatization; scheduling work–rest cycles according to work intensity and climate; and maintaining hydration
- Treatment of heatstroke victims should be initiated immediately by cooling the body with copious amounts of cool or tepid water. Most heatstroke victims survive if treated properly
- Dehydration and hyponatremia are preventable conditions if one follows proper hydration guidelines
- The time it takes for cold adaptation has not yet been well defined; behavioral adaptation, including modification of shelter, clothing, caloric and fluid intake, are most significant in reducing the hazards of cold
- Intensive treatment of deep hypothermia can be life-threatening in and of itself; definitive treatment should be commenced at a medical center equipped with intensive care facilities

Introduction

As travelers become more adventurous, exposure to climatic and environmental extremes has almost become the norm. For these travelers, education about the importance of preparation has become an important part of the pre-travel consult. In order to do this, the health advisor should understand the basic concept of homeostasis, which requires stability of the 'inner environment' of the human body. Body temperature and water are among the main factors that must be constantly controlled to achieve this stability. The human body, being homeothermic, maintains a fairly constant internal temperature, regardless of environmental temperature, by adjusting the rate of heat loss to the environment to the rate of heat generated by metabolic processes.[1] The volume of total body fluids is also regulated within very narrow limits.[2]

Maintaining constant body temperature requires the involvement of several thermoregulatory mechanisms. The most important is the vasomotor regulatory system, through which blood flow to the skin is regulated. When vasomotor activity alone cannot regulate body temperature, other physiological mechanisms are recruited, such as shivering when body temperature is reduced or sweating when body temperature is elevated.

'Normal' Body Temperature

The phrase 'normal' body temperature, although commonly used, is a misnomer. Body temperature is dependent on various factors, such as site of measurement, metabolic state, time of day, age, and for women, the time during the ovulatory cycle. At rest, body-core temperature ranges from 36° to 37.5°C (96.8–99.5°F). The limits for body temperature to maintain efficient thermoregulation are 35–40°C (95–104°F). Frequently, outdoor activities in a warm climate under high solar radiation may result in hyperthermia. It is noteworthy that exhaustive exercise, even under mild environmental conditions, may result in an increased core temperature.[3] Likewise, exposure to cold environments may cause body temperature to equilibrate at the lower end of the acceptable limit.[4]

Monitoring Body-Core Temperature

Overall, the status of the thermoregulatory system can be determined by measuring body-core temperature. This requires an accurate measuring instrument and the measuring site should reflect actual body-core temperature.[5]

Measuring Instruments

The mercury-in-glass and liquid crystal thermometers commonly in use have a number of disadvantages, including a long equilibrium time, a tendency to break, loss of accuracy over time, poor readability, and unsuitability for monitoring extreme hyperthermia or even mild hypothermia because of their upper, and especially lower, limits. 'Tympanic' infrared thermometers that have become very popular respond very quickly, but they usually do not accurately reflect body-core temperature because the aural canal temperature is influenced by environmental conditions. Digital clinical thermometers are simple, available commodities and may be used with relatively high precision (± 0.1°C) in the range of 32–42°C (89.6–107.6°F). At extreme temperatures, however, especially at the lower range, measurements tend to be inaccurate and should be regarded as such. The advantages of electronic thermometers, which use thermistors or thermocouples as sensors, are that they contain an easily read digital display, which reduces operator error. They also tend to have shorter equilibration times than mercury-in-glass thermometers. Electronic thermometers

©2012 Elsevier Inc
DOI: 10.1016/B978-1-4557-1076-8.00041-7

have the requisite degree of wide range accuracy, are very flexible, and are easily applied.

Measurement Sites

Non-invasive measurement sites, including the axilla, oral cavity, and forehead, reflect surface temperatures and are highly influenced by the environment. Minimally invasive sites, including rectal, esophageal, and tympanic (not aural canal), accurately reflect body-core temperature; however, tympanic and esophageal temperatures are far less convenient to obtain.

Under emergency conditions (heatstroke, hypothermia), which require continuous accurate monitoring of body-core temperature, it is advisable to measure rectal temperature (at around 10 cm beyond the anal sphincter) using an electronic thermometer.

Thermoregulation

Heat Balance

A delicate balance between heat accumulation in the body and its dissipation determines body heat content and consequently body-core temperature. Ambient conditions (dry air temperature, mean radiant temperature, and water vapor pressure, as well as clothing) affect the heat flux to and from the body by their influence on dry (sensible) heat exchange and wet (insensible) heat loss.

Dry Heat Exchange

Dry heat exchange occurs through conduction, convection, and radiation. Conduction is heat exchange between two surfaces in direct contact. Since the contact areas are usually small (e.g., feet contact with the ground), heat exchange by conduction is relatively low. It becomes significant when one lies uninsulated on cold ground, especially if under the influence of vasodilating drugs or alcohol. Convection refers to heat transferred from a surface to a gas or liquid. For example, during cold-water immersion heat loss occurs at a faster rate than when standing nude in cold air, because of the much higher heat capacity and the higher thermal conductivity of water as opposed to air. Radiation refers to the transfer of heat by electromagnetic waves (at the spectrum of infrared wavelength). Radiant heat transfer is very much dependent on the insulation from the environment. A major source of heat gain in hot climates is solar load, which can be significantly reduced (by >50%) by wearing light clothing. Radiation is the major way of losing heat in the cold.

Evaporative Heat Exchange (Sweating)

In a thermally neutral environment sweating is minimal and evaporation accounts for only 15% of total heat loss. Of this, approximately half is due to evaporation from the respiratory tract. When the body is unable to maintain thermal equilibrium by dry heat exchange, sweating ensues, permitting heat loss by vaporization of water.

Evaporation of sweat is the major means of dissipating excessive heat accumulated in the body, but evaporation is limited by environmental conditions. Ambient air, humidity, clothing vapor resistance, and wind velocity determine the maximal evaporative capacity of the environment.[1] In practice, under the same ambient temperature, the lower the humidity, the higher the evaporation; the higher the clothing permeability, the higher the evaporative capacity.

Environmental Conditions Assessment

The ability to work in a hostile environment is inversely related to the prevailing environmental climatic stress: the greater the environmental

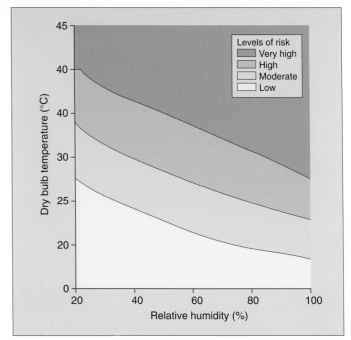

Figure 41.1 Risk of heat exhaustion or heatstroke during intense work in the heat. (Adjusted to the ACSM Position Stand: the prevention of thermal injuries during distance running[7]). Under the level of moderate risk, a rest period of 15 min should be scheduled for every hour of activity. Under the level of high risk, 20–30 min rest should be scheduled. When climatic conditions indicate a level of very high risk, all physical exertion should be avoided.

stress, the shorter the tolerance time and the greater the risk for injury. Therefore, safety regulations concerning work intensity, duration, and work–rest cycles in a hostile climate depend on proper assessment of the environmental stress.

Heat Stress

Ambient temperature by itself does not provide enough information about the prevailing climatic stress. This is better determined by a combination of temperature, solar radiation, and humidity.[6] Noteworthy, solar radiation adds ~5° C to the operative temperature. Accordingly, for an ambient temperature of 30°C the operative temperature would be 35°C.

A simple measurement is called the Discomfort Index (DI), which is easier and more practical to calculate than others[6] and combines only ambient temperature and wet-bulb temperature (an estimate of ambient humidity). Based on this, safety guidelines have been issued regarding the risk encountered while working in the heat (Fig 41.1).[7,8] It is advisable that work–rest cycles during periods of physical activity be scheduled according to work intensity and environmental heat stress.

Cold Stress

Determination of cold stress is more complex than assessment of heat stress. Ambient temperature, wind velocity, and precipitation are variables in this respect. The wind chill index, which estimates the convective cooling power of the environment, is used to assess cold intensity. The calculated 'equivalent temperature', which reflects the lowering effect of wind on ambient temperature, is the link to the perception of cold (Fig. 41.2). Often, weather reports will state the true temperature as well as that calculated using the wind chill factor. Levels of cold intensity may vary according to adaptation and acquaintance

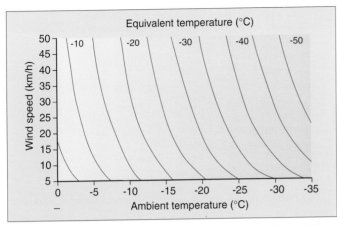

Figure 41.2 The wind chill index chart. The chilling effect of the wind in combination with a low temperature is expressed as the 'equivalent temperature'. Health risk is related to habituation to cold, and thus thresholds are defined as follows:

	Habituated	Non-habituated
Low	−10°C	−5°C
Moderate	−25°C	−10°C
High	−45°C	−25°C
Extreme	−60°C	−35°C

with the hazards of cold. Wind chill warnings should therefore be monitored more carefully by those who are less accustomed to the cold than by those who are more adapted to the cold.[9,10]

Acclimatization

When an individual undergoes prolonged exposure to a stressful environment (heat, cold, or altitude), the subsequent repeated stress creates adaptive changes. These changes reduce the physiological strain, increase tolerance to the stressful environment, and reduce the dangers to health.

Heat Adaptation

Acclimatization to heat is specific to the climatic conditions to which a person is exposed, and can be achieved within a few weeks of exposure. (Acclimatization to heat can, under controlled laboratory conditions, be attained within 5–10 days by a 2 h daily exposure to exercise-heat stress).[11] There are some differences in the dynamics of acclimatization to hot/wet and hot/dry climates. While in hot, dry climates, sweating is the predominant effector mechanism; in hot, wet climates, it is the cardiovascular system. There are also gender differences in the ability to acclimatize: males tend to acclimatize better to hot/dry conditions and females acclimatize better to hot/wet climatic conditions. The traditional hallmarks of heat acclimatization are lower thermal and cardiovascular strain, manifested primarily by reduced body-core temperature and heart rate, and an increase in sweating following exercise-heat stress. Acclimatization to heat has been found to be very effective in alleviating symptoms related to heat stress. To prevent excessive heat stress and guard against heat injuries, the non-acclimatized individual should remember the following:[8,12]

- Acclimatization to heat is time dependent. Working in the heat should be graded in terms of duration and intensity

- During the first few days a sense of fatigue, headache, and lassitude will be present. These are 'warning signs'. Rest periods should be lengthened and fluid consumption should be enhanced
- Within a few days symptoms abate, and more physical work can be done
- Depending on physical fitness and age, acclimatization to heat at a level that enables adequate performance will take 5–10 days
- Acclimatization to a hot/wet climate takes longer than acclimatization to a hot/dry climate.

Cold Adaptation

The most common observation with regard to adaptation to cold is the great drop in body-core temperature before the onset of shivering. It is possible that increased heat production can occur by a shift later from shivering to non-shivering. This is less well understood and the time course to achieve cold adaptation has not yet been defined; it may indeed prove to be long. The practical advantages provided by adaptation in terms of conservation of body heat are questionable. Behavioral adaptation (e.g., seeking shelter, proper clothing, adjusting caloric and fluid intake, and building fires) is much more significant in reducing the hazards of cold.[10,13]

Fever

Normally, body temperature is determined by the delicate balance between heat gain and heat loss, which is described in thermodynamic terms by the heat balance equation. Fever, in contrast, represents a state in which the body temperature 'set point' has been reset from its base value of circa 37°C (98.6°F) to a higher value.

The effect of pathogens on regulated temperature occurs through the interaction of components within the immune system. This interaction stimulates the production of cytokines, which in turn induce the release of prostaglandin E_2 (PGE_2), leading to an increase in the body's 'set point' temperature. As a result, the body responds by elevating metabolic heat production (shivering).[14]

Most antipyretics (i.e., acetaminophen, aspirin) work by inhibiting the enzyme cyclo-oxygenase in the hypothalamus and reducing the levels of PGE_2. Other agents reduce the proinflammatory mediators, enhance anti-inflammatory signals, or boost antipyretic messages within the brain.[15] This in turn shifts the 'set point' temperature 'to the left,' back to its natural value, and the body responds by enhancing heat dissipation (sweating). Therefore, antipyretic therapy, which may prove to be effective in febrile conditions, is totally ineffective in reducing body-core temperature that results from a thermodynamic imbalance. It is noteworthy that in the case of heatstroke, when the liver becomes extremely vulnerable, treatment with antipyretic drugs (e.g., acetaminophen) is dangerous and life-threatening.[16]

Steam Baths and Saunas

Steam baths and saunas are traditional forms of public bathing, recognized for over 2000 years. They have become very popular in the modern era at leisure facilities, among travelers visiting those areas where this is still considered part of the traditional way of life, and for health-seeking travelers.

The common belief that sauna bathing has a therapeutic application, besides being a short-term muscle relaxation, has not been established. On the contrary, the severe heat stress in the sauna (≈100°C, 212°F); ≈40% relative humidity) and the steam bath (≈50°C, 122°F); ≈100% relative humidity) results in a significant physiological strain, especially to the cardiovascular system. This is exhibited by an increase in heart rate, stroke volume, and blood pressure. In addition, a steep increase in body-core temperature is evident and the excessive sweating enhances the danger of dehydration.[17]

For most people saunas and steam baths are safe unless misused or abused. Those who wish to bathe in a sauna or in a steam bath should be aware of the potential risk involved. Cardiac patients, hypertensive patients, pregnant women, and children are especially vulnerable. Others should:

- Limit the exposure to <15 min
- Drink water to reduce dehydration
- Not bathe immediately after physical exertion
- Not consume alcohol during bathing (alcohol increases the risk of arrhythmia and hypotension).

Heat-Related Illnesses

Heatstroke

Heatstroke is the most serious of the syndromes associated with excess body heat. It is defined as a condition in which body temperature is elevated to such levels that body tissue damage occurs, giving rise to a characteristic multiorgan clinical and pathological syndrome. The severity depends on the degree of hyperthermia and its duration. Heatstroke is a medical emergency that can be fatal if not diagnosed and treated promptly.[8,18,19]

The literature differentiates between two entities of heatstroke: exertional heatstroke (EHS) and classic heatstroke. EHS occurs when excess heat, generated by muscular exercise, exceeds the body's ability to dissipate it. Patients are typically young and very active physically. Its occurrence is sporadic.[12,18] Classic heatstroke, which will not be discussed in this chapter, is a common disorder of the elderly during heat waves and occurs in the form of an epidemic.[20]

Pathophysiology

Heatstroke usually occurs when extreme heat stress leads to marked hyperthermia after thermoregulation is subordinated to circulatory and metabolic demands. Collapse occurs because of central nervous system and other secondary non-cardiovascular effects of severe hyperthermia. The latter, such as erythrocyte alterations and disseminated intravascular coagulation (DIC), result in microthrombosis and coagulative necrosis, causing diffuse neurological and other damage leading to death.[21]

Early Presentation

The presentation of EHS is usually acute. The prodrome, occurring in about 25% of casualties, consists of dizziness, weakness, nausea, confusion, disorientation, drowsiness, and irrational behavior; this may last from minutes to hours. Failure to recognize these first signs can result in dire consequences.

The early clinical signs of heatstroke are non-specific; therefore, any systemic disease or condition that presents with an increase in body temperature and manifestation of brain dysfunction should be considered only after heatstroke is excluded (Table 41.1).

Diagnosis

Exertional heatstroke should be the working hypothesis in any case of collapse during exercise or immediately after exercise of a young, apparently healthy individual whose body-core temperature is high (≈40°C, 104°F) and who presents with neurological signs (from aggressiveness to coma). Prolonged exertion, warm climate, very high body-core temperature (above 40.6°C, 105.08°F), and dry skin are typically linked with EHS, but are misleading yardsticks.[12,18]

Table 41.1 Differential Diagnosis of Heatstroke

Dehydration
Encephalitis, meningitis
Coagulopathies
Cerebrovascular accidents (e.g., hypothalamic hemorrhage)
Seizures
Hypoglycemia
Drug intoxication
Animal poisoning or stings (snakes, bees)

The performance of strenuous physical exercise in the heat has been notorious as a cause of heatstroke. In many instances, however, EHS occurs within the first 2 h of exercise and not necessarily at a high ambient temperature.

Body-core temperature of 40.6°C (105.08°F), as a critical temperature to define heatstroke, is arbitrary. In many instances lower temperatures are recorded because the first measurements are delayed, performed by untrained individuals, or measured incorrectly.

At the stage of collapse profuse sweating is still likely to be present, unless heatstroke develops in an already anhydrous subject. Dry skin might be evident either in situations where the climate is very dry and sweat evaporates very easily, or when heatstroke coincides with a severe degree of dehydration.

Clinical Picture

The clinical manifestations of heatstroke usually follow a distinct pattern of events:[8]

- *The hyperthermic phase*: Central nervous system disturbances are present in all cases of heatstroke, as the brain is extremely sensitive to hyperthermia. Signs of depression in the central nervous system often appear simultaneously in the form of coma, stupor, or delirium, irritability and aggressiveness. Seizures occur in approximately 60–70% of cases
- *The hematological and enzymatic phase*: Hematological and enzymatic disorders peak usually 24–48 h after the collapse (but might be present already at an earlier stage). Typical, although not pathognomonic, is a marked elevation in plasma CPK activity, which resembles rhabdomyolysis
- *Renal and hepatic phase*: Manifests 2–5 days after collapse and is characterized by serious disturbances in renal (acute renal failure) and hepatic function (markedly elevated liver enzymes).

Treatment

Treatment of heatstroke is supportive (Table 41.2). Cooling should be initiated vigorously immediately upon collapse and only minimally delayed for vital resuscitation measures. Any time-consuming examinations should be postponed until body temperature is controlled.

The most practical and efficient method of cooling is the use of large quantities of tap water, which is readily available and does not require any complicated logistic arrangements. It eliminates the hazard of cold-induced vasoconstriction that reduces the efficiency of heat dissipation. The victim should be placed in the shade and any restrictive clothing must be removed. The patient's skin must be kept wet and the body should be continually fanned. Cooling should be continued until body temperature reaches 38°C (100.4°F); otherwise there is a danger of overcooling and entering a state of hypothermia and undesirable shivering.[22] This should not, however, delay the rapid evacuation of the patient to the nearest medical facility, which is of the utmost importance.

Table 41.2 Treatment for Exertional Heatstroke

Cooling	Tap water (large quantities) (Antipyretics are ineffective and dangerous)
Seizures	Diazepam (titration i.v. 10 mg) until seizure ceases
Rehydration	2 L/1st h, then after according to water deficit
Oliguria	Mannitol (0.25 mg/kg) Furosemide (1 mg/kg)
Clotting	Fresh frozen plasma Cryoprecipitate Platelet concentrate
Brain edema	Dexamethasone

Acid–base balance, electrolytes, and glucose levels usually correct spontaneously after cooling and rehydration.

Table 41.3 On Admission, and at 12 h Intervals, the Following Should be Checked

ECG
Muscle enzymes
Transaminases and liver function
Renal function
Coagulation indices
Acid–base balance
Electrolytes
Glucose

No drug is effective in reducing body temperature. Dantrolene is not effective, since in EHS there is no involvement of the calcium channels as there is in malignant hyperthermia. Antipyretics are also ineffective, since the thermoregulatory 'set point' is not affected in heatstroke. Antipyretics might be harmful, as they cannot be metabolized in the heat-affected liver.

To confirm the diagnosis and, afterwards, the effectiveness of cooling, a rectal temperature must be measured and vital signs monitored.

Usually, not more than 2 L of Ringer's lactate or saline should be infused in the first hour, after which fluids should be administered in accordance with the state of hydration. Overhydration might result in hyponatremia and brain edema.

Some of the clinical manifestations of heatstroke may develop during the second or third day after collapse. Therefore, it is imperative that any suspected case of heatstroke be followed for at least 48 h. During this period, and at 12 h intervals, laboratory and clinical evaluations should be carried out (Table 41.3).

Prognosis

Survival rate from EHS is <95% if diagnosed and treated properly. The noxious effect on the tissues caused by heatstroke is directly and closely correlated with the duration of the high-temperature phase. Therefore, misdiagnosis, lack of appropriate or aggressive treatment, and delay in evacuation are the major causes for deterioration in the patient's condition. Predictors of poor prognosis include prolonged body temperature >42°C (107.6°F), prolonged coma, hyperkalemia, oliguric renal failure, and continuous hepatic dysfunction. The vast majority of cases of heatstroke patients recover with no long-term sequelae.[8] Neurological deficits may persist in some patients, usually for only a limited period, in the form of cerebellar deficits, hemipare-sis, aphasia, and mental deficiency. In rare cases, neurological impairment may be chronic.

Prevention

Most heatstroke patients are motivated, but relatively untrained subjects who exert themselves beyond their physiological capacity. Therefore, EHS frequently occurs during relatively short exertions. Early collapse during exercise may point to the possibility that, besides over-motivation, other underlying factors compromise the individual's thermoregulation. For the young and healthy, four factors are of relevance: poor physical fitness, lack of heat acclimatization, acute febrile illness, and dehydration.[12]

Following some simple guidelines and providing proper health education can easily prevent EHS:[8,12,18]

- Only healthy, fit subjects should participate in strenuous physical activity. Exercise should be commensurate with the individual's fitness level
- Rest periods should be incorporated into long periods of activity (a proper night's rest is also imperative)
- Physical exertion should not be undertaken during the hottest hours of the day
- Adequate hydration is essential. Water should be readily available and used freely during activity (Fig. 41.3). Adhering to guidelines regarding fluid replacement will eliminate dehydration.

Other Heat-Related Concerns

Several other conditions associated with exertion outdoors in the heat warrant attention. They are not considered medical emergencies and can be easily prevented.[23]

Heat Exhaustion

Heat exhaustion lies on a continuum with heatstroke. The term 'heat exhaustion' is used to describe the inability to continue exercising in situations of heat stress. Symptoms are milder than those expected for heatstroke and include dizziness, confusion, nausea, muscle cramps, and mild elevation in body-core temperature. Major neurological impairment is absent.

Treatment is similar to that for heatstroke, and includes removal of the patient to a shaded area, cooling with copious amounts of water, and continuously monitoring body-core temperature. Fluid replacement by drinking or by infusion should be according to the patient's clinical condition and hydration status.

Heat Cramps

The term 'heat cramps' is a misnomer because heat itself does not cause them; rather, they occur in muscles subjected to intense activity and fatigue. Heat cramps are described as painful spasms of skeletal muscles that usually involve the arms, legs, or abdominal muscles. Because heat cramps tend to occur more in physically conditioned subjects, it is difficult to differentiate them from other muscle pains related to physical activity. The etiology is not fully clear but is probably related to sodium depletion. Sodium replacement in the diet is effective in preventing this syndrome.

Heat Syncope

Episodes of orthostatic hypotension may result from prolonged standing in the heat or a sudden change in postural position from lying to standing. It occurs because of the massive peripheral vasodilatation, reduction in venous return and, consequently, inadequate cardiac output. Treatment consists of placing the patient in a supine position with legs elevated.

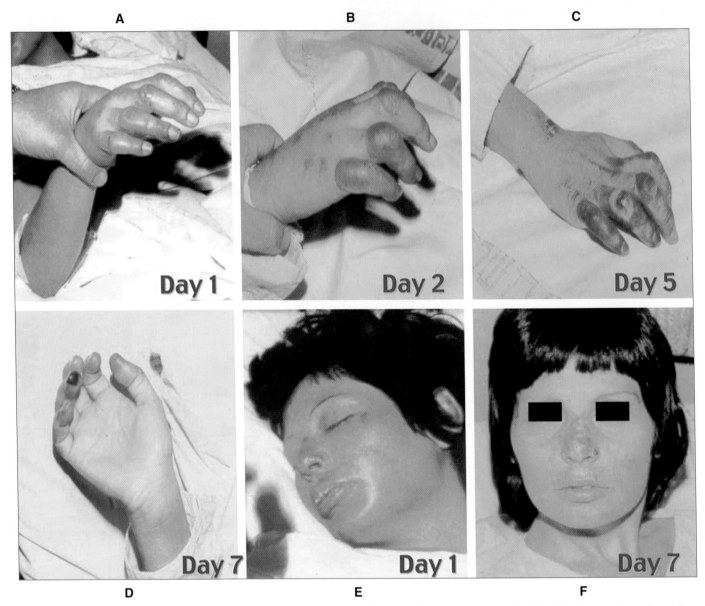

Figure 41.3 Recovery from combined hypothermia and frostbite. An 18-year-old girl was exposed to a snow blizzard for 24 h in a remote rural area. She was not dressed properly and became fatigued and dehydrated after she left her car in an attempt to reach rescue. Two other people who accompanied her died from hypothermia. The girl was rescued with a body-core temperature of 27°C (80.6°F). **(A)** Day 1, third-degree frostbite; **(B)** day 2, seemingly the condition worsens after re-warming in a warm bath of 42°C (107.6°F), three times daily (chlorhexidine gluconate solution added to bath water). Re-warming continued until day 10; **(C)** day 5; **(D)** day 7, the proximal flange of the fourth finger is necrotic. This flange was amputated on day 10; **(E)** the hypothermic, waxy, edematous face of the unconscious patient on admission to the ER. The patient was treated by immersion in a warm bath of 42°C (107.6°F); **(F)** day 7, post trauma.

Heat Edema

Heat edema is typically mild and is occasionally seen during the early stages of heat exposure, especially in the unconditioned subject. It results from plasma volume that expands to compensate for the increased need for thermoregulatory blood flow. This condition has no clinical significance and will resolve itself spontaneously. Diuretic therapy is not necessary.

Cold Injuries

Cold injuries occur when the body is unable to protect itself from the environment, and heat loss from the body exceeds heat gain. Cold injuries are subdivided into peripheral injuries (chilblains, trench foot, and frostbite) and systemic injury (hypothermia). Cold injuries result mainly because of inappropriate behavior (Table 41.4), and can be significantly reduced by following simple guidelines (Table 41.5).

Hypothermia

Hypothermia is defined as a body-core temperature of <35°C (95°F).[9] It occurs when massive body heat is lost to the environment and exceeds metabolic heat production. Scientific literature differentiates between 'urban hypothermia' and 'accidental hypothermia', based on the etiology and the population at risk. 'Urban hypothermia', which is not the focus of this chapter, is characteristic of cold exposure in

Table 41.4 Factors that Increase the Risk for Cold Injuries

Hypothermia
    Low ambient temperatures (high cold intensity)
    Improper insulation of clothing and equipment
    Wet clothing
    Fatigue
    Dehydration
    Poor food intake
    Inactivity
    Lack of knowledge or inappropriate risk taking
    Alcohol intake
Peripheral injuries
    Improper, constricting, and wet clothing
    Cold intensity
    Immobilization
    Smoking
    Hypothermia
    Vasoconstrictive drugs

Table 41.5 Cold Injuries are Preventable by Following Simple Guidelines

Staying in shelters that protect from wind and rain/snow
Matching outdoor activities with cold intensity
Wearing multilayered, unrestrictive dry clothing
Performing light–moderate work to prevent sweating
Adjusting layers of clothing to work rate in order to eliminate wearing wet items
Eating high-calorie diets and eliminating alcohol consumption

the elderly suffering from poor health and poor nutrition, and cold exposure in alcoholics, and drug users. Young children from lower socioeconomic strata are also at risk. The population at risk for 'accidental hypothermia' is usually the young and active, e.g., winter sport participants, hikers, travelers, military personnel, and adventurers.

Diagnosis

The diagnosis of hypothermia is dependent solely on body-core temperature. Accordingly, it is classified as mild, moderate, or severe. All organ systems are affected by hypothermia. This should be kept in mind during re-warming. During the hypothermic stage, however, the central nervous system and the cardiovascular system are the most sensitive.[9,10,24]

- *Mild hypothermia*: Body temperature falls in the range of 35–32°C (95–89.6°F). The patient may be slightly cool and pale, but is usually shivering and conscious. Central nervous system reactions are slowed. Cardiovascular changes include initial tachycardia, which is secondary to catecholamine release, followed by bradycardia. Common in this stage are shivering, confusion, disorientation and dysarthria.

- *Moderate hypothermia*: Body temperature falls in the range of 32–28°C (89.6–82.4°F). Shivering ceases and the patient becomes unconscious to varying degrees. Myocardial irritability is evident by the appearance of atrial fibrillation and changes in the ECG complex. A characteristic, although not pathognomonic, deflection at the junction of the QRS complex and ST segment, known as J-waves (Osborn waves) appears.

- *Severe hypothermia*: Body temperature < 28°C (82.4°F). In this condition, arrhythmias in the form of ventricular fibrillation are common. Unconsciousness, waxy pale skin, the absence of corneal reflexes, and undetectable breathing, pulse rate, and blood pressure often mislead providers into thinking that the patient is dead.

In the management of hypothermia, the working hypothesis should always be '*no patient is dead until warm and dead*'. Asystole usually is seen at body temperature of 18°C (64.4°F). The lowest known survival temperature for adults is 16°C (60.8°F), and for infants 15°C (59.0°F).

Treatment

Hypothermia is a condition that can also be life-threatening during the treatment stage. Therefore, intensive treatment should be commenced at a medical center equipped with intensive care facilities.[25]

- *In the field*: During all stages of hypothermia the patient should be evacuated to a dry shelter and all wet clothing removed. Passive external heating, by covering the patient with dry blankets, sleeping bags, etc., is the safest first-aid treatment until evacuation to a hospital is possible. The low metabolic rate associated with hypothermia actually has a protective effect on the body's vital organs and function. Therefore, when treated properly, individuals, especially children, have been successfully resuscitated after prolonged severe hypothermia.

- *In the hospital*: Active re-warming should be initiated, concomitant with continuous monitoring of body-core temperature by an electronic thermometer. Aggressive, active re-warming can be accomplished by several means, e.g., warm water bottles, radiant heat, hot-water immersion (42–43°C; 107.6–109.4°F), warm inhalation (43°C; 109.4°F), gastrointestinal irrigation or peritoneal dialysis with warm fluids (42–43°C; 107.6–109.4°F), and cardiopulmonary bypass (37°C; 98.6°F); the last is probably the safest and most effective treatment. Mild hypothermia will resolve itself regardless of the re-warming technique. For moderate and severe hypothermia, aggressive re-warming should be initiated. The re-warming stage, however, might be associated with severe complications, especially for moderate and severe cases of hypothermia.

Advanced life support protocols, especially defibrillation, may be ineffective when body-core temperature is low (moderate and severe hypothermia). Defibrillation should be tried and medications given only when body temperature is >32°C (89.6°F).[24,25]

Complications Associated with Re-Warming

The associated complications from re-warming result from abrupt changes in the metabolic rate and effective blood volume.

- *After-drop*: Despite re-warming, body temperature continues to fall. This phenomenon is related to the return of cold blood from the periphery to the central circulation. After-drop may be significant if re-warming is not sufficiently aggressive. Immersion in hot water and cardiopulmonary bypass result in the lowest after-drop

- *Re-warming shock*: During aggressive re-warming, effective peripheral circulation increases, resulting in low cardiac output and a state of shock

- *Arrhythmias*: During re-warming, as cold blood returns from the periphery to the central circulation, arrhythmias may develop. Atrial fibrillations may spontaneously convert to sinus rhythm, but ventricular fibrillation is often resistant and does not respond to conventional medications. Bretylium tosylate may be helpful

- *Hypoglycemia*: Re-warming abruptly increases metabolic rate. This requires the recruitment of any available energy source, which, in turn, will cause hypoglycemia. A continuous infusion of 5% dextrose in isotonic sodium chloride solution should be the treatment of choice.

Frostbite

Frostbite is the most serious peripheral cold injury. It occurs when unprotected tissue is exposed to sub-zero cold environments, even for relatively short periods. The tissues in the affected area freeze, and ice crystals form within the cells, causing them to rupture.

Frostbite is divided into four levels depending on the severity of the injury, but it may be more useful to classify it as superficial (levels I–II) and deep (levels III–IV).[26,27]

- *Level I (frostnip) –II*: The skin surface freezes. It begins with itching and pain; then, when blood supply to the skin decreases because of extensive vasoconstriction, sensation is lost and the area becomes numb. Because only the top skin layers are affected, healing is short, usually without subsequent problems. Hard blisters may form that can take up to a few months to resolve. Cold sensitivity may result.
- *Levels III–IV*: The muscles, tendons, blood vessels, and nerves of the affected area are frozen. The area feels hard, woody, and numb. The affected area appears red, deep purple, or blackened with blisters usually filled with blood. Often it takes months to determine the extent of the damage. Amputation of extremities is usually required, but is delayed until it is ascertained which tissues are viable.

Treatment

Treatment should be commenced only at a medical installation under conditions that ensure that the affected area will not re-freeze. The proper way to treat frostbite and trench foot is to re-warm the affected area in warm water (40–42°C; 104–107.6°F), usually for 15–30 min. This should be done 3–4 times/day until thawing is complete.[10,27] In addition:

- The patient should be kept in a warm environment
- The affected area should be kept dry and clean under sterile sheets, and should not be dressed
- Blisters should not be opened or manipulated
- Analgesia should be administered
- A broad-spectrum antibiotic should be administered.

'Trench Foot' (Immersion Foot)

The term 'trench foot' was derived from the cold injury that occurred in soldiers living in the trenches during the First World War. It occurs when a part of the body, usually the feet, is exposed to non-freezing cold and wet environments for prolonged periods (>10 h). The feet are especially vulnerable, since boots restrict proper blood flow to the feet, thereby worsening the condition. The affected area is pale, cold, swollen, and painful; deep blisters may develop.[10,28]

Treatment

The treatment of trench foot is similar to that of frostbite.

Chilblains

These are the most common cold injuries. Chilblains occur when there is exposure of the skin, especially the fingers, to dry, non-freezing cold. The affected area may itch, appear reddish-blue, and be swollen and painful. Blisters containing clear fluid may form after some time, and the area may become sensitive to cold in the future. Usually there is no permanent damage.[13]

Treatment

Prevention is the best treatment. This includes protecting fingers and toes with dry gloves, dry socks, and boots. Affected areas should be kept warm and dry.

Preventing Cold Injuries

The physiological ability of humans to adapt to cold is limited, but behavioral measures can minimize the risks associated with exposure to cold. These include: dressing in proper clothing, consuming an energy-rich diet, maintaining hydration, and staying in a dry shelter.

- *Clothing* – The single most important way to protect the body from excessive heat loss is by wearing properly insulated clothing. Dressing in multiple layers of clothing allows air to be trapped and serves as insulation. This will also enable one to adjust the insulation according to environmental conditions and activity levels. Most important is to keep the skin dry; thus, the innermost layer must have wicking properties that allow water vapor to be transmitted to the outer layers. The outer shell of the clothing ensemble should be water resistant to eliminate the saturation of clothing. The insulating effect of wet clothing is reduced by 50–85% and so conductive heat loss increases substantially (Table 41.6)
- *Diet* – Energy expenditure in cold weather is higher than in thermoneutral conditions, both at rest and during exercise. This results from a higher basal metabolic rate and increased energy expenditure while shivering or walking on harsh terrain (i.e., snow). Food consumption should be increased by approximately 25–50% depending on the weather conditions and activity level. The key to cold weather nutrition is ingestion of hot, palatable food and beverages and eating healthy snacks. This helps by providing a warm sensation and improves morale
- *Hydration* – A cold-induced diuresis can lead to dehydration, a blunted sensation of thirst and sweating. Drinking should be regularly scheduled even if no sense of thirst exists. Daily fluid intake in cold weather should be 5–6 L/day if active, and about 4 L if less active

Table 41.6 The Acronym COLD for Proper Dressing in Cold Weather

C	Clean	Keep clothing clean. Fumes and other organic substances reduce clothing insulation
O	Open	Avoid overheating by keeping openings in clothing to ensure sweat evaporation
L	Loose and in layers	Dress in layers. The air trapped inside clothing serves as an insulator
D	Dry	Keep clothing dry. Wet clothing loses about 85% of its insulation

- *Shelter* – The risks of cold-weather injuries vary with temperature, wind speed, and duration of exposure, as well as with moisture, altitude, and the individual's physical condition and health. Rest breaks taken in a closed warm environment during activity will help in preventing unnecessary exposure. One should take care to leave an opening to secure proper ventilation in the shelter in order to eliminate the hazard of accumulation of carbon dioxide.

Dehydration and Fluid Consumption

Euhydration is represented by a sinusoidal wave indicating the normal, daily body water content fluctuations that expand and contract within very narrow limits (total body water volume within ±0.22% of body weight and plasma volume within ±0.7%).[2] Steady-state conditions of increased and decreased body water content are defined as hyperhydration and hypohydration, respectively.

Hypohydration

The adverse effects of hypohydration occur via the impairment of the thermoregulatory and cardiovascular systems, which results in reduced performance and compromised body temperature control. Impairment in physical performance is noticed already at 1% dehydration (600–800 mL water loss), and total collapse is evident when water loss is at around 7% of body weight. The dehydrated subject is described as an apathetic, listless, plodding person straining to finish a given task that he previously performed easily. Cognitive performance is also adversely influenced by body water deficits.[29]

Voluntary Dehydration

Thirst is an adequate stimulus for total fluid replacement when at rest. During physical activity or exercise-heat stress thirst does not appear to be a sufficient stimulus for maintaining body water levels. Spontaneous drinking occurs only after a considerable amount of water loss (>2% of body weight). In addition, when water is not readily available, or if the water is unpalatable, salty, or warm, drinking is also reduced.[2]

The slowdown in voluntary fluid intake is termed 'voluntary dehydration'. That is, individuals will drink to temporary satiety, but a water deficit remains. Voluntary dehydration is considered the main cause for dehydration during exercise.[2]

Although physical activity accentuates voluntary dehydration, leisure reduces it. Therefore, a water deficit accumulated between meals is usually restored during meals. Awareness of the need for fluid replenishment increases voluntary fluid intake and reduces voluntary dehydration.

Overhydration and Hyponatremia

Hyponatremia is commonly defined as sodium plasma concentrations <135 mEq/L. Clinical symptoms of hyponatremia are not expected to appear unless sodium blood concentrations are <130 mEq/L. Whereas subclinical exercise-induced hyponatremia (EH) may be common during long (>8 h) exertion in heat when sweating is excessive, in the young active population clinically significant EH is a rare condition.[30]

Hyponatremia can result from either excessive loss of sodium in sweat, which is not compensated for by proper salt intake while the extracellular compartment is replenished by adequate water intake, or because of overhydration with hypotonic fluids (e.g., water).

In practice, for a healthy individual maintaining a normal diet, to develop a salt deficiency is extremely difficult, perhaps impossible, regardless of the environment and the amount of exercise performed.

Cumulative data suggest that in healthy individuals, symptomatic hyponatremia develops mainly because of gross fluid overload. Therefore, for individuals who maintain normal sodium levels in the diet, electrolyte supplementation may be needed only in rare cases for exercising subjects who (1) lose >8 L of sweat; (2) skip meals; (3) experience a caloric deficit of <1000 kcal/day; or (4) are ill with diarrhea.[2]

Isotonic Fluids ('Sport Drinks')

A debated topic is 'appropriate' fluid replacement during physical activity, especially in the heat. Some advocate that water is not enough and that it should be enriched with carbohydrates and electrolytes. 'Sport drinks' are commercial or homemade beverages that contain carbohydrates ('to enhance performance') and electrolytes ('to prevent hyponatremia'). In general, the benefit of ingesting sports drinks appears to be their enhanced palatability, which increases fluid consumption.[29]

Most sport drinks contain a low concentration of sodium in order to maintain a hypotonic or isotonic solution so as not to hamper gastric emptying. Therefore, under normal conditions, the use of electrolyte-carbohydrate beverages offers no advantages over water. Consumption of these beverages may be indicated only under conditions of long physical exertions with caloric restriction.

Rehydration

At rest and thermal comfort, urination is the major cause for loss of body water (around 1.5 L/day). During physical activity or in hot environments, a considerable amount of body water is lost through sweat secretion, enabling evaporative cooling of the body. Sweat secretion can vary considerably, depending on environmental conditions, work intensity, clothing, gender, age, state of acclimatization, and fitness.

The general concept that prevails is that during prolonged intermittent exercise, the optimal rate of fluid replacement appears to be the rate which most closely matches the rate of sweating (Fig. 41.4). On average, sweat rates of 1–1.5 L/h during exercise in the heat are common.[2,29]

To reduce the rate of voluntary dehydration without exposing the individual to the dangers involved in dehydration or overhydration, the following should be remembered:

- One should not assume that unlimited quantities of water can be consumed
- Fluids should be palatable and consumed at regular intervals at a rate sufficient to replace water loss through sweating
- Fluid intake should be at frequencies and in quantities that will be ingested with ease; volumes of 200–250 mL should be consumed each time
- Hyponatremia is a potential risk only for activities lasting longer than 8–10 h. There is little physiological basis for the adding of salt to fluid if it is sufficiently available in the diet.

Summary

Environmental conditions may restrict travelers. Lack of behavior modification during adverse climatic conditions and improper

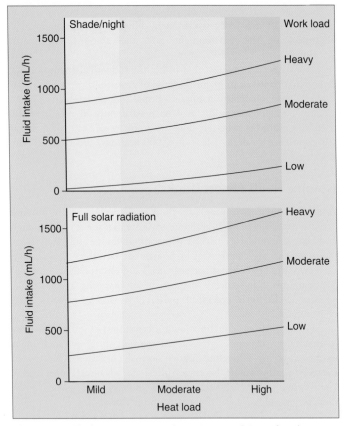

Figure 41.4 Fluid requirements under various conditions of work intensity and heat load. (Levels of heat load are depicted in Fig. 41.1.) How to calculate daily fluid requirements:

Heat load	Work load	Length (h)	mL/h	Total (L)
Moderate (+)	Moderate	6	750	4.5
Moderate (−)	Rest	8	100	0.8
Mild	Moderate	4	500	2.0
Total				7.3

+, With solar radiation; −, without solar radiation.

preparedness may result in heat- or cold-related injuries. Preventing these potentially life-threatening problems is possible by adherence to some simple guidelines:

- Only fit, healthy, acclimatized individuals should conduct physical exercise in adverse climatic conditions
- Physical exertion should be performed within the individual's capacity; over-exertion can be life-threatening
- Work–rest cycles should be planned and adhered to
- Fluid intake should compensate fluid loss. Euhydration should be maintained
- Clothing should be suitable to the climatic conditions and work intensity
- Casualties of heat or cold weather should be treated vigorously. The sooner body temperature returns to its normal range, the better the prognosis.

References

1. Gagge AP, Gonzalez RR. Mechanisms of heat exchange: biophysics and physiology. In: Fregly MJ, Blatteis CM, editors. Handbook of Physiology. Section 4: Environmental Physiology. Vol. 1. Oxford: Oxford University Press; 1996. p. 45–84.
2. Epstein Y, Armstrong LE. Fluid-electrolyte balance during labor and exercise: concepts and misconceptions. Int J Sport Nutr 1999;9:1–12.
3. Cheuvrout SN, Haynes EM. Thermoregulation and marathon running: biological and environmental influences. Sports Med 2001;31:743–62.
4. Young AJ. Human adaptation to cold. In: Pandolf KB, Sawka MN, Gonzalez RR, editors. Human Performance Physiology and Environmental Medicine at Terrestrial Extremes. Cooper Pub Group; 1988. p. 401–34.
5. Moran DS, Mendel L. Core temperature measurements – methods and current insights. Sports Med 2002;32:879–85.
6. Epstein Y, Moran DS. Thermal comfort and the heat stress indices. Indust Health 2006;44:388–98.
7. Armstrong LE, Epstein Y, Greenleaf JE, et al. ACSM position stand: heat and cold illnesses during distance running. Med Sci Sports Exerc 1987;19:529–33.
8. Shapiro Y, Seidman DS. Field and clinical observations of exertional heat-stroke patients. Med Sci Sports Exerc 1990;22:6–14.
9. Hamlet MP. Prevention and treatment of cold injury. Int J Circumpolar Health 2000;59:108–13.
10. Mills WJ. Cold injury [a collection of papers]. Alaska Med 1993;35:6–140.
11. Wenger CB. Human heat acclimatization. In: Pandolf KB, Sawka MN, Gonzalez RR, editors. Human Performance Physiology and Environmental Medicine at Terrestrial Extremes. Carmel: Cooper; 1988. p. 153–98.
12. Epstein Y, Moran DS, Shapiro Y, et al. Exertional heat stroke: a case series. Med Sci Sports Exerc 1999;31:224–8.
13. Burr RE. Medical aspects of cold weather operations: a handbook for medical officers. USARIEM Report TN3–4, 1993.
14. Stitt JT. Fever versus hyperthermia. Fed Proc 1979;38:39–43.
15. Aronoff DM, Neilson EG. Antipyretics: mechanisms of action and clinical use in fever suppression. Am J Med 2001;111:304–15.
16. Helled Y, Rav-Acha M, Shani Y, et al. The 'golden hour' for heatstroke treatment. Milit Med 2004;169:184–6.
17. Hannuksela ML, Ellahham S. Benefits and risks of sauna bathing. Am J Med 2001;110:118–26.
18. Shibolet S, Lancaster MC, Danon Y. Heat stroke: a review. Aviat Space Environ Med 1976;47:280–301.
19. Boucham A, Knochell JP. Heat stroke. NEJM 2002;346:1978–88.
20. Bouchama A, Debbi M, Mohamed G, et al. Prognostic factors in heat wave-related deaths: a meta-analysis. Arch Intern Med 2007;167:2170–6.
21. Epstein Y, Roberts WO. The pathophysiology of heat stroke: an integrative view of the final common pathway. Scand J Med Sci Sports 2011;21:742–8.
22. Makranz C, Heled Y, Moran DS. Hypothermia following exertional heat stroke treatment. Eur J Appl Physiol 2011;111:2359–62.
23. Armstrong LE. Exertional heat illnesses. Human Kinetics; 2003.
24. Danzl DF, Pozos RS. Current concepts: accidental hypothermia. NEJM 1994;331:1756–60.
25. Kempainen RR, Brunette DD. The evaluation and management of accidental hypothermia. Resp Care 2004;49:192–205.
26. Reamy BV. Frostbite: a review and current concepts. J Am Board Fam Pract 1998;11:34–40.
27. Murphy JV, Banwell PE, Roberts HN, et al. Frostbite: pathogenesis and treatment. J Trauma 2000;48:171–8.
28. Lloyd EL. ABC of sports medicine. Temperature and performance. I: cold. BMJ 1994;309:531–4.
29. Convertino VA, Armstrong LE, Coyle EF, et al. ACSM position stand: Exercise and fluid replacement. Med Sci Sports Exerc 1996;28:1–5.
30. Montain SJ, Sawka MN, Wenger LB. Hyponatremia associated with exercise: risk factors and pathogenesis. Exerc Sports Sci Rev 2001;29:113–7.

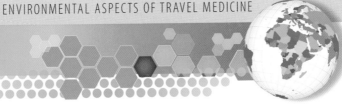

Jet Lag

Susan L.F. McLellan

Key points

- The suprachiasmatic nucleus acts as our primary internal timekeeper and regulates diurnal variations in body temperature and the release of melatonin, cortisol, and growth hormone, which are important in maintaining circadian rhythm
- The time required to reset the internal clock is generally agreed to be about 1 day per time zone crossed
- Jet lag tends to increase with age and number of time zones crossed, and eastward travel is generally more difficult than westward travel
- Melatonin has been shown to reduce symptoms of jet lag in most studies, appears to be safe, and is recommended by an expert panel. Issues remain with regard to its effects in the very old and the very young, use in combination with other strategies, and quality control of commercially available products
- Light therapy with sleep time adjustment can help speed the resolution of circadian dyssynchronism: an eastward traveler should seek light in the morning, and a westward traveler in the afternoon/evening. Phototherapy, with or without melatonin, can be used before travel to advance circadian rhythms

Definition

'Jet lag' is a condition well known to travelers since the introduction of passenger jet aircraft. The term is commonly used, but the condition manifests itself differently between individuals. Simply defined, it is a combination of malaise, fatigue, derangement of the sleep–wake cycle, and poor performance, which occurs when travelers cross several time zones rapidly and attempt to follow the time schedule of the new destination.

Physiology

The condition known as jet lag is due primarily to the forced recalibration of the body's natural clock, or circadian rhythms. 'Circadian rhythms' are those innate synchronizations of physiologic processes to natural time cycles, which occur in all animals. These rhythms are present at the cellular level, so that periodicity of firing can be observed in dissected neurons from the suprachiasmatic nuclei of neonatal animals.[1]

In most mammalian species circadian rhythms are synchronized with the 24 h duration of the earth's rotation and the associated pattern of day and night. The suprachiasmatic nucleus (SCN) of the hypothalamus acts as the primary internal timekeeper and cycles on a schedule which is close to, but usually not exactly, 24 hours long. Any dyssynchrony of the schedule of the SCN with the 24-hour environmental cycle is corrected on a daily basis by signals from the environment (*zeitgebers*), including light, food availability, activity, and social cues, in a process called entrainment. It has recently been recognized that 'clock genes' in other parts of the brain and in peripheral organs also create cycles which are coordinated with each other and the environment by the SCN.[2]

Light, specifically outside daylight, is the major cue for the adjustment of the SCN's 'internal clock' in humans. This clock regulates the release of melatonin, the secretion of which is associated with sleepiness. Darkness is also required for the secretion of melatonin; daylight levels of light suppress the release of melatonin from the pineal gland. Furthermore, melatonin also provides feedback to the SCN, thereby controlling its own production and contributing to the modulation of other circadian variables.[3] Other rhythms that appear to be controlled by the SCN are diurnal variations in body temperature and the release of cortisol and growth hormone.[4] A circadian rhythm of cortisol secretion has been identified in infants from the time of birth.[5]

When a traveler crosses several time zones, or meridians, in a short timespan, these circadian rhythms initially continue to operate on the 'home' schedule. The process of re-entrainment takes a certain amount of time, generally agreed to be approximately 1 day per time zone crossed. During this period the traveler experiences what is known as jet lag, or circadian dyssynchronism. Typically, after eastward travel it is difficult to fall asleep at the new bedtime, and consequently very difficult to arise in the morning; after westward travel the main complaint is waking in the early hours of the morning. The result is lost total sleep time as well as sleep irregularity. For most persons, westward travel results in less dysynchronism than eastward because the SCN cycle of most persons, without entrainment from zeitgebers, is bit longer than 24 hours.[6] In addition, there is evidence that the mild hypoxia resulting from the incomplete pressurization of transoceanic aircraft (typically equivalent to an altitude of 8000–12 000 ft) results

DOI: 10.1016/B978-1-4557-1076-8.00042-9

Table 42.1 Behavioral Methods of Adjusting Circadian Rhythm

Method	Pros	Cons	Efficacy
Sleep schedule	Inexpensive, easily available	Inconvenient, especially for longer time changes	Good, if able to achieve adjustment
Sunlight exposure	Inexpensive, easily available	Requires scheduling	Good
Phototherapy	Convenient	Some devices are bulky, expensive	Good
Exercise	Inexpensive, easily available Other health benefits	Requires scheduling, effort	Inconclusive data
Diet	Inexpensive, easily available	Inconvenient, requires careful planning	Recent studies suggest little benefit

in reduced nocturnal melatonin secretion, and may therefore contribute to the fatigue and other symptoms of jet lag.[7] Contributing to the 'jet lag syndrome' are the conditions that are often associated with preparing for and undertaking long-distance travel. Stress, lack of sleep, culture shock, and the interruption of regular mealtimes and exercise routines may increase the traveler's sense of discomfort and disorientation. There is some disagreement about the extent to which dehydration occurs during a long flight, but certainly reduced mobility and less-than-spacious seating can be a factor. In addition, travelers often indulge in excessive alcohol and/or caffeine, both of which may compound the effects of jet lag.

The consequences of the jet lag syndrome extend beyond the loss of vacation time for pleasure-seeking travelers. The decline in cognitive and athletic function has obvious consequences for politicians, diplomats, soldiers, businesspeople, and professional athletes.

Effects

The most obvious evidence of jet lag for most travelers is inability to sleep during destination night and remain alert during destination day. Additional symptoms include headache, gastrointestinal complaints, clumsiness, irritability, difficulty concentrating, and reduction in cognitive and athletic functioning. Individuals vary considerably in their susceptibility to these symptoms. Studies in shift workers, who suffer repeated episodes of dyssynchrony, suggest more severe consequences, including increased rates of cancer, cardiovascular disease, and female reproductive problems.[8] Jet lag tends to be worse for older travelers, while infants appear to be less affected. Not surprisingly, the symptoms increase with the number of time zones crossed; as mentioned above, eastward travel is usually more problematic than westward.

Treatments

A multitude of therapeutic interventions have been promoted to reduce or eliminate jet lag, with varying degrees of scientific evidence to support them. The best studies use clearly defined measures of cognitive performance and functioning, but the protocols vary among investigators. In 2007, the American Academy of Sleep Medicine

published guidelines on the management and treatment of circadian rhythm disorders based on peer-reviewed published literature through October 2007,[9] and the degree to which the following management approaches are recommended by the guidelines will be noted in the following discussion. Strategies to reduce the effects of jet lag can be classified according to their ability to achieve one or more of three goals: resetting the internal 'clock', promoting sleep at destination bedtime, and promoting alertness during destination day. Behavioral methods of adjusting circadian rhythm are summarized in Table 42.1.

Resetting the Clock

Pre-Travel Sleep Schedule Adjustment

Many travelers find it useful to attempt adjusting their sleep and awakening times by an hour per day for several days before travel in an attempt to coincide with destination time. This approach is recommended as an option for travelers by the AASM guidelines. Obviously this approach carries little risk, but it does require considerable diligence on the part of the traveler. As noted below, pre-travel sleep schedule adjustment can be combined with light therapy to try to increase the effect.

Sleep Schedule on Arrival

Planning sleep times on arrival is also important. An overall sleep deficit is common in travelers, due to pre-travel preparations, stress, and loss of sleep during transit. Short daytime naps of 45 min or less may be surprisingly helpful in maintaining alertness,[10] and may be most beneficial at the time which would be the body's temperature nadir (~4 am home time). Longer naps can be beneficial, but should be scheduled so as not to delay the adjustment of the internal clock. If traveling westward, it is preferable to delay sleeping until bedtime at the destination. It is generally felt to be more difficult to advance sleeping time when traveling eastward. In fact, for eastward travel over more than nine time zones, the body's response is often to delay the internal clock rather than advance it, as if a longer westward shift had occurred. Travelers may find themselves more easily able to adjust to a new time zone after traveling eastward, for example over 10 time zones, if they plan their sleep recalibration to delay the body clock by 14 hours rather than try to advance it by 10 hours.

Light Therapy

It is clear that light exposure is the strongest stimulus to circadian re-entrainment in mammals, including humans.[4] Deliberate exposure to bright light at the appropriate time can therefore help to speed the resolution of circadian dyssynchronism. The efficacy of this approach depends on timing the light exposure around the nadir of the body temperature, which typically occurs at about 4–5 am home time. Hence bright light in the internal clock's morning will cause a phase advance, and bright light in the evening will cause a phase delay. An eastward traveler should therefore seek light in the morning (05:00–11:00 h), and a westward traveler in the evening (22:00–04:00 h), based on home time. Exposure to bright light should be avoided at times that will produce a phase shift opposite in direction to what is desired, and judicious use of sunglasses may be helpful. For travelers passing more than eight or so time zones, the above recommendations for light exposure might, for example, result in morning light actually causing a phase delay if the light exposure occurs prior to the home time nadir of the body temperature. Light avoidance may be necessary for the first few days in order to prevent re-entrainment in the wrong direction.[11] Some studies have found that prior to travel, circadian rhythms can be successfully advanced with a combination of advancing sleep schedules by 1 hour per day in conjunction with exposure to early morning bright light. Attempting to advance by 2 hours per day was less successful.[12]

For most travelers, sunlight will provide an adequate light source. Even on a cloudy day, daylight is much brighter than most inside lighting. However, although early studies indicated that only bright levels of light similar to daylight were adequate to affect the internal clock, there is now evidence to suggest that even lower levels of light, such as those in offices and homes, may also play a role in resynchronization.[13] More interestingly, a study at Cornell showed that the application of a 3-hour pulse of light behind the knee to subjects otherwise kept in low ambient light succeeded in generating a phase response of up to 3 hours over a 4-day period compared to controls, suggesting a response to extrapineal and extraocular light sensors.[14] However, this study has not been replicated and extraocular light exposure is not mentioned in the AASM guidelines.

A number of commercial products are also available to help travelers use light exposure to adjust to a new time zone. Computer programs to create the appropriate exposure schedule and caps that shine light on the eyes both have their adherents. A quick internet search using 'light therapy' or 'phototherapy' will reveal multiple sources for phototherapy aids. To what extent such devices are practical for travelers or an improvement over natural light sources is unclear. One study found that although a head-mounted light visor providing either bright white or dim red light resulted in a circadian shift as measured by salivary dim light melatonin onset, this effect was not accompanied by any improvement in jet lag symptoms or improvements in sleep or performance.[15] The AAMS guidelines do not specifically endorse any product.

Diet

Adjustment of diet has been recommended by some researchers for amelioration of jet lag. One technique which has been described is a 'feast then fast' strategy, alternating days of high caloric intake with days of fasting for the 4 days prior to departure. The hypothesis behind this diet plan is that high-protein meals increase tyrosine concentrations, promoting an increase in the levels of norepinephrine and dopamine, therefore increasing alertness. High-carbohydrate meals elevate tryptophan concentrations, resulting in higher serotonin levels, thought to have a role in sleep regulation and acting as a precursor to melatonin. Hence high-protein breakfasts and high-carbohydrate dinners are recommended. Formal research has not confirmed the efficacy of this diet. A study in military reservists suggested good efficacy, but that study was hampered by lack of blinding and self-selection of participants, so the placebo effect may have played a significant role.[16] This approach is not mentioned in the AASM guidelines.

Exercise

For some individuals, vigorous exercise after arrival is helpful in alleviating jet lag. Experiments in hamsters have suggested that exercise can help adjust the internal clock, but its true effect on humans is less clear.[17] Exercise is not mentioned in the AAMS guidelines. Exercise may help by forcing a state of alertness, promoting more restful sleep, or by actually inducing arousal in the central nervous system and affecting the suprachiasmatic nuclei.

Melatonin – as Resetting the Clock

Endogenous melatonin is secreted normally in a regular rhythm coinciding with nighttime, from approximately 21:00 h to 08:00 h. The hormone appears to directly affect the internal clock, thereby altering other circadian rhythms. Among these is the temperature rhythm: melatonin has a temperature-lowering effect. The ingestion of exogenous melatonin appears to help induce sleep and to induce a phase

shift. There is also an apparent hypnotic effect of melatonin, the mechanism of which is not completely clear, but may be due to its action in lowering temperature, resetting the internal clock, and/or other mechanisms. Blind persons, who have what is termed 'free-running' circadian rhythms which tend to oscillate on a schedule slightly longer than 24 h, often have sleep disorders. Melatonin has been found to help 'reset' these rhythms and reduce sleep problems in some blind persons.[18] The drug has been evaluated for the alleviation of symptoms of jet lag, and in most studies appears to show some benefit.[11,19] A Cochrane review, which included a meta-analysis of four randomized trials as well as reviews of other literature, concluded that melatonin will help one out of two adults reduce the symptoms of jet lag. Doses between 0.5 and 5 mg appear to be equally effective in reducing daytime sleepiness, although the hypnotic effect may be stronger with the higher doses. Taking the drug before the travel date did not seem to confer any benefit.[20]

As with light exposure, when using melatonin to induce a phase shift, the timing of ingestion must be scheduled to advance or delay the internal clock appropriately.[13] The optimal dose amount and dosing regimen have not been determined. Most studies have focused on eastward travel, with a dose given at bedtime for several days after arrival to cause a phase advance. Another recommendation suggests that the timing of melatonin ingestion for a situation where phase advance is desired would be 1 hour earlier each day until 15:00 home time is reached, by which time no further adjustment should be necessary. For a phase delay melatonin would be taken 1 hour later each day until the dose falls at 06:00 home time. However, for westward travelers melatonin at bedtime may not confer much benefit; melatonin administration after endogenous release has already occurred may not have much effect.[11] Regarding the amount to give, a dose of 2–5 mg is typically recommended, although doses of from 0.5 to 8 mg have been used and appear to be similarly effective. A 2 mg controlled-release formulation was shown to be less effective than even the lower-dose immediate-release formulation.[21] Agomelatine is a melatonin agonist in development which may also be effective in promoting phase shift and has been evaluated in older adults, who are more susceptible to jet lag.[22]

Combining melatonin with phototherapy may potentiate the phase-shifting effects. A combination of afternoon melatonin with early morning light exposure was shown to be effective in advancing circadian rhythm by 1 hour per day over a 3-day treatment period.[23] Some authors propose carefully calculated adjustment of both light exposure and melatonin administration, based on the direction and extent of time zones crossed.[11,24]

Getting to Sleep (see Table 42.2)

Melatonin – in Getting to Sleep

As has been mentioned, not only does melatonin have an effect upon the circadian clock, it has a direct hypnotic effect. It has been compared in a clinical trial with midazolam for pre-operative premedication and found to confer anxiolysis and sedation without affecting the quality of recovery, whereas the midazolam caused some degree of impairment of cognitive and psychomotor skills.[25] A study on travelers flying from the USA to Switzerland showed that zolpidem was more effective in promoting sleep than melatonin (which was more effective than placebo), but again, more side-effects were noted with the zolpidem and almost none with melatonin.[26] However, at least one study showed adverse effects on vigilance and mental performance after doses of melatonin if the subjects were not allowed to sleep.[27]

Melatonin is sold as an unregulated herbal supplement in the USA and Hong Kong. As such, it has not been formally studied for safety,

Table 42.2 Pharmacologic Options for Jet Lag Therapy

Product	Action	Side-Effects	Availability
Melatonin	Induces sleep, resets circadian clock	Inappropriate drowsiness may occur	Over the counter in USA, Hong Kong and perhaps elsewhere; by prescription only in Europe and Canada; further restrictions may exist in some countries
Sedatives	Induce sleep	Inappropriate drowsiness, 'hangover', addictive potential	By prescription
Caffeine	Promotes alertness	Jitteriness, hypertension, tachycardia, dependence, may prevent normal sleep	Easily available in various over-the counter forms
Armodafinil, modafinil	Promotes alertness without interfering with sleep	Slow onset of action, many drug interactions	By prescription
Amphetamines	Promote alertness	May reduce decision-making capability; hypertension, tachycardia, addictive potential, may prevent normal sleep	By prescription
Nicotinamide	Promotes alertness, mental clarity, though very limited data	Few reported	Available over the counter as a nutritional supplement (NADH)

especially with long-term use, and the standards and quality of available preparations are uncontrolled. However, in the many years in which melatonin has been in common use in the United States, the medical literature reveals little evidence of adverse events. Based on its apparent safety and the relatively large amount of supportive efficacy data, the use of melatonin receives the strongest recommendation of any intervention for jet lag by the AAMS.[9]

In many European countries and in Canada, the use of melatonin is strictly regulated or entirely prohibited. In some cases the importation of even small amounts for personal use may be illegal. Healthcare providers and travelers should check local regulations before recommending or transporting melatonin.

Sedatives

Sedatives such as benzodiazepines can be used to help induce sleep at the appropriate hour in the new time zone but may cause residual drowsiness on awakening. The shorter-acting sedatives, such as zolpidem or temazepam, are less likely to produce such a 'hangover', but certain individuals will have untoward effects.[26] Whether the sedatives have any specific effect on the internal clock remains unclear. GABA type A receptors exist in the suprachiasmatic nuclei, so benzodiazepines may have some direct effect, but animal studies are inconclusive and there are no data on humans. Concern has been raised over the use of any sedative while still on a plane, as a sedated sleeper may be less mobile and more prone to deep venous thrombosis (the same, of course, applies to alcohol). The AAMS guidelines recommend the short-term use of sedatives as optional, with cautions that side-effects are a concern and that although sleep onset is improved, there is no evidence to support improvement of daytime symptoms of jet lag.

Staying Awake (See Table 42.2)

Stimulants
Caffeine

Caffeine clearly has the ability to promote alertness and delay sleep. It does, however, have just as clearly recognized side-effects, including tachycardia and the development of a degree of dependence (resulting in the development of the 'caffeine withdrawal headache' upon

discontinuation). As caffeine is also a diuretic, there are concerns that over-consumption of the stimulant may promote dehydration, even when taken as a drink. Heart arrhythmias have been reported in some cases. Caffeine is the only stimulant which is discussed by the AAMS guidelines as an option for the treatment of daytime jet lag symptoms, with the caution that it may disrupt sleep and that its use should be monitored.[9] Long-acting pharmaceutical preparations of caffeine are available for those who do not enjoy the beverages. The long-acting preparation has been shown to be effective, but may affect sleep quality.[28]

Amphetamines

Amphetamines are effective in promoting alertness, but there remain concerns about their addictive potential and capacity for abuse. There is also some evidence that amphetamines may reduce decision-making ability and psychomotor performance, rather than enhance it.[13] Although they have been studied by the military, they are not currently recommended.

Modafinil and Armodafinil

Modafinil, and its longer-acting isomer armodafinil, are non-amphetamine stimulants approved for the treatment of narcolepsy and sleepiness due to shift work disorder and sleep apnea. Their action involves the presynaptic activation of dopamine transmission in promoting wakefulness and the amplification of cortical serotonin release.[29,30] They appear to have minimal side-effects, low abuse potential, and do not interfere with normal sleep. Modafinil has been used therapeutically in patients with narcolepsy for several years without the development of tolerance, and has been investigated by the military.[31] It has also been shown to have memory-enhancing effects.[32] The drugs have a slow onset of action and a fairly long half-life; they also have significant interactions with other medications, including anti-seizure medications, some cardiac medications, and oral contraceptives. However, the safety profile appears to be good. Armodafinil has been studied specifically for jet lag and appears to have efficacy,[33] but has not been FDA approved for that indication. Of note, pharmacokinetic studies show that the elderly develop higher plasma concentrations of the drug, so although the rate of side-effects was not increased, caution may be warranted.[34]

NADH

Nicotinamide adenine dinucleotide (NADH) is a co-enzyme required for the production of energy in cells. Its effects include the stimulation of dopamine, noradrenaline, and serotonin receptors, by which mechanism it is thought to increase mental alertness and clarity and improve concentration. In small preliminary studies it has been investigated for jet lag as well as Alzheimer's, Parkinson's, and chronic fatigue syndrome. In the jet lag study, subjects who received NADH had significantly better cognitive performance and a trend toward reduced sleepiness on the first post-flight day than controls, and a smaller pilot study showed similar trends lasting through the second day.[35] A stabilized form for oral consumption is marketed as a nutritional supplement, and therefore, like melatonin, is not under FDA regulation.

Conclusion

Jet lag is an essentially unavoidable consequence of rapid travel, and there are no highly effective therapies, although several management strategies appear to confer some benefit. The prepared traveler will plan the journey with the expectation of having to make some accommodations for this condition. Most experts recommend ensuring adequate sleep for the several nights prior to travel, given that some sleep deficit is almost sure to occur after arrival. Immediately resetting one's watch to destination time upon boarding the plane for a flight across several time zones may provide an additional mental cue to adjust sleep and eating times. During the flight, moderation is recommended with regard to food, alcohol, and caffeine, and of course the respective sedative and stimulating effects of the latter two must be kept in mind when trying to adjust sleep patterns. For many, taking flights that arrive at destination bedtime is a helpful maneuver. Schedules for work or play for the first few days after arrival should be devised taking into account the internal clock's home 'night' and 'day'; important meetings or performances should if possible be scheduled at the time of maximal alertness, or delayed until the traveler has adjusted. For very short trips it may be easier to remain on home time rather than attempt to adjust. For longer trips in which no important activities are scheduled for the first several days, a few days of decreased performance may not be an issue.

Whether or not to use more specific therapeutic interventions such as those outlined above will depend on the traveler's needs and itinerary. Of note, of the above therapies, the AAMS guidelines give their strongest recommendation to the use of melatonin as a standard therapy based on high levels of evidence. Adjustment of sleep schedules, light therapy, the use of caffeine, and the short-term use of hypnotics are considered 'options', based on inconclusive or conflicting evidence or expert opinion.[9] Other stimulants, homeopathic remedies, and diet therapy are not addressed. The use of interventions, especially pharmacologic compounds, that have not been rigorously studied should be considered only with careful attention to the safety of the product and potential side-effects. Most travelers will find it useful to consider the possible approaches and select or modify those therapies that will fit their personal requirements.

References

1. Hastings M. The brain, circadian rhythms, and clock genes. BMJ 1998;317(7174):1704–7.
2. Kyriacou CP, Hastings M. Circadian clocks: genes, sleep, and cognition. Trends Cogn Sci 2010;14(6):259–67.
3. Arendt J. Melatonin and the Mammalian Pineal Gland. London: Chapman & Hall; 1995.
4. Sack RL. The pathophysiology of jet lag. Travel Med Infect Dis 2009;7:102–10.
5. Seron-Ferre M, Riffo R, Valenzuela GJ, et al. Twenty-four-hour pattern of cortisol in the human fetus at term. Am J Obstet Gynecol 2001;184(6):1278–83.
6. Wever RA. Light effects on human circadian rhythms: a review of recent Andechs experiments. J Biol Rhythms 1989;4(2):161–85.
7. Coste O, Beaumont M, Batejat D, et al. Hypoxic depression of melatonin secretion after simulated long duration flights in man. J Pineal Res 2004;37(1):1–10.
8. Mahoney MM. Shift work, jet lag, and female reproduction. Int J Endocrinol 2010; Article ID 813764, 9 pages. Epub 2010, March 8.
9. Morgenthaler TI, Lee-Chiong T, Alessi C, et al. Practice parameters for the clinical evaluation and treatment of circadian rhythm sleep disorders. Sleep, 2007;30:1445–59.
10. Naitoh P, Kelly TL, Babkoff H. Napping, stimulant, and four-choice performance. In: Broughton RJ, Ogilvie RD, editors. Sleep, Arousal, and Performance: Problems and Promises. Cambridge, MA: Birk Hauser Boston; 1992. p. 198–219.
11. Sack RL. Jet lag. N Engl J Med 2010;362:440–7.
12. Eastman CI, Gazda CJ, Burgess HJ, et al. Advancing circadian rhythms before eastward flight: a strategy to prevent or reduce jet lag. Sleep 2005 Jan 1;28(1):33–44.
13. Waterhouse J, Reilly T, Atkinson G. Jet-lag. Lancet 1997;350(9091):1611–6.
14. Campbell SS, Murphy PJ. Extraocular circadian phototransduction in humans. Science 1998;279(5349):396–9.
15. Boulos Z, Macchi MM, Sturchler MP, et al. Light visor treatment for jet lag after westward travel across six time zones. Aviat Space Environ Med 2002 Oct;73(10):953–63.
16. Reynolds NC, Montgomery R. Using the Argonne diet in jet lag prevention: deployment of troops across nine time zones. Mil Med 2002;167(6):451–3.
17. Reebs S, Mrosovsky N. Effects of induced wheel-running on the circadian activity rhythm of Syrian hamsters: entrainment and phase-response curve. J Biol Rhythms 1994;4:39–48.
18. Sack RL, Brandes RW, Kendall AR, et al. Entrainment of free-running circadian rhythms by melatonin in blind people. N Engl J Med 2000;343(15):1070–7.
19. Brzezinski A. Mechanisms of disease: melatonin in humans. N Engl J Med 1997;336(3):186–95.
20. Herxheimer A, Petrie KJ. Melatonin for the prevention and treatment of jet lag. The Cochrane Library, Copyright 2005, The Cochrane Collaboration Volume (4), 2005.
21. Suhner A, Schlagenhauf P, Johnson R, et al. Comparative study to determine the optimal melatonin dosage form for the alleviation of jet lag. Chronobiol Int 1998;15:655–66.
22. Leproult R, Van Onderbergen A, L'hermite-Baleriaux M, et al. Phase-shifts of 24-h rhythms of hormonal release and body temperature following early evening administration of the melatonin agonist agomelatine in healthy older men. Clin Endocrinol 2005 Sep;63(3):298–304.
23. Revell VL, Burgess HJ, Gazda CJ, et al. Advancing human circadian rhythms with afternoon melatonin and morning intermittent bright light. J Clin Endocrinol Metabol 2006 Jan;91(1):54–9.
24. Kolla BO, Augur RR. Jet lag and shift work sleep disorders: how to help reset the internal clock. Cleve Clin J Med 2011 Oct;78(10):675–84.
25. Naguib M, Samarkandi AH. The comparative dose-response effects of melatonin and midazolam for premedication of adult patients: a double-blinded, placebo-controlled study. Anesth Analg 2000;91(2):473–9.
26. Suhner A, Schlagenhauf P, Hofer I, et al. Effectiveness and tolerability of melatonin and zolpidem for the alleviation of jet lag. Aviat Space Environ Med 2001;72:638–46.
27. Zhdanova I, Wurtman R, Lynch H, et al. Sleep inducing effects of low doses of melatonin ingested in the evening. Clin Pharm Ther 1995;57:552–8.
28. Beaumont M, Batejat D, Pierard C, et al. Caffeine or melatonin effects on sleep and sleepiness after rapid eastward transmeridian travel. J Applied Physiol 2004 Jan;96(1):50–8.
29. Nishino S, Mao J, Sampathkumaran R, et al. Increased dopaminergic transmissin mediates the wake-promoting effects of CNS stimulants. Sleep Res Online 1998;1(1):49–61.

30. Ferraro L, Fuxe K, Tnaganelli S, et al. Amplification of cortical serotonin release: a further neurochemical action of the vigilance-promoting drug modafinil. Neuropharmacology 2000;39(11): 1974–83.

31. Lyons TJ, French J. Modafinil: the unique properties of a new stimulant. Aviat Space Environ Med 1991;62(5):432–5.

32. Turner DC, Robbins TW, Clark L, et al. Cognitive enhancing effects of modafinil in healthy volunteers. Psychopharmacology (Berl) 2003 Jan;165(3):260–9.

33. Rosenberg RP, et al. A Phase 3, double-blind, randomized, placebo-controlled study of armodafinil for excessive sleepiness associated with jet lag disorder. Mayo Clin Proc 2010;85(7):630–8.

34. Darwish M, Kirby M, Hellriegel ET, et al. Systemic exposure to armodafinil and its tolerability in healthy elderly versus young men. Drugs Aging 2011;28(2):139–50.

35. Birkmayer GD, Kay GG, Vurre E. [Stabilized NADH (ENADA) improves jet lag-induced cognitive performance deficit]. [German] Wien Med Wochenschr 2002;152(17–18):450–4.

Motion Sickness

Susan M. Kuhn and Beth Lange

Key points

- In most people, if there is sustained motion (as on a cruise ship), habituation will occur in 3–4 days
- Women are more likely to suffer from motion sickness, particularly around menses and during pregnancy
- Young children and the elderly are less likely to suffer from motion sickness
- Acupressure has not been shown to be effective in the prevention or treatment of motion sickness
- In general, anti-motion sickness medications are more effective if taken prior to exposure; a major adverse event is drowsiness

Introduction

To travel is to move – so what condition is potentially more relevant to the traveler than motion sickness? In fact, virtually anyone can suffer from this malady, given the right – or more accurately the *wrong* – circumstances. The frequency and severity vary, but for some travelers the impact is significant and may ruin a long-awaited and expensive holiday. The secret is to 'be prepared.' The travel health professional must gather sufficient information about an individual's general health, motion susceptibility, and trip itinerary to identify situations in which motion sickness will be a potential risk. For some travelers, counseling on the topic may consist of suggesting the inclusion of an anti-motion sickness medication in a medical kit. For others who will be sailing to the Antarctic, crossing the Sahara on camel-back, or for the scuba-diver with severe motion sensitivity, discussing preventive and treatment strategies may be an important component of the pre-travel consultation. Therefore, it is essential that the travel health professional has a clear understanding of motion sickness and how it can be prevented or treated.

Triggers of Motion Sickness

Motion sickness results from exposure to movement or visual suggestion of movement.[1] Traveling through water, on land, and in air may all trigger motion sickness, although seasickness is the most common and notorious form of this condition. Provocative environments include a variety of mechanical vehicles, such as ships, planes, cars, buses, trains, carnival rides, and spinning chairs. Tilting trains in Europe have been a recent addition to the list of problematic transportation.[2] Riding on the back of an animal can also be a powerful stimulus, particularly those that cause a lot of swaying or rocking (e.g., camels). Self-propelled motion such as gymnastics or downhill skiing during white-out conditions, or even motion in a state of weightlessness during spaceflight or floating in water, may also be a trigger. Scuba-diving or snorkeling in rough water, for example, results in turbulent movement in the absence of both the orienting influence of gravity and a visual frame of reference. Luckily, sustained exposure to constant motion over 3–4 days results in habituation in most individuals.[3] Habituation is thought to be the result of central nervous system compensation, but the exact mechanism has yet to be elucidated. Unfortunately, this tolerance is lost within a similar time frame if the motion stops or changes.

Similar symptoms can also result when the movement to which the person has adapted suddenly stops – a kind of 'anti-motion' sickness. The most common example is the transient 'landsickness' sometimes experienced after disembarking from a ship. An unusual and persistent condition known as *mal de débarquement* syndrome (MDD) is literally an 'illness of disembarkment'. Those who suffer from MDD are usually asymptomatic during the journey, which may include travel by ship, train, or even in space. Symptoms of this form of post-motion vertigo include a sense of disequilibrium along with sensations of swaying or rocking, lasting from a month to years. Recent data suggest that those who are prone to MDD may have an overreliance on the somatosensory system for balance relative to vestibular and visual inputs.[4] MDD that does not typically respond to first-line anti-motion sickness medications[5] may respond to benzodiazepines or selective serotonin reuptake inhibitors (SSRIs).[6]

Visual suggestion of movement when the individual is stationary is an equally strong trigger for motion sickness. 'Vection', or illusory self-motion, is created with rotating drums around a stationary patient for laboratory studies.[6] It is also encountered in many real-life situations such as flight simulators, computer games, and movies (e.g., often prompted by sitting close to the screen or three-dimensional films).

What is Motion Sickness?

Motion sickness typically consists of a progression of symptoms.[1] The individual initially feels a vague abdominal discomfort sometimes

©2012 Elsevier Inc
DOI: 10.1016/B978-1-4557-1076-8.00043-0

referred to as 'stomach awareness', followed by malaise and nausea which may culminate in vomiting. These gastrointestinal symptoms are associated with measurable changes in gastric muscle activity. Electrogastrography (EGG) in laboratory settings reveals increased and/or un-coordinated muscle activity known as gastric tachyarrhythmia.[7]

In addition to these gastrointestinal effects, other symptoms may include a sense of body warmth, lightheadedness, tachypnea, sighing, yawning, headache, drowsiness, increased salivation, and frequent swallowing. Pallor and sweating is often observed.[1] Lethargy, fatigue and mental slowness that persists after resolution of the gastrointestinal symptoms in some patients has been labeled the 'Sopite syndrome'. Electroencephalography (EEG) monitoring reveals slowing of α waves over the frontal areas for about 2 hours after severe motion sickness, and correlates with this drowsiness and loss of performance.[8]

Who is Likely to Get Motion Sickness?

Although motion sickness can occur in virtually anyone given sufficiently rough conditions, a small proportion of the population is highly resistant while a similar number are very susceptible. In the latter group this tendency does not seem to decrease with exposure.[9] The condition is also related to gender and age, and may be influenced by other personal and environmental factors. Women are more likely than men to suffer,[10] particularly near menses and during pregnancy, suggesting a hormonal influence. Symptoms such as nausea and vomiting are uncommon in children under the age of 2, but susceptibility increases thereafter until about 12–15 years of age, and then declines steadily and is least common among the elderly.[10] Those who suffer from migraine headaches are more likely to be sensitive to motion. Persons with an inner ear disturbance, especially a recent one, may be more intolerant of movement in general. Persons with rare, central nervous system disorders of the part of the brain that processes signals from the inner ear may also be unusually susceptible to motion sickness. Other underlying conditions or medications that cause nausea may mimic or increase the severity of motion sickness as well.

What is the Mechanism of Motion Sickness?

'Motion sickness' is a normal response to an abnormal stimulus, namely conflicting information from the sensory systems that detect and interpret motion with respect to one's surroundings.[11] Contributing input comes from the vestibular, proprioceptive, and visual systems, although past experience or memory of motion sickness may also influence this reaction. Individuals can suffer as a result of a visual perception of movement in the absence of a corresponding vestibular sensation, or when there is a sensation of body movement with contradictory visual cues. Processing of this sensory input occurs in the central nervous system, and results in a complex physical response via the autonomic nervous system.

The Vestibular System

Studies comparing persons with normal vestibular systems with those who have bilateral peripheral vestibular deficiencies (e.g., labyrinthectomy) clearly show the inability of the latter to suffer motion sickness.[12] On the other hand, blindness does not confer immunity against the condition. Therefore, it appears that a functioning vestibular system is probably essential for the development of motion sickness. Different types of real or perceived movement may trigger motion sickness, including both linear and angular head acceleration. A very powerful stimulus combines these movements with rotation around a vertical axis and movement in the sagittal plane, known as the Coriolis effect.[1]

The vestibular or balance system works to maintain the physical self in appropriate alignment with the earth (gravity) and to respond to changes in position in space. The semicircular canals and the vestibule are contiguous and filled with a fluid called endolymph (Fig. 43.1). The three semicircular canals are perpendicular to each other; rotational movement in any direction can be detected as the endolymph shifts and stimulates ciliae of the ampullae of the appropriate canal(s) (Fig. 43.2). Hence the semicircular canals provide information about non-linear acceleration. The vestibule is a fluid-filled space occupied by two sensory membranes perpendicular to each other called the utricle and the saccule. The membrane surfaces are made up of hair cells covered by a gelatinous layer in which microscopic particles (otoliths) are embedded. The mass of the latter can be affected by linear movements as well as by gravity in the absence of motion. Therefore, the signals from the utricle and saccule provide information with respect to head orientation as well as detecting linear acceleration in those planes (Fig. 43.3).[1]

The central physiology of motion sickness is less clear, but appears to involve a complex interplay between all levels of the brain and vestibular, visual, proprioceptive, and autonomic centers (Fig. 43.4). This may explain why medications with a variety of mechanisms of action can ameliorate symptoms.[8] Along with the clinical symptoms resembling an adrenalin-like 'fight or flight' response, there is laboratory evidence of sympathetic nervous system and sympathoadrenal–medullary system activation. Both epinephrine and norepinephrine levels rise in subjects reporting motion sickness. Cortisol and β-endorphin levels do not rise but are elevated at baseline prior to exposure to the stimulus in those who develop motion sickness, possibly suggesting anticipation based on past experience.[7]

Non-Medicinal Prevention and Treatment Options

Most environmental preventive approaches have had little evaluation to determine efficacy, particularly in real-life situations. Positioning oneself in the most stable part of the vehicle is commonly recommended, and while it may benefit in some situations, it has been shown to have little impact in severe conditions.[13] Exaggerated movement of the head and upper body appears to be strongly linked to symptoms, possibly greater in certain planes of movement than in others. If the person is firmly restrained across the upper body, motion sensitivity is reduced or prevented.[10] Assuming a recumbent position presumably has a similar ameliorating or preventive effect and is commonly advised. Minimizing conflicting visual input is another strategy found useful by those who suffer motion sickness, including avoidance of fixation on close objects (such as reading), and instead focusing on a distant point. Although consumption of large meals or certain foods, drinking alcohol, and exposure to poor ventilation or noxious odors have been noted to increase the risk, data to confirm some of these claims are contradictory or sparse. One simple intervention that appears to have some impact in mildly nauseogenic motion is that of controlled breathing, consisting of a natural, comfortable breathing rate and depth, principally through the nose. Subjects reported reduction in nausea, a longer tolerance of motion before nausea occurred, and a shorter recovery time after motion stopped.[14] Personal experience with exacerbating and relieving factors may prove to be the most useful guide for individual travelers.

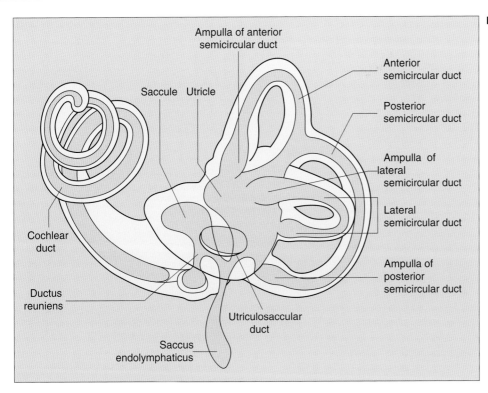

Figure 43.1 Anatomy of the Labyrinth.

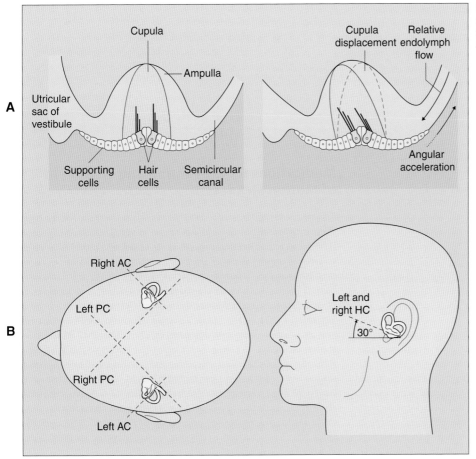

Figure 43.2 The Crista. **(A)** Organ of crista of semicircular canals. **(B)** Orientation of semicircular canals in skull. HC, horizontal canal; AC, anterior canal; PC, posterior canal.

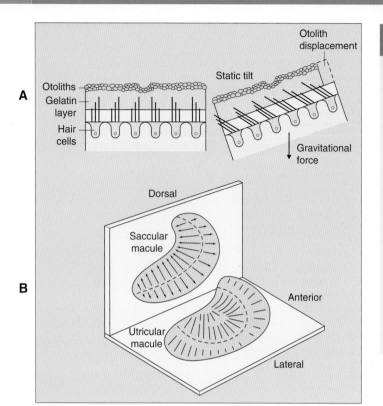

A

Otoliths
Gelatin layer
Hair cells

Static tilt

Otolith displacement

Gravitational force

B

Dorsal

Saccular macule

Anterior

Utricular macule

Lateral

Figure 43.3 **(A)** Macule within saccule and utricle. **(B)** Orientation of saccule and utricle in skull.

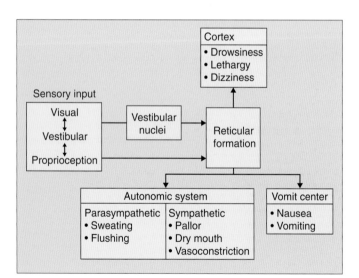

Cortex
• Drowsiness
• Lethargy
• Dizziness

Sensory input

Visual
⇅
Vestibular
⇅
Proprioception

Vestibular nuclei

Reticular formation

Autonomic system

Parasympathetic
• Sweating
• Flushing

Sympathetic
• Pallor
• Dry mouth
• Vasoconstriction

Vomit center
• Nausea
• Vomiting

Figure 43.4 Proposed Neural Pathway Resulting in Motion Sickness.

Acupressure has been claimed to be an efficacious treatment for motion sickness and other nauseating situations. A variety of acupressure products are marketed commercially for this purpose. The theory behind wrist bands is that stimulation or pressure at the P6 or Neiguan point (located three finger-widths proximal from the wrist crease between the palmeris longus and flexor carpi radialis tendons) reduces symptoms of nausea. However, a placebo-controlled study using a commercial band as recommended suggested minimal to no impact on motion sickness, at least in males subjected to very provocative

Table 43.1 Behavioral Strategies to Prevent or Reduce Motion Sickness

Select seating in most stable area of vehicle with good visibility
    Mid-ship, near center of vessel
    Over wings of aircraft
Front seat of car, or front section of train or bus
    Minimize upper body and head movement
    Lie recumbent
    Use seat restraint
    Lean against head-rest
Maintain visual orientation
    Fix gaze on distant object or horizon
    Take over driving of car
    Close eyes
    Avoid reading
Personal adjustments
    Eat small, frequent meals
    Avoid alcohol and smoking
    Controlled breathing
    Sit in well-ventillated area or open a window
    Avoid or remove odors that exacerbate symptoms

rotational stimuli.[9] Insufficient pressure applied at this point during stimulation may explain this negative result, but also suggests the potential for incorrect use and, at best, variable results.[1] Another item proposed is a user-worn see-through display, which has been experimented with to enhance vestibular rehabilitation. This involves an eyewear-mounted visual display that projects a stable artificial horizon.[15] These are not commercially available.

Habituation has been used to successfully reduce motion sensitivity in the military.[16] A commercial home-exercise protocol (The Puma Method; www.pumamethod.com) has also been developed by a former flight surgeon, and is advocated by some clinicians, although it has not been scientifically evaluated. Therefore, additional strategies or medications should be offered for situations where motion sickness is very likely or severe (Table 43.1).

Medications for Prevention and Treatment of Motion Sickness

Unfortunately, no new medications have come into use for the prevention or treatment of motion sickness. However, in its management it is better to anticipate and prevent motion sickness rather than attempt to treat it after it occurs. There are a number of different classes of medications used for motion sickness, although many have similar central effects leading to the reduction or relief of symptoms. The chemoreceptor trigger zone and the emetic center are thought to play key roles, therefore the major categories include antihistamine (H1), anti-muscarinic, and anti-dopaminergic medications. Stimulants are sometimes added to counteract the adverse effects of the other agents. Benzodiazepines are also effective, and are believed to suppress vestibular nuclei via gamma-aminobutyric acid (GABA) receptors.[1, 17] A variety of other agents have also been studied or used empirically. Not all of the medications discussed are available in all countries, but the travel health practitioner should become familiar with other products since travelers sometimes seek out remedies in the country they are visiting (Table 43.2).

Table 43.2 Medications for the Prevention or Treatment of Motion Sickness

Drug	Oral Dose (mg)	First dose (Prophylaxis)	Dosing Interval (Hours)	Route(s) of Administration	Comments	Common Adverse Effects	Availability
Dimenhydrinate (Gravol®, Dramamine®)	Adult: 50–100 Child (yrs): >12: 50 6–12: 25–50 2–6: 12.5–25	1–2 hr prior	>12 yrs: 4–6 <12 yrs: 6–8	Oral, i.m., suppository	Not in pregnancy or < 2 yrs	Drowsiness (moderate), vertigo	US, Canada, Europe, Australia, S. Africa
Meclizine (Bonine®, Bonamine®, Antivert®)	Adult: 25–50	1–2 hr prior	12–24	Oral	Not in pregnancy	Drowsiness (mild)	US, Canada (limited), Europe
Cinnarizine (Sturgeon®)	Adult: 30 initially, 15 thereafter Child 5–12 yrs: 15 initially, 7.5 thereafter	1–2 hrs prior	6–8	Oral	Not in pregnancy. Dose < 5 yrs unknown	Drowsiness (varies)	Europe, S. Africa
Cyclizine (Marezine®, Marzine®, Valoid®)	Adult: 50 Child: 6–12 yrs: 25	1–2 hrs prior	4–6	Oral or i.m.	Not in pregnancy	Drowsiness	US (oral), Canada (i.m.)
Buclizine (Buclizin-S Softabs®)	Adult: 50 mg	1 hr prior	4–6	Oral	Not in pregnancy or children	Drowsiness	Europe
Promethazine (Phenergan®)	Adult: 25–50 Child: ≥2 yrs 0.25–0.5 mg/kg (max 25 mg)	2 hrs prior	6–12	Oral, i.m.	May be used in pregnancy. Avoid < 2 yrs	Severe drowsiness, impaired mental performance	US, Canada, Europe, Australia
Scopolamine hydrobromide (Hyoscine ®)	Adult: 0.4–0.8	1 hr prior	4–6	Oral or i.m.	Not in childhood, or with glaucoma. Avoid in elderly, with urinary obstruction, or sedatives	Dry mouth, drowsiness, blurred vision	Europe, Australia
Scopolamine (Transderm-Scop®, Transderm-V®)	Adult: 1.5 in topical form	≥ 4 hrs prior	72	Topical patch behind ear (wash hands after applying)			US, Canada, Europe, S.Africa
Lorazepam (Ativan®)	Adult: 0.5–2.0 mg	1–2 hrs prior	4–6	Sublingual, i.m., i.v.	Useful if vomiting or with MDD Syndrome	Mild drowsiness, impaired memory, addiction	US, Canada, Europe, Australia
Dextroamphetamine (Dexedrine®, Dextrostat®)	Adult: 5–10	1–2 hrs prior	8	Oral	Reserved for extreme conditions, usually in combination with other drugs	Restlessness, potential for abuse	US, Canada, Europe; illegal to prescribe for motion sickness in some areas
Ephedrine	Adult: 25–50	1–2 hrs prior	8	Oral	Less effective than dextroamphetamine but not a controlled drug	Restlessness, tachycardia	US, Canada, Europe, Australia

There are a large number of potential agents in use around the world. Examples of antihistamines include dimenhydrinate, cinnarazine, cyclizine, buclizine and meclizine. The most common phenothiazine used is promethazine, which blocks both dopamine and histamine receptors. Metoclopromide can also be used and is particularly effective in reducing gastrointestinal symptoms, although it is not indicated for motion sickness in some countries. The most common anti-muscarinic medication used is scopolamine. Benzodiazepines such as lorazepam and clonazepam are also effective.[17] Product presentations for all of these medications vary, in some cases including oral (liquid, tablets, chewables), sublingual, suppositories, topical (skin patches), and injectable formulations.

These drugs have varying degrees of adverse effects. Drowsiness is common with all, but tends to be most pronounced with dimenhydrinate, scopolamine, and promethazine. Addiction and impaired memory are potential problems with benzodiazepines.[17] For the other medications, dry mouth, blurred vision, tachycardia, headache, vertigo, restlessness, euphoria, hallucinations, constipation, urinary retention, and rash may occur. Scopolamine should be strictly avoided with conditions such as prostatic hypertrophy and glaucoma. Concomitant use of alcohol or other CNS-depressants should be avoided to prevent potentially life-threatening additive effects. These adverse effects may reduce the utility of these medications in situations where mental alertness is essential, although they may be partly counteracted by the addition of stimulants, which, for example, may be incorporated into regimens for space travel.

Avoidance of anti-motion sickness medications is usually advised in pregnancy and infancy. For the latter this may not be a frequent issue in view of their relative resistance to the effects of movement. The best option for children less than 2 years of age is probably judicious use of dimenhydrinate. On the other hand, pregnant women are at increased risk of motion sickness. If the instigating conditions cannot be avoided or modified, it may become necessary to use medication for prophylaxis or treatment. Most antihistamines, including meclizine, and dimenhydrinate are considered category B substances with no evidence of risk in humans. These, along with scopolamine, have been used safely in pregnancy.[18] A risk–benefit discussion should be undertaken to plan a course of action for the pregnant individual. Particular caution should be exercised with the elderly, in whom adverse effects such as hallucinations and confusion may be exaggerated, especially as motion sickness is less likely in this age group.

There is a plethora of studies comparing different agents with each other and with placebo. Although some studies have found certain drugs to be more efficacious than others, a 2008 study examining seven different products in field conditions found no significant differences in reported symptoms of motion sickness during a sea voyage.[19] Generally, promethazine and scopolamine are considered more effective in extreme conditions than the antihistamines. The side-effect profile is also an important guide to the selection of one class of agents over another.[8] A more recent Cochrane evaluation of 35 studies looking specifically at scopolamine and comparing it to other agents, found that it is either superior or equivalent (vs. antihistamines) as a preventive. Evidence comparing it to cinnarizine or combinations of scopolamine and ephedrine were equivocal or minimal.[20]

It is important to point out that while reduction of the symptoms of motion sickness is appealing, in doing so these medications are interfering with the normal CNS response to conflicting vestibulovisual input. As a result, adaptation is slowed, and therefore it may actually take longer to adjust to motion if medication is used than if it is not.[3]

Treatment of Established Motion Sickness

It is preferable to prevent rather than treat motion sickness; however, this may become necessary when the degree of motion is not anticipated, or if the preventive medication proves inadequate. Oral medications are often not tolerated owing to established nausea and vomiting, so alternative routes of administration are necessary. Suppositories (dimenhydrinate) and sublingual (lorazepam) are options, but in some circumstances intramuscular injections may be necessary.

Intramuscular (i.m.) dimenhydrinate is less effective than i.m. promethazine or scopolamine for treatment of motion sickness. Promethazine has a longer duration of action, but time to onset of action is slightly longer than scopolamine by this route. All three can cause marked drowsiness and decreased performance.[21] Caution must be exercised if such medications are taken after prophylactic drugs fail, given the potentially additive adverse effects.

Adjunctive, New and Experimental Agents

Other categories of medications and foods have been investigated for their utility in the prevention of motion sickness. Stimulants such as caffeine or ephedrine are sometimes combined with other agents to counter side-effects such as drowsiness. Amphetamines such as dextroamphetamine sulfate also have a direct effect on motion sickness[8] via inhibition of vestibular nuclei activity,[1] which may be synergistic when used with drugs such as scopolamine or promethazine.[22] Ginger powder has shown variable efficacy, although it may be more useful to counter the gastrointestinal rather than the central effects.[19] Similarities between the EEG activity seen in motion sickness and seizures led to the discovery that the anticonvulsant phenytoin reduces motion-induced nausea.[23] Phenytoin affects a wide variety of sites in the central nervous system, including vestibular nuclei. Blood level monitoring and potentially significant side-effects mean it has limited applications for most travelers. Potent anti-emetics such as the 5-HT3 antagonist ondansetron may prevent vomiting but not other symptoms of motion sickness.[24,25] Calcium channel antagonists such as cinnarizine (also an antihistamine) and flunarizine have been reported to be effective.[17]

Individualized Recommendations for Prevention or Treatment of Motion Sickness

Pharmacologic differences between anti-motion sickness drugs result in variable efficacy, onset, and duration of activity, as well as adverse effects. Therefore, medication selection is based on an assessment of the likelihood and severity of motion sickness, the time before it is expected to occur, the anticipated duration of exposure, as well as the traveler's underlying age and health characteristics. For some occupational travelers, efficacy must be balanced with the impact of adverse effects on job performance. In these cases, combination with sympathomimetic drugs should be considered (Table 43.3).

Conclusion

Motion sickness need not be the bane of the traveler's existence. Armed with sufficient knowledge about both the traveler and their itinerary, the travel health professional should be able to offer advice on appropriate behavioral and pharmacologic options that may prevent and/or treat motion sickness. Unfortunately, none of the pharmacologic options come without adverse effects, which may

Table 43.3 Selection of Anti-Motion Sickness Medications

Traveler	Duration of motion	Time prior to departure (for prophylaxis)	Preventive drug options	
			Mild to moderate conditions	**Moderate to severe conditions**
Healthy adult or teenager	≤6 hrs	1 hr or more	Antihistamines* or lorazepam	Promethazine ± amphetamine, dimenhydrinate, scopolamine (oral)
Healthy adult or teenager	> 6 hrs	8 hrs or more	Antihistamines or or lorazepam or scopolamine patch	Scopolamine patch, promethazine ± amphetamine, dimenhydrinate
Elderly	Any	Any	Nil	Consider antihistamine
Pregnant woman	Any	Any	See text	See text
Child 2–12 yrs	Any	1 hour or more	Meclizine, cyclizine, cinnarizine (>5 yrs), dimenhydrinate (>2 yrs)	Dimenhydrinate, promethazine
Child < 2yrs	Any	Any	Nil	Dimenhydrinate (0.5 mg/kg) if necessary

*Meclizine, cyclizine, cinnarizine, buclizine, dimenhydrinate.

significantly impair the traveler. Travel health providers need to continue to look to those investigating methods of managing nausea and vomiting in the postoperative period, during chemotherapy, and for space travel for innovative ways of handling the challenge of motion sickness.

References

1. Baloh R. Dizziness, Hearing Loss, and Tinnitus. Philadelphia: FA Davis; 1998.
2. Neimer JES, Ventre-Dominy J, Darlot C, et al. Trains with a view to sickness. Curr Biol 2001;2001(11):2.
3. Wood CDSJ, Wood MJ, Struve FA, et al. Habituation and motion sickness. J Clin Pharmacol 1994;34:7.
4. Nachum ZSA, Ietichevsky V, Ben-David J, et al. Mal de debarquement syndrome and posture: Reduced reliance on vestibular and visual cues. Laryngoscope 2004;114:6.
5. Hain RCHP, Rheinberger MA. Mal de debarquement. Arch Otolaryngol Head Neck Surg 1999;125:6.
6. Cha YHBJ, Ishiyama G, Sabatti C, et al. Clinical features and associated syndrom of mal de debarquement. J Neurol 2008;255:7.
7. Koch KLSR, Vasey MW, Seaton FJ, et al. Neuroendeocrine and gastric myoelectric responses to illusory self-motion in humans. Am J Physiol 1990;258:7.
8. Wood CDSJ, Wood MJ, Manno BR, et al. Therapeutic effects of antimotion sickness medicatons on the secondary symptoms of motion sickness. Aviat Space Environ Med 1990;61:5.
9. Warwick-Evans LAMI, Redstone SB. A double-blind placebo controlled evaluation of acupressure in the treatment of motion sickness. Aviat Space Environ Med 1991;62:13.
10. Mills KL, Griffin MJ. Effect of seating, vision and direction of horizontal oscillation on motion sickness. Aviat Space Environ Med 2000;71(10):996–1002.
11. Eyeson-Annan MPC, Brown B, Atchinson D. Visual and vestibular components of motion sickness. Aviat Space Environ Med 1996;67:8.
12. Cheung BSKHI, Money KE. Visually-induced sickness in normal and bilaterally labyrinthine-defective subjects. Aviat Space Environ Med 1991;62:5.
13. Gahlinger PM. Cabin location and the likelihood of motion sickness in cruise ship passengers. J Travel Med 2000;7:120–4.
14. Yen Pik Sang FDGJ, Gresty MA. Suppression of sickness by controlled breathing during mildly nauseogenic motion. Aviat Space Environ Med 2003;74(9):5.
15. Krueger WW. Controlling motion sickness and spatial disorientation and enhancing vestibular rehabilitation with a user-worn see-through display. Laryngoscope 2011 Jan;121(Suppl. 2):S17–35.
16. Cheung BHK. Desensitization to strong vestibular stimuli improves tolerance to simulated aircraft motion. Aviat Space Environ Med 2005;76(12):5.
17. Hain TCYD. Pharmacologic treatment of persons with dizziness. Neurol Clin 2005;23:23.
18. Carroll IDWD. Pre-travel vaccination and medical prophylaxis in the pregnant traveler. Travel Med Infect Dis 2008;6:17.
19. Schmid RST, Steffen R, Tschopp A, et al. Comparison of seven commonly-used agents for prophylaxis of seasickness. J Travel Med 1994;1:4.
20. Spinks A, Wasiak J. Scopolamine for preventing and treating motion sickness. Cochrane Database Syst Rev 2011 June 15;(167), CD002851.
21. Wood CDSJ, Wood MJ, Mims ME. Effectiveness and duration of intramuscular antimotion sickness medications. J Clin Pharmacol 1992; 32:5.
22. Dobie TGMJ. Cognitive-behavioral management of motion sickness. Aviat Space Environ Med 1994;65:20.
23. Knox GWWD, Chelen W, Ferguson R, et al. Phenytoin for motion sickness: Clinical evaluation. Laryngoscope 1994;104:5.
24. Levine MECM, Stern RM, Knox GW. The effects of serotonin (5-HT3) receptor antagonists on gastric tachyarrhythmia and the symptoms of motion sickness. Aviat Space Environ Med 2000;71:4.
25. Muth EREA. High dose ondansetron for reducing morion sickness in highly susceptible subjects. Aviat Space Environ Med 2007;78(7):7.

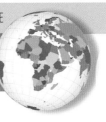

The Aircraft Cabin Environment

Michael Bagshaw and Deborah N. Barbeau

Key points

- Although the occupant density, noise and vibration, and relative immobilization may cause physical and/or emotional stresses, the modern commercial aircraft cabin is maintained with adequate environmental control for the safety and comfort of most healthy individuals
- Transmission aboard aircraft of illnesses, such as tuberculosis, influenza and other respiratory diseases, has been reported but infrequently documented. There is no evidence of disease transmission via the environmental control system, with recirculated air being passed through HEPA filters
- Sophisticated equipment, such as automated defibrillators and telemedicine, has saved the lives of critically ill passengers. Nonetheless, a passenger's fitness to fly is the responsibility of the traveler, with advice from his or her healthcare providers
- Pre-flight notification of special needs and assistance will reduce the stress of a journey and enhance the standard of service delivered by the airlines

Introduction

Although the physiology of the human being is optimized for existence at sea level, most fit and healthy individuals can ascend to around 10 000 feet (3048 m) above sea level before lack of oxygen (hypoxia) begins to have ill effects and reduces performance.

With increasing altitude there is a fall in the atmospheric pressure, together with a decrease in density and temperature. The pressure at sea level in the standard atmosphere is 760 mmHg (29.92 inHg, or 1013.2 mb) and this falls to half at 18 000 ft (5486 m), where the ambient temperature is about −20°C. The composition of the atmosphere remains constant up to the tropopause (approximately 36 000 ft or 10 973 m), the most abundant gases being nitrogen (78%) and oxygen (21%), with the remaining 1% being argon, carbon dioxide, neon, hydrogen, and ozone.

The relationship between the oxygen saturation of hemoglobin and oxygen tension minimizes the effect on the human of the reduction in partial pressure of oxygen. Whereas ascent to an altitude of 10 000 ft (3048 m) produces a fall in the partial pressure of oxygen in the alveoli, there is only a slight fall in the percentage saturation of hemoglobin with oxygen. However, once altitude exceeds 10 000 ft (3048 m) the percentage saturation of hemoglobin falls quickly, resulting in hypoxia with a decrease in an individual's ability to perform complex tasks.[1]

Figure 44.1 shows the oxygen dissociation curve of blood.

The concentrations of physically dissolved and chemically combined oxygen are shown separately and the curve illustrated is the average for a fit young adult. The actual shape of the curve will be influenced by factors such as age, state of health, tobacco abuse, and ambient temperature.

Normal healthy individuals can tolerate altitudes up to about 10 000 ft (3048 m) with no harmful effects. However, elderly people or individuals suffering from some diseases of the respiratory or circulatory system are less able to tolerate the mild hypoxia at even this altitude. In an ideal world, the aircraft cabin would be pressurized to simulate sea level conditions. However, to achieve this would require an extremely strong and heavy aircraft structure with severe implications on load-carrying capacity, fuel consumption, and resulting effects on the external environment. As a result, a compromise has to be struck and airworthiness regulations[2] state that 'pressurized cabins and compartments to be occupied must be equipped to provide a cabin pressure altitude of not more than 8,000ft at the maximum operating altitude of the aeroplane under normal operating conditions'.

The Pressurized Cabin

In most aircraft, pressurization is achieved by tapping bleed air from the engine compressors and passing this flow of air through the air-conditioning packs into the cabin. The outside air is very dry and cold and the temperature is controlled via the air-conditioning packs. The cabin pressure is maintained at the desired level by regulating the flow of air overboard. Figure 44.2 illustrates typical ambient and cabin altitudes for a typical flight. Figure 44.3 shows how the air circulates in the cabin in the case of twin-aisle aircraft.

As a result of the change in cabin pressure during climb and descent, it is possible for individuals to suffer discomfort as a result of expansion of gas trapped within the body. In particular, gas can be trapped within the gut and within the middle ear and sinuses. Normally this trapped gas is able to escape without any problem, but there may be occasions when this is not so. In particular, the human ear is

DOI: 10.1016/B978-1-4557-1076-8.00044-2

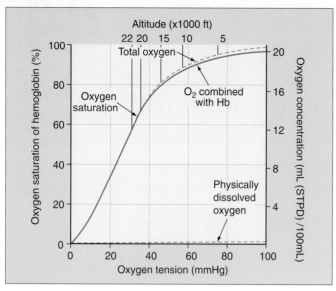

Figure 44.1 The Oxygen Dissociation Curve of Blood.

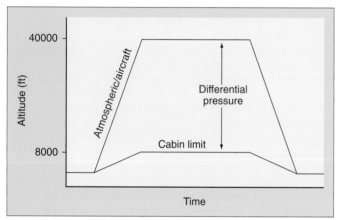

Figure 44.2 Typical Cabin Pressure Flight Profile.

very sensitive to rates of pressure change. In the human ear the cavity of the middle ear is separated from the outer ear by the tympanic membrane. It communicates with the nasopharynx and hence the atmosphere by way of the eustachian tube, the proximal two-thirds of which has soft walls which are normally collapsed. During ascent to altitude, the gas in the middle ear cavity expands and escapes along the eustachian tube into the nasopharynx, thereby equalizing the pressure across the tympanic membrane. The pharyngeal portion of the eustachian tube acts as a one-way valve, allowing expanding air to escape easily to the atmosphere. This can be sometimes felt as a 'popping' sensation as air escapes from the tube during ascent.

During descent, air from the nasopharynx must enter the middle ear to maintain equilibrium. In some individuals the one-way valve mechanism of the eustachian tube can prevent passive flow of air back into the middle ear cavity. This causes a relative increase of pressure on the outside of the tympanic membrane, pushing it into the middle ear cavity, and may cause a sensation of fullness, a decrease in hearing acuity and eventually pain. It is possible to perform active maneuvers to open the eustachian tube, such as swallowing, yawning, and jaw movements. However, in some people these simple maneuvers are not effective and it may be necessary to occlude the nostrils and raise the pressure in the mouth and nose in order to force air into the middle ear cavities. This increase in pressure can usually simply be achieved by raising the floor of the mouth with the glottis shut, while other individuals raise the pressure in the lungs and the respiratory tract by contracting the expiratory muscles (Valsalva's maneuver).

As well as regulating the airflow rate required to pressurize the aircraft, the environmental control system controls the flow rate of outside air required to remove contaminants and control the temperature in the cabin. This is facilitated by the recirculation of approximately 50% of the cabin air, achieved by extracting air from the cabin and mixing it with conditioned outside air. Recirculation provides two benefits: it allows the total airflow rate to be higher than the flow rate of the outside air, so good circulation in the cabin can be maintained independently of the outside airflow; and the conditioned air is mixed with comparatively warm recirculated air before being introduced into the cabin. Consequently, the conditioned air is supplied at a much

Figure 44.3 Examples of Air Flow Patterns in the twin-aisle Cabin.

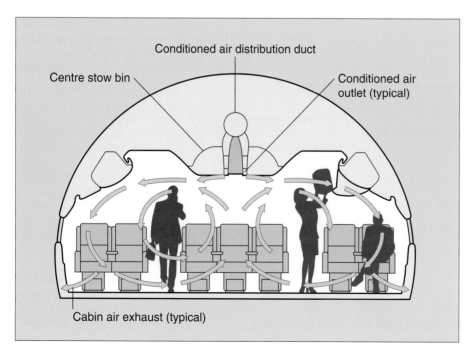

lower temperature without causing discomfort from cold draughts. Also, the recirculated air will have picked up moisture from the cabin occupants and the cabin activities, hence the humidity level is improved. In older generation jet aircraft, all the air supplied to the cabin came from outside air, without the benefits of recirculation (leading to perceived draughts and reduced humidity). This practice was inefficient, with a substantial energy cost.

In modern jet aircraft the recirculated air is passed through high-efficiency particulate (HEPA) filters which have an efficiency of 99.97% for 0.3 μm particles. They are effective in removing bacteria and viruses from the recirculated air, thus preventing their spread through the cabin by this route. Air filters are changed during routine aircraft maintenance, as specified by the manufacturer in the servicing schedule.

Recirculated air is obtained from the area above the cabin or under the floor; air from the cargo bay, lavatories, and galleys is not recirculated. The flow rate of outside air per seat ranges from 3.6 to 7.4 L/s (7.6 to 15.6 cubic feet per minute), with the percentage of recirculated air distributed to the passenger cabin being of the order of 30–55% of the total air supply.[3] The result of filtering the recirculated air is a significant improvement in cabin air quality by the removal of particles and biological microorganisms. It is not necessary to pass the compressed air from outside through HEPA filters, since the outside air at altitude is bacteriologically clean.

The use of recirculation has been common in the design of building environmental control systems for many years. Building environmental systems are commonly designed and operated with up to 90% of recirculated air, compared to the maximum recirculated air flow in aircraft of 55%.

The air supply to the flight deck (or cockpit) is delivered at a slightly higher pressure than the air supplied to the cabin. This ensures a positive pressure differential to prevent the ingress of smoke or fumes to the flight deck in the event of a fire or similar in-flight emergency. The flow rate of the flight deck air supply is also slightly higher than that to the cabin because this supply is used to cool the avionics and other electronic equipment.

Concerns have been expressed that oil fumes may be present in cabin air as a result of leakage into the engine bleed air. Independent research has so far failed to confirm adverse health effects caused by cabin air contamination.[4,5]

Humidity

Humidity is the concentration of water vapor in the air. Relative humidity is the ratio of the actual amount of vapor in the air to the amount that would be present if the air was saturated at the same temperature, expressed as a percentage. Saturated air at high temperature holds more water vapor than at low temperature, and if unsaturated air is cooled, it becomes saturated. Humidity in the aircraft cabin is controlled both for human comfort and for aircraft safety. High humidity can lead to passenger and crew discomfort when it is accompanied by high temperature. High humidity can cause condensation, dripping and freezing of moisture on the inside of the aircraft shell, which can lead to a variety of safety problems, including corrosion. Condensation can give rise to biological growth, thus causing adverse effects on cabin air quality.

At a typical aircraft cruising altitude of 30 000 ft (9144 m), the outside air temperature is in the region of −40°C and is extremely dry, typically containing about 0.15 g/kg of moisture. For pressurized aircraft flying at these levels, the conditioned air entering the cabin has a relative humidity of <1%. Exhaled moisture from passengers and crew, together with moisture from galleys and toilet areas, increases the humidity to an average of 6–10%, which is below the 20% normally accepted as comfort level.[6]

Research has shown that the maximum additional water lost from an individual during an 8-hour period in zero humidity, compared to normal day-to-day loss, is around 100 mL. The sensation of thirst experienced by healthy individuals in the low-humidity environment is due to local drying of the pharyngeal membranes, and this itself may lead to the spurious sensation of thirst. There is no evidence that exposure to a low-humidity environment itself leads to dehydration, although local humidity can cause mild subjective symptoms, such as dryness of the eyes and mucous membranes.[7]

No significant effect has been shown on reaction time or other measures of psychomotor performance, although there can be some changes in the fluid regulatory hormones.[7] It is unlikely that low humidity has any long- or short-term ill effects, provided overall hydration is maintained by drinking adequate amounts of fluid. The body's homeostatic mechanisms ensure that central hydration is maintained, although the peripheral physical effects can lead to discomfort. Dry skin can be alleviated by using aqueous moisturizing creams, particularly just before flight, and dry eye irritation can be alleviated by the use of moisturizing eye drops. Individuals prone to develop dry eyes are advised not to wear contact lenses during long flights in pressurized aircraft.[8]

Although the aircraft cabin environment is similar to many other indoor environments, such as homes and offices, in that people are exposed to a mixture of external and recirculated air, the cabin environment is also different in many respects: the high occupant density, the inability of the occupants to leave at will, and the need for pressurization. In flight there is a combination of environmental factors, including low air pressure and low humidity, as well as low-frequency vibration and constant background noise. Although the noise and vibration can contribute to fatigue, the levels are all below those which are accepted as potentially harmful to hearing.[8,9]

Ozone

Ozone is a highly reactive form of oxygen found naturally in the upper atmosphere. It is formed primarily above the tropopause as a result of the action of UV light on oxygen molecules. The amount and distribution of natural ozone in the atmosphere varies with latitude, altitude, season, and weather conditions. The highest concentrations in the northern hemisphere are generally found at high altitude over high-latitude locations during the winter and spring.

The effects of high ozone concentration on human beings can include eye irritation, coughing due to irritation of the upper respiratory system, nose irritation and chest pains. As a result of this, the airworthiness regulatory authorities require that transport category aircraft operating above 18 000 ft (5486 m) must show that the concentration of ozone inside the cabin will not exceed 0.25 parts per million (ppm) by volume (sea level equivalent) at any time, and a time weighted value of 0.1 ppm by volume (sea level) for scheduled segments of more than 4 hours.[10] For this reason, long-haul transport jet aircraft are equipped with ozone catalytic converters which break down or 'crack' the ozone before it enters the cabin air circulation.

Cosmic Radiation

Natural radiation consists of cosmic rays from outer space (galactic radiation) and the gamma rays from rocks, earth and building materials. Cosmic radiation is produced when primary photons and α particles from outside the solar system interact with components of the earth's atmosphere. A second source of cosmic radiation is the release of charged particles from the sun, which become significant during periods of solar flare ('sun storm'). Cosmic radiation is an ionizing radiation, as are radiation sources such as X-rays and that from radio-active materials. Ionizing radiation is a natural part of the environment in which we live and is present in the earth, buildings, the food we eat, and even in the bones of our bodies.

The other type of radiation is known as non-ionizing radiation and this includes ultraviolet light, radio waves, and microwaves. Humans, animals, and plants have all evolved in an environment with a back-ground of natural radiation and, with few exceptions, it is not a sig-nificant risk to health.

The amount of cosmic radiation that reaches the earth from the sun and outer space varies: its energy is effectively absorbed by the atmosphere and is also affected by the earth's magnetic field. The effect on the body will depend on the latitude and altitude at which the individual is flying, and also on the length of time in the air.

Cosmic radiation may be measured directly using sophisticated instruments, as was done routinely in the Concorde supersonic trans-port, or it can be estimated using a computer program. These pro-grams look at the route, time at each altitude, and the phase of the solar cycle and calculate the radiation dose received by the aircraft occupant for a particular flight. A number of airlines and research organizations have compared actual measurements taken on board an aircraft with the computer estimations, and the two are very similar.[11] Effective doses of cosmic radiation are in fact very low.

The International Commission for Radiological Protection (ICRP) recommends maximum mean body effective dose limits of 20 mil-liSieverts (mSv) per year (averaged over 5 years) for workers exposed to radiation as part of their occupation (including flight crew), and 1 mSv/year for the general population, with an additional recommen-dation that the equivalent dose to the fetus should not exceed 1 mSv during the declared term of pregnancy.

On ultra-long-haul flights at high latitudes, such as a Boeing 747–400 flying between London Heathrow and Tokyo Narita, the effective dose rate at cruising altitude is around 5 μSv (microSieverts)/h. On short-haul commercial operations the effective dose rate in Europe and in the American land mass is in the region of 1–3 μSv/h.

For typical annual flight schedules, crew members accumulate around 4 or 5 mSv/year on long-haul operations, and between 1 or 2 mSv/year on European short-haul operations from cosmic radiation.

For airline passengers, the ICRP recommended limit for the general public of 1 mSv/year equates to about 200 flying hours per year on the trans-equatorial routes. There are essentially two types of airline passenger: the occasional social traveler and the frequent business traveler. The public limit (1 mSv/year) will be of no consequence to the social traveler but could be of significance to the frequent business traveler. The 1 mSv annual public limit would be exceeded if the busi-ness traveler was flying more than eight trans-Atlantic or five antipo-dean return journeys per year. However, business travelers are exposed as an essential part of their occupation, and it is entirely logical to apply the occupational limit of 20 mSv/year to this group.

Cosmic radiation is of no significance at altitudes below about 25 000 ft (7620 m) because of the attenuating properties of the earth's atmosphere. There is no evidence from epidemiological studies of flight crew of any increase in incidence of cancers linked to ionizing radiation exposure, such as leukemia.

While it is known that there is no level of radiation exposure below which effects might not occur, all the evidence indicates that there is an extremely low probability of airline passengers or crew suffering any abnormality or disease as a result of exposure to cosmic radiation.

Pesticides in the Cabin

The use of pesticides in the aircraft cabin is important for the control of vector-borne diseases, but controversy remains about the potential adverse health effects on passengers and crew members.[12] A detailed review released by the World Health Organization (WHO) in 1995 concluded that no toxicological hazard was attributable to any chemi-cals or methods recommended for use in aircraft disinfection.[13] A variety of agents and a variety of methods are used for this. Require-ments may be found at http: ostpxweb.dot.gov/policy/safetyenergyenv/disinsection.htm. The issue remains controversial: some advocate non-pesticide methods of disinfection, and WHO is currently re-evaluating the safety of chemicals in use and proposed for use in aircraft.

Air-borne Disease in the Cabin

People are the primary source of air-borne bacteria and are the most important reservoirs of infectious agents on aircraft. Most microorgan-isms that have been isolated from occupied spaces, including aircraft cabins, are human in source, including bacteria which have been shed from exposed skin and scalp and from the nose and mouth.[14] These microorganisms are found normally on the human body (normal flora) and very rarely cause infections. Studies have shown no statisti-cally significant differences in concentrations of bacteria and fungi sampled:

- between different aircraft, airlines or flight durations
- between aircraft cabins and other types of public transport vehicles
- between aircraft cabins and typical indoor and outdoor urban environments.

There has been increasing concern over the respiratory spread of infections during air travel, via droplet and air-borne transmission. Droplet transmission may occur whenever a person coughs, sneezes, or talks.[15] Droplets are relatively large particles (>5 μm) that can travel only a short distance through the air; they do not remain suspended. Infection occurs when microorganisms within the droplets come into contact with the conjunctiva, nasal mucosa, or mouth of a susceptible person. In air-borne transmission, smaller respiratory particles (≤5 μm), called droplet nuclei, are inhaled by a susceptible host. These particles remain suspended in air indefinitely and may spread over long distances, depending on environmental factors.

There is no evidence that the pressurized cabin itself makes trans-mission of disease any more likely. The risk of exposure to infectious individuals is highest for the passengers seated closest to a source person, typically within 3 ft.[15] Microorganisms suspended in cabin air will be removed by the HEPA filters during air recirculation, but these filters provide no protection from the cough or sneeze emitted by an infected neighbor. Fortunately, the natural or acquired immunity of most individuals prevents the development of infectious disease.

Limited data are available on the true risk of disease transmission during air travel. Studies of potential infectious disease transmission on aircraft have considered tuberculosis, influenza, measles, meningo-coccal disease, SARS, and acute respiratory infections, such as the common cold.

Tuberculosis

The transmission of *Mycobacterium tuberculosis* (TB) during air travel has been most extensively studied.[16] The risk of TB transmission on a commercial aircraft remains low. Mathematical models estimate that the chance of acquiring TB during air travel while sitting near a highly infectious source is approximately 1 in 1000. Few studies have documented conversion from a negative to a positive tuberculin skin reaction as a result of exposure during air travel; no cases of active TB resulting from transmission during air travel have been reported. In light of the emergence of multidrug- and extensively drug-resistant TB, WHO updated its guidance for the prevention and control of TB during air travel in 2008 and will do so again in 2013: http://www.who.int/tb/publications/2008/WHO_HTM_TB_2008.399_eng.pdf.[17]

Influenza

There is little well-documented evidence for the transmission of influenza during air travel.[18] The last decade has seen growing concern over the importance of air travel in the spread of influenza, especially pandemic influenza strains. Since 1997, a new strain of avian influenza virus (H5N1) has been responsible for a number of outbreaks involving birds, and infrequently, humans. Between December 2003 and June 2011, 562 laboratory-confirmed human infections with 329 deaths were reported worldwide to the WHO.[19] Then in 2009, a novel strain of influenza H1N1 was identified, causing approximately 400 000 confirmed cases worldwide and almost 5000 deaths, leading the WHO to declare the first influenza pandemic in 40 years. Although air travel was strongly associated with the importation of cases to other countries, actual transmission during air travel was often suspected, but difficult to document.[20–22]

Measles

Measles is a highly contagious viral disease that is spread by air-borne transmission. A person infected with measles is contagious from the first onset of vague symptoms (up to 4 days before the rash appears) to approximately 4 days after the development of rash; therefore, the potential for disease transmission during air travel exists. Because of the occasional outbreaks of measles not only in developing countries, but also in the developed world due to lower than desirable immunization rates, this continues to be a concern, as imported cases of measles are increasing in many countries. Cases of measles continue to be identified as a direct result of in-flight exposure.[23,24]

Guidelines exist to assist flight crew in the management of ill passengers and can be accessed from www.who.org, www.cdc.gov, or www.iata.org. In general, good respiratory and hand hygiene practices should always be encouraged, and people with febrile illnesses should postpone air travel.

Passenger Health

Flying as a passenger should be no problem for the fit, healthy, and mobile individual, but for the passenger with certain pre-existing conditions or developing an acute medical problem in flight, the cabin environment may be a challenge and may even exacerbate the problem.

In-flight medical problems can result from the exacerbation of a pre-existing medical condition, or can be an acute event occurring in a previously fit individual. Although the main problems relate to the physiological effects of hypoxia and expansion of trapped gases, it should be remembered that the complex airport environment, and even transport from home to the airport, can be stressful and challenging to the passenger, leading to problems before even getting airborne.

Although passengers with medical needs require medical clearance from the airline, passengers with disabilities do not. However, disabled passengers do need to notify the requirement for special needs, such as wheelchair assistance or assignment of seats with lifting armrests, and this should be done at the time of booking, or at least several days prior to needing the assistance.

Pre-flight Assessment and Medical Clearance

The objectives of medical clearance are to provide advice to passengers and their medical attendants on fitness to fly, and to prevent delays and diversions to the flight as a result of deterioration in the passenger's wellbeing. It depends upon self-declaration by the passenger, and upon the attending physician having an awareness of the flight environment and how this might affect the patient's condition.

Most major airlines provide services for passengers who require extra help, and most have a medical adviser to assess the fitness for travel of those with medical needs. Individual airlines work to their own guidelines, but these are generally based on those published by the Aerospace Medical Association on fitness for travel.[25]

The International Air Transport Association (IATA) publishes a recommended Medical Information Form (MEDIF) for use by member airlines.[26] The MEDIF can be downloaded from the website of most airlines; it should be completed by the passenger's medical attendant and passed to the airline, or travel agent, at the time of booking to ensure timely medical clearance.

Medical clearance is required when:

- Fitness to travel is in doubt as a result of recent illness, hospitalization, injury, surgery, or instability of an acute or chronic medical condition;
- Special services are required, e.g., oxygen, stretcher, or authority to carry or use accompanying medical equipment such as a ventilator or a nebulizer.

Medical clearance is *not* required for carriage of an invalid passenger outside these categories, although special needs (such as a wheelchair) must be notified to the airline at the time of booking. Cabin crew members are unable to provide individual special assistance to invalid passengers beyond the provision of normal in-flight service. Passengers unable to look after their own personal needs during flight (such as toileting or feeding) must travel with an accompanying adult who can assist.

It is vital that passengers remember to carry with them any essential medication, and not pack it in the baggage checked in for the hold.

Deterioration on holiday or on a business trip of a previously stable condition such as asthma, diabetes, or epilepsy, or accidental trauma, can often give rise to the need for medical clearance for the return journey. A stretcher may be required, together with medical support, and this can incur considerable cost. It is thus important for all travelers to have adequate travel insurance, which includes provision for the use of a specialist repatriation company to provide the necessary medical support where necessary.

Assessment Criteria

In determining the passenger's fitness to fly, a basic knowledge of aviation physiology and physics can be applied to the pathology. Any trapped gas will expand in volume by up to 30% during flight, and consideration must be given to the effects of the relative hypoxia encountered at a cabin altitude of up to 8000 feet above mean sea level. The altitude of the destination airport may also need to be taken into account in deciding the fitness of an individual to undertake a particular journey.

The passenger's exercise tolerance can provide a useful guide on fitness to fly: if unable to walk a distance greater than about 164 ft

(50 m) without developing dyspnea, there is a risk that the passenger will be unable to tolerate the relative hypoxia of the pressurized cabin. More specific guidance can be gained from knowledge of the passenger's blood gas levels and hemoglobin value. Information is available on the websites of the Aerospace Medical Association (AsMA)[27] and the International Air Transport Association (IATA),[28] but it should be remembered that individual cases might require individual assessment by the attending physician.

Deep Vein Thrombosis

The prolonged period of immobility associated with long-haul flying can be a risk for those individuals predisposed to develop deep venous thrombosis (DVT). Pre-existing risk factors include:

- Blood disorders and clotting factor abnormalities
- Cardiovascular disease
- Malignancy
- Recent major surgery
- Lower limb/abdominal trauma
- DVT history
- Pregnancy
- Estrogen therapy (including oral contraception and hormone replacement therapy)
- Age >40
- Immobilization
- Pathological body fluid depletion.

Although many airlines promote lower limb exercise via the in-flight magazine and encourage mobility within the cabin, those passengers known to be vulnerable to DVT should seek guidance from their attending physician on the use of compression stockings and/or anticoagulants. There is currently no evidence that flying, per se, is a risk factor for the development of DVT, but those at high risk should always have medical guidance prior to any form of prolonged travel or immobility.

Considerations of Physical Disability or Immobility

As well as the reduction in ambient pressure and the relative hypoxia, it is important to consider the physical constraints of the passenger cabin. A passenger with a disability must not impede the free egress of the cabin occupants in case of emergency evacuation.

There is limited leg space in an economy class seat and a passenger with an above-knee leg plaster or an ankylosed knee or hip may simply not fit in the available space. The long period of immobility in an uncomfortable position must be taken into account, and it is imperative to ensure adequate pain control for the duration of the journey, particularly following surgery or trauma. Even in the premier class cabins, with more available legroom, there are limits on space.

To avoid impeding emergency egress, immobilized or disabled passengers cannot be seated adjacent to emergency exits, despite the availability of increased leg room at many of these positions. Similarly, a plastered leg cannot be stretched into the aisle because of the conflict with safety regulations.

There is limited space in aircraft toilet compartments, and if assistance is necessary a traveling companion is required.

The complexities of the airport environment should not be underestimated, and must be considered during the assessment of fitness to fly.[29]

The formalities of check-in and departure procedures are demanding and can be stressful, and this can be compounded by illness and disability as well as by language difficulties or jet lag.

The operational effect of the use of equipment such as wheelchairs, ambulances and stretchers must be taken into account, and the possibility of aircraft delays or diversion to another airport must be considered. It may be necessary to change aircraft and transit between terminals during the course of a long journey, and medical facilities will not easily be available to a transiting passenger.

There is often a long distance between the check-in desk and the boarding gate. Not all flights depart from or arrive to jet-ways, and it may be necessary to climb up or down stairs and board transfer coaches. It is therefore important for the passenger to specify the level of assistance required when booking facilities such as wheelchairs.

Oxygen

In addition to the main gaseous system, all commercial aircraft carry an emergency oxygen supply for use in the event of failure of the pressurization system or during emergencies such as fire or smoke in the cabin. The passenger supply is delivered via drop-down masks from chemical generators or an emergency reservoir, and the crew supply is from oxygen bottles strategically located within the cabin. The drop-down masks are automatically released en masse (the so-called 'rubber jungle') in the event of the cabin altitude exceeding a predetermined level of between 10 000 and 14 000 ft (3048–4267 m). This passenger emergency supply has a limited duration if provided by chemical generators – usually in the region of 10 minutes. The flow rate is between 4 and 8 L (NTP – Normal Temperature and Pressure conditions) per minute, and is continuous once the supply is triggered by the passenger pulling on the connecting tube. Oxygen supplied from an emergency reservoir is delivered to the cabin via a 'ring main', and in some aircraft it is possible to plug a mask into this ring main to provide supplementary oxygen for a passenger.

Sufficient first-aid oxygen bottles are carried to allow the delivery of oxygen to a passenger in case of an in-flight medical emergency, at a rate of 2 or 4 L (NTP) per minute. However, this cannot be used to provide a premeditated supply for a passenger requiring it continuously throughout a journey, as it would then not be available for emergency use.

If a passenger has a condition requiring continuous ('scheduled') oxygen for a journey, this must be pre-notified to the airline at the time of booking. Most airlines make a charge to contribute to the cost of its provision. One major British international airline charges £100 (US$163, € 113) per sector, whether the supply is derived from gaseous bottles or via a mask plugged into the ring main. For US carriers, a fee of approximately US$100 (€ 61) is charged for providing oxygen during flight. Some carriers allow passengers to use their own portable oxygen concentrators, provided the unit meets regulatory specifications. An additional charge may be levied for medical clearance by airline representatives. Airlines provide an oxygen service only during the flight and not during the time spent in the airport terminal. Arrangements need to be made for oxygen to be provided at the passenger's destination and, if necessary, during connections to other flights.

Some airlines do not allow passengers to supply their own oxygen. Oxygen bottles, regulators, and masks must meet minimum safety standards set by the regulatory authorities, and the oxygen must be of 'aviation' quality, which is a different specification with respect to water content from 'medical' quality.[26,27]

In-flight Medical Emergencies

An in-flight medical emergency is defined as a medical occurrence requiring the assistance of the cabin crew. It may or may not involve the use of medical equipment or drugs, and may or may not involve a request for assistance from a medical professional traveling as a passenger on the flight. Thus it can be something as simple as a headache or a vasovagal episode, or something major such as a myocardial infarction or impending childbirth.

The incidence is comparatively low, although the media impact of an event can be significant. One major international airline recently reported 3022 incidents occurring in something over 34 million passengers carried in 1 year.

Any acute medical condition occurring during the course of a flight can be alarming for the passenger and crew owing to the remoteness of the environment. The cabin crew receive training in advanced first aid and basic life support and the use of the emergency medical equipment carried on board the aircraft. Many airlines give training in excess of the regulatory requirements, particularly when an extended range of medical equipment is carried. Although the crew are trained to handle common medical emergencies, in serious cases they may request assistance from a medical professional traveling as a passenger. Such assisting professionals are referred to as Good Samaritans. Cabin crew members attempt to establish the bona fide of medical professionals offering to assist, but much has to be taken on trust.

Responsibility for the conduct of the flight rests with the aircraft captain, who makes the final decision as to whether or not an immediate unscheduled landing or diversion is required for the wellbeing of a sick passenger. The captain has to take into account operational factors as well as the medical condition of the passenger. In making the decision whether or not to divert, the captain will take advice from all sources. If a Good Samaritan is assisting, he or she has an important role to play, perhaps in radio consultation with the airline's medical adviser.

Telemedicine

Many airlines use an air-to-ground link which allows the captain and/or the Good Samaritan to confer with the airline's medical adviser on the diagnosis, treatment, and prognosis for the sick passenger.[30] The airline operations department is also involved in the decision-making process. Some airlines maintain a worldwide database of medical facilities available at or near the major airports; others subscribe to a third-party provider giving access to immediate medical advice and assistance with arranging emergency medical care for the sick passenger at the diversion airport.

The link from the aircraft is made using radio-telephone voice or data link (VHF or ACARS), high-frequency radio communication (HF) or a satellite communication system (satcom). Satcom is installed in newer long-range aircraft, and is gradually replacing HF as the industry norm for long-range communication. The advantage is that Satcom is unaffected by terrain, topography, or atmospheric conditions, allowing good transmission of voice and data from over any point on the globe.

Digitization and telephone transmission of physiological parameters is a well-established practice, particularly in remote areas of the world.

An aircraft cabin at 37 000 ft (11 278 m) can be considered a remote location in terms of the availability of medical support, and the digital technology used in satcom is similar to that used in modern ground-to-ground communication. The advent of satcom has enabled the development of air-to-ground transmission of physiological parameters to assist in diagnosis. Pulse oximetry and ECG are examples of data which can assist the medical adviser to give appropriate advice to the aircraft captain, although the cost–benefit analysis has to be weighed very carefully.

Aircraft Emergency Medical Equipment

National regulatory authorities stipulate the minimum scale and standard of all equipment to be carried on aircraft operating under their jurisdiction. This includes the emergency medical kit (EMK) and associated equipment. The FAA requires an EMK on all aircraft of carriers operating under Part 121, for which at least one flight attendant is required. In Europe, the European Aviation Safety Authority (EASA) is assuming responsibility for aviation regulation and has adopted the requirements of the Joint Aviation Authorities (JAA), which are similar to the FAA. These regulations stipulate the minimum requirement, although in practice many airlines carry considerably more equipment.[31]

Resuscitation Equipment

Although basic cardiopulmonary resuscitation (CPR) techniques are an essential part of cabin crew training, the outcome of an in-flight cardiac event may be improved if appropriate resuscitation equipment is available. This can range from a simple mouth-to-mouth face guard, to a resuscitation bag and mask and airway, to an endotracheal tube and laryngoscope, to an automatic external defibrillator (AED).

As well as meeting regulatory requirements, a cost–benefit analysis has to balance the cost of acquisition, maintenance, and training against the probability of need and the expectation of the traveling public.

The European Resuscitation Committee and the American Heart Association endorse the concept of early defibrillation as the standard of care for a cardiac event both in and out of the hospital setting. However, the protocol includes early transfer to an intensive care facility for continuing monitoring and treatment, which is not always possible in the flight environment. Despite this inability to complete the resuscitation chain, it has become increasingly common for commercial aircraft to be equipped with AEDs and for the cabin crew to be trained in their use. This has been mandated in the USA by the FAA for all aircraft of air carriers operating under Part 121 with a maximum payload capacity of >7500 lb and with at least one flight attendant.[32]

Experience of those airlines which carry AEDs indicates that there may be benefits to the airline operation as well as to the passenger. Some types of AED have a cardiac monitoring facility, and this can be of benefit in reaching the decision on whether or not to divert. For example, there is no point in initiating a diversion if the monitor shows asystole, or if it confirms that the chest pain is unlikely to be cardiac in origin.

Lives have been saved by the use of AEDs on aircraft and diversions have been avoided, so it could be argued that the cost–benefit analysis is weighted in favor of carrying AEDs as part of the aircraft medical equipment. Nonetheless, it is important that unrealistic expectations are not raised. An aircraft cabin is not an intensive care unit, and the AED forms only a part of the first-aid and resuscitation equipment.

The regulatory authorities decree that EMKs and AEDs are 'no-go' items and must be carried as indicated on the Minimum Equipment List.

Many airlines have in place a procedure for the follow-up of crew members involved in a distressing event, such as a serious medical emergency. This can be valuable in avoiding long-term post-traumatic stress disorder, and also in reinforcing the training the crew member has undergone.

Conclusions

The pressurized aircraft cabin provides protection against the hostile environment encountered at cruising altitudes.

- Although the partial pressure of oxygen is less than at sea level, it is more than adequate in a pressurized aircraft cabin for normal healthy individuals
- The cabin air, although dry, does not cause systemic dehydration and harm to health. However, dry skin and eyes can lead to discomfort, which can be alleviated by the use of moisturizing creams and eye drops
- Although up to half of the air in modern pressurized aircraft is recirculated, the amount of fresh air available to each occupant exceeds that available in airconditioned buildings. Recirculating the air has the advantage of reducing cold draughts and increasing the humidity
- In modern aircraft, all the recirculated air is passed through high-efficiency particulate filters which remove >99% of particles, including bacteria and viruses
- There is an extremely low probability of airline passengers or crew suffering any abnormality or disease as a result of exposure to cosmic radiation

The passenger cabin of a commercial airliner is designed to carry the maximum number of passengers in safety and comfort, within the constraints of cost-effectiveness. It is incompatible with providing the facilities of an ambulance, an emergency room, an intensive care unit, a delivery suite, or a mortuary.

The ease and accessibility of air travel to a population of changing demographics inevitably means that there are those who wish to fly who may not cope with the hostile physical environment of the airport, or the hostile physiological environment of the pressurized passenger cabin. It is important for medical professionals to be aware of the relevant factors, and for unrealistic public expectations to be avoided.

Most airlines have a medical adviser who may be consulted prior to flight to discuss the implications for a particular passenger. Such pre-flight notification can prevent the development of an in-flight medical emergency which is hazardous to the passenger concerned, inconvenient to fellow passengers and expensive for the airline.

For those with disability, but not a medical problem, pre-flight notification of special needs and assistance will reduce the stress of the journey and enhance the standard of service delivered by the airline.

Finally, the importance of adequate medical insurance cover for all travelers cannot be over-emphasized.

References

1. Ernsting J, Nicholson AN, Rainford DJ. Aviation Medicine (Third edition). Butterworth-Heinemann; 1999.
2. http://rgl.faa.gov/Regulatory_and_Guidance_Library/rgFAR.nsf/0/FED94F31539484AB852566720051AA5D?OpenDocument.
3. Lorengo D, Porter A. 1986. Aircraft ventilation systems study. Final report. DTFA-03-84-C-0084. DOT/FAA/CT-TN86/41-I. Federal Aviation Administration, US Department of Transportation. September 1986.
4. http://dspace.lib.cranfield.ac.uk/handle/1826/5305
5. www.nap.edu/catalog.php?record_id=10238 pp180–1.
6. de Ree H, Bagshaw M, Simons R, et al. Ozone and relative humidity in airliner cabins on polar routes: measurements and physical symptoms. In: Nagda NL, editor: Air Quality and Comfort in Airliner Cabins, ASTM STP 1393. West Conshocken, PA: American Society for Testing and Materials; 2000. p. 243–58.
7. Nicholson AN. Dehydration and long haul flights. Travel Med Int 1998;16:177–81.
8. Campbell RD, Bagshaw M. Human Performance and Limitations in Aviation (Third edition). Blackwell Science; 1999.
9. Bagshaw M, Lower MC. Hearing loss on the flight deck – origin and remedy. Aeronaut J 2002;106(1059):277–89.
10. http://rgl.faa.gov/Regulatory_and_Guidance_Library/rgFAR.nsf/0/fc2dab7134678df9852566ef006da773!OpenDocument
11. Bagshaw M. Cosmic Radiation measurements in airline service. Radiat Prot Dosim 1999;86:333–4.
12. Gratz NG, Steffen R, Cocksedge W. Why aircraft disinsection? Bull of WHO 2000;78:995–1004.
13. Report on the Informal Consultation on Aircraft Disinsection. Geneva, 6–10 November 1995. Geneva: World Health Organization; 1995 (WHO/PCS/ 95.51). Available at http://whqlibdoc.who.int/hq/1995/WHO_PCS_95.51_Rev.pdf
14. The Airliner Cabin Environment and the Health of Passengers and Crew (2001). Report of the National Research Council. Washington DC: National Academy Press; December 2001.
15. US Department of Health and Human Services. Guidelines for environmental infection control in health-care facilities, Online. Available: http://www.cdc.gov/hicpac/pubs.html; 2003.
16. Abubakar I. Tuberculosis and air travel: a systematic review and analysis if policy. Lancet Infect Dis 2010;10:176–83.
17. Martinez L, Thomas K, Figueroa J. Guidance from WHO on the prevention and control of TB during air travel. Travel Med Infect Dis 2010;8:84–9.
18. Mangili A, Gendreau MA. Transmission of infectious diseases during commercial air travel. Lancet 2005;365:989–96.
19. WHO. Global Alert and Response. Confirmed Human Cases of Avian Influenza A(H5N1) – 22 June 2011. Available at http://www.who.int/csr/disease/avian_influenza/country/en
20. Khan K, Arino J, Hu W, et al. Spread of a novel influenza A (H1N1) virus via global airline transportation. NEJM 2009;361:212–4.
21. Baker MG, Thornley CN, Mills C, et al. Transmission of pandemic A/H1N1 2009 influenza on passenger aircraft: retrospective cohort study. BMJ 2010;340:c2424. doi: 10.1136/bmj.c2424.
22. Mukherjee P, Lim PL, Chow A, et al. Epidemiology of travel-associated pandemic (H1N1) 2009 infection in 116 patients, Singapore. Emerg Infect Dis 2010;16:22–6.
23. Amornkul PN, Takahashi H, Bogard AK, et al. Low risk of measles transmission after exposure on an international airline flight. J Infect Dis 2004;189:S81–5.
24. CDC. Notes from the field: Multiple cases of measles after exposure during air travel – Australia and New Zealand, January 2011. Morb Mortal Wkly Rep 2011;60(25):851.
25. www.asma.org/publications/paxguidelines.doc
26. http://www.iata.org/ps/publications/Documents/Medical-Manual%20 3rd-edition.pdf
27. www.medaire.com
28. www.airsep.com
29. Bagshaw M, Byrne NJ. La sante des passagers. Urgence Pratique 1999;36:37–43
30. Bagshaw M. Telemedicine in British Airways. Journal of Telemedicine and Telecare 1996;2(1):36–8
31. http://rgl.faa.gov/Regulatory_and_Guidance_Library/rgAdvisoryCircular.nsf/list/AC%20121–33B/$FILE/AC121–33B.pdf
32. http://rgl.faa.gov/Regulatory_and_Guidance_Library/rgAdvisoryCircular.nsf/list/AC%20121–33B/$FILE/AC121–33B.pdf

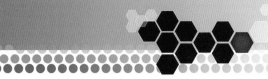
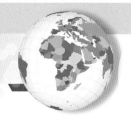

45

Bites, Stings, and Envenoming Injuries

Michael Callahan

Key points

- Pre-travel counseling should include destination-specific advice on avoiding hazardous animals, the principles of first aid and basic steps to prevent wound infection during pre-hospital transport
- Animal attack injuries can be prevented by avoiding behaviors that attract or threaten dangerous species
- Travelers with allergies to bee, wasp, and ant stings (Hymenoptera) should be trained and equipped for self-treatment with epinephrine auto-injection devices (e.g., Epipen or similar).
- Treatment of jellyfish stings requires the removal of nematocysts from skin with seawater or acetic acid; fresh water, hot water, and alcoholic beverages may stimulate remaining nematocysts to fire, increasing the severity of the sting injury
- Venom-laden spine injuries from marine animals such as stingrays should be treated with warm (120°F/50°C) water immersion and prompt removal of retained spine fragments and irrigation to remove venomous mucus
- Care of venomous injuries should prioritize rapid transport to the nearest qualified medical facility; transport should not be delayed by any field treatment (exception: compression wrap bandages for krait, mamba, coral snake, and all Australian land snakes)
- Severe venomous injuries require antivenin immunotherapy; challenges to therapy include matching antivenins to offending species, and avoiding antivenin preparations that are expired, improperly stored or counterfeit
- Mobile field communication is now common, allowing clinicians to send and receive information and images that help guide assessment and treatment

Introduction

In recent years the growth of adventure travel, eco-tourism, extreme dive tours and wilderness safaris has increased opportunities for travelers to encounter dangerous land and marine species. Competition among tour operators has driven some to offer packages specifically designed for encounters between paying clients and dangerous species

©2012 Elsevier Inc

DOI: 10.1016/B978-1-4557-1076-8.00045-4

(Fig. 45.1). This chapter is divided into three sections: non-venomous injuries resulting from blood-feeding arthropods and animal attacks; venomous injuries from arthropods and reptiles; and traumatic or traumatic envenoming injuries from dangerous marine fauna. Each section includes methods for avoiding encounters, principles of first aid and hospital-based care, and the prevention and management of wound infection during pre-hospital and hospital management.

The first step in injury prevention is education of the traveler prior to departure. An attempt should be made to identify those travelers with itineraries and activities that increase the risk of animal encounters, and to provide destination-specific advice. For example, travelers to Cambodia should be counseled against feeding long-tail monkeys, a large species which frequent local temples and are commonly implicated in severe bites. Divers visiting Cape Town should be discouraged from paying to dive 'cage-free' with the region's great white sharks. Travelers to remote destinations should receive safety education that includes principles of first aid for animal bite and puncture wounds and sting injuries. Travelers with high-risk itineraries should carry global communication devices and be provisioned with basic wound care supplies and standby antibiotics for treating high-risk wounds. Clinicians requiring additional information should consult more detailed references.[1]

Non-Venomous Injuries

Arthropod Bites

Bites from hematophagous arthropods, including insects, ticks, and mites, can cause sequelae ranging from minor pruritic bites to devastating vector-borne illness.

Prevention of Arthropod Bites

Strategies for avoiding blood-feeding species include chemical repellents and pesticides, forgoing brightly colored clothing (or in the case of black-flies and mosquitoes, dark colors), and locating camps on high, dry, cool, and sparsely vegetated terrain far from insect havens (Table 45.1). A layered deterrent strategy consisting of topical DEET or picaridin (icaridin) repellents, proper clothing and use of insecticide-treated ground barriers and bed-nets together dramatically reduces the likelihood of phlebotamine bites. For example, the probability of being bitten by many species of *Anopheline* mosquito, which transmit malaria, is greatest at night, whereas *Aedes*

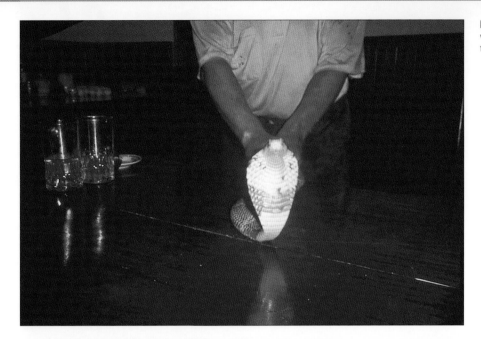

Figure 45.1 Travelers should avoid high-risk wildlife encounters, such as 'workshops' that teach tourists how to handle cobras.

Table 45.1 Important Hematophagous Insects, Recommended Deterrents and Treatments

Insect	Indicators	Deterrents/Treatments
Mosquito	Mosquitoes fly up CO_2 gradients until they are close enough to rely on thermal and visual senses.	Minimize CO_2 and heat-emitting sources such as generators. Maintain air movement to disrupt CO_2 and heat gradients. Wear light-colored clothing. Use repellents containing extended-release preparations of DEET (30–45%): picardin (>20%) or wear permethrin-impregnated clothing.
True flies	Horseflies and tsetse flies rely on vision, whereas sand flies and black flies use CO_2 and thermal detection to locate warm-blooded prey.	Light blue clothing attracts tsetse flies in Sub-Saharan Africa. Many biting flies preferentially land on dark-colored clothing.
Fleas	Fleabites occur when the preferred host animal is unavailable. Eggs lie in ground cover and may last for weeks so pesticides need to be repeated at 4–6 week intervals.	Long-lasting pesticides help with infestations. Diethyltoluamide (DEET) and permethrin are effective for all but the most voracious species.
Lice	Lice are highly specific for certain animal species. *Anthrophilic* species spend their entire life in human hair. Egg cases ('nits') are resistant to many insecticides; repeated applications are often required.	Mild infestations in adults may be treated with benzene hydrochloride. Heavy infestations will need topical 1% permethrin or 0.5% malathion. Children should be treated with care.
Chiggers (mite larvae)	Trombiculid mites are small arachnid larva (200 μm–1m) that feed on epithelial cells and secrete digestive enzymes, which cause hypersensitivity reactions. Soft tissue edema and severe pruritus are typical and unremitting.	DEET and permethrins are both effective for prevention. Pruritic papules are treated with antihistamines or topical corticosteroids.
Scabies	*Sarcoptes scabiei* are transmitted under crowded pestilent conditions. Patients become sensitized to digested secretions leading to characteristic itching. Infections are identified by distinctive linear tracks, which may be highlighted with dilute povidone-iodine or gentian violet.	Infested areas should be monitored for infection. Scabicidal agents include topical 5% permethrin or ivermectin. Treatment of close contacts is recommended.

mosquitoes, which transmit dengue and yellow fever, are most active between dawn and dusk. One newly developed strategy to protect travelers sleeping in infested settings makes use of 4 mm polypropylene cord impregnated with 3–5% permethrin, which is used to encircle the sleeping area. These 'bug cords' are effective deterrents for ground-crawling arthropods such as reduviid bugs (the vector of Chagas' disease), ticks, bed bugs, spiders, and centipedes. These inexpensive, easily prepared cords are effective for up to 90 days when stored in a reclosable plastic bag.

Treatment of Arthropod Bites

Local reactions to the bite of hematophagous insects vary with species and the sensitivity of the individual. Local reactions include delayed blood clotting at the bite site due to salivary anticoagulant (e.g., black flies), inflammatory pruritic lesions (e.g., chiggers), persistent granulomas (e.g., hard ticks) and immediate hypersensitivity reactions. Bites terminated by the slap of a hand or other action that tears the insect from its feeding position may cause mouthparts to be retained in the bite wound. Improper removal of attached ticks, tumba fly larvae, and

Table 45.2 Annual Human Deaths from Animal Attack (1978–2007)

Species	Fatalities	Comments
Venomous snakes	~100 000	Annual deaths are increasing with improved reporting; however, actual numbers are likely decreasing with habitat destruction
Tiger and lion	750	Attacks are decreasing; the majority of attacks are due to elderly and rogue cats that become human predators
Crocodile	600–800	Worldwide, attacks are decreasing; however, in Australasian saltwater and Nile crocodile attacks are increasing with human encroachment, river rafting and anti-poaching laws
Elephant	250	The leading non-predator killer. Attacks by elephants are increasing along game park boundaries. Young solitary males are key offenders
Hippopotamus	130	Decreasing. There is a high encounter to attack ratio, an indication that attack may occur with little provocation
Cape buffalo	85	Previously one of the leading African killers; attacks have dropped in recent years due to population reductions from droughts
Hyena	40	Unattended children are the primary victims
Feral and wild pig	20	Wounded animals are the primary threat
Bear	11	Polar bears are the most dangerous species. Food stresses on polar bears have increased marauding, invasion of villages, and predation of humans
Shark	11	Regional increases in attacks associated with coastal recreation activities; many attacks in developing regions go unreported
Alligator/Caiman	4	Attacks are increasing as protected animals grow to full maturity
Python/Anaconda	<2	Large captive snakes are responsible for fatalities
Rhinoceros	2–3	Decreasing quickly as animals are extirpated

chigger fleas also commonly results in retained insect parts. Close inspection of all feeding wounds using an illuminated magnifying glass, and prompt removal of any foreign body reduces inflammation and secondary infection. Chronic inflammatory reactions to arthropod bites may persist for months after exposure. Antihistamines and topical steroids are helpful; systemic steroids should be avoided. A list of important hematophagous insects and recommended deterrents is provided in Table 45.1.

Several large insects are capable of defending themselves with spines, powerful claws, or chelicerae. Species that can cause painful bites or pinches include African driver or *siafu* ants (*Dorylus*), American leaf-cutter ants, staghorn beetles, and large praying mantises. Although many species are capable of drawing blood, wound management requires little more than inspection for retained mouthparts, routine wound care, updating of tetanus prophylaxis, and monitoring for secondary bacterial infection.

Animal Attack Injuries

A compilation of annual animal attack fatalities over a 30-year period is provided in Table 45.2. Much of the literature on animal bite injuries, in particular factors that influence secondary wound infection, is derived from retrospective series of dog bites.[2,3] However, international travelers may be bitten by a wide variety of exotic, feral, and domestic animals, and injuries from many of these species result in a combination of crush, shear, and puncture wounds. Until recently, bite wound infections were categorized as 'secondary infections'; however, several monitor lizards have been shown to have adapted oral microbial ecologies which favor colonization with virulent bacteria that cause fast-moving sepsis in bitten prey animals.[4,5] Among travelers, the majority of bite wounds are caused by dogs (51%), monkeys (21%), and cats (8%).[6,7] The recent canine rabies epidemic in Bali has caused a surge in travelers presenting for rabies prophylaxis after receiving bites, including monkey bites, at that destination.[8]

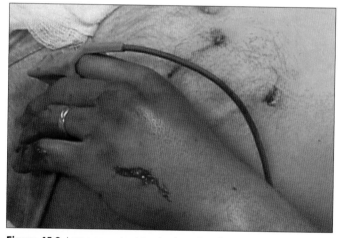

Figure 45.2 Large opportunist animals such as bears are attracted to messy, odoriferous campsites. This hunter was bitten on the abdomen and hand by a male grizzly bear. (*Courtesy Dr Luanne Freer.*)

Injuries resulting from animal attack vary with circumstance and species, and predictably are most significant when involving large animals. Among these, injuries resulting from attempted predation, which include virtually all polar bear attacks, are more severe than injuries from the defensive attacks of, for example, a sow bear defending her cubs. Wounds inflicted by large ungulates such as moose and cape buffalo are often a combination of fractured bones, punctures, avulsions, abrasions, and crush injuries (Fig. 45.2), the last of which may not be apparent until compartment syndrome or rhabdomyolysis develops. Injuries caused by horned ungulates are a combination of massive blunt and penetrating trauma, usually with disastrous amounts of soil contamination and complex polymicrobial bone and tissue infections.

Prevention of Animal Attack

Back-country travelers, wildlife photographers, naturalists, and others who anticipate close contact with dangerous animals should learn about the dangerous fauna of foreign ecosystems prior to travel. Travelers intent on avoiding dangerous species should be aware that many species travel beyond the jungle edge, trespassing into resorts and popular tourist attractions.

The victim's defensive response to animal attack must adapt with the situation and the offending species. The most important determinant is whether the animal is attacking in self-defense or predation. Many unprovoked attacks occur when the predator mistakes the victim, or a part of the victim, for prey. For example, divers may be bitten on the hands by barracuda and sharks, which are attracted to shiny rings, watches, and bracelets, particularly when underwater visibility is poor. If attack resulted from an animal's attempts to defend itself, the traveler needs to adopt non-threatening behaviors (backing away quietly, moving slowly, playing dead). However, if the animal intends to eat the traveler, as suggested by stealthy tracking behaviors by bears, great cats, and crocodiles, the traveler should portray themselves as a large and unpleasant target. Deterrents for predators include making loud noises, appearing larger by unzipping coats and holding them open, holding packs overhead, standing upright, and throwing rocks and sticks. Small children, who are preferential targets for hyenas and the great cats, should be picked up and carried. Running from predators is known to trigger a chase response and exposes the unprotected backside to attack; running is ill advised unless sanctuary is within immediate reach. Large predators such as the great cats direct the attack at the head and neck of human victims in a manner similar to the killing bites used on normal prey. Victims of cat attack should protect the cervical vertebrae and anterior neck. Several cat attack victims interviewed by the author report being 'saved' by bicycle helmets and water hydration packs, which interfered with bites to the cervical spine. Wild and feral pigs are dangerous when injured or protecting piglets; javelina, boar, and feral pigs account for a significant number of bite and tusk injuries in developing regions.[9] In many Asian temples and beach resorts monkey bites often result from attempts to recover pilfered food or possessions from human-habituated primates. In several developing regions crocodile attack is increasing as protection of threatened species allows more animals to reach adult size. Crocodile and caiman attack injuries can be horrific and commonly include crush and shear injuries, and many of the victims will suffer from near drowning.[10]

Factors and injuries compiled from 577 wild animal attacks are listed in Table 45.3.

Table 45.3 Factors Influencing Animal Attack	
Attack Unlikely (Favorable)	**Attack Likely (Unfavorable)**
Omnivore/herbivore	Carnivore
Female	Female with young
Young	Male (breeding season or rut)
	Young adult (recently displaced)
	Territorial species
Plentiful food	Starvation/debilitation
	Prior human predation (man-eater cats; riverine bull sharks)
Wild (fearful of humans)	Habituated to humans (e.g., temple monkey, camp bear; raccoons)

Any activity that places dangerous animals and travelers in close proximity should be avoided. Examples from recent attacks include paying for 'extreme encounters' such as free-swimming with dangerous species of shark, feeding large crocodiles in Africa and Asia, spear-hunting peccary in Amazonia, and free-handling venomous snakes in India. Travelers should also avoid behaviors that attract predators or their prey; examples include improper storage of food, cooking within the campsite, and use of fragrant deodorants or toothpastes in the back country.

Treatment of Animal Attack Injuries

Protecting the victim from the attacking animal while minimizing the risk for additional injuries is the first priority. Initial medical care should be basic, cause no harm, and not delay transport to advanced medical care. Medical considerations for treatment of animal attack victims are shown in Table 45.4.[5–8] One development that has transformed field care is the proliferation of data-enabled satellite phones that allow quick access to consultation with appropriately qualified clinicians; however, many emergency calls go to international medical assistance services and insurance providers, which lack appropriate expertise or which neglect peer-reviewed principles for initial care (see Table 45.4). All phone recommendations should address immediate priorities such as control of bleeding and protection of neurovascular structures and efforts to reduce shock. When appropriate, wounds should be inspected, thoroughly irrigated, and closely monitored. High-risk wounds such as those to the hand, foot, or joint capsule should not be closed in the field. Contaminated and poorly vascularized wounds should be packed open with a sterile dressing and covered with a clean bandage during pre-hospital transport. If evacuation is prolonged the wound and peripheral pulses should be regularly reassessed for evidence of infection or ischemia. All patients with risky wounds should receive prophylactic antibiotics while awaiting more definitive medical care or repatriation (see below).

Infection from Animal Attacks

Wounds from bites, horns, and hooves become infected when microflora from the animal's mouth, or remnants of horn and avulsed teeth, are introduced into the wound. The resulting wound infection is polymicrobial and frequently involves unfamiliar species.[11–14]

In all cases, prompt, aggressive wound decontamination has been shown to reduce infection and hasten healing.[8] The dentition of the offending species, location of the wound, vaccination history and immune status and splenic function of the victim all influence the likelihood of infection. Bites caused by species with needle-like teeth, such as arboreal bird-eating snakes, felines, mongooses, and members of the weasel family, are particularly prone to infection owing to bacteria being inoculated deeply into tissues. Bites to joints may result in tenosynovitis or septic arthritis. Asplenic patients bitten by carnivores are at risk of severe infection from *Bartonella*, *Pasteurella*, and *Capnocytophaga* spp. The septicemia-inducing bite of one monitor lizard, the Komodo dragon (*V. komodoensis*) found on the islands of Komodo, Flores, and Java, causes fast-moving infections which disable prey animals in as little as 14 hours. Komodo dragons also secrete a weak venom which further complicates management of these bite injuries. Other animals associated with atypical bite wound infections include sheep and horses, both of which have been implicated in *Actinobacillus* infections.[11] Rat bites in the Americas are associated with infection by *Streptobacillus moniliformis*, whereas *Spirillum minus* is responsible for rat bite infections in continental Asia, particularly during the cane harvest. Domestic and feral dogs continue to cause more bite injuries than any other animal – except for other humans – and many of these are associated with infections by *Capnocytophaga canimoris*[12] and

Table 45.4 Emergency Care of Animal Attack Victims

Pre-Hospital Management	
Get victim away from animal	Use noise, distraction, lights and pepper sprays to drive off animal.
ABCs	If unconscious, assess airway, breathing, circulation (ABCs) and presence of shock.
Bleeding control	Control hemorrhage with direct and indirect pressure and elevation. Traumatic amputations are often ragged, and accompanied by spasm of arterial structures, the result of which is less than expected hemorrhage. Bleeding is likely to be adequately controlled using direct pressure rather than tourniquets.
Irrigation	Wounds should be irrigated as soon as possible. In the field, filtered or boil-sterilized water may be used but isotonic fluids produce less tissue damage. Puncture wounds should be irrigated under pressure. Appropriate irrigation pressures may be delivered using an improvised pressure governor made from a 20 mL syringe with 22 gauge 1.5 inch angiocatheter. Open wounds contaminated with dirt may be washed with warm water containing a gentle dirt flocculent such as baby shampoo.
History	After emergency care is performed, the clinician should obtain an accurate history including the circumstances of the bite, description of the offending animal, documentation and description of first aid received, and changes in wound appearance over time.
Foreign body	Carefully remove any teeth, retained viper fangs, spines, and organic matter. Stingray and sea urchin spine injuries are notoriously contaminated with spine fragments.
Wound immersion	Wash contaminated wounds in warm water with dilute soap, shampoo, or disinfectant (full strength disinfectant applied to the wound can damage tissue).
Wound dressing	Cover wound with absorbent sterile dressing or clean cloth.
Wound closure	Do not close hand and foot injuries or bites in the field. Contaminated wounds should be packed open and covered with a sterile dressing. Low risk wounds – aside from hand and foot wounds – may be closed by a skilled clinician.
Immobilize	Envenomed and severely injured extremities should be bandaged, splinted in a functional position and patient transported to a local qualified medical facility.
Prophylactic antibiotics	Antibiotics should be started for all high-risk bites, stings and penetrations, and any bites to immunocompromised/asplenic patients. High-risk bites include those to joints, hands and feet, and to extremities with chronic edema. Bites from humans, monkeys, cats, rats, and monitor lizards, marine spine injuries and those contaminated by organic matter should all receive antibiotics (see Discussion).
Hospital management	
Culture	Wounds that present >6 h after attack and those with evidence of infection should be cultured. The laboratory should be instructed to culture for aerobic, anaerobic, atypical and fastidious microorganisms. Many laboratories require special notification regarding non-tuberculous mycobacteria and marine species.
Radiographs	X-rays should be obtained for all suspicious wounds and bites to joints.
Debridement	Devitalized tissue should be debrided until a clear base and margins are observed.
Wound approximation	The minority of bite wounds, all low-risk and seen early, may be closed. Select wounds may have edges loosely approximated with sterile closure strips. Skin glue should not be used.
Antibiotics	Treatment should cover anaerobes, such as *Prevotella*, *Pasteurella* and routine species, such as *S. aureus*. Oral antibiotics such as amoxicillin-clavulanic acid 875/125 g b.i.d. (Augmentin) may be used for mild infections. Penicillin-allergic patients will require mixed antibiotic regimens.[5,6] Travelers bitten by old-world monkeys should be treated with valacyclovir to prevent transmission of herpes B virus.[7]
Post-exposure immunization	All patients with severely contaminated wounds should receive a tetanus booster. Non-immunized patients should undergo the primary series and be treated with anti-tetanus immunoglobulin. The risk of rabies should be considered using revised risk criteria for animal bites and bat contact (see Ch. 12).

Staphylococcus intermedius.[13] Herpes B virus is enzootic in old-world monkeys (macaques) and in the majority of primate species remains asymptomatic. In humans, infection can lead to a life-threatening encephalitis, which occurs when humans are bitten, scratched, or contaminated by saliva from infected primates (Figs 45.3, 45.4).[14,15] Animal wounds associated with increased risk of infection are listed in Table 45.5.

Venomous Bites and Stings

The process of delivering venom, or 'envenoming', may involve the use of a caudal stinger, as in the case of scorpions and the Hymenoptera (bees and wasps); fangs, as in reptiles, centipedes, and spiders; or spines, as in certain caterpillars, stingrays, sea urchins, and the

duck-billed platypus. Treatment of envenomation varies with the offending species, the amount, location, and toxicity of venom injected, and the sensitivity of the patient. In the case of envenoming by certain lethal species of snake, spiders, and marine species, definitive treatment is only possible using genus- or species-specific antivenin. When the traveler is envenomed in remote regions, antivenin is often difficult to locate, of dubious quality when available, and prone to significant side-effects when administered (see Treatment).

Clinicians who are advising a patient over the phone or internet will need to sort through the patient's description of the offending animal, the circumstances of the event, and the progression of early symptoms. This information will need to be cross-referenced using an appropriate data resource with clinical presentations of venoms from medically significant species native to that region to determine whether significant envenoming has occurred. This will avoid unnecessary

Table 45.5 Animal Wounds at High Risk of Infection

Wounds to joints, hands, feet, tendons, and ligaments

Deep puncture injuries

Older age of victim

Certain medical conditions (diabetes, cirrhosis, solid organ transplant)

Marine and estuarine injuries

Contaminated wounds, including those treated with traditional remedies

Retained teeth, spines, mouthparts

Carnivores, particularly feline, monkey, and monitor lizards

Delay in wound treatment

Inappropriate (e.g., early) wound closure

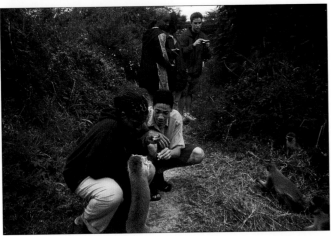

Figure 45.3 Many bites result from attempts to feed or pet semi-wild animals. Monkeys are a frequent and dangerous cause of bites to tourists.

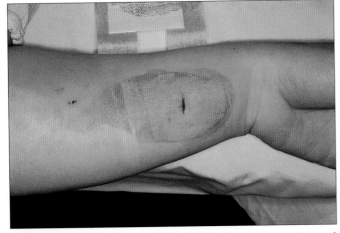

Figure 45.4 Monkey bite to wrist. Monkey bites have a high incidence of bacterial infection and bites from old-world species also risk transmission of herpes B virus, a zoonotic virus associated with fatal cases of encephalitis.

antivenin treatment by eliminating the probability of dangerous species by region; the use of pre-hospital images to identify species which in turn guide decisions on compression bandages; the need for whole blood clotting assays (discussed below); selection of antivenin; and use of adjunct anticholinesterase therapy.

Table 45.6 Prevention of Venomous Injuries

Venomous arthropods	Bees, wasps (Hymenoptera)	Do not wear bright colored clothing, perfumes and aromatic sprays. Avoid trash cans, flowers, and rotting fruit. Keep wasps away from opened soft drinks.
	Centipedes (*Scolopendra*)	Ensure permethrin-treated bed-nets touch the floor but that bed sheets do not. Encircle sleeping pads with permethrin impregnated ground cord. Avoid sandals; shake out shoes before wearing.
Venomous arachnids	Spiders: Widow spiders (*Latrodectus*), Banana leaf spiders (*Phoneutria*), Violin spiders (*Loxosceles*), Funnel web	Avoid webs; Use permethrin cord and keep bed-nets from touching floor. Use insecticide to reduce prey species. Inspect privies before sitting (widow (*Atrax*) spiders).
	Scorpions: *Tityus, Buthus, Centruroides*	Check tub before entering (scorpions). Use UV light wands at night (scorpions).
Venomous reptiles	Snakes: Cobras (Naja), mambas, Australian elapids and vipers.	Do not attract rodents (which attract snakes that feed on them). Do not handle unknown species, even if 'dead'. Use a flashlight and walking stick after dark. Shake out boots and clothing. Avoid sleeping on the ground.
	Lizards	Do not handle Gila monsters or Beaded lizards even if they are 'tame'.

If envenoming is likely, the patient must first be directed to appropriate in-country medical services *even when international medical evacuation services are immediately available.* For many snake, spider and scorpion envenomings prompt access to in-country care by skilled clinicians and access to appropriate antivenins is more important to patient outcome than hasty medical evacuation to homeland hospitals, as these facilities lack both the bedside expertise and access to the appropriate antivenins that improve patient outcomes.

Prevention of Venomous Bites and Stings

Methods for preventing encounters with venomous arthropods, reptiles, and marine animals are listed in Table 45.6.

Venomous Arthropods

Venom may be introduced by specialized fangs, caudal stingers, or dorsal spines and seta. Envenoming often results from the defensive actions – usually the final actions – of a spider, wasp, or scorpion that has been swatted or stepped on.

Hymenoptera

The most medically significant venomous arthropods belong to the order Hymenoptera, which include bees, wasps, and stinging ants. Together the Hymenoptera account for the greatest number of sting injuries, considerable morbidity and death from venom effects, or more commonly, hypersensitivity reactions.[16] The most dangerous Hymenoptera is the Central American bullet ant (*Paraponera clavata*), named after a sting so painful that it has been compared with a gunshot wound by victims unlucky enough to make the comparison.[17] Most Hymenoptera venom contains serotonin, histamine, and in some tropical hornets, acetylcholine. The sting injuries cause immediate pain, which tends to decrease over 30 minutes in the case of honeybees (*Apidae*) or hours in the case of large hornets (*Vespidae*). Africanized honeybees, also known as 'killer bees', have venom comparable to that of domesticated honeybees. The species is, however, irritable and prone to swarming attacks; victims may be chased considerable distances before the bees give up. Local reactions to Hymenoptera stings include a raised papule, often with the stinger-wound in the center, erythema, and edema at the bite site.

Honeybees have a barbed stinger. When the bee attempts to fly away, it is eviscerated, leaving the stinger and the contracting venom gland behind. When present, the stinger–gland complex should be quickly removed with minimal regard to method, as even minor delays will increase the amount of venom that is delivered. In contrast to earlier recommendations, grasping the gland has not been shown to force more venom into the wound.[18] A reasonable method of removal makes use of a fine-toothed comb to gently lever the stinger–gland from the wound. Additional care of bee stings includes wound cleansing, verifying tetanus immunization, and monitoring for infection. Oral non-steroidal anti-inflammatory agents (NSAIDs) such as ibuprofen are effective in reducing pain and swelling. Oral antihistamines are effective at reducing post-sting pruritus and cold packs help relieve pain; cold packs should not be used on stings from unknown species.

Treatment of hypersensitivity reactions should be initiated *as soon as* systemic symptoms appear. The most effective therapy is prompt treatment with 1 : 1000 epinephrine hydrochloride (0.25–0.5 mL subcutaneous). The injection site should be massaged to speed drug absorption. Patients with severe reactions are likely to need a second injection. In recent years, handheld preloaded epinephrine autoinjectors (e.g., EpiPen) have simplified self-treatment; however, travelers should practice with the sham device supplied before using them under emergency circumstances. Sting injuries on the lower extremities have a higher likelihood of becoming infected. Sting injuries that develop pain, erythema, and lymphadenopathy should be treated with antibiotics active against Gram-positive skin flora.

Spiders and Scorpions

Some spider species, such as the hobo spider (*Tageneria*), the violin spider group (violin or recluse spiders; *Loxosceles*), and sac spiders (*Chiarcanthium*) possess venom capable of causing necrotic skin lesions. In the case of *Loxosceles* spiders, tissue necrosis may be severe. Systemic effects of *Loxosceles* spiders include renal failure, hepatic insufficiency, and hemolysis. No FDA-approved polyvalent antivenin is available for *Loxosceles* envenoming, and treatment remains

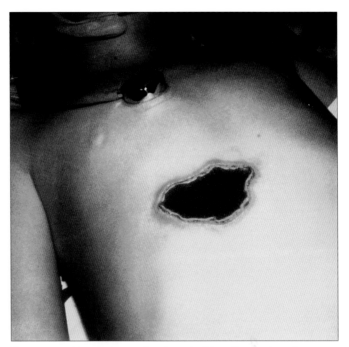

Figure 45.5 Necrotic loxoscelism from the bite of *Loxosceles reclusa*, or violin spider, in an 8-year-old boy. The child developed acute renal failure, hepatic insufficiency and hemolysis requiring transfusion and prolonged support.

supportive (Fig. 45.5). A promising new *Loxosceles* antivenin is being produced by immunizing horses with recombinant sphingomyelinases cloned from three South American *Loxosceles* spiders, but clinical studies demonstrating efficacy have not been completed.[19]

Widow spiders (*Latrodectus*) have a worldwide distribution and are responsible for a significant number of neurotoxic bites. All widow spiders are web-dwelling species and only female spiders bite, usually when webs are disturbed. Widow spiders prefer to build webs where insects congregate, such as near windows, trashcans, refuse piles, and latrines. Bites by widow spiders cause instant pain which escalates with onset of cramping and muscular spasms, particularly in the abdominal musculature. Small children are at increased risk of both envenoming and death. Highly effective antivenins against widow spider bites are produced in Australia, South Africa, and the United States. The unrelated South American banana spiders (*Phoneutria*), in particular one Brazilian spider (*P. nigriventer*), are a common neurotoxic species capable of fatal envenoming. Unlike widow spiders, the foraging behaviors of the *Phoneutria* spiders bring them into contact with humans. An antivenin with activity against *Phoneutria* species is produced in Brazil. The most dangerous neurotoxic spiders belong to the genus *Atrax*, typified by the Sydney funnel web spider (*Atrax robustus*), which is found on the East coast of Australia. The majority of funnel web spider bites occur during summer months when male spiders roam searching for a mate. These spiders are significantly venomous and possess large fangs capable of penetrating thick clothing and footwear. An antivenin is made in Australia.

Scorpions are responsible for a significant number of fatalities in Central America, India, and North Africa, mostly among small children and debilitated patients. Travelers are frequently stung when they step on scorpions that have fallen into the shower or tub. Scorpions often seek shelter in footwear or between folded clothing, leading to many stings. Some species favor sand beaches in Latin America. Antivenin is produced against many toxic species, notably

Table 45.7 Representative Venomous Arachnids

	Type/Species	Range
Spiders	Widow spiders (*Latrodectus*)	Worldwide
	Violin spiders (*Loxosceles*)	Western hemisphere
	Banana spiders (*Phoneutria*)	Tropical Americas
	Sac spiders (*Cheiracanthium*)	Worldwide
	Funnel web spiders (*Atrax*)	Australia
	Hobo spiders (*Tegeneria*)	Europe, Asia, Northwest USA
Scorpions	Amazon yellow (*Tityus*)	South America
	African scorpions (*Leiurus*; *Buthus*)	N. Africa
		N. Africa, Spain
	Indian scorpions (*Buthotus*)	India, Sri Lanka, Bangladesh
	American bark scorpions (*Centruroides*)	S. USA to Colombia

Table 45.8 Representative Venomous Snakes by Region

Range	Species	
Europe	Vipers	European asp (*Vipera berus*)
Africa	Elapids	Cobra (*Naja, Walterinnesia*)
		Mambas (*Dendroaspis*)
		African coral snakes (*Aspidelaps*)
	Vipers	Gaboon viper/puff adder (*Bitis*)
		Forest vipers (*Aetheris*)
	Ground vipers	Stiletto snakes/burrowing asps (*Atractaspis*)
	Rear fanged colubrids	Boomslang (*Dispholidus*)
Americas	Pit vipers	Rattlesnakes (*Crotalus*)
		Cottonmouth/copperhead (*Agkistrodon*)
		Central/Southern pit vipers (*Bothrops*)
	Elapids	Coral snakes (*Micrurus*)
Asia/Australia	Elapids	Asian coral snakes (*Maticora/Caliophus*)
		Kraits (*Bungarus*)
		Cobras (*Naja*)
		Australian elapids (*Notechis, Oxyuranus, Pseudechis*)
		Sea snakes (*Enhydrina*)
	Vipers	Daboia (*Daboia russelli*)
		Saw-scale vipers (*Echis*)
		Sand vipers (*Cerastes*)
	Pit vipers	Green tree viper group (*Trimeresurus*)
		Malayan pit viper (*Calloselasma*)

the Middle Eastern *Leiurus* and American *Centruroides*. In addition to antivenin, neurotoxic bites and stings may be treated with a compression bandage as with neurotoxic snake envenoming (see Venomous reptiles; snakebite). Medically important spiders and scorpions are listed in Table 45.7.

Venomous Reptiles

Snakebite accounts for the majority of severe envenomings in tropical developing countries. Snakebite experts generally agree that although elapids (cobras and kraits) account for the greatest number of deaths, vipers account for the greatest number of bites. Viper venom is rich in enzymes, which cause local pain, swelling, tissue damage, coagulopathy, and for several species, damage to the kidneys, adrenals, and even the pituitary gland.[20] Contrary to classic teaching, the venom of many cobra species is in fact profoundly destructive, whereas other cobras possess venom that is purely neurotoxic (e.g., Cape cobra; Philippine cobra). The venom of the majority of species possesses different mixtures of neurotoxic and complex dermatomyonecrotic enzymes. Early death from cobra bite is usually the result of respiratory failure. Table 45.8 lists representative species of venomous snakes and their geographic distribution.

Human anatomy plays a role in the severity and time course of snakebite. When bites are delivered to the back of the hand or other sites where superficial veins make intravenous injection likely, death may occur quickly. It is important to note that between 25% and 40% of defensive snakebites result in negligible or trivial envenoming and may be treated conservatively; the clinician is warned, however, that neurotoxic findings may be delayed for many hours after the bite. The majority of viper and cobra venoms cause local pain, swelling and erythema. Bites from kraits, mambas, coral snakes, the Cape (Africa) Philippine (Mindanao Island) and King cobras (rural Southeast Asia) and several Australian species are highly neurotoxic and cause negligible local symptoms. Bites from these species may initially appear to be 'dry', but if not treated promptly death from respiratory paralysis can occur quickly (Fig. 45.6). Indeed, cryptic envenoming by kraits in particular may go unrecognized until neurotoxic symptoms such as ptosis or bulbar paralysis appear. In the case of vipers, coagulopathy is common and is usually first noted at the bite site, where unclotted blood drains from fang marks. Local necrosis may be significant following bites by most vipers and many species of cobra (Fig. 45.7).

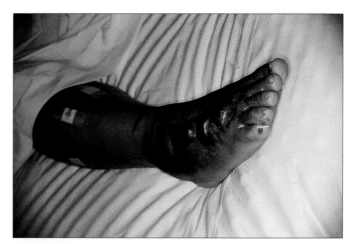

Figure 45.6 Bites by vipers and many cobras cause local pain, swelling and ecchymosis, as in the case of this Thai woman bitten on the foot by a 1 m long Daboia (*Daboia russelli*) viper. The patient infarcted her pituitary gland, resulting in endocrine abnormalities.

Death more than 12 hours after viper bite usually is related to defibrination-related coagulopathy and shock. In developing regions, patients may succumb days to weeks after the bite, owing to complications such as renal failure, secondary wound infection, or failure of manual ventilation due to operator fatigue, or in the case of mechanical ventilation, to power outages.

Snake envenoming is a medical emergency until proved otherwise. No other treatment priority, including air-evacuation to a developed western medical system, is more important than immediate access to effective antivenin and clinicians with experience in treating bites from local species. Most snake bites cause local pain, swelling and erythema, making the decision to treat obvious; however, the near absence of local findings following bites by mambas, coral snakes, and kraits requires these patients to be observed until they are symptom free for

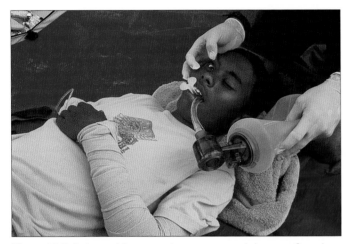

Figure 45.7 Patients with neurotoxic symptoms and those confirmed to be bitten by neurotoxic species should be treated with compression dressings and monitored closely. This 8-year-old boy presented 9 hours after being bitten by a krait (*Bungarus*) with diplopia, bulbar palsy, and respiratory difficulty. The patient was intubated and treated with compression dressings while waiting for antivenin. Note disconjugate gaze.

at least 18 hours. First aid for snakebite is supportive, not therapeutic, and is no substitute for antivenin therapy.

Pre-hospital care includes removal of rings, watches, and other potentially constrictive items, splinting the bitten limb at or below heart level, and the judicious use of compression dressings (pressure bandages) for neurotoxic species.[21,22] There is growing evidence that compression bandages are contraindicated for virtually all viper bites.[23] In the author's experience, compression bandages exacerbate local tissue damage when applied to bites from certain species of cobra with highly myonecrotic venoms (e.g., *Naja kaouthia*). Compression wraps are applied by wrapping an elasticized bandage or gauze bandage around the bitten extremity, moving centripetally from the fang marks. Patients treated with compression wraps require close supervision as increasing pain forces the patient to unwrap the dressing, releasing sequestered venom and the products of tissue destruction into the systemic circulation. Venom extraction devices, cauterization, stun guns, and native remedies (hot rocks, liniments, raw meat poultices) have not been shown to be efficacious and may complicate assessment and treatment.

Venom coagulopathy may be crudely assessed by obtaining 5–6 mL of whole blood by peripheral venipuncture and leaving it undisturbed to clot; after 20–30 minutes the tube should be decanted and the presence of unclotted blood noted. Unclotted blood indicates consumptive coagulopathy, which is typical of viper venoms, or defibrination from the venom of certain rear-fanged arboreal snakes such as *Rhabdophis*. The author has had success adapting this technique to the field by placing 3–4 drops of blood (100 µL) on a clean glass microscope slide and monitoring for clot formation by tipping the slide after 15 minutes. The point is reiterated that patients bitten by a neurotoxic species require close monitoring for the development of paralysis. Early symptoms include agitation followed by diplopia, ptosis, and bulbar palsy (Fig. 45.8). Evidence of neurologic abnormalities that cannot be attributed to other causes (i.e., anxiety, hyperventilation, narcotic analgesia, etc.) is an indication for immediate treatment with antivenin effective against local neurotoxic species. Many snakes of the same species have venom that may vary in potency and clinical effects across that species' range. Polyvalent antivenins, developed to protect against the venom of several species, are commonly used in

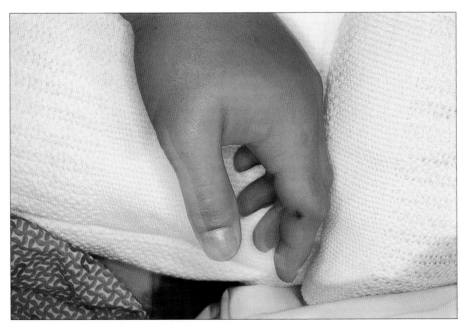

Figure 45.8 Patients envenomed by members of the stonefish group, such as this 19-year-old man who received a single spine injury to the hand, experience intense pain.

sub-Saharan Africa, Asia, and the tropical Americas. The majority of these antivenins will be unfamiliar to western medical consultants and none are FDA or EMA approved. Antivenin supplies in rural hospitals are often stored without refrigeration, are out of date or in limited supply. If the patient is critically envenomed and no alternatives exist, unrefrigerated and expired antivenin should be used. The challenge of treatment is now even more complicated owing to an increasing prevalence of counterfeit antivenins, especially in Africa.

Antivenin is stored as either hyperimmune serum or as lyophilized powder, which must be reconstituted prior to IV infusion. Attempts to give antivenin by arterial infusion may prove catastrophic in the patient with coagulopathy. Intramuscular and local injection of antivenin is not recommended. The first vial of antivenin should be given slowly and at dilute concentrations if possible. Although potency varies between manufacturers, antivenin is generally administered in 1–2 vial aliquots over 10–20 minutes. Pain, paralytic symptoms, and blood clotting abnormalities often improve transiently after antivenin, but re-treatment is usually necessary. Antivenin therapy may be stopped when no further progression of pain, swelling, or erythema is noted, or when coagulation dyscrasias are stabilized. If neurotoxicity of bulbar or respiratory muscles is noted, anticholinesterases such as edrophonium may be administered to delay the onset of respiratory failure and allow time for antivenin to work. Multiple studies have failed to demonstrate benefit from pre-medicating patients prior to systemic antivenin therapy. [24]

Following successful resuscitation and antivenin treatment, patients should be monitored for sequelae of envenoming, such as tissue necrosis, renal failure, endocrinopathies, and serum sickness reactions from antivenin. Wound care includes debridement of necrotic tissues until clean margins are observed, and daily wound care as for burn injuries. Travelers envenomed by dangerous species should be transported (when stable) to an appropriate medical center for wound evaluation and initiation of physical therapy. Important points regarding snake envenoming are highlighted in Table 45.9.

Two New World lizards, the Gila monster and the Mexican beaded lizard (*Heloderma*), are venomous. These species possess mandibular

Table 45.9 Clinical Pearls for Snake Envenoming

Local pain, swelling, and erythema are the hallmarks of viper and most cobra envenomations

Venoms frequently possess both hemotoxic and neurotoxic activity

The venom of most cobras causes significant tissue injury as well as neurotoxicity

The venom of most vipers causes significant tissue injury, and often, systemic coagulopathy

The venom of several colubrids causes minimal local reaction but may cause severe coagulopathy (e.g., *Rhabdophis*, Asian keel back)

Persistent bleeding from the fang marks (after 15 in) suggests coagulopathy

Bites from kraits, mambas, the Philippines cobra, and all coral snakes can cause life-threatening neuroparalysis with minimal local symptoms

Cryptic envenomation by vipers and the majority of cobras is rare in the absence of local symptoms

Neurotoxic effects of mambas and many cobras can be reversed with antivenin; in contrast, kraits bites cannot be reversed by antivenin once symptoms are present. Krait paralyzed patients may need to be ventilated for weeks

In certain elapid bites anticholinesterases may delay the onset of respiratory paralysis and buy time for antivenin to work

venom glands which secrete moderately toxic venom into the wounds made by grooved teeth. Deaths from lizard envenoming are rare but have occurred with captive lizards. No antivenin is available for bites by *Heloderma* lizards.

Marine Animal Bites and Stings

Sea urchins, spiny starfish, and fire corals cause many more injuries than do marine predators. Sharks are frequently associated with marine attack injuries on humans, but fewer than 100 attacks and fewer than 10 fatalities occur each year. Bites from sharks and other predatory fish often occur in conditions suggesting that the predator mistook the victim for more typical prey. Other marine species implicated in human bites include groupers, triggerfish, bluefish, billfish, and large eels. Wounds caused by shark attack often result in extensive loss of soft tissue, fractures, and massive hemorrhage. Bite wounds from other species, albeit less traumatic, may still result in significant blood loss and tissue damage.

Marine envenomings may be caused by vertebrates such as sea snakes and venomous fish; or by invertebrates, such as anemones, sea plumes, fire corals, and cone shells, which possess a harpoon that injects venom into prey or naïve beachcombers. The blue-ringed octopus, which is found in Indonesian and Australian waters, secretes the potent neurotoxin tetrodotoxin in its saliva. Bites, which may go unnoticed, may cause systemic neurotoxic symptoms, including respiratory paralysis and death. As its name suggests, the octopus has indigo blue-colored rings along the head and tentacles which flash brightly when disturbed. Some marine species, such as sea cucumbers, secrete crinotoxins that may be absorbed by the unwary handler.

Prevention of Marine Animal Stings and Attacks

The majority of marine invertebrates responsible for injuries reside in tropical reef habitats. Humans who wade, surf, snorkel, and scuba dive in these ecosystems should be careful where they sit, step, or place their hands. Many venomous corals and anemones are distinctive in appearance, allowing them to be identified and avoided with ease. Many stinging species, such as the harpoon-equipped conus snails, are beautifully patterned. Stingray injuries frequently result from waders stepping on or swimming above large rays. Many travelers and treating physicians are surprised by the frequency and severity of freshwater stingray injuries. Stingray injuries may be avoided by shuffling the feet or by taking care while swimming in shallow water. Protective footwear provides reasonable protection against sharp corals and the smaller venomous creatures.

Swimmers, snorkelers, and surfers should remain vigilant for jellyfish, which often cluster in large numbers. Jellyfish, like the anemones and soft corals, deliver venom through a specialized structure known as a nematocyst. Large jellyfish may possess hundreds of thousands of nematocysts, sometimes millions per tentacle, leading to severe envenoming injuries when the victim becomes entangled and struggles to get free. Nematocysts on detached tentacles are capable of delivering venom for many weeks after being severed. The box jellyfish (*Chironex fleckeri*) is generally considered to be the most dangerous species. [25] The box jellyfish is a mid-sized species that appears seasonally along Australia's north coast and the tropical Indo-Pacific. The mortality rate for patients envenomed by box jellyfish ranges from 15% to 20%, a rate that has improved following the development of highly effective antivenin. Box jellyfish victims may lose consciousness within 2–3 minutes of being stung; patients have lost consciousness before reaching shore. Death is due to hypotension, respiratory paralysis, and cardiac arrest.

Venomous injuries from marine fish are increasing with the popularity of reef diving and snorkeling. These venoms are delivered through specialized caudal or dorsal spines. Several tropical reef fish species, such as the stonefish and scorpionfish, are particularly toxic; pain associated with envenoming is said to be extreme and intractable.

Treatment of Marine Bites, Stings and Attacks

First aid for severe marine injuries focuses on management of ABCs, control of bleeding, and prompt transport to a hospital. Wound care for marine bites and stings prioritizes irrigation, removal of foreign bodies, use of appropriate dressings and splinting injured extremities in a functional position and, where appropriate, treatment with antivenin. Bite and puncture wounds, and virtually all wounds on hands, feet and other complex structures, should be left open to reduce the likelihood of infection. For jellyfish and soft coral envenoming, attached nematocysts need to be quickly removed before further venom is injected. Adhered tentacles may be removed with an instrument or gloved hand, or by washing with seawater. Fresh water should never be used as the hypotonic environment stimulates intact nematocysts to discharge their venom. Nematocysts may also be deactivated by topical application of alcohol, weak acid solutions, and weak basic solutions. Although recommendations vary with region, there is good clinical experience inactivating the nematocysts of most species (*Chironex, Chrysaora, and Cyanea*) using household vinegar (5% acetic acid) or isopropyl alcohol (50–70%).[25–26] The value of ethyl alcohol, which is often present on the beaches where these stings occur – and often contributes to the stinging misadventures in the first place – is controversial. Vinegar should not be used to inactivate nematocysts of the unrelated Portuguese Man o' War jellyfish *Physalia physalis*, because this may cause discharge of nematocysts.

Urchin and starfish spine wounds should initially be treated with warm water immersion (120°F/50°C) for 30–60 minutes as tolerated or until pain dissipates. In the author's experience, pain invariably returns as the soft tissue around the injury cools to body temperature. Urchin spines should be removed as soon as possible, as venom will continue to leach from the spine integument. The first-aid provider should be cautioned that the spines are fragile and should be removed in precisely the reverse direction as the trajectory of the entrance wound. Severe envenoming from marine fish also shows benefit from hot water immersion. The principal difference between stingray injuries and marine fish stings is that the trauma is greater from stingray injuries and severity greater from scorpionfish and stonefish stings (Fig. 45.8). Retained spines and spine fragments should be quickly removed and the affected area immersed in hot water as described above. If a skilled medical provider is present and circumstances permit, the wound may be irrigated with sterile warm water and inspected for spine fragments.[27] The victim of marine fish envenoming will require thorough wound exploration, probable radiographic studies, and prophylactic antibiotics. Owing to the severity of infections associated with these injuries, travelers should be advised to seek evaluation while overseas, rather than waiting until they return home.

Marine Infections

Wound infection is common following traumatic marine injuries; however, the range of responsible microorganisms differs from those observed in terrestrial wounds. Although staphylococcal and streptococcal wound infections are still common, marine and estuarine infections also include a large number of Gram-negative species, such

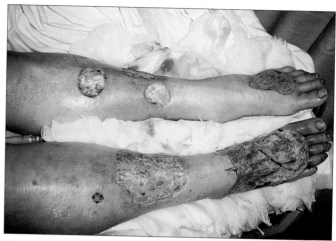

Figure 45.9 Debilitated patients are at increased risk of severe infections by *Vibrio vulnificus* and related species. This 56-year-old patient with cirrhotic liver disease developed *V. vulnificus* septicemia and widely scattered hemorrhagic bullae requiring debridement.

as *Vibrio, Aeromonas, Halomonas, Erysipelothrix, Edwardsiella,* and *Chromobacterium*.[28–31]

Indolent nodular lesions at the site of prior marine injury suggest *Mycobacterium marinum*, a difficult-to-treat infection that presents weeks after the original wound has healed. Injuries caused by fish spines and broken seashells may result in *Erysipelothrix rhusiopathiae* infection, a species that causes a distinctive erythematous cellulitis which spreads quickly from the site of infection. Patients who are immunosuppressed, and those with liver or renal disease, are at risk of severe infection from marine vibrios *V. carchariae, V. vulnificus,* and *V. parahaemolyticus*. In these patients, the appearance of fast-moving cellulitis, darkening skin and hemorrhagic bullae should prompt immediate administration of appropriate intravenous antibiotics and emergency consultation with infectious disease physicians and surgeons (Fig. 45.9).

The likelihood of infection following marine wounds is reduced by careful inspection and removal of foreign bodies, irrigation, and monitoring for pain, swelling, and lymphangitis. Injuries from stingrays deserve special mention because the wound often contains deeply embedded remnants of the spine's outer sheath, which if retained virtually ensures infection. Culture of marine wounds should be reserved for cases presenting with evidence of infection. As with other high-risk wilderness wounds, marine and estuarine wounds should receive antibiotic prophylaxis. Antibiotics should be effective against Gram-negative microorganisms unless culture and Gram stain and special stains suggest otherwise. Appropriate antibiotics include ciprofloxacin and the extended-spectrum fluoroquinolones, trimethoprim-sulfamethoxazole, and third-generation cephalosporins. If *Aeromonas* infections are suspected, aminoglycosides may be added.

References

1. Auerbach P. Wilderness Medicine. 6th ed. Philadelphia: Mosby (Elsevier); 2012.
2. Talan DA, Citron DM, Abrahamian FM, et al. Bacteriologic analysis of infected dog and cat bites. Emergency Medicine Animal Bite Infection Study Group. N Engl J Med 1999;340:85–92.
3. Sudarshan MK, Mahendra BJ, Madhusudana SN, et al. An epidemiological study of animal bites in India: results of a WHO sponsored national multi-centric rabies survey. J Commun Dis 2006;38:32–9.
4. Montgomery JM. Aerobic salivary bacteria in wild and captive Komodo dragons. J Wildl Dis 2002 Jul;38(3):545–51.

5. Bull JJ, Jessop TS, Whitely M. Deathly drool: evolutionary and ecological basis of septic bacteria in Komodo dragon mouths. PLoS One 2010 Jun 21;5(6):e11097.

6. Gautret P, Schwartz E, Shaw M, et al. Animal-associated injuries and related diseases among returned travelers: a review of the GeoSentinal Surveillance Network. Vaccine 2007;25:2656–63.

7. Goldstein EJC. Bite wounds and infection. Clin Infect Dis 1992;14:633–40.

8. Gautret P, Lim PL, Shaw M, Leder K. Rabies post-exposure prophylaxis in travelers returning from Bali, Indonesia, November 2008 to March 2010; Clin Microbiol Infect 2011;17:445–7.

9. Barss P, Ennis S. Injuries caused by pigs in Papua New Guinea. Med J Aust 1988;149:649–56.

10. Caldicott DG, Croser D, Manoser C, et al. Crocodile attack in Australia: an analysis of its incidence and review of the pathology and management of crocodilian attacks in general. Wilderness Environ Med 2005;16:143–59.

11. Goldstein Citron DM, Merkin TE, et al. Recovery of an unusual Flavobacterium IIb-like isolate from a hand infection following pig bite. J Clin Microbiol 1990;28:1709–81.

12. Peel NM, Hornridge KA, Luppino M, et al. Actinobacillus spp. and related bacteria in infected wounds of humans bitten by horses and sheep. J Clin Microbiol 1991;29:2535–8.

13. Talan DA, Goldstein EJC, Staatz D, et al. Staphylococcus intermedius: Clinical presentation of a new human dog bite pathogen. Ann Emerg Med 1989;18:410–3.

14. Holmes GP, Hilliard JK, Klontz KC, et al. B virus (Herpesvirus simiae) infection in humans: epidemiologic investigation of a cluster. Ann Intern Med 1990;112:833–9.

15. Cohen JI, Davenport DS, Stewart JA, et al. B Virus Working Group. Recommendations for prevention of and therapy for exposure to B virus (Cercopithecine herpesvirus 1). Clin Infect Dis 2002;35:1191–203.

16. Nall TM. Analysis of 677 death certificates and 169 autopsies of stinging insect deaths. J Allergy Clin Immunol 1990;75:185.

17. Schmidt JO. Hymenopteran venoms: striving toward the ultimate defense against vertebrates. In: Evans DL, Schmidt JO, editors. Insect Defenses, Adaptive Mechanisms and Strategies of Prey And Predators. Albany: State University of New York Press; 1990. p. 387–419.

18. Visscher PK, Vetter RS, Camazine S. Removing bee stings. Lancet 1996;348:301–2.

19. de Almeida DM, Fernandes-Pedrosa Mde F, de Andrade RM, et al. A new anti-loxoscelic serum produced against recombinant sphingomyelinase D: Results of preclinical trials. Am J Trop Med Hyg Sept 2008;79(3):463–47.

20. Tun Pe, Phillips RE, Warrell DA, et al. Acute and chronic pituitary failure resembling Sheehan's syndrome following bites by Russell's viper in Burma. Lancet 1987:763–7.

21 Warrell DA. Treatment of bites by adders and exotic venomous snakes. BMJ 2005;331:1244–7.

22. Hack JB, Deguzman JM, Brewer KL, et al. A localizing circumferential compression device increases survival after coral snake envenomation to the torso of an animal model. J Emerg Med 2011 Jul;41(1):102–7.

23. Seifert S, White J, Currie BJ. Pressure bandaging for North American *snake bite*? No! Clin Toxicol; Dec; 2011;49(10):883–5.

24. Habib AG. Effect of pre-medication on early adverse reactions following antivenom use in snakebite: a systematic review and meta-analysis. Drug Saf 2011 Oct 1;34(10):869–80.

25 Tibballs J. Australian venomous jellyfish, envenomation syndromes, toxins and therapy. Toxicon 2006;48:830–59.

26. Fenner PJ, Williamson JA, Burnett JW, et al. First aid treatment of jellyfish stings in Australia: response to a newly differentiated species. Med J Aust 1993;158:498.

27. Clark RF, Girard RH, Rao D, et al. Stingray envenomation: a retrospective review of clinical presentation and treatment in 119 cases. J Emerg Med 2007 Jul;33(1):33–7.

28. Lehane L, Rawlin GT. Topically acquired bacterial zoonoses from fish: a review. Med J Aust 2001;174:480–1.

29. Pavia AT, Bryan JA, Maher KL, et al. Vibrio carchariae infection after a shark bite. Ann Intern Med 1989;111:85–6.

30. Howard RJ, Burgess GH. Surgical hazards posed by marine and freshwater animals in Florida. Am J Surg 1993;166:563–7.

31. Domingos MO, Franzolin MR, Dos Anjos MT, et al. The influence of environmental bacteria in freshwater stingray wound-healing. Toxicon 2011 Aug;58(2):147–53.

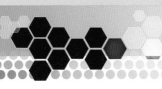 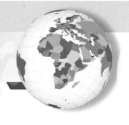

46

Food-Borne Illness

Vernon Ansdell

Key points

- Travelers to the Caribbean and Indo-Pacific Ocean regions should be aware of the risk of ciguatera poisoning and avoid consumption of large carnivorous reef fish such as grouper, snapper, amberjack, and barracuda. The toxin survives normal cooking procedures
- Paralytic shellfish poisoning occurs after ingestion of contaminated bivalve mollusks such as clams, mussels, oysters, and scallops. The toxin survives normal cooking procedures
- Toxic and unfamiliar mushrooms abound in destination countries. Cooking generally (but not always) inactivates the toxins

Ciguatera

It is estimated that there are over 50 000 new cases of ciguatera poisoning worldwide every year, making it one of the commonest causes of marine poisoning from a food toxin (Table 46.1). It is widespread in tropical and subtropical waters between the latitudes of 35° North and 35° South, and is particularly common in the Pacific and Indian Oceans and the Caribbean Sea (Fig. 46.1).[1,2] Recent evidence suggests that the incidence, especially in the Pacific, and worldwide distribution of ciguatera poisoning is increasing. Newly recognized areas of risk include the Canary Islands, the western Gulf of Mexico and the eastern Mediterranean. Most cases follow the ingestion of coral reef fish containing potent toxins such as ciguatoxin or maitotoxin that originate in dinoflagellates found in coral reefs. Average annual incidence rates for ciguatera fish poisoning vary from 5 to 50/100 000 in major endemic areas, with rates of up to 1500/100 000 or even higher in some areas of the South Pacific during certain years. Of particular relevance to scuba divers is the fact that many of the symptoms of ciguatera poisoning may closely mimic those of decompression sickness.

The toxins that cause ciguatera poisoning originate from dinoflagellates such as *Gambierdiscus toxicus* which are found on marine algae usually attached to dead coral reefs. Dinoflagellates are ingested by herbivorous fish and the toxins are concentrated as they pass up the food chain to large (usually >6 lb) carnivorous fish and finally to humans.[3]

Ciguatoxin (CTX) and maitotoxin are among the most lethal natural substances known and may be concentrated up to 50–100 times in parts of the fish such as the liver, gastrointestinal tract, roe, and head. The toxins do not affect the appearance, texture, smell, or taste of the affected fish and are not destroyed by gastric acid, cooking, or other fish-processing methods such as canning, drying, freezing, smoking, salting, or pickling. CTX has recently been completely characterized and synthesized,[4] which may lead to advances in the understanding of its mechanism of action and potential therapies. Pacific Ocean, Caribbean, and Indian Ocean CTX appear to be structurally different.[5]

Over 400 species of fish have been implicated in ciguatera poisoning. They are mainly carnivorous reef fish, such as grouper, snapper, barracuda, jack, sturgeon, sea bass, and moray eel. Certain herbivorous or omnivorous reef fish, such as surgeonfish and parrotfish, may also be responsible. Open ocean pelagic fishes such as tuna and mahi-mahi have not been associated with ciguatera poisoning.

Ciguatera-like illnesses were known in ancient Egypt. Some of the earliest recorded cases in travelers were in the crews sailing with European explorers such as Christopher Columbus and James Cook[6] (Table 46.2). Captain Bligh and his followers apparently developed ciguatera poisoning after the historic mutiny aboard *HMS Bounty*, and it has been speculated that Alexander the Great refused to let his troops eat fish because of concerns regarding ciguatera poisoning.

A wide range of symptoms has been reported, but, typically, there is an acute gastrointestinal illness followed by neurologic symptoms and, rarely, cardiovascular collapse. The onset of symptoms is usually within 1–3 h of eating contaminated fish, but may occur within 15–30 min or be delayed for up to 30 h. Most symptoms resolve within 1–4 weeks. Gastrointestinal symptoms occur in most cases and include diarrhea, nausea, vomiting, and abdominal pain. They usually occur 1–3 h after eating affected fish and may last for 1–2 days. Neurologic symptoms tend to occur later and may be delayed for up to 72 h. They may last for several months or even years. Neurologic symptoms include cold allodynia (dysesthesia when touching cold water or objects). This is very characteristic of ciguatera poisoning but is not pathognomonic, as it may also occur in neurotoxic shellfish poisoning. Other neurologic symptoms include paresthesias involving the arms, legs, perioral area, tongue, and throat. About one-third of patients report pain in the teeth or a sensation that the teeth are numb or loose. Visual symptoms include blurred vision and transient blindness. Chronic neuropsychiatric symptoms may be very disabling and include malaise, depression, headaches, myalgias, and fatigue.[7]

©2012 Elsevier Inc
DOI: 10.1016/B978-1-4557-1076-8.00046-6

Table 46.1 Summary of Seafood Toxins

Syndrome	Toxin	Origin of Toxin	Seafood Vehicle	Geographic Distribution	Typical Symptoms	Typical Onset
Scombroid	Histamine	Histidine converted to histamine by enzyme action	Inadequately refrigerated, histidine-rich fish, e.g., mahi-mahi, tuna, mackerel, skipjack	Worldwide	Flushing, headache, nausea, vomiting, diarrhea, urticaria	10–60 minutes
Ciguatera	Ciguatoxin Maitotoxin	Dinoflagellates. *Gambierdiscus toxicus* and others	Large carnivorous tropical and subtropical reef fish (e.g., barracuda, grouper, moray eel, snapper, jack, sea bass)	Tropical and subtropical waters between 35° North and 35° South. Commonest in the Caribbean and South Pacific Islands	Gastroenteritis followed by neurologic symptoms (e.g., dysesthesia, temperature reversal, pruritus, weakness). Rarely, bradycardia and hypotension	GI Symptoms: 1–3 hours Neurological Symptoms: 3–72 hours
Pufferfish poisoning	Tetrodotoxin		Pufferfish, porcupine fish and rarely ocean sunfish	Worldwide. Commonest in Japan, Indo-Pacific oceans	Perioral paresthesiae, nausea, dizziness followed by weakness, numbness, slurred speech, incoordination, respiratory failure	10 minutes–4 hours
Paralytic shellfish poisoning	Saxitoxin	Dinoflagellates, *Alexandrium* species and others	Bivalve shellfish	Worldwide. Commonest in temperate coastal waters	Paresthesiae of face and limbs, gastroenteritis. Rarely, dysphonia, ataxia, weakness, respiratory failure	30–60 minutes
Neurotoxic shellfish poisoning	Brevetoxins	Dinoflagellates. *Gymnodinium breve*	Bivalve shellfish	Rare. Gulf of Mexico and New Zealand	Gastroenteritis and neurologic symptoms (e.g., paresthesiae, temperature reversal, vertigo, ataxia). Respiratory and eye irritation in the presence of aerosol	15 minutes–8 hours
Diarrheic shellfish poisoning	Okadaic acid and others	Dinoflagellates. *Dinophysis* species	Bivalve shellfish	Japan, Europe (France), Canada, New Zealand and S. America	Gastroenteritis	30 minutes–6 hours
Amnesic shellfish poisoning	Domoic acid	Diatoms. *Pseudonitzschia* species	Mussels	Extremely rare, NE Canada only	Gastroenteritis followed by neurologic symptoms (e.g., amnesia, cognitive impairment, headache, seizures)	GI Symptoms: <24 hours Neurological Symptoms: <48 hours

Cardiac manifestations include bradycardia (possibly due to cholinesterase inhibition), tachycardia, and other arrhythmias. Hypotension in the absence of hypovolemia may be due to the hypotensive properties of maitotoxin. Persistent symptomatic hypotension has been described and is probably due to an increase in parasympathetic tone and impaired sympathetic reflexes. Hypertension has also been described. The cardiac effects of ciguatera poisoning may be serious, but usually resolve within 5 days of onset.

General symptoms include profound weakness, chills, sweating, arthralgias, myalgias, and a metallic taste in the mouth. Pruritus, particularly involving the palms and soles, occurs 2–5 days after ingestion of contaminated fish and has been reported in 5–89% of cases. It seems to be more common in the Pacific than the Caribbean and is particularly common in New Caledonia, where ciguatera poisoning is known as 'la gratte' or 'the itch.' Deaths result from respiratory or cardiac failure and are most common in patients who have eaten parts of the fish known to contain high levels of toxin, such as the liver, intestines, or roe. The case-fatality rate is usually 0.1–1%, depending on geographic location.

Disturbances to reef systems and the subsequent proliferation of toxic dinoflagellates have been shown to have an important impact on the incidence of ciguatera poisoning, although there is often a

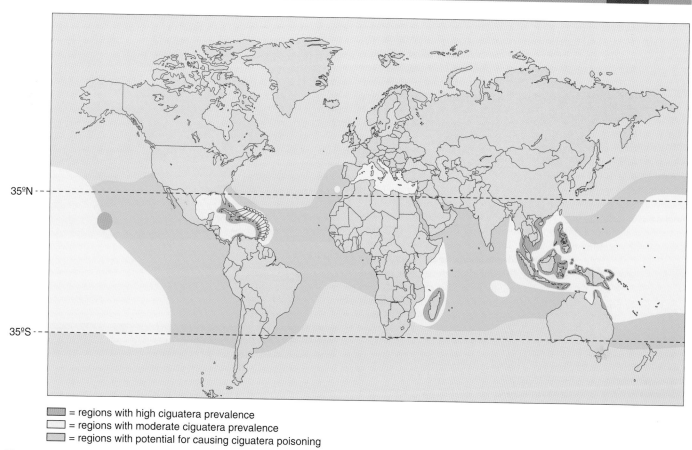

= regions with high ciguatera prevalence
= regions with moderate ciguatera prevalence
= regions with potential for causing ciguatera poisoning

Figure 46.1 Worldwide distribution of ciguatera. Pink indicates coral reef regions located between 35° North and 35° South latitudes; lilac indicates disease-endemic areas of ciguatera; red circle indicates Canary Islands (latitude 28°06' North, longitude 15°24' West. *(With permission from Patricia A. Tester, et al. Smithsonian Contributions to the Marine Sciences; Ciguatera Fish Poisoning in the Caribbean; 38: 301)*

Table 46.2 Excerpt from the Journals of Captain James Cook's Voyage in the South Pacific in 1774

The Night before we came out of Port, two Red fish about the Size of large Bream and not unlike them were caught with hook and line of which Most of the officers and Some of the Petty officers dined the next day. In the Evening every one who had eat of these fish were seiz'd with Violant pains in the head and Limbs, so as to be unable to stand, together with a kind of Scorching heat all over the Skin, there remained no doubt but that it was occasioned by the fish being of a Poisoness nature and communicated its bad effects to every one who had the ill luck to eat of it even to the Dogs and Hogs, one of the latter died in about Sixteen hours after and a young dog soon after shared the same fate: and it was a week or ten days before all the gentlemen recovered.

6–24-month time lag. Reef systems may be disrupted by natural disasters such as hurricanes, tidal waves, heavy rains, and earthquakes, or manmade activities such as underwater nuclear explosions, coastal construction projects, dredging, shipwrecks, or golf-course run-off. There are concerns that ciguatera poisoning may increase as more coral reefs die as a result of global warming, nutrient run-off and construction.

Several factors have been shown to influence the severity of ciguatera poisoning. These include the amount of fish eaten and the consumption of parts known to contain high levels of toxin, such as the head, liver, intestine, and roe, or soup made from those parts. Previous exposure to ciguatera also increases the severity of poisoning, probably as a result of accumulation of toxin or immune sensitization.

Medical management is mainly symptomatic and supportive. If patients are seen within 3 h of ingestion of contaminated fish, emetics such as ipecac or gastric lavage followed by activated charcoal may be indicated. In theory, antiemetics and antidiarrheals should be avoided because they may prolong toxin contact time. Bradycardia responds to atropine. Intravenous fluids are indicated if there is volume depletion and hypotension. Hypotension in the absence of volume depletion is treated with pressors such as dopamine or dobutamine. Intravenous calcium gluconate 10% can be used to treat the inhibited calcium uptake caused by ciguatoxin. Treatment of prolonged orthostatic hypotension may require sodium and fluid replacement, fludrocortisone acetate, and lower-extremity support stockings. Lidocaine or mexiletine have been used to treat ventricular arrhythmias. Treatment options for specific symptoms include cyproheptadine or hydroxyzine for pruritus, acetaminophen or nifedipine for headache,[8] and non-steroidal anti-inflammatory agents (NSAIDs) for musculoskeletal pains. Amitriptyline[9] appears to be effective in treating depression associated with ciguatera poisoning and may also be effective in treating other neuropsychiatric symptoms, such as dysesthesias. Chronic fatigue associated with ciguatera poisoning has been treated successfully with fluoxetine (Prozac).[10] There is limited evidence that cholestyramine, an ion exchange resin, may relieve some of the symptoms of chronic ciguatera poisoning by binding ciguatoxins in the intestine.[11]

Intravenous mannitol (1 g/kg over 30 min) has been reported to reduce the severity and duration of neurologic symptoms, particularly if given within the first 24 h of poisoning.[12] A double-blind randomized controlled trial found no significant difference between intravenous mannitol and intravenous saline.[13] Clinical opinion is divided on the use of mannitol in ciguatera poisoning, but many experts strongly recommend using it in the acute phase.[14] If used, it should be given with caution and only after ensuring adequate hydration. A potential mechanism of action has not been established. Recent case reports suggest that gabapentin (Neurontin), a drug occasionally used to treat neuropathic pain, may be useful in relieving symptoms late in the illness.[15]

Travelers to endemic areas, particularly the Caribbean and Indo-Pacific regions, should be warned about the risk of ciguatera poisoning and should avoid or limit consumption of reef fish, particularly carnivorous fish weighing over 6 lb.[16,17] The risk of ciguatera fish poisoning in local populations on some endemic Pacific Island populations has been estimated at 2% per year. Particularly high-risk fish such as tropical moray eels or barracuda should never be eaten. Travelers should be reminded that it is important to avoid parts of the fish known to contain large amounts of toxin, such as the head, liver, intestine, and roe, or soup made from these parts, and not to consume large reef fish weighing more than 6 lb.

Radioimmunoassays or enzyme-linked immunosorbent assays have been developed to investigate ciguatera poisoning, and a commercial immunoassay has recently become available for the identification of toxic fish (Cigua-Check, Oceanit Test Systems Inc., Honolulu). The test is easy to perform and very sensitive, but is relatively expensive (approximately US$10/test). It will probably have limited value for travelers to endemic areas.

Any patient with a history of ciguatera poisoning should avoid consumption of reef fish, fish sauces, shellfish, alcoholic beverages, caffeine, nuts, and nut oils for at least 6 months, as they may provoke recurrent symptoms.

Diagnosis of ciguatera poisoning is usually made on clinical grounds. If a portion of the fish is still available, it should be frozen and, if possible, submitted to a laboratory that can test for the presence of toxin.

In a survival situation, organ meat should be fed to susceptible animals such as dogs, cats, or mongooses. If the animals show no sign of illness, then the flesh of the fish is probably safe for human consumption.

Scombroid

Scombroid is one of the most common fish poisonings and occurs worldwide in both temperate and tropical waters. The illness often resembles a moderate to severe allergic reaction and occurs after eating improperly refrigerated or preserved fish containing high levels of histamine. Fish that cause scombroid include dark- or red-muscled fish belonging to the family Scombridae, such as albacore, bluefin and yellowfin tuna, mackerel, saury, skipjack, and bonito. Various non-scombroid fish may also be responsible, including mahi-mahi (dolphinfish) (Fig. 46.2), sardine, pilchard, anchovy, herring, bluefish, amberjack, and black marlin.[1,18,19] Cases of fish poisoning closely resembling scombroid were described by Captain Edmund Fanning while sailing in the North Atlantic in 1797 (Table 46.3).

Fish that cause scombroid have high levels of the amino acid histidine in the flesh. As a result of improper handling and storage after catch, histidine is converted to histamine and other scombrotoxins by bacteria with high histidine decarboxylase activity. These bacteria

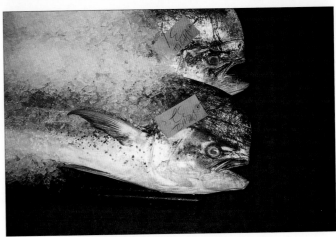

Figure 46.2 Mahi-mahi (dolphinfish), a common cause of scombroid poisoning. Prompt refrigeration, using ice as shown here, will prevent poisoning. *(Photograph courtesy of David Ansdell.)*

Table 46.3 Excerpt from the Journals of Captain Edmund Fanning's Voyage in the North Atlantic 1797

'During this period we caught, with hook and grains, as many of the Spanish mackerel, or bonetos, as were wished for; shoals of these fish, as well as the dolphin, being all around us; … On eating of the dolphin and mackerel, almost all on board were affected with a severe pain in the head, which shortly after was much inflamed; the eyes became red, and these distressing symptoms were attended with violent vomiting. Those who were thus affected, were evidently poisoned; the head and some of the limbs began also to swell, which swelling increased, until they had attained a most disagreeable form, having at the same time, a reddish cast over the head and limbs thus swollen … whenever the fish, on being taken out of the water, was immediately cooked, and then eaten, no evil or unpleasant sensation was experienced; …'

occur as normal surface flora or secondary contaminants and include *Morganella morganii*, *Klebsiella pneumoniae*, *Escherichia coli*, *Aerobacter aerogenes*, and *Plesiomonas shigelloides*.

Conversion of histidine to histamine and other scombrotoxins occurs optimally at 20–30°C, and scombroid typically occurs in fish that have not been promptly refrigerated after capture. Histamine and other scombrotoxins are resistant to freezing, cooking, smoking, or canning.

Symptoms of scombroid poisoning usually appear abruptly 10–60 min after eating contaminated fish, although they may appear within a few minutes of ingestion or be delayed for several hours. Untreated, symptoms typically last for an average of 4 h, but may persist for up to 24 h. Symptoms often resemble an acute IgE-mediated allergic reaction and are frequently misdiagnosed as an allergy to fish. Affected fish often have a peppery, sharp, metallic or bitter taste, but may be normal in taste and appearance. There are several characteristic symptoms of scombroid poisoning.[1] Flushing of the skin resembling sunburn with a sharply demarcated edge confined to the face and upper body may be present. Pruritus is common, and there may be urticaria or angioneurotic edema. A throbbing headache is often present. Gastrointestinal symptoms include nausea, vomiting, abdominal cramps, and diarrhea. Other clinical features may include perioral paresthesiae, burning of the mouth and gums, conjunctival suffusion, palpitations, blurred vision, and diaphoresis. Scombroid is usually a benign, self-limited illness; rarely, however, it may produce a more serious illness with respiratory compromise, malignant arrhythmias, and hypotension requiring hospitalization. Serious illness seems to be more likely in the elderly and asthmatics. Patients who are already taking isoniazid may have a severe reaction because the drug inhibits histamine metabolism. Deaths are extremely rare, and none have been reported in recent years. As expected, persons already taking antihistamines tend to have fewer symptoms.

Diagnosis is usually made on clinical grounds. There may be a clustering of cases, which helps to exclude the possibility of fish allergy. The diagnosis can be confirmed by measuring histamine levels in any leftover fish.

Treatment with H_1 antagonists (e.g., diphenhydramine) given orally or parenterally provides symptomatic relief. Newer, second-generation, non-sedating H_1 antagonists (e.g., astemizole) have not yet been proved to be as effective. H_2 antagonists (e.g., cimetidine) given orally or parenterally may shorten the course of illness and have been particularly useful in controlling headache.[20] A combination of H_1 and H_2 antagonists may be particularly valuable, but rarely may cause hypotension. Steroids have not been shown to be of any benefit. In severe scombroid poisoning intravenous fluids, inhaled bronchodilators, oxygen, and pressor agents may be indicated. Gastric lavage or catharsis may be worthwhile if large quantities of contaminated fish have been consumed within the previous few hours.

The most important preventive measure is to chill the fish promptly after capture and maintain adequate refrigeration until the fish is prepared for consumption. Fish kept at ≤15–20°C prior to cooking should be safe for consumption.

Pufferfish (Fugu) Poisoning

Pufferfish or fugu poisoning occurs after ingestion of fish containing tetrodotoxin, a potent neurotoxin. Potentially toxic fish are distributed widely throughout the world and include pufferfish, porcupine fish, and ocean sunfish.[1] The toxin is usually concentrated in the ovaries, liver, intestines, and skin of the fish. Pufferfish poisoning has been recognized since ancient Egyptian times. One of the earliest recorded outbreaks of pufferfish poisoning in travelers may have involved Captain Cook and members of his crew, who became ill after eating pufferfish liver while sailing in the South Pacific during their second voyage around the world in 1774 (Table 46.4).

Most cases of pufferfish poisoning occur in Japan, where pufferfish or fugu is eaten as a very expensive and prized delicacy. The fugu is filleted, thinly sliced, and then arranged in traditional patterns such as a crane. The fugu experience is characterized by tingling of the lips and tongue, a sensation of generalized warmth and flushing, and a feeling of euphoria and exhilaration. Over the 78-year period from 1886 to 1963, there were 6386 cases of fugu poisoning in Japan, with an approximately 59% mortality. Increased awareness of fugu poisoning and strict regulation and training of licensed fugu chefs has resulted in far fewer cases and lower mortality in recent years. For example, in the 10-year period from 1967 to 1976 there were 1105 cases and 372 deaths (34% mortality), and from 1983 to 1992 there were only 449 cases and 49 deaths (11% mortality).[21] Nowadays, all cooks and restaurants handling fugu must be licensed, and most cases of pufferfish poisoning occur in inexperienced fishermen who prepare their own food. In 1996, three cases of fugu poisoning occurred in San Diego in chefs who ate pre-packaged, ready-to-eat fugu illegally imported from Japan.[22]

Table 46.4 Excerpt from the Journals of Captain James Cook's Voyage in the South Pacific in 1774

This afternoon a fish being struck by one of the natives near the watering place, the Captain's clerk purchased it, and sent it to him after his return on board. It was of a new species, something like a sun-fish, with a large, long, ugly head. Having no suspicion of its being of a poisonous nature, they ordered it to be dressed for supper; but, very luckily, the operation of drawing and describing took up so much time that it was too late, so that only the liver and roe were dressed, of which the two Mr. Fortsters and the Captain did but taste. About three o'clock in the morning they all found themselves seized with an extraordinary weakness and numbness all over their limbs. The Captain had almost lost the sense of feeling; nor could he distinguish between light and heavy bodies, of such as he had strength to move; a quart pot full of water and a feather being the same in his hand. They each took an emetic, and after that a sweet, which gave them much relief. In the morning, one of the pigs which had eaten the entrails was found dead.

Tetrodotoxin is a heat-stable, water-soluble, non-protein toxin that is 50 times more potent than strychnine. It acts by binding to sodium channels and blocking axonal nerve transmission, and results in ascending paralysis and respiratory failure. In addition to pufferfish, porcupine fish and ocean sunfish, tetrodotoxin has been found in other marine animals, such as the blue-ringed octopus, starfishes, flatworms, various crabs, and mollusks.

Levels of toxin are usually highest in the ovaries, liver, intestine, and skin. The toxin does not alter the taste or appearance of the fish, and it is not destroyed or inactivated by cooking, canning, freezing, or smoking.

The onset of symptoms of pufferfish poisoning may occur within 10 min of ingestion of toxic fish or be delayed for up to 4 h or longer. Severe cases are usually associated with ingestion of large amounts of toxin and early onset of symptoms. Initial symptoms include perioral paresthesiae and numbness, nausea, and dizziness. Later, there may be more generalized paraesthesia and numbness, dysarthria, ataxia, ascending paralysis, and a variety of other symptoms, such as headache, hypersalivation, diaphoresis, vomiting, abdominal pain, and diarrhea. In the most severe cases there is widespread paralysis, respiratory failure, bradycardia and other arrhythmias and hypotension. Most deaths are due to respiratory failure and occur within the first 6 h. In patients who survive the first 24 h the prognosis is usually excellent.

Diagnosis is made on clinical grounds. There is no specific antidote for tetrodotoxin and treatment is aimed at limiting absorption of toxin and treating the adverse effects. Absorption of toxin can be limited by gastric lavage, which is indicated if patients are seen within 3 h of ingestion of toxic fish. Emetic agents such as ipecac should probably be avoided because of the risk of aspiration. In severe cases, intravenous fluids, vasopressors, endotracheal intubation, and ventilatory support may be indicated. Bradycardia may respond to atropine. As a general rule, all cases of pufferfish poisoning should be admitted to hospital for observation. Moderate or severe poisonings should be admitted to an intensive care unit.[23]

It is impossible to guarantee that fish are free from toxins, and travelers should be advised to avoid any potentially toxic fish even when prepared by trained chefs in licensed restaurants. In life-threatening (survival) situations, travelers should take advantage of the water-soluble properties of the toxin. Viscera and skin must not be eaten under any circumstances, but the muscle of the fish can be shredded into small pieces, kneaded, and soaked in water for at least 4 h in an attempt to remove toxin prior to consumption.

Paralytic Shellfish Poisoning

Paralytic shellfish poisoning (PSP) has been recognized for over 200 years. The first recognized outbreak in travelers was in 1793 and was reported in Captain George Vancouver's *A Voyage of Discovery to the North Pacific Ocean and Round the World*. PSP is the most common and most serious form of shellfish poisoning and occurs after eating contaminated bivalve mollusks (clams, cockles, mussels, oysters, and scallops) containing saxitoxin and other potent neurotoxins produced by dinoflagellates (e.g., *Alexandrium* sp.). Saxitoxin, like ciguatoxin and tetrodotoxin, causes paralysis by blocking sodium channels in nerve cell membranes. It is 50 times more potent than curare. Saxitoxin and other toxins that cause PSP are heat stable and survive normal cooking procedures.

As in other forms of shellfish poisoning, outbreaks of PSP often follow dinoflagellate blooms. In the past, most cases of PSP occurred in cold, temperate waters above latitude 30° North and below latitude 30° South. Recently, outbreaks in tropical and subtropical waters have become more frequent, with cases reported from countries such as Guatemala, El Salvador, Mexico, Thailand, Singapore, Malaysia, Papua New Guinea, India, and the Solomon Islands.

Because the main toxins that produce pufferfish poisoning (tetrodotoxin) and paralytic shellfish poisoning (saxitoxin) are very similar, the clinical effects are almost indistinguishable. Symptoms of PSP usually occur within 30–60 min of eating toxic shellfish but can be delayed for 3 h or longer. Early symptoms include paresthesiae of the face, lips, and tongue, and later the arms and legs. Affected persons may complain of lightheadedness or a floating sensation. Other symptoms may include headache, increased salivation, nausea, vomiting, and diarrhea. Hypertension may be an important finding. Severe cases are usually associated with ingestion of large doses of toxin and clinical features, such as ataxia, dysphagia, and mental status changes. Flaccid paralysis occurs in the most severe cases, with respiratory insufficiency as a result of paralysis of the diaphragm and chest wall muscles. Deaths are typically caused by respiratory failure and tend to occur within 12 h of eating toxic shellfish. For patients who survive past 12 h the prognosis is good. Recovery usually occurs within a week, but may occasionally be prolonged for several weeks.[24]

Case fatality rate averages 6% but may be as high as 44%. Mortality is higher in children, who seem to be particularly sensitive to the effects of the toxin. Travelers to developing countries who are tempted to eat shellfish should be reminded that the highest mortality from PSP occurs in areas with poor access to good-quality medical care.

Diagnosis is usually made on clinical grounds, although in special circumstances it can be confirmed by a standard mouse bioassay method.

There are no antidotes for PSP, but saxitoxin and other toxins that cause PSP bind well to charcoal and, if safe, oral charcoal should be given. Victims should be observed for at least 24 h for respiratory insufficiency. Mechanical ventilation may be necessary.

PSP can be prevented by avoiding potentially contaminated shellfish. This is particularly important in children, who are at greater risk of fatal illness. It is important to emphasize that the presence of the toxin does not affect the appearance, smell, or taste of the shellfish, and cooking will not destroy the toxin. Because of the lack of sophisticated medical facilities for resuscitation and mechanical ventilation, it is prudent for all travelers to developing countries always to avoid potentially toxic shellfish.

Neurotoxic Shellfish Poisoning

Neurotoxic shellfish poisoning (NSP) occurs after eating bivalve mollusks (e.g., oysters, clams, scallops, and mussels) contaminated by heat-stable brevetoxins produced by the marine dinoflagellate *Gymnodinium breve*. *G. breve* is an important cause of red tides and has been responsible for the deaths of large numbers of fish, seabirds, and even marine mammals, such as manatees.

NSP usually presents as gastroenteritis, accompanied by neurologic symptoms, and often resembles mild paralytic shellfish poisoning or ciguatera poisoning. No deaths have been reported in humans. Inhalation of aerosolized brevetoxins from the seaspray associated with a red tide may cause an acute respiratory illness often referred to as aerosolized red tide respiratory irritation (ARTRI).

NSP was first described on the west coast of Florida in 1844. Since then, it has been reported from the Gulf of Mexico, the east coast of Florida, the North Carolina coast, and New Zealand. It is expected to be reported from other areas of the world in the future.

Symptoms of NSP may develop within 15 min of ingestion of contaminated shellfish or be delayed for up to 18 h. Gastrointestinal symptoms include abdominal pain, nausea, vomiting, and diarrhea. There may be myalgias and dizziness. Neurologic symptoms include circumoral paresthesias, paresthesias of the arms and legs, temperature reversal, vertigo, and ataxia. Symptoms may last for several hours or a few days. Symptoms of ARTRI occur almost immediately after exposure and include a non-productive cough, wheezing, conjunctivitis, and rhinorrhea. Asthmatics are particularly susceptible, and there is some anecdotal evidence of long-term pulmonary symptoms following ARTRI in the elderly or those with pre-existing lung disease.

Treatment of NSP and ARTRI is symptomatic and supportive. Preventive measures include avoiding shellfish associated with red tides and limiting coastline exposure to red tides and aerosolized brevetoxins. Particle masks can be used to prevent inhalation of aerosolized toxins.

Diarrheic Shellfish Poisoning

Diarrheic shellfish poisoning (DSP) results from ingestion of contaminated bivalve mollusks (clams, mussels, and scallops) containing okadaic acid and other toxins produced by various marine dinoflagellates.

Historically, DSP was reported predominantly from Japan and European countries, such as The Netherlands, Italy, and Spain. As a result of increased global spread of toxic dinoflagellates, however, outbreaks have recently been reported from Canada, South America, Australia, New Zealand, and Indonesia. As in other shellfish poisonings, outbreaks tend to follow red tides or dinoflagellate blooms. Okadaic acid triggers sodium release by intestinal cells and produces diarrhea. Symptoms usually appear 30 min to 6 h after ingestion of contaminated shellfish, although onset may be delayed for up to 12 h. Typically, symptoms last for up to 4 days and include diarrhea, abdominal cramps, nausea, vomiting, weakness, and chills. The severity of symptoms is usually related to the amount of toxin ingested. No fatalities have been reported. Diagnosis is usually made on clinical grounds and treatment is symptomatic and supportive.

Amnesic Shellfish Poisoning

Amnesic shellfish poisoning (ASP) is a recently described toxic encephalopathy. It was first identified in 1987 after an outbreak involving over 100 Canadians who had eaten mussels contaminated

Table 46.5 Mushroom Poisoning

Syndrome	Incubation	Clinical Features	Mushrooms Involved	Treatment
Gastrointestinal (multiple)	Usually 1–2 h; Rarely >4 h	Nausea, vomiting, abdominal pain, diarrhea	Multiple	Symptomatic and supportive. Fluid and electrolytes. Gastric lavage, catharsis
Hallucinations (psilocybin, psilocin)	15–30 min (30–60 min)	Resembles alcohol intoxication. Hallucinations, euphoria, loss of time sensation, tachycardia, hypertension	*Psilocybe, Panaeolus, Gymnopilus* species	Symptomatic and supportive
Anticholinergic (muscarine)	15–30 min	Salivation, sweating, lacrimation, urination, GI symptoms. Bradycardia, hypotension, constricted pupils	*Amanita, Inocybe, Clitocybe* species	Symptomatic and supportive. Fluid and electrolytes, atropine for bradycardia or to control secretions
Delirium (ibotenic acid, muscimol)	<30 min (20–90 min)	Delirium, hyperactivity, alteration in visual perception, ataxia, seizures, muscle twitching	*Amanita* and other species	Symptomatic and supportive. Antiseizure medications
Disulfiram-like (coprine)	2–6 h, symptoms 15–30 min after alcohol	Nausea, vomiting, headache, flushing, palpitations. Resembles alcohol-disulfiram (antabuse) reaction	*Coprinus* species	Symptomatic and supportive fluid and electrolytes. Avoid alcohol
Renal	2–20 days	Thirst, nausea, paresthesias, taste impairment, renal failure	*Cortinarius* species	Symptomatic and supportive. Fluid and electrolytes. Dialysis and renal transplantation
Hepatorenal (amatoxins, phallotoxins)	4–16 h	Nausea, vomiting, abdominal pain, diarrhea. Hepatic and renal failure	*Amanita phalloides* and other species	Symptomatic and supportive. Fluid and electrolytes. Thioctic acid. Dialysis, renal/liver transplantation

by domoic acid harvested off Prince Edward Island. Domoic acid is a heat-stable toxin produced by diatoms, such as *Nitzschia pungens*. High levels of toxin have been demonstrated in shellfish in areas such as the Pacific Northwest, the Gulf of Mexico, and off the west coast of Scotland, although no clinical cases have been reported from those areas.

In the Prince Edward Island outbreak, symptoms of ASP developed within 15 min to 38 h (median 6 h) of ingestion of contaminated mussels. Acute gastrointestinal symptoms were very common and included nausea, vomiting, abdominal cramps, and diarrhea. Neurologic features occurred in over one-third of patients and included headaches, short-term memory loss, confusion, disorientation, dizziness, seizures, and comas. Several patients developed long-term cognitive dysfunction. There were four deaths, all in patients over 70 years of age.

Treatment for ASP is symptomatic and supportive. Potentially contaminated shellfish, particularly those associated with red tides, should never be eaten.

Mushroom Poisoning

Mushroom poisoning is a rare but potentially very serious hazard for travelers. Since facilities for the diagnosis and treatment of mushroom poisoning may be unavailable or inadequate in many foreign

– particularly developing – countries or in wilderness regions, there is an increased risk of a complicated or even fatal outcome in travelers in those areas.

A variety of toxins have been extracted from mushrooms. Most are heat labile, but may not be completely destroyed by cooking.

Toxins in mushrooms cause a variety of clinical syndromes (Table 46.5) and a history of recent mushroom ingestion should always be sought in travelers who present with suspicious symptoms. Onset of illness is usually within a few hours of ingestion of toxic mushrooms, and cases in returned travelers are most likely to be seen if they have brought back mushrooms and consumed them after returning. Since some of the non-gastrointestinal symptoms may last for several days, however, certain travelers may not present until after returning home.

Most toxic mushrooms cause gastrointestinal symptoms – nausea, vomiting, abdominal pain, and diarrhea – beginning 1–2 h after ingestion and resolving in 6–12 h. Occasionally, symptoms may be severe enough to require fluid and electrolyte replacement. In general, if gastrointestinal symptoms are delayed for 4 h or more after ingestion, there is an increased chance that one of the highly toxic mushrooms, such as *Amanita phalloides* or death cap mushroom, is responsible, and a complicated or even fatal outcome is more likely. General symptoms of mushroom poisoning often include chills, myalgias, and headache. Mushroom toxins may also produce a variety of neurologic, renal, or hepatic syndromes (Table 46.5) that can be difficult to diagnose unless there is a high index of suspicion.[25]

Unless very experienced, travelers should not attempt to identify mushrooms that are considered safe to eat. Not uncommonly, non-toxic mushrooms in Europe and North America closely resemble highly toxic mushrooms found in other parts of the world, and vice versa. There have been a number of tragic deaths in immigrants from SE Asia as a result of misidentifying and ingesting highly toxic mushrooms such as *Amanita phalloides* or death cap mushroom.

References

1. Skinner MP, Brewer TD, Johnstone R, et al. Ciguatera fish poisoning in the Pacific Islands (1998 to 2008). PLoS Negl Trop Dis 2011;5:e1416.
2. Lewis RJ. The changing face of ciguatera. Toxicon 2001;39:97–106.
3. Glaziou P, Legrand AM. The epidemiology of ciguatera fish poisoning. Toxicon 1994;32:863–73.
4. Hirama M, Oishi T, Uehara H, et al. Total synthesis of ciguatoxin CTX3C. Science 2001;294:1904–7.
5. Hamilton B, Hurbungs M, Vernoux JP, et al. Isolation and characterisation of Indian Ocean ciguatoxin. Toxicon 2002;40:685–93.
6. Doherty M. Captain Cook on poison fish. Neurology 2005;65:1788–91.
7. Bagnis R, Kuberski T, Langier S. Clinical observations on 3009 cases of ciguatera fish poisoning in the South Pacific. Am J Trop Med Hyg 1979;28:1067.
8. Calvert GM, Hryhorczuk DO, Leikin JB. Treatment of ciguatera fish poisoning with amitriptyline and nifedipine. J Toxicol Clin Toxicol 1987;25:423–8.
9. Davis RT, Villar LA. Symptomatic improvement with amitriptyline in ciguatera fish poisoning. N Engl J Med 1986;315:65.
10. Berlin RM, King SL, Blythe DG. Symptomatic improvement of chronic fatigue with fluoxetine in ciguatera fish poisoning. Med J Aust 1992;157:567.
11. Palafox NA, Buenconsejo-Lum LE. Ciguatera fish poisoning: Review of clinical manifestations. J Toxicol – Toxin Reviews 2001;20(2):141–60.
12. Palafox NA, Buenconsejo-Lum L, Riklon S, et al. Successful treatment of ciguatera fish poisoning with intravenous mannitol. JAMA 1988;259:2740.
13. Schnorf H, Taurarii M, Cundy T. Ciguatera fish poisoning: a double-blind randomized trial of mannitol therapy. Neurology 2002;58:873–80.
14. Isbister GK, Kiernan MC. Neurotoxic marine poisoning. Lancet Neurol 2005;4:219–28.
15. Perez CM, Vasquez PA, Perret CF. Treatment of ciguatera poisoning with gabapentin. N Engl J Med 2001;344:692–3.
16. Develoux M. A Case of Ciguatera fish poisoning in a French traveler. Eurosurveillance 2008;Nov 6:1–2.
17. Arnett MV, Lim JT. Ciguatera fish poisoning: Impact for military health care provider. Mili Med 2007;172, 9:1012–5.
18. Hungerford JM. Scombroid poisoning: A review. Toxicon 2010;56:231–43.
19. Lavon O, Lurie Y, Bentur Y. Scombroid fish poisoning in Israel, 2005–2007. IMAJ 2008:789–92.
20. Blakesley ML. Scombroid poisoning; prompt resolution of symptoms with cimetidine. Ann Emerg Med 1983;12:104.
21. Kaku N, Meier J. Clinical toxicology of fugu poisoning. In: Meier J, White J, editors. Handbook of Clinical Toxicology of Animal Venoms and Poisons. 1st ed. Boca Raton: CRC Press; 1995. p. 75–83.
22. Centers for Disease Control. Tetrodotoxin poisoning associated with eating pufferfish transported from Japan-California 1996. MMWR 1996;45:389–91.
23. Sobel J, Painter J. Illness caused by marine toxins. Clin Infect Dis 2005;41:1290–6.
24. Gessner BD, Middaugh JP. Paralytic shellfish poisoning in Alaska: a 20-year retrospective analysis. Am J Epidemiol 1995;141:766.
25. Schneider S, Donnelly M. Toxic mushroom ingestions. In: Auerbach PS, editor. Wilderness Medicine. 6th ed. St Louis: Mosby; 2011. p. 1276–1301.

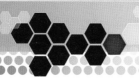
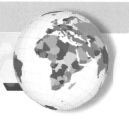

47

Injuries and Injury Prevention

Stephen Hargarten and Tifany Frazer

Key points

- Injuries are a more significant cause of travel-related mortality and morbidity than infectious diseases
- Road traffic crashes are the leading causes of injury mortality and can be prevented by traveling in safe vehicles with seat belts, driven by someone else. Motorcycles and bicycles should be avoided. Pedestrians are highly vulnerable in unfamiliar environments
- Death by drowning can be avoided by use of personal flotation devices, abstention from alcohol during water-related activities and close supervision of children. Fences and safety barriers are often absent overseas
- Data deficiencies and discrepancies in the manner of reporting cause of death have made it difficult to create a profile of injury risk based upon type of tourist, nationality, destination and travel activity. Better data on injury mortality to travelers (and all causes of mortality) should be maintained by respective embassies and governmental organizations

Introduction

Injuries are one of the leading causes of travel-related mortality worldwide, accounting for up to 25 times more deaths than infectious disease.[1] Researchers from several different countries have reported that non-infectious causes of travel-related deaths, especially injury, pose a serious health risk to travelers.[2–10] Injuries to tourists are also a significant burden to hospitals and healthcare systems, both at the tourist destination, during transport, and in terms of continuing care when the patient returns home.[11–14] Travel medicine specialists and government agencies have traditionally used comprehensive infectious disease information to promote immunization against infectious agents to protect travelers. Advice, however, on injury precautions during travel has received much less attention.[2] It is believed that tourists tend to be more at risk for an injury because they frequently find themselves in unfamiliar environments, participating in unfamiliar activities.[15]

It should be emphasized that injuries are not accidents or random events, though common usage sometimes favors the term 'accident'

to describe many injuries and their unexpected outcomes.[1] Injuries are predictable and preventable.[16] It is important for travel medicine specialists, tourism professionals, and government agencies issuing travel health advisories to create and communicate evidence-based injury prevention messages tailored for travelers, travel activities, and travel destinations. This chapter reviews the types of fatal and non-fatal injuries most frequently experienced by travelers, and provides evidence-based prevention and control recommendations.

Fatal Injury

Injury is a leading cause of travel-related mortality worldwide. Most mortality studies report that travelers most frequently die in road traffic crashes and drownings.[2–8] Other causes of travel-related injury death, though less common, include violent events, natural disasters such as tsunamis and earthquakes, airplane crashes, extreme environmental exposures, and animal or marine life bites and stings.[2–8]

The World Health Organization has estimated that road traffic crashes take the lives of nearly 1.3 million people every year, injure 20–50 million more, and have become the leading cause of death for people aged 15–29 years.[17] Nearly half (46%) of those dying on the world's roads are vulnerable road users: pedestrians, cyclists, and motorcyclists.[17] In addition to the grief and suffering they cause, road traffic crashes result in considerable economic losses to victims, their families, and nations as a whole, costing most countries 1–3% of their gross national product.[17]

The precise number of deaths and proportion of injury deaths to travelers worldwide is not known. From 2004 to 2006, 2361 US tourist deaths were due to injury, compared to a total for the years 1998, 2000 and 2002, in which there were 2011 deaths due to injury.[18] Injuries to US citizens traveling internationally occur at a higher proportion than to citizens residing in the United States.[18] Injury was reported to be the cause of 23% of deaths among visitors to the US.[19]

Injury deaths occur most commonly in low- to middle-income America (50.4%), followed by Europe and Eastern Mediterranean countries.[18] In each of these regions, US citizens have a greater proportion of injury mortality compared to host county nationals.[18] Overwhelmingly, young males tend to be at greater risk for an injury leading to death during travel.[3]

There is no uniform way to report deaths to travelers and no one agency is responsible for compiling these deaths. Mortality studies are

©2012 Elsevier Inc

DOI: 10.1016/B978-1-4557-1076-8.00047-8

expensive, time-consuming and difficult to conduct. Some government agencies, such as the US State Department, are working towards more complete reporting and categorization of the causes of non-natural death for their citizens who die while traveling or living in another country. This information is published on the internet and includes numbers, causes, and location of non-natural deaths to US citizens abroad, by year.[20]

The difficulty in counting and categorizing the causes of death among international travelers was highlighted by the 2004 tsunami disaster in the Indian Ocean and the 2011 Japanese earthquake and tsunami. The precise mortality count for both locals and travelers from these events may never be known. Each government had a different way to count their citizens' deaths. Many people, especially travelers, could be counted twice because of dual citizenship, and apart from obtaining a visa, travelers tend not to register their trip itinerary with their appropriate home government agency. Numbers have been pieced together from individual government counts, with news and relief agencies compiling overall counts.

Albeit challenging, mortality studies remain an important source of information about the seriousness of the injury problem for travelers in order to advise future travelers. Mortality surveillance is useful to travel medicine professionals as it provides a research-based foundation for the design of pre-travel advice tailored by destination, type of travel, and activity.

Non-Fatal Injuries

Studies focusing on non-fatal health incidents are also important to gain a more complete understanding of the larger travel injury problem. Morbidity studies often rely on data captured by hospital inpatient admissions or emergency department data in a specific geographic locale. This can be a rich source of data, as it routinely includes consistently coded information on the type of injury, the external causes, and the diagnostic and procedures codes. These types of study can reveal an interesting injury pattern for a given location, depending upon type of tourist and popular tourist activities at the destination.

A review of hospital records in Jamaica showed that injury was the main cause of hospitalization for international tourists, especially among tourists younger than 40 years.[21] In Australia, many of the presenting fractures, lacerations, sprains, and dislocations in tourists are the result of falls.[11] Another study of seven coastal hospitals in Australia found decompression illness associated with scuba diving to be the second most frequent reason for overseas visitor hospital admissions.[12] In contrast, reviewing visitor hospital admissions in New Zealand, tourist injuries were most frequently associated with skiing, mountaineering, and trekking.[22]

Data from morbidity studies also provide insight into how causes of non-fatal injury vary between local residents and tourists. A study conducted on the Greek island of Crete showed that left-side-driving country nationals were at greater risk for crashes than right-side-driving counterparts.[23] When comparing residents to tourists in Australia, injuries to tourists were higher for water-related activities only, especially decompression illness associated with scuba diving.[13]

Morbidity studies can be useful to develop location-specific community-based injury prevention recommendations. A study investigating 276 ocean sports-related injuries in Hawaii found that swimming, board surfing, and scuba diving were the main activities associated with injury, while lacerations, stings, and decompression illness were the primary diagnoses for treatment. Based on their identification of groups at risk for injury, they were able to recommend

specific research-based injury prevention initiatives, including improved warning signs on beaches and targeted education for both tourists and local residents.[24] Similarly, a study conducted in Australia reported on 1183 outpatient clinic visits by tourists. Following this study, island management purchased sandshoes for hotel guests on guided and unaccompanied reef walks in order to prevent coral stings. Similarly, the study findings on bites and stings led to several large wasps' nests being removed from the resort golf course, while information on marine stingers was specifically included in guest orientation briefings.[25]

A Global Public Health Approach for Travel Medicine

The public health approach describes the problem, identifies risk factors, and helps to develop and evaluate research-based interventions. Haddon's event-phase matrix is a tool commonly used to deconstruct a specific event to identify salient risk factors and develop prevention or risk reduction strategies.[26] In Table 47.1 an example using malaria, an infectious disease that frequently affects travelers in tropical destinations, has been compared to a child drowning and a motor vehicle crash. Research has demonstrated that injuries have three phases: the pre-event, the event and the post-event phases.[26] The pre-event phase describes events leading up to the injury or illness and relates to the development of primary prevention strategies; the event phase describes the actual injury or illness incident and efforts to control the damage of the event once it has occurred; and the post-event phase focuses on describing the consequences following the event and controlling the damage.

Increasingly, the effectiveness of injury prevention strategies requires travel medicine leadership to engage and partner in broader, global efforts. The World Report on Road Traffic Injury Prevention requests that governments make road safety a political priority with regard to policy legislation, law enforcement, and improved road conditions. May 2011 marked the official launch of the Decade for Action for Road Safety (2011–2020).[27] The World Health Organization has begun to work with governmental and non-governmental partners worldwide to raise the profile of the preventability of road traffic injuries and promote good practices related to helmet and seatbelt wearing, not drinking and driving, not speeding, and being visible in traffic.

Injury Prevention Recommendations

International travelers should know the address and phone number of their nearest embassy, and register their trip itinerary with that embassy. Trip registration can be done easily using the internet. It is important that travelers make their presence in the country and their specific whereabouts known in case of an emergency. Registration of travelers' itineraries also helps to improve governments' surveillance of injury events. Travelers' fatality data can be used to better inform future travelers about potential risks in a given destination.

It is also recommended that travelers purchase international travel insurance that includes emergency evacuation to adequately cover an urgent departure from their intended destinations. This will help to ensure that healthcare received by injured or ill travelers will be at international standards. Travelers' insurance will also help to bridge the gap should cultural and language barriers exist, provide ambulances or other means of patient transport, and support for a travel companion to assist if they need to be hospitalized for a long period of time (Table 47.2).[2,28–30]

Table 47.1 Phase-Factor Matrix

Injury/Illness	Pre-Event		Event		Post-Event	
	Description	Strategy	Description	Strategy	Description	Strategy
Malaria	Traveler visits area with endemic malaria	Avoid travel to destination with malaria Chemoprophylaxis Avoid contact with mosquitoes that transmit malaria	Mosquito bites traveler during high-risk hours and transmits malaria	DEET Protective clothing Avoid mosquito during peak hours Chemoprophylaxis	Traveler becomes ill with malaria; has fevers associated with malaria	Access to quality medical care, treatment of fever to reduce severity Access to appropriate drugs
Motor vehicle crash	Travel requires motor vehicle transportation between cities	Rent a well-equipped vehicle with a qualified driver who is not under the influence of alcohol or drugs Drive during daytime hours Travel by bus during daytime hours	Vehicle crashes	Seat belts Child safety seats Airbags	Passengers inside vehicle are injured	Access to emergency medical services and quality healthcare Proximity to major trauma center and acceptable blood products Travelers' health insurance
Drowning	Child staying in poolside hotel room	Four-sided isolation fencing around pool	Child wanders to pool unsupervised	Lifeguard-approved personal flotation devices	Child falls into pool and near drowning occurs	CPR Lifeguard is monitoring pool – prompt emergency response system

Table 47.2 General Injury Prevention Recommendations for Travelers

1. Review travel warnings and travel alerts of the destination.[45]
2. Learn about the common travel safety concerns, health risks and travel health notices related to the destination as some locations are prone to certain natural disasters.[35,45]
3. Understand local laws and culture of the destination.[45]
4. Purchase international travel and medical evacuation insurance appropriate for the destination.[28,45]
5. Register the travel itinerary with the appropriate government agency or embassy in order to get assistance should an emergency situation arise or natural disaster occur. Governments cannot assist their citizens if they do not know their whereabouts.[28,45]
6. Develop an emergency response plan, know the name and location of the nearest major medical center and embassy and whether or not it is safe to receive blood products in their country/ies of destination.[28,45]
7. Consume alcohol responsibly and in moderation when in an unfamiliar environment. Alcohol should be avoided if one is operating a vehicle, boat, machinery, or supervising children around water. Alcoholic beverages should not be consumed if one is planning to be in or around the water.[2,29,30,45]

Road Traffic Safety

Road traffic injuries are the leading cause of injury death worldwide and among all travelers.[1,3,19] The World Health Organization estimates that approximately 1.17 million deaths occur each year worldwide.[27] The majority of these crashes (90%) occur in low- or middle-income countries, and the majority of road crash victims in developing countries are *not* the motor vehicle occupants, but pedestrians, motorcyclists, bicyclists, and other non-motorized vehicle occupants.[31,32]

Road traffic crashes, including motor vehicles, pedestrians, and other non-motorized transportation, such as bicycles and rickshaws, consistently emerge from the travel medicine literature as the most common cause of injury death for tourists.[3,5,7,19,33–34] According to US Department of State data, road traffic crashes are also the leading cause of injury death to US citizens while traveling internationally and the leading cause of death to healthy US travelers. Recent estimates show that 745 US citizens were killed in road traffic crashes from 2007 through 2009.[35] Approximately 13% of these road traffic deaths involved motorcycles and 5% involved pedestrians.[35] While much progress has been made in making motor vehicles, roads, and drivers safer worldwide, there has been very little focus specifically on the risk to international travelers. Road traffic injuries were also the leading cause of death for travelers visiting the US, accounting for 37% of deaths of non-residents.[4] The Australian tourism and transport authorities found that the rate of tourist deaths on Australian roads was double that for all Australians.[33]

Seatbelts and Child Safety Seats

The advantage of road travel in more developed countries is that rental vehicles and public roads tend to be maintained at a reasonably safe standard according to government regulations. In countries with less familiar local customs governing driving, smaller means to support road maintenance and infrastructure, and possibly with fewer regulations governing road safety, a traveler may choose to be a passenger rather than a driver. Only 15% of countries have comprehensive laws relating to five key risks: speeding, drinking and driving, and the

Table 47.3 Road Traffic Safety Recommendations for Travelers

1.	*Wear a seatbelt* no matter where they are seated in any vehicle. Parents need to bring appropriate car seats or communicate with the vehicle rental agency about availability. Guidelines about use of car seats are as follows: [38,40–46] 　Children birth to age 1 and at least 20 pounds need to be in a rear-facing child safety seat in the rear of the vehicle. 　Children ages 1 and 20 pounds until age 4 and 40 pounds should be in a front-facing car seat in the rear of the vehicle. 　Children ages 4–8 years should be placed in a booster seat in the rear of the vehicle unless they are taller than 4′ 9″. 　Children older than 8 years and taller than 4′ 9″ should use a seatbelt and sit in the rear of the vehicle. 　Children 12 and younger should always ride in the rear of the vehicle.
2.	Avoid driving if possible.[45]
3.	Look for a reputable company through the embassy, hotel concierge or other reliable source that employs certified and trained drivers familiar with the driving culture, laws, and roads. Avoid driving at night and with drivers who may be under the influence of drugs or alcohol.[29]
4.	Avoid alcohol, fatigue, jet lag, all night-driving, and learn local road signs, roads, driving customs, and laws. Check with the embassy in country of destination to understand the requirements for license, road permits, auto insurance, local road rules, driving culture, and road conditions.[30]
5.	Rent a vehicle (with or without driver) equipped with seatbelts for all seats (rear and front), air bags, and the LATCH (lower anchors and tethers for children) System if traveling with small children that require child safety seats.[37,39]
6.	Choose commonly available cars when renting (with or without driver), and request that any obvious rental car markings be removed. Travelers should request a map, directions, list of local traffic signs and laws pertaining to road travel and a full familiarization of their rental vehicle from staff of the rental agency prior to their departure. Take time to inspect the tires, breaks, lights, airbags, and seatbelts.[28]
7.	Carry a mobile phone and know how to initiate an emergency response in the travel destination should a crash occur. Do not talk on the phone while driving.[46]
8.	Avoid riding on or driving a moped or motorbike while traveling. If travelers rent mopeds, motorbikes, or bicycles *helmets should be worn by adults and children.* Travelers may need to bring appropriately fitting helmets, especially for children, if they plan to rent bicycles or motorized vehicles.[41]
9.	Be aware of possible car-jacking schemes and hotspots locally, and keep the doors of the vehicle locked at all times.[28]

non-use of helmets, seat-belts and child restraints.[17] In most cases, hiring a vehicle with a driver is recommended as a safer way to travel than driving yourself. In many countries seatbelts are not required to be fitted in motor vehicles, or may only be required in the front seats.[36,37] Despite local laws, travelers should demand vehicles with the appropriate safety equipment for themselves and their companions, especially if traveling with young children. Research has shown that seatbelts, when properly worn, are the most effective way to survive a road traffic crash with minimal injury.[38,39] The same is true for young children: appropriately sized car seats have been shown to be effective in reducing deaths and injuries to children in car crashes.[39,40] Appropriately sized child safety seats should be rented or brought with the tourist family.

Helmets

Because of the non-protective nature of the vehicle, along with other factors such as speed and relative lack of visibility, motorcycle crash victims make up a high percentage of those killed or injured in road traffic crashes worldwide. The number of travelers injured or killed by motorcycle crashes is not yet known. Helmets reduce the risk of head injury mortality in riders who crash.[41]

Head injury also poses the greatest risk to bicyclists. In the US, for example, about 900 people die as a result of a bicycle crash each year.[42] A global estimate for the number of travelers affected by bicycle-related injury is not known. What is known is that bicycle helmets reduce the risk of head and brain injury for riders of all ages by 75%. Bike helmets have also been shown to reduce the number of facial injuries among riders by 65%.[42]

Travelers should be encouraged to rent helmets if renting bicycles, mopeds, or motorcycles. It should not be assumed that helmets will

be available: if tourists are planning to participate in this type of activity, they might consider bringing helmets along, especially for children.

Evidence-based road traffic safety recommendations for travelers are summarized in Table 47.3.[28,29,32,37,38,40–46]

Water-Related Injuries

Drowning is a serious but mostly preventable injury problem, particularly among international travelers. About 450 000 people drown worldwide each year.[47] The exact number of travelers who drown or experience a near-drowning is not known.[48] Drowning accounts for 14% of deaths of US citizens abroad.[47] Limited data exist to describe drowning during travel, but also lacking is a clear and accurate description of how international travelers drown.[2]

Many popular travel destinations are situated in warmer climates near oceans or lakes, or have elaborate pools and feature water-related activities such as surfing, scuba diving, snorkeling, boating, parasailing, and water-skiing. US citizens traveling to Central America, the Caribbean, Oceania, and Mexico have significantly higher proportions of death due to drowning than US residents.[6,19]

Drowning is consistently reported as a leading cause of injury death among tourists, while near-drowning or non-fatal submersion commonly appears as a cause of injury in non-fatal data.[2,6–8,11,12,42] The risk factors have not been clearly defined, but are most likely related to unfamiliarity with local water currents and water conditions, as rip tides can be especially dangerous, as are sea animals, such as urchins, jellyfish, coral, and sea lice.[47] In low- to middle-income American, drowning accounts for 13.1% of injury deaths to US tourists but only 4.6% to native citizens.[35,47] Drowning remains the leading cause of injury death to US tourists in island nations.[18,35] A study of British children traveling abroad over an 8-year period found that 74% of deaths occurred in a swimming pool, with the highest rates of drowning occurring in the US as a travel destination.[48]

Swimming in an unfamiliar environment can present difficulties for even the best swimmers, let alone some tourists who may have no background, skills, or ability in the water. Primary and secondary prevention measures are extremely important for near-drowning and drowning. Treatment measures in an intensive care unit or medical unit have limited effect on the outcome for those admitted to hospital because of near-drowning.[50]

Supervision of children around the water deserves special attention. Select lodgings that do not allow direct access by your child to a body of water in which the child could potentially drown. Ideally, swimming pools at the destination should be completely surrounded by a 4-ft climb-proof fence with a self-closing, self-latching gate.[51] The responsibility of supervising children around the water should be delegated only to experienced adults who practice 'touch supervision' with their full attention focused on the child, who know CPR, how to initiate an emergency response plan, and have not and will not be consuming alcohol. Even children who may be considered excellent swimmers need supervision in and around the water.[52]

Table 47.4 has a summary of evidence-based recommendations for water safety.[52–57]

Table 47.4 Water Safety and Drowning Prevention Recommendations for Travelers

1. Bring personal flotation devices (PFDs) along if you think they will not be available, especially for adult non-swimmers and children, and *use them* when in and around the water. Select a proper sized and coastguard-approved PFD by looking at the label to ensure a safe and proper fit. Use PFDs when water skiing or during towed activities, on personal watercraft, during white water boating, sail boarding and on moving vessels of <26 ft. Children under 13 years of age should use them at all times. Identify their location when on board a yacht or cruise ship.[53,54]

2. Learn cardio-pulmonary resuscitation (CPR) prior to departure. CPR is critical in improving the outcome should a near-drowning occur.[50,54]

3. If traveling with children, inquire whether there is 4-foot climb-proof isolation fencing around the pools and/or if there is a barrier between your place of lodging/hotel room and any body of water in which your child may drown.[51]

4. Limit alcoholic consumption to one beverage, preferably none if planning to be in or around the water or on a boat. Alcohol should be avoided when adults are supervising children around the water.[30]

5. Swim in designated swimming areas, preferably that provide a trained and certified lifeguard. The presence of lifeguards will improve the outcome should a near-drowning occur.[55]

6. Learn about animal-related risks and other environmental risks in and near the water in your travel destination. Be aware of signs posting surf and weather conditions or other environmental risks that may be present in natural bodies of water.[52]

7. When diving or participating in more strenuous water-related activity than normal, a re-assessment of physical, mental, and medical fitness is recommended prior to travel, at regular intervals and following an illness or injury.[54]

Alcohol as a Risk Factor

Alcohol use during travel is one of the most serious risk factors for travel-related injury. Travelers tend to consume more alcohol while on vacation than in their home environments.[35] Alcohol is a major risk factor for road traffic crashes, and injury in general.[29,30] In the Greek island of Crete, alcohol is reported as primary cause of crashes more often among tourists than residents.[23] Alcohol also contributes to drowning and boating crashes and is thought to be involved in 30–50% of adult and adolescent drownings.[47,56,57] A case–control study revealed that boaters with a blood alcohol level ≥100 mg/dL had a 16-fold greater risk of drowning than those with no alcohol in their blood, and that this risk increases as blood alcohol level increases.[30]

Physicians and travel medicine professionals should address alcohol as a risk factor for injury when advising their patients. It is highly recommended that travelers do not drink alcohol while driving motorized vehicles, driving or riding on motorcycles or motorbikes, operating or riding in a boat, swimming, supervising children around the water or in and around the water in general.[2,29,30,54]

Summary

The World Tourism Organization recommends that every country should develop a national policy on tourism safety to address and prevent injury to tourists.[58] All destinations have a major responsibility to protect their visitors, and, in turn, their reputation. Similarly, governments have a responsibility to protect their citizens traveling internationally. The World Health Organization's resolution to advance emergency care requested the Director-General to raise awareness of low-cost ways to reduce mortality through improved organization and planning of the provision of trauma and emergency care, and to organize regular expert meetings to further technical exchange and build capacity in this area.[17]

Travel medicine practitioners, along with embassies, governmental agency health, tourism, and transportation partners, need to monitor the risk of injury according to geographic location in order to provide up-to-date evidence-based pre-travel advice. The World Health Organization Global Burden of Disease Study database shows that great improvements in reporting, coding, and classification of injury mortality have been made, but significant challenges remain.[59] Injury prevention recommendations need to be communicated effectively to travelers along with other travel health-related advice, preferably prior to departure, by travel medicine professionals, family physician, travel agent, or through government travel health advisories.

References

1. Hargarten SW, Güler Gürsu K. Travel-related injuries, epidemiology, and prevention. In: DuPont HL, Steffen R, editors. Textbook of Travel Medicine and Health. Hamilton: BC Decker; 1997. p. 258–61.
2. Cortes LM, Hargarten SW, Hennes H. Recommendations for water safety and drowning prevention for travelers. J Travel Med 2006;13:21–34.
3. McInnes RJ, Williamson LM, Morrison A. Unintentional injury during foreign travel: a review. J Travel Med 2002;9:297–307.
4. Sniezek JE, Smith SM. Injury mortality among non-US residents in the United States 1979–1984. Int J Epidemiol 1991;20:225–9.
5. Baker TD, Hargarten SW, Guptill KS. The uncounted dead – American civilians dying overseas. Public Health Rep 1992;107:155–9.
6. Guptill KS, Hargarten SW, Baker TD. American travel deaths in Mexico. Causes and prevention strategies. West J Med 1991;154:169–71.
7. Hargarten SW, Baker TD, Guptill K. Overseas fatalities of United States citizen travelers: an analysis of deaths related to international travel. Ann Emerg Med 1991;20–6.

8. Paixao ML, Dewar RD, Cossar JH, et al. What do Scots die of when abroad? Scott Med J 1991;36:114–16.

9. Shilm DR, Gallie J. The causes of death among trekkers in Nepal. Int J Sports Med 1992;13(Suppl. 1):S74–6.

10. MacPherson DW, Guerillot F, Streiner DL, et al. Death and dying abroad: the Canadian experience. J Travel Med 2000;7:227–33.

11. Walters J, Fraser HS, Alleyne GAO. Use by visitors of the services of the Queen Elizabeth Hospital, Barbados. WI. WI Med J 1993;42:13–17.

12. Nicol J, Wilks J, Wood M. Tourists as inpatients in Queensland regional hospitals. Aust Health Rev 1996;19:55–72.

13. Cossar JH. Travelers' health: a medical perspective. In: Clift S, Page SJ, editors. Health and the International Tourist. London: Routledge; 1996. p. 23–43.

14. Petridou E, Gatsoulis N, Dessypris N, et al. Imbalance of demand and supply for regionalized injury services: a case study in Greece. Int J Qual Health Care 2000;12:105–13.

15. Page SJ, Meyer D. Injuries and accidents among international tourists in Australia: scale, causes and solutions. In: Clift S, Grabowski P, editors. Tourism and Health: Risks, Research and Responses. London: Pinter; 1997. p. 61–79.

16. Grossman DC. The history of injury control and the epidemiology of child and adolescent injuries. Future Child 2000;10:23–52.

17. World Health Organization, Sixteenth World Health Assembly WHA 60.22, Health Systems: emergency-care system, Eleventh plenary meeting, Agenda item 12.14, 23 May 2007.

18. Tonellato D, Guse C, Hargarten S. Injury deaths of US citizens abroad: new data source, old travel problem. J Trav Med 2009:16:304–10.

19. Guse CE, Cortés LM, Hargarten SW, et al. Fatal injuries of US citizens abroad. J Travel Med 2007;14:279–87.

20. US Department of State. Non-natural deaths of US Citizens Abroad. Online. Available: http://travel.state.gov/family/family_issues/death/death_594.html (accessed Jul 15, 2011).

21. Thompson DC, Ashley DV, Dockery-Brown CA, et al. Incidence of health crises in tourists visiting Jamaica, West Indies, 1998 to 2000. J Travel Med 2003;10:79–86.

22. Bentley T, Meyer D, Page S, et al. Recreational tourism injuries among visitors to New Zealand: an exploratory analysis using hospital discharge data. Tourism Manage 2001;22:373–81.

23. Petridou E, Askitopoulou H, Vourvahakis D, et al. Epidemiology of road traffic accidents during pleasure travelling: the evidence from the Island of Crete. Accid Anal Prev 1997;29:687–93.

24. Hartung GH, Goebert DA, Taniguchi RM, et al. Epidemiology of ocean sports-related injuries in Hawaii: 'Akahele O Ke Kai'. Hawaii Med J 1990;49:52, 54–6.

25. Wilks J, Walker S, Wood M, et al. Tourist health services at tropical island resorts. Aust Health Rev 1995;18:45–62.

26. Wilson MH, Baker SP, Teret SP, et al. Saving Children. A Guide to Injury Prevention. New York: Oxford University Press; 1991.

27. World Health Organization, Saving Millions of Lives, 2011. Online. Available: http://www.who.int/roadsafety/decade_of_action (accessed Jul 15, 2011).

28. US State Department website. Online. Available: www.travel.state.gov/travel/tips/safety/ssafety_1179.htm(accessed Jul 15, 2011).

29. Heng K, Hargarten S, Layde P, et al. Moderate alcohol intake and motor vehicle crashes: the conflict between health advantage and at-risk use. J Alcohol 2006;41(4):451–4.

30. Smith GS, Keyl PM, Hadley JA, et al. Drinking and recreational boating fatalities, a population-based case control study. JAMA 2001;286:2974–80.

31. Sharma BR. Road traffic injuries: a major global public health crisis. Public Health 2008;122:1399–406.

32. Peden M. Global collaboration on road traffic injury prevention. Int J Inj Contr Saf Promot 2005;12:85–91.

33. Wilks J, Watson B, Hansen R, editors. International Visitors and Road Safety in Australia. A Status Report. Canberra: Australian Transport Safety Bureau; 1999.

34. Wilks J, Watson B, Hansen J. International drivers and road safety in Queensland, Australia. J Tourism Stud 2000;11:36–43.

35. US Department of State. Death of US citizens abroad by non-natural causes. Washington, DC: US Department of State; 2010. Online. Available: http://travel.state.gov/law/family_issues/death/death_600.html. (accessed Jul 15, 2011).

36. Wilks J, Watson B, Faulks IJ. International tourists and road safety in Australia: developing a national research and management programme. Tourism Manage 1999;20:645–54.

37. Hargarten SW. Availability of safety devices in rental cars: an international survey. Travel Med Int 1992;10:109–10.

38. Allen S, Zhu S, Sauter C, et al. A comprehensive statewide analysis of seatbelt non-use with injury and hospital admissions: new data, old problem. Acad Emerg Med 2006;13(4):427–34.

39. NHTSA website. Online. Available: http://www.nhtsa.dot.gov/people/injury/childps/ParentGuide2005/pages/WhenDoYou.htm) (accessed Jul 15, 2011).

40. Zaza S, Carande-Kulis VG, Sleet DA, et al. Task force on community preventive services. Methods for conducting systematic reviews of the evidence of effectiveness and economic efficiency of interventions to reduce injuries to motor vehicle occupants. Am J Prev Med 2001;21:S23–30.

41. Lui B, Ivers R, Norton R, et al. Helmets for preventing injury in motorcycle riders. Cochrane Database Syst Rev 2004;2:CD004333.

42. Thompson DC, Rivara FP, Thompson R. Helmets for preventing head and facial injuries in bicyclists. Cochrane Database Sys Rev 2000;2:CD001855.

43. Zaza S, Thompson RS, editors. The guide to community prevention services: reducing injuries to motor vehicle occupants. Systematic reviews of evidence, recommendations from the task force on Community Preventive Services and Expert Commentary. Am J Prev Med 2001;21:whole issue.

44. Dihn-Zarr TB, Sleet DA, Shultz RA, et al. Task force reviews of evidence regarding interventions to increase the use of safety belts. Am J Prev Med 2001;21:S48–65.

45. US State Department. Online. Available: www.travel.state.gov/travel/tips/safety/ssafety_1179.htm (accessed Jul 15, 2011).

46. McEvoy SP, Steventson MR, McCartt AT, et al. Role of mobile phones in motor vehicle crashes resulting in hospital attendance: a case-crossover study. BMJ 2005;331:428.

47. CDC. The Yellow Book, Health Information for International Travel. New York: Oxford University Press; 2012.

48. Peden M, Mc Gee K, Sharma G. The Injury Chart Book: A Graphical Overview of the Global Burden of Injuries. Geneva: World Health Organization; 2002.

49. Cornall P, Howie S, Mughal A, et al. Drowning of British children abroad. Child Care Health Dev 2005;31(5):611–13.

50. Kyriacou DN, Arcinue EL, Peek C, et al. Effect of immediate resuscitation on children with submersion injury. Pediatrics 1994;94:137–42.

51. Thompson DC, Rivara FP. Pool fencing for preventing drowning in children. Cochrane Database Sys Rev 2000;2:CD001855.

52. Brenner RA, Committee on Injury and Violence and Poison Prevention. Prevention of drowning in infants, children and adolescents. Pediatrics 2003;112:440–5. Online. Available: http://www.pediatrics.org/cgi/content/full/112/440 (accessed Jul 15, 2011).

53. US Coast Guard website. Online. Available: http://www.uscgboating.org/regulations/Nasbla_Ref_Guide6.pdf (accessed Jul 15, 2011).

54. World Congress on Drowning Resolutions. Online. Available: www.drowning.nl (accessed Jul 15, 2011).

55. Branche CM, Stewart S, editors. Lifeguard Effectiveness: A Report of the Working Group. Atlanta: Centers for Disease Control and Prevention, National Center for Injury Prevention and Control; 2001.

56. American Academy of Pediatrics. Prevention of drowning in infants, children and adolescents. Pediatrics 2003;112:437–9.

57. Driscoll TR, Harrison JA, Steenkamp M. Review of the role of alcohol in drowning associated with recreational aquatic activity. Inj Prev 2004;10:107–13.

58. UNWTO World Tourism Organization. Tourist safety and security: practical measures for destinations, 1996, Madrid, Spain. Online. Available: http://pub.world-tourism.org:81/epages/Store.sf/?ObjectPath=/Shops/Infoshop/Products/1023/SubProducts/1023–1 (accessed Jul 15, 2011).

59. Chandran A, Hyder AA, Peek-Asa C. The global burden of unintentional injuries and an agenda for progress. Epidemiol Rev 2010;32:110–20.

48

Psychiatric Disorders of Travel

Thomas H. Valk

Key points

- Traveling and living overseas involve unique stressors, and frequent international travel may correlate with increased need for mental health services
- There are no data on the epidemiology of psychiatric disorders in the population of international travelers, much less on any subtypes
- An inquiry into past psychiatric history and treatment should always be a standard part of any pre-travel consultation
- The international traveler and expatriate population generally suffer from the same range of serious mental disorders as seen in clinics or hospitals
- The clinical operating environment overseas provides clinicians with many challenges, given the wide variation from country to country in the availability of culturally compatible clinicians, hospital and laboratory facilities, and medications. Improvised outpatient approaches may be necessary

Introduction

International travel is a stressful experience. Travelers face separation from family and familiar social supports, and must deal with the impact of foreign cultures and language, jet lag, and bewildering, unfamiliar threats to health and safety. Having to accomplish even the most mundane tasks of everyday living while overseas can become a major challenge, leading to a loss of the sense of active mastery over the environment. Under the stress of travel, pre-existing psychiatric disorders can be exacerbated and predispositions towards illness may emerge for the first time. Reflecting these stressors, international business travelers have been found to file insurance claims at higher rates than non-traveling counterparts. This effect was greatest for claims for psychological disorders, and increased with the frequency of travel.[1] Streltzer, in his study of psychiatric emergencies in travelers to Hawaii, estimated an incidence of emergencies of 220/100 000 population per year for tourists, 2250/100 000 per year for transient travelers, i.e., those who arrived in Hawaii with no immediate plans to leave, and a rate of 1250/100 000 per year for the non-traveling population.[2] Diagnostically, the problems seen, in order of decreasing

frequency, were schizophrenia, alcohol abuse, anxiety reactions, and depression.

Despite the clear stress involved, international travelers generally suffer from the same range of disorders as seen in a clinic or hospital. Rather than deal with all possible psychiatric disorders, this chapter will focus on a discussion of the psychotic patient, the assessment of the suicidal patient, and some further examination of brief psychotic disorder, schizophrenia, mania, major depression, and selected substance use disorders as they relate to international travel. Sections on initial assessment of the traumatic event victim and pre-travel counseling are included.

Types of International Traveler

Typologies of international travelers have been proposed based on conscious and unconscious motivations for travel.[3,4] However, these classifications are unlikely to be clinically useful and would be difficult to define operationally for the purposes of research. Classification based on the overtly stated reason for travel, e.g., tourism, study overseas, business and expatriate travel, is widely used if also not known to be clinically relevant.

Epidemiologic data based on population surveys of the rates of psychiatric disorder by type of traveler are non-existent. Anecdotal and clinical evidence points to possible differences, but more study is necessary to establish incidence and prevalence rates. Business and expatriate executives are almost certainly less likely to suffer from the more debilitating, chronic mental disorders, such as schizophrenia, if only because such a disorder is incompatible with high office in the workplace, and because the disorder usually begins in younger patients. Such would not necessarily be true of expatriates' family members.

Pre-Travel Screening

Given the potential consequences of a psychiatric emergency in the overseas environment, as discussed in this chapter, an inquiry into past psychiatric history and treatment should always be a standard part of any pre-travel consultation. Any condition that has involved a psychotic or manic state, a major depression, a history of danger to self or others, psychiatric hospitalization, or substance abuse, dependence or withdrawal would be of substantial concern. Circumstances worthy of particular attention include individuals with bipolar I disorder, especially if they have not been stable on medications for a substantial

©2012 Elsevier Inc
DOI: 10.1016/B978-1-4557-1076-8.00048-X

period (of the order of years), individuals with recurrent major depressions that have not been stabilized on appropriate medication and/or who have evinced psychotic symptoms or significant suicide risk, and either practicing substance abusers or those who have only recently recovered and are in early sobriety. In general, it is not advisable to generate a list of disorders that should preclude international travel. At least in the United States, such would be precluded if tied to employment decisions by the Americans with Disabilities Act, as amended. Rather, each patient should be considered in terms of severity of illness, the long-term stability of treatment and the availability of psychiatric resources and medications that may be necessary in the overseas environment in question.

To aid in overcoming reluctance to discuss mental health issues, it might be helpful as preface to talk about the fact that international travel is known to be uniquely stressful, mental health care is highly variable, and the consequences of a psychiatric emergency overseas can be considerable. Having elicited a psychiatric history, the degree of risk involved depends upon a number of factors, including the diagnosis; the degree of stability and likelihood of recurrence; the duration of intended travel; the availability of required psychotropic medications and of culturally compatible mental health providers and facilities, including reliable laboratories, as needed. For any complicated condition, or if there is any doubt as to the diagnosis, stability of treatment, or availability of appropriate treatment in destination countries, it would be a good idea obtain a specialty consultation with a psychiatrist familiar with the vicissitudes of international travel.

Particular situations of note would be the patient on lithium (Eskalith). Even on the same dose, blood levels will vary with ambient temperature, exercise, diet, and hydration. Travelers should be educated carefully on the signs and symptoms of toxicity, and the availability of reliable laboratory facilities for the measurement of blood levels should be ascertained. Patients on MAO inhibitors, a class of antidepressants, should be educated carefully on dietary restrictions to avoid foods with high tyramine content, which may be difficult when presented with new or exotic foods overseas. Adequate treatment facilities for hypertensive crisis should also be available. If abuse of drugs is suspected, a careful explanation of the large variation in the legal status of drug abuse from country to country should be undertaken, noting that penalties for drug use can be severe. For alcohol or drug abusers who are currently sober, the availability of language-compatible Alcoholic or Narcotic Anonymous meetings is important. Sexual activity should also be frankly discussed, particularly as it relates to exposure to STDs, including HIV.[5]

Clinical Operating Environments Overseas and Their Vicissitudes

Although travelers present with the usual range of disorders, the clinician tending to this population will find many challenges in the clinical operating environment overseas. Countries, and even cities within countries, vary enormously in a number of parameters that affect dealing with psychiatric emergencies. Some countries do not have well-developed mental health systems. Hospital facilities for the psychiatric patient may be lacking, and culturally compatible clinicians may be rare or non-existent. Nurse staffing, training, and practices can differ enormously from country to country. Cross-cultural problems arise, as examined by Fennig et al. in their paper on the Arab nurse and the Jewish psychotic patient, and by Westermeyer in his discussion of cross-cultural diagnosis.[6,7] The range of psychotropic medications available locally may be limited and of unknown quality. Laboratory

Table 48.1 Challenges Found in Some Clinical Operating Environments Overseas

Lack of well-developed mental health system

Inpatient facilities either not available or not culturally compatible

Nursing practices, scope of duty, and training vary widely

Culturally compatible mental health clinicians rare or not present

Locally available psychotropic medications limited or of unknown quality

Laboratory facilities for serum levels of psychotropic medications not available or of unknown reliability

Wide variations in the legal environment, affecting commitment and treatment of drug abuse

facilities to determine blood levels of frequently used mood stabilizers may not be reliable or available.

The legal environment within which a clinician practices can also vary widely, a fact especially relevant when facing a patient in imminent danger to self or others. Local commitment laws vary widely from country to country, and some countries may not have any laws dealing with such matters.[8] Laws dealing with illicit substance use vary considerably, and in some countries can be quite severe.

As a result of these mental health and legal infrastructure differences, which are summarized in Table 48.1, the first decision a clinician may have to make is the strategic one of whether or not a given patient can be managed in place or requires evacuation. Having decided this key issue, clinicians frequently will have to be creative in their management. Problems that normally would require hospitalization, such as the psychotic, manic, or suicidal patient, may have to be handled on an outpatient basis, using friends, family and/or private duty nurses to monitor and contain the patient pending medical evacuation. In some countries, psychiatric problems are normally handled on general medical wards. If hospital facilities are present, but of questionable quality, safety, or cultural compatibility, the treating physician will have to balance the relative benefits of containment in hospital versus some more ad hoc arrangement outside. The same balance will have to be made in countries with no or few legal provisions for commitment of the dangerous patient. The physician will need to be familiar with the legal situation and how the laws, if any, are enforced, in order to make a good decision to invoke commitment.

Based upon the author's experience and an internet review of consular services offered by English-speaking countries to their citizens (US, UK, Canada and Australia), clinicians should not rely upon direct medical or evacuation services from embassies' Consular Service sections, although checking with a particular patient's embassy would be reasonable. US, Canadian, and Australian consular services do provide their respective citizens with lists of local doctors, and some US embassies maintain downloadable lists that can be accessed through their websites. These lists may also include local facilities, and are usually accompanied with the caveat that being on the list does not imply endorsement or guarantee of quality. None of the consular services reviewed offer financial help with medical evacuation or in-country treatment.

The Psychotic Patient

A psychotic state is a major break with reality and can be characterized by delusions, hallucinations, and thought disorder, either alone or in some combination. Hallucinations may or may not be accompanied by insight into their not being real. Thought disorder is a disruption of the normal train of thought such that sequential ideas are not connected. It can be mild to severe in nature, such as in 'word salad', where the patient is seemingly stringing words together without any connection at all. Severe changes in behavior, including disorganization and catatonia, can be present.

The psychotic patient is a psychiatric emergency regardless of causation. Psychosis may be present in a number of psychiatric conditions, including mania, major depression, schizophrenia, substance use disorders, and brief psychotic disorder. Where possible, such a patient should be hospitalized, preferably in a psychiatric closed ward. If hospitalization is not available, then the clinician should use a safe, contained, and quiet environment that allows for frequent monitoring.

The following section reviews the general treatment of the psychotic patient, with special emphasis on stabilization and appropriate attention to differential diagnosis.

Treatment

When presented with a psychotic patient, the clinician must stabilize with appropriate medication while simultaneously searching diligently for medical etiologies. Organic causes of psychosis are numerous and include cerebral malaria or other systemic or CNS infection, brain tumors, dementia, intoxication with stimulants or hallucinogens, alcohol and/or minor tranquilizer withdrawal, use of mefloquine (Lariam) and a number of other medications. The presence of visual, tactile, or olfactory hallucinations suggests an organic cause, as do delirium, tremors, altered sensorium, disorientation, fever, or neurological findings. A general medical evaluation is imperative and should include appropriate laboratory tests for detection of substance use. Attention to suicidal ideation is important.

The use of antipsychotic medications will almost always be necessary. In some settings immediate-release (i.m.) forms may be necessary for rapid control of symptoms, especially if agitation or aggressive behavior is present. Haloperidol (Haldol), an older, high-potency typical antipsychotic is often available and is effective. The i.m. form can be used in doses of 1–5 mg every 30–60 minutes until sedation is achieved. The oral form can be used in doses of 1–15 mg/day p.o. on a q.d. or b.i.d. dosing schedule. Higher doses of up to 40 mg/day may be used, although safety has not been established for does >100 mg/day, and in the author's experience such a dose is rarely necessary. Caution in patients with Parkinson's disease, dementia or severe cardiovascular diseases should be exercised.[9,10] Side-effects are common and include extrapyramidal symptoms that can mimic Parkinson's disease, with bradykinesia, tremor, and muscular rigidity. These may be treated with a reduction in dose of the antipsychotic, if possible, followed by the use of anticholinergic agents such as benztropine (Cogentin) 0.5–2 mg/day, t.i.d. Akathisia also occurs, can be quite uncomfortable, and can be mistaken for an increase in agitation. It is experienced as a continuous restlessness and may lead to pacing and an inability to sit down. This side-effect may respond to a dose reduction of the antipsychotic, followed, if necessary, by the introduction of a β-blocker such as propranolol (Inderal) 20–40 mg p.o. t.i.d. Acute dystonias occur, sometimes with the first dose, and can be treated with diphenhydramine (Benadryl) 25 mg i.m.[11]

The newer atypical antipsychotics may be available and offer some advantages over the typical antipsychotics, including few extrapyramidal side effects and better general tolerability. Olanzapine (Zyprexa) in an initial i.m. dose of 10 mg and a second dose of 5–10 mg in 2 hours, with no more than 3 i.m. doses per day, may be used in patients in need of rapid control. Oral doses of 5–10 mg/day p.o. initially and up to 20 mg/day may be used in a q.d. dosing schedule. Olanzapine's sedative side-effect may be of particular use in this setting. Contraindications include unstable medical conditions, prostatic hypertrophy and narrow-angle glaucoma. Other atypical antipsychotics are also effective. Aripiprazole (Abilify) 5.25–9.75 mg i.m. with repeat injections every 2 hours and a maximum daily dose of 30 mg may be used. Initial oral doses of 10–15 mg/day on a q.d. schedule may be used, with a maximum daily dose of 30 mg. Caution should be used in patients with a history of seizure.[9]

Adjunctive treatment with benzodiazepines can be helpful, especially given agitation or sleep deprivation. Lorazepam (Ativan) may be given i.m. using 4 mg with a repeat dose in 10–15 minutes to a maximum of 10 mg/day. The oral form may be used at 2–6 mg in divided doses. When given in conjunction with an antipsychotic, benzodiazepines may lower effective doses of both medications, with resultant likely decrease in side-effects. However, benzodiazepines are not recommended with olanzapine (Zyprexa), because of the possibility of a hypoventilatory syndrome.[9]

Some mention of the potential for violence in the psychotic patient is necessary, even though it does not occur frequently and in fact is not strongly associated with mental illness. Patients responding to paranoid delusions or to command auditory hallucinations may be more prone to violence, as are patients intoxicated on certain drugs, including stimulants or PCP. Manic patients may become violent on occasion. Observation for severe agitation and inquiry into any history of violence, including recent violent behavior, combat experience and violence in the family of origin, can help determine the risk. Approaching a violent patient is, of course, hazardous, and a general rule is that a display of force can often obviate the need for force. Using adequate staff in dealing with a violent patient is, therefore, essential. Use of physical restraints may be tightly governed by local law in some countries and should be regarded as an absolute last resort to be monitored very carefully.

The Suicidal Patient

Suicide potential can be present with any psychiatric disorder, and the first rule of thumb is to ask all patients if they have suicidal ideation, suicide plans, or a past history of attempts.

Assessment of Suicide Risk

Careful assessment of suicide risk should be carried out in a forthright manner for every psychiatric patient. Assessment should include the following:

- Frequency and persistence of suicidal ideation (SI): frequent SI with a ruminative quality indicates higher risk
- Ascertainment of any suicide plans: the presence of plans, especially realistic, non-contingent ones, indicates a higher risk
- Access to lethal means for an attempt: assess access to firearms, medications, knives, tall buildings, etc.
- Assessment of intent: how serious or 'close' to attempting suicide is the patient? A clear wish to die indicates a very high risk
- Personal history of suicide attempts and their exact nature: e.g., if prior attempts, were they conducted in a lethal manner with low chance of discovery? Such would indicate high risk
- Family history of suicide or suicide attempts
- The presence of psychotic features and/or any substance use or abuse greatly increases risk

- Command hallucinations, if present, can imply substantial risk, depending on their nature
- The presence of any major adverse life events or their anniversaries, such as the death of a spouse, parent, or significant other.

Although the above points represent a reasonable first assessment, the reader is referred to any general psychiatric text for a complete discussion of all known risk factors and associations.

The risk of suicide should always be taken seriously and, when there is any doubt, treated with an abundance of caution. Should the risk appear to be substantial, immediate hospitalization is best. If not available, then evacuation to the nearest adequate facility is the next best option. While waiting for evacuation, the clinician should implement such appropriate suicide prevention steps as can be done under the circumstances and begin treatment of the underlying disorder. These may include arranging for a 24/7 continuous watch of the patient by family, private duty nurses, or others; removal of any obvious means of suicide, such as firearms, medications, knives, ropes, belts, ties, razors, etc.; and frequent checks on the patient's status. If the patient has been actively using substances, access should be removed if at all possible, and careful watch kept for withdrawal symptoms.

Other Disorders of Interest in International Travel

Brief Psychotic Disorder

The essence of a brief psychotic disorder is a rapid onset of one or more of the symptoms of psychosis, a relatively brief duration of the order of days to a month, and return to a full level of functioning.[12] As discussed above, psychotic states can occur as a result of depression or mania, substance use disorders, or schizophrenia. These conditions, as well as causative general medical conditions or medications, must be excluded in order to make the diagnosis.

Psychotic states are frequently cited in the literature as being associated with travel, and some of these may fulfill the criteria of brief psychotic disorder. The author found that 6.2% of psychiatric evacuations within the US Foreign Service involved a psychotic state, exclusive of mania or hypomania.[13] In an outpatient population of US Foreign Service personnel and dependents living overseas, brief psychosis accounted for 1.6% of adult patients.[14] Episodes of acute situational psychosis have been reported in tourists to Nepal and in American expatriates in South Vietnam.[15,16] Flinn and Singh have commented upon transient psychotic reactions associated with long travel. Flinn in particular cited isolation of long-distance travel, increased alcohol intake, irregular food and fluid intake, and insomnia as contributing factors.[17,18] Acute psychotic reactions have been reported in Japanese honeymooners traveling to Honolulu. These cases appeared to occur with greater frequency among honeymooners than among non-honeymoon Japanese tourists, and the authors speculated that arranged marriages and other cultural factors might be at play.[19] In many of these reported situations the psychotic state evolved rapidly, there was no prior history of such problems, and symptoms resolved quickly with treatment. Given all the various stressors from international travel, and the fact that brief psychotic disorder is recognized to be associated with significant life stresses, this presentation may be one of the psychiatric disorders truly related to travel in all its vicissitudes.

Treatment is as discussed in the section on the psychotic patient, although lower doses of antipsychotic medications may suffice.

Schizophrenia

Schizophrenia is a chronic, debilitating mental illness that often begins in the teens or early adulthood and can last for years. It is characterized by psychotic symptoms that can wax and wane over time and, with treatment, may be absent for extended periods. Negative symptoms, such as flat affect, amotivation, and poverty of thought and speech, are also present for extended periods of time, even in the absence of psychosis. There are a number of recognized subtypes and each emphasizes a specific set of symptoms. Subtypes include: paranoid, disorganized, catatonic, and undifferentiated. The residual type is where the symptoms of psychosis are not prominent but negative symptoms continue.

Relation to International Travel

It is abundantly clear that individuals with schizophrenia travel internationally. Numerous authors have found this disorder in travelers at international airports, in Hawaii, and in Jerusalem.[2,20–22] In the author's experience, and that of a number of US consular officers, individuals who probably meet the criteria for schizophrenia are known to wander about internationally, occasionally showing up at embassies for some form of assistance. These individuals may constitute an international form of chronically mentally ill, homeless persons. The prevalence of this disorder in the internationally traveling population is not known. Given its nature, schizophrenia is less likely to be seen in the business traveler or the expatriate employee.

Treatment

Individuals with schizophrenia can have coexisting substance use disorders that can complicate treatment considerably. In assessing patients, it is important to obtain as clear a history of substance use as possible. Due attention to substance intoxication and withdrawal states may be necessary. Appropriate laboratory tests, if available, are warranted. Since some of these patients have been wandering internationally for extended periods, a general medical examination is advisable. Treatment depends primarily upon the patient's status upon first contact. If the patient is compliant with medication and there are few prominent psychotic symptoms, hospitalization may not be necessary. Psychotic symptoms, however, should be treated with antipsychotic medications, such as those enumerated in the section on the psychotic patient. Frequently, the patient can tell the physician which medications have been of most benefit in the past, and these should be reinstituted if possible. The presence of suicidal ideation should be assessed. Individuals at high risk of suicide should be hospitalized, if possible, or contained as well as can be arranged. Given stabilization, individuals should be sent home to family or their country of origin, although they may not comply despite admonition.

Mania

Although relatively rare, mania is one of the most difficult problems to handle overseas. The manic state occurs as part of bipolar I disorder. Bipolar I disorder is a form of bipolar or manic–depressive disorder in which episodes of mania predominate, although patients with this disorder also may have major depressive episodes.

Patients with mania frequently present with a truly vexatious combination of inflated self-esteem, even grandiosity; abundant energy; and heightened libido; all coupled with poor judgment and negligible insight into the nature of their illness. These symptoms can continue for weeks and can lead to ruinous loss of fortune, numerous and indiscreet sexual contacts, and even loss of career. In the author's experience, a single manic patient can completely paralyze a sponsoring overseas organization until such time as either the symptoms

Table 48.2 Clinical Vignette of Typical Features of a Patient with Mania Overseas

Mr A was a businessman traveling overseas for a temporary posting in a developing nation. His sponsoring company did a pre-travel medical evaluation without any specific screening for mental health problems. As a result, Mr A's first, relatively mild hypomanic episode, occurring some time before his transfer, and for which he did not receive treatment, went unnoticed.

Over the course of a few weeks, Mr A began to display an elevated and expansive mood along with seemingly endless amounts of energy, albeit applied to projects in an uneven, haphazard manner. Uncharacteristically, he soon required only a few hours of sleep at night. His colleagues noticed increasingly rapid and pressured speech and sometimes had problems following Mr A's train of thought. Even more disturbing, however, was Mr A's deteriorating business and social judgment. He began talking about and attempting to implement highly questionable business deals and was very easily irritated at any questioning of his plans. Socially, Mr A at first became the life of every party, but soon began making increasingly bothersome and overt sexual advances towards women. His colleagues finally approached the company's medical division when Mr A started singing loudly in the office, convinced that he was a world-class, albeit undiscovered, baritone, and talking about the fact that he was receiving direct, divine guidance and that as a result his business schemes could not fail.

The company medical division had a consultant physician in the country. Fortunately, this physician suspected a manic episode, although substance abuse could not be entirely ruled out. As this was a developing country, however, hospital facilities for psychiatric treatment were poorly staffed and were judged to be potentially worse for Mr A than his disorder. Culturally compatible psychiatric care was also not available. As Mr A had virtually no insight into his condition and would not acknowledge the fact that he was ill, and since he had made no threats to himself or to others, the lack of inpatient facilities and specialists was a moot point as he refused treatment anyway.

There began several weeks of increasingly difficult and embarrassing incidents, damaging both to Mr A's and the sponsoring company's reputation, and colleagues and finally, Mr A's home country supervisor exerted considerable pressure upon Mr A to accept medication and return to his home country for care. The company's business came to a standstill for the duration. Eventually, having been told by the company that he would be summarily dismissed if he did not accept the recommended medical care, Mr A accepted haloperidol, the most appropriate medication available on the local market. It was never clear, however, if his acceptance was the result of the gradual diminution of his symptoms with time or the pressure from multiple sources. Lithium carbonate was available, but laboratory facilities for monitoring serum lithium levels were judged to be unreliable. After being sufficiently stabilized to fly, Mr A was flown to his home country with a colleague and a male nurse as escorts. He was not allowed to return to his assignment overseas.

subside, the patient spirals into incoherence allowing hospitalization or other immediate care, or the patient consents to effective treatment or evacuation. To compound the problem, commitment under criteria of imminent danger to self or others is not always possible, and the patient's lack of insight can make voluntary consent to treatment difficult to achieve. Frequently, some sort of leverage or pressure from family or sponsoring organization is necessary to obtain the patient's cooperation. Table 48.2 is a clinical vignette which is illustrative of the presentation and problems encountered in dealing with a person with a manic episode overseas. The vignette is a composite of typical features and is not based upon any actual patient.

Incidence, Prevalence and Relation to Travel of Bipolar I Disorder

Incidence and prevalence data for bipolar I disorder are not available for international travelers. In the US Foreign Service population studied by the author, manic and hypomanic states accounted for 2.8% of all psychiatric medical evacuations.[13] Hypomanic states are less serious versions of mania that usually do not require hospitalization. With regard to a specific link to travel, some investigators have found a tendency towards more hypomanic or manic symptoms in travelers who had transited time zones in the eastbound direction.[20,23] These studies also found the opposite effect: there were more depressive symptoms associated with westward travel. Methodological limitations preclude a definitive statement, however, and the question of illness causing travel versus travel causing illness is not clearly answered. Nevertheless, sleep deprivation has been thought to have an antidepressant effect and to precipitate elevated moods.[24,25] The question is, then, does the phase advance of the sleep–wake cycle of eastbound travel particularly induce manic or hypomanic episodes in susceptible individuals, in contrast to the general sleep deprivation often associated with any extended travel?

Diagnosis and Differential

A manic episode is characterized by an abnormally elevated, euphoric or irritable mood that persists for days or weeks. Other features include grandiosity, a dramatically decreased need for sleep, and a marked increase in energy and libido, sometimes resulting in inappropriate sexual adventures. Often, there is a lack of insight such that the patient is not aware that anything is wrong. As a consequence, patients may resist attempts at treatment or hospitalization. Speech can become quite rapid and can be difficult to follow. This mix of signs and symptoms can have disastrous financial, social, and career consequences.

Occasionally, symptoms will progress to florid psychosis with incoherence, delusions, and hallucinations. In these instances, the episode may be mistaken for an acute or schizophreniform psychosis that only prior history or subsequent course will clarify. Substance abuse can produce manic symptoms, especially stimulants such as amphetamines or cocaine. Alcohol use during episodes occurs and may or may not be part of a comorbid alcohol abuse or dependence disorder. Thus, prior or current drug use is important to establish. In addition, there are a number of medical conditions and medications that can produce manic symptoms. Medical conditions include various brain lesions, infections producing encephalitis, hyperthyroidism, and Cushing's disease. In practice, these are not frequently encountered although they can be catastrophic if missed. Medications of particular note include virtually any antidepressant. The reader is referred to any general psychiatric textbook for a more complete list. A general medical examination should be conducted at the first opportunity and should include testing for substance abuse.

Treatment

Treatment is frequently aimed at either hospitalization, if possible, or stabilization pending medical evacuation. Use of an antipsychotic medication is frequently the first step in order to gain some control of the situation in the least amount of time. In fact, in the absence of laboratory facilities to monitor blood levels of the various mood stabilizers, such medication may be the practitioner's only choice. Medications should be used as discussed in the section on the psychotic patient.

Table 48.3 Clinical Vignette of Typical Features of a Patient With Major Depression Overseas

Mrs B was the wife of an expatriate employee. She was in her early 30s and posted overseas to a developing country. Over the course of several months, her fellow expatriate spouses noted increasing withdrawal from the usual active expatriate social life. At home, over the course of weeks, her husband noted an unrelentingly depressed outlook and mood, worse in the mornings, frequent crying spells, a complete lack of interest in sexual relations, and unremitting fatigue. She began to be unable to keep up with managing the household and staff, spending much of her time either in bed or walking aimlessly around the house in her night-clothes. Mrs B also began to show little interest in personal care and dress, and was consistently waking up in the early hours of the morning, unable to return to sleep. Her appetite fell and she lost 15 pounds, which was over 10% of her initial body weight.

Mrs B's husband brought his wife to the company-approved, host-country physician shortly after she began to talk openly of having suicidal thoughts, albeit without specific plans or apparent intent. On evaluation, she was noted to be disheveled and dressed in a bathrobe and pyjamas. She complained of being depressed, and had nothing good to say about herself or her situation in life. The future looked bleak to her and her affect was noted to be invariant and depressed in nature. Although she was oriented in all spheres, her speech was noticeably slowed, as were all her motor movements. She was unable to concentrate. On direct questioning she admitted to having daily, frequent suicidal thoughts of a fleeting nature, but denied current plans or intent. She denied any hallucinations or delusions, and none were evident. There was no history or evidence of substance abuse. She had no prior history of a psychiatric disorder, or suicide attempts, although there was a family history of depression. There was no significant medical history and no particular findings on physical examination, except those related to the weight loss and her slowed motor movements.

The physician suspected a major depression, first episode. There were no adequate or culturally compatible psychiatric inpatient facilities or specialists available. Also, many of the newer antidepressants were not available on the local market. Because of the suicidal ideation, which was judged to be serious, if not of immediate danger over the next several days, it was arranged for Mrs B to fly to her home country the next day, with her husband and a female nurse as escorts. Although Mrs B did not believe she could be helped, she reacted passively and did not resist these arrangements. Immediate psychiatric evaluation was arranged upon their arrival and she was hospitalized for several weeks, during which she responded rapidly to antidepressant medications. Extended outpatient follow-up over the next month found continued improvement to the point of remission of symptoms. Working with her psychiatrist, the company's medical department and the host-country consulting physician, a plan was devised for her return to her husband's overseas posting. The psychiatrist was willing to maintain telephone contact both with the consulting physician and with Mrs B and her husband on a regular basis. Both Mrs B and her husband were agreeable to regular follow-up visits to the consultant physician and to a follow-up visit to the psychiatrist in several months. Arrangements were made to ship Mrs B's medication to her via overseas post. In all, it was felt that a return was safe. In making this judgment, multiple factors were considered: (1) Mrs B's suicidal ideation had never progressed to a point of imminent danger and she had no history of prior attempts; (2) her symptoms evolved over a matter of months, allowing for timely intervention in the event of recurrence; (3) she displayed good insight into and acceptance of the fact that she had had a major depression; (4) her husband was both understanding and supportive of her; (5) she responded quickly to medication and was both motivated in treatment and compliant; (6) she did not have any psychotic symptoms; and (7) this had been her first episode and there was no personal or family history to suggest bipolar disorder.

In the long term, patients with mania frequently lack the insight to comply with treatment, even after acute symptoms have subsided. This tendency and the natural history of the disorder suggest that further travel or residence overseas is not in the patient's best interests until the pattern of recurrence is known, they achieve a good degree of insight into their illness accompanied by compliance with treatment, and stability is achieved.

Major Depression

The other mood disorder of particular note for the overseas clinician is major depression. Of all the types of depression, this one is the most serious. Since it can take a matter of weeks to develop, the disorder itself is not the proximate cause of a psychiatric emergency. Unlike the manic patient, patients with major depression are relatively inactive, anergic, and unmotivated. The emergent problem is frequently the risk of suicide and/or psychotic symptoms. Table 48.3 is a clinical vignette which is illustrative of the presentation and problems encountered in dealing with a person with a major depressive episode overseas. The vignette is a composite of typical features and is not based on any actual patient.

Incidence, Prevalence, and Relationship to Travel

As with other disorders in the population of international travelers, incidence and prevalence data are lacking. In the US Foreign Service population, depression of all sorts, including major depression, accounted for 20% of all psychiatric medical evacuations from overseas, second only to alcoholism.[13] In a clinical population of US

Foreign Service personnel and dependants living overseas, 9.5% of patients suffered from major depression.[14] The stressors of international travel or overseas residence, the isolation from family and familiar social supports, reactions to a foreign culture and language, all likely contribute to depression, major or otherwise, at least in the susceptible individual.

Diagnosis and Differential

Major depression can occur as a single episode, as recurrent episodes, or as part of bipolar or manic–depressive disorder. It is characterized by persistent depressed mood over a number of weeks. Associated symptoms can include insomnia, especially terminal insomnia, but sometimes hypersomnia, a distinct lack of energy, and a hopeless or at least grim outlook. Appetite may be decreased with associated, significant weight loss, but can be increased in some. There may be a loss of interest or loss of pleasure in usually pleasurable activities, along with significant feelings of worthlessness. Suicidal ideation or thoughts of death are often present. Signs may include either psychomotor retardation or agitation, loss of concentration, and some impairment of short-term memory.

A number of medical conditions can cause depression of this sort, including pancreatic cancer, hypothyroidism, sleep apnea, and a number of infectious and inflammatory diseases, to name a few. Some medications have been associated with major depression, such as reserpine (Serpalan) and propranolol (Inderal). The reader is referred to a textbook of general psychiatry for a complete listing. A general medical evaluation is recommended. A personal or family history of prior episodes or of bipolar illness may help clarify the diagnosis. Substance abuse does occur with major depression, and patients with a primary diagnosis of alcohol dependence can appear severely depressed. Patients may also use alcohol, stimulants, or marijuana concurrently with major depression, either to alleviate symptoms or because of concurrent substance abuse disorders. Evaluation should include a substance use history. Major depressive episodes can also occur with psychotic features such as delusions or hallucinations, which are usually mood congruent. Psychotic features usually mean that the patient will be more difficult to treat.

Treatment

Treatment of major depression should be aimed at preventing suicide and treatment of any psychosis prior to evacuation or hospitalization. Psychotic features should be treated aggressively with antipsychotic medications, as discussed in the section on the psychotic patient. If the patient has had particular difficulty sleeping, judicious use of a benzodiazepine may be useful.

The patient should be started on an antidepressant unless there is a history of manic or hypomanic episodes. If such a history exists, it would be best not to start antidepressant medications in the overseas environment. Given the fact that virtually any antidepressant has a delayed response effect of the order of weeks, such may not be of immediate benefit. However, in the seriously ill patient, time is of the essence. Choice of antidepressant depends upon local availability. Certainly, if the patient has had previous episodes and has responded to a particular antidepressant, then that is the drug of choice. In general, the newer antidepressants are preferable to either the older tricyclics or the MAO inhibitors because of their better side-effect profiles and safety in overdose situations. A reasonable place to start would be one of the specific serotonin reuptake inhibitors (SSRI), such as fluoxetine (Prozac) 20 mg p.o. q.d., sertraline (Zoloft) 200 mg p.o. q.d., or paroxetine (Paxil) 20 mg p.o. q.d. Titration upwards to their maximum dose and following manufacturers' recommendations is recommended. Many of the SSRI medications have significant effects on hepatic enzyme systems, and careful attention to possible drug–drug interactions is important.

Substance Use Disorders

Virtually any mind-altering, intoxicating or addicting substance has a corresponding substance use disorder. A complete account of all possible substances is beyond the scope of this chapter and the reader is referred to general psychiatric textbooks or specific works on addictions. Rather, some specific circumstances that are likely to culminate in emergencies are discussed, along with more general information concerning substance use disorders and their consequences overseas.

Most substances of abuse have both a dependence and an abuse diagnostic category. For either category, the affected individual continues to use the substance despite repeated, serious problems associated with its use. For abuse, these problems do not include either the development of tolerance or withdrawal symptoms. Rather, the emphasis is upon continued use despite substance-related social, family, work, or legal problems, and repeated use in hazardous situations (e.g., driving while intoxicated). Dependence includes the possibility of developing either tolerance or withdrawal for many substances, along with a range of cognitive and behavioral symptoms. These include consumption of the substance in larger amounts than anticipated, attempts or a desire to cut down on use, continued use despite adverse medical or psychiatric consequences, and a loss of social or other activities due to continued use.[12]

Relationship to International Travel

Virtually any substance of abuse is encountered in the international traveler population. In the US Foreign Service population, substance use disorders of any type were the leading cause of psychiatric medical evacuation, accounting for 28% of the total, with alcohol abuse or dependence accounting for the majority of these evacuations and 22.9% of the total.[13] In a clinical population of expatriate US Foreign Service personnel and dependents, 12.5% of patients were alcohol dependent and 1.6% had cannabis abuse.[14] Heavy alcohol use or dependence among international travelers has also been reported by a number of authors in a variety of settings, as has the use of other addictive or illicit substances.[2,4,16,17,21,26]

Given the number of years it takes to develop alcohol dependence, it is unlikely that travel is a causative factor. Anecdotally, for alcoholics or other substance abusers in remission, international travel and/or expatriation with their inherent stressors can threaten sobriety. In some countries, minor tranquilizers and even stimulants are readily available on the open market, are legal, and can be purchased without prescription. This is an open invitation to self-medication, which certainly occurs and can lead to abuse and dependence.

When does substance abuse or dependence become a psychiatric emergency? Usually, alcohol intoxication by itself does not become a psychiatric emergency unless the patient becomes violent or suicidal. The vast majority of cases of alcohol intoxication never come to medical attention. However, intoxication with stimulants, hallucinogens, phencyclidine, inhalants, and cannabis can result in psychotic states that can present as a psychiatric emergency.[12] Treatment of these psychotic states should include careful observation for overdose, and evaluation for use of multiple substances and coexisting medical conditions. Laboratory tests for the detection of substances of abuse are imperative, as is a general medical evaluation.[9]

Treatment of Intoxication States

In general terms, treatment of intoxication states will involve use of antipsychotic and anxiolytic medications to control psychotic symptoms and severe agitation, respectively. Judicious use of restraints may be necessary to control potentially violent patients, and quiet, minimally stimulating environments are best. Particularly in the treatment of opioid and sedative–hypnotic intoxication, overdose should always be suspected and appropriate support of vital functions undertaken. Reversal of opioid intoxication should be undertaken immediately using naloxone (Narcan). Three i.v. doses of this medication may be given, each separated by a 15 min period of observation, beginning at 0.8 mg i.v., then 1.6 mg i.v., and finally 3.2 mg i.v. The dosing escalation is halted at any point at which reversal is observed. If reversal is not observed after the final dose, then an alternative diagnoses should be entertained. If reversal is obtained at any point, naloxone (Narcan) should be continued at 0.4 mg/h i.v.[11] The reader is referred to any text on the treatment of psychiatric emergencies or addiction disorders for a more complete discussion of substances and symptoms that can result in intoxication.

Given the complexity of treating these states of intoxication, hospitalization, or at least treatment in an emergency room over the course of hours, is preferred. The immediate goal is to support the patient as necessary, deal with acute agitation and psychotic symptoms, and prevent injury to the patient and staff, as well as morbidity or mortality from overdose. If hospitalization is not available or adequate, the physician may need to set up treatment in a controlled environment with 24-h monitoring using private duty nurses or other personnel as available. After the acute phase is treated, longer-term treatment for substance abuse or dependence that relies upon abstinence should be recommended. Such treatment may involve return to the country of origin. Clinicians and patients should be mindful that in some countries laws regarding illicit drug use are quite severe, and that relapse risk is generally felt to be higher if long-term treatment of those with substance abuse or dependence is not undertaken.

Alcohol Withdrawal

Withdrawal states seen in patients who are substance dependent can also present as psychiatric emergencies. Alcohol, opioid, and sedative, hypnotic, and anxiolytic withdrawals can lead to hallucinations, delusions, agitation, and delirium that may prompt psychiatric attention. Of these substances, alcohol is frequently the culprit in the overseas travel-oriented environment, at least in some expatriate populations. For the specifics of management of opioid and sedative, hypnotic and anxiolytic withdrawal states, the reader is referred to a general textbook of psychiatry or addiction medicine.

Alcohol withdrawal is characterized by autonomic hyperactivity, hand tremor, insomnia, anxiety, and agitation. It can include illusions, hyperacusis, hallucinations, and grand mal seizures. In about 5% of alcohol-dependent individuals delirium tremens occurs, marked by delirium, severe autonomic hyperactivity, vivid auditory, visual, tactile and/or olfactory hallucinations, delusions that are frequently paranoid, severe tremor, and agitation. Seizures may develop and occur before the delirium. Treatment of withdrawal states can prevent progression to delirium tremens, which can be lethal in 5–10% of treated patients, with an even higher mortality rate in untreated patients.[9]

As with the other substance abuse disorders, patients presenting with alcohol withdrawal should always be evaluated for concurrent medical conditions and for concurrent use of other substances. Medical conditions to be especially considered are those associated with prolonged alcohol intake, such as cirrhosis, gastritis, GI bleeding, pneumonia, subdural hematomas, and dehydration. A thorough medical evaluation is imperative. History should include any prior episodes of withdrawal and the signs and symptoms thereof.

Treatment of medically complicated cases, those with significant amounts of agitation, hallucinations, or delirium tremens, is best carried out in a hospital, if available. In any event, individuals will need to be in a well-lit environment with minimal stimulation and frequent monitoring. Concurrent medical problems will need to be treated. Suicidal ideation should be assessed.

The standard treatment for alcohol withdrawal is the benzodiazepines, which are cross-tolerant with alcohol. Tremor, mild to moderate agitation and/or increased vital signs, including temperature, pulse or blood pressure can be treated with chlordiazepoxide (Librium) 25–100 mg p.o. The initial dose may be repeated every 2 h until the patient is calm. After that, the dose may be given every 4–6 h. In setting the dose and schedule, the clinician must walk the line between alcohol withdrawal symptoms on the one hand and benzodiazepine intoxication, as indicated by ataxia or slurred speech, on the other. The former state favors an increased dose, while the latter situation leads to a decrease. Once a patient is stabilized, chlordiazepoxide should be tapered at a rate of 20% every 5–7 days. In cases involving extreme agitation or delirium tremens, chlordiazepoxide may be given i.v. 0.5 mg/kg at 12.5 mg/min until the patient is calm, with individual titration thereafter. Antipsychotics should be used with caution and only if the patient is psychotic despite adequate doses of a benzodiazepine. Haloperidol (Haldol) may be considered as it is less likely to result in seizures. Other medications that should be used routinely are thiamine 100 mg p.o. q.d. to t.i.d., folic acid 1 mg p.o. q.d., and one multivitamin daily.

In patients with a history of withdrawal seizures, magnesium sulfate 1 g i.m. q. 6 h for 2 days is recommended.[11]

Any patient with alcohol withdrawal disorder is virtually certain to be alcohol dependent. Thus, after withdrawal is completed, patients should undergo longer-term treatment aimed at abstinence, with the inpatient basis being preferred. Travel to undertake such treatment may well be necessary, and careful thought should be given following successful treatment as to the possible impact upon sobriety of a return to international travel or posting overseas. Insight, however, can be quite variable in alcohol dependence, and compliance with recommended treatment, even after a stormy withdrawal, or serious medical complications, may not occur.

Initial Assessment of Travelers Exposed to Traumatic Events

International travelers are exposed to a wide range of potentially traumatic events, including motor vehicle accidents, civil disturbances, terrorist incidents, and natural disasters, to name a few. The travel medicine clinician may well be confronted with making an initial assessment of such travelers and, for the most part, should be familiar with the concept of post-traumatic stress disorder (PTSD) and its subclinical presentations. It is not suggested that travel medicine clinicians diagnose or treat such maladies, but they should be able to discern the symptoms and refer appropriately if significant symptoms exist. Since symptoms of PTSD can occur months to even years after the event, education about symptoms that may occur is probably the single most important activity. Subclinical symptom complexes in which symptoms do not rise to the level of a standard diagnosis, but are nevertheless of significance and warrant treatment, do occur. It should also be noted that not all persons exposed to traumatic events subsequently develop PTSD. The incidence of PTSD after exposure to any trauma is 8% in males and 20% in females.[27]

Although the diagnosis of PTSD has been controversial, the basic elements include exposure to an incident that involved actual or threatened death or serious injury along with an emotional reaction of intense fear, helplessness, or horror. Symptoms involve a combination of re-experiencing the event, persistent avoidance of stimuli associated with the event, and increased arousal. Re-experiencing could include the following symptoms: recurrent and intrusive recollections of the event; recurrent distressing dreams of the event; or acting or feeling as if the event was recurring. Avoidance symptoms can include: efforts to avoid thoughts, feelings, conversations, activities, places or people that lead to recollections of the event; feelings of detachment from others; an inability to recall some important aspect of the event; or diminished interest in significant activities. Arousal symptoms can include: difficulty sleeping or concentrating; irritability or anger outbursts, hypervigilance; or an exaggerated startle response.[12] Victims of traumatic events with any of these symptoms would best be referred to a psychiatrist for further assessment. As suicidal ideation can be associated with PTSD, suicide assessment should be undertaken. As substance abuse issues can also be frequently associated, inquiries into substance use and sequelae should also be performed.

References

1. Liese B, Mundt KA, Dell LD, et al. Medical insurance claims associated with international business travel. Occup Environ Med 1997;54:499–503.
2. Streltzer J. Psychiatric emergencies in travelers to Hawaii. Compr Psychiatry 1979;20:463–8.
3. Cohen E. A phenomenology of tourist experiences. Sociology 1979;13:179–201.

4. Heltberg J, Steffen R. Psychiatric and psychological problems in travellers. Paper presented to the First Scandinavian Symposium on Travel Medicine and Health, Uppsala, 21–22 May, 1992.

5. Valk T. Psychiatric and psychosocial counseling of the international traveler and expatriate family. Shoreland's Travel Medicine Monthly 1998;2:1, 3–5, 10.

6. Fennig S, Tevesess I, Gaber K, et al. The Arab nurse and the Jewish psychotic patient in the closed psychiatric ward. Int J Soc Psychiatry 1992;38:228–34.

7. Westermeyer J. Clinical considerations in cross cultural diagnosis. Hosp Community Psych 1987;38:160–5.

8. Rodgers TA. Involuntary commitment of the mentally ill: The overseas experience. Paper delivered to the psychiatrists of the US Department of State, New York City. May 1990.

9. Riba MB, Ravindranath D, editors. Clinical Manual of Emergency Psychiatry. Washington DC: American Psychiatric Publishing, Inc; 2010.

10. Stahl SM, editor. Stahl's Essential Psychopharmacology. 4th ed. Cambridge: Cambridge University Press; 2011.

11. Sadock BJ, Sadock VA, editors. Pocket Handbook of Clinical Psychiatry. 4th ed. Philadelphia: Lippincott Williams & Wilkins; 2005.

12. American Psychiatric Association. Diagnostic and Statistical Manual of Mental Disorders. 4th ed. Washington, DC: American Psychiatric Association; 2000.

13. Valk TH. Psychiatric medical evacuations within the Foreign Service. Foreign Serv Med Bull 1988;268:9–11.

14. Valk TH. Psychiatric practice in the Foreign Service. Foreign Serv Med Bull 1990;280:6–11.

15. Shlim DR. Personal communication, 11 January, 2002.

16. Talbot JA. The American expatriate in South Vietnam. Am J Psychiatry 1969;126:555–60.

17. Flinn DE. Transient psychotic reactions during travel. Am J Psychiatry 1962;119:173–4.

18. Singh HA. A case of psychosis precipitated by confinement in long distance travel by train. Am J Psychiatry 1961;117:936–7.

19. Langen D, Streltzer J, Kai M. 'Honeymoon psychosis' in Japanese tourists to Hawaii. Cult Divers Ment Health 1997;3:171–4.

20. Jauhar P, Weller MPI. Psychiatric morbidity and time zone changes: a study of patients from Heathrow airport. Br J Psychiatry 1982;140:213–35.

21. Shapiro S. A study of psychiatric syndromes manifested at an international airport. Compr Psychiatry 1976;17:453–6.

22. Bar-el I, Witztum E, Kalian M, et al. Psychiatric hospitalizations of tourists in Jerusalem. Compr Psychiatry 1991;32:238–44.

23. Young DM. Psychiatric morbidity in travelers to Honolulu, Hawaii. Compr Psychiatry 1995;36:224–8.

24. Wehr TA. Improvement of depression and triggering of mania by sleep deprivation. JAMA 1992;267:548–51.

25. Wehr T, Goodwin F, Wirz-Justice A, et al. 48-hour sleep-wake cycles in manic-depressive illness: naturalistic observations and sleep deprivation experiments. Arch Gen Psychiatry 1982;39:559–65.

26. Paz A, Sadetzki S, Potazman I. High rates of substance abuse among long–term travelers to the tropics: an interventional study. J Travel Med 2004;11:75–81.

27. Benedec D, Wynn G, editors. Clinical Manual for Management of PTSD. Washington DC: American Psychiatric Publishing, Inc.; 2011.

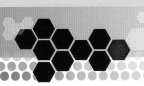
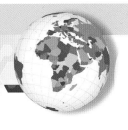

49

Travelers' Thrombosis

Suzanne C. Cannegieter and Frits R. Rosendaal

Key points

- A long-haul flight increases the risk of venous thrombosis about threefold. In absolute terms the risk is about 1 in 4500 long-haul passengers over a period of 8 weeks
- Several high-risk groups are known, i.e. tall, short, and obese people, as well as people with a genetic predisposition (e.g., Factor V Leiden – FVL) and oral contraceptive users. People with a history of venous thrombosis are considered to be a particularly high-risk group
- All travelers should remain well hydrated, exercise their legs regularly in flight, and avoid any use of sedatives
- For those with a moderately strong risk factor for venous thrombosis, properly fitted compression stockings (providing 15–30 mmHg of pressure at the ankle) and aisle seating for flights of more than 8 hours are recommended
- For high-risk patients (those with a history of venous thrombosis, major surgery within 6 weeks, and known malignancy) a low molecular weight heparin injection before departure is recommended
- Aspirin alone is never recommended as prophylaxis, as there is no evidence showing substantial benefit, whereas it does increase the risk of major hemorrhage

Introduction

Travel was not established as a risk factor for venous thrombosis until the year 2000. Case reports have appeared from the days when commercial aircraft became a regular undertaking (1950s) linking long-haul flights to a subsequent thrombosis, but a causal relation could not be derived from these individual descriptions.[1] Only since the year 2000 have controlled studies on this association been published.[2] The reason for this sudden interest was the tragic death of a young, healthy woman in the UK, who died of a pulmonary embolism shortly after arriving at Heathrow airport from a long-haul flight. This event was widely covered in the media, which led to questions in the House of Lords and eventually to a large-scale investigation into this issue, carried out under the auspices of the WHO, the so-called WRIGHT project (WHO Research Into Global Hazards of Travel). The results of this project, as well as of other studies published since then, have led to a better insight into the association between air travel and thrombosis, into the magnitude of this risk, into high-risk groups and the mechanism of thrombosis after air travel.

Venous Thrombosis

Venous thrombosis (VT) manifests as deep vein thrombosis (DVT) with or without pulmonary embolism (PE). The leg veins are the most common site of DVT, accounting for about 90% of cases; other locations include arm and abdominal veins. It is a common disease with an annual incidence of 2/1000, and is hence the third most common vascular disease after myocardial infarction and ischemic stroke. The incidence varies strongly with age, with 0.1 in adolescence to 8 per 1000 in those over the age of 80.[3] The occurrence of VTE has shown a slow but steady increase over recent decades. In the USA, this has led to the recent publication of a 'call to action' by the surgeon general. (http://www.surgeongeneral.gov/topics/deepvein/). Venous thrombosis is an important and often underestimated healthcare problem, with considerable mortality, morbidity, and resource expenditure. Mortality in non-cancer patients is about 4% within 30 days and 13% within 1 year.[3] Furthermore, surviving patients are at high risk of recurrent venous thrombosis, with a cumulative incidence of about 25% at 5 years and 30% at 10 years.[4] About 20–50% of patients suffer from chronic post-thrombotic syndrome, which has important clinical and socioeconomic consequences.[5] In two recent prospective studies, chronic thromboembolic pulmonary hypertension developed in 1–4% of patients after a first episode of PE.[6,7] Recurrent DVT and PE are associated with a several-fold increased likelihood of post-thrombotic syndrome and chronic thromboembolic pulmonary hypertension, respectively.

In 1856 Rudolf Virchow, a 19th century pathologist, postulated his triad, which consists of three major components of thrombogenesis: stasis of the blood, changes in the vessel wall, and altered blood coagulability. Indeed, most risk factors known today are related either to immobilization (bed rest, plaster cast) or to hypercoagulability, owing, for example, to inherited thrombophilia, hormone use, pregnancy, or cancer. Over the past decades, knowledge on the etiology of VT has expanded rapidly, with dozens of genetic or acquired risk factors currently known. As venous thrombosis is a multicausal disease, a set of risk factors has to be present before a clinical event will occur.[8]

DOI: 10.1016/B978-1-4557-1076-8.00049-1

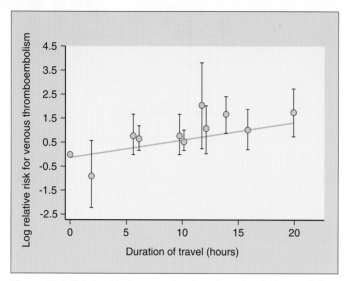

Figure 49.1 Relationship between duration of travel and relative risk for venous thromboembolism. *(From: Chandra D, Parisini E, Mozaffarian D. Meta-analysis: travel and risk for venous thromboembolism. Ann Intern Med 2009;151:180–90.)*

Size of the Risk after Travel

The first controlled study providing a link between air travel and VT was published before the year 2000, i.e. in 1986.[9] This study was not primarily focused on the relationship between travel and thrombosis risk, but was carried out to review causes of sudden death at a large international airport. To this end, the author noted numbers and causes of death separately by arrival and departure halls at London's Heathrow airport. It turned out that PE occurred much more often in the arrival hall (18%) than in the departure hall (4%), whereas one would expect these numbers to be more or less the same, which was the case for all other causes of death. Therefore, the difference had to be attributed to the air travel itself.

After the year 2000 many reports have published results of case–control, follow-up, and intervention studies on the association between air travel and VT. A recent meta-analysis summarized the results of 14 studies (11 case–control, two cohort and one cross-over), with a total of 4055 cases of thrombosis.[2] The pooled relative risk of thrombosis in all travelers was 2.8 (95% confidence interval 2.2–3.7). In addition, the risk increased by 26% for every 2-hour increase in duration of travel. Such a dose–response relationship is suggestive of a causal association (Fig. 49.1). Although fewer data are available on travel by other means, the meta-analysis also summarized these results separately, which led to a pooled relative risk of 1.4 (05% CI 1.0–2.1).

Although a relative risk is useful to demonstrate the strength of an association, an estimate of the absolute risk of disease is required for questions with clinical, individual, or public health relevance. Knowledge of the probability of thrombosis for an individual per flight is particularly relevant for passengers, clinicians, and airlines. This can be assessed in cohort studies, two of which studied the occurrence of PE immediately after arrival at the airport.[10,11] Both studies found a risk of about 0.1 per million passengers for short flights, which greatly increased with duration of travel, to up to 5 per million passengers for a flight of more than 10 000 km. However, these results were not a useful measure of the absolute risk, as neither thromboses of the arms or legs, or PEs that occurred after leaving the airport, had been taken into account. In another study design, 964 passengers were systematically screened by ultrasound for the presence of asymptomatic VT after a long-haul flight.[12] In 1213 non-traveling controls

the same procedure was performed. The risk of asymptomatic clots was 0.7% in the travelers and 0.2% in the control group. While these results are useful to show an effect of air travel itself, they are less informative as an estimate of the absolute risk, as the relevance of asymptomatic clots is not clear.

In the WRIGHT project, another cohort study was carried out to estimate the absolute risk of thrombosis after air travel.[13] Nearly 9000 frequently flying employees from international companies and organizations were followed over a period of 5 years. During this time, they made more than 100 000 flights of more than 4 hours' duration, and 53 confirmed venous thromboses occurred. This led to a risk estimate of 1 per 4656 travelers (95% CI 1/7526–1/3163). For long-haul travel compared to not flying the risk of thrombosis remained 3.2 times increased over an 8-week time window, after which time the risk returned to normal levels. The risk of thrombosis increased sharply with the duration of the flight, up to 1 per 1200 travelers for flights over 16 hours. Those who made several flights within the 8-week time window also had increased risks.

Factors Influencing the Risk

Passenger-Related Risk Factors

As venous thrombosis is a multicausal disease, it occurs due to a specific set of risk factors that are present simultaneously in an individual, with each of these factors affecting the probability of disease. Hence, the term 'travelers' thrombosis' is not really appropriate, as an event occurring after air travel will have been caused in part by the flight, but other risk factors must also have been present, otherwise air travel would lead to thrombosis in every passenger. Therefore, it can be useful to study additional risk factors in passengers, with the aim of identifying high-risk groups.

The first to describe two of these high-risk groups were Martinelli et al. in 2003, who found a 16-fold increased risk in subjects with Factor V Leiden (a common genetic risk factor for VT), and a 14-fold increased risk for women using oral contraceptives, all compared to non-flying subjects without these risk factors.[14]

In the WRIGHT project a large case–control study was carried out in which high-risk groups could be identified. Among 1906 patients with a first DVT or PE and 1906 controls, an additionally increased risk was again found in subjects with FVL and in contraceptive pill users.[15] Furthermore, it was found that in tall individuals (>1.90 m) the risk of thrombosis after air travel was increased ninefold compared to individuals of average height who did not travel. This finding can be explained by the fact that tall people are subjected to even more cramped seating. Interestingly, short people also had a fivefold increased risk compared to people of average height. This finding is also biologically plausible because these people's feet generally cannot touch the floor of the cabin when seated, which leads to extra compression of the popliteal veins (Table 49.1). In the same study it was described that certain combinations of risk factors strongly increased the risk of VT: overweight women using oral contraceptives, for example, had a 60-fold increased risk after a long-haul flight, compared to non-flying women without these risk factors (Table 49.2; please note that the odds ratios in this table are calculated from flying subjects. To determine the risk compared to non-flying individuals, the results should be multiplied by the relative risk of air travel, i.e., 2–3).[16]

Travel-Related Risk Factors

In the same case–control study the effect of external circumstances and behavior during air travel was studied.[17] Window seating turned

Table 49.1 The Combined Effect of Other Risk Factors and Travel on The Risk of Venous Thrombosis (DVT, PE and Both; 1906 Pairs)

Risk Factor	Subcategory	Travel by Car, Bus, or Train	Or	95% ci	Air Travel	Or	95% ci
Factor V Leiden	–	–	1		–	1	
	–	+	2.2	1.3–3.7	+	2.0	1.0–3.9
	+	–	3.1	2.3–4.1	–	3.0	2.3–4.0
	+	+	8.1	2.7–24.7	+	13.6	2.9–64.2
Prothrombin 20210A	–	–	1		–	1	
	–	+	1.9	1.3–3.7	+	2.2	1.3–3.6
	+	–	2.6	1.6–4.1	–	2.7	1.7–4.4
	+	+	3.1	0.3–36.6	+	7.9	0.9–67.2
BMI (kg/m^2)	<25	–	1		–	1	
		+	1.5	0.8–2.6	+	2.0	1.0–4.1
	25–30	–	1.4	1.2–1.7	–	1.4	1.2–1.7
		+	3.6	2.1–6.3	+	2.1	1.0–4.4
	>30	–	1.7	1.4–2.1	–	1.7	1.3–2.1
		+	9.9	3.6–27.6	+	2.6	1.0–6.4
Height (m)	1.60–1.90	–	1		–	1	
		+	2.3	1.5–3.7	+	1.5	0.9–2.8
	<1.60	–	0.7	0.5–0.9	–	0.7	0.5–0.9
		+	1.0	0.3–2.8	+	4.9	0.9–25.6
	>1.90	–	0.9	0.7–1.1	–	0.9	0.7–1.2
		+	4.7	1.4–15.4	+	6.8	0.8–60.6

Travel indicates journey by train, car, bus, or airplane lasting more than 4 h within the 8 wk before venous thrombosis, or corresponding index for control individuals.
DOI: 1.0.1371/journal.pmed.0030307.t003
From: Cannegieter SC, Doggen CJ, Houwelingen HC, et al. Travel-related venous thrombosis: Results from a large population-based case control study (MEGA Study). PLoS Med 2006;3:e307.

Table 49.2 Odds Ratios for Venous Thrombosis for Combinations of Risk Factors

	FII	FVIII	FVL*	OC*	BMI	Fam†
FII	2.2 (1.3–3.7)					
FVIII	7.9 (3.4–18.3)	6.2 (3.6–10.5)				
FVL	17.5 (2.3–135)	24.7 (4.4–139)	4.5 (1.9–10.4)			
OC	4.6 (1.1–19.8)	51.7 (5.4–198)	18.3 (2.0–171)	5.0 (2.1–12.1)		
BMI	9.5 (3.6–25.1)	18.6 (7.0–49.9)	20.5 (2.5–170)	31.4 (3.0–334)	1.9 (1.4–2.7)	
Fam†	2.4 (0.9–6.1)	8.7 (3.5–21.7)	4.7 (1.7–16.5)	10.7 (1.5–75.6)	2.4 (1.0–5.8)	1.7 (1.0–2.9)

*FVL indicates Factor V Leiden mutation; OC, oral contraceptive use; BMI, body mass index >26.9 kg/m^2 compared to a BMI of <23.7 kg/m^2. For each combination, the odds ratio for the presence of both risk factors compared to absence of both factors is presented. In the boxes. Where the risk factor in the column is the same as in the row, the odds ratio for presence of only that risk factor is given.
†Fam indicates a positive family history, meaning at least one thrombotic event in a brother, sister, or parent.
Copied from: Kuipers S, Cannegieter SC, Doggen CJ, et al. Effect of elevated levels of coagulation factors on the risk of venous thrombosis in long-distance travelers. Blood 2009;113:2064–9.

out to increase the risk twofold compared to an aisle seat. In combination with obesity (body mass index >30 kg/m^2), the risk was sixfold increased. Anxiety or sleeping during flying slightly increased the risk, but drinking alcohol did not. Traveling business class appeared to be associated with a slightly reduced risk, which can obviously be attributed to the less cramped conditions.

Mechanism

Immobilization and venous stasis lead to thrombosis owing to impairment of the function of the calf musculature in pumping the blood upstream. Circumstances related to immobilization, such as bed rest and plaster casts, are well known risk factors for thrombosis, but the contribution of general disease or damage to veins after a fracture will

also have an effect. Immobilization as a risk factor per se has been described in the Second World War, when an increased incidence of pulmonary embolism was observed during the bombardment of London, when people sought shelter in the underground railway system, where they sat in chairs for long periods.[18] A more recent case of thrombosis related to immobilization was described as 'e-thrombosis', in a young man with a serious PE without any known risk factor for VT, who appeared to spend more than 12 hours per day sitting at his computer.[19]

That immobilization is an important explanation for travel-related thrombosis can be inferred from the finding that traveling by other modes (car, bus, train) also increases the risk, although to a lesser extent. Furthermore, the additionally increased risk observed in tall, short, and obese people is also most likely due to impaired flow in cramped conditions. Nevertheless, it has been suggested that other factors may attribute to the increased risk, such as dehydration, or the hypobaric circumstances in the cabin. In a Norwegian study at high altitude (similar to levels in an airplane) an effect of hypobaric hypoxia on the coagulation system was described for the first time,[20] although later studies disputed these results.[21,22]

In the WRIGHT project the effect of an actual flight on the coagulation system was studied. Seventy-one young volunteers were exposed to an 8 hour flight with two control exposure situations, i.e., 8 hours' immobilization in a cinema and 8 hours in a daily life situation, separated by 2 weeks or more.[23] The volunteers had been selected in such a way that a substantial proportion had FVL, half of whom also took oral contraceptives. Thrombin formation (the end product of the coagulation system) could be demonstrated in 17% of the participants after the flight, whereas this was the case in only 3% and 1% in the cinema and the daily life situation, respectively. Of the persons in whom such coagulation activation could be demonstrated, the largest part had the FVL mutation and used oral contraceptive pills.

The results of this experiment suggest that circumstances in the airplane contribute to thrombus formation. Although other studies found opposing results, one of these circumstances could be hypobaric hypoxia, as it is possible that hypobaric hypoxia only has an effect in subjects in whom a slight procoagulant tendency is already present, such as people with FVL and oral contraceptive pill users. The other studies were all performed in subjects without risk factors. The effect of other cabin-related factors, such as stress, dehydration, virus infection, or air pollution, was also studied in the WRIGHT project. With respect to dehydration, no association was found between the amount of non-alcoholic beverages that the volunteers had drunk and hematocrit, or with osmolality.[24] Furthermore, changes in parameters of fluid loss during the flight were not different in volunteers with an activated clotting system from those without. Overall, the results of several laboratory markers suggested that hypoxia was a more likely explanation than any of the others.[25]

Prevention

Although the absolute risk of a symptomatic thrombotic event is only moderately increased (1 in 4500 passengers), many travelers will still develop thrombosis; considering the large yearly number of air travelers (over 2 billion per year), this leads to a total of 150 000 extra cases per year. Since each case of thrombosis is associated with considerable morbidity and a risk of death of several percent, attempts to prevent this complication should be worthwhile. However, preventive measures will be effective in only a very small proportion of travelers: based on a risk of 1 in 4500, 4500 people need to be treated to prevent one event, using a treatment that is 100% efficacious (number needed to treat). For this reason, preventive measures with side-effects should not be considered for indiscriminate use. This means that prevention by pharmacologic means (such as by low molecular weight heparin (LMWH) or aspirin, which all carry a bleeding risk) is not advisable as a general preventive strategy.

An alternative is mechanical prevention by the use of elastic stockings or calf compression devices. Elastic stockings prevent edema and have been shown in other risk situations to reduce thrombotic risk. From a biologic viewpoint, however, it is unlikely that stockings have much effect in the absence of leg muscle movement. Several studies focused on asymptomatic clots detected by ultrasound and observed a decrease in such clots occurring in those wearing elastic stockings.[26,27] However, in one study grade I elastic stockings also caused symptomatic superficial thrombosis in 3% of patients.[27] So, elastic stockings are not without potential side-effects. Elastic stockings should exert a pressure that is graded from distal to proximal, and therefore should be fitted individually. It is highly implausible that the one-size-fits-all 'traveler socks' that are sold over the counter at airports have any effect in preventing thrombosis.

An alternative to offering preventive measures to all passengers is to focus only on high-risk groups. This would lead to smaller numbers to treat and a better risk–benefit ratio. Some high-risk groups have already been identified, but no intervention studies have been performed to determine whether prevention of a thrombotic event outweighs the bleeding risk. In the absence of such evidence, caution should be used in prescribing any prophylaxis beyond exercise. However, although this has not been studied, patients who have a history of venous thrombosis are at the highest risk of thrombosis during air travel, considering their risk of recurrence of 3% per year.[4] In these patients, prophylaxis with low molecular weight heparin may be justified on theoretical grounds.

There are guidelines, such as those that have been published by the British Thoracic Society, that include so-called 'common sense advice', i.e., avoidance of alcohol, liberal intake of non-alcoholic beverages, and regular exercise of the legs.[28] As it is not very likely that dehydration plays a role in the development of thrombosis, the liberal intake of beverages probably has no major effect on prevention. However, it is plausible that regular movement of the legs will be beneficial. Exercise is obviously also without a risk of side-effects. Guidelines published by the American College of Chest Physicians[29] additionally advise properly fitted compression stockings (providing 15–30 mmHg of pressure at the ankle) and aisle seating for flights of more than 8 hours in the presence of a moderately strong risk factor for VT. For high-risk patients (those with a history of VT, major surgery within 6 weeks and known malignancy) both guidelines recommend or provide consideration for LMWH injection before departure. LMWH is not necessary in those already on oral anticoagulants. Aspirin alone is never recommended as prophylaxis, as there is no evidence showing substantial benefit, while it does increase the risk of major hemorrhage.

Conclusions and Recommendations

A long-haul flight increases the risk of venous thrombosis about three-fold. In absolute terms the risk is about 1 in 4500 long-haul passengers over a period of 8 weeks. The risk becomes higher with increasing duration of the flight and with making several flights in a short time frame. Several high-risk groups are known, i.e., tall, short, and obese people, as well as people with a genetic predisposition (e.g., Factor V Leiden) and oral contraceptive users. People with a history of venous thrombosis are considered to be a particularly high-risk group on theoretical grounds.

In most passengers, prevention can be limited to encouraging exercise and discouraging behavior that will restrict movement, such as excessive alcohol intake and any use of sleeping medication, which tends to keep passengers immobile for 5 hours or more. There is a need for studies into the efficacy and safety of preventative measures in high-risk individuals. Until such data are available, patients perceived to be at high risk (subjects with a history of venous thrombosis, known malignancy, or recent surgery) may benefit from a short period (1–3 days) of LMWH therapy starting 6–12 hours before the flight.

References

1. Kuipers S, Schreijer AJM, Cannegieter SC, et al. Travel and venous thrombosis: a systematic review. J Intern Med 2007;262:615–34.
2. Chandra D, Parisini E, Mozaffarian D. Meta–analysis: travel and risk for venous thromboembolism. Ann Intern Med 2009;151:180–90.

3. Naess IA, Christiansen SC, Romundstad P, et al. Incidence and mortality of venous thrombosis: a population-based study. J Thromb Haemost 2007;5:692–9.

4. Christiansen SC, Cannegieter SC, Koster T, et al. Thrombophilia, clinical factors, and recurrent venous thrombotic events. JAMA 2005;293: 2352–61.

5. Ashrani AA, Heit JA. Incidence and cost burden of post-thrombotic syndrome. J Thromb Thrombolysis 2009;28:465–76.

6. Becattini C, Agnelli G, Pesavento R, et al. Incidence of chronic thromboembolic pulmonary hypertension after a first episode of pulmonary embolism. Chest 2006;130:172–5.

7. Pengo V, Lensing AW, Prins MH, et al. Incidence of chronic thromboembolic pulmonary hypertension after pulmonary embolism. N Engl J Med 2004;350:2257–64.

8. Rosendaal FR. Venous thrombosis: a multicausal disease. Lancet. 1999;353(9159):1167–73.

9. Sarvesvaran R. Sudden natural deaths associated with commercial air travel. Med Sci Law 1986;26:35–8.

10. Lapostolle F, Surget V, Borron SW, et al. Severe pulmonary embolism associated with air travel. N Engl J Med 2001;345:779–83.

11. Perez-Rodriguez E, Jimenez D, Diaz G, et al. Incidence of air travel-related pulmonary embolism at the Madrid-Barajas airport. Arch Intern Med 2003;163:2766–70.

12. Schwarz T, Siegert G, Oettler W, et al. Venous thrombosis after long-haul flights. Arch Intern Med 2003;163:2759–64.

13. Kuipers S, Cannegieter SC, Middeldorp S, et al. The absolute risk of venous thrombosis after air travel: a cohort study of 8,755 employees of international organisations. PLoS Med 2007;4:e290.

14. Martinelli I, Taioli E, Battaglioli T, et al. Risk of venous thromboembolism after air travel: interaction with thrombophilia and oral contraceptives. Arch Intern Med 2003;163:2771–4.

15. Cannegieter SC, Doggen CJ, van Houwelingen HC, et al. Travel–related venous thrombosis: Results from a large population–based case control study (MEGA Study). PLoS Med 2006;3:e307.

16. Kuipers S, Cannegieter SC, Doggen CJ, et al. Effect of elevated levels of coagulation factors on the risk of venous thrombosis in long–distance travelers. Blood 2009;113:2064–9.

17. Schreijer AJ, Cannegieter SC, Doggen CJ, et al. The effect of flight–related behaviour on the risk of venous thrombosis after air travel. Br J Haematol 2009;144:425–9.

18. Simpson K. Shelter deaths from pulmonary embolism. Lancet 1940;ii:744.

19. Beasley R, Raymond N, Hill S, et al. eThrombosis: the 21st century variant of venous thromboembolism associated with immobility. Eur Respir J 2003;21:374–6.

20. Bendz B, Rostrup M, Sevre K, et al. Association between acute hypobaric hypoxia and activation of coagulation in human beings. Lancet 2000;356:1657–8.

21. Toff WD, Jones CI, Ford I, et al. Effect of hypobaric hypoxia, simulating conditions during long-haul air travel, on coagulation, fibrinolysis, platelet function, and endothelial activation. JAMA 2006;295:2251–61.

22. Crosby A, Talbot NP, Harrison P, et al. Relation between acute hypoxia and activation of coagulation in human beings. Lancet 2003;61:2207–8.

23. Schreijer AJ, Cannegieter SC, Meijers JC, et al. Activation of coagulation system during air travel: a crossover study. Lancet 2006;367:832–8.

24. Schreijer AJ, Cannegieter SC, Caramella M, et al. Fluid loss does not explain coagulation activation during air travel. Thromb Haemost 2008;99:1053–9.

25. Schreijer AJ, Hoylaerts MF, Meijers JC, et al. Explanations for coagulation activation after air travel. J Thromb Haemost 2010;8:971–8.

26. Clarke M, Hopewell S, Juszczak E, et al. Compression stockings for preventing deep vein thrombosis in airline passengers. Cochrane Database Syst Rev 2006;2:CD004002.

27. Scurr JH, Machin SJ, Bailey-King S, et al. Frequency and prevention of symptomless deep-vein thrombosis in long- haul flights: a randomised trial. Lancet 2001;357:1485–9.

28. Ahmedzai S, Balfour-Lynn IM, Bewick T, et al; British Thoracic Society Standards of Care Committee. Managing passengers with stable respiratory disease planning air travel: British Thoracic Society recommendations. Thorax 2011 Sep;66(Suppl. 1):i1–30.

29. Kahn SR, Lim W, Dunn AS, et al. American College of Chest Physicians. Prevention of VTE in nonsurgical patients: Antithrombotic Therapy and Prevention of Thrombosis. 9th ed. American College of Chest Physicians Evidence-Based Clinical Practice Guidelines. Chest 2012;141(2 Suppl): e195S–226S.

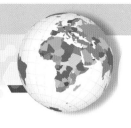
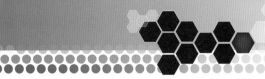
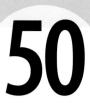

50

Healthcare Abroad

William L. Lang

Key points

- Travelers should leave with a prepared plan on how to access medical care at the destination, should the need arise
- The Joint Commission International is certified as a World Health Organization Collaborating Center and accredits approximately 450 medical facilities around the world outside the US/Canada/Europe
- Evacuation or repatriation to the home country may not be preferable in cases of serious illness when adequate local care that can be accessed immediately may be available
- For those with complex medical problems, storing medical records with an internet vendor or on a portable USB thumb drive may prove life-saving, especially in settings with language differences
- A list of physicians at many destinations is available from non-profit entities such as embassies, the International Society of Travel Medicine, www.istm.org, and IAMAT, www.iamat.org
- Many hospitals do not accept insurance and require sizeable upfront cash payment prior to admission
- Medical insurance for long-stay travelers should be renewable from abroad, include hospitalization coverage with direct payments to the facility, cover pre-existing conditions, include repatriation of mortal remains, and include evacuation
- Counterfeit medications are common abroad

Introduction*

International travelers place themselves at greater risk for illness or injury than those remaining at home living their normal lives.[1] Whether destination related, due to inadequate preparation, connected to risky behavior, or all of the above, the traveler usually views travel-related illness as surprising, uninvited, and intrusive. The frightening qualities of any medical event can be greatly

*This chapter is adapted from the similar chapter in the earlier edition by Dr. Nicholas Riesland.

©2012 Elsevier Inc
DOI: 10.1016/B978-1-4557-1076-8.00050-8

amplified in an unfamiliar country, particularly if the traveler does not speak the local language and is not conversant with local health beliefs, customs, or expectations. Consequently, their first reaction to anything other than minor illness is often to try to 'get home'. When problems do occur during international travel, however, even in less-developed countries, travelers (or long-term expatriates) need not assume they must return home to receive adequate medical care. As our world is changing, even in poor countries well-equipped private (frequently 'cash-upfront') medical facilities with well-trained staff often exist to serve an affluent minority. Overlooking or pre-judging such readily available options may be dangerous and costly. Still, assessing these possibilities can prove a daunting task, even for experienced expatriate healthcare professionals working in such environments. In developed nations, the familiar mechanisms in place to access care have caused many to neglect to consider the entire spectrum of care available to them. In international locations, the availability of parts of this spectrum can be vastly different, so it is important to keep in mind the entire range of sources of care, from self-care all the way to medical evacuation, in determining where to seek care when care is needed (Box 50.1). The challenges are to understand the capabilities and limitations of available medical resources, make timely and informed decisions about using them, and always keep in mind the optimal time and situation for returning the traveler to their itinerary, to their home, or to an intermediate destination for higher levels of care.

Changes in the Last Decade

As of June 2012, The Joint Commission International, founded in 1999 and certified as a World Health Organization Collaborating Center, accredits approximately 450 programs around the world (which does not include major international health destinations such as the United States, Canada, and the United Kingdom).[2] Not only does the Joint Commission International accredit specific programs, but it works with healthcare organizations, ministries of health, and global organizations in over 80 countries to push for greater acceptance of and adherence to common quality measures worldwide.[3] This does not mean that high-quality care is available throughout the world, but it does mean that there is an effective global effort to promote high-quality care, so travelers should not assume that they must travel to the more traditionally recognized locations to obtain good care.

BOX 50.1   Spectrum of Acute Care Available Overseas

- Self-care
  First aid to oneself administered using supplies and medications that are either brought with the traveler or available 'over-the-counter'
- Buddy care
  Similar to self-care, but involving a traveling companion to obtain and administer first-aid or comfort care
- Remote medical advice
  Still using self-transported or locally available over-the-counter supplies and equipment to deliver care based on the assessment and recommendation of a healthcare professional remote from the traveler
- Tele-health
  Itself a spectrum of services, but generally involving some degree of tele-presence (video-teleconferencing, remote diagnostic equipment, telemetry) enhancing the ability of the remote healthcare provider to diagnose health issues and direct treatment
- Primary care provider
  Office (or mobile)-based care with ability to provide physical exam and, usually, basic laboratory services, but with limited treatment ability beyond prescribing medications and simple treatment modalities
- Rural 'hospital'
  Typically staffed by primary care physicians but with the addition of (often limited) nursing services. Diagnostic and treatment capabilities are extremely variable, but typically very limited in developing nations
- Multispecialty clinic or polyclinic
  Typically a fee-for-service private clinic with multiple specialties and diagnostic (laboratory/imaging) capabilities located either on-site or close by. Usually do not have inpatient capabilities but often have treatment areas for managing minor injuries or stabilizing acute medical conditions
- Community hospital
  'Generalist'- based hospital focused on general internal medicine and general surgery for syndromes requiring surgical or inpatient care. Typically with a primary care-based emergency room or urgent care facility
- General hospital
  Greater availability of specialists, but limited, if any subspecialty services. Specialized emergency department typically available. Capable of stabilizing most illness or injury not requiring immediate subspecialty intervention (e.g., invasive cardiology, neurosurgery)
- Medical center
  Highest level of care. Greatest degree of subspecialist availability, including definitive management or, at least, intermediate stabilization of all medical, surgical, or traumatic emergencies

Growth of Medical Tourism

The last decade has seen significant shifts in healthcare services available internationally. In some ways reversing the trend whereby residents of what were traditionally considered 'medically underserved' countries would travel to North America and Europe, increasing numbers of travelers from developed nations are traveling abroad for services. While there are always disputes in the absolute numbers of 'medical tourists' internationally, ranging from under 100 000/year to over 1 000 000/year, what is clear is that quality of care is a prime determinant when a patient chooses to seek care abroad.[4–7] It is important to note, however, that even larger numbers of patients seek care abroad for outpatient services such as dentistry and cosmetic procedures, so this is a significant under-representation of the total number of medical tourists. The demand generated by medical tourism is a major driver of demand for increased quality of care measured against common health-quality metrics worldwide (e.g., access, infection rates, etc.). See Chapter 36 for an expanded discussion on medical tourism.

Risks of Needing Care Abroad

The epidemiology of travel-related illness is covered in Chapter 2 and in a number of careful studies over the past several decades.[6–16] Travel destination is an important determinant of risk. The developing world, especially, is associated with travel-related illness and risk of injury compared with travel elsewhere. Duration of travel in poorer countries is also linked to increasing travel-related illness.

Situations Requiring Care

A basic concept about the need for care while traveling is that 'common things happen commonly'. Robust data indicate that three of the four most common issues are gastroenteritis, upper respiratory disease, and dermatologic inflammatory processes. They all lend themselves well to care at the lower end of the care spectrum (self-care, remote consultation), at least initially. The use of these care modalities is predicated on pre-travel planning to have an appropriate medical kit at hand and, possibly, access to an appropriate source of remote care.

The fourth major syndrome is systemic febrile illness, which in some areas of the world, including sub-Saharan Africa and Southeast Asia, is the most common syndrome group.[7] These febrile syndromes can often, but not always, require more complex diagnostic or therapeutic activities than can be accomplished by self-care or remote care, although remote diagnostics are changing this for initial management.

The two most important categories of deaths abroad, which are a proxy for serious conditions requiring advanced care, are consistently shown to be cardiovascular events and trauma.[8,9] While initial care for these critical situations is limited to what is available in the vicinity of the event, given that time is of the essence in both situations, it is important to know the best local source of care for each condition. Additionally, pre-travel preparation for obtaining medical evacuation to a source of higher level care is critical.

Critical Differences in Approaches to Healthcare Abroad

The need for urgent healthcare is stressful, and this is compounded by having to interact with systems that are unfamiliar. While globalization is slowly bringing greater commonalities to healthcare systems around the world, there are still significant differences, especially in the developing world. The traveler who understands some of these differences will be less stressed should they need to seek care.

Cultural Differences

An important consideration in obtaining care abroad is the importance of language and culture. A large body of research has demonstrated the importance of effective communication to effective care.[10] In the US, when English-speaking providers care for 'low English proficiency' patients, care is demonstrably inferior.[11] Internationally, however, English has increasingly become the lingua franca of medicine, so the language effects are somewhat mitigated for English speakers traveling throughout the world. It is important to recognize, however, that this typically only applies to the physician staff delivering care, as nursing and ancillary support staff – critical members of the care team – do not as commonly speak English in non-English speaking countries. Additionally, even when the language barrier is successfully addressed, there are still cultural issues that can affect the quality of the medical communication. For all but the most straightforward medical situations, travelers are best served by a medically bilingual translator, followed closely by a general bilingual translator, and only as a last resort by a translator-of-convenience.[12]

Nursing Care

In developed nations there is a ratio of approximately 1000 nurses to 100 000 population. This ratio drops to only 20 per 100 000 in developing nations of Africa.[13] Even discounting the educational differences in nursing training in developed versus developing nations, patients should not expect to receive similar access to nursing care in developing nations. In many of these countries the nursing profession is plagued by lack of prestige, support, education, and resources, resulting in inability to attract smart, motivated students. Nurses are often actively discouraged or even prohibited from challenging physicians' orders, even if known to be inappropriate. Sometimes cultural views on confrontation and 'face' may contribute to this behavior. A similar dynamic also may exist among younger, less experienced physicians, wherein it is simply not acceptable to question a professor even though the professor may be in error or teaching obsolete medical doctrine. This means that patients and family members have to pay closer attention to the directions of the physician staff and be prepared to deliver more self-care and self-monitoring. Even where nurses are available, 'universal precautions' for the prevention of infectious disease are not necessarily universal, as running water, gloves, and sterile supplies may not be as routinely available. In fact, not uncommonly, the availability of quality nursing care is an important determinant in making medical evacuation decisions.[14]

No 'Right to Care'

Outside the developed world there is typically no perceived 'right' to urgent healthcare. In overtaxed and resource-limited communities, patients, including travelers, will often be turned away at the door to the emergency department if they cannot provide upfront payment or proof of ability to pay. Conversely, foreigners who are able to pay in hard currency or the equivalent are often shuttled to a specialized 'foreigners' clinic, where the ambience is often much more relaxed than the busy general receiving ward. While many travelers express an ethical discomfort with receiving 'special treatment' that locals do not receive, they should understand that the additional funding they provide by paying for care keeps the medical staffs paid and enables better care in the general areas.

General Categories of Services Available

As noted earlier, the systems available for healthcare support of travelers have changed greatly in the past decade. At the same time, the available systems are extremely variable around the world, although there are some general categories of sources of care of which travelers should be aware.

Self- or buddy-care is an important source of care when abroad. In many places in the world, entering the formal care system can be

---

BOX 50.2   Medical Kit for Travelers

- Medications
  - Analgesics (acetaminophen or aspirin). Also consider taking a stronger painkiller and anti-inflammatory such as ibuprofen
  - Antidiarrheal agents such as loperamide
  - Antibiotics for treating diarrhea
  - Oral rehydration packets
  - Antihistamine tablets for hay fever, itching, and other allergies
  - Sting relief spray or hydrocortisone cream for insect bites
  - Calamine lotion for sunburn and other skin rashes
  - Eye drops for sore eyes
  - DEET- or picaridin-containing insect repellent
- Optional medications/supplies
  - Hypnotics such as zolpidem or zopiclone for time-zone travel and jetlag
  - Melatonin for time-zone travel and jetlag
  - Anti-motion sickness remedies
  - Soluble fiber for constipation
  - Medication to prevent altitude sickness
  - Condoms
- Simple first-aid kit
  - Thermometer
  - Scissors
  - Tweezers to remove splinters and ticks
  - Adhesive bandages of various sizes
  - Gauze swabs and adhesive tape
  - Bandages and safety pins to fasten them
  - Non-adhesive dressings (such as Telfa or Melolin)
  - Antiseptic powder or solution (e.g., povidone-iodine), antiseptic wipes
  - Wound closure strips (Steri-strips) or butterfly strips
- Additions for long journeys, trekking, or camping
  - A course of broad-spectrum antibiotics for infections of the chest, ear, skin, etc.
  - Antibiotics to treat cystitis and a treatment for vaginal yeast infection
  - Antibiotics drops for eyes and ears
  - Topical antifungal cream or powder
  - Elasticized support bandage or crepe bandage
  - Triangular bandage for making an arm sling
  - Dental first-aid kit
  - Sterile kit, including needles, syringes, suture kit, intravenous cannula for IV fluids
- Additions for highly malarious regions
  - Permethrin to treat clothes and bed-nets
  - Course of standby treatment for malaria if more than 24 hours from medical care

---

difficult and time-consuming and can be fraught with infectious disease dangers. Where it is appropriate to care for oneself, either directly or with the assistance of remote medical advice, this important option should not be overlooked. Often international medical/evacuation insurance (see insurance discussion, later) comes with access to nurse or physician advice services, but these interventions will be much more effective if the traveler has access to basic diagnostic and treatment items from a basic travel medical kit (Box 50.2).

Local physician offices/clinics. In many parts of the world the best place to obtain other-than-emergency care is a local physician's office, as long as you have a way of knowing which of the available physicians is reliable. In many cases, local physicians group themselves into polyclinics, which can function almost as small hospitals. Catering to paying patients, these multispecialty polyclinics are frequently equipped to manage or stabilize minor trauma and medical urgencies. These clinics can often be identified through local residents or hotels. In many cases embassies can provide listings of providers with whom they have had acceptable interactions in the past, although for obvious political and diplomatic reasons, the embassies are very careful not to recommend one source of care over another.[15] Instead, they will quietly omit from their list sources of care that have had reported problems in the past.

For-profit international healthcare organizations. As the international travel market has grown, so too has the demand for healthcare in a manner similar to what travelers would find at home. Responding to this market, for-profit international medical assistance organizations, including both insurance-based providers and companies typically thought of as evacuation providers, have established clinics focusing on care for travelers from developed nations. Although these services are designed for patients who have pre-subscribed to their traveler programs, they are typically willing to take any patient willing to pay cash. These clinics provide an atmosphere akin to a developed nation health clinic, have providers who are either expatriates or trained in a developed nation environment, and who have specialized local knowledge of local health systems and key people so that higher levels of care can be facilitated. In some cases, agreements with local health authorities require that the actual hands-on care must be delivered by local staff, but even in these situations the close involvement of international staff, both at the clinic level and in helping to monitor and coordinate more advanced care, can help provide an effective outcome.[16]

Foreigners' Clinics. Many hospitals abroad, especially in major cities, have emergency departments that are overwhelmed by the volume of local patients seeking care, many of whom do not have resources to pay for care. Recognizing the importance of international business travel and tourism, as well as the need for paying patients, in many developing nations major hospitals have clinical areas, and in some cases full hospitals, dedicated to caring for international (paying) patients. In most cases, these clinics will provide more attentive care than is provided to the general population, but they often suffer from the same limits on resources as the general emergency department. Additionally, providers in these clinics are usually local and focus on managing any problems locally, without early consideration of evacuation as possibly the best option. It is very difficult to make general statements about the use of these clinics, as some can be very good whereas others are simply whitewash on a very under-resourced capability. Pre-travel research addressing which facilities are more acceptable, or pre-travel establishment of access to just-in-time medical facility/provider information, is critical to making the right decision should care be needed.

A related caveat addresses 'VIP' clinics, which were a staple of socialized medicine in communist countries and are often still present serving government leadership and paying patients. In many cases these clinics are entirely isolated from the general population, and albeit much higher-end in appearance, can suffer from the same problems as the 'foreigner's clinics', with the added problem of low volume leading to atrophy of skills, expiration of pharmaceuticals, and obsolescence (or poor maintenance) of equipment that is rarely used.

Hospital Care. The developed world has seen a consolidation of hospitals in the past 20 years, with a significant reduction in 'boutique' facilities and smaller hospitals.[17] This has meant that many travelers from developed nations are accustomed to going to any hospital and expecting to be able to receive urgent or emergency care. In the developing world and former communist nations, however, there is still a significant presence of specialty hospitals. Often, these specialty hospitals cannot provide urgent or emergency care services. Additionally, the presence of the specialty hospital system can result in a 'balkanization' of care, such that the specialists see problems only through their own lens. One illustration from the experience of a previous author of this section comes from a large city in the former Soviet Union involving a 58-year-old man with chest pain. He was taken by ambulance to a large cardiology hospital, diagnosed as having an acute coronary syndrome and started on thrombolytic therapy (streptokinase). During treatment he developed gastrointestinal hemorrhage, severe enough to require transfer to a gastrointestinal hospital. The bleeding was adequately treated, but he developed a fever and was sent to an infectious disease hospital. Owing to blood loss, however, renal failure ensued and he was then taken to a nephrology center on the other side of town. After several days, he became progressively dyspneic and was diagnosed with heart failure, prompting transfer back to the cardiology hospital where care had been initiated. The important message here is that patients should attempt to ensure they have someone overseeing their care with the '50 000 foot' view of the clinical progress, all of the resources available locally, and the options for evacuation to more comprehensive sources of care.

Pharmacy and Medication Issues

The combination of the international 'war on drugs' and the recognition of problems caused by overuse of antibiotics has caused a general tightening of restrictions internationally on pharmaceuticals. Japan, for example, prohibits the importation of some over-the-counter medicines commonly used in most countries, including inhalers and some allergy/sinus medications. Specifically, products that contain stimulants (e.g., pseudoephedrine, contained in medications such as Actifed, Sudafed, and Vicks inhalers) or codeine (contained in medications such as Tylenol 3) are prohibited.[18] Additionally, common medication such as insulin cannot be imported into many countries, Japan included, without lengthy procedures to obtain a specialized importation permit, even for personal use. While travelers who are on medications will generally have no issues with bringing personal use quantities of medications with them on international travel, travelers should make sure that the medications are packed in their original prescription bottles and that they carry a copy of the prescription with them. Although generally prescriptions from foreign providers are invalid in most countries, having a valid prescription lessens the risk of confiscation at border crossings, and will facilitate obtaining a local prescription from a local provider should it become necessary to obtain resupply of an important medication. At the other end of the spectrum, in many countries no prescription is required for medications other than narcotics. In this case, possession of a prescription from home will still assist the pharmacist in determining the closest locally available match to the required medication.

Travelers should also be aware of the prevalence of counterfeit medications and poor quality control of medications in many countries around the world. A first consideration is using, whenever possible, trusted pharmacies identified by sources such as an international clinic or an international medical assistance provider. Second, attempt to ensure that medications are from international providers rather than local manufacturers, although in many areas this is not possible. Third, examine packaging carefully for signs of tampering or poorly executed 'safety seals' designed to approximate the real product (manufacturers' websites often have detailed descriptions and pictures of their packaging, and tamper-control seals to aid users in confirming that the medication is not counterfeit). Finally, as with any product, if the price appears to be too good to be true, it is a red flag, although developing world prices for legitimate medications are often lower than in developed nations.

Evacuation Issues

Local Evacuation Issues

The past decade has seen a great increase in the availability of '911' systems in major international cities, including much of the developing world. Dialing the local equivalent of 911 (which varies throughout the world), however, does not reliably call a well-trained emergency medical technician or paramedic. In much of the developing world, ambulances are strictly transport vehicles with minimal stabilization or resuscitation equipment/capability. The main advantage of an ambulance may simply be that they know the best way to get to a hospital, and may have better luck in negotiating traffic. Advance awareness of the ambulance capabilities of a destination city, and how to call for emergency assistance, including the phone number to dial (using pre-travel research tools such as Travax) will help a traveler to know whether to call and wait for an ambulance or to use a transport-of-convenience such as a private auto or a taxi.

Long-Distance Evacuation

With the diversity of quality and quantity of care available around the world, in the case of a significant injury or illness many travelers from developed nations desire to get to the highest possible level of care as rapidly as possible. Consequently, air evacuations from developing nations to developed home countries fall into two primary categories: first, urgent evacuation required because local care is unable to fully stabilize a patient, or the risk of local procedures is perceived to be higher than the risk of moving the patient; and second, elective evacuation after the patient is stabilized, but recovery and longer-term management are more desirable at or near home. In either case, close involvement of physicians with extensive experience in the management of evacuation decisions that balance risk/benefit/cost are critical to the decision process. Providers with patients considering evacuation should be familiar with these issues and be careful not to let the emotions of the situation dictate over the careful consideration of the options.[19,20,21,22] Commercial airlines meet the vast share of overseas medical evacuation needs. Air ambulances are used much less frequently. In 2004, among a population of approximately 50 000 travelers residing abroad, the US government authorized nearly 1300 medical evacuations. Air ambulances were only used approximately 2% of the time.[23] Airlines may accept seriously ill patients as stretcher cases, although procedures and policies among carriers differ widely. Each airline determines whom they will transport and under what conditions. Commercial carriers will uniformly not transport someone who is not medically stable, or who may present a risk to other passengers or crew members.

Planning Ahead

With a basic familiarity with the risks of requiring healthcare abroad, the differences that may be found in the way care is delivered, and the types of care that may be available in any given location, the importance of advance planning for the specific travel destination becomes evident. Box 50.3 outlines teaching points about healthcare abroad to be discussed during the pre-travel consultation.

BOX 50.3 Teaching Points about Healthcare Abroad to be Discussed during the Pre-Travel Consultation

- Understand differences in insurance between:
  Standard health insurance
  Travel health insurance
  Evacuation insurance
  Medical evacuation
  Security evacuation
- Know types of places to seek care abroad:
  'Accident and emergency' (A&E) wards of hospitals
  Foreigners' wards of hospitals
  Stand-alone 'foreigners' clinics'
  Doctors' offices
- Know how to find reliable sources of care and limitation of each method:
  Referrals from insurance companies
  Embassy physician lists
  Commercial subscription services (e.g., Travax)
  Hotel referrals
- Medication Issues:
  Have copy of prescription
  Carry medicines in original pharmacy containers
  Be aware of any importation restrictions (e.g., narcotics, decongestants)
  Be wary of counterfeit medications

At the most basic level, travelers to medically underserved areas should prepare for as much self-care as is reasonable, given their risk tolerance, experience, and the availability of communications to reliable medical consultation. The ideal preparation consists of a standardized medical kit (see Box 50.2) containing basic first-aid materials, topical anti-inflammatories and disinfectants, and limited oral agents, including anti-inflammatories, antipyretics, antidiarrheals, and possibly antibiotics. This kit is ideally coordinated with a source of care that is experienced in remote management of common international health issues, and familiar with the contents of the kit. While international communications have become reliable and relatively low-cost over the past decade, communications are only effective if the source of care is available around-the-clock. For this reason, many travelers choose to subscribe to medical assistance plans that combine 24-hour care call-in lines with aid in managing more complex care, including access to care and evacuation assistance.

If a traveler elects not to use a medical assistance organization, or plans to use their home-based care organization, for assistance, they still need to have a mechanism for identifying higher level sources of care should self-care or assisted self-care be inadequate. Although embassy clinics are usually not accessible to non-government travelers, embassies can still provide valuable information about local health risks and available healthcare resources for foreigners. For example, the American Citizen Services branch of embassy consular sections keeps and makes available upon request updated lists of local medical facilities and clinics deemed reliable. Usually these lists do not indicate which facilities or consultants are preferred, however.

Lists of potential sources of care are often available via internet searches. Travelers and providers must be careful about relying too heavily on the recommendations found on the internet, as it is very easy to 'plant' favorable or unfavorable comments about certain facilities or providers. Some global organizations maintain medical capability databases, drawing from their collective assessments of and experiences with local medical facilities and providers throughout the world. Proprietary publishing companies such as Shoreland, Inc. market products, such as Travax, that facilitate such information exchange among selected subscribers. Medical assistance companies such as International SOS, EuropeAssistance, Healix, and BUPA have access to their own databases for subscribers' benefit, with similar valuable information. These tools help determine whether or not an inpatient or ambulatory medical care provider in a particular overseas city is 'adequate' or 'preferred' for a specific diagnosis. Such data can assist in deciding where to go for initial care, when local resources are likely to be exceeded, whether resources should be committed to medical evacuation and, if so, help determine the closest suitable destination.

Sometimes travelers try to access missionary clinics. These are not generally intended for affluent travelers and so do not usually operate on a fee-for-service basis, though increasingly some do so in major tourist areas. Nonetheless, medical providers in these facilities often go to great lengths to assist travelers with severe problems. Other local clinics with less predictable quality often accept foreign travelers and are frequently used by budget travelers. Hotel doctors, whose main qualifications may be political or via family connections, often have tenuous reputations among peers in the local healthcare system. Still, in serious medical situations they may be able to move things in the proper direction. Note, however, that hotel doctors often receive some type of 'referral fee' when they send a well-insured traveler to an underfunded clinic or hospital, so there is often a risk of inappropriate hospitalization or use of a less-than-optimal facility when using the hotel physician. Finding oneself in a local hospital at the hands of a young or inexperienced doctor, it is often worth asking for an 'international representative' who can assist with translation and coordination. Asking for the chief of the service or 'professor' is also a useful strategy. Senior physicians often speak better English and may have more experience and training in Western-style medicine.

Paying for Care

A final consideration surrounding international healthcare is how to pay for care obtained abroad. For residents of the European Economic Area (EEA) (European Union plus Iceland, Liechtenstein, Norway, and Switzerland) traveling within the EEA, a European Health Insurance Card entitles the traveler to the same level of public-access care as a national of that country, not including pre-existing conditions.[24] Outside of that, however, travelers should assume in most cases that cash – or in some cases a credit card guarantee – will be required before care is rendered. Before traveling, travelers should ask their insurance carrier three questions: (1) Does my policy apply when I'm outside my home country? (2) Will it cover emergencies such as a trip to a foreign hospital? (3) Does my policy provide for medical evacuation if needed? In most cases the answer to the first two questions is 'yes' (with limitations, especially for health-maintenance organization (HMO)-based policies) but 'no' to the evacuation question. Even when home-based health insurance will cover the cost of care, it is often only retrospectively after the submission of detailed bills (translated, at patient expense, where needed).[25] Because of this, many travelers obtain supplemental travel health insurance that has mechanisms in place to guarantee payment to foreign providers. Travelers must remember, however, that guarantees only work if the provider accepts the guarantee. A good checklist addressing travel health insurance is provided by the Canadian government agency Foreign Affairs and International Trade Canada (Box 50.4).[26]

BOX 50.4   Assessing Travel Insurance Policies

When assessing a travel health insurance plan, ask if it:
- provides continuous coverage before departure and after return;
- offers coverage renewable from abroad and for the maximum period of stay;
- has an in-house, worldwide, 24-hour/7-day emergency contact number in your native language and/or translation services for healthcare providers in your destination country;
- pays for foreign hospitalization for illness or injury and related medical costs (treatment for some injuries may exceed $250,000) and, if so, whether it has provision to pay up front (or guarantee payment) or expects you to pay and be reimbursed later;
- provides coverage for doctor's visits and prescription medicines;
- provides direct payment of bills and cash advances abroad so you don't have to pay out of your own pocket;
- covers pre-existing medical conditions (when in doubt, get an agreement in writing that you're covered). Otherwise, you could find your claim 'null and void' under a pre-existing condition clause;
- provides for medical evacuation to your home country or the nearest location with appropriate medical care;
- pays for a medical escort (healthcare provider) to accompany you during evacuation. This service can cost as much as $100,000 if it is not included;
- covers premature births and related neonatal care, as needed;
- clearly explains deductible costs (plans with 100 percent coverage are more expensive but may save money in the long run);
- covers preparation and return of your remains to your home country if you die abroad (in most cases, costs will exceed plan coverage);
- covers emergency dental care;
- covers emergency transportation, such as ambulance services; and
- does not exclude or significantly limit coverage for certain regions or countries you may visit.

Importantly, neither home-based health insurance nor standard travel health insurance typically covers evacuation. Because medical evacuation can cost multiple tens of thousands of dollars (US), many travelers choose to obtain evacuation insurance. Almost as important as paying for evacuation, purchase of this insurance carries with it access to physicians experienced in determining the method and provider of evacuation, given the specific situation and in working with local facilities to ensure stability for travel. In most cases, evacuation insurance can be obtained in two levels. The first level covers only medical situations, while a higher level (typically double the cost) will also provide for evacuation in the case of an urgent security situation, such as political unrest or terrorist activity that places the insured traveler at risk. A routinely updated list of evacuation and evacuation insurance providers can be found at the US Department of State's International Travel advisory website.[27] Insurance policies require that ill travelers must be inpatients in order for evacuation to be covered. Travelers must be aware that evacuation insurance will provide medical evacuation in situations where that is the only option for obtaining required inpatient care at a level comparable to what would be available in the traveler's home country. Specific policies can vary greatly, but issues that can be adequately managed with a short stay at a local facility that has limited but adequate capability will not result in a paid evacuation. An example might be an acute appendicitis, when a local facility has a competent surgeon and good record of outcomes. In this case, the insurer may determine that the best medical outcome would result from local care and return home by standard commercial flight following an adequate recovery period. Many variables go into this decision process, which is why travelers must understand the specifics of their policy, including who has the final say on when and what type of evacuation is appropriate.

References

1. Liese B, Mundt KA, Dell LD, et al. Medical insurance claims associated with international business travel. Occup Environ Med 1997;54:499–503.

2. Joint Commission International. Retrieved July 23, 2011, from www.jointcommissioninternational.org/JCI-Accredited-Organizations.

3. Joint Commission International. About the Joint Commission. Retreived July 23, 2011 from http://www.jointcommissioninternational.org/About-JCI.

4. Ehrbeck T, Guevara C, Mango P. Mapping the Market for Medical Travel. McKinsey Quarterly. May 2008 (monograph).

5. Youngman I. Medical tourism statistics: Why McKinsey has got it wrong. Int Med Travel J 2009.

6. Rack J, Wichmann O, Kamara B, et al. Risk and spectrum of diseases in travelers to popular tourist destinations. J Travel Med 2005;12:248–53.

7. Freedman DO, Weld LH, Kozarsky PE, et al. for the GeoSentinel Surveillance Network. N Engl J Med 2006;354:119–30.

8. Redman CA, MacLennan A, Walker E. Causes of death abroad: Analysis of data on bodies returned for cremation to Scotland. J Travel Med 2011;18:96–101.

9. Groenheide AC, van Genderen PJ, Overbosch D. East and West, home is best? A questionnaire-based survey on mortality of Dutch travelers Abroad. J Travel Med 2011;18:141–4.

10. Lee S. A Review of Language and Other Communication Barriers in Healthcare. US Department of Health and Human Services. April 2003.

11. Flores G. The impact of medical interpreter services on the quality of healthcare: A systematic review. Med Care Res Rev 2005 Jun;62(3):255–99.

12. Baker DW, Hayes R, Fortier JP. Interpreter use and satisfaction with interpersonal aspects of care for Spanish-speaking patients. Med Care 1998;36:1461–70.

13. 'Nursing Shortage Knows No Boundaries.' Editorial. The Baltimore Sun. September 13, 2010.

14. Teichman PG, Dnochin Y, Kot RJ. International aeromedical evacuation. N Engl J Med 2007;356:262–70.

15. For example, see http://travel.state.gov/travel/tips/emergencies/emergencies_1195.htmll (US); http://www.fco.gov.uk/en/travel-and-living-abroad/when-things-go-wrong/ (UK); Most developed nations' consular services can provide similar information through their embassies.

16. Wilde H, Roselieb M, Hanvesakul R, et al. Expatriate clinics and medical evacuation companies are a growth industry worldwide. J Travel Med 2003;10:315–7.

17. Vogt W. Hospital Market Consolidation: Trends and Consequences. Expert Voices (newsletter). National Institute for Healthcare Management, Nov 2009.

18. US Department of State, Japan Country Specific Information, travel.state.gov (accessed August 10, 2011).

19. Teichman PG, *op cit.*

20. Greuters S, Christiaans HMT, Veenings B, et al. Evaluation of repatriation parameters: Does medical history matter? J Travel Med 2009;16:1–6.

21. Duchateau F-X, Verner L, Cha O, et al. Decision criteria of immediate aeromedical evacuation. J Travel Med 2009;16:391–4.

22. Jorge A, Pombal R, Peixoto H. et al. Preflight medical clearance of ill and incapacitated passengers: 3-year retrospective study of experience with a European airline. J Travel Med 2005;12:306–11.

23. US Department of State. Office of Medical Services, 2005.

24. European Commission, Employment, Social Affairs, and Inclusion. The European Health Insurance Card. http://ec.europa.eu/social/main.jsp?catId=559. Accessed September 4, 2011.

25. US Department of State. Bureau of Consular Affairs. Medical Insurance. http://travel.state.gov/travel/cis_pa_tw/cis/cis_1470.html. Accessed September 4, 2011.

26. Foreign Affairs and International Trade Canada. Travel Insurance FAQ. http://www.voyage.gc.ca/faq/insurance_assurance-eng.asp. Accessed September 4, 2011.

27. US Department of State. Bureau of Consular Affairs. http://travel.state.gov/travel/cis_pa_tw/cis/cis_1470.html. Accessed September 4, 2011.

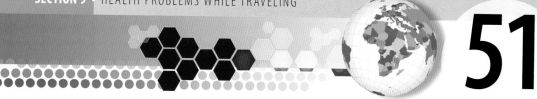

Personal Security and Crime Avoidance

David O. Freedman

Introduction

Crimes and violent acts against the person occur with some regularity while traveling. Because tourists and business travelers are perceived to be both wealthy and possibly carrying large sums of money and valuables, they are often the specific targets of criminals. Despite this, little formal research has been done to prioritize or rank personal protection measures, or even to define which of a long list of frequently given recommendations have any real benefit at all. Nevertheless, security experts agree that a large proportion of criminal occurrences are avoidable if travelers adhere to a number of these commonsense guidelines. The 'key points' (see above) should be reviewed during the pre-travel consultation and the rest given in an easy to follow written format for the traveler to carry with them.

The cornerstone of personal safety is situational awareness. Every city, no matter whether in a rich or a poor country, has unsafe zones of varying size, where personal risk is high. Most individuals know where these zones are in their own home city; the same level of knowledge should be obtained by all travelers prior to or as soon as possible after arrival at any destination. Once the high-risk zones and high-risk activities are identified, avoid them.

Travelers must not only be constantly aware of the general environment in the destination city or town, but also stay constantly alert to the ongoing minute-by-minute situation in their immediate personal proximity as they move through the day. Travelers should know the country's history, its culture, and follow current events for the destination in the media prior to departure and during the stay. This can be accomplished by use of Consular Information Sheets (Table 51.1), corporate or organizational security reports, and reports from threat assessment consultancies (Table 51.2). However, good statistical data on crime and violent events are often not kept in many countries. In those places where data are kept, for political and economic reasons the information is often not easily available to foreign consulates, consultants, or international authorities. Thus, in many cases the most accurate and timely advice on districts, regions, or situations to avoid may be from friends, colleagues, clients, tour operators, or the hotel concierge. Such advice is usually based on recent real experiences of other travelers and should be sought immediately on arrival. In addition, embassies usually monitor incidents involving their own citizens and can provide useful guidance when asked.

The second over-riding crime avoidance principle is to not be a creature of habit. This applies as much to the short-stay hotel guest as to the higher-profile corporate expatriate. Jogging at the same time each early morning and following the same route from a well-known business hotel identifies a potential target just as easily as the expatriate who leaves the house vacant each Saturday morning to go grocery shopping.

Complex security issues that are beyond the scope of the typical travel clinic patient interaction are not covered here. These include hostile surveillance, kidnapping and hostage situations, hijackings, surviving in hostile situations during armed conflict, humanitarian work in troubled areas, and recognition of land mine/unexploded ordnance risks. A number of highly experienced risk consultancies, usually staffed by former law enforcement, espionage, and military personnel, are available to provide appropriate risk management, threat assessment, and training packages to organizations and corporations (see Table 51.2). The basics of many of these issues are covered elsewhere.[1-3]

Larger organizations and corporations that may contract out their travel medicine needs to outside clinics often have corporate security departments which will have already provided destination-specific risk ratings and written security reports to employees and expatriates on an ongoing basis. This will include very specific information on safe and unsafe districts within a destination city, and lists of hotels and residential areas considered to be the most desirable and safe. Country- and city-specific security reports are available from most of the risk consultancies (Table 51.2). (Personal safety as pertains to injury

©2012 Elsevier Inc
DOI: 10.1016/B978-1-4557-1076-8.00051-X

Table 51.1 Consular Websites with Comprehensive Security and Risk Information

US Department of State Travel Warnings and Consular Information
http://travel.state.gov/travel/travel_1744.html
Citizens register at: https://travelregistration.state.gov/

UK Foreign and Commonwealth Office Country Advice
http://www.fco.gov.uk/en/travel-and-living-abroad/travel-advice-by-country/
Citizens Register at: http://www.fco.gov.uk/en/travel-and-living-abroad/staying-safe/Locate/

Canada Department of Foreign Affairs & International Trade Travel Reports
http://www.voyage.gc.ca/countries_pays/menu-eng.asp
Citizens Register at: https://www.voyage2.gc.ca/Registration_inscription/Register_Inscrire/Login_ouvrir-une-session-eng.aspx?fwd=true&hash=p0V4sJhYtXNnDsAOImpW8w6161

Australia Department of Foreign Affairs and Trade Travel Advice by Country
http://www.smartraveller.gov.au/zw-cgi/view/Advice/Index
Citizens Register at: https://www.orao.dfat.gov.au/orao/weborao.nsf/homepage?Openpage

US Department of State Overseas Security Advisory Council (OSAC), Daily Global News Bulletins
http://www.osac.gov

Table 51.2 Major Consultancies Specializing in Risk Management and Security

Kroll Inc. Risk Consulting
www.kroll.com
Control Risks
www.crg.com
iJet Travel Intelligent Risk Systems
www.ijet.com
International SOS Assistance
www.internationalsos.com

prevention, motor vehicle crash protection, and prevention of drowning is covered in Ch. 47.)

Before Departure

Before departing, or sometimes before booking, travelers should seek advice from their own country's consular website regarding local safety and political stability. The most comprehensive English-language consular websites are shown in Table 51.2. These countries all have consular personnel on the ground in most destinations, so can provide detailed situational information. These consular reports contain much street- and district-specific information, so are best printed and carried during travel. More than one national website should be checked when assessing a destination, as language used in reports from one country may reflect political influences or threat situations targeted only at the citizens of that particular reporting country. In recent years, the trend for consular reports has been away from blanket 'go' or 'no-go' labels for entire destination countries and more towards an enumeration of risk in specific parts of those countries. In addition, risk levels have been introduced into the reports, so that leisure travelers may be advised to avoid travel, but essential travel may be sanctioned within certain geographic limits. In addition, for specific situations or enhanced information, citizens can usually telephone or e-mail their own embassy at the destination and obtain details from the security attaché or consul that may be too sensitive or complex to post on the public consular reports.

Priorities Upon Arrival

Unfortunately, the initial airport arrival constitutes one of the highest threat situations of the entire trip for the typical leisure traveler. Travelers are tired from the journey, unfamiliar with the surroundings, the arrivals lobby is usually crowded and noisy, and directions and signs may be in a foreign language. This is a natural magnet for criminals in any country. An advance plan needs to be in place. Travelers who are to be met at the airport in a high-risk destination by an individual, tour company representative, or driver not personally known to them should be instructed not to leave the arrivals lobby with anyone who does not know a pre-arranged verbal recognition code. Company signboards as well as a traveler's name are easily copied by anyone in the arrivals area. Missed pick-ups often occur, no matter how meticulous the arrangements were. Travelers should always know the address of exactly where they are supposed to get to on arrival, and also have phone numbers for appropriate local contact people.

Many airports have kiosks in the terminal rented by reputable taxi concessionaires where prepaid taxi rides can be purchased and where travelers will be then led to a waiting car. Next best is to look for an organized taxi rank with cars lined up, accepting passengers in sequence, and located within the airport perimeter. At all costs avoid individuals on foot soliciting for passengers solo in the airport arrivals area. In any country, many criminals purport to be taxi drivers or taxi operators.

Travelers should put a system into place to always ensure that someone knows where they are and what the expected schedule is at all times. Given the ease of modern communication this may include someone in the home country. If staying for any length of time, travelers should register with their country's embassy, something that is now done only via the internet. Travelers should be familiar with appropriate modes of contact should emergency situations arise.

Unless otherwise mandated by law (uncommon), passports should be locked in a safe at home or in the hotel and a photocopy of the face page carried at all times on the traveler's person. The photocopy should include any necessary visa as well as the legal entry stamp to the country, as authorities are usually on the lookout for individuals who entered illegally. Additional photocopies, or at least passport number and issue details, should be kept in a separate place. A scanned copy of the passport that can be e-mailed later can be left at home or can be e-mailed to the traveler's own e-mail address prior to departure for later access.

Travelers should learn telephone-dialing sequences even for short stays immediately on arrival, and certainly before an emergency situation arises. Travelers should be aware of the dial sequence necessary to access both local and long-distance circuits from their hotel room, residence, place of business, and/or locally on leased or personal mobile phone. They should ascertain all emergency phone numbers, including police, fire, ambulance, as well as neighbors, key business colleagues, and the hotel if applicable. These should be posted prominently in the home, if applicable, and carried on the person at all times. Organizations with local operations often have laminated wallet cards with key contact points regularly made up, and these can be delivered to all arriving employees or visitors right at the airport.

The hotel desk or colleagues should be questioned upon arrival about common local scams and distraction techniques used by pickpockets and thieves. Thieves often work in groups of two or more, one to distract and the others to take.

Mobile Phones and Electronic Devices

Even the poorest countries generally have a high-quality mobile phone service. Efficient and rapid communication with sources of potential help when a traveler finds him/herself in a high-risk situation can provide solutions to that particular situation or can help to minimize the time the traveler is exposed to that threat.

A locally purchased or leased mobile phone is best, because of ease of dialing local numbers and the ease with which local people can dial the traveler. A mobile phone should ideally have local emergency and consulate numbers programmed at the earliest chance. In most countries, cheap handsets with a local number and costing less than 20 dollars can be purchased on arrival and charged from prepaid cards. Organizations or companies that have short-term visitors or staff coming in from other countries can consider providing a local mobile phone upon arrival. Alternatively, frequent travelers should carry their own GSM band phone so that they can roam on the local network. GSM band service is the most prevalent in the world and is available in almost every country (except Japan), although the majority of US mobile phones still use a different standard. GSM frequencies in the Americas differ from other parts of the world, but tri- and quad-band GSM handsets that automatically detect the ambient GSM signal are available from all GSM operators worldwide.

Mobile phones, laptop computers, tablet computers, mobile readers, and other personal electronic devices frequently contain sensitive financial or personal data and are easily lost or stolen. All devices should be secured with locking password access software and encrypted if possible.

In the Hotel

In high-threat countries, hotel locations should be carefully selected using advance knowledge and ideally located in proximity to planned activities. Rooms on floors three to six are generally regarded as optimal for safety and security. They are harder to break into from the outside of the hotel, but are accessible to firefighting equipment. Travelers should look for fire safety instructions in the room upon arrival, and also familiarize themselves with escape routes. Travelers may consider counting doors in the corridor in order to find exits in case of poor visibility due to dark or smoke.

The hotel room door should be locked at all times. For those anticipating stays in budget accommodations, compact locking and door opening blocking devices are cheap and readily available. Doors should not be opened to strangers, and a call to the front desk can be made to confirm the identity of someone knocking at the door. Leave shower curtains open upon leaving the room to discourage intruders from hiding there. Room safes are less secure than individual safe deposit boxes at the front desk but may be preferable, depending on model type, to a large hotel safe readily accessible to many hotel employees.

Room numbers should not be disclosed to any but the closest personal friends and colleagues. Meet visitors in the lobby. Room keys that identify the room number together with the hotel should be left with the concierge upon leaving the building. Hotel business cards with address and phone number in the local language should be carried on the person at all times.

Disagreement exists about the wisdom of informing the hotel desk about expected time of return to the hotel. This is probably unwise in general, but may be considered if a traveler is to be returning late at night and no one else is aware of the anticipated destination and schedule.

Out and About

Travelers should radiate confidence and know exactly where they are going. Situational awareness requires planning ahead before venturing out. If the terrain and routes are already familiar, little planning time will be required. However, all travelers need to have good knowledge of high-risk areas and potentially high-risk situations. Methods for ascertaining these have been described above, but it is important to remember that high-risk areas can change with time, so even frequent travelers need to do an assessment on each visit. Consult local media regularly to keep up with current events and potentially volatile situations. Routes should be decided either mentally or using a map before setting out. Maps or mobile devices should not be studied in the street as this broadcasts vulnerability.

Travelers should not wear expensive clothing or jewelry or carry expensive cameras or electronics. They should dress to blend in as much as possible, and definitely avoid clothing that declares their nationality or any indication of local or global political beliefs. Travelers should always carry either a mobile phone or whatever phone cards or coins are needed to operate a public telephone.

Carry only the cash required for the outing. Anything more than a small amount should always be in a secure money belt or inside zippered pocket. Take only one credit or debit card at a time. Do not carry details of financial accounts with you. Familiarize yourself quickly with the local currency and the appearance of the banknotes or coins: substitution using worthless notes or coins is always a risk.

Travelers should be constantly attentive to surroundings and be wary of any stranger who engages them in any form of conversation or touches their person in any way, no matter how accidental the contact may appear to be. Travelers should never accept any sort of food or drink from strangers on the street, in bars, or from taxi drivers: drugging is common in many places. Drinks should never be left unattended at the bar. While out on foot, travelers should always have one hand free to protect themselves and their valuables. Specific targets for thieves are shoulder bags, outside pouches of backpacks, and cameras that hang from straps. Valuables should be slung across the chest and preferably under a jacket or shirt, so that they are less accessible to thieves. Pants and jackets with zippered compartments inside major pockets can provide an extra level of protection against pickpockets. Valuables are best split into more than one location, especially if a passport or relatively large amounts of currency must be carried. Luggage or personal belongings should never be given to anyone who cannot be directly supervised or observed.

Even if the area is familiar, travelers need always use extra caution in tourist sites, market places, elevators, crowded subways, train stations, and at festivals. Isolated beaches should always be avoided, and even popular and safe beaches should be avoided after dark and in the early morning. Joggers are at risk of losing even shoes and clothing whose brand names may have high value in many countries. Curiosity is dangerous, and political gatherings and any sort of crowd should always be avoided, particularly in potentially unstable civil environments. Travelers should be aware of special dates and anniversaries on which any public place is best avoided.

Travelers should never withdraw money from ATMs or change money at a money-changing establishment after dark. Darkness makes it simple for potential assailants to observe discreetly from a relatively short distance. After obtaining cash, travelers should verify carefully that they are not being followed.

In any country, many criminals pose as willing sex partners. The set-up may entail a sex-for-hire scenario or may appear as a casual or accidental meeting in a hotel, bar, restaurant, or even on the street. Whether the liaison moves on to the traveler's hotel/apartment or a location of the criminal's choice carries an equal risk of a poor outcome. Potentially intimate encounters with host-country nationals should be avoided at all times. Travelers should avoid being intoxicated at night on the street, and taxis should be used even for short distances in this situation.

Long-stay travelers should be constantly alert to their immediate environment and make mental notes of the usual neighborhood and work environments. This makes anomalies, out-of-place persons, and suspicious situations more instantly obvious.

Taxis and Public Transport

The taxi situation varies greatly by country and the guidelines here will often need to be adapted to local conditions. In general, travelers should use only 'registered' taxis, but the guidelines for identifying these require local knowledge that must be ascertained upon arrival.

For day-to-day use, radio taxis are always the safest, although in many countries with a well-enforced system of registration, taxis found in marked ranks may be equally safe. Local colleagues can usually inform as to the phone numbers of reputable radio taxi operators. If it is possible to adequately communicate with the radio dispatcher when ordering the taxi, travelers should obtain the car number or license plate number of the taxi that has been dispatched. If the situation requires the taxi driver to ring up over an apartment block intercom, a pre-arranged recognition signal should be requested from the telephone dispatcher.

The fare should always be fixed before entering any taxi, even if sign language must be used. Travelers anticipating taxi travel should always have local money in small denominations, as change for large bills is never available even if it is on board. Taxis should never be shared with unknown passengers.

Hotels often have their own vehicles and drivers for hire. These are usually very overpriced but generally safe and reliable. However, travelers need to beware of hotel doormen who, when asked for a taxi, will put the traveler into a taxi operated by an accomplice who will at best just overcharge and at worst rob the traveler. Warning signs would include a taxi parked to a side away from a marked taxi line or rank, or a taxi apparently taken out of turn.

Public transportation, particularly if overcrowded, presents many safety risks that are detailed in Chapter 47. In addition, public vehicles present a situation where foreigners will both stand out and will be relatively stationary targets for a fixed period of time. Travelers should ride public transportation in pairs if possible. Thieves often work in pairs or groups, so travelers should avoid continuing to move in the direction of anyone that suddenly appears and is positioned in a way to be blocking the path forward. Gangs in crowded vehicles or trains may work to restrain arms while others search for valuables; wallets and belts under the clothes are most effective in these situations. Public transportation should be avoided late at night at all costs. Travelers should never sit in a train car that is otherwise empty of other passengers.

Car Travel

Travelers should never drive themselves or travel by private car at night in a foreign country, particularly in rural areas. Of all the recommendations in this chapter, this is the one that has the strongest support from the literature and by consensus of security experts. This has to do as much with crime avoidance as with the injury prevention issues covered elsewhere in this book. Local travel at night in the company of trusted and close colleagues may be unavoidable and is perhaps somewhat safer, but out of town travel even under these circumstances is still usually extremely dangerous. After an appropriate period of acclimatization, driving in a personal automobile at night to familiar local venues in non-high-risk neighborhoods can be considered, but this still represents some increase in the chance of being a victim of a crime.

Whether traveling locally or between cities by car in a destination country, efficient communications can greatly reduce exposure time and risk of attack in case of getting lost or breakdowns. Even if not carried on a day-to-day basis, a mobile telephone should be borrowed or leased for out of town travel.

Where appropriate, travelers should consider hiring a local driver who is familiar with the terrain, the road rules, and the driving customs, and has been personally recommended. This is especially important for remote areas and where language is an issue. The sobriety of the driver should be verified each time the car is entered. Because of prevailing wages in poorer countries, the cost of a car and driver is usually similar to the cost of renting the car itself. When renting a car or car and driver, travelers should avoid those with any sort of rental markings.

En route, car doors should be kept locked at all times and the windows should be kept closed as much as is feasible. In hot climates air-conditioned cars should be sought for this reason. As at home, travelers should not pick up hitchhikers. Travelers need to be alert at all times even as a passenger. Car-jacking and grab-and-run thefts happen when stopped at gas stations, parking lots, or in slow city traffic.

Learn Local Regulations Early

Travelers should make efforts to learn, in advance, the rules and regulations of the destination country. Procedures to follow when involved in a motor vehicle incident need to be known. Penalties for breaking the law can be surprisingly severe. An embassy can help ensure legal representation but cannot over-rule local laws. Some countries have a 'zero tolerance' policy, with severe penalties for those driving under the influence of alcohol or other drugs. Drug violations, firearms possession, photography of government or military installations, and antiques purchases are frequent causes of detention by local authorities.

Conclusion

All experts agree that travelers should give up valuables without a struggle once confronted. Money and passports can be replaced; human lives cannot.

References

1. Various authors. Operational Security Management in Violent Environments (Revised Edition). Good Practice Review 8. London: Overseas Development Institute; December 2010. <http://www.odihpn.org/report.asp?id=3159>
2. Generic Security Guide for Humanitarian Organizations. European Commission. *ec.europa.eu/echo/policies/evaluation/files-en/pdf-en/guide-en.pdf*; 2004.
3. Roberts DL. Staying Alive: safety and security guidelines for humanitarian volunteers in conflict areas. Geneva: ICRC; 2006. www.icrc.org

52

Post-Travel Screening

J. Clerinx, D. H. Hamer, and A. Van Gompel

Key points

- Medical history taking is the cornerstone of post-travel screening
- Asymptomatic short-term travelers rarely need a post-travel medical examination unless they have been exposed to a particular risk
- Long-term travelers, expatriates, and highly adventurous travelers need a thorough medical interview to assess potential exposures to a wide array of infections
- Minimal laboratory tests comprise a total blood count, WBC differential count, liver transaminases, blood urea nitrogen (BUN), and creatinine levels as well as serological markers according to type of exposure

Introduction

Many travel clinics provide pre-travel counseling as well as post-travel screening and care. Pre-travel screening focuses on preparation for residence in or travel to a different physical environment, and on preventing common infectious diseases by means of vaccination, chemoprophylaxis, self-treatment, and behavioral counseling. During the post-travel screening of asymptomatic travelers, the physician estimates the risk of having acquired occult travel-related infections, both tropical and cosmopolitan, and their potential impact on the traveler's health.[1] Additionally, older long-term travelers and expatriates may benefit most from an assessment of common non-infectious conditions such as cardiovascular disease, neoplasia and complications of trauma. For those intending to travel again in the future, the post-travel consultation offers an ideal opportunity to provide advice on personal precautions, and to review immunization status and chemoprophylaxis.

The medical history – the cornerstone of the post-travel screening process – focuses on infectious diseases transmitted by various routes.[2,3] Laboratory tests, although indispensable, are often insensitive and non-specific and may not be available for diagnosis of latent conditions in their preclinical stage (e.g., malaria). Qualitative diagnostic tests are useful to detect infection, but (semi)quantitative tests are essential to determine the 'parasite load'. This is important for malaria, schistosomiasis, and some filarial infections.

The cost–benefit analysis of post-travel screening activities in asymptomatic travelers is questionable. Post-travel screening by itself will hardly have an impact on morbidity or mortality. Its effect on health status is probably comparable with health check-ups for cardiovascular and neoplastic diseases, and with the periodic medical examinations in occupational medicine.[1,4] Relying too heavily on laboratory results alone leads quite often to control visits to test the validity of the results, rather than focusing on morbidity. One may rightly question the cost-effectiveness of investigating too thoroughly, especially for infections whose associated morbidity is minimal.[5]

Who and When to Screen?

A post-travel medical examination is not required for all travelers. Potential benefits can be assessed according to demographic factors (age, gender, socioeconomic status), travel characteristics (duration, destination), and specific disease exposure. Immigrants, refugees, and adopted children from tropical countries constitute a particular subgroup that is not specifically dealt with in this chapter. Moreover, this category of travelers often visits friends and relatives in their country of origin ('VFRs'), but only rarely consults for post-travel screening if asymptomatic.[6]

Travelers should be advised to have a medical examination on their return if they:

- suffer from a chronic disease, such as cardiovascular disease, diabetes mellitus, chronic respiratory disease, or autoimmune disorders
- have acquired immunosuppression, either through HIV infection or medically induced
- experience illness within 3 months after returning, particularly if fever, persistent diarrhea, nausea, vomiting, weight loss, jaundice, urinary disorders, skin disease, or genital infection occurs
- consider that they have been exposed to a potentially severe infectious disease while traveling
- have spent >3 months in a developing country.

A medical examination is therefore advisable after a long stay in the tropics and for travelers with a chronic disease. It is not necessary for asymptomatic short-term travelers who had only minor health problems such as travelers' diarrhea or transient fever. To be useful, a post-travel examination has to be able to rule out, rather than confirm, a latent (subclinical) disease. This requires knowledge of the

DOI: 10.1016/B978-1-4557-1076-8.00052-1

incubation period of suspected infectious diseases and awareness of the shortcomings of many laboratory procedures to detect correctly indolent but still active infections.

Probing for exposure to infection may be concise and limited to food- and water-borne contamination, arthropod exposure, fresh water contact and sexual contacts. Screening for sexually transmitted infections (STI) deserves special consideration. Rapid diagnosis may prevent further spread, often of emerging multiresistant strains.[7]

There is still some uncertainty about when to conduct a post-travel medical examination. Infections with a long incubation period may be overlooked if the screening process is carried out soon after exposure. Therefore, a medical visit up to 3 months later may be required in order to avoid missing infections with a potential community health impact, such as tuberculosis (TB) or HIV. The traveler must be informed about disease manifestations that may occur at a much later stage (e.g., benign tertian malaria). Meanwhile travelers should have urgent access to specialized medical care, especially when fever may herald the onset of diseases with potentially severe consequences, such as malaria, amebic liver abscess, acute schistosomiasis (Katayama fever), or acute HIV seroconversion.

Targeted Populations

Asymptomatic Short-Term Traveler

Asymptomatic short-term travelers, whether tourists or professionals, rarely need medical post-travel screening, as long as they have been aware of the health risks and do not report a particularly hazardous exposure. This assumes that travelers have been correctly instructed before traveling.

Routine post-travel screening is probably redundant in short-term travelers who had a self-limiting illness. It can be restricted to individuals with chronic underlying medical conditions.

For some professional corporate travelers, a post-travel screening procedure constitutes an integral part of the (often compulsory) periodic medical evaluation in occupational medicine.

Asymptomatic Long-Term Traveler or Expatriate

This group benefits from a more thorough medical interview to assess exposure to a wide array of chronic subpatent infections: air-borne diseases (tuberculosis), arthropod-borne diseases (e.g., malaria, filariasis, and trypanosomiasis), water-borne infections (schistosomiasis), soil-transmitted helminths (strongyloidiasis, hookworm, and other intestinal helminths), food-borne parasites (amebiasis, giardiasis, intestinal helminths), and some STIs. If a specific exposure is identified, one has to estimate the risk of being infected and/or of the infective load incurred.

Expatriates and long-term travelers should have a general health assessment for more common medical problems, as these services are often lacking in the country of residence. This includes cardiovascular disorders, hypertension, and diabetes mellitus, and preventive screening for malignancies including prostate, breast and colon cancer, according to national guidelines or practices.

Asymptomatic Adventurous Traveler

Adventurous travelers frequently adopt lifestyles similar to those of the indigenous peoples in the countries visited, and hence present a greatly increased risk for unusual infections. Eating raw meat and fish, undercooked food, exotic foods such as reptiles, or unpasteurized diary products or drinking unpurified water, are potential sources of infections such as anisakiasis, gnathostomiasis, paragonimiasis, trichinosis, sarcocystosis, brucellosis, and porocephalosis.

Exposure to specific biotopes, such as contact with fresh water while bathing or swimming in lakes, ponds, or rivers, or when wading through flooded areas (schistosomiasis, leptospirosis), bat-infested caves (histoplasmosis: rare, but specific high-risk environment), game parks infested with tsetse flies (East African trypanosomiasis: very rare, but serious mortality risk), walking safaris (African tick-bite fever, frequent but benign), equatorial forests (loiasis and onchocerciasis in west and central Africa: occasional), and marine environment (stings or bites of fish, mollusks, coelenterates, and contact with coral reefs: tissue inflammation and necrosis, neurotoxic poisoning, streptococcal and mycobacterial infections) may cause specific disease manifestations.

Travelers with Self-Identified Risk Factors and/or Disease Symptoms during Travel

This group of travelers frequently consult because they may be worried about the outcome or seek to have confirmed a diagnosis established elsewhere, or want proof of a complete cure. For frequent travelers, the physician can provide information on important disease manifestations and presumptive treatment strategies associated with a particular exposure. Some travelers are mistakenly convinced that a previous disease episode makes them more susceptible to re-infection, e.g., with malaria or amebic disease, or may be unduly worried about complications when re-infected during future travel, e.g., after a first dengue episode. Fear of contaminating others is another incentive to consult. This applies to certain occupations where air-borne contamination (TB), fecal–oral transmission (salmonellosis), or direct skin contact (scabies) with vulnerable groups of people may occur (elderly, institutions for mentally retarded, immunocompromised patients, food industry, etc.), and to STIs.

Post-travel screening thus provides an opportunity to establish a definite retrospective diagnosis, to confirm complete cure, and to provide information about the consequences regarding transmission and future travel.

General Screening

Medical Interview

A medical interview by an experienced physician is the cornerstone of the post-travel screening process. It identifies exposure to specific infections and estimates the magnitude of risk. Risk perception in travelers often differs considerably from what health professionals perceive.

For a correct travel risk assessment in asymptomatic travelers, the questions must include a basic set of standard items (Tables 52.1–52.3). Using a concise intake questionnaire on a printed form will speed up the general risk assessment. This will ultimately steer clinical examination, paraclinical investigations, and counseling.

Physical Examination

In asymptomatic travelers a physical examination is usually of limited value. However, unsuspecting individuals may present with lymphadenopathy, splenomegaly, hypertension, cardiopulmonary dysfunction, or a skin disorder that may require attention. If medical history reveals a specific complaint, carrying out a physical examination often yields useful information and reassures patient and physician alike. The extent of examination should be guided by the nature of the ailment.

General Paraclinical Tests

General Laboratory Tests

A basic set of tests comprises a total blood count, a WBC differential count, determination of liver transaminases, BUN, creatinine, and

Table 52.1 Self-Administered Questionnaire in Post-Travel Screening

Demographic Factors	Age, Gender
Travel characteristics	Destination, duration of stay and date of return
Vaccinations	(Note down year of last dose) Polio, diphtheria, tetanus Hepatitis A and B Yellow fever Typhoid fever Meningococcal meningitis type A, C, W and Y Japanese encephalitis Other (rabies, tick-borne encephalitis)
Malaria chemoprophylaxis	Drug scheme used and duration of intake

Table 52.2 Interactive Post-Travel Screening Questionnaire

Basic medical information	Weight change, tobacco, alcohol and psychotropic drug use, concomitant medication
Travel intentions	Holiday, professional travel, visiting friends and relatives (VFR), adventure sports, etc.
Physical environment	Destination, duration, transport means, travel route, type of accommodation, altitude
Specific environment	Freshwater contact (rivers, lakes, flooded areas), caves, marine environment, forests, game parks, etc.
Food intake habits	Exposure to raw meat and fish, undercooked food, unusual ingredients, unpurified water, unpasteurized dairy products
Previous disease history	Chronic diseases and allergic conditions (asthma, eczema, urticaria), potentially interfering with screening procedures
Malaria protection	Physical protection, type of anti-malaria drugs, dosage, and duration of intake
STD risk	Protective measures, contact with risk groups
Blood-borne risks	IVDU, needle-prick accidents, trauma, blood transfusion
Diseases during travel	Febrile, intestinal and skin diseases, STDs

Table 52.3 Specific Exposure Risks for Tropical Infectious Diseases

Physical Environment (Exposure)	Disease Risk
Urban environment	Dengue[b,c]
Fresh water contact (swimming, wading, rafting)	Schistosomiasis Leptospirosis
Estuaries, rivers (borders)	Soil-transmitted helminths Onchocerciasis Leptospirosis Cutaneous larva migrans West-African sleeping sickness[a]
Tropical forests	Filariasis (blood) Viral hemorrhagic fevers
Caves, speleology	Histoplasmosis
African game parks (tsetse infested)	East-African sleeping sickness[a]
Tropical grassland (walking safaris)	Tick bite fever[a] Tsutsugamushi fever[c]

[a]Africa.
[b]Central and South America.
[c]SE Asia.

Blood Eosinophil Count

This screening test is a pivotal parameter to suspect active parasitic infection, especially with nematodes or trematodes, but not with cestodes. Eosinophilia is more marked when blood or tissue migration occurs, as in strongyloidiasis, schistosomiasis, blood filariasis and intestinal helminths (*Ascaris*, hookworm), but less so in lymphatic filariasis.

However, in most individuals harboring subclinical helminth infections the eosinophil count is normal.[8] A low cut-off level (500 eosinophils/mm^3) considerably reduces its specificity as a screening marker for helminth infection.[5] Its predictive value is greater in travelers with particularly high eosinophil counts (absolute count >1000/mm^3), suggesting that further etiologic work-up should be restricted to this subpopulation. Likewise, extremely high levels of IgE in long-term travelers or expatriates may suggest a past or present helminthic infection, and do not merely reflect an allergic constitution.

Abdominal Ultrasound

At present ultrasound may only be considered as a secondary diagnostic procedure in asymptomatic travelers presenting with abnormal liver and urinary tract function tests, or as part of a screening strategy for prostate disorders in the elderly. The latter applies specifically to long-term expatriates and missionaries without access to quality healthcare in their country of residence.

Resting Electrocardiogram (ECG)

A resting ECG can help identify individuals with the 'long QT' syndrome, who are at risk for a specific malignant ventricular tachycardia ('torsade de pointes') when treated with drugs that promote QT prolongation. Lumefantrine, part of the fixed antimalarial combination artemether-lumefantrine (Riamet and Coartem) (AL), is structurally related to halofantrine, an antimalarial that causes QT prolongation. Although lumefantrine is not associated with measurable QT prolongation in currently recommended dosages, caution is warranted in persons with long QT syndrome, or if AL is used in association with other drugs causing QT prolongation.

C-reactive protein (CRP). These tests provide essential information on infection, systemic inflammation, liver and kidney function.

Urinalysis, including urine microscopy and proteinuria, is essential when urinary schistosomiasis is suspected, but will usually fail to detect light infections, as is often the case in travelers. It does not necessarily yield reliable information on renal disease, bladder cancer, or urinary tract infection in asymptomatic persons.

Determining fasting blood glucose levels and blood lipids as a marker for diabetes and cardiovascular disease risk is optional, but certainly recommended as part of a general health screening in long-term expatriates.

Specific Screening Tests

The main objective of these tests is to provide information on occult infection with TB, STIs, hepatitis, and both intestinal and extraintestinal parasitic diseases (Table 52.4).

Screening for Latent Tuberculosis

Infection with TB usually happens in a confined space protected from sunlight and air flow, when one inhales infected droplets from an index case with active pulmonary TB. In contrast, the risk of infection outdoors is comparatively negligible. Risk will thus be minimal in short-term travelers, but increases substantially in long-term travelers and expatriates. The TB incidence rate in the latter is comparable to that of the indigenous population, and was estimated at 2.8 per 1000 person-months in a Dutch study, a >100-fold increase in baseline risk. Nevertheless, at 0.6/1000 person-months, the risk remains relatively modest in absolute figures.[9] However, healthcare workers are at much higher risk (7.9 per 1000 person-months), rendering strict follow-up with tuberculin reaction and chest X-ray before and after exposure a highly recommended option.

Whether screening for latent TB should be performed in all long-term travelers and residents in the tropics is debatable. The American Thoracic Society advocates tuberculin testing only for persons likely to have been recently infected, particularly those who have been in close contact with a known infectious case. Although post-exposure prophylaxis averts progression to active disease in most cases, detection and treatment of clinically apparent TB is currently the most cost-effective strategy.[10]

Chest X-ray

Routine chest X-ray is both non-specific and insensitive in detecting latent TB. In industrialized countries with low levels of TB endemicity, mass chest X-ray as a means of controlling TB have long been abandoned. Consequently, a chest X-ray cannot be recommended as a routine screening procedure for TB in asymptomatic travelers. If considered, it should be restricted to expatriates or adventurous travelers with a positive tuberculin reaction, especially if there has been exposure to a known or strongly suspected pulmonary TB index case in the household or at the workplace.

Tuberculin Skin Testing (TST) and Interferon-γ Release Assay (IGRA)

TST (skin reaction after intradermal injection of 1–5 IU PPD) is the preferred option to detect latent TB infection. A conversion from a negative skin reaction before travel to positive after return is definite proof of recent infection. The tuberculin reaction turns positive typically 6 weeks after TB exposure, but conversion can take longer, sometimes up to 4 months.

As a diagnostic test, the TST requires reading and interpretation within a 72-hour interval, necessitating two visits. Indeterminate reactions frequently occur. The intradermal injection and reading the reaction must be performed correctly by experienced personnel to avoid false-negative results. TST is less sensitive in pregnancy, old age, diabetes, corticosteroid treatment, and unreliable in immunodeficient individuals. BCG (Bacille Calmette–Guérin) vaccination during childhood usually results in a positive skin test for many years afterwards.

The recently developed IGRAs specifically detect infection with *M. tuberculosis*. These are unresponsive in persons vaccinated with BCG or infected with non-tuberculous mycobacteria. IGRAs have an internal positive control that produces less indeterminate results. There is no need for a follow-up visit. Although promising as an alternative to TST, IGRAs share similar limitations: they do not discriminate between latent and active TB, nor between recent, past, or treated TB, and sensitivity is impaired in immunodeficient persons. On the other hand, previous TST has no impact on IGRA results. So far, performance is best in targeted populations with a relatively high risk of TB exposure.[11] Its specific role in post-travel screening has yet to be defined.

Sexually Transmitted Infections (STIs)

Travelers have a surprisingly high rate (5–50%) of unprotected sexual contacts with new partners, primarily with persons from the countries visited.[12] STIs have become a pivotal part of post-travel screening, largely due to the HIV pandemic. Therefore, counseling on sexual practices and STI risk must be reinforced during post-travel screening. For travelers running an occupational or recreational risk for HIV infection, the modalities of post-exposure antiretroviral prophylaxis should be discussed prior to travel.

Screening for STIs serves a dual purpose: limiting secondary transmission through prevention and treatment, and reassuring the asymptomatic traveler. It should involve detection of HIV, syphilis, gonorrhea and chlamydia, genital herpes, and condylomata. HIV and syphilis are conveniently detected by serum detection methods. On the other hand, screening for gonorrhea and chlamydia involves sampling of the urethra and/or cervix by means of either bacterial culture, antigen tests or polymerase chain reaction (PCR), or indirectly from the detection of an abnormal number of white blood cells in a first pass of urine. Direct sampling may be unacceptable to asymptomatic patients, particularly women, and may be reserved for travelers engaging in high-risk sexual behavior, i.e., frequent unprotected sex with multiple partners.[12]

Screening for HIV may prevent further transmission and may improve personal infection management, though the potential benefit of antiretroviral treatment soon after HIV seroconversion remains undetermined. The current combined HIV antigen (p24 or PCR detection) and antibody assays are highly specific and sensitive, even in recent infection. It allows reliable screening of any traveler with a history of sexual contact with a new partner within a time lapse of 3 weeks to 3 months after exposure.[13] In syphilis, seroconversion (VDRL or RPR) may take some time after disappearance of the primary chancre, which may go totally unnoticed, and must be repeated if suspected. Therefore, in asymptomatic travelers with a low-risk profile, STI screening may be preferentially conducted 3 months after exposure.

To prevent transmission of STDs during the period before seroconversion, safe sexual practices, primarily through condom use, are strongly recommended.

Screening for HIV and syphilis, but also for hepatitis B and C, and for American trypanosomiasis (Chagas' disease) may be indicated for recipients of blood transfusions in developing countries where blood screening procedures are often less complete and reliable. During the incubation period, blood recipients need to adopt safe sexual practices.

Viral Hepatitis

Hepatitis B, which may be considered an STI and/or a tropical infection, has its place in post-travel screening. The prevalence of chronic active hepatitis B in many populations from developing countries is high even though infection is often asymptomatic. Vaccination offers satisfactory protection in most people. In unvaccinated travelers who

Table 52.4 Diagnosis of Exposure to Common Travel-Related Infections

Infection	Incubation Period	Diagnostic Procedure	Use of Test	Time Lapse After Which Asymptomatic Infection Becomes Very Unlikely
Amebiasis	1 day–>6 months	Stool microscopy Stool antigen test[a] Serum antibody test[a]	Infection E.histolytica/E.disar Infection (E. histolytica) tissue invasion E.histolytica	6 months, but may be longer, even years
Malaria (P. falciparum)	9–35 days	Thick film, antigen test Serum antibody test[a]	Active infection/disease Postinfection confirmation Chronic suppressed infection	Non-immunes: 3 months Semi-immunes: 4 years
Malaria (benign tertian-quartan)	10 days–>1 year	Thick film, (antigen test) Serum antibody test[a]	Active infection/disease Postinfection confirmation	Benign tertian: 2–4 years Quartan: >10 years
Typhoid	7–45 days[a]	Blood culture Stool, urine culture[a] Serum antibody test (Widal)	Active disease Convalescent carrier state Postinfection (controversial, not reliable)	2 months
Tuberculosis	>30 days	Tuberculin test[a]	Asymptomatic infection Active infection/disease	2–4 months N/a – risk lifelong
Schistosomiasis	21–>60 days	Serum antibody tests[a] Microscopy stools, urine[a] Microscopy rectal snips[a] Antigen in stool, urine[a]	Asymptomatic infection Katayama syndrome Active infection/disease	3–6 months, exceptionally longer
Intestinal helminths	3–>60 days	Stool microscopy[a]	Active infection	2 months
Filariasis (bancroftian)	?–>1 year	Serum antibody tests[a] Serum antigen test[a] (Nocturnal) microfilaremia	Exposure Active infection Active infection	Up to 2 years
Filariasis (onchocercosis)	3–>15 months	Serum antibody tests[a] Cutaneous, ocular microfilaria[a]	Exposure (low sensitivity) Active infection	Up to 2 years
Filariasis (loiasis)	?–>12 months	Serum antibody tests[a] Microfilaremia	Exposure Active infection	Up to 2 years
Strongyloidiasis	7–>21 days	Serum antibody tests[a] Stool microscopy (concentration)[a]	Exposure, active infection Active infection	1 month
HIV	14–>90 days	Serum antigen/antibody test (HIV-ELISA)[a] HIV-WB[a]	Active infection: screening Active infection: confirmation	3–6 months
Syphilis	9–>90 days	RPR and VDRL[a] TPHA, FTA[a]	Active infection Confirmation Postexposure, post-treatment	3 months
Hepatitis B	1–6 months	Serum antibody tests[a]	Active or latent infection/disease	6 months
Hepatitis C	2 weeks–6 months	Serum antibody tests[a]	Active or latent infection/disease	6 months
Trypanosoma gambiense	>14 days	Serum antibody test	Active infection	Up to several months or even years
Trypanosoma cruzi (Chagas' disease)	5–14 days	Serum antibody test	Latent or active infection	To be followed-up serologically until 6 months after possible exposure
Visceral leishmaniasis	2–6 months	Serum antibody test	Active infection	Up to several months or even years

[a]Useful in asymptomatic travelers.

have been recently exposed to unprotected sex with a partner likely to be chronically infected with hepatitis B, or who have received injections or tattoos, testing for hepatitis B surface antigen will detect recent infection or carrier state. Testing for both hepatitis B surface and core antibodies provides information on past exposure and seroconversion, or on previous vaccination.

Screening for hepatitis A (HAV) still may be indicated for the non-vaccinated in view of future travel. Not all travelers are immunized, and few of the younger generation have been naturally infected.

Although hepatitis C prevalence is relatively high in some developing country populations, heterosexual practices do not play an important role in its transmission. Systematic screening of asymptomatic travelers is probably not cost-effective. Screening for hepatitis C could be restricted to travelers who have received blood products, with a history of IDU or with high-risk sexual behavior. It should also be part of the routine screening in travelers and expatriates involved in healthcare work.

Dengue

It is tempting to seek confirmation of a past dengue infection in asymptomatic travelers returning to an endemic area, to ascertain whether there is increased risk for hemorrhage and/or vascular collapse if re-infected. However, routine serology is not the best of tools to achieve that goal. Interference with other (flavi)virus vaccinations (yellow fever, Japanese encephalitis, tick bite encephalitis) or infections (West Nile virus) frequently produces false-positive test results. Dengue serological response wanes over time. It is noteworthy that in travelers, many dengue infections remain asymptomatic.

Parasitic Diseases

Although parasitic infections other than malaria in travelers are not rare, only a handful are relatively common and may cause potentially serious morbidity: schistosomiasis, strongyloidiasis, and invasive amebiasis.[14]

Schistosomiasis

Infection with human schistosomes has to be suspected in any traveler who has been in contact with potentially infected fresh water in endemic regions, primarily in sub-Saharan Africa. This includes swimming, bathing, or wading in rivers, lakes, ponds, or irrigated wet rice fields, but also wading through seasonally flooded areas with runoffs from contaminated freshwater sources. Even when parasite burden is light, schistosome infection may sometimes cause severe neurological impairment, most notably transverse myelitis following embolization of schistosomal eggs or adult worms in the spinal cord.[15]

The first stage of infection usually passes unnoticed, though a pruriginopapulous rash ('swimmer's itch') can sometimes appear soon after infection. Primary infection with all human schistosome species may cause a febrile hypersensitivity reaction with fever, cough, and/or abdominal pain when schistosomules mature to adults and start producing eggs – the so-called 'Katayama syndrome'. There is marked hypereosinophilia during the active disease, and it occurs from 3 weeks to 3 months after infection. Schistosome antibodies do not appear until at least 2–8 weeks after the onset of the febrile episode, and it may take longer before schistosome eggs appear in stool or urine. Long-term residents in endemic regions rarely incur heavy parasite loads. Therefore, late-stage latent disease manifestations such as periportal liver fibrosis, extensive colitis (Schistosoma mansoni) or irreversible urinary tract lesions (S. haematobium) are hardly ever seen in this risk group.

Infection with S. haematobium causes a non-specific urinary tract inflammation involving the urether and bladder wall, sometimes associated with pseudopolyps and obstruction. This results in microscopic hematuria in the unsuspecting traveler. Urinary schistosomiasis is often a surprise diagnosis when patients undergo cystoscopy for suspicion of bladder malignancy.[16] Direct stool or urine microscopy lacks sensitivity to detect schistosome ova. Fecal and urine concentration methods greatly facilitate detection, even in light infections. The 'rectal snip' technique is even more sensitive and requires four to six superficial rectal biopsies, squeezed between microscopy slides, to observe at low magnification the characteristic eggs containing a viable miracidium, embedded in the mucosa.

In asymptomatic travelers, latent infection is routinely detected by schistosome antibody tests. Seroconversion usually occurs within 3 months, but may take up to 1 year. Antibody detection is both sensitive and specific, but does not provide information about the worm load. Antibody titers remain detectable many years after successful eradication. Molecular tests amplifying schistosome DNA are currently being developed as a diagnostic tool for use with feces and urine, but it is as yet unclear whether these assays are more sensitive than stool and urine microscopy. A serum PCR assay may be a useful early marker of infection. Further testing is required to assess its potential as a quantitative marker of parasite load in infected travelers.[15]

Strongyloidiasis

Strongyloidiasis may persist lifelong through its endogenous re-infection cycle and may produce a potentially lethal disseminated hyperinfection in patients on high-dose steroids or immunosuppressants, or in immunocompromised persons. Eosinophilia is often absent (20–60%) or only mildly elevated. Suspicion of infection should be high in patients with a history of intermittent itching with serpiginous urticaria ('larva currens'), hypereosinophilia, and/or a positive antibody test.[8]

In patients excreting rhabditidiform larvae, serologic assays are reported to be highly sensitive and specific, although not necessarily in asymptomatic carriers with negative stool tests. There is little cross-reactivity with other helminth species. Sensitivity of single stool microscopy after concentration for the detection of rhabditoid larvae is low. It increases markedly by repeating stool examinations (20–30% for a single examination and up to 100% after seven stool examinations). Specific concentration methods such as the 'Baermann' concentration or the S. stercoralis culture test are more sensitive, but are time-consuming and thus not cost-effective. As a screening test, detecting S. stercoralis antigen using an ELISA or by PCR offers a useful, more sensitive and specific alternative.

Invasive Amebiasis

Detection of amebic infection remains problematic. Amebic colitis and liver abscess are by far the most important clinical manifestations of invasive amebiasis, but infection may remain asymptomatic for many months.

Stool microscopy is not a reliable test for Entamoeba histolytica infection. The vast majority of asymptomatic amebic cyst passers in fact harbor the non-pathogenic E. dispar strain (>90%), indistinguishable by microscopy from the potentially invasive E. histolytica.[17] A PCR-DNA amplification test has been developed to differentiate both species in a stool sample, and this is currently the preferred diagnostic tool. PCR tests can be performed on both formalin-fixed and frozen stool samples.[18] Furthermore, E. histolytica coproantigen tests on a fresh stool sample have been developed for commercial use, with sensitivity and specificity exceeding 95% in patients with active amebic colitis.[17,18] Sensitivity may be considerably lower in asymptomatic cyst passers.

Serum antibody tests for *E. histolytica* have proven value in amebic liver abscess, and are more sensitive than serum amebic lectin antigen tests.[17] It is an unreliable marker for amebic colitis, and also for microinvasive infection in asymptomatic cyst carriers, because antibodies persist for many months and even years after eradication.

It is unclear whether treatment with non-absorbed 'contact' amebicides will suffice in asymptomatic *E. histolytica* carriers. A positive serum antibody test in an asymptomatic traveler probably indicates subclinical invasion and might warrant combination treatment with 'tissue' amebicides, whereas this may not readily apply in immigrants.

Neurocysticercosis

In asymptomatic travelers, testing with an enzyme-linked immuno-electrotransfer blot (EITB) assay with purified glycoprotein antigens for cysticercosis reveals the problems with screening. It is not yet clear whether a positive serological test is associated with active disease that may one day become symptomatic. Although a seroprevalence of 8.2% has been reported in Peace Corps volunteers in Madagascar, exploring seropositive asymptomatic travelers thoroughly may be an expensive exercise that may create more anxiety than tangible benefits.[19]

Other Intestinal Parasites

Other intestinal nematode infections (*Ascaris lumbricoides*, *Trichuris trichiura*, hookworm) rarely achieve parasite burdens that lead to significant symptoms in chronically infected adult travelers and expatriates, with the exception of the occasional aberrant migration of adult ascarids into the biliary or pancreactic ducts.[20] Occasionally peptic ulcer-like symptoms may appear, even in light infections.

In asymptomatic travelers, microscopy of a single stool sample subjected to a concentration method for ova and cysts is sufficiently sensitive to detect the majority of clinically significant nematode infections (*A. lumbricoides*, *T. trichiura*, *A. duodenale*, *N. americanus*) and pathogenic intestinal protozoa, but is insufficient for *S. stercoralis* (see above).

In asymptomatic travelers *Giardia lamblia* is the most common intestinal protozoon. It can be reliably detected by means of microscopy of a single concentrated stool sample stained with Lugol.[21] Occasionally, *Isospora belli*, *Cyclospora cayetanensis*, and rarely, *Cryptosporidium* spp. are found in stools of asymptomatic travelers. The latter requires specific staining methods. A growing array of coproantigen tests has been introduced in recent decades. Currently available antigen tests for *G. lamblia* and *Cryptosporidium* spp. perform at least as well as microscopy, and are less time-consuming. Likewise, PCR tests that amplify the DNA of several intestinal nematodes and protozoa in fecal samples are under development. Real-time PCR tests, using DNA probes to a panel of chosen parasites ('multiplex PCR'), may be interesting alternatives because of their excellent sensitivity and specificity.[22] Because of the costs involved, it would be advisable to restrict coproantigen screening to the 'big five' intestinal parasites (hookworm, *S. stercoralis*, *Schistosoma* spp., *E. histolytica*, and *G. lamblia*).

Infections with Blood- or Tissue-Dwelling Parasites

For many parasitic diseases, serum antibody tests still provide the main diagnostic screening tool to detect exposure or latent infection in asymptomatic travelers. Most techniques currently used are based on an ELISA or immunofluorescent antibody assay.

The tests are relatively easy to standardize and to perform, and therefore quite convenient, but sensitivity or specificity are often uncertain in asymptomatic or light infections. Serum antibody tests do not provide information on parasite activity nor on parasite burden, and antibody response may persist many years after exposure and curative treatment (e.g., in schistosomiasis and amebiasis). Whether molecular PCR-based tests might supplant the current antibody tests depends on the specific diagnostic aim for each parasite.

Malaria

Many travelers who have been treated for malaria during travel are anxious to have the diagnosis confirmed. Malaria antibody response against the blood-stage parasites persists for at least 2 months after treatment, and may be of use in the retrospective diagnosis of malaria in non-immune travelers.[23] Extensive cross-reactivity between malaria species exists. A negative *P. falciparum* antibody titer practically rules out malaria in travelers who have reported several febrile episodes.

Malaria antigen tests targeting histidine-rich protein-2, which is specific for *P. falciparum*, can be used to confirm a recent infection in retrospect; a positive result may persist for more than 4 weeks after successful treatment. PCR tests using *Plasmodium* species-specific DNA probes are excellent to identify the incriminating species in an ongoing infection or in chronic asymptomatic semi-immune carriers.

Leishmaniasis

In visceral leishmaniasis the pre-patent period may be protracted. In the disease stage, antibody detection is both sensitive and specific. However, as antibody production depends on disease activity, serology is not able to reliably diagnose infection during the asymptomatic incubation period. PCR-based molecular detection techniques may have a role in assessing cryptic infection in immunocompromised patients.[24]

Filariasis

The risk of acquiring a filarial infection is very low in short-term travelers.[8,25] Onchocerciasis, lymphatic filariasis, and loiasis are nearly exclusively seen in immigrants and long-term expatriates. Occasionally, relatively mild symptoms may occur periodically in loiasis (Calabar swellings, superficial ocular migration) and in onchocercosis (itching) a long time after exposure.

In asymptomatic travelers, antibody tests using *Dirofilaria immitis* antigens as a substrate are the first-line procedure to detect filarial infection. Sensitivity is high for loiasis and lymphatic filariasis but low in onchocerciasis. Specific antibody tests are not available for routine use, and lack sensitivity.

Blood microfilaria may sometimes be found in a 'thick film' from unsuspecting travelers infected with *Mansonella perstans*, and occasionally in those with *Loa loa*. Case reports of lymphatic filariasis in asymptomatic travelers are scarce. Detection requires either microfilaria concentration techniques or provocation tests (DEC-test). Nighttime sampling for microfilaria in bancroftian filariasis (*Wuchereria bancrofti*) has been largely supplanted by filarial antigen detection using monoclonal antibodies.

Diagnosis of cutaneous filariasis with *Onchocerca volvulus* requires detection of microfilaria in skin snips or in exudate from superficial scarifications of the affected skin. Ophthalmologic examination of the cornea and the anterior chamber may reveal microfilaria, or its characteristic corneal lesions (punctate keratitis).

Recently developed PCR-based diagnostic tests may supplant blood concentration techniques in microfilaremic disease, and are more sensitive than skin snip microscopy in onchocerciasis. Expert advice should be sought for further species differentiation in case filarial antibody tests are found to be positive, as treatment differs according to species.

Trypanosomiasis

Serological screening for American trypanosomiasis (*T. cruzi*) and West African trypanosomiasis (*T. gambiense*) should be restricted to adventurous travelers and immigrants exposed to triatomid bugs in poor housing facilities in endemic areas of South America, or to the occasional long-term resident and missionary in Africa who reports tsetse fly exposure in areas known for intense transmission. Infection may go unnoticed in most individuals infected with *T. cruzi*, and may not be suspected in persons infected with West African trypanosomiasis. In contrast, East African trypanosomiasis (*T. rhodesiense*) has a short incubation period (<14 days) and always starts off as an acute febrile disease with detectable parasitemia.

Serological tests are highly sensitive and may therefore be an ideal tool to exclude infection. No firmly established guidelines are available to determine how often and when a screening test has to be conducted. Expert advice should be sought for further work-up in case serology is found positive.

Conclusions

Although probably not cost-effective in terms of morbidity reduction, post-travel screening in asymptomatic travelers is popular and widely practiced. A careful itinerary-specific history with detailed questioning about potential risky exposures, ranging from food, water, and human contact, is the cornerstone of the post-travel evaluation. A concise physical examination focused on specific signs and symptoms, and a selected array of laboratory tests is helpful to detect subclinical infections and assert the immune status against common pathogens. Its main benefit may lie in its preventive counseling potential with respect to future travel.

References

1. McLean JD, Libman M. Screening the returning travelers. Inf Dis Clin Trav Med 1998;12(2):431–43.
2. Whitty CJ, Carroll B, Armstrong M, et al. Utility of history, examination and laboratory tests in screening those returning to Europe from the tropics for parasitic infection. Trop Med Int Health 2000;5(11):818–23.
3. Carroll B, Dow C, Snashall D, et al. Post-tropical screening: how useful is it? BMJ 1993;307(6903):541.
4. Carlos Franco-Paredes. Asymptomatic Post-Travel Screening. In: http://wwwnc.cdc.gov/travel/yellowbook/2012/chapter-5-post-travel-evaluation/asymptomatic-post-travel-screening.htm
5. Wintour K, Jones ME. Routine Medical Evaluation of Expatriate Volunteers – Retrospective Analysis of 613 Patients. 7th Conference of the International Society of Travel Medicine (CISTM7), Innsbruck, 27–31 May 2001: Abstract FC09.03
6. WHO. International Travel and Health. Geneva 2005. Yearly update: www.who.int/ith.
7. Jakopanec I, Borgen K, Aavitsland P. The epidemiology of gonorrhoea in Norway, 1993–2007: past victories, future challenges. BMC Infect Dis 2009;9:33.
8. Baaten GG, Sonder GJ, van Gool T, et al. Travel-related schistosomiasis, strongyloidiasis, filariasis, and toxocariasis: the risk of infection and the diagnostic relevance of blood eosinophilia. BMC Infect Dis 2011;11:84.
9. Cobelens FG, Deutekom H van, Draayer-Jansen IW, et al. Risk of infection with *Mycobacterium tuberculosis* in travelers to areas of high tuberculosis endemicity. Lancet 2000;356(9228):461–5.
10. Rieder HL. Risk of travel-associated tuberculosis. Clin Infect Dis 2001;33(8):1393–6.
11. Guidelines for using the QuantiFERON-TB test for diagnosing latent *Mycobacterium tuberculosis* infection. Centers for Disease Control and Prevention. MMWR Recomm Rep 2003;52(RR-2):15–8.
12. Matteelli A, Carosi G. Sexually transmitted diseases in travelers. Clin Infect Dis 2001;32(7):1063–7.
13. Chang D, Learmonth K, Dax EM. HIV testing in 2006: issues and methods. Expert Rev Anti Infect Ther 2006;4(4):565–82.
14. Libman MD, MacLean D, Gyorkos TW. Screening for schistosomiasis, filariasis, and strongyloidiasis among expatriates returning from the tropics. Clin Infect Dis 1993;17:353–9.
15. Clerinx J, Van Gompel A. Schistosomiasis in travelers and migrants. Travel Med Infect Dis 2011;9:6–24.
16. Harries AD, Fryatt R, Walker J, et al. Schistosomiasis in expatriates returning to Britain from the tropics: a controlled study. Lancet 1986;86(i):86.
17. Tanyuksel M, Petri Jr WA. Laboratory diagnosis of amebiasis. Clin Microbiol Rev 2003;16(4):713–29.
18. Visser LG, Verweij JJ, Van Esbroeck M, et al. Diagnostic methods for differentiation of *Entamoeba histolytica* and *Entamoeba dispar* in carriers: performance and clinical implications in a non-endemic setting. 1. Int J Med Microbiol 2006;296:397–403.
19. Leuscher P, Andriantsimahavandy A. Cysticercosis in Peace Corps volunteers in Madagascar. N Engl J Med 2004;350:311–2.
20. Gilles HM. Soil-transmitted helminths. In: Cook GC, Zumla A, editors. Manson's Tropical Diseases. 21st edn. London: WB Saunders – Elsevier Science Ltd; 2003. p. 1527–60.
21. Farthing MJ, Cevallos AM, Kelly P. Intestinal protozoa. In: Cook GC, Zumla A, editors. Manson's Tropical Diseases. 21st edn. London: WB Saunders – Elsevier Science Ltd; 2003. p. 1373–410.
22. Taniuchi M, Verweij JJ, Noor Z, et al. High throughput multiplex PCR and probe-based detection with Luminex beads for seven intestinal parasites. Am J Trop Med Hyg 2011;84(2):332–7.
23. Jelinek T, Sonnenburg F von, Kumlien S, et al. Retrospective immunodiagnosis of malaria in nonimmune travelers returning from the tropics. J Travel Med 1995;2(4):225–8.
24. Colomba C, Saporito L, Vitale F, et al. Cryptic *Leishmania infantum* infection in Italian HIV infected patients. BMC Infect Dis 2009;9:199.
25. Lipner EM, Law MA, Barnett E, et al. Filariasis in travelers presenting to the GeoSentinel Surveillance Network. PLoS Negl Trop Dis 2007;1(3):e88.

53

Fever in Returned Travelers

Mary Elizabeth Wilson, Eli Schwartz, and Philippe Parola

Key points

- Predominant causes of fever vary by different geographic areas of exposure
- Malaria is the most common overall cause of systemic febrile illness in travelers returning from tropical areas; dengue is the most common cause in travelers to some regions
- The approach to a febrile patient must consider travel and exposure history, incubation period, mode of exposure, and impact of pre-travel vaccination
- Initial symptoms of self-limited and life-threatening infections may be similar; focal signs and symptoms can help to limit the differential diagnosis
- Routine laboratory results can provide clues to the final diagnosis

Introduction

Fever in a returned traveler demands prompt attention. While fever may be the manifestation of a self-limited, trivial infection, it can also presage an infection that could be rapidly progressive and lethal. International travel expands the list of infections that must be considered but does not eliminate common, cosmopolitan infections. Initial attention should focus most urgently on infections that are treatable, transmissible, and that cause serious sequelae or death.[1,2] The characteristics of the places visited and the recency of travel will affect the urgency and extent of the initial work-up. This chapter will focus on identifying the cause of fever in a returned traveler. The reader should refer to other sources for the specifics of therapy.

Epidemiology of Fever in Travelers

How Common is Fever in Returning Travelers?

Fever in the absence of other prominent findings has been reported in 2–3% of European and American travelers to developing countries. Among 784 American travelers who traveled for 3 months or less to developing countries, 3% reported fever unassociated with other illness.[3] These results are similar to those reported in classic studies by Steffen et al.[4] in which 152 of 7886 (almost 2%) of Swiss travelers

with short-term travel to developing countries reported 'high fevers over several days' on questionnaires completed several months after return. Of those with fever, 39% reported fever only while abroad, 37% had fevers while abroad and at home, and 24% had fevers at home only.

Analysis of the GeoSentinel surveillance network database found that 28% of ill returned travelers seeking care at a GeoSentinel clinic had fever as a chief reason for seeking care.[5] Among patients with travel-related hospitalization, febrile illnesses predominated, accounting for 77% of admissions in a study from Israel.[6]

Causes of Fever in Returned Travelers

Findings from eight studies, each with at least 100 cases, that examined causes of fever after tropical travel are shown in Table 53.1.[5–13] The geographic region of exposure helps to explain the marked differences in the relative likelihood of various diagnoses, as has been shown in a study by Freedman et al.[14] Malaria was the most common diagnosis among those requiring hospitalization for fever in most recently published series. In the GeoSentinel study 33% of the 12 deaths in febrile returned travelers were caused by malaria; in the study by Bottieau and colleagues[9] falciparum malaria was the only tropical disease that was fatal (n = 5). In the GeoSentinel study 17% of febrile illnesses were caused by infections that are preventable with vaccines or specific chemoprophylaxis (e.g., falciparum malaria). Common cosmopolitan infections were found in 34% of returned febrile travelers in the Bottieau study. Infections, such as respiratory tract infections, hepatitis, diarrheal illness, urinary tract infections and pharyngitis, with a broad or worldwide distribution, account for more than half of fevers in some series,[8] and the cause of fever remained undefined in about one-quarter of cases.[5,9,10] While, overall, malaria is the most common specific infection causing systemic febrile illness, dengue fever, mononucleosis, rickettsial infections, and enteric fever are also important infections. Their relative rank varies by geographic location, with dengue common after travel to Southeast Asia, enteric fever one of top three diagnoses after travel to South Central Asia, and rickettsial infections the second only to malaria after travel to sub-Saharan Africa. Leptospirosis is likely underrecognized because of difficulty in confirming the diagnosis in many laboratories. The major increase in chikungunya virus infections in Indian Ocean Islands and Asia has been reflected in an increase in cases in travelers to those regions (and even local spread of infection introduced by travelers in Europe).[15]

DOI: 10.1016/B978-1-4557-1076-8.00053-3

Table 53.1 Summary Data from Major Studies of Fever in Returned Travelers

Study	Patient Population (Location)	Most Common Specific Infections	Most Frequently Visited Regions
Wilson et al. 2007[5]	24 920 ill returned travelers, 6957 of whom had fever (Multicenter, Global)	Malaria (21%) Acute TD (15%) RTI (14%) Dengue (6%) Dermatologic illness (4%) Enteric fever (2%) Rickettsioses (2%) Acute UTI (2%) Acute hepatitis (1%)	Sub-Saharan Africa (37%) Southeast Asia (18%) Latin America / Caribbean (15%) South Central Asia (13%) North Africa (3%)
Bottieau et al. 2006[9]	1743 outpatients presenting with fever after tropical travel (Belgium)	Malaria (27.7%) RTI (10.5%) Bacterial enteritis (6.2%) Mononucleosis-like syndrome (3.9%) Skin/soft-tissue infection (3.6%) GU infection/STD (3.4%) Rickettsioses (3.3%) Dengue (3%)	Sub-Saharan Africa (68%) Southeast Asia (12%) Latin America (7%) Indian subcontinent (6%) North Africa (4%)
Doherty et al. 1995[10]	195 inpatients presenting with fever after tropical travel (United Kingdom)	Malaria (42%) Non-specific viral syndrome (25%) Dengue (6%) Bacterial dysentery (5%) RTI (4%) Hepatitis A (3%) UTI (2%) Typhoid (1.5%)	Sub-Saharan Africa (60%) Indian subcontinent (13%) Far East (8%) South America (3%) Europe (0.5%)
O'Brien et al. 2001[11]	232 inpatients admitted for management of fever after overseas travel (Australia)	Malaria (27%) RTI (24%) Gastroenteritis (14%) Dengue (8%) Typhoid (3%) Hepatitis A (3%) Rickettsioses (2%) Tropical Ulcer (2%)	Asia (61%) The Pacific (20%) Africa (15%) Latin America (2%)
Antinori et al. 2004[12]	147 inpatients admitted for fever after tropical travel (Italy)	Malaria (48%) Presumptive viral illness (12%) Viral hepatitis (9%) Gastroenteritis (5%) Schistosomiasis (5%) Typhoid (4%) Dengue (3%) RTI (3%) UTI (1%)	Africa (61%) Asia (22%) Central and South America (13%) Oceania (2%) Middle East (2%)
Parola et al. 2006[13]	613 inpatients admitted for fever after tropical travel (France)	Malaria (75%) RTI (4%) Food / water-borne infection (4%) Dengue (2%) Viral hepatitis (1%)	Indian Ocean (55%) West Africa (22%) Central Africa (9%) Southeast Asia (4%) Indian subcontinent (3%) North Africa (2%) Central America/Caribbean (0.5%)

Table 53.1 Summary Data from Major Studies of Fever in Returned Travelers—cont'd

Study	Patient Population (Location)	Most Common Specific Infections	Most Frequently Visited Regions
West and Riordan, 2003[8]	162 pediatric inpatients admitted with fever following travel to tropics and subtropics (United Kingdom)	Viral illness (34%) Diarrheal illness (27%) Malaria (14%) Pneumonia (8.5%) Hepatitis A (5%) UTI (4%) Enteric fever (3%)	Indian subcontinent (82%) Middle East (6%) Africa (4%) Southeast Asia (2%)
Siikamaki et al., 2011[7]	462 febrile adults returned from malaria-endemic area; emergency room of tertiary hospital; 54% hospitalized (Finland)	Diarrheal disease (27%) Systemic febrile illness (21%) [sepsis 3%; enteric fever and other bacteria 3.7%; dengue 3%; other viral including EBV and HIV 5%; rickettsiosis 1.3%] RTI (15%) UTI (4%) Other GI (3%)	Sub-Saharan Africa (42%) Southeast Asia (28%) Central Asia and Indian subcontinent (20%) South and Central America and Caribbean (6%) Other (6%) Unknown (1%)
Steinlauf et al. 2005[6]	211 inpatient adults after tropical travel, of whom 163 were febrile (Israel)	Malaria (33%) Dengue (17%) RTI (6%) Diarrhea (6%) Enteric fever (3%) Hepatitis (2%)	East Asia (48%) Sub-Saharan Africa (34%) Latin America (16%)

RTI, respiratory tract infection; TD, traveler's diarrhea; UTI, urinary tract infection; GU, genitourinary; STD, sexually transmitted disease.
Adapted from reference 2: Wilson M, Boggild A. Fever and systemic symptoms. In: Guerrant R, Walker D, Weller P, editors. Tropical Infectious Diseases: Principles, Pathogens and Practice. 3rd ed. Edinburgh: Saunders Elsevier; 2011. p. 925–38.

Differences Between Travelers and Local Residents

Important differences exist between short-term travelers to developing countries and residents or long-term visitors in the types of infection commonly seen and in clinical manifestations. These differences reflect differences in the likelihood of exposure to infections and the age and intensity of exposure. For example, melioidosis (caused by the Gram-negative soil- and water-associated bacterium *Burkholderia pseudomallei*) is a common cause of community-acquired sepsis in northern Thailand, yet is rarely seen in short-term travelers. In many developing countries hepatitis A is not viewed as an important problem. Clinical disease is largely unknown because most children are infected at a young age when infection is mild and often unrecognized. Older children and adults are immune, but the virus regularly contaminates food and water and poses a threat to non-immune travelers who enter the area. Katayama syndrome, an immunologically mediated disease, is seen in travelers and persons newly infected with schistosomiasis, but not in residents of endemic areas who have been repeatedly exposed to the parasite.[16]

Approach to the Patient with Fever

The Travel and Exposure History

The fever pattern and clinical findings for many infections are similar. A detailed history of where a person has lived and traveled (including intermediate stops and modes of travel), dates of travel and time since return, as well as activities during travel (such as types of accommodation, food habits, exposures, including sexual exposures, needle and blood exposures, animal and arthropod bites, water exposures), and vaccinations and other preparation before travel and prophylaxis or treatment during or after travel are essential in developing a list of what infections are possible based on potential exposures and usual incubation periods. Relevant exposures can also occur in transit, e.g., on an airplane flight or cruise ship.[17]

During the work-up the clinician should keep in mind that fever after exotic travel may reflect infection with a common, cosmopolitan pathogen acquired during travel or after return home. At the same time, it should be noted that unfamiliar infections can be acquired in industrialized countries (such as plague, Rocky Mountain spotted fever, tularemia, Lyme disease, and hantavirus pulmonary syndrome in North America, and visceral leishmaniasis, hemorrhagic fever with renal syndrome and other hantaviral infections, and tick-borne encephalitis in Europe).

A detailed review of the clinical course, supplemented by the physical examination and laboratory data, will help to determine more likely causes and also to identify any infections that might require urgent interventions, hence expedited diagnostic studies. The process involved in the evaluation can be summarized in the following questions:

- What diagnoses are possible based on the geographic areas visited?
- What diagnoses are possible based on the time of travel, taking into account incubation periods?
- What diagnoses are more likely based on activities, exposures, host factors, and clinical and laboratory findings?
- Among the possible diagnoses, what is treatable, transmissible, or both?

Table 53.2 Common Infections, by Incubation Periods

Disease	Usual Incubation Period (Range)	Distribution
Incubation <14 days		
Malaria, *P. falciparum*	6–30 days	Tropics, subtropics
Dengue	4–8 days (3–14 days)	Topics, subtropics
Chikungunya	2–4 days (1–14 days)	Tropics, subtropics (Eastern Hemisphere)
Spotted fever rickettsiae	Few days to 2–3 weeks	Causative species vary by region
Leptospirosis	7–12 days (2–26 days)	Widespread; most common in tropical areas
Enteric fever	7–18 days (3–60 days)	Especially in Indian subcontinent
Malaria, *P. vivax*	8–30 days (often >1 month to 1 year)	Widespread in tropics/subtropics
Influenza	1–3 days	Worldwide; can also be acquired en route
Acute HIV	10–28 days (10 days to 6 weeks)	Worldwide
Legionellosis	5–6 days (2–10 days)	Widespread
Encephalitis, arboviral (e.g., Japanese encephalitis, tick-borne encephalitis, West Nile virus, other)	3–14 days (1–20 days)	Specific agents vary by region
Incubation 14 days to 6 weeks		
Malaria, enteric fever, leptospirosis	See above incubation periods for relevant diseases	See above distribution for relevant diseases
Hepatitis A	28–30 days (15–50 days)	Most common in developing countries
Hepatitis E	26–42 days (2–9 weeks)	Widespread
Acute schistosomiasis (Katayama syndrome)	4–8 weeks	Most common after travel to sub-Saharan Africa
Amebic liver abscess	Weeks to months	Most common in developing countries
Incubation >6 weeks		
Malaria, amebic liver abscess, hepatitis E, hepatitis B	See above incubation periods for relevant diseases	See above distribution for relevant diseases
Tuberculosis	Primary, weeks; reactivation, years	Global distribution; rates and levels of resistance vary widely
Leishmaniasis, visceral	2–10 months (10 days to years)	Asia, Africa, S. America

Adapted from Centers for Disease Control and Prevention. CDC Health Information for International Travel 2012. New York: Oxford University Press; 2012.

Incubation Period

Incubation time is a valuable tool in evaluating a febrile patient. Knowledge of the incubation periods can allow one to exclude infections that are not biologically plausible. For example, dengue fever typically has an incubation of 3–14 days. Thus fever that begins more than 2 weeks after return from Thailand is not likely to be related to dengue fever. Remote travel is sometimes relevant, but most severe, acute life-threatening infections result from exposures that have occurred within the past 3 months. Important treatable infections that may occur more than 3 months after return include malaria, amebic liver abscess, and visceral leishmaniasis. In the study by O'Brien et al.[11] analyzing patients hospitalized with fever after travel, 96% were seen within 6 months of return from travel; in the study by Bottieau et al.[9] of patients referred for fever after tropical travel, fever occurred during travel or within1 month of return home in 78%. Although the initial focus should be on travel within the past 3–6 months, the history should extend to include exposures a year or more earlier, if the initial investigation is unrevealing. More than a third of malaria-infected travelers in a study from Israel and the USA had illness that developed more than 2 months after return from endemic areas.[18] Onset of illness more than 6 months after return occurred in 2.3% of malaria patients

reported to the CDC in 2009.[19] Table 53.2 lists many of the infections seen in travelers by time of onset of symptoms relative to the exposure and the initial clinical presentation. In assessing potential incubation period one must take into account the duration of the trip (and points of potential exposure during travel) and time since return.

Mode of Exposure

Infections that can be acquired by a single bite of an infective arthropod, ingestion of contaminated food or beverages, swimming in contaminated water, or from direct contact with an infected person or animal are most often seen in short-term travelers. Casual sexual contact with new partners is common in travelers (5–50% among short-term travelers) and inquiry about sexual exposures should be included as part of the history of an ill traveler. A Canadian study found that 15% of travelers reported sex with a new partner, or potential exposure to blood and body fluids through injections, dental work, tattoos, or other skin-perforating procedures during international travel.[20] This history is important to review even in returned travelers who are not acutely ill. In many instances travelers will be unaware of exposures. For example, patients with mosquito and tick-borne infections may not recall any bites. In contrast, patients who have had freshwater exposure (such as swimming, wading, bathing, or rafting) that places them at risk for schistosomiasis will typically recall the exposure with focused questioning, though they may have been unaware that the exposure carried any risk for infection. The provider should also inquire about medical care during travel. Travel for the purpose of seeking medical care (medical tourism) has expanded; travelers may undergo extensive surgery including cardiac surgery and organ transplantation overseas. In the course of medical care, patients may become colonized or infected with bacteria that are extremely resistant to usual antibiotic therapy, as has recently been reported with the New Delhi metallo-β-lactamase resistance mechanism,[21] or they may have other hospital-acquired infections.

Impact of Pre-Travel Vaccination

The history should include a review of pre-travel vaccines, including dates of vaccination, types of vaccines received, and number of doses for multidose vaccines. Vaccines vary greatly in efficacy, and knowledge of vaccine status can influence the probability that certain infections will be present. For example, hepatitis A and yellow fever vaccines have high efficacy and only rare instances of infection have been reported in vaccinated travelers. In contrast, the typhoid fever vaccines (oral and parenteral) give incomplete protection.[22] The protective efficacy with the available typhoid vaccines was estimated to be 60–72% in field trials in endemic regions.[23]

Clinical Presentations

Many febrile infections are associated with focal signs or symptoms, which may help to limit the differential diagnosis. Undifferentiated fever can be more challenging. The following sections discuss common clinical presentations, with focus on more common diseases causing each. Other chapters provide more detailed discussions of diarrhea, skin diseases, and respiratory diseases.

Undifferentiated Fever

Always Look for Malaria

Malaria remains the most important infection to consider in anyone with fever after visiting or living in a malarious area. In non-immune travelers falciparum malaria can be fatal if not diagnosed and treated urgently. Although most patients with malaria will report fever, as many as 40% or more may not have fever at the time of initial medical evaluation.[24] Risk of malaria varies greatly from one endemic region to another, but in general risk is highest in parts of sub-Saharan Africa; most severe and fatal cases in travelers follow exposure in this region. Tests to look for malaria should be done urgently (same day) and repeated in 8–24 h if the initial blood smears are negative. In recent years rapid diagnostic tests for malaria have become valuable tools for the diagnosis of malaria in both endemic and non-endemic areas.[25] Infected erythrocytes may be sequestered in the deep vasculature in patients with falciparum malaria, so few parasites may be seen on a blood smear even in a severely ill patient.

Prompt evaluation is most critical in persons who have visited areas with falciparum malaria in recent weeks. In the USA in 2009, 81% of reported patients with acute falciparum malaria had onset of symptoms within a month of return to the USA; another 15% had onset of illness before arriving in the USA.[19] Use of chemoprophylaxis may ameliorate symptoms or delay onset. No chemoprophylactic agent is 100% effective, so malaria tests should be done even in persons who report taking chemoprophylaxis. Many antimicrobials (e.g., TMP-SMX, azithromycin, doxycycline, clindamycin) have some activity against plasmodia. Taking these drugs for reasons unrelated to malaria may delay the onset of symptoms of malaria or modify the clinical course.

Although fever and headache are commonly reported in malaria, gastrointestinal and pulmonary symptoms may be prominent and may misdirect the initial attention toward other infections. Thrombocytopenia and absence of leukocytosis are common laboratory findings. A prospective study of 335 travelers and migrants with suspected malaria found WBC count <10 000 cells/L, platelet count < 150 000/μL, hemoglobin <12 g/dL and eosinophils <5% to be associated with malaria parasitemia.[26]

Dengue

Dengue, a mosquito-transmitted flavivirus that exists in four serotypes, is the most common arbovirus in the world. It is increasing in incidence in endemic areas and is an increasingly common cause of fever in returned travelers.[27,28] Dengue is found in tropical and subtropical regions throughout the world. Among travelers, dengue is seen most often in visitors to Southeast Asia and Latin America (including the Caribbean) and infrequently in travelers to Africa – though infections may be under-recognized.[29] Because humans are the main reservoir for the dengue virus, which is transmitted primarily by the *Aedes aegypti* mosquito that inhabits urban areas and lives in close association with humans, travelers visiting only urban areas can become infected. Symptoms of dengue, also known as breakbone fever, typically begin 4–7 days (range 3–14 days) after exposure. Common findings are fever, frontal headache, and myalgia. Approximately 50% of patients have skin findings, which can be a diffuse erythema or a maculopapular or petechial eruption. Intense itching may be present toward the end of the febrile period. Leukopenia, thrombocytopenia, and elevated transaminases are common laboratory findings. The most serious forms of infection – dengue hemorrhagic fever (DHF) and dengue shock syndrome (DSS) – in many studies have been observed more often in persons who have a second dengue infection with a different serotype. In a well-characterized outbreak in Cuba, 98.5% of DHF/DSS cases were in persons with a prior dengue infection. The attack rate of DHF/DSS was 4.2% in persons with prior dengue infection who became infected with a new serotype.[30] Other factors also influence the severity of disease, including virus serotype and genotype and genetics and age of the host. Severe and complicated infection can occur in travelers and has been observed in travelers with primary infection, as discussed in a recent review.[31]

Supportive care, including IV fluids, can be life-saving in severe dengue. Diagnosis is usually confirmed by serologic tests; viral isolation or detection of viral RNA by PCR is available in some laboratories. Because specific IgM antibodies take several days to develop (usually present by day 5 of illness), serologic diagnosis may not be possible in the early febrile period.[32] IgG antibody response can be difficult to interpret because of extensive cross-reactions with other flaviviruses (e.g., yellow fever, Japanese encephalitis, West Nile). In recent years, several diagnostic methods, including real-time RT-PCR and NS1 antigen detection, have been proposed to optimize the early diagnosis of DENV in travelers.[32] However, it is likely that only a minority of cases that occur in travelers are documented. A recent prospective study of Dutch travelers found that seroconversion to dengue virus occurred in 1.2% (incidence was 14.6 per 1000 person-months).[27] In the GeoSentinel database, confirmed or probable dengue fever was the most common specific diagnosis in patients with febrile systemic illness who had traveled to tropical and subtropical areas in the Caribbean, South America, south central and Southeast Asia.[14]

In 2009, dengue was the second most frequent cause of fever among 6392 patients with travel-associated health complaints seen in

GeoSentinel European sites (no dengue hemorrhagic fever/dengue shock syndrome), a significant increase over 2008.[33] Dengue infections in travelers can vary seasonally, reflecting the oscillations in the endemic regions.[34]

Chikungunya

Chikungunya (CHIK) fever is a tropical arboviral disease responsible for acute polyarthralgia, which can last for weeks to months. After half a century of focal outbreaks in Africa and Asia, the disease has emerged or re-emerged in many parts of the world in the past decade, and has unexpectedly spread, with large outbreaks in Africa and around the Indian Ocean and rare autochthonous transmission in temperate areas. It has now become an important global public health problem, with several ongoing outbreaks occurring worldwide.[35] Since the beginning of this outbreak, several million cases of chikungunya virus disease have occurred in autochthonous populations and in travelers who were diagnosed after they returned home from epidemic areas. CHIKV, usually transmitted by *Aedes aegypti* mosquitoes, has now been repeatedly associated with a new vector, *Aedes albopictus* (the 'Asian tiger mosquito'), which has spread into tropical areas previously occupied predominantly by *A. aegypti*.[36] Introduction into Europe and spread has been described.[37]

Rickettsial Infections

Rickettsial infections are widely distributed in developed and developing countries and often named for a geographic region where they are found, though names can mislead. Rickettsial diseases are increasingly being recognized among international travelers. A recent study of ≈7000 returnees with fever as a chief reason to seek medical care suggested that 2% of imported fevers are caused by rickettsioses and that 20% of these patients are hospitalized.[5] Most infections are acquired in sub-Saharan Africa, where spotted fever group (SFG) rickettsioses are second only to malaria as the most commonly diagnosed diseases in returnees with systemic febrile illness.[14]

Rickettsia rickettsii, the cause of Rocky Mountain spotted fever in the USA, is found throughout the Americas from Canada to Brazil. Rickettsial infections such as African tick-bite fever (*R. africae*), Mediterranean spotted fever (*R. conorii*), and murine or endemic typhus (*R. typhi*) are important treatable infections in travelers.[38] Many additional rickettsioses have emerged throughout the world. These are being increasingly recognized in travelers, probably reflecting increased travel to high-risk areas, such as southern Africa, and increased awareness among clinicians.[39,40] Diagnosis is usually confirmed with serologic tests or molecular tools such as PCR-based assay on skin biopsies or after eschar swabbing.

Clinical presentations of the rickettsial infections are varied, depending on the species. Most rickettsial infections are transmitted by arthropods, such as ticks and mites, and an eschar may mark the inoculation site. Eschars are often small (<1 cm in diameter), asymptomatic, and may be overlooked. In South African tick-bite fever eschars are often multiple (>50% of cases). Rashes may be present, but many rickettsial infections (even among the spotted fever group) are spotless. *R. australis, R. africae*, and rickettsialpox can cause a vesicular rash that may be mistaken for varicella, monkeypox, or even smallpox. High fever, headache, and normal or low white blood cell count and thrombocytopenia are characteristic. Lymphadenopathy may be present. Infections may be confused with dengue fever. *Rickettsiae* multiply in and damage endothelial cells and cause disseminated vascular lesions. Without treatment, the illness may persist for 2–3 weeks. Response to tetracyclines is generally prompt. Patients with suspected rickettsial infections should be treated empirically while awaiting laboratory confirmation.

Other tick-borne infections, human monocytic ehrlichiosis, and human granulocytic ehrlichiosis (granulocytotropic anaplasmosis),[41] are most commonly diagnosed in the USA but are also found in Europe, Africa, and probably Asia. Clinical findings include prominent fever and headache. These infections may also be associated with leukopenia and thrombocytopenia, and respond to treatment with tetracyclines.

When epidemiologic and clinical aspects of rickettsial diseases were investigated in 280 international travelers reported to the GeoSentinel surveillance network during 1996–2008, 231 (82.5%) had spotted fever (SFG) rickettsiosis, 16 (5.7%) scrub typhus, 11 (3.9%) Q fever, 10 (3.6%) typhus group (TG) rickettsiosis, 7 (2.5%) bartonellosis, 4 (1.4%) indeterminable SFG/TG rickettsiosis, and 1 (0.4%) human granulocytic anaplasmosis; 197 (87.6%) of SFG rickettsiosis cases were acquired in sub-Saharan Africa and were associated with higher age, male gender, travel to southern Africa, late summer season travel, and travel for tourism.[42]

Enteric Fever

Enteric fever (typhoid and paratyphoid fever) is another infection that causes fever and headache and can be associated with an unremarkable physical examination, though a faint rash (rose spots) may appear at the end of the first week of illness. Laboratory findings include a normal or low white blood cell count, thrombocytopenia, and elevation (usually modest) of liver enzymes. Gastrointestinal symptoms such as diarrhea, constipation, and vague abdominal discomfort may be present, as well as dry cough. In contrast to the abrupt onset of fevers in dengue and rickettsial infections, the onset of typhoid fever may be insidious. Leukocytosis in a patient with typhoid fever should raise suspicion of intestinal perforation or other complication. Diagnosis should be confirmed by recovery of *Salmonella typhi* (or *S. paratyphi*) from blood or stool.[43] Culture of bone marrow aspirate may have a higher yield than blood or feces but is generally not favored by clinicians and patients. Serologic tests lack sensitivity and specificity. Increasing resistance of *S. typhi* to many antimicrobials makes it important to isolate the organism and to do sensitivity testing. The emergence of multidrug resistance and decreased ciprofloxacin susceptibility in *Salmonella enterica* serovar *typhi* in South Asia have rendered older drugs, including ampicillin, chloramphenicol, trimethoprim sulfamethoxazole, ciprofloxacin, and ofloxacin, ineffective or suboptimal for typhoid fever.[44]

Multiple studies have identified the Indian subcontinent as a destination with relatively high risk for enteric fever in travelers, especially VFRs.[45]

The efficacy of typhoid vaccines in published studies varies widely depending on the type of vaccine, number of doses, and population studied. As noted above, the efficacy of commonly used vaccines may be 60–70%.[23] The important observation for clinicians evaluating returned travelers is that typhoid fever remains a concern (albeit lower) in persons who have received a typhoid vaccine. Infections with *S. paratyphi* may be relatively more common as a cause of typhoid fever in vaccinated populations because vaccine protects mainly against *S. typhi*.[43] Notably, the course of *S. paratyphi* A was not found to be milder than that of *S. typhi* infection.[45]

Leptospirosis

Although leptospirosis has a broad geographic distribution, infections in humans are more common in tropical and subtropical regions. Recreational activities of travelers, including white water rafting in Costa Rica and other sports involving water exposures, have been associated with sporadic cases and large outbreaks.[46] Among 158 competitive swimmers in the Eco-Challenge in Malaysia in 2000, 44% met the case definition for acute leptospirosis.[47] Although clinical manifestations may be protean, common findings include fever, myalgia, and headache. Among 353 cases reported from Hawaii, 39% had jaundice and 28% conjunctival suffusion.[48] Other findings such as meningitis, rash, uveitis, pulmonary hemorrhage, oliguric renal failure, and refractory shock may be present. A summary of 72 sporadic leptospirosis cases in travelers from Europe and Israel shows that the majority were reported from SE Asia, were male (84%), the disease was associated with water activities in 91%, and 90% were hospitalized with no mortality.[49] Multiple different serovars exist, and clinical presentation and severity vary with infecting serovar. In Israeli travelers 55% had severe leptospirosis, usually associated with ictero-hemorrhagic serogroup.[50]

Owing to lack of sensitive and specific diagnostic tests to confirm infection early in the course in most institutions, early empiric therapy is recommended for suspected infection, especially if severe. Agents used include doxycycline (and other tetracyclines), penicillins, and ceftriaxone.

Acute Schistosomiasis

Acute schistomaisis (Katayama syndrome) follows exposure to fresh water infested with cercariae that penetrate intact skin. The disease, seen primarily in non-immunes, manifests 3–8 weeks after exposure. Clinical manifestations include high fever, myalgia, lethargy, and intermittent urticaria.[51] Dry cough and dyspnea, sometimes with pulmonary infiltrates, are noted in the majority of patients.[52] Eosinophilia, often high grade, is usually present. In one outbreak involving 12 travelers the median duration of fever was 12 days (range 4–46 days) and 10 of 12 had eosinophilia during the first 10 weeks of infection.[51] In most cases the disease is acquired in Africa (not only sub-Saharan); however, in the last decade an important focus was documented in Laos with infection due to *S. mekongi*.[53]

Amebic Liver Abscess

An amebic abscess can cause fever and chills that develop over days to weeks. Although focal findings may not be prominent, 85–90% of patients will report abdominal discomfort and about 70–80% will have right upper quadrant tenderness on examination.[54] Extension of infection to the diaphragmatic surface of the liver may lead to cough, pleuritic or shoulder pain, and right basilar abnormalities on chest X-ray, which may initially suggest a pulmonary process. The abscess can be seen on ultrasound and serology for *Entamoeba histolytica* is usually positive.

Hemorrhagic Fevers

Several infections in addition to exotic infections such as Ebola and Marburg can cause fever and hemorrhage in travelers and many are treatable. Leptospirosis, meningococcemia, and other bacterial infections can cause hemorrhage. Rickettsial infections can produce a petechial rash or purpura, and severe malaria may be associated with disseminated intravascular coagulation. Many viral infections, in addition to dengue, can cause hemorrhage. Most are arthropod-borne (especially mosquito or tick) or have rodent reservoir hosts. Among those reported in travelers are dengue fever (DHF), yellow fever, Lassa fever, Crimean Congo hemorrhagic fever, Rift Valley fever, hemorrhagic fever with renal syndrome (and other hantavirus-associated infections), Kyasanur Forest disease, Omsk hemorrhagic fever, and several viruses in South America (Junin, Machupo, Guanarito, Sabia). Other geographically focal infections can cause hemorrhagic fever and would be expected primarily in travelers who visit rural or remote areas. Lassa fever responds to ribavirin therapy if started early. Several

of the viruses can be transmitted during medical care, so it is important to institute barrier isolation in a private room pending a specific diagnosis. Identification of viral agents causing hemorrhage may require the assistance of staff working in special laboratories, such as one available at CDC. (Assistance is available through the Special Pathogens Branch, Division of Viral and Rickettsial Diseases, CDC, Atlanta, GA 404 639 1511 and other specialized laboratories). Even when specific treatment is not available, good supportive care can save lives.

Fever and CNS Changes

Neurological findings in the febrile patient indicate the need for prompt work-up. High fever alone or in combination with metabolic alternations precipitated by systemic infections can cause changes in the mental status in the absence of CNS invasion. One must consider common, cosmopolitan bacterial, viral, and fungal infections that cause fever and CNS changes. Additional considerations in travelers include Japanese encephalitis, rabies, West Nile, polio, tick-borne encephalitis, and a number of other geographically focal viral infections, such as Nipah virus.

Outbreaks of meningococcal infections (meningococcemia and meningitis) have been associated with the annual *Hajj* pilgrimage to Mecca in Saudi Arabia. Beginning in 2000, for the first time ever, infection with *Neisseria meningitidis* serogroup W-135 caused outbreaks of meningococcal disease in pilgrims and subsequently in their contacts in multiple countries. Pilgrims vaccinated with the quadrivalent meningococcal vaccine (serogroups A, C, W-135 and Y) can still carry *N. meningitidis* in the nasopharynx. Dengue fever can cause neurological findings that mimic Japanese encephalitis. In a study in Vietnam, dengue-associated encephalopathy was found in 0.5% of 5400 children admitted with DHF.[55] Meningitis may be present in leptospirosis. The parasite *Angiostrongylus cantonensis* causes sporadic infection in many countries and was responsible for an outbreak of eosinophilic meningoencephalitis in travelers to Jamaica in 2000.[56] African trypanosomiasis (sleeping sickness), transmitted by an infective tsetse fly, initially causes a non-specific febrile illness. A chancre marks the site of the bite. If untreated, trypanosomes can infect the CNS and cause lethargy. Several cases have been seen in travelers after exposures, especially in Tanzania and Kenya. Patients with malaria, typhoid fever, and rickettsial infections often have severe headache, but CSF is typically unremarkable in these infections. Cerebral malaria causes altered mental status and can progress to seizures and coma. Mefloquine taken for malaria chemoprophylaxis has rarely been associated with seizures and other neuropsychiatric side-effects, but fever typically is absent. Neuroschistosomiasis can be seen in travelers, but fever usually is not present at the time of the focal neurological changes, caused by tissue reaction to ectopic schistosome egg deposition in the nervous system.

Sexually transmitted infections such as HIV and syphilis, whether acquired at home or during travel, can involve the CNS. Lyme and ehrlichiosis are other treatable infections that can cause prominent neurological findings. Other treatable infections that are unfamiliar to clinicians in many geographic areas include Q fever, relapsing fever, brucellosis, bartonellosis, anthrax, and plague.

Persistent and Relapsing Fevers

Diagnoses to be considered in patients with persistent or relapsing fevers include malaria, typhoid fever, tuberculosis, brucellosis, CMV, toxoplasmosis, relapsing fever, melioidosis, Q fever, visceral leishmaniasis, histoplasmosis (and other fungal infections), African trypanosomiasis, and infections that may be unrelated to exposures during travel, such as endocarditis.

For fever with prominent respiratory symptoms please refer to references 57–62 and Chapter 56.

Laboratory Clues

Routine Laboratory Studies

Results of routine laboratory findings may provide clues to the diagnosis in the febrile traveler. An elevated white blood cell count may suggest a bacterial infection, but a number of bacterial infections, such as uncomplicated typhoid fever, brucellosis, and rickettsial infections, are associated with a normal or low white blood cell count.

Elevated Liver Enzymes

In the past hepatitis A virus was the most common cause of hepatitis after travel to developing regions. With the wide use of the hepatitis A vaccine, acute hepatitis A now is seen primarily in persons who failed to receive vaccine (or immunoglobulin) before travel. Hepatitis B remains a risk for unvaccinated persons. Hepatitis E, transmitted via fecally contaminated water or food, clinically resembles acute hepatitis A. Cases have been reported in travelers.[63] Mortality may be 20% or higher in women infected during the third trimester of pregnancy.

Many common as well as unusual systemic infections cause fever and elevation of liver enzymes. Among those that may be a concern, depending on geographic exposures, are yellow fever, dengue and other hemorrhagic fevers, typhoid fever, leptospirosis, rickettsial infections, toxoplasmosis, Q fever, syphilis, psittacosis, and brucellosis. Transaminases are often elevated in these infections. Parasites that directly invade the liver and bile ducts (e.g., amebic liver abscess and liver flukes) often cause right upper quadrant pain, tender liver, and elevated alkaline phosphatase. Drugs and toxins (sometimes found in herbal drugs or nutritional supplements) can damage the liver, so a careful review of these agents should be part of the history.

Fever and Eosinophilia

Eosinophilia is sometimes an incidental finding on laboratory testing. When it is found in a person who has visited or lived in tropical, developing countries, it is a clue that should suggest several specific parasitic infections.[64] Before beginning an extensive work-up to look for parasites, however, it is important to carefully review the general medical history for other processes that may be associated with eosinophilia, and to review drug history (including drugs received during travel, over-the-counter drugs, and drugs that may have been given by injection during travel). Many parasitic infections are not associated with eosinophilia or may be associated with eosinophilia only during one stage of development. Infections that can cause both eosinophilia and fever include acute schistosomiasis (Katayama syndrome), trichinosis, fascioliasis, opisthorchiasis, gnathostomiasis, lymphatic filariasis, tropical pulmonary eosinophilia, toxocariasis, opisthorchiasis, and loiasis.[1] Many of these helminthic infections are seen primarily in persons with prior residence or prolonged stays in tropical developing countries. Acute coccidioidomycosis, resolving scarlet fever, and a few other non-helminthic infections may also be associated with eosinophilia, but in these infections eosinophilia usually is not high grade or persistent. The protozoan infections, malaria, amebiasis, giardiasis, and leishmaniasis, are not associated with eosinophilia.

Initial Diagnostic Work-Up

A careful, complete physical examination should be carried out, looking with special care for rashes or skin lesions, lymphadenopathy, retinal or conjunctival changes, enlargement of liver or spleen, genital lesions, and neurological findings. The initial laboratory evaluation in a febrile patient with a history of tropical exposures should generally include all or most of the following:

- Complete blood count with a differential and estimate of platelets
- Liver enzymes
- Blood cultures
- Blood smears for malaria or rapid diagnostic tests for malaria
- Urinalysis and urine culture
- Chest radiograph.

If malaria is suspected, it is essential not only to request the appropriate tests for malaria but also to make certain that tests are done expeditiously and by knowledgeable persons. In patients with diarrhea or GI symptoms (or if enteric fever is suspected), stool culture should be requested. In a patient with persisting fever a repeat physical examination will sometimes identify new findings (e.g., new rash, splenomegaly) that can provide useful clues to the diagnosis. Table 53.3 lists

Table 53.3 Common Clinical Findings and Associated Infections

Common Clinical Findings	Infections to Consider after Tropical Travel
Fever and rash	Dengue, chikungunya, rickettsioses, enteric fever (skin lesions may be sparse or absent), acute HIV infection, measles, acute schistosomiasis
Fever and abdominal pain	Enteric fever, amebic liver abscess
Undifferentiated fever and normal or low white blood cell count	Dengue, malaria, rickettsial infection, enteric fever, chikungunya
Fever and hemorrhage	Viral hemorrhagic fevers (dengue and others), meningococcemia, leptospirosis, rickettsial infections
Fever and eosinophilia	Acute schistosomiasis; drug hypersensitivity reaction; fascioliasis and other parasitic infections (rare)
Fever and pulmonary infiltrates	Common bacterial and viral pathogens; legionellosis, acute schistosomiasis, Q fever, meliodosis
Fever and altered mental status	Cerebral malaria, viral or bacterial meningoencephalitis, African trypanosomiasis
Mononucleosis syndrome	Epstein–Barr virus, cytomegalovirus, toxoplasmosis, acute HIV
Fever persisting >2 weeks	Malaria, enteric fever, Epstein–Barr virus, cytomegalovirus, toxoplasmosis, acute HIV, acute schistosomiasis, brucellosis, tuberculosis, Q fever, visceral leishmaniasis (rare)
Fever with onset >6 wk after travel	Vivax malaria, acute hepatitis (B, C, or E), tuberculosis, amebic liver abscess

Adapted from Health Information for International Travel, 2012.

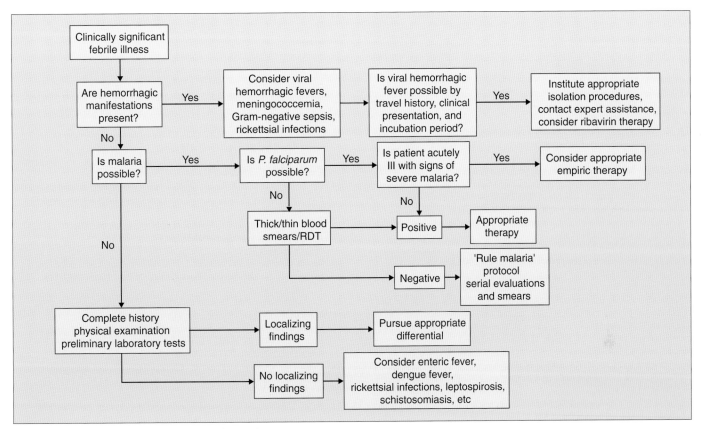

Figure 53.1 Flowchart for the Management of a Febrile Patient.

tests used to diagnose common infections in febrile returned travelers.

The process of travel may lead to medical problems. The immobility associated with travel may predispose to deep vein thrombosis; sinusitis may flare up during or after air travel, related to changes in pressure during ascent and descent. Non-infectious disease causes of fever, such as drug fever, and pulmonary emboli, should also be considered if initial studies do not confirm the presence of an infection. In the study by Bottieau et al.[9] non-infectious causes accounted for 2.2% of the fevers.

Management

Prompt diagnosis and urgent treatment may be necessary to save the patient's life. Figure 53.1 provides an algorithm for the approach to a febrile patient following travel. Useful algorithms based on expert opinion and review of published literature are also available.[65] During the evaluation and treatment, the clinician should also keep in mind the public health impact. Outside resources, such as CDC or other reference laboratories with special expertise, may be needed to provide diagnostic studies or other support. Familiar infections (e.g., salmonellosis, campylobacteriosis, gonorrhea) may be caused by multidrug-resistant organisms. It is especially important to recognize the potential for multidrug resistance in infections, such as typhoid fever, that can be lethal. Absence of response to what should be appropriate treatment should lead the clinician to consider drug resistance, the possibility of the wrong diagnosis, or the presence of two infections. A number of case reports document the simultaneous presence of malaria and typhoid fever, amebic liver abscess and hepatitis A, and other dual infections.[66,67]

Sources of Current Information and Assistance

Knowledge of the epidemiology of infections in a given geographic area is valuable, but detailed, up-to-date information about a specific location may be unavailable. Electronic databases are a useful source of current information about disease outbreaks and alerts about antimicrobial resistance patterns.

References

1. Ryan ET, Wilson ME, Kain KC. Illness after international travel. N Engl J Med 2002 Aug 15;347(7):505–16.
2. Wilson M, Boggild A. Fever and systemic symptoms. In: Guerrant R, Walker D, Weller P, editors. Tropical Infectious Diseases: Principles, Pathogens and Practice. 3rd ed. Edinburgh: Saunders Elsevier; 2011. p. 925–38.
3. Hill DR. Health problems in a large cohort of Americans traveling to developing countries. J Travel Med 2000 Sep–Oct;7(5): 259–66.
4. Steffen R, Rickenbach M, Wilhelm U, et al. Health problems after travel to developing countries. J Infect Dis 1987 Jul;156(1):84–91.
5. Wilson ME, Weld LH, Boggild A, et al. Fever in returned travelers: results from the GeoSentinel Surveillance Network. Clin Infect Dis 2007 Jun 15;44(12):1560–8.
6. Stienlauf S, Segal G, Sidi Y, et al. Epidemiology of travel-related hospitalization. J Travel Med 2005 May–Jun;12(3):136–41.
7. Siikamaki HM, Kivela PS, Sipila PN, et al. Fever in travelers returning from malaria-endemic areas: don't look for malaria only. J Travel Med 2011 Jul–Aug;18(4):239–44.
8. West NS, Riordan FAI. Fever in returned travelers: a prospective review of hospital admissions for a 2½ year period. Arch Dis Child 2003 May 1;88(5):432–4.

9. Bottieau E, Clerinx J, Schrooten W, et al. Etiology and outcome of fever after a stay in the tropics. Arch Intern Med 2006 Aug 14–28;166(15):1642–8.

10. Doherty JF, Grant AD, Bryceson ADM. Fever as the presenting complaint of travelers returning from the tropics. Quart J Med 1995 Apr 1;88(4):277–81.

11. O'Brien D, Tobin S, Brown GV, et al. Fever in returned travelers: review of hospital admissions for a 3-year period. Clin Infect Dis 2001 Sep 1;33(5):603–9.

12. Antinori S, Galimberti L, Gianelli E, et al. Prospective observational study of fever in hospitalized returning travelers and migrants from tropical areas, 1997–2001. J Travel Med 2004 May–Jun;11(3):135–42.

13. Parola P, Soula G, Gazin P, et al. Fever in travelers returning from tropical areas: prospective observational study of 613 cases hospitalised in Marseilles, France, 1999–2003. Travel Med Infect Dis 2006 Mar;4(2):61–70.

14. Freedman DO, Weld LH, Kozarsky PE, et al. Spectrum of disease and relation to place of exposure among ill returned travelers. N Engl J Med 2006 Jan 12;354(2):119–30.

15. Rezza G, Nicoletti L, Angelini R, et al. Infection with chikungunya virus in Italy: an outbreak in a temperate region. Lancet 2007 Dec 1;370(9602):1840–6.

16. de Jesus AR, Silva A, Santana LB, et al. Clinical and immunologic evaluation of 31 patients with acute schistosomiasis mansoni. J Infect Dis 2002 Jan 1;185(1):98–105.

17. Olsen SJ, Chang HL, Cheung TY, et al. Transmission of the severe acute respiratory syndrome on aircraft. N Engl J Med 2003 Dec 18;349(25):2416–22.

18. Schwartz E, Parise M, Kozarsky P, et al. Delayed onset of malaria–implications for chemoprophylaxis in travelers. N Engl J Med 2003 Oct 16;349(16):1510–6.

19. Mali S, Tan KR, Arguin PM. Malaria surveillance–United States, 2009. MMWR Surveill Summ 2011 Apr 22;60(3):1–15.

20. Correia JD, Shafer RT, Patel V, et al. Blood and body fluid exposure as a health risk for international travelers. J Travel Med 2001 Sep–Oct;8(5):263–6.

21. Kumarasamy KK, Toleman MA, Walsh TR, et al. Emergence of a new antibiotic resistance mechanism in India, Pakistan, and the UK: a molecular, biological, and epidemiological study. Lancet Infect Dis 2010 Sep;10(9):597–602.

22. Schwartz E, Shlim DR, Eaton M, et al. The effect of oral and parenteral typhoid vaccination on the rate of infection with Salmonella typhi and Salmonella paratyphi A among foreigners in Nepal. Arch Intern Med 1990 Feb;150(2):349–51.

23. Levine MM, Ferreccio C, Cryz S, et al. Comparison of enteric-coated capsules and liquid formulation of Ty21a typhoid vaccine in a randomised controlled field trial. Lancet 1990 Oct 13;336(8720):891–4.

24. Dorsey G, Gandhi M, Oyugi JH, et al. Difficulties in the prevention, diagnosis, and treatment of imported malaria. Arch Intern Med 2000 Sep 11;160(16):2505–10.

25. Bronner U, Karlsson L, Evengard B. Evaluation of rapid diagnostic tests for malaria in Swedish travelers. APMIS 2011 Feb;119(2):88–92.

26. D'Acremont V, Landry P, Mueller I, et al. Clinical and laboratory predictors of imported malaria in an outpatient setting: an aid to medical decision making in returning travelers with fever. Am J Trop Med Hyg 2002 May;66(5):481–6.

27. Baaten GG, Sonder GJ, Zaaijer HL, et al. Travel-related dengue virus infection, The Netherlands, 2006–2007. Emerg Infect Dis 2011 May;17(5):821–8.

28. Wilder-Smith A, Schwartz E. Dengue in travelers. N Engl J Med 2005 Sep 1;353(9):924–32.

29. Amarasinghe A, Kuritsk JN, Letson GW, et al. Dengue virus infection in Africa. Emerg Infect Dis 2011 Aug;17(8):1349–54.

30. Guzman MG, Kouri G, Valdes L, et al. Epidemiologic studies on dengue in Santiago de Cuba, 1997. Am J Epidemiol 2000 Nov 1;152(9):793–9.

31. Meltzer E, Schwartz E. A travel medicine view of dengue and dengue hemorrhagic fever. Travel Med Infect Dis 2009 Sep;7(5):278–83.

32. Huhtamo E, Hasu E, Uzcategui NY, et al. Early diagnosis of dengue in travelers: comparison of a novel real-time RT-PCR, NS1 antigen detection and serology. J Clin Virol 2010 Jan;47(1):49–53.

33. Odolini S, Parola P, Gkrania-Klotsas E, et al. Travel-related imported infections in Europe, EuroTravNet 2009. Clin Microbiol Infect 2012;18(5):468–74.

34. Schwartz E, Weld LH, Wilder-Smith A, et al. Seasonality, annual trends, and characteristics of dengue among ill returned travelers, 1997–2006. Emerg Infect Dis 2008 Jul;14(7):1081–8.

35. Simon F, Savini H, Parola P. Chikungunya: a paradigm of emergence and globalization of vector-borne diseases. Med Clin North Am 2008 Nov;92(6):1323–43.

36. Simon F, Javelle E, Oliver M, et al. Chikungunya virus infection. Curr Infect Dis Rep 2011 Jun;13(3):218–28.

37. Grandadam M, Caro V, Plumet S, et al. Chikungunya virus, southeastern France. Emerg Infect Dis 2011 May;17(5):910–13.

38. Parola P, Paddock CD, Raoult D. Tick-borne rickettsioses around the world: emerging diseases challenging old concepts. Clin Microbiol Rev 2005 Oct 1;18(4):719–56.

39. Jensenius M, Fournier PE, Vene S, et al. African tick bite fever in travelers to rural sub-Equatorial Africa. Clin Infect Dis 2003 Jun 1; 36(11):1411–7.

40. Raoult D, Fournier PE, Fenollar F, et al. Rickettsia africae, a tick-borne pathogen in travelers to sub-Saharan Africa. N Engl J Med 2001 May 17;344(20):1504–10.

41. Olano JP, Walker DH. Human ehrlichioses. Med Clin North Am 2002 Mar;86(2):375–92.

42. Jensenius M, Davis X, von Sonnenburg F, et al. Multicenter GeoSentinel analysis of rickettsial diseases in international travelers, 1996–2008. Emerg Infect Dis 2009 Nov;15(11):1791–8.

43. Shlim DR, Schwartz E, Eaton M. Clinical importance of Salmonella paratyphi A infection to enteric fever in Nepal. J Travel Med 1995 Sep 1;2(3):165–8.

44. Butler T. Treatment of typhoid fever in the 21st century: promises and shortcomings. Clin Microbiol Infect 2011 Jul;17(7):959–63.

45. Connor BA, Schwartz E. Typhoid and paratyphoid fever in travelers. Lancet Infect Dis 2005 Oct;5(10):623–8.

46. Centers for Disease Control and Prevention. Outbreak of leptospirosis among white-water rafters–Costa Rica, 1996. MMWR Morb Mortal Wkly Rep 1997 Jun 27;46(25):577–9.

47. Centers for Disease Control and Prevention. Update: outbreak of acute febrile illness among athletes participating in Eco-Challenge-Sabah 2000–Borneo, Malaysia, 2000. MMWR Morb Mortal Wkly Rep 2001 Jan 19;50(2):21–4.

48. Katz AR, Ansdell VE, Effler PV, et al. Assessment of the clinical presentation and treatment of 353 cases of laboratory-confirmed leptospirosis in Hawaii, 1974–1998. Clin Infect Dis 2001 Dec 1;33(11):1834–41.

49. Leshem E, Meltzer E, Schwartz E. Travel-associated zoonotic bacterial diseases. Curr Opin Infect Dis 2011 Oct;24(5):457–63.

50. Leshem E, Segal G, Barnea A, et al. Travel-related leptospirosis in Israel: a nationwide study. Am J Trop Med Hyg 2010 Mar;82(3):459–63.

51. Visser LG, Polderman AM, Stuiver PC. Outbreak of schistosomiasis among travelers returning from Mali, West Africa. Clin Infect Dis 1995 Feb;20(2):280–5.

52. Schwartz E, Rozenman J, Perelman M. Pulmonary manifestations of early schistosome infection among nonimmune travelers. Am J Med 2000 Dec 15;109(9):718–22.

53. Leshem E, Meltzer E, Marva E, et al. Travel-related schistosomiasis acquired in Laos. Emerg Infect Dis 2009 Nov;15(11):1823–6.

54. Hughes MA, Petri Jr WA. Amebic liver abscess. Infect Dis Clin North Am 2000 Sep;14(3):565–82.

55. Cam BV, Fonsmark L, Hue NB. Prospective case-control study of encephalopathy in children with dengue hemorrhagic fever. Am J Trop Med Hyg 2001 Dec;65(6):848–51.

56. Slom TJ, Cortese MM, Gerber SI, et al. An outbreak of eosinophilic meningitis caused by Angiostrongylus cantonensis in travelers returning from the Caribbean. N Engl J Med 2002 Feb 28;346(9):668–75.

57. Miller JM, Tam TW, Maloney S, et al. Cruise ships: high-risk passengers and the global spread of new influenza viruses. Clin Infect Dis 2000 Aug;31(2):433–8.

58. Mutsch M, Tavernini M, Marx A, et al. Influenza virus infection in travelers to tropical and subtropical countries. Clin Infect Dis 2005 May 1;40(9):1282–7.

59. Cairns L, Blythe D, Kao A, et al. Outbreak of coccidioidomycosis in Washington state residents returning from Mexico. Clin Infect Dis 2000 Jan;30(1):61–4.

60. Centers for Disease Control and Prevention. Update: outbreak of acute febrile respiratory illness among college students–Acapulco, Mexico, March 2001. MMWR Morb Mortal Wkly Rep 2001 May 11;50(18):359–60.

61. Panackal AA, Hajjeh RA, Cetron MS, et al. Fungal infections among returning travelers. Clin Infect Dis 2002 Nov 1;35(9):1088–95.

62. Salomon J, Flament Saillour M, De Truchis P, et al. An outbreak of acute pulmonary histoplasmosis in members of a trekking trip in Martinique, French West Indies. J Travel Med 2003 Mar–Apr;10(2):87–93.

63. Emerson SU, Purcell RH. Running like water–the omnipresence of hepatitis E. N Engl J Med 2004 Dec 2;351(23):2367–8.

64. Schulte C, Krebs B, Jelinek T, et al. Diagnostic significance of blood eosinophilia in returning travelers. Clin Infect Dis 2002 Feb 1;34(3):407–11.

65. D'Acremont V, Ambresin AE, Burnand B, et al. Practice guidelines for evaluation of fever in returning travelers and migrants. J Travel Med 2003 May;10(Suppl. 2):S25–52.

66. Gopinath R, Keystone JS, Kain KC. Concurrent falciparum malaria and Salmonella in travelers: report of two cases. Clin Infect Dis 1995 Mar;20(3):706–8.

67. Schwartz E, Piper-Jenks N. Simultaneous amoebic liver abscess and hepatitis A infection. J Travel Med 1998 Jun;5(2):95–6.

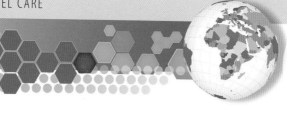

54

Skin Diseases

Eric Caumes

Key points

- Dermatoses are the third most common health problem in travelers
- Skin problems occurring while abroad are cosmopolitan; most of these dermatoses are related to an infectious origin, insect bites, envenomization, or solar exposure
- The dermatoses occurring after return are usually of infectious origin; some of these are tropical diseases

Epidemiological Data

Prospective questionnaire-based studies show that skin diseases are a leading cause of health impairments during travel abroad. In the 1980s a study showed that sunburns and insect stings were reported by respectively 10% and 3% of 2665 Finnish travelers worldwide.[1]

Today, dermatoses are considered the third most common cause of health problems in travelers, after diarrhea and respiratory tract infection. Indeed, they have been reported during travel by 8% of 784 American travelers worldwide.[2] Most of the 63 dermatoses observed in this cohort were related to insect bites or stings, sun exposure, contact allergy, and infectious agents.

Dermatoses Diagnosed Abroad

Similarly, on-site studies of health impairment during travel showed that dermatoses were one of the three main reasons for consultation in travelers abroad. In Nepal, three studies showed that dermatoses were the third to fourth most frequent presenting illness among tourists: skin diseases accounted for 12% of 860 health impairments among 838 French tourists in 1984, 8.7% of health impairments among 276 French tourists in 2001,[3] and in another report for 10% of 19 616 presentations of patients of all nationalities at a private clinic.[4] Bacterial and fungal skin infections as well as scabies infestation were the most common travel-associated dermatoses in Nepal in 1984, accounting for 4.35%, 1.86%, and 2%, respectively, of 860 health impairments in French tourists. In 2001, dermatoses were due to bacteria (40% of the dermatoses), fungi (25%), and frostbite (16%), whereas scabies was no more observed.[3]

Moreover, in the Maldives and Fiji, dermatoses were the most frequent presenting illnesses in tourists, with sunburns and superficial injuries documented most often.[5] In Fiji, injuries (including those due to contact with marine creatures) and skin rash (frequently related to sunburn) each accounted for 10% of clinic visits by tourists, while skin infections accounted for 13%.[5] In the Maldives, superficial injuries (usually caused by contact with corals and shells) and 'sun allergies' accounted for 14% and 13%, respectively, of health impairments among tourists.[6] Dermatoses were also the most frequent reason for consultation in US military troops in Thailand, accounting for 19% of 1299 patient visits to three military clinics during a 33-day exercise.[7]

In Ouagadougou (Burkina Faso), among 100 westerners (93% expatriates) presenting with 106 skin diseases, the main dermatoses identified through a telemedicine network were bacterial infections (18%), arthropod-induced pruritic dermatitis (15%), fungal infections (13%), contact dermatitis (12%), and viral infections (8%). Parasitic dermatoses were not observed in westerners in contrast to Burkinabes nationals. Among westerners, fungal dermatoses were only observed in long-term residents.[8]

Dermatoses Diagnosed Upon Return

Results of studies of travelers returning from tropical countries show that dermatoses are the third cause of health impairment in this setting, after fever and diarrhea. Three studies have helped to identify more specifically the spectrum of travel-associated dermatoses observed after return.[9–11] These studies carry the same message. The most common causes of skin consultations are skin and soft tissue infections, consequences of insect bites or stings and hookworm-related cutaneous larva migrans (Table 54.1).

Therefore, the spectrum of travel-related dermatoses seems to be closely related to the geographic location visited and the onset of signs and symptoms relative to the date of return. Sunburns, arthropod-related reactions and superficial injuries are most often seen during the patient's stay abroad and are prominent in hot seaside areas. Skin infections, most particularly pyoderma, are ubiquitous and are a common cause of dermatoses abroad and after return. Infectious cellulitis is certainly the most severe dermatosis to be encountered by travelers.

Tropical Dermatoses in the Traveler

Tropical dermatoses are usually seen after the traveler returns, given the prolonged incubation period of these diseases. The part occupied

DOI: 10.1016/B978-1-4557-1076-8.00054-5

Table 54.1 The Top Nine Travel Associated Dermatoses Diagnosed in Returning Travelers

Year	1995	2007	2008
First Author	9	10	11
Study type	Observational monocentric prospective study	Observational monocentric prospective study	Observational multicentric retrospective study
Study site	France	France	31 GeoSentinel sites worldwide
Study period	1991–1993 (2 years)	2002–2003 (6 months)	1997–2006 (10 years)
Number of patients	269	165	4594
Patients	Tourists (76%), business (24%)	Tourists (44.8%), VFRs (30.9%), expatriates (16.4%), business (7.9%)	Tourists (69.1%), VFRs (10.9%), business (10.4%), expatriates (9.4%)
Top nine diagnoses	– HRCLM (24.9%) – Pyodermas (17.8%) – Arthropods-related pruritic dermatitis (9.7%) – Myiasis (9.3%) – Tungiasis (6.3%) – Urticaria (5.9%) – Rash with fever (4.1%) – Cutaneous leishmaniasis (3%) – Scabies (2.2%)	– Infectious cellulitis (13%) – Scabies (10%) – Pruritus of unknown origin (9%) – Pyoderma (8%) – Myiasis (7%) – Dermatophytosis (6%) – Filariasis (5%) – HRCLM (4.8%) – Urticaria (4.8%)	– HRCLM (9.8%) – Insect bite (8.2%) – Skin abscess (7.7%) – Superinfected insect bites (6.8%) – Allergic rash (5.5%) – Rash, unknown etiology (5.5%) – Dog bite (4.3%) – Superficial fungal infection (4%) – Dengue (3.4%)
Diagnosis related to imported tropical diseases	53%	33.9%	24%

VFRs, travelers visiting friends and relatives; HRCLM, hookworm-related cutaneous larva migrans.

by tropical diseases within the spectrum of travel associated dermatoses varies from 24% to 53%.[9,11] However, these studies probably overestimate it. Indeed, studies of health impairments occurring during travel show a more cosmopolitan pattern of skin diseases. In addition, the fact that these studies took place in tropical disease units may have biased the patient recruitment, and may explain why relatively few non-infectious dermatoses were diagnosed.

The most common tropical skin conditions include hookworm-related cutaneous larva migrans, tungiasis, myiasis, and localized cutaneous leishmaniasis.[9–11] Limited knowledge of tropical dermatoses among Western physicians can delay the diagnosis and effective treatment. This is well illustrated by a study of cutaneous leishmaniasis where the median time interval from when the lesions were first noticed to when treatment was instituted was 112 days (range 0–1032 days).[12] Similarly, 55% of 64 patients with cutaneous larva migrans had already consulted a general practitioner or a dermatologist (mean number of consultations: two; range: 1–6) before the correct diagnosis was made.[13]

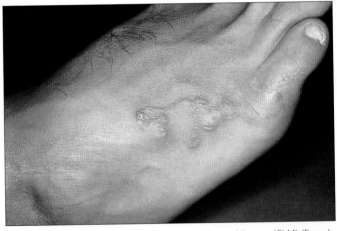

Figure 54.1 Serpiginous Track of Cutaneous Larva Migrans (CLM) (French West Indies).

Hookworm-Related Cutaneous Larva Migrans

Hookworm-related cutaneous larva migrans (HRCLM) (also called creeping eruption, creeping verminous dermatitis, clam-digger's itch, sandworm eruption, plumber's itch) is the most frequent travel-associated skin disease of tropical origin. HRCLM is caused most often by the larvae of hookworms (*Ancylostoma braziliense*) of dogs, cats, or other mammals. It is widely distributed in tropical and sub-tropical countries. HRCLM is acquired by skin contact with infective larvae in the soil, usually while landing or walking on the beaches in hot seaside areas.

Two outbreaks have been observed in travelers. In a group of 32 Canadians who acquired CLM (25% of exposed persons) in Barbados, risk factors for developing the illness were younger age (39 versus 41 years, p = 0.014) and less frequent use of protective footwear while

walking on the beach (risk ratio of 4 for people who never wear sandals to and on the beach).[14] Interestingly, 90% of travelers reported seeing cats, whereas only 5% of the group noticed dogs on the beach and around the hotel area. The other outbreak involved a group of 13 (87% of exposed persons) British military personnel who acquired CLM during a training exercise in Belize.[15]

HRCLM has recently been exhaustively reviewed.[16,17] The incubation period of CLM is usually a few days and rarely goes beyond 1 month. The eruption usually lasts between 2 and 8 weeks, but has been reported to last up to 2 years. Apart from pruritus, the most frequent clinical sign of CLM is an erythematous, linear, or serpiginous lesion that is approximately 3 mm wide and may be up to 15–20 cm in length (Fig. 54.1). The mean number of lesions per patient varies from one to three. The most frequent anatomic locations of

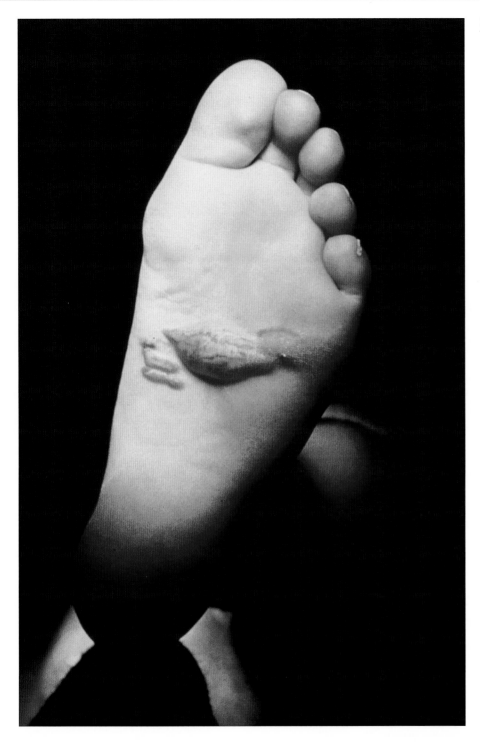

Figure 54.2 Vesiculobullous Lesion Over CLM Track (Brazil).

HRCLM lesions are the feet, followed by the buttocks and trunk. The larva advances a few millimeters to a few centimeters daily. Vesiculobullous lesions (Fig. 54.2) and to a lesser extent impetiginization (Fig. 54.3) are common. Superinfection has been estimated at 8% in one study.[13] Edema and vesiculobullous lesions are observed in approximately 10% of patients.[16,17] In the Canadian outbreak all the lesions were located on the feet, and a more significant number (40%) of patients reported bullous lesions.[14] Systemic signs and symptoms such as erythema multiforme, dry cough, wheezing, and eosinophilic pneumonitis have been rarely reported.

Blood eosinophilia may be increased.[16,17] Nonetheless, blood tests are not necessary to assess the diagnosis, which is usually based on the characteristic clinical findings and a history of possible exposure. The differential diagnoses include the other dermatoses that give rise to serpiginous or linear migrating cutaneous lesions (see creeping eruptions, cutaneous larva migrans).

There is a particular form of HRCLM, known as hookworm folliculitis, which usually occurs on the buttocks (Fig. 54.4). The largest series includes seven patients.[18] The diagnosis is made clinically when the serpiginous tracks are seen among the lesions of folliculitis, or relies on histopathological and parasitological grounds when the hookworm larva is found in the sebaceous follicular canal.

The treatment of choice for HRCLM was the topical application of a 15% liquid suspension (or ointment) of thiabendazole, but

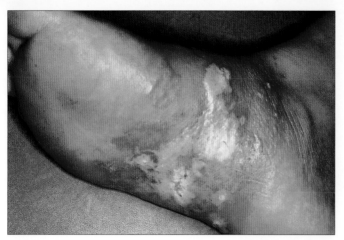

Figure 54.3 Super Infection of CLM of the Foot (Senegal).

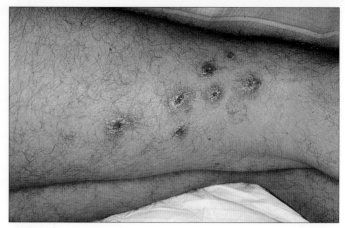

Figure 54.5 Localized Cutaneous Leishmaniasis (LCL), Papular form (Saudi Arabia).

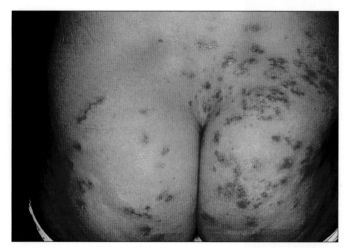

Figure 54.4 Hookworm Folliculitis (Senegal).

thiabendazole is no longer marketed and oral treatment has become the first-line treatment.[16] Of all the efficient oral antihelminthic agents, ivermectin has the advantage of being well tolerated, with high efficacy when taken in a single dose, the cure rate being >94%.[16] Oral albendazole (400–800 mg/day) for 3 consecutive days is also effective and well tolerated. A single 12 mg oral dose of ivermectin was significantly more efficacious in a prospective comparative study than a single 400 mg oral dose of albendazole (100% versus 46%; p = 0.017).[19]

Treatment of HRCLM is challenging when oral ivermectin and albendazole are contraindicated, because thiabendazole is no longer marketed. In this setting, a 10% albendazole ointment twice a day for 10 days is a safe and effective treatment for cutaneous larva migrans.[16]

To avoid HRCLM on tropical beaches frequented by dogs and cats, it is best to wear shoes, to use a mattress, or to lie on sand washed by the tide.

Localized Cutaneous Leishmaniasis

Localized cutaneous leishmaniasis (LCL) occurs in tropical and warm temperate countries and is transmitted by sandflies. Old World LCL (caused primarily by *L. major* and *L. tropica*) occurs mainly in travelers to the sub-Saharan and North Africa, the Mediterranean basin, and the Middle East. The Indian subcontinent and China seem to be less at risk. New World LCL (caused primarily by the species of *L. braziliensis* and *L. mexicana* complexes) occurs mainly in travelers to the

forested parts of Latin America. Workers in the Amazon forest are particularly at risk.

There are four series of LCL imported in to western countries by travelers.[12,20–22] LCL has also recently been exhaustively reviewed.[23,24] Of all the clinical forms of cutaneous leishmaniasis, LCL occurs more often in travelers than in immigrants. Of the 59 cases of cutaneous leishmaniasis reported to the National Institutes of Health from 1973 to 1991, there were 42 cases of LCL (23 Old World, 19 New World), four cases of recurrent cutaneous leishmaniasis (RCL), two cases of mucosal leishmaniasis (ML) and 10 cases of diffuse cutaneous leishmaniasis (DCL).[20] LCL was essentially observed in American travelers, whereas RCL, ML and DCL occurred mainly in immigrants to the USA. In Germany, of the 26 cases of imported leishmaniasis reported to the German surveillance network for imported infectious diseases from January 2001 to June 2004, there were 23 cases of LCL and three cases of mucous forms.[21] Between 1985 and 1990, the CDC provided a pentavalent derivative of antimony for 59 American travelers with New World LCL. A total of 26 (46%) of those treated were expatriates and 23 (39%) were tourists.[12] Of the 15 (26%) patients who had stayed in a forest region for ≤1 week, at least six were exposed for no more than 2 days. LCL has been shown to be more frequent among people traveling for professional reasons than among tourists, and among men rather than women.[9,10] Small outbreaks are observed among travelers, with attack rates of 17–42% in a group of students in Guatemala and Belize and 15–23% in a group of tourists in Peru.[12] These attack rates may go up to 100% for workers in the Amazon forest.[9] The incidence of LCL has been estimated at 1/1000 travelers to Surinam and 1/million travelers to Mexico.[12] In the French series of 39 patients with LCL, 13 had already consulted general practitioners, and the diagnosis was missed in five cases (38%). Five clusters were identified.[22]

The incubation period varies from a few days to a few months. The median interval between return from the tropics and the onset of imported cutaneous lesions has been estimated to be 15 days (range 7–30 days) in one American study,[20] 52 days (7–104 days) in a French study,[9] and 22 days (1–150 days) in another French study,[22] whereas the median maximum possible incubation period was 30 days (range 1 day to 5 months) in another report.[10] In the German series the median time to a definitive diagnosis was 61 days in cases of cutaneous/mucocutaneous leishmaniasis, reflecting the unfamiliarity of German physicians with leishmanial infections.[21]

The clinical forms of LCL include papule (Fig. 54.5), nodule (Fig. 54.6), plaque (Fig. 54.7), ulcer (Fig. 54.8) or nodular lymphangitis (Fig. 54.9).

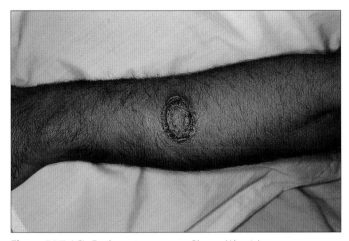

Figure 54.6 LCL, Nodular form (Ethiopia).

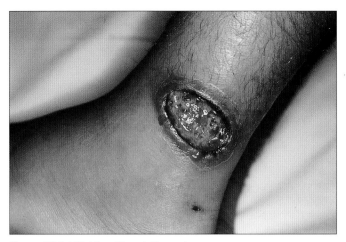

Figure 54.8 LCL, Ulcer (French Guyana).

Figure 54.7 LCL, Erythematosquamous Plaque (Algeria).

Cutaneous ulcer is the most frequent clinical presentation (at least in the New World)[22] and is commonly characterized by a well-circumscribed border, a crusted base and the absence of pain. The average number of cutaneous lesions varies from one to three and rarely exceeds 10/patient. Usual features of LCL include the anatomic location on exposed skin (face, arms, legs), absence of pain, chronicity (>15 days' duration), and failure of antibiotics (which are often prescribed, given that it often looks like pyoderma).

Late destructive ML is rather more frequently observed in immigrants than in travelers.[20] Nonetheless, it has been described in immunocompromised persons who have traveled to endemic areas in the past and have been infected with a *Leishmania* species (e.g., *L. braziliensis*) that has the potential for mucous involvement. The differential diagnosis of LCL includes pyoderma, anthrax, myiasis, arthropod bite or sting, tick eschar, and sporotrichosis, mostly in the case of nodular lymphangitis (see Nodular lymphangitis).

Diagnosis is usually made by evaluating a slit skin smear of the cutaneous lesion stained with Giemsa under light microscopy.[23,24] Skin biopsy from the edge of the ulcer may reveal the characteristic amastigotes within macrophages but is less sensitive than culture. *Leishmania* species may be cultured on various media (e.g., Novy–MacNeal–Nicolle). DNA and monoclonal antibodies may also be used for *Leishmania* antibody analyses and species identification. The PCR technology allows rapid and high-sensitivity diagnosis with determination of most identified species, thereby permitting

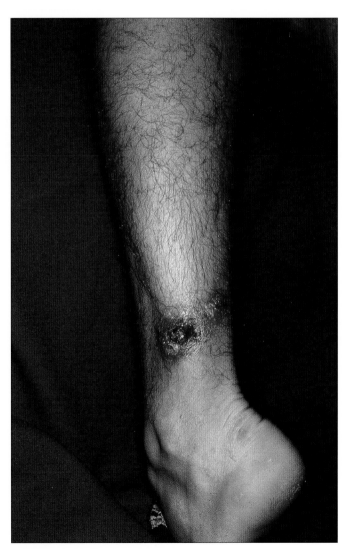

Figure 54.9 LCL, Nodular Lymphangitis (French Guyana).

immediate species-orientated treatment, but this technology is not yet available everywhere.

At least six drugs have showed significant efficacy in the treatment of LCL in placebo-controlled trials (most of them coming from the New World).[23–25] The mainstay of treatment is pentavalent antimonial agents given intramuscularly in New World LCL, and intralesionally in Old World LCL. Other treatments include pentamidine salts, fluconazole, ketoconazole, miltefosine, liposomal amphotericin B, and topical treatment with paromomycin (15%) and gentamicin (0.5%), which have been evaluated in a few species only. In case of failure, liposomal amphotericin B seems to be of great interest. In some instances, mainly cases originating from the Old World, lack of treatment may be considered, given that the cutaneous lesions heal spontaneously in nearly all patients within 1 year.

Myiasis

Cutaneous myiasis is the infestation of human tissues by *Diptera* fly larvae. According to the results of three series of imported cases in Western countries, various forms of cutaneous myiasis are observed in travelers. In a series of 25 cases imported in France, 20 were due to *Cordylobia anthropophaga* (the tumbu fly), four to *Dermatobia hominis* (the human botfly), and one to *Cochliomyia hominivorax*.[9] In a series of 19 cases imported in England, nine were due to *C. anthropophaga*, four to *D. hominis*, one to *C. hominivorax* and one to *Oestrus ovis*.[26] In a series of 13 cases imported in Germany, six were infected with *C. anthropophaga*, six with *D. hominis* and one with *Hypoderma lineatum*.[27]

Furuncular myiasis is caused primarily by *C. anthropophaga* in sub-Saharan Africa and *D. hominis* in Central and South America. Depending on which fly is involved (the tumbu fly or the botfly), the presentation of myiasis differs by the place of acquisition, duration of maturation, number and anatomic location of cutaneous lesions, and the ability to manually extract the larvae (Table 54.2). *C. anthropophaga* larvae penetrate the skin after hatching from eggs deposited on clothing and bedlinen hung to dry outdoors and which have not been ironed. Infestations by *D. hominis* larvae develop from fly eggs carried to the human by a biting mosquito. In both cases the larvae develop by successive molts. The incubation period varies from days to weeks (7–10 days for the tumbu fly and 15–45 days for the botfly).

The cutaneous lesion is a 1–2 cm furuncle-like lesion with a central punctum through which serosanguineous or purulent fluid discharges (Figs 54.10 and 54.11). Importantly, the patient complains of a crawling sensation within the lesion, and movements of the larvae may be seen within the central punctum. *C. anthropophaga* lesions are more commonly multiple, whereas *D. hominis* lesions usually number from one to three. Indeed, the number of maggots removed from the skin was markedly higher in six patients infected with the tumbu fly (average of five) compared with the six with botfly (average of 1.7).[27] *C. anthropophaga* lesions are usually located on areas of the body covered by clothing (such as the trunk), whereas *D. hominis* lesions are commonly located on exposed areas such as the scalp, face, forearms, and legs. The largest number of lesions ever reported was 94 in a child from Ghana infected by *C. anthropophaga*.[28]

The diagnosis of myiasis is made by the identification of the larva from the lesion. The differential diagnosis primarily includes pyoderma, LCL, and tungiasis. Treatment is the removal of the larvae. It is important to avoid breaking the larvae, as incomplete removal may result in a hypersensitivity or foreign body reaction to the larvae. In the case of *C. anthropophaga*, manual pressure to the lateral aspects of the lesion easily allows the expression of the maggot. With *D. hominis*, extraction is facilitated by placing an occlusive agent (e.g., paraffin, petrolatum, pork fat, toothpaste cap) onto the lesion, which may cause the larva to migrate to the skin surface.[29]

Tungiasis

Tungiasis is the infestation by the female sand flea, *Tunga penetrans* (also called chigoe flea, jigger flea). It is widely distributed throughout Latin America, the Caribbean, Africa, and Asia, up to the west coast of India.[29] The sand flea penetrates human skin, feeds on blood, and produces eggs within its abdomen. In the largest study of 17 imported cases, the median lag time between return and onset was 5 days (range 2–10 days) and the median lag time between return and presentation was 12 days (range 5–40 days).[9] This confirms that the time of exposure to the onset of cutaneous lesions is short and that the flea may survive >1 month. The cutaneous lesion is a black papule (at the site of penetration) that develops into a nodule through which the eggs of the flea are expelled (Fig. 54.12). There is a limited number of nodules

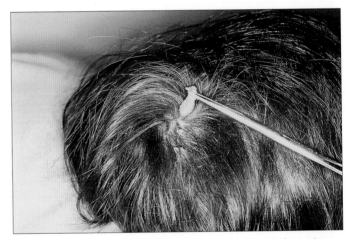

Figure 54.10 Cutaneous Myiasis Due to *D. hominis* (French Guyana).

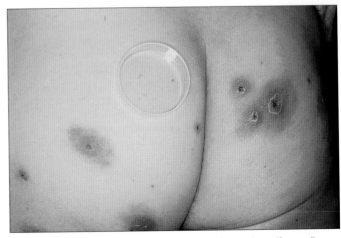

Figure 54.11 Cutaneous Myiasis Due to *C. anthropophaga* (Senegal).

Table 54.2 Furuncular Myiasis		
Diptera (Fly)	**Cordylobia anthropophaga (Tumbu Fly)**	**Dermatobia hominis (Human Botfly)**
Distribution	sub-Saharan Africa	Latin America
Duration	9 days	6–12 weeks
Localization	Covered areas	Uncovered areas
Number of lesions	1–94[30]	1–3
Removal	Local pressure	Extraction

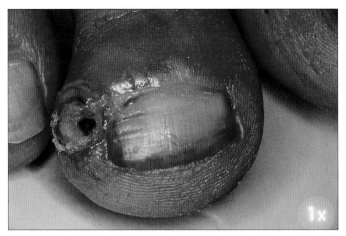

Figure 54.12 Tungiasis of the Toe (Ivory Coast).

(most commonly one), which are usually located on the feet (subungual, sole, toe) and lower extremities.[30] The diagnosis relies on clinical findings and is confirmed by the morphology of the flea. The differential diagnosis includes myiasis, pyoderma, and foreign body reaction. The treatment is removal of the flea by excision and curettage[29].

Cutaneous Gnathostomiasis

Cutaneous gnathostomiasis is increasingly reported in travelers returning from endemic countries.[29] The largest series of imported cutaneous gnathostomiasis includes five patients returning from southeast Asia.[31] The cutaneous lesions appeared within a mean period of 62 days (range 10–150 days) after return. They consisted of creeping eruptions in three patients, migratory swellings in two, papules and nodules in one. The mean eosinophilic count was 1556/mm³ (range 398–3245/mm³). The diagnosis relied on positive serological tests in two patients and seroconversion in two, and was confirmed by identification of *Gnathostoma hispidum* in one biopsy specimen. The treatment of cutaneous gnathostomiasis consisted of repeated courses of albendazole or ivermectin. Recurrence may occur up to 20 months after apparent cure without re-infection.[29]

Ciguatera

Ciguatera is a significant cause of pruritus, which may last months after the initial event.[32] This is a fish poisoning, which is acquired by the consumption of certain tropical marine reef fish in tropical and subtropical regions (also see Ch. 46). The diagnosis relies on the history of fish consumption, other cases in travelers sharing the same food habit, a short incubation period (2–30 h), and the association with gastrointestinal signs and symptoms, fatigue, myalgias (particularly of the lower extremities), pruritus, and neurosensory manifestations (perioral and distal extremity paresthesias and altered temperature sensation). The reversal of temperature sensation (i.e., cold beverages and objects are described as feeling hot) is unique to ciguatera. There may be cardiovascular impairment. Whereas gastrointestinal symptoms resolve within a few hours, myalgias, pruritus, and neurosensory symptoms last longer. Treatment is essentially supportive.

Other Tropical Dermatoses of Interest for Travelers

Many other tropical dermatoses (e.g., acute filariasis, loiasis, onchocerciasis, West and East African trypanosomiasis, mucosal leishmaniasis, genital amebiasis, Buruli's ulcer, cutaneous anthrax) have been observed in travelers.[29]

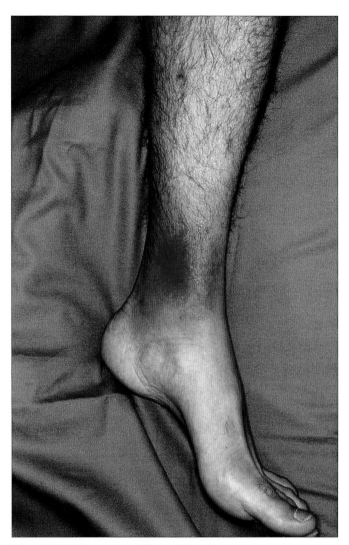

Figure 54.13 Trypanosomal Chancre (Congo).

African trypanosomiasis as well as schistosomiasis may often be revealed by dermatological manifestations. Cutaneous signs are possible at all the phases of these two diseases. In both instances recognition of the early cutaneous sign may allow a rapid diagnosis. African trypanosomiasis, which is on the rise, may be revealed by trypanosomal chancre (Fig. 54.13). Cases of acute onchocerciasis acquired in West or Central Africa and responsible for limb lymphedema (Fig. 54.14) have been reported.[33]

Numerous cases (including clusters) of tropical diseases which cause febrile rash (e.g., rickettsial diseases, dengue fever, acute schistosomiasis) have been reported in travelers (see Febrile rash).

Cosmopolitan Dermatoses

Pyodermas

Skin and soft tissue infections (SSTI) are the first cause of skin consultations in returning travelers.[29] The lesions usually appear while the patient is still abroad. The clinical spectrum is broad-ranging, from impetigo (Fig. 54.15) and ecthyma to erysipelas and necrotizing cellulitis.[9,10,34] The most common bacterial species involved are *Staphylococcus aureus* and *Streptococcus pyogenes*. Whereas ecthyma, with subsequent transmission of the infection on returning home have been reported, travel becoming the primary source of PVL-positive staphylococcal infections in the family and the community. Both methicillin-resistant *Staphylococcus aureus* (MRSA) and methicillin-sensitive *Staphylococcus aureus* (MSSA) can carry the gene of the PVL, a cytotoxin that confers higher morbidity. Travelers exposed to exotic strains of *Staphylococcus aureus* may also be at risk of acquiring staphylococcal strains with an unusual profile of resistance to antibiotics. Unsurprisingly, importation of MRSA has been linked to returning travelers in Sweden.[35]

Most of the cases of SSTI are secondary to an insect bite.[9,10,11,34] This points towards the importance of insect protection in the prevention of pyodermas. In addition, travel first-aid kits should include antibiotics effective against bacterial infections, at least in susceptible persons (history of erysipelas or infectious cellulitis, presence of venous or lymphatic insufficiency).

Dermatophytosis

Dermatophytosis, or tinea, is a worldwide cutaneous infection but its incidence is higher in the tropics and subtropics. Tinea infections rank among the most common skin diseases observed during travel abroad.[3,8]

According to the at-risk exposure during travel, all the forms of tinea may be described: tinea corporis, tinea barbae, tinea cruris, tinea axillaris, and tinea unguium.[29] Tinea of the feet is probably the most common dermatophytic infection to be encountered in travelers who are not going barefoot or wearing sandals. The predominant agent of tinea pedis is *T. rubrum*. Three clinical varieties may be described: the intertriginous type, the vesicular, bullous or vesiculobullous type, and the squamous or hyper-keratotic type.

Scalp ringworm is a common variety of dermatophytosis in children coming back from visiting friends and relatives in Africa.

Tinea versicolor is a chronic, superficial yeast infection of the epidermal stratum corneum.[29] It is worldwide, but extremely common in the tropics and subtropics. Tinea versicolor is caused by the hyphal form of *Malassezia furfur*. The characteristic clinical lesion is a well-defined round or oval macule covered with adherent fine scales. The macules may remain isolated, but have a tendency to coalesce, and cover large areas of the body on the chest, shoulders, back and neck. Usually asymptomatic, the eruption may become pruritic in hot climates. The diagnosis is evoked on the distribution, shape and appearance of the patches and the fingernail test, which demonstrates the fine scales, limited to affected spots. The final diagnosis relies on the microscopic examination of a scotch tape.

Arthropod-Related Dermatoses

Exposure to an arthropod (see Ch. 45) is a common cause of skin lesions in travelers.[9–11] Attempts to identify the implicated arthropod are often difficult in that arthropods of different species may give rise to similar dermatologic manifestations. Nonetheless, epidemiological exposures suggested by history are useful.

The clinical picture varies according to the nature of the skin injury (e.g., traumatic injury, local envenomation, hypersensitivity reaction). The predominant feature of the arthropod reaction is prurigo, an eruption of intensely pruritic erythematous and excoriated papules (Fig. 54.16). This reaction is considered to be an evolutive stage of papular urticaria related to a hypersensitivity reaction to the bites of insects such as fleas, bedbugs, and less commonly, mosquitoes, chiggers, and mites. Arthropod bites may also result in vesiculobullous lesions and papular urticaria. Cutaneous lesions are self-limited.

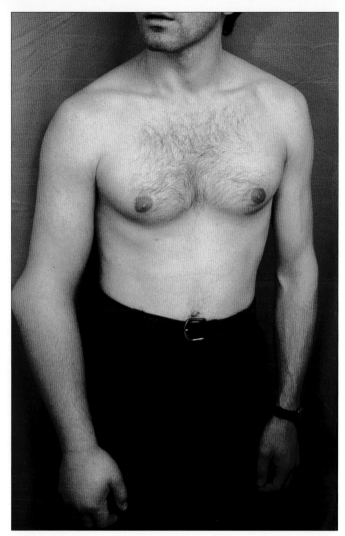

Figure 54.14 Limb Lymphedema Related to Onchocerciasis (Cameroon).

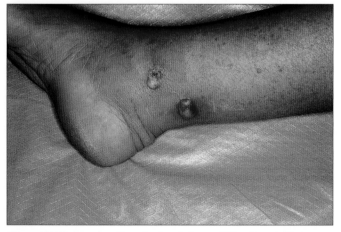

Figure 54.15 Impetigo Complicating Arthropod Bites (French West Indies).

erysipelas and cellulitis are more likely to be due to *Streptococcus* sp., others such as impetigo, folliculitis, carbuncles, and abscesses are more related to *Staphylococcus aureus*.[34] Cutaneous lesions may act as a portal of entry for septicemia. Cases of Panton Valentine leukocidine (PVL)-positive *Staphylococcus aureus* infections acquired abroad

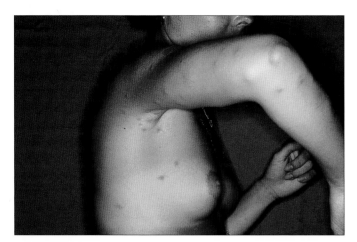

Figure 54.16 Prurigo after Exposure to Trombiculidae (Brazil).

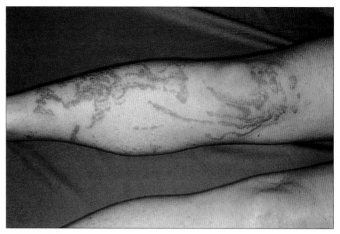

Figure 54.17 Erythematous Flagellations after Contact with Jellyfish (Thailand).

Oral antihistamines and topical corticosteroids may improve the symptoms.

Scabies

Scabies is the most common cause of generalized pruritus in travelers.[8,9] Scabies is acquired by skin-to-skin contact. Clinically, the patient complains of pruritus within 4 weeks of contact in cases of primary exposure.[29] In patients with a history of previous scabies exposure, pruritus may occur within a few days. The more specific skin findings include burrows, papulonodular genital lesions, and pustules on the hands. Other skin changes are secondary to pruritus and include excoriation, lichenification, and impetiginization.

The diagnosis is made by the microscopic identification of the *S. scabiei var. hominis* mite, eggs, or feces on skin scrapings of a cutaneous lesion. Treatment includes permethrin cream 5%, lindane 1% (γ-benzene hexachloride), benzyl benzoate (in Europe), and ivermectin. Bedding and clothing must be laundered or removed from contact for at least 3 days. Personal and household contacts must also be treated.

Cercarial Dermatitis

Cercarial dermatitis (also called clam-digger's dermatitis, schistosome dermatitis, sedge pool itch, swimmer's itch) is caused by the infestation of the skin by cercariae (larvae) of non-human schistosomes whose usual hosts are birds and small mammals.[34] Cercarial dermatitis is acquired by skin exposure to fresh and, to a lesser -extent, salt water. The cercariae penetrate intact human skin within a few minutes. Cercarial dermatitis occurs in swimmers and those with occupations that include water exposure. There are sporadic reports and few outbreaks reported from all continents.

The time from exposure to onset of symptoms varies from a few minutes to a maximum of 24 h after exposure.[34] A prickling sensation during or shortly after exposure to infested water may be reported. Typically, and approximately 1 h later, the cutaneous lesions begin as a pruritic macular erythematous eruption that progresses to a papular, papulovesicular, and urticarial eruption. The eruption typically covers skin surfaces that are exposed to water, but the skin surfaces that are covered by swimwear are not spared. The eruption peaks in 1–3 days and lasts 1–3 weeks. In cases of previous contact the clinical findings may begin sooner, with increased severity and a prolonged course.

The diagnosis is made by history of exposure and the characteristic clinical findings.[34] The differential diagnosis includes sea-bather's eruption, contact dermatitis (secondary to marine plants, hydroids and corals), and insect bites. Cercarial dermatitis is self-limited. Oral antihistamines and topical steroids reduce the symptoms.

Sea-Bather's Eruption

Sea-bather's eruption (also called sea lice) is acquired by skin exposure to salt water inhabited by larvae of sea anemone and jellyfish.[36] Sea-bather's eruption is caused by the larvae discharging toxin from nematocysts into human skin. Sea-bather's eruption has been reported on the Atlantic coast of the USA, the Caribbean, Central and South America, and in SE Asia. It probably exists worldwide in tropical and subtropical marine environments.

The time from exposure to onset of symptoms is usually a few minutes to 24 h. Individuals with a history of previous exposures may develop a prickling or stinging sensation or urticarial lesions while in the water. The clinical features include pruritic, erythematous macules, that progress to papules, vesicles, and urticarial lesions. The anatomic distribution typically includes skin surfaces covered by swimwear and uncovered skin surfaces where there is friction (e.g., axillae, medial thighs, surfer's chest). The eruption is more pronounced in areas that are more confined (e.g., waistband). The eruption can last from 3 days to 3 weeks.

The diagnosis is made by the characteristic clinical findings and history of exposure. The differential diagnoses include cercarial dermatitis, contact dermatitis (secondary to marine life inhabitants) and insect bites. Sea-bather's eruption is self-limited. Oral antihistamines and topical steroids may reduce the symptoms.

Marine Life Dermatitis

Dermatoses associated with contact with a marine creature (see Ch. 45) are one of the most frequent causes of disease in travelers to tropical islands.[5,6]

The most dangerous creatures are the coelenterates, which are found worldwide in tropical and subtropical waters.[37] Contact with Portuguese Man-of-War, fire coral, jellyfish, and sea anemone immediately produces a stinging sensation that varies from a slight burning sensation to excruciating pain. The cutaneous lesions appear at the site of exposition within a few minutes, begin as macules and papules, and may progress to vesicles, bullae, and ulceration (Fig. 54.17). Contact with a jellyfish may result in systemic symptoms such as hypotension, muscle spasm, and respiratory paralysis, and may be fatal.[38] Sea urchins and other echinoderms may produce similar cutaneous and systemic symptoms as observed with coelenterates.

Other dangers of the marine environment include shark and Moray eel bites, stonefish and firefish stings, sea leech burns, and coral cuts and scratches.

Photosensitivity and Photo-Induced Disorders

Ultraviolet irradiation has both acute and chronic effects on the skin. In the traveler, skin changes due to acute sun exposure are common, including sunburn, phototoxic reactions, both drug induced and plant induced (phytophotodermatitis), photoallergic reactions, solar urticaria, polymorphic light eruption, actinic prurigo, and hydroa vacciniforme.

Chronic sun exposure over the years results in dermatoheliosis, including chronic actinic dermatitis, lentigines, actinic keratoses, and skin cancer.

Other Cosmopolitan Infections of Interest to Travelers

Hypersensitivity reaction to drugs, not only daily medications but also prophylaxis, must always be considered in the differential diagnosis of urticaria and exanthema in travelers. Adverse cutaneous reactions are a treatment-limiting effect of antimalarial drugs. In a prospective study of the tolerability of malaria chemoprophylaxis in 623 non-immune travelers to sub-Saharan Africa, the incidences of moderate or severe skin problems were 8% among persons receiving chloroquine-proguanil versus 3% for doxycycline, 2% for atovaquone-proguanil and 1% for mefloquine.[39]

Mycobacterial cutaneous infections are a possible complication of medical tourism. Indeed, a growing number of Westerners undergo plastic surgery in developing countries. As an example, 20 US 'lipotourists' have been infected with *Mycobacterium abscessus* after abdominoplasty in the Dominican Republic, highlighting the risks of traveling abroad for surgery.[40]

Exacerbation of chronic diseases such as acne, atopic dermatitis, lupus erythematosus, dermatomyositis, pemphigus foliaceus, and several of the porphyries may occur, and some of them result from sun exposure. Other dermatoses of interest include miliaria rubra, frostbite, plant-related dermatoses, and contact dermatitis.

Diagnosis of A Skin Lesion in the Traveler

The evaluation of a traveler with skin lesions first includes an extensive history with a focus on possible epidemiologic exposures.[29] The differential diagnosis is broadened. It depends on factors such as geographic location visited, length of stay, and many other entities (Table 54.3).

Complete physical examination will focus on the appearance of cutaneous lesions because dermatologic diseases are classified according to their morphologic characteristics, for example type (e.g., macule, papule, nodule, vesicle, ulcer), color (e.g., skin colored, red, brown, blue, black, hyperpigmented, hypopigmented, depigmented), shape or configuration (e.g., round, oval, annular, serpiginous, linear, zosteriform, reticulated), and distribution (e.g., localized, generalized, limited to a specific anatomic location).

Further diagnostic studies such as blood tests and serologies, skin biopsy and cultures, and imaging techniques may be warranted according to the results of clinical examination.

Table 54.3 Relevant Historical Data in the Evaluation of Skin Lesions in the Traveler

Travel history
Duration of travel
Duration of time since return
Geographic locations visited
Recent outbreaks of disease in locations visited
Fellow travelers with similar signs and symptoms
Means of transportation
Housing and lifestyle, dietary habits
Clothing and shoes worn
Exposures: beach, fresh or salt water, rural, plants, insects, animals, sexual contacts
Medications: therapeutic and prophylactic
Use of personal preventive measures: insect repellent, mosquito net
Previous medical care
Immunization against tetanus

Dermatological history
Underlying skin diseases
Alteration of skin integrity during travel
Time of onset relative to potential exposures
Time of onset relative to return
Description of initial presentation and anatomic distribution of lesion(s)
Description of progression of lesion(s)

Diseases with dermatological manifestations that are encountered by travelers are listed according to the type of cutaneous lesion and history in Table 54.4. In addition, some symptoms, signs or syndromes warrant further consideration given their frequency in travelers.

Pruritus

The diagnosis of a pruritic dermatosis relies mainly on the location of the symptoms and the presence of more specific cutaneous signs (Table 54.5). Generalized pruritus usually orients towards scabies, one of the most common causes of skin disease in travelers. Another significant cause of pruritus is ciguatera fish poisoning. Pruritus of unknown origin (PUO) is more frequently seen in immigrants and elderly patients. It is a leading reason for consultation. In a series of 60 dermatoses observed among foreign immigrants in France (92% from Africa), pruritus was the cause of consultation in 21 cases (35%), including 10 cases (16.7%) of PUO. PUO in this setting could be due to acclimatization. Self-limited and localized pruritus orients towards an allergic reaction to insect bites or stings.

Creeping Eruption, Cutaneous Larva Migrans

Creeping eruption is a clinical sign defined by a linear or serpiginous cutaneous track, slightly elevated, erythematous, and mobile. This eruption must be distinguished from other non-creeping dermatoses that give rise to serpiginous or linear cutaneous lesions. The numerous causes of creeping eruption have been reviewed recently.[41] Most of them are of parasitic origin (Table 54.6).

Cutaneous larva migrans is a syndrome defined clinically (and parasitologically) by subcutaneous migration of a non-human nematode's larva making the infected human a dead-end host. The hallmark

Table 54.4 Dermatoses Encountered by Travelers According to the Type of Cutaneous Lesion and Nature of Exposure

Clinical Presentation	Short-Term Traveler	Long-Term Traveler and Immigrant
Papules and nodules	Adverse drug reaction, acne exacerbation, miliaria rubra, sea urchin granuloma	Leprosy, tuberculosis, mycetoma, pinta, bartonellosis, glanders, yaws
	Arthropod bites, tungiasis, myiasis, tick granuloma, lice	Orf, milker's nodules
	Pyodermas, mycobacterial infection	Onchocerciasis, cysticercosis, schistosomiasis, dirofilariasis, sparganosis, trypanosomiasis
	Leishmaniasis, scabies, cercarial dermatitis, gnathostomiasis, sea-bather's eruption	Paracoccidioidomycosis, paragonimiasis, chromomycosis, West African histoplasmosis, lobomycosis
	Sporotrichosis	
Erythematous plaque	Bacterial cellulitis, pyoderma, Lyme disease	African trypanosomiasis
	Leishmaniasis	
	Dermatophytosis (tinea)	
Vesicles and bullae	Sunburn, blister beetle dermatitis, contact dermatitis, irritant dermatitis, phytophotodermatitis, miliaria rubra, fixed drug eruption	Varicella infection
	Arthropod bites	Dracunculiasis
	Bullous impetigo	
	Herpes simplex infection	
	Cutaneous larva migrans, cercarial dermatitis, sea-bather's eruption	
Ulcers	Spider bite	Cupping
	Ecthyma, pyodermas, tache noire (tick eschar)	Mycetomas, anthrax, tuberculosis, mycobacterial infection, cutaneous diphtheria, glanders, melioidosis, plague[a], yaws[a], tularemia[a]
	Herpes simplex infection	Cutaneous amebiasis, dracunculiasis
	Leishmaniasis	West African histoplasmosis, North American blastomycosis, paracoccidioidomycosis, chromomycosis
	Sporotrichosis	

Any of the diseases listed above that may affect the short-term traveler may also affect the long-term traveler and immigrant and vice versa.
[a]Primary inoculation site.

Table 54.5 Causes of Pruritus in Travelers

Localized pruritus	Contact dermatitis, irritant dermatitis, phytophotodermatitis, arthropod bite, lice, sea-bather's eruption
	Cercarial dermatitis, cutaneous larva migrans, enterobiasis (perianal), gnathostomiasis, loiasis, strongyloidiasis (larva currens)
Generalized pruritus	Adverse drug reactions, ciguatera fish poisoning, atopic dermatitis exacerbation
	Varicella (in adult)
	Scabies
	Loiasis, onchocerciasis, African trypanosomiasis
	Schistosomiasis, ascariasis, hookworm, trichinellosis and strongyloidiasis (in association with urticarial rash during invasive phase)

Table 54.6 Causes of Creeping Eruption

Nematode: larva	Strongyloidiasis (larva currens)
	Hookworm-related cutaneous larva migrans
	Gnathostomiasis
	Dirofilariasis
Trematode larva	*Fasciola gigantica*
Nematode: adult	Loiasis
	Dracunculiasis
Maggot	Myiasis (due to *Gasterophilus* spp.)
Mites	Human scabies
	Pyemotes ventricosus

is a creeping eruption. This syndrome is due to subcutaneous larval migration of various animal nematodes such as hookworms (hookworm-related cutaneous larva migrans), *Gnathostoma* spp (gnathostomiasis), *Pelodera strongyloides* (and various zoonotic species of *Strongyloides*), *Dirofilaria* sp. and *Spirulina* sp.[1] By definition, this syndrome does not include diseases in which creeping eruption is due to the subcutaneous migration of a human nematode's larva (*Strongyloides stercoralis*, i.e., larva currens), a trematode larvae (*Fasciola gigantica*), fly's maggot (migratory myiasis), adult nematode (*Loa loa*,

Dracunculus medinensis), or mites (human scabies due to *Sarcoptes scabiei*, *Pyemotes* dermatitis due to *Pyemotes ventricosus*). The same applies to parasites whose larvae do not give rise to migratory signs when they travel through the skin (onchocerciasis, human hookworms whose larva are just in transit through the skin, i.e., ground itch).[41]

Urticaria

Acute urticaria is a common reason for consultation. The causes of urticaria are numerous (Table 54.7). The travel history may provide epidemiologic clues, such as exposure to fresh water (Katayama fever associated with acute schistosomiasis), ingestion of fish (anisakiasis),

Table 54.7 Causes of Urticaria in Travelers or Expatriates

Adverse drug reaction
Hepatitis A infection
Invasive phase of helminthic diseases: schistosomiasis, ascariasis, hookworm, strongyloidiasis, and fascioliasis
Chronic phase of helminthic disease where man is a dead-end host: trichinellosis, toxocariasis
Rupture of cyst during hydatidosis

Table 54.8 Causes of Fever and Rash in Travelers

Adverse drug reaction
Meningococcemia (purpura), typhoid fever, syphilis, rat-bite fever, leptospirosis, trench fever, rickettsial infections, brucellosis
Measles, rubella, Epstein–Barr virus, HIV and cytomegalovirus primary infection, dengue, chikungunya, West Nile and other arboviral infections, viral hemorrhagic fever
African trypanosomiasis, trichinellosis, toxoplasmosis

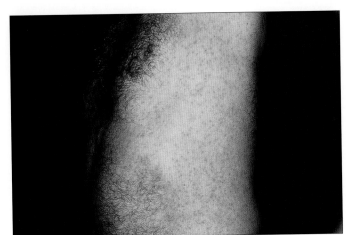

Figure 54.19 Febrile Rash in Dengue Fever (Thailand).

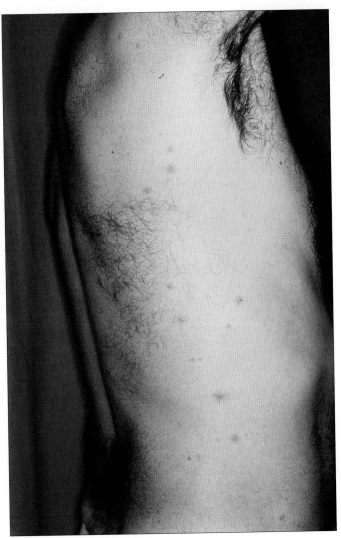

Figure 54.18 Febrile Rash in African Tick Bite Fever (South Africa).

undercooked meats (trichinellosis) and raw vegetables (ascariasis), or walking barefoot (hookworm, strongyloidiasis).[29] Adverse drug reactions must also be considered in the differential diagnosis of urticaria.[29]

Febrile Rash

The occurrence of febrile maculopapular rash warrants immediate attention. Indeed, the association of rash and fever may herald a life-threatening infectious disease such as hemorrhagic viral fever, meningococcemia, rickettsial infections (Fig. 54.18), or typhoid fever.[29]

Otherwise, it points to adverse drug reaction or viral infection (Table 54.8). The most frequent cause of febrile rash in travelers is probably dengue (Fig. 54.19), with a frequency estimated at 30%.[42] The development of a rash within 10 days after return is suggestive of arboviral infection, mostly in cases of mucous membrane involvement. The skin manifestations of dengue fever infection are remarkably similar to those described for chikungunya, with a diffuse, sometimes pruritic, macular or maculopapular exanthema in which small islands of normal skin are spared.[42]

Alternatively, the high prevalence of measles and the low vaccine coverage, especially (but not only) in developing countries, can be a problem for non-immune travelers and can be responsible for measles importation in Western countries, with subsequent outbreaks.[29]

Edema

Localized edematous plaque anywhere on the body surface is always suggestive of infectious cellulitis when inflammatory, and of a reaction to arthropod (cellulitis-like reaction) when pruritic. When localized to a limb, it points to acute lymphatic filariasis, lymphedema of onchocerciasis, or Calabar swelling of loiasis. It may also suggest gnathostomiasis when located elsewhere, and American trypanosomiasis or trichinellosis when located on the face.[29]

Nodular Lymphangitis

Nodular lymphangitis is defined by an eruption of nodules along the lymphatic vessels of a limb, usually the arm or forearm, thus conferring the so-called sporotrichoid pattern.[43] This condition primarily suggests cutaneous leishmaniasis and sporotrichosis. However, this sign has been linked to many other causes, such as tularemia, cat-scratch disease, pyogenic or mycobacterial infection.

Sexually Transmitted Infections

Travel is a major factor contributing to the spread of sexually transmitted infections (STI), as it can remove many of the social taboos that normally restrict sexual behavior.[44] Between 5% and 51% of short-term travelers engage in casual sex while abroad. Moreover, it is estimated that between 25% and 75% of travelers do not use condoms when they have casual sex abroad. In Finnish travelers, 39% of round-the-world travelers and 30% of tourists to Thailand reported having had 'high-risk' behavior.[2]

Sexually transmitted diseases (STD) are particularly frequent in travelers. STDs were the sixth cause of consultation, accounting for 3.5% of the 637 diseases diagnosed in travelers returning from the tropics to Paris. The spectrum of STDs presumably acquired during travel has been found to be broad.[45] The main diagnoses of STDs are gonococcal urethritis, herpes simplex virus-2 infection, and *Chlamydia trachomatis* infection; primary syphilis and primary human immunodeficiency infection may also be diagnosed.

Gonococcal infection is the most frequent cause of STDs in travelers. STDs contracted in tropical areas may be unusual (donovanosis, lymphogranuloma venereum) or have a different antibiotic susceptibility profile from that seen in Western countries. Genital ulceration suggests primary syphilis, herpes and chancroid, possibly donovanosis and rarely lymphogranuloma venereum. A genital discharge points to gonococcal, *Chlamydia trachomatis*, or *Mycoplasma genitalium* infections. Inguinal suppurative bubo suggests chancroid when it is close to a genital ulcer (Fig. 54.20) and lymphogranuloma venereum when it follows a self-healing genital lesion. When these pathogens are acquired abroad, it is preferable to test for antimicrobial susceptibility as most strains are resistant to common antibiotics.

Conclusion

Travelers abroad must be instructed to take precautions to prevent the most common skin diseases during travel. They must be appropriately vaccinated against tetanus before departure and specifically instructed to avoid arthropods bites, sun overexposure and STIs. They should be informed of the risk of acquiring localized cutaneous leishmaniasis, hookworm-related cutaneous larva migrans, tungiasis, pyoderma, and STIs. Travel first-aid kits should include antibiotics effective against bacterial skin infection, oral antihistamines and corticosteroid ointments.

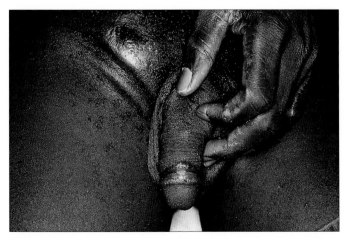

Figure 54.20 Genital ulcer Associated with Inguinal Bubo, Chancroid (Mali).

References

1. Peltola H, Kironseppa H, Holsa P. Trips to the south; a health hazard. Morbidity of Finnish travelers. Scand J Infect Dis 1983;15:375–81.
2. Hill DR. Health problems in a large cohort of Americans traveling to developing countries. J Travel Med 2000;7:259–66.
3. Hochedez P, Vinsentini P, Ansart S, et al. Changes in the pattern of health disorders diagnosed among two cohorts of French travelers to Nepal, 17 years apart. J Travel Med 2004;11:341–6.
4. Shlim DR. Learning from experience: travel medicine in Kathmandu. Travel medicine 2. Proceedings of the Second Conference on International Travel Medicine. Atlanta: International Society of Travel Medicine; 1992.
5. Raju R, Smal N, Sorokin M. Incidence of minor and major disorders among visitors to Fiji. Travel medicine 2. Proceedings of the Second Conference on International Travel Medicine. Atlanta: International Society of Travel Medicine; 1992.
6. Plentz K. Nontropical and noninfectious diseases among travelers in a tropical area during five year period (1986–1990). Travel medicine 2. Proceedings of the Second Conference on International Travel Medicine. Atlanta: International Society of Travel Medicine; 1992.
7. Sanchez JL, Gelnett J, Petruccelli BP, et al. Diarrheal disease incidence and morbidity among United States military personnel during short-term missions overseas. Am J Trop Med Hyg 1998;58:299–304.
8. Caumes E, Le Bris V, Couzigou C, et al. Dermatoses associated with travel to Burkina Faso and diagnosed by means of teledermatology. Br J Dermatol 2004;150:312–6.
9. Caumes E, Carrière J, Guermonprez G, et al. Dermatoses associated with travel to tropical countries: a prospective study of the diagnosis and management of 269 patients presenting to a tropical disease unit. Clin Infect Dis 1995;20:542–8.
10. Ansart S, Perez L, Jaureguiberry S, et al. Spectrum of dermatoses in 165 travelers returning from the tropics with skin diseases. Am J Trop Med Hyg 2007;76:184–6.
11. Lederman ER, Weld LH, Elyazar IR, et al. Dermatologic conditions of the ill returned traveler: an analysis from the GeoSentinel Surveillance Network. Int J Infect Dis 2008;12:593–602.
12. Herwaldt BL, Stokes SL, Juranek DD. American cutaneous leishmaniasis in US travelers. Ann Intern Med 1993;118:779–84.
13. Bouchaud O, Houzé S, Schiemann R, et al. Cutaneous larva migrans in travelers: a prospective study, with assessment of therapy with Ivermectin. Clin Infect Dis 2000;31:493–8.
14. Tremblay A, MacLean JD, Gyorkos T, et al. Outbreak of cutaneous larva migrans in a group of travelers. Trop Med Intern Health 2000;5:330–4.
15. Green AD, Mason C, Spragg PM. Outbreak of cutaneous larva migrans among British Military Personnel in Belize. J Travel Med 2001;8:267–9.
16. Hochedez P, Caumes E. Hookworm-related cutaneous larva migrans. J Travel Med 2007;14:339–46.
17. Heukelbach J, Feldmeier H. Epidemiological and clinical characteristics of hookworm-related cutaneous larva migrans. Lancet Infect Dis 2008;8:302–9.
18. Caumes E, Ly F, Bricaire F. Cutaneous larva migrans with folliculitis: report of seven cases and review of the literature. Br J Derm 2002;146:1–3.
19. Caumes E, Carrière J, Datry A, et al. A randomized trial of ivermectin versus albendazole for the treatment of cutaneous larva migrans. Am J Trop Med Hyg 1993;49:641–4.
20. Melby PC, Kreutzer RD, McMahon-Pratt D, et al. Cutaneous leishmaniasis: review of 59 cases seen at the National Institutes of Health. Clin Infect Dis 1992;15:924–37.
21. Weitzel T, Muhlberger N, Jelineck T, et al. Imported leishmaniasis in Germany 2001–2004: data of the SIMPID surveillance network. J Eur Clin Microbiol Infect Dis 2005;24:471–6.
22. El Hajj L, Thellier M, Carriere J, et al. Localized cutaneous leishmaniasis imported into Paris: a review of 39 cases. Int J Dermatol 2004;43:120–5.
23. Blum JA, Hatz CF. Treatment of cutaneous leishmaniasis in travelers 2009. J Travel Med 2009;16:123–31.
24. Schwartz E, Hatz C, Blum J. New world cutaneous leishmaniasis in travelers. Lancet Infect Dis 2006;6:342–9.
25. Wortmann G, Zapor M, Ressner R, et al. Lipsosomal amphotericin B for treatment of cutaneous leishmaniasis. Am J Trop Med Hyg 2010;83:1028–33.

26. McGarry JW, McCall PJ, Welby S. Arthropod dermatoses acquired in the UK and overseas. Lancet 2001;357:2105–6.

27. Jelinek T, Nothdurft HD, Rieder N, et al. Cutaneous myiasis: review of 13 cases in travelers returning from tropical countries. Int J Derm 1995;34:624–6.

28. Biggar RJ, Morrow H, Morrow RH. Extensive myiasis from tumbu fly larvae in Ghana, West Africa. Clin Pediatr 1980;19:231–2.

29. Hochedez P, Caumes E. Common skin infections in travelers. J Travel Med 2008;15:223–33.

30. Veraldi S, Valsecchi M. Imported tungiasis: a report of 19 cases and review of the literature. Int J Dermatol 2007;46:1061–6.

31. Menard A, Dos Santos G, Dekumyoy P, et al. Imported cutaneous gnathostomiasis: report of five cases. Trans R Soc Trop Med Hyg 2003;97:200–2.

32. Bavastrelli M, Bertucci P, Midula M, et al. Ciguatera fish poisoning: an emerging syndrome in Italian travelers. J Travel Med 2000;8:139–42.

33. Nozais JP, Caumes E, Datry A, et al. A propos de cinq nouveaux cas d'oedème onchocerquien. Bull Soc Path Exot 1997;90:335–8.

34. Hochedez P, Canestri A, Lecso M, et al. Skin and soft tissue infections in returning travelers. Am J Trop Med Hyg 2009;80:431–4.

35. Helgason KO, Jones ME, Edwards G. Panton-Valentine leukocidin-positive Staphylococcus aureus and foreign travel. J Clin Microbiol 2008;46:832–3.

36. Freudenthal AR, Joseph PR. Seabather's eruption. N Engl J Med 1993;329:542–4.

37. Auerbach PS. Marine envenomations. N Engl J Med 1991;325:486–95.

38. Fenner PJ, Lippmann J, Gershwin LA. Fatal and nonfatal severe jellyfish stings in Thai waters. J Travel Med 2010;17:133–8.

39. Schlagenhauf P, Tschopp A, Johnson R, et al. Tolerability of malaria chemoprophylaxis in non-immune travelers to sub-Saharan Africa: multicentre, randomised, double blind, four arm study. BMJ 2003;327:1078.

40. Furuya EY, Paez A, Srinivasan A, et al. Outbreak of *Mycobacterium abscessus* wound infections among 'lipotourists' from the United States who underwent abdominoplasty in the Dominican Republic. Clin Infect Dis 2008;46:1181–8.

41. Caumes E. Creeping eruption, a sign, has to be distinguished from hookworm-related cutaneous larva migrans, a disease. Dermatology 2006;4:659–60.

42. Hochedez P, Canestri A, Guihot A, et al. Management of travelers with fever and exanthema notably dengue and chikungunya infections. Am J Trop Med Hyg 2008;78:710–13.

43. Kostman JR, DiNubile MJ. Nodular lymphangitis: a distinctive but often unrecognized syndrome. Ann Intern Med 1993;118:883–8.

44. Matteelli A, Carosi G. Sexually transmitted diseases in travelers. Clin Infect Dis 2001;32:1063–7.

45. Ansart S, Hochedez P, Perez L, et al. Sexually transmitted diseases diagnosed among travelers returning from the tropics. J Travel Med. 2009;16:79–83.

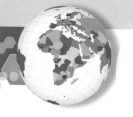

55

Eosinophilia

Amy D. Klion

Key points

- Eosinophilia, as defined by ≥450 blood eosinophils/μL, occurs in up to 10% of travelers
- It may be caused by a variety of conditions, including allergies and asthma, drug hypersensitivity, infection, neoplasm, and other miscellaneous disorders
- One-third of returned travelers with eosinophilia are asymptomatic at the time of presentation, and helminth infection, notably schistosomiasis, filariasis, strongyloidiasis, and hookworm infection, is the most common treatable cause
- An accurate exposure history is crucial to the evaluation of eosinophilia
- The utility of screening tests, including liver function tests, IgE levels, and chest radiography, remains controversial in asymptomatic returned travelers

Introduction

Eosinophilia, as defined by ≥450 blood eosinophils/μL in the peripheral blood, occurs in up to 10% of travelers[1] and may be caused by a variety of conditions, including allergies and asthma, drug hypersensitivity, infection, neoplasm, and other miscellaneous disorders (Table 55.1). Although the utility of screening for eosinophilia in returned travelers remains controversial, eosinophilia may be the first (or only) indication of a condition associated with potentially serious sequelae, such as schistosomiasis or strongyloidiasis, and is often useful in guiding the diagnostic evaluation in symptomatic patients. In this chapter, the causes of eosinophilia in travelers will be reviewed and a systematic approach to patients with eosinophilia in the presence and absence of symptoms will be presented.

Eosinophil Biology

Eosinophils are bone marrow-derived leukocytes that are found predominantly in peripheral tissues that interface with the environment, such as the lungs, skin, and gastrointestinal tract. Whereas eosinophil levels in the peripheral blood are normally ≤450/mm³, eosinophil numbers can increase dramatically in certain disease states, including

acute helminth infection and hypereosinophilic syndrome, reaching levels of >20 000/mm³. In these situations, blood eosinophils may undergo characteristic morphologic and functional changes that have been associated with 'cellular activation' and eosinophil-induced tissue damage, including endomyocardial fibrosis and peripheral neuropathy.

Peripheral blood eosinophil levels exhibit diurnal variation, with the highest levels occurring in the early morning when endogenous corticosteroid levels are low. Levels may be decreased (eosinopenia) in acute bacterial and viral infections, acute malaria, pregnancy, and in response to certain medications, including corticosteroids, epinephrine, and estrogens. Conversely, the use of β-adrenergic blockers can result in a mild increase in eosinophil counts.

The development of eosinophilia in response to a particular stimulus (e.g., helminth infection, allergen exposure) is dependent not only on the nature of the offending agent, but on the host immune response to that agent. In the case of helminth infection, the stage of parasite development, the location of the helminth within the host and the parasite burden are important determinants of the host immune response, and consequently of the degree of eosinophilia. Although tissue invasion by the parasite tends to be associated with a pronounced peripheral blood eosinophilia, the eosinophil response may be restricted to the involved tissues. Finally, eosinophilia is more pronounced in travelers to helminth-endemic areas (i.e., individuals not previously exposed to helminth infections) than in residents of those areas.[2,3]

Causes of Eosinophilia

Overview

Although the list of potential etiologies of eosinophilia is overwhelming, the most commonly identified cause of eosinophilia in returned travelers is unquestionably helminth infection. It should be noted, however, that the absence of eosinophilia does not exclude helminth infection. Allergic diseases, including drug hypersensitivity, account for the second largest group of travelers with eosinophilia in most studies. Consequently, although the initial evaluation of travelers with eosinophilia should include screening for the most common helminth infections, non-infectious causes of eosinophilia should be considered before an extensive evaluation for unusual parasitic causes of eosinophilia is undertaken.

©2012 Elsevier Inc
DOI: 10.1016/B978-1-4557-1076-8.00055-7

Table 55.1 Conditions Associated with Eosinophilia[a]

Allergic Disorders

Asthma

Atopic dermatitis

Allergic rhinitis

Drug Hypersensitivity (see Table 55.2)

Infection

Parasitic

    Helminth

    Ectoparasite (scabies, myiasis)

    Protozoan (*Isospora belli*, sarcocystis)

Bacterial (resolving scarlet fever, chronic tuberculosis)

Fungal (coccidiomycosis, allergic bronchopulmonary aspergillosis)

Viral (human immunodeficiency virus)

Neoplasm

Eosinophilic leukemia (rare)

Myelogenous leukemia

Lymphoma, especially Hodgkin's

Adenocarcinoma of the bowel, lung, ovary or other solid organs

Connective Tissue Disorders

Churg–Strauss vasculitis

Systemic lupus erythematosus

Rheumatoid arthritis

Primary Eosinophilic Disorders

Idiopathic hypereosinophilic syndrome

Eosinophilic gastroenteritis

Chronic eosinophilic pneumonia

Familial hypereosinophilia

Episodic angioedema and eosinophilia

Kimura's disease

Other

Hypoadrenalism

Sarcoid

Ulcerative colitis

Radiation

Cholesterol embolization

[a]Lists are not exhaustive.

A definitive diagnosis is found in 16–45% of travelers with eosinophilia,[1,4] and the likelihood of a definitive diagnosis increases with the duration of travel and the degree of eosinophilia (>60% in patients with ≥16% eosinophils[1]). Surprisingly, the presence or absence of symptoms does not appear to influence the diagnostic yield.[4]

Allergic Disorders/Asthma

Allergic disorders, including allergic rhinitis, atopic disease, and asthma, are extremely common in the general population and are a common cause of mild eosinophilia. Changes in the external environment associated with travel can lead to an exacerbation (or improvement) in allergic disease; however, marked eosinophilia (≥3000 eosinophils/mm[3]) is rare in the absence of another cause (e.g., helminth infection, drug hypersensitivity).

Drug Hypersensitivity

Among non-infectious causes of eosinophilia in travelers, drug-related hypersensitivity reactions are among the most common, accounting for up to 20% of cases of eosinophilia in some studies.[5] Although any drug has the potential to cause eosinophilia, some are more likely to do so,

Table 55.2 Common Drugs Associated with Eosinophilia in Travelers

Clinical Manifestation	Drug(s)[a]
Asymptomatic or skin rash	Antibiotics, including penicillins, cephalosporins, quinolones, quinine and quinine derivatives, macrolides
Pulmonary infiltrates	Non-steroidal anti-inflammatory agents; sulfa-containing drugs
Hepatitis	Tetracyclines; semi-synthetic penicillins
Interstitial nephritis	Cephalosporins; semi-synthetic penicillins
Asthma, nasal polyps	Aspirin

[a]*Note*: this list is limited to common drugs that may be used in the treatment and prevention of travel-related illnesses, such as malaria, travelers' diarrhea, skin and upper respiratory infections.

including many of the agents used to prevent or treat malaria and travelers' diarrhea (i.e., quinine, quinolones, tetracyclines, and sulfonamides). Prescription and non-prescription drugs, as well as dietary supplements and herbal medications, have been implicated (Table 55.2).

In many instances, drug-induced eosinophilia is entirely asymptomatic. End-organ involvement, such as pulmonary infiltrates, interstitial nephritis, hepatitis, or rash, can occur, however, and may be suggestive of hypersensitivity to a particular agent. In addition, some drugs are associated with specific syndromes, such as tryptophan-induced eosinophilia myalgia syndrome.

Infection

Helminths

Helminth infections are the most commonly identified cause of eosinophilia in travelers, accounting for 30–60% of cases, depending on the study.[5,6] Although intestinal nematode infection, filariasis, strongyloidiasis, and schistosomiasis comprise the majority of cases in most studies, the precise causes depend on the particular population studied, and the location and duration of travel. It is important to remember that although helminth infection is a common cause of eosinophilia, not all patients with documented helminth infection have eosinophilia. In one study of 1107 travelers with schistosomiasis, only 44% had eosinophilia.[7] Similar findings have been reported in other helminth infections, including strongyloidiasis and hookworm infection.[8] In addition, helminths that do not invade tissues at all during their lifecycle, such as *Trichuris* and *Enterobius*, rarely cause eosinophilia.

Marked eosinophilia tends to be associated with tissue invasion and is seen in a relatively limited number of infections (Table 55.3). In some infections, including ascariasis and hookworm infection, marked eosinophilia is seen only in the early phase of infection, when developing larvae migrate through the lungs or other tissues and come into contact with the cells of the host immune system. In most instances, eosinophilia gradually resolves over time with or without anthelminthic treatment. However, chronic eosinophilia does occur in some infections (Table 55.4).

Ectoparasites

Scabies infestation occurs worldwide and is an unusual, but treatable, cause of eosinophilia in travelers.[9] Sensitization to the mites and their eggs typically produces intense itching, rash and erythema, which is accompanied by mild to moderate eosinophilia in up to 10% of cases. Although data regarding eosinophilia and other common ectoparasite infestations are lacking, hypersensitivity reactions can occur in response to flea, bedbug, and tick bites. Rare cases of hypereosinophilic syndrome secondary to myiasis (infestation by fly larvae) have been reported, with complete resolution following removal of the larvae.[10]

Protozoa

Protozoan infections, including giardiasis and amebiasis, are not associated with eosinophilia. Consequently, the identification of protozoa in the stool should prompt further search for an underlying cause. Infection with the intestinal coccidian parasite *Isospora belli*, which causes diarrhea and malabsorption, is a rare exception to this rule and has been associated with eosinophilia in a minority of cases.[11] The parasite may be detected in the stool by modified acid-fast stain, or in intestinal biopsies. Sarcocystis has also been associated with outbreaks of acute symptomatic eosinophilic myositis.[12]

Other

Bacterial, fungal and viral infections typically cause eosinopenia and may suppress eosinophilia from other causes. An important exception is HIV infection. Numerous studies have demonstrated an increased risk of sexually transmitted diseases, including HIV, in travelers. Increased eosinophil counts in HIV-infected individuals may be the direct result of immune dysregulation produced by the HIV infection itself, or may occur secondary to drug hypersensitivity or hypoadrenalism.[13] Peripheral blood eosinophilia may also accompany eosinophilic pustular folliculitis, a chronic pruritic dermatosis seen in advanced HIV disease. Other notable exceptions include coccidioidomycosis[14] and chronic tuberculosis,[15] which can be acquired during travel and are associated with eosinophilia in a minority of cases.

Other Causes

Eosinophilia can be seen in a variety of common disorders associated with dysregulation of the immune response, including neoplasms, connective tissue diseases, sarcoidosis,[16] and ulcerative colitis.[17] Less frequent etiologies include hypoadrenalism, irradiation, and a variety of primary eosinophilic disorders (Table 55.2). Although these disorders are unlikely to be caused by travel, eosinophilia arising from any of these conditions may first be detected during a post-travel evaluation.

Clinical Syndromes

Skin/Soft Tissue Involvement

Dermatologic problems (Table 55.5) are among the most frequent complaints in returning travelers and are commonly associated with eosinophilia.[9,18] In a prospective study of returning French travelers, cutaneous larva migrans, myiasis, filariasis, urticaria, and scabies, all of which can be associated with eosinophilia, were among the 10 most frequent dermatologic diagnoses.[9] Of note, exacerbations of

Table 55.3 Helminth Infections Associated with Eosinophilia

Mild to moderate eosinophilia (≤3000/mm³)	
Anisakiasis[a]	Echinostomiasis
Capillariasis[a]	Enterobiasis
Coenurosis	Heterophyiasis
Cysticercosis	Hymenolepiasis
Dicrocoeliasis	Metagonimiasis
Dirofilariasis	Sparganosis
Dracunculiasis	Trichuriasis
Echinococcosis	

Marked eosinophilia (>3000/mm³)	
Angiostrongyliasis[a]	Mansonellosis
Ascariasis[a]	Onchocerciasis
Clonorchiasis[a]	Opisthorchiasis[a]
Fascioliasis[a]	Paragonimiasis[a]
Fasciolopsiasis	Schistosomiasis[a]
Gnathostomiasis	Strongyloidiasis[a]
Hookworm infection[a]	Trichinosis[a]
Loiasis	Visceral larva migrans
Lymphatic filariasis	

[a]Eosinophilia predominantly during acute phase of infection.

Table 55.4 Helminthic Causes of Eosinophilia of >2 Years' Duration

Cysticercosis[a]	Mansonellosis
Clonorchiasis	Onchocerciasis
Echinococcosis[a]	Opisthorchiasis
Fascioliasis	Paragonimiasis
Gnathostomiasis	Schistosomiasis
Hookworm infection	Strongyloidiasis
Loiasis	Visceral larva migrans
Lymphatic filariasis	

[a]Intermittent eosinophilia due to cyst leakage.

Table 55.5 Evaluation of Eosinophilia with Dermatologic Manifestations

Clinical Manifestation	Most Common Etiologies	Diagnostic Tests
Urticaria	Helminth infection Drug hypersensitivity Idiopathic	Stool for ova and parasites, serology
Chronic pruritic dermatitis	Onchocerciasis Scabies Drug hypersensitivity	Skin snips, serology Skin scraping
Subcutaneous nodules	Onchocerciasis Myiasis	Skin snips, excisional biopsy, serology Visual inspection
Migratory angioedema	Loiasis Gnathostomiasis	Serology, midday blood filtration for microfilariae Serology, excision of parasite
Serpiginous lesions	Cutaneous larva migrans Strongyloidiasis	Visual inspection Serology, stool for larvae

Helminth infections that commonly cause urticaria include ascariasis, fascioliasis, gnathostomiasis, hookworm infection, filariasis, paragonimiasis, schistosomiasis, strongyloidiasis, trichinosis, and visceral larva migrans.

pre-existing skin conditions, such as atopic dermatitis, eczema and psoriasis, can be precipitated by tropical climates and should be included in the differential diagnosis of travel-related dermatologic disorders.[18] Although skin biopsy (or skin snips in suspected onchocerciasis) may be necessary in some cases, many dermatologic causes of eosinophilia can be identified by observation alone.

Urticaria is a frequent symptom in the general population and may be idiopathic or related to a variety of allergies. In travelers with eosinophilia, urticaria may signal the presence of a drug allergy or a helminth infection. Transient pruritic skin rashes also occur in response to a variety of stimuli, including but not limited to the penetration of the skin by a variety of helminth larvae, such as hookworm species, *Strongyloides*, and schistosomes. The differential diagnosis of persistent or recurrent dermatitis and eosinophilia is more restrictive, with onchocerciasis, scabies, and hypersensitivity reactions among the most common causes in travelers.

Subcutaneous nodules may be present in a number of infections commonly associated with eosinophilia, including onchocerciasis, dirofilariasis, paragonimiasis, fascioliasis, trichinosis, echinococcosis, cysticercosis, coenurosis, sparganosis, and myiasis. In many of these infections, including onchocerciasis and cysticercosis, subcutaneous nodules are painless and easily overlooked. Since excisional biopsy of such nodules can be diagnostic, a careful skin and soft tissue examination should be undertaken if one of these infections is suspected. Over time, with the death of the parasite, nodules may calcify and become detectable in soft tissue films.

Invasion of the skin by larval maggots of the *Diptera* species (myiasis) typically produces painful nodules that may be confused with a furuncle. Visible movement of the maggot within the characteristic central punctum is diagnostic. Painful subcutaneous nodules that migrate are the hallmark of sparganosis, a disease caused by migration of tapeworm larvae of *Spirometra* species through the subcutaneous tissues of humans or other paratenic hosts.[19]

Localized, intermittent, migratory angioedema is characteristic of loiasis, a filarial infection that is endemic in Central and West Africa. Infective *Loa loa* larvae are transmitted through the bite of infected *Chrysops* flies and develop into adult worms that migrate through the subcutaneous tissues, provoking a hypersensitivity reaction (Calabar swelling).[2] Swellings are most common on the extremities and face and typically resolve within a few days, only to recur weeks to months later. Eyeworm (migration of the adult worm across the subconjunctiva) occurs in up to 20% of infected patients and, when present, is diagnostic of loiasis. Peripheral eosinophilia is present with rare exception and is frequently marked (>3000 eosinophils/mm^3). Complications, including endomyocardial fibrosis and encephalitis, are uncommon and are thought to be due to the host immune response to the parasite. In the absence of demonstrable parasites in the peripheral blood or subcutaneous tissues, a presumptive diagnosis can be made in the setting of eosinophilia, positive serology, and an appropriate exposure history.

Migrating *Gnathostoma* larvae can cause migratory angioedema indistinguishable from that of loiasis, although localized pain, pruritus and erythema are more frequent and the swellings tend to last longer (1–2 weeks).[20] Migration of larvae to deeper tissues and organs (visceral gnathostomiasis) can occur, producing a wide variety of symptoms. Endemic in parts of SE Asia, Central and South America, gnathostomiasis is usually acquired by ingestion of the parasite in inadequately cooked freshwater fish or other intermediate hosts. As in loiasis, symptoms may appear months to years after infection, and eosinophilia is often striking. Whereas recovery of the parasite is necessary for a definitive diagnosis of gnathostomiasis, positive serology in a traveler with migratory subcutaneous

Table 55.6 Causes of Eosinophilia with Pulmonary Manifestations

Transient infiltrates
    Ascariasis, hookworm infection, strongyloidiasis, drug hypersensitivity, acute eosinophilic pneumonia

Chronic infiltrates
    Tropical pulmonary eosinophilia, strongyloidiasis, drug hypersensitivity reactions, hypereosinophilic syndrome, chronic eosinophilic pneumonia, Churg–Strauss vasculitis

Eosinophilic pleural effusion
    Helminths (toxocariasis, filariasis, paragonimiasis, anisakiasis, echinococcosis, strongyloidiasis)
    Other infections (coccidiomycosis, TB)
    Other causes (malignancy, hemothorax, drug reactions, pulmonary infarct, rheumatologic disease, pneumothorax)

Parenchymal invasion with or without cavitation
    Paragonimiasis, tuberculosis, allergic bronchopulmonary aspergillosis, echinococcosis (rare)

swellings, eosinophilia and an appropriate exposure history is highly suggestive of the diagnosis.

Cutaneous larva migrans, or creeping eruption, results when the larval stages of animal hookworms inadvertently penetrate human skin. The appearance of the intensely pruritic, reddened serpiginous track, found most commonly on the feet or buttocks, is diagnostic.[21] Larva currens, the serpiginous skin lesions seen in chronic strongyloidiasis, can be easily distinguished from creeping eruption by the evanescent nature of the lesions and the speed with which they migrate (5–10 cm/h).[22] Whereas eosinophilia is present in a minority of patients with creeping eruption, it is common in patients with strongyloidiasis and may be the first clue to the diagnosis.

Pulmonary Manifestations

Migration of helminth larvae through the lung can cause eosinophilia and migratory pulmonary infiltrates, or Loeffler's syndrome (Table 55.6).[23] The most common cause of Loeffler's syndrome is infection with *Ascaris lumbricoides*, an intestinal nematode that is worldwide in distribution. Patients typically present with non–productive cough and substernal burning occurring 1–2 weeks after ingestion of embryonated eggs on contaminated foodstuffs. The symptoms resolve once larval migration is finished (within 5–10 days), but chest X-ray abnormalities and eosinophilia may persist for weeks. Diagnosis is complicated by the fact that eggs may not be apparent in the stool for months, at which time the eosinophilia has generally resolved. Consequently, the detection of *Ascaris* eggs in the stool of a traveler with marked eosinophilia should prompt a search for another cause of the eosinophilia.

Acute schistosomiasis may present with eosinophilia, cough, and transient pulmonary infiltrates; however, the presence of concomitant gastrointestinal and constitutional symptoms helps distinguish this from Loeffler's syndrome.[24] Although hookworm and *Strongyloides* larvae also pass through the lungs early in infection, this is rarely associated with pulmonary symptoms.

Unlike the transient migratory infiltrates of Loeffler's syndrome, the pulmonary infiltrates of tropical pulmonary eosinophilia, a hyperreactive form of lymphatic filariasis, persist in the absence of anthelminthic therapy.[25] Nocturnal cough or wheezing is characteristic, and the eosinophilia is accompanied by extremely high levels of serum IgE and antifilarial antibodies. A similar syndrome can be seen in strongyloidiasis.[26] Other causes of pulmonary infiltrates recurring over a period of weeks to months include drug reactions and several rare idiopathic disorders (e.g., hypereosinophilic syndrome, chronic eosinophilic pneumonia, and Churg–Strauss syndrome).

Eosinophilic pleural effusions have been described in the setting of numerous helminth infections, including echinococcosis, paragonimiasis and disseminated strongyloides infection. Fungal and mycobacterial infections, hypersensitivity reactions, malignancy, pulmonary infarct, and hemothorax have also been implicated.[27]

Relatively few infections give rise to eosinophilia and lesions of the pulmonary parenchyma. Although tuberculosis should be considered in any traveler with a cavitary lesion, eosinophilia in tuberculosis is exceedingly uncommon. Other infections to consider in the appropriate epidemiologic setting include paragonimiasis, which can present with cavitary infiltrates and hilar adenopathy, and pulmonary echinococcosis, which typically presents as a solitary cystic lesion.

Gastrointestinal Symptoms

Gastrointestinal symptoms are the most frequent complaint in returned travelers presenting to travel clinics.[28] When accompanied by peripheral blood eosinophilia, they are most often indicative of a helminth infection, although the onset of a non-infectious gastrointestinal disorder associated with eosinophilia, such as inflammatory bowel disease or eosinophilic gastroenteritis, may coincide with travel.

Transient gastrointestinal symptoms, including nausea, diarrhea, vomiting, and abdominal pain, occur in the early stages of a number of helminth infections, including trichinosis, schistosomiasis, paragonimiasis, and hookworm infection. These symptoms may precede the characteristic clinical manifestations of the infection, as in trichinosis, where abdominal pain and diarrhea, if present, develop in the first week after ingestion of contaminated pork (or other meats) as the larvae migrate to the intestine. The well-recognized syndrome of eosinophilia, myalgia, fever, and periorbital edema typically does not appear until 1–2 weeks later as new larvae migrate through the tissues and encyst in the muscle.[29] Diagnosis in these early-stage infections can be difficult, as serologic tests are often negative and production of larvae and/or eggs may not have been initiated.

Although liver fluke infections are uncommon in travelers, they do occur and need to be considered in the differential diagnosis of recurrent cholangitis and eosinophilia in travelers. Obstruction of the biliary system by an echinococcal cyst or aberrant migration of an adult *Ascaris* worm has also been reported. In *Fasciola* infection, migration of the fluke larvae through the liver parenchyma causes an acute syndrome of eosinophilia, abdominal pain, fever, and variable hepatomegaly that can last for up to 4 months.[30] Multiple small tunnel-like hypodense lesions can be seen in CT scans of the liver, and represent microabscesses. Other helminth infections, including toxocariasis,[31] can produce a similar clinical syndrome.

Neurologic Disease

Neurologic syndromes (Table 55.7) associated with eosinophilia are relatively infrequent in travelers, but include eosinophilic meningitis, seizures, focal neurologic deficits, peripheral neuropathy, transverse myelitis, and eosinophilic myeloencephalitis.

The most common cause of eosinophilic meningitis in travelers is infection with the rat lungworm, *Angiostrongylus cantonensis*, although infection with other helminths,[32] fungal infections, drug hypersensitivity, and other non-infectious causes should also be considered. *Angiostrongylus* infection is most prevalent in SE Asia and the Pacific,

Table 55.7 Evaluation of Eosinophilia with Neurologic Manifestations

Clinical Manifestation	Most Common Etiologies	Diagnostic Tests
Headache and meningeal signs	Angiostrongylus Gnathostomiasis Coccidioidomycosis Drug hypersensitivity Neoplasm, esp. Hodgkin's lymphoma	Lumbar puncture[a], serology
Headache and/or seizures	Cysticercosis Echinococcosis Schistosomiasis Paragonimiasis Fascioliasis Trichinosis Toxocariasis Sparganosis	CT, MRI, serology
Transverse myelitis	Schistosomiasis	Spine MRI, serology (serum and CSF), stool or urine exam for ova, rectal snip
Peripheral neuropathy	Loiasis	Serology, midday blood filtration for microfilariae

[a]Larvae of *Angiostrongylus* may be detected in the CSF.

but is present in other tropical areas worldwide, including the Caribbean.[33] Infection occurs following ingestion of an infected mollusk, vegetables, or other uncooked foods contaminated with mollusk slime. Whereas gastrointestinal symptoms may occur soon after ingestion of the larvae, the most common presenting complaint is an intermittent excruciating headache occurring after an incubation period of 2–30 days. Cranial nerve palsies may also be present. Lumbar puncture reveals an elevated opening pressure, pleocytosis with ≥10% eosinophils, elevated protein, and normal glucose. Infection is self-limited as larvae do not reach maturity in the human host, and treatment is supportive. Peripheral eosinophilia is marked early in infection but decreases as the infection resolves.

Headache and/or seizures in a patient with eosinophilia may be the presenting symptom of a number of helminth infections that affect the central nervous system, including cysticercosis, schistosomiasis, and echinococcosis. Focal neurologic findings may also be present. Many of these infections have a characteristic appearance on imaging studies that may facilitate diagnosis. For example, the presence of both cystic lesions with surrounding edema and calcifications in the brain parenchyma is highly suggestive of cysticercosis, whereas soap-bubble cystic lesions in a grape-like cluster with calcification are characteristic of *Paragonimus* infection, and septate lesions with daughter cysts are typical of echinococcal disease. In contrast, the mass lesions with surrounding edema that can occur in the brain and spinal cord in schistosomiasis are indistinguishable from the mass lesions of other causes.

Other neurologic syndromes that occur in association with eosinophilia include peripheral neuropathy secondary to nerve compression by angioedema in loiasis, transverse myelitis in schistosomiasis, and potentially fatal eosinophilic myeloencephalitis due to gnathostomiasis.

Fever

Because fever can suppress eosinophilia, it is not surprising that the potential etiologies of fever and eosinophilia are few. Drug hypersensitivity should be excluded in all patients. The possibility of a parasitic infection, such as acute schistosomiasis, visceral larva migrans, trichinellosis, fascioliasis, or gnathostomiasis, should also be considered, depending on the exposure history.

Asymptomatic Eosinophilia

As many as one-third of returned travelers with eosinophilia are asymptomatic at the time of presentation.[1] Helminth infection, notably schistosomiasis, filariasis, strongyloidiasis, and hookworm infection, is listed as the most frequently identified treatable cause in most studies.[1,6,34]

Schistosomiasis

Endemic in 74 countries in Africa, Asia, Central and South America, schistosomiasis is acquired when infective larvae (cercariae) swimming in fresh water penetrate the skin. A mild dermatitis at the site of penetration is sometimes seen within a few hours to 1 week after exposure. Acute schistosomiasis (Katayama fever) may occur 2–12 weeks after exposure and is characterized by fever, headache, myalgias, right upper quadrant pain, bloody diarrhea, pulmonary symptoms, and marked eosinophilia.[24] Although the acute symptoms resolve without treatment within 3–4 months after exposure, the eosinophilia may persist for many years. Central nervous system involvement is uncommon in travelers, but can lead to permanent deficits,[35] underlining the importance of early diagnosis and treatment.

The gold standard for the diagnosis of schistosomiasis remains the detection of viable parasite eggs in the stool, urine, or a tissue biopsy. However, as many as 50% of patients with chronic schistosomiasis,[36] and most patients with acute schistosomiasis,[24] will not have eggs detected in stool or urine. Serologic tests are more sensitive and can detect infection prior to the appearance of eggs in the stool or urine, but do not distinguish between active and past infection, which limits their utility in the detection of infection in long-term residents of endemic countries and travelers with a history of prior infection.

Filarial Infection

One of the most frequently identified causes of eosinophilia in long-term travelers returning from Africa is *Loa loa* infection. Although symptoms, including urticaria, myalgias, arthralgias, migratory angioedema (Calabar swellings), and eyeworm, are common, some travelers and most residents of endemic areas remain asymptomatic despite microfilariae detectable in the peripheral blood.[2]

Endemic in parts of Africa and Central and South America, onchocerciasis is the second most common filarial infection that afflicts travelers.[37] Infection typically presents with a pruritic papular dermatitis and eosinophilia, although asymptomatic infection does occur.[3] Palpable subcutaneous nodules, when present, are useful from a diagnostic standpoint, but are uncommon in travelers, who generally have light infections. The keratitis and blindness that characterize onchocerciasis in some regions of Africa are rarely, if ever, seen in temporary residents of these areas.

Lymphatic filariasis is estimated to affect 120 million people worldwide, but is a relatively uncommon cause of eosinophilia in travelers. Although acute clinical manifestations, including adenolymphangitis, fever, and recurrent swelling of the extremities or genitalia, may be seen in travelers, progression to chronic lymphedema or elephantiasis is rare. Other filariae that occasionally infect travelers include *Mansonella perstans*, which is endemic in Africa and parts of the Caribbean, *Mansonella streptocerca*, which is endemic in Western and Central Africa, and *Mansonella ozzardi*, which is found in Central and South America and on some Caribbean islands.

A definitive diagnosis of filarial infection can be made by the detection of microfilariae or their DNA in the blood or skin, identification of an adult worm, or, in the case of lymphatic filariasis due to *Wuchereria bancrofti*, by the demonstration of circulating antigen in the peripheral blood. Serology may be useful in making a presumptive diagnosis in visitors to endemic areas who have suggestive clinical symptoms or unexplained eosinophilia.

Strongyloidiasis

In most series *Strongyloides* infection accounts for a high percentage (up to 38%) of unexplained eosinophilia in travelers and immigrants.[8,38] Worldwide in distribution, *Strongyloides* infection is acquired by penetration of exposed skin by infective-stage larvae. Early in infection the developing larvae migrate through the lungs, and pulmonary symptoms may predominate. Later, infection may be associated with intermittent creeping eruption (larva currens), urticaria, or gastrointestinal symptoms, but is often asymptomatic. Because of the capacity of the third-stage larvae to reinvade the intestinal mucosa or skin of the infected host, untreated strongyloidiasis can persist for decades.[39] More importantly, life-threatening dissemination may occur in the setting of immunosuppression.

Stool examination is an insensitive means of diagnosis in strongyloidiasis, as larvae are often shed sporadically and in very low numbers. Eosinophilia is present in 40–80% of immunocompetent patients with strongyloidiasis and may be the only clue to the diagnosis.[40] However, the eosinophilia generally decreases over time and may or may not be present during hyperinfection syndromes. Serologic tests remain the most sensitive and specific method of diagnosis in travelers. Although antibody levels decrease following treatment and may be a useful marker of response to therapy, levels remain positive for long periods of time after treatment, limiting their use as a screening tool in previously infected populations.

Hookworm Infection

Although some patients with chronic hookworm infection complain of vague abdominal pain or nausea, most are asymptomatic. Eosinophilia is usually mild, but may exceed 3000/mm^3 in some cases.[41] Since hookworm infection is self-limited in the absence of treatment, eosinophilia rarely persists for >3 years.

Evaluation of Patients with Eosinophilia

Eosinophilia (Fig. 55.1) should always be confirmed with an absolute eosinophil count (eosinophils/µL blood), since an increased percentage of eosinophils may reflect a decrease in the number of non-eosinophil leukocytes (e.g., neutropenia) rather than a true increase in eosinophils. Once eosinophilia has been established, the next problem is to establish the etiology. Because the potential causes of eosinophilia are many, and the diagnostic tests required to distinguish between them are extensive, a careful history and physical examination are essential. Pre-travel eosinophil counts, if available, are useful in determining whether the eosinophilia is travel related. Similarly, pre-existent medical problems (e.g., asthma, atopic disease) associated with eosinophilia should be excluded. A detailed drug history, including over-the-counter medications, vitamins, and dietary supplements,

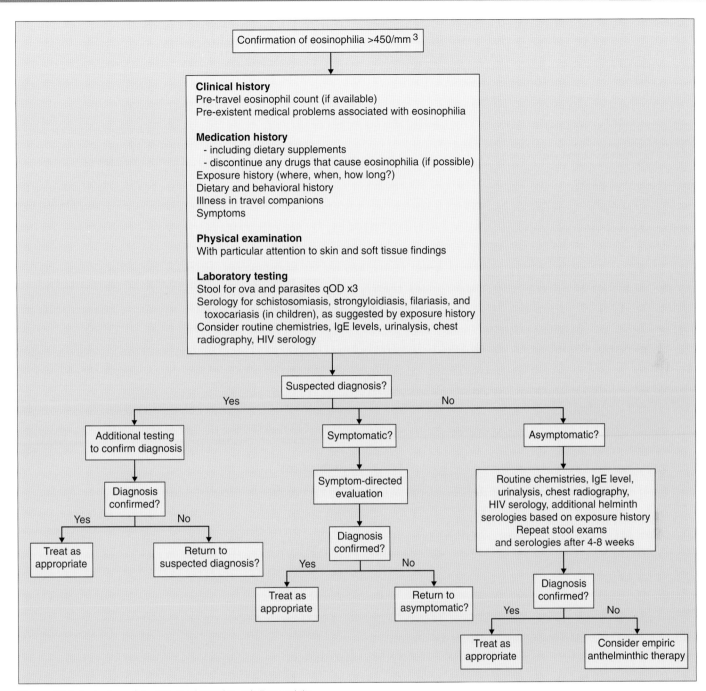

Figure 55.1 Evaluation of the Returned Traveler with Eosinophilia.

should be obtained, and drugs or other agents associated with eosinophilia should be discontinued if possible.

An accurate exposure history is crucial to the evaluation of eosinophilia. Since many infectious agents have restricted geographic distribution, or a limited lifespan, a detailed review of recent and past travel can narrow the differential diagnosis significantly.[42] For example, eosinophilia and migratory angioedema in a patient who has traveled only to SE Asia would suggest gnathostomiasis, whereas identical symptoms in a patient from West Africa would likely be due to loiasis. Similarly, abdominal symptoms and eosinophilia occurring in a traveler whose last potential exposure was 3 years prior to evaluation is not likely to be due to ascariasis (lifespan 1–2 years), but could be indicative of hookworm (lifespan ≤6 years) or *Strongyloides*

infection (lifespan in decades). The duration of exposure is also helpful, as some helminth infections, such as filariasis, paragonimiasis, and cysticercosis, are uncommon in short-term travelers, whereas others, such as schistosomiasis or trichinosis, require only a single exposure.

Most studies have demonstrated an increased incidence of certain infections, including schistosomiasis and HIV, in travelers who report risk-taking behavior; however, the absence of such a history does not exclude infection.[4] Nevertheless, significant exposures, such as a history of swimming in Lake Malawi or ingestion of raw pork, may prompt a more thorough search for a particular etiologic agent. Up-to-date information with respect to recent outbreaks or epidemics in the regions visited should be sought, since unusual causes of eosinophilia may be more likely in these settings (e.g., the outbreak of eosinophilic meningitis caused by *Angiostrongylus* in a group of students visiting the Caribbean[33]). A history of illness in travel companions can be extremely helpful, as some infections may occur in clusters as a result of exposure to a common contaminated source (e.g., schistosomiasis in a group of rafters on the Omo River in Ethiopia,[43] or trichinosis diagnosed in 13 travelers on a cruise to Alaska[44]).

A detailed symptom history should be elicited, including symptoms that occurred during or soon after travel but have since resolved, as they may provide important clues to the underlying diagnosis. Similarly, a careful physical examination should be performed, with particular attention to the dermatologic examination, since skin and soft tissue findings, such as larva currens (the fleeting serpiginous rash of strongyloidiasis) and the mild unilateral limb swelling due to early lymphatic filariasis, are easily missed.

Although the exposure history, symptoms and signs may help to narrow down the possible etiologies of eosinophilia in travelers and guide the diagnostic evaluation, specific features of the eosinophilia can also be useful. For example, intermittent eosinophilia is characteristic of echinococcosis and cysticercosis, and reflects the inflammatory response to leakage of cyst contents. Marked eosinophilia ($\geq 3000/mm^3$) is most commonly associated with tissue-invasive helminth infections and drug hypersensitivity reactions.

If the history and physical examination do not point to a specific diagnosis, three stool specimens collected 48 h apart should be obtained to look for ova and parasites. Specimens should be examined by direct smear and using a concentration technique. In patients with potential exposure to *Schistosoma haematobium*, urinalysis and examination of three midday urine specimens for ova and parasites should also be performed.

Whereas routine stool examination will detect most helminths with an intestinal phase in their lifecycle, their sensitivity is poor in the detection of strongyloidiasis, a common infection that may be asymptomatic, prolonged (up to several decades) and associated with potentially life-threatening complications. Tissue parasites, including schistosomiasis, filariae, *Trichinella* and agents of visceral larva migrans, will also be missed. Consequently *Strongyloides* serology is indicated in the assessment of all travelers with unexplained eosinophilia, and serology for the most common helminth infections (schistosomiasis, strongyloidiasis, and filariasis) is recommended, as suggested by the exposure history.

The utility of additional screening tests, including liver function tests, IgE levels and chest radiography, remains controversial in asymptomatic returned travelers. These tests, as well as other diagnostic procedures, including biopsies, radiologic studies, and specific serologic tests, should be guided by the patient's symptoms and exposure history. For example, the initial evaluation of a returned traveler with jaundice and eosinophilia following a trip to rural China should include stool examination for ova and parasites, liver function studies, and abdominal imaging, as well as serologies for schistosomiasis, toxocariasis, and the liver flukes. In contrast, evaluation of the same traveler complaining of dyspnea and cough should include a chest X-ray, sputum for larvae, eggs and acid-fast bacilli, and serologic studies for schistosomiasis, strongyloidiasis, and filariasis.

Because of the long pre-patent period characteristic of some helminth infections, eosinophilia may occur at a time when parasitologic diagnosis is not possible, e.g., prior to egg secretion or antibody positivity. The clinical manifestations of early infection may be markedly different from those occurring later, further obscuring the diagnosis (e.g., acute schistosomiasis). Repeat stool examinations and/or serology should be considered in 4–8 weeks.

Approach to the Patient with Undiagnosed Eosinophilia

Despite extensive evaluation, up to 50% of cases of eosinophilia remain undiagnosed.[6,8,42] In such cases, empiric anthelminthic therapy with albendazole (400 mg p.o. b.i.d. for 3 days) should be considered prior to beginning an extensive evaluation for non-infectious etiologies.[6,42] If serology is not available, the addition of ivermectin and/or praziquantel may be warranted to treat occult strongyloidiasis and/or schistosomiasis, respectively. In patients with persistently elevated eosinophil counts $\geq 1500/mm^3$, evaluation for eosinophil-related end-organ damage is warranted, as well as a comprehensive evaluation for non-infectious etiologies of eosinophilia, including myeloproliferative disorders.

Conclusion

Although screening for eosinophilia may not be appropriate in all cases, it can be a useful tool in the evaluation of returned travelers, particularly those with potential exposure to helminth infections. Because of the wide spectrum of causes of eosinophilia, a careful exposure and symptom history is crucial to narrow down the diagnostic possibilities. The initial evaluation of all travelers with eosinophilia should include screening for the most common helminth infections to which they may have been exposed, since several of these, including strongyloidiasis, schistosomiasis, and filariasis, are associated with potentially serious long-term sequelae. Non-infectious causes should be considered, however, before an extensive evaluation for unusual parasitic causes of eosinophilia is undertaken.

References

1. Schulte C, Krebs B, Jelinek T, et al. Diagnostic significance of blood eosinophilia in returned travelers. Clin Infect Dis 2002;34:407–11.
2. Klion AD, Massougbodji M, Sadeler B-C, et al. Loiasis in endemic and non-endemic populations: immunologically mediated differences in clinical presentation. J Infect Dis 1991;163:1318–25.
3. McCarthy JS, Ottesen EA, Nutman TB. Onchocerciasis in endemic and nonendemic populations: differences in clinical presentation and immunologic findings. J Infect Dis 1994;170:736–41.
4. Whitty CJM, Carroll B, Armstrong M, et al. Utility of history, examination and laboratory tests in screening those returning to Europe from the tropics for parasitic infection. Trop Med Int Health 2000;5:818–23.
5. Van den Ende J, van Gompel A, van den Enden E, et al. Hypereosinophilia after a stay in tropical countries. Trop Geogr Med 1994;46:191.
6. Harries AD, Myers B, Bhattacharyya D. Eosinophilia in Caucasians returning from the tropics. Trans R Soc Trop Med 1986;80:327–8.
7. Whitty CJ, Mabey DC, Armstron M, et al. Presentation and outcome of 1107 cases of schistosomiasis from Africa diagnosed in a non-endemic country. Trans R Soc Trop Med Hyg 2000;94:531–4.
8. Libman MD, MacLean JD, Gyorkos TW. Screening for schistosomiasis, filariasis, and strongyloidiasis among expatriates returning from the tropics. Clin Infect Dis 1993;17:353–9.
9. Ansart S, Perez L, Jaureguiberry S, et al. Spectrum of dermatoses in 165 travelers returning from the tropics with skin diseases. Am J Trop Med Hyg 2007;76:184–6.
10. Starr J, Pruett JH, Yuninger JW, et al. Myiasis due to Hypoderma lineatum infection mimicking the hypereosinophilic syndrome. Mayo Clin Proc 2000;75:755–9.
11. Junod C. Isospora belli coccidiosis in immunocompetent subjects (a study of 40 cases seen in Paris). Bull Soc Pathol Exot 1988;81:317–25.
12. Centers for Disease Control and Prevention (CDC). Notes from the field: acute muscular sarcocystosis among returning travelers – Tioman Island, Malaysia, 2011. MMWR Morb Mortal Wkly Rep 2012;61:37–8.
13. Skiest DJ, Keiser P. Clinical significance of eosinophilia in HIV-infected individuals. Am J Med 1997;102:449–53.

14. Harley WB, Blaser MJ. Disseminated coccidioidomycosis associated with extreme eosinophilia. Clin Infect Dis 1994;18:627–9.

15. Flores M, Merino Angulo J, Tanago JG, et al. Late generalized tuberculosis and eosinophilia. Arch Intern Med 1983;143:182.

16. Renston JP, Goldman ES, Hsu RM, et al. Peripheral blood eosinophilia in association with sarcoidosis. Mayo Clin Proc 2000;75:586–90.

17. Keene WR. Uncommon abnormalities of blood associated with ulcerative colitis. Med Clin North Am 1966;50:535–41.

18. Kain K. Skin lesions in returned travelers. Med Clin North Am 1999;83:1077–102.

19. Sarma DP, Weilbaecher TG. Human sparganosis. J Am Acad Dermatol 1986;15:1145–8.

20. Rusnak JM, Lucey DR. Clinical gnathostomiasis: case report and review of the English-language literature. Clin Infect Dis 1993;16:33–50.

21. Jelinek T, Maiwald H, Nothdurft HD, et al. Cutaneous larva migrans in travelers: synopsis of histories, symptoms, and treatment of 98 patients. Clin Infect Dis 1994;19:1062–6.

22. von Kuster LC, Genta RM. Cutaneous manifestations of strongyloidiasis. Arch Dermatol 1988;124:1826–30.

23. Loeffler W. Transient lung infiltrations with blood eosinophilia. Int Arch Allergy Appl Immunol 1956;8:54.

24. Hiatt RA, Sotomayor ZR, Sanchez G, et al. Factors in the pathogenesis of acute schistosomiasis mansoni. J Infect Dis 1979;139:659–66.

25. Boggild AK, Keystone JS, Kain KC. Tropical pulmonary eosinophilia: a case series in a setting of non-endemicity. Clin Infect Dis 2004;39:1123–8.

26. Rocha A, Dreyer G, Poindexter RW, et al. Syndrome resembling tropical pulmonary eosinophilia but of non-filarial aetiology: serological findings with filarial antigens. Trans R Soc Trop Med Hyg 1995;89:573–5.

27. Krenke R, Nasilowski J, Korczynski P, et al. Incidence and aetiology of eosinophilic pleural effusion. Eur Resp J 2009;34:1111–17.

28. Ryan ET, Wilson ME, Kain KC. Illness after international travel. N Engl J Med 2002;347:505–16.

29. McAuley JB, Michelson MK, Schantz PM. Trichinella in travelers. J Infect Dis 1991;164:1013–6.

30. Arjona R, Riancho JA, Aguado JM, et al. Fascioliasis in developed countries: A review of classic and aberrant forms of the disease. Medicine (Baltimore) 1995;74:13–23.

31. Schantz PM, Glickman LT. Toxocaral visceral larva migrans. N Engl J Med 1978;298:436–9.

32. Diaz JH. Recognizing and reducing the risks of helminthic eosinophilic meningitis in travelers: differential diagnosis, disease management, prevention and control. J Travel Med 2009;16:267–75.

33. Slom TJ, Cortese MM, Gerber SI, et al. An outbreak of eosinophilic meningitis caused by Angiostrongylus cantonensis in travelers returning from the Caribbean. N Engl J Med 2002;346:668–75.

34. Meltzer E, Percik R, Shatzkes J, et al. Eosinophilia among returning travelers: a practical approach. Am J Trop Med Hyg 2008;78:702–9.

35. Scrimgeour EM, Gadjusek DC. Involvement of the central nervous system in Schistosoma mansoni and S haematobium infection: review. Brain 1985;108:1023–38.

36. Harries AD, Fryatt R, Walker J, et al. Schistosomiasis in expatriates returning to Britain from the tropics: a controlled study. Lancet 1986;1:86–8.

37. Lipner EM, Law MA, Barnett E. Filariasis in travelers presenting to the GeoSentinel Surveillance Network. PLoS Negl Trop Dis 2007;1:e88.

38. Nutman TB, Ottesen EA, Ieng S, et al. Eosinophilia in Southeast Asian refugees: Evaluation at a referral center. J Infect Dis 1987;155:309–13.

39. Pelletier LL, Baker CB, Gam AA, et al. Diagnosis and evaluation of treatment of chronic strongyloidiasis in ex-prisoners of war. J Infect Dis 1988;157:573–6.

40. Loutfy MR, Wilson M, Keystone JS, et al. Serology and eosinophil count in the diagnosis and management of strongyloidiasis in a non-endemic area. Am J Trop Med Hyg 2002;66:749–52.

41. Maxwell C, Hussain R, Nutman TB, et al. The clinical and immunologic responses of normal volunteers to low dose hookworm (Necator americanus) infection. Am J Trop Med Hyg 1987;37:126–34.

42. Checkley AM, Chiodini PL, Dockrell DH. Eosinophilia in returning travelers and migrants from the tropics: UK recommendations for investigation and initial management. J Infect 2010;60:1–20.

43. Istre GR, Fontaine RE, Tarr J, et al. Acute schistosomiasis among Americans rafting the Omo River, Ethiopia. JAMA 1984;251:508–10.

44. Singal M, Schantz PM, Werner SB. Trichinosis acquired at sea – report of an outbreak. Am J Trop Med Hyg 1974;25:675–81.

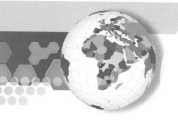

56

Respiratory Infections

Alberto Matteelli, Nuccia Saleri, and Edward T. Ryan

Key points

- Respiratory tract infections (RTIs) are among the most common illnesses reported by travelers. The estimated monthly incidence of acute febrile respiratory tract infections is 1261/100 000 travelers
- Most RTIs are viral in nature, involve the upper respiratory tract, and do not require specific diagnosis or treatment
- Lower respiratory tract infections, including pneumonia, often require antimicrobial therapy
- High-risk groups such as infants, small children, the elderly and subjects with chronic tracheobronchial or pulmonary disease are at increased risk of developing severe clinical consequences should infection occur
- Influenza is often considered the most important travel-related infection. Travelers play an integral role in the yearly and global spread of influenza
- All travelers 6 months of age and older should receive yearly influenza vaccination, and travelers should be instructed in hand-hygiene and sneeze and cough hygiene
- All travelers should be up to date on any indicated vaccines that prevent RTIs, including measles, pneumococcal diseases, Hib, meningococcal disease, diphtheria, and pertussis
- Travelers may be at increased risk of geographically restricted RTIs, and clinicians should be familiar with the major manifestations of these illnesses

Introduction

Respiratory diseases are a frequent[1-3] and potentially life-threatening[4] health problem in travelers. Travelers may be at increased risk of certain respiratory tract infections (RTIs) due to travel itself (mingling and close quarters in airports, airplanes, cruise ships and hotels, and risk of influenza, legionella, and tuberculosis) and due to unique exposure at travel destinations (melioidosis, plague, Q fever, and coccidioidomycosis). Travel-related respiratory infections can lead to importation and secondary transmission, as occurred during the global SARS (severe acute respiratory syndrome) outbreak in 2003, and have occurred repetitively with influenza and tuberculosis.[5,6] This chapter reviews causative agents, clinical manifestations, and management approaches for travel-related RTIs.

Causative Agents and Clinical Presentation

Respiratory infections may manifest as upper tract disease (rhinitis, sinusitis, otitis, pharyngitis, epiglottitis, tracheitis), lower tract disease (bronchitis, pneumonia), or both. Systemic manifestations may include fever, headache, and myalgia. The vast majority of RTIs are caused by agents with global distribution.

The usual causative agents of acute upper respiratory tract infections are listed in Table 56.1. Most upper RTIs are caused by viruses, evolve as uncomplicated disease, and resolve without specific treatment. Acute coryzal illness, traditionally referred to as a 'common cold', manifests as nasal discharge and obstruction, sneezing and sore throat, and is most commonly caused by viruses, including rhinovirus, parainfluenza virus, influenza virus, respiratory syncytial virus, adenovirus, enterovirus (especially coxsackievirus A21), coronaviruses, and metapneumonia virus. Acute laryngitis is characterized by hoarseness of voice with a deepened pitch, with possible episodes of aphonia. Often these signs are associated to those of coryza and pharyngitis. Common causes of laryngitis include parainfluenza virus, rhinovirus, influenza virus, and adenovirus. Less frequently, laryngitis can be caused by bacteria including *Corynebacterium diphtheriae*, *Branhamella catarrhalis*, and *Haemophilus influenzae*. Pharyngitis is also most commonly viral in origin, although streptococcal disease accounts for a significant minority. Other causes of pharyngitis include Epstein–Barr virus (EBV) and the human immunodeficiency virus (HIV).

Lower respiratory infections (LRTIs) are characterized by bronchial and/or pulmonary parenchymal involvement. The most common etiologic agents of pneumonia are listed in Table 56.2. Viruses commonly occur, but bacteria are responsible for a significant proportion of community-acquired cases of LRTI, and include *Streptococcus pneumoniae* and *Haemophilus influenzae*, as well as *Mycoplasma* spp. and *Chlamydia* spp., *Legionella* spp., and mycobacteria (tuberculosis). Fungal and parasitic involvement of the lung is also well recognized in travelers. Young children may sometimes be affected by severe forms of tracheobronchitis and croup, characterized by the stridorous croup-cough. The majority of these cases are due to viruses.

Travel destination, exposure, and activities should be considered in returned travelers with an RTI, as shown in Table 56.3. A list of common manifestations and complications of RTIs is presented in Table 56.4.

DOI: 10.1016/B978-1-4557-1076-8.00056-9

Epidemiology

Steffen et al. estimated the monthly incidence of acute febrile RTIs to be 1261/100 000 travelers.[1] In that analysis, RTI ranked third after travelers' diarrhea and malaria among all infectious problems of travelers. However, that rate, which is equivalent to 0.2 episodes/person/year, is much lower than the incidence of common respiratory diseases among adults in the USA, which approximates four episodes per person per year.[7] The difference is likely to be attributable to under-reporting among travelers, because a large proportion of RTIs are mild, not incapacitating, are not reported, and do not require hospital care.

The incidence of RTI is similar in developing and developed nations. In a classic study comparing incidence rates in travelers to different areas, RTI occurred in 3.7/1000 travel days to Latin America, 3.5/1000 to Oceania, and 3.1/1000 to the Caribbean.[8]

In the literature, there are large variations in the proportion of respiratory infections among all causes of illness in returning travelers. Comparison among studies, however, is difficult, and differences are likely to reflect diverse diagnostic procedures and definitions of syndromes rather than true epidemiologic differences. Still, RTIs consistently rank among the most frequently diagnosed and/or reported conditions among travelers. Attack rates in reported studies have ranged from 5% to 40%.[9–15]

In a large database of ill travelers from all continents within the GeoSentinel Surveillance System, Freedman described a frequency of respiratory disorders of 77 per 1000 ill returned travelers, ranging from 45/1000 in the Caribbean to 97/1000 in Southeast Asia.[2] In that analysis, respiratory disorders that prompted the seeking of medical care were less commonly reported than systemic febrile illnesses, acute diarrhea, dermatologic disorders, chronic diarrhea, and non-diarrheal gastrointestinal disorders.[2] Using the same database, Leder and colleagues found that 7.8% of ill travelers seeking medical care through GeoSentinel sites reported a respiratory illness.[16] In that series, of 1719 patients with respiratory infection, approximately 65% had an upper RTI, 75% of which were labeled as 'non-specific' and 20% were categorized as pharyngitis. Approximately 35% of all RTIs were characterized as lower tract infection, with 35% of these classified as pneumonia and over 50% being classified as bronchitis.[16] Prolonged travel, travel involving visiting friends and relatives, and travel during the northern hemisphere winter increased the likelihood of influenza and lower respiratory tract infections in this cohort.[16]

O'Brien et al. studied a group of 232 sick travelers at a tertiary hospital in Australia who had largely traveled through Asian countries: RTIs were second after malaria, accounting for 24% of cases.[17] In that series, lower tract infections accounted for 50% of all RTIs, and were almost equally distributed between bacterial pneumonia and influenza.[17] Bacterial pneumonia was significantly more common in patients aged >40 years, with an odds ratio (OR) of 5.5. One-quarter of upper tract infections were due to group A *Streptococcus*. In a multicenter hospital study in Italy, of 541 travelers with fever, 8.1% of the

Table 56.1 Most Common Etiologic Agents of Upper Respiratory Tract Infections

	Viral	Bacterial
Coryzal syndrome	Rhinovirus Parainfluenza virus Influenza virus Respiratory syncytial virus Enterovirus Coronavirus Metapneumonia virus Measles	
Laryngitis	Influenza virus Parainfluenza virus Rhinovirus Adenovirus	*Corynebacterium diphtheriae* *Haemophilus influenzae* *Branhamella catarrhalis*
Pharyngitis	Rhinovirus Adenovirus Coronavirus Enterovirus Influenza virus Parainfluenza virus Respiratory syncytial virus Epstein-Barr virus Herpes Simplex Virus Human Immunodeficiency Virus type 1	*Streptococcus pyogenes* Group C β-hemolytic Streptococci *Corynebacterium diphtheriae* *Mycoplasma pneumoniae* *Chlamydia pneumoniae*

Table 56.2 Most Common Etiologic Agents of Pneumonia and/or Pulmonary Involvement

Bacterial	Fungal	Viral	Other
Streptococcus pneumoniae	*Histoplasma capsulatum*	Influenza A	*Mycobacterium tuberculosis*
Staphylococcus aureus	*Coccidioides immitis*	Influenza B	*Coxiella burnetii*
Haemophilus influenzae	*Aspergillus* spp.	Adenovirus type 4 and 7	*Yersinia pestis*
Mixed anaerobic bacteria	Cryptococcus neoformans	Hantavirus	*Francisella tularensis*
Klebsiella pneumoniae	Paracoccidioides brasiliensis	Coronavirus	*Burkholderia pseudomallei*
Pseudomonas aeruginosa			*Bacillus anthracis*
Legionella spp.			*Leptospira* spp.
Mycoplasma pneumoniae			*Schistosoma* spp. (acute)
Chlamydia pneumoniae			*Ascaris lumbricoides*
Chlamydia psittaci			*Strongyloides stercoralis*
			Hookworm
			Paragonimus westermani
			Wuchereria bancrofti (Tropical pulmonary eosinophilia)

Table 56.3 Diagnostic Possibilities Based on The Region of Travel

	Africa	Asia	Central and South America	Europe	North America
Bacteria	Tuberculosis, plague	Tuberculosis, melioidosis, plague	Tuberculosis, plague	Legionellosis	Plague
Viruses	Hemorrhagic fever viruses, influenza	Hemorrhagic fever viruses, influenza	Hantavirus pulmonary syndrome, influenza	Influenza	Hantavirus pulmonary syndrome, influenza
Parasites	Paragonomiasis, schistosomiasis, strongyloidiasis, tropical eosinophilia	Paragonomiasis schistosomiasis strongyloidiasis tropical eosinophilia	Schistosomiasis, strongyloidiasis, tropical eosinophilia		
Fungi	Histoplasmosis		Histoplasmosis, coccidioidomycosis	Histoplasmosis, coccidioidomycosis	

Modified by Gluckman SJ, Chest 2008;134;163–171.

Table 56.4 Common Manifestations and Complications of Respiratory Tract Infections and Common Etiologic Agents of Otitis Media

Complications	Agents of Otitis Media
Otitis media	Streptococcus pneumoniae
Sinusitis	Streptococcus Group A
Epiglottitis	Staphylococcus aureus
Mastoiditis	Haemophilus influenzae
Periorbital cellulitis	Branhamella catarrhalis
Peritonsillar abscess	
Retropharyngeal abscess	
Adenitis	

patients had a respiratory syndrome, one-third of whom had pneumonia. TB was responsible for 29% of pneumonia cases in this cohort. Among cases with RTI and no signs of pneumonia, malaria was the underlying disease in 11 of 27.[18]

In a recent analysis of GeoSentinel data on ill children after international travel, approximately 86% of ill children who were brought by their parents for medical care had four major syndromes: 28% had a diarrheal process; 25% had a dermatologic disorder; 23% had a systemic febrile illness; and 11% had a respiratory disorder. Upper respiratory tract infections (38%), hyperactive airway disease (20%), and acute otitis media (17%) accounted for the majority of the cases of respiratory syndrome in these children.[19]

Risk Factors

In the GeoSentinel Surveillance System, women were more likely than men to present with upper respiratory tract infection associated with travel (OR 1.3).[10] Prolonged travel, travel involving visiting friends and relatives, and travel during the northern hemisphere winter increased the odds of being diagnosed with influenza and lower respiratory tract infection rather than upper tract disease in this cohort, and male gender was associated with twofold increased risk odds of pneumonia compared with female gender.[10]

Air travel itself is not a major risk factor for transmission of RTI owing to the high cabin air exchange rate, air filtering, and relatively laminar-down pattern air flow active during flight,[20] although sitting in close proximity to a person who is highly infectious can result in infection.[21–23] Sitting for a prolonged period in a confined air cabin not in flight and not with air flow can also markedly increase the risk of infection.[24] The reduced pressure of inspired oxygen found on airline flights or at high-altitude destinations may adversely affect infants' breathing patterns.[25]

Respiratory and intestinal infections are the most common diagnosis for passengers and crew seeking medical care on board ships,[26] and cruise travelers are at increased risk for legionellosis, influenza, and pneumococcal disease.[4] Reasons for increased susceptibility of cruise ship travelers to respiratory infections may include contaminated ventilator-cooling systems and spas, common points-of-fomite contact (e.g., salad bars), as well as passenger factors such as age, underlying illnesses, and physical condition.[27]

Infants, small children, the elderly, and subjects with chronic tracheobronchial or cardiopulmonary diseases are at increased risk of developing severe clinical consequences from RTIs.

Transmission

The spread of agents such as streptococci or meningococci is by direct, person-to-person contact, and via large droplets. These droplets usually fall to the ground within 1 m (3 ft) of an infectious person.

Other pathogens are transmitted by tiny droplet nuclei (<10 μm in diameter) that can be dispersed widely and randomly, can remain viable in the air for hours, and may be inhaled and pass easily through the narrow bronchioles. These agents can lead to infection in a large number of people, presenting as 'clusters' or disease outbreaks of disease among those exposed. Measles and *M. tuberculosis* can disseminate in this way. Influenza is transmitted by droplets and fomites.

Legionellosis is a respiratory disease with a unique chain of transmission. It is a bacterium that multiplies in water systems, often within free-living ameba, forming biofilms in cooling towers, water-pipe fittings, and showers. *Legionella* can be disseminated in the aerosols generated by showerheads, whirlpools, and cooling systems. Such transmission contributes to outbreaks in hotels and cruise ships.

Management of the Respiratory Syndrome

An example of a decision algorithm for approaching patients with a RTI is presented in Figures 56.1 and 56.2. A syndromic management algorithm should effectively differentiate upper from lower respiratory tract infections, incorporating probable causative agents to guide treatment decisions. It should also assist in identify complications that

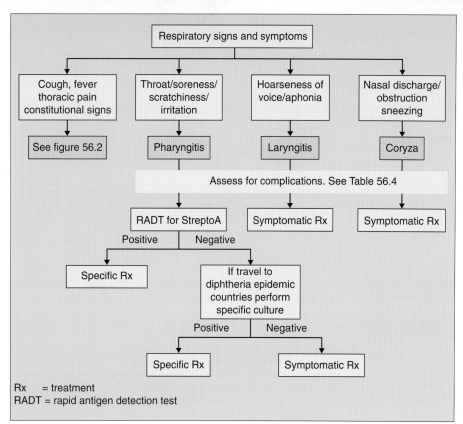

Figure 56.1 Decision algorithm for acute upper respiratory tract infections.

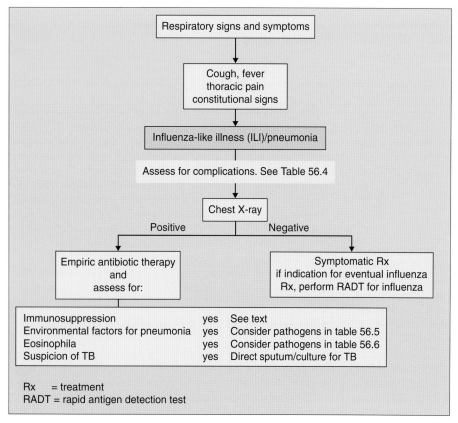

Figure 56.2 Decision algorithm for acute lower respiratory tract infections.

require specific treatment approaches. For practical purposes, a cough with rhinorrhea, or either of these with headache, fever, or shortness of breath can be used to generally define a RTI.

Among upper respiratory tract infections (Fig. 56.1), the isolated coryzal syndrome is rarely a cause of medical consultation. No additional diagnostic procedures are required and treatment is usually supportive. The diagnosis of laryngitis is also clinical, and treatment is usually supportive. Although the diagnosis of pharyngitis is also clinical, it is important to identify individuals with pharyngitis caused by group A streptococcal infection from other causes to lessen the likelihood of subsequent sequelae, including glomerulonephritis and rheumatic fever. Bacterial pharyngitis is reportedly associated with more severe pharyngeal pain, odynophagia, and higher fever, with grayish-yellow exudate on the tonsils and enlarged cervical lymph nodes. However, clinical criteria are unreliable to identify bacterial pharyngitis/tonsillitis because a typical presentation occurs in <50% of cases. Rapid antigen detection tests are available with a specificity >90% and sensitivity of 60–95%, and should generally be performed in patients ill enough to seek medical care for pharyngitis, especially in young children, in whom the risk of streptococcal disease is highest. The need to perform a bacterial culture if a rapid test is negative is debated. A treatment course with penicillin or amoxicillin for 10 days is appropriate to treat pharyngitis due to *S. pyogenes*. Diphtheria is a rare cause of pharyngitis, with a potentially fatal outcome. It is characterized by a thick and gray pharyngeal and tracheal membrane that bleeds upon attempted removal. Diagnosis is based on clinical recognition and culture isolation of a toxigenic strain of *Corynebacterium diphtheriae*. The mainstay of therapy is diphtheria antitoxin, associated with antibiotic treatment with penicillin or macrolides. Vaccination effectively eliminates the risk of travel-related pharyngeal diphtheria.

Otitis media and sinusitis can complicate air travel secondary to barotrauma. Viral and bacterial causes are common, and empiric treatment usually involves some combination of supportive care and hydration, with or without antibiotics. If an antibiotic is prescribed, it should primarily target an *S. pneumoniae* infection. Upper RTIs can occasionally be complicated by peritonsillar and retropharyngeal abscess formation. Treatment usually involves mechanical drainage and antibiotics.

Clinical signs suggestive of pneumonia include productive cough, thoracic pain, and shortness of breath. Examination usually discloses pulmonary crepitation, rhonchi, and adventitial sounds. Chest imaging should be used to further characterize and define pulmonary involvement. Complications of pneumonia include pulmonary cavitation, pneumothorax, and empyema formation. In many facilities, it is now standard to collect nasopharyngeal swabs or washings from patients with severe RTIs and pneumonia, and to apply rapid antigen tests to assess for common respiratory viruses, including influenza, parainfluenza, respiratory syncytial virus, adenovirus, and metapneumonia virus. Although the majority of cases with radiologic evidence of pneumonia may still have a viral infection, the proportion of cases due to bacteria is high enough to usually warrant systematic antibacterial treatment, especially if a viral screen is unrevealing. The chest film is not helpful in making a specific etiologic diagnosis; however, lobar consolidation, cavitation, and large pleural effusions support a bacterial cause. Pneumococcal disease is often characterized by abrupt onset of fever, cough, rapid respiration, and lobar consolidation on chest film. Atypical pneumonias caused by *M. pneumoniae* and *C. pneumoniae* may be characterized by gradual onset of symptoms, cough progressive from dry to productive, chest film worse than symptoms, and normal peripheral white blood cell counts. Overall, however, the clinical presentation is not specific enough to make an etiologic diagnosis, and effective methods to recognize the causative agent of

Table 56.5 Important Environmental Factors in Respiratory Tract Infections

Pneumonia	
Melioidosis	Travel to endemic areas, usually in SouthEast Asia
Brucellosis	Exposure to cattle, unpasteurized dairy products
Plague	Travel to endemic areas and contact with rats
Anthrax	Exposure to husbandry or animal hide or hair products
Tularemia	Hunting or other exposure to wild animals
Psittacosis	Exposure to birds
Leptospirosis	Exposure to rat or animal infested water
Coccidioidomycosis	Travel to dry-arid endemic areas
Histoplasmosis	Exposure to bird or bat droppings, spelunking
Q fever	Exposure to infected animals
Legionnaires' disease	Ship trip or enclosure in epidemic foci
Hantavirus	Exposure to rodents
Pharyngitis	
Diphtheria	Travel to epidemic countries, unimmunized status

Table 56.6 Causes of Pulmonary Involvement and Eosinophilia

Acute Ascaris lumbricoides infection (Loeffler's syndrome)
Strongyloides stercoralis infection (Loeffler's syndrome)
Acute Hookworm infection (Loeffler's syndrome)
Mycobacterium tuberculosis
Coccidioides immitis
Paragonimus spp.
Visceral larva migrans
Acute Schistosoma spp. infection (Katayama fever)
Dirofilaria immitis
Tropical pulmonary eosinophilia (lymphatic filariasis)

pneumonia are not available. The sputum Gram stain is a simple, quick, and inexpensive procedure, but its helpfulness in establishing a specific etiologic diagnosis is uncertain. The utility of the sputum culture is also unclear, since the procedure is insensitive: only half of patients with pneumonia produce sputum and contamination occurs in one-third. An advantage of routine sputum Gram stain and culture is that these procedures would capture rare causes of pneumonia such as tuberculosis and melioidosis in travelers. Because the cause of pneumonia cannot be determined on the basis of any specific clinical, radiographic, or laboratory parameter, antibiotic therapy is usually begun empirically. Treatment should be effective on *S. pneumoniae*, the most frequently responsible agent, and on agents of atypical pneumonia: *M. pneumoniae*, *C. pneumoniae*, and legionella infections.

A thorough travel and exposure history (Table 56.5) can also help identify diagnostic possibilities, for example legionella, and the differential in immunocompromised patients can be quite broad.

Pneumonia or pulmonary findings with eosinophilia in a traveler may also suggest specific diagnoses (Table 56.6).[28,29]

Table 56.7 Prevention of Respiratory Tract Infections in Travelers

Prevention strategy	Preventable condition
Hand-washing Alcohol-based hand sanitizers Soap and water	Influenza Respiratory viruses Bacterial fomite transmission
Vaccine	Influenza Measles *Streptococcus pneumoniae* *Haemophilus influenzae* Diphtheria
Early presumptive treatment	Influenza
Public health interventions	Influenza → Guidelines for international response Legionellosis → Alert networks (EWGLI) → Guidelines for safe water systems
Behavioral interventions	Influenza and respiratory viruses → Handwashing Paragonimiasis → Avoid eating raw crabs or crayfish Histoplasmosis → Avoid bat caves Leptospirosis → Avoid adventurous travel Plague → Avoid contacts with rodents Anthrax/Q fever → Avoid contact with cattle and sheep

Prevention in Travelers

Prevention of RTIs in the traveler as in all individuals usually relies on behavioral changes (hand-washing and avoidance of close contact with sick individuals), vaccination, and rarely chemoprophylaxis (example, anti-influenza medication during an outbreak) (Table 56.7).

Influenza, measles, diphtheria, pertussis, as well as pneumococcal and Hib-associated infections are vaccine-preventable diseases. All travelers should be up to date with anti-measles, anti-influenza, anti-diphtheria and anti-pertussis vaccines (example Tdap: tetanus, anti-diphtheria, acellular pertussis vaccine). All children should be up to date with anti-*H. influenzae* B immunization (Hib) and pediatric pneumococcal polyvalent vaccine. Travel itself is not an indication for adult pneumococcal vaccination, but all adults 65 years of age or older, or with certain indications, should be up to date for adult pneumococcal vaccination.[30] All travelers should be up to date for immunization against influenza.[31,32]

Control measures for legionellosis are based on the application of guidelines for maintaining safe water systems in international tourist locations and cruise ships.[33] These include proper disinfection, filtration and storage of source water, avoidance of dead ends in pipes, proper cleaning and maintenance of spas, and periodic replacement of devices likely to amplify or disseminate the organism.

The early recognition of outbreaks is exceedingly important in the management of individual cases of diseases such as legionellosis. The European Working Group for Legionella Infections (EWGLI) is a network created to report legionella cases diagnosed in patients who have been traveling within the likely incubation period of 2 weeks, together with geographic location of suspected source of transmission. Members of the group report cases of Legionnaires' disease to the coordinating center, which then notifies all EWGLI members of any disease cluster. Other international global and regional surveillance networks, including GeoSentinel, TropNet, and EuroTravNet play a pivotal role in early detection and public warning of travel-related epidemics.[34,35]

International health authorities may impose and have imposed public health interventions during worrisome outbreaks (example, H5N1 and H1N1 influenza and SARS), including animal culling, travel restrictions, screening at airports and points of arrival and departure, and quarantine in efforts to limit the spread of respiratory infections.

Infections of the Respiratory Tract Associated With Epidemics

SARS

Although SARS is no longer an ongoing public health threat, it can serve as a paradigm infection that underscores the risk and consequences of international travel, and the role that travelers can play in the global, rapid and lethal spread of a highly pathogenic RTI. In November 2002, reports from Guangdong Province in Southern China suggested that more than 300 cases of a mysterious, highly contagious pneumonia had occurred. This severe atypical pneumonia appeared to be particularly prevalent among healthcare workers and their families. As the condition began to spread from China, on 13 March 2003 the World Health Organization issued a global alert about the outbreak and subsequently named this condition severe acute respiratory syndrome (SARS). The virus spread among travelers, with a focused outbreak radiating out from a single Bangkok hotel to a number of countries, with subsequent ongoing spread. From November 2002 to July 2003, 8098 cases and 774 deaths were reported from 28 countries, with a fatality rate of 9.6%.[36] A global public response was initiated. Fortunately, since April 2004 not a single case of SARS has been reported worldwide.

A novel coronavirus distinct from those previously reported in animals and humans caused SARS.[37,38] The virus was thought to have emerged in the animal and food markets of Asia, and after introduction into a human, was transmitted person-to-person by inhalation of droplets, although aerosol transmission may have occurred in 'super spreaders' patients who are severely ill and excreting large viral loads. Some 60% of SARS cases occurred among healthcare workers who had not been adequately protected.[39] The incubation period of SARS was 3–11 days, with a median of 5 days. The syndrome often began with a prodrome of headache, myalgia, and fatigue, progressing a day later to fever >38°C and subsequently to a non-productive cough and/or shortness of breath. Patients presented with fever and non-specific symptoms 1–3 days before respiratory symptoms began. Gastrointestinal symptoms (nausea, vomiting, and diarrhea) occurred in approximately 20% of patients.[40] In the series of 144 patients seen in Toronto hospitals, the chest X-ray was normal in 25% on admission.[41] Unilateral and bilateral infiltrates were observed in 46% and 29% of the patients, respectively. Most patients eventually developed multifocal opacities. Laboratory investigations typically showed lymphopenia and to a lesser extent thrombocytopenia; during hospitalization many patients developed hypocalcemia, hypomagnesemia, hypokalemia, and hypophosphatemia.

The diagnosis of SARS was based on a case definition, which included a possible contact history, fever, and respiratory symptoms. Although not available for use by routine laboratories, serology and PCR used for viral RNA detection were used more and more widely during the epidemic.[42] The treatment of SARS was largely supportive. Corticosteroid therapy and the antiviral drug ribavirin were used, with little certainty of efficacy. Most patients recovered in spite of not receiving these drugs, but the mortality rate from SARS had a median of 10%. Those with the highest mortality rate were the elderly (>60 years) and those with underlying comorbid conditions such as diabetes and chronic lung disease.

Avian Influenza

Since 2005, highly pathogenic H5N1 influenza A virus endemic in avian populations in SE Asia has been tracked by the WHO and related agencies. H5N1 has resulted in millions of poultry infections, several hundred recognized human cases, and a high case-fatality rate. Human cases continue to accumulate. Currently, avian influenza H5N1 virus continues to circulate in poultry in some countries, especially in Asia and northeast Africa. In June 2011, Egypt and Indonesia confirmed their 150th and 178th human cases of avian flu, respectively. Of the 150 cases confirmed in Egypt, 52 have been fatal, compared to 146 of 178 in Indonesia.[43] Large amounts of the virus are known to be excreted in the droppings shed by infected birds. Transmission requires direct contact with birds or their droppings. Populations in affected countries are advised to avoid contact with dead birds or birds showing signs of disease. Human-to-human transmission has fortunately been very sporadic thus far, and limited to very close contacts. However, should the virus mutate to become steadily transmissible in the human community, a new deadly pandemic influenza could emerge. Human cases of avian influenza are characterized by severe pneumonia, which is frequently rapidly fatal. Evidence suggests that some antiviral drugs, notably oseltamivir, can reduce the duration of viral replication and improve survival.[44]

Influenza

Influenza is the most important viral respiratory infection of travelers and non-travelers.

Travelers acquire influenza both as sporadic cases and as clusters from common sources aboard ships, airplanes, and in tour groups. All described outbreaks are caused by the type A virus, and are characterized by involvement of a large proportion of the population at risk, and the explosive nature of outbreaks. In 1998, approximately 40 000 tourists and tourism workers were affected by an influenza outbreak in Alaska and the Yukon Territory.[45] Influenza is a common infection also among *Hajj* pilgrims, with 24 000 estimated cases per *Hajj* season.[46]

Influenza is a self-limited disease that produces high morbidity and is responsible for lethal cases, most commonly among the youngest and eldest. The hallmark of the clinical presentation of influenza is a febrile illness with cough. Fever characteristically lasts 3–5 days, but dry cough may persist for much longer. Pneumonia is the most frequent complication, either from direct viral involvement or bacterial suprainfection, the latter most comonly caused by *S. pneumoniae*, *H. influenzae*, group A *Streptococcus*, and *Staphylococcus aureus*. Otitis media and sinusitis are other serious complications. Complications are more frequent and severe among patients with chronic diseases of the lung or heart.

Diagnosis is usually based on clinical criteria during an outbreak. Rapid diagnostic antigen-based tests are being increasingly used. Viral isolation (which is the method of reference) and antibody determination are seldom used in clinical care. Treatment is symptomatic in most cases. For severe cases and for patients at highest risks of complications and severe disease, anti-influenza therapy with neuraminidase inhibitors can be used. In many countries, yearly influenza vaccination is now indicated for all individuals 6 months of age or older. A live attenuated nasal vaccine is available for use in healthy young individuals 2–49 years of age. Parenteral inactive vaccines are available for use in all those over 6 months of age. All travelers should receive the current year's influenza vaccine.[32] Northern and southern hemisphere influenza vaccine may be different. Influenza in the northern hemisphere occurs mainly from October to February; influenza in the southern hemisphere predominantly occurs in April–August. As one approaches the Equator influenza circulates year-round. Travelers are at high risk of influenza year-round, since they are often mingling with other travelers from current influenza zones, or traveling directly to those zones.

Legionellosis

Legionella infections occur worldwide as sporadic cases. Endemic legionellosis is responsible for approximately 2% of community-acquired pneumonia; the highest incidence is in people over 40 years of age, but only a fraction of cases are recognized. According to the CDC, 20% of patients hospitalized with Legionnaires' disease in the United States acquired their infection while traveling.[47]

A European Working Group on *Legionella* Infection involving 35 countries was started in 1987. During 2008, a total of 866 travel-associated Legionnaires' cases were reported. Travel outside Europe was reported in 12% of the cases. The scheme identified 108 new clusters in 2008, the largest cluster (six cases) being associated with travel to Spain.[48] Countries whose tourist industries are expanding appear to have higher rates of infection. The Mediterranean region in Europe has been the origin of most reported outbreaks, but no area is excluded from risk, as exemplified by the identification of a cluster of cases associated with a hotel in Bangkok.[49]

Transmission is air-borne, but the source of infection is the environment, rather than other persons.

The incubation period is classically considered as 2–10 days, although 16% of 188 cases described in a recent large outbreak in The Netherlands reported incubation periods exceeding 10 days.[50] The clinical spectrum is wide, ranging from subclinical to lethal manifestations. The overt picture of legionellosis is that of a lobar pneumonia with abrupt onset characterized by high fever, severe headache, and confusion.[51] Patchy infiltrates are often present bilaterally. Mortality may be as high as 20% if diagnosis and antibiotic treatment are delayed. Diagnosis is usually based on detection of antigen in urine (for *L. pneumophila* type 1, which accounts for 85% of cases). Culture can also be employed. Treatment is often empiric: macrolides are the treatment of choice. Co-trimoxazole and fluoroquinolones are also effective.

Tropical and Geographically Restricted Respiratory Infections

Travelers may be at risk of a number of geographically restricted respiratory infections, as well as those associated with travel to resource-limited areas.

Melioidosis

Melioidosis is caused by a Gram-negative rod, *Burkholderia pseudomallei*. Cases usually occur within 20° north to 20° south of the Equator, with the vast majority of cases being reported in Southeast Asia and northern Australia. The bacterium is free-living in soil and water, and humans can become infected through inhalation or through direct contact (wounds). Melioidosis remains a risk for travelers to endemic areas, especially those with exposure to wet-season soils and surface water.[52,53] *B. pseudomallei* was one of the more frequent isolates from travelers and patients affected by the 2005 Asian tsunami.[54] Reactivated melioidosis has been reported among tourists, immigrants, and Vietnam veterans decades after leaving endemic regions. Risk factors for clinical disease include diabetes, chronic alcoholism, chronic lung disease, and chronic renal disease.

Cellulitis, abscess formation, pneumonia and septicemia are the most frequent manifestations. Lung involvement consists of acute necrotizing pneumonia or chronic granulomatous or fibrosing lung disease mimicking tuberculosis. The diagnosis of pulmonary melioidosis is difficult. It might be suspected in travelers from endemic areas, though cases have also been reported from areas not typically considered endemic.[55] The diagnosis can be confirmed by Gram stain and culture of respiratory specimen and/or blood. The presumptive diagnosis of melioidosis may be based on a positive IHA or ELISA serology in the appropriate clinical setting.[56,57] IHA titers above 1 : 80 are suggestive of active infection, but can also be seen in asymptomatic subjects in endemic regions.[57] Current therapy recommendations are ceftazidime or imipenem plus trimethoprim-sulfamethoxazole, doxycycline or amoxicillin-clavulanic acid for a period of 2–6 weeks. Maintenance therapy for 3–6 months using either trimethoprim-sulfamethoxazole, doxycycline or amoxicillin-clavulanic acid is also necessary. A vaccine against melioidosis is not available, and there is no role for chemoprophylaxis.

Leptospirosis

Pulmonary involvement in leptospirosis is not rare, and usually manifests as a dry cough, or occasionally as a cough with blood-stained sputum.

Leptospirosis is due to several serovars of a spirochetal bacterium, often *Leptospira interrogans*, and is a zoonosis. Transmission occurs by accidental contact with water or soil contaminated with the urine of an infected animal, often a rodent. Outbreaks have occurred among adventure travelers on group tours,[58] and leptospirosis with pulmonary hemorrhage has been noted with increasing frequency.[59,60] Clinical manifestation of leptospirosis may vary from asymptomatic infection to fulminant disease. Severe cases are characterized by liver and renal failure, with mortality as high as 30% in untreated cases. Pulmonary complications often contribute to the fatal outcome: they include extensive edema and alveolar hemorrhages in the context of an ARDS episode. The radiologic findings are those of ARDS. The diagnosis requires the isolation of the bacteria from blood or urine samples, but this is rarely performed. The diagnosis usually rests on clinical recognition and serology.

Prevention of leptospirosis is difficult, especially in tropical areas where the disease is not limited to high-risk groups. Prevention of rodent–human contacts is important. A human vaccine and the use of tetracycline chemoprophylaxis (200 mg/week) are available but are rarely indicated.

Anthrax

Cutaneous disease is the most commonly observed form of human anthrax. Pulmonary anthrax is less common but more deadly, and is caused by inhalation of *Bacillus anthracis* spores. Naturally acquired anthrax may occur in developing countries, where the risk is still significant in rural parts of Asia, Africa, Eastern Europe, South and Central America as a result of contact with contaminated soil or animal products; a few cases of anthrax have been described in travelers who import souvenirs.

Inhalation anthrax is notable for its absence of pulmonary infiltrate on chest imaging, but the presence of extensive mediastinal lymphadenopathy, pleural effusions, and severe shortness of breath, toxemia, and sense of impending doom. The incubation period is 2–5 days, but spores can germinate up to 60 days after exposure. Pathogenesis is mediated by a toxin responsible for hemorrhage, edema, and necrosis. The presenting symptoms are non-specific, with mild fever, malaise, and a non-productive cough. After a period of a few days in which the patient's condition apparently improves, a second phase begins with high fever, respiratory distress, cyanosis, and subcutaneous edema of the neck and thorax. Crepitant rales are evident on auscultation. Inhalation anthrax is almost invariably fatal with a very short time between the onset of the second phase, mediastinal signs, and death. The diagnosis of inhalation anthrax is extremely difficult outside of epidemic conditions. Direct examination and Gram stain of the sputum specimen are unlikely to be positive. A serologic ELISA test is available, although a significant increase in titer is usually obtained only in convalescent subjects who survive. The most useful bacteriologic test in case of suspicion, however, is a blood culture demonstrating *B. anthracis*. Treatment of inhalation anthrax should be as early as possible and usually involves a carbapenem, penicillin, doxycycline, and fluoroquinolone such as ciprofloxacin. Ancillary treatment to sustain vascular volume, cardiac, pulmonary, and renal functions is essential.

Plague

Plague is caused by *Yersinia pestis*, a Gram-negative coccobacillus. It is considered a re-emerging disease because of the increase in the number of reported cases worldwide, the occurrence of epidemics (such as the one in India in 1994), and the gradual expansion in areas of low endemicity (including the US). The most heavily affected African countries are the Democratic Republic of Congo, Madagascar, Mozambique, Uganda, and the United Republic of Tanzania. The Central Asian region has active plague foci in the Central Asian desert, affecting Kazakhstan, Turkmenistan, and Uzbekistan. Plague foci are distributed in 19 provinces and autonomous regions of China, and the incidence has been increasing rapidly since the 1990s. Permanent plague foci exist in the Americas among native rodent and flea populations in Bolivia, Brazil, Ecuador, Peru, and the USA.[61] The 1994 Indian epidemic, where a total of 5150 suspected pneumonic or bubonic cases occurred in a 3-month period, caused travel and trade disruption and resulted in severe economic repercussions.[62] Travelers are rarely affected by plague while visiting endemic areas: for example, no visitors were affected during the 1994 epidemic in India. Campers or visitors staying in rodent-infested lodges are exposed to the highest risk of infection.

In humans, pneumonia may follow septicemia or may be a primary event in the case of air-borne transmission (though pneumonic plague is currently very rare). Plague should be suspected in febrile patients who have been exposed to rodents or other mammals in known endemic areas. The presence of buboes in this setting is highly suspicious. The bacterium may be isolated on standard bacteriologic media from culture samples of blood or bubo aspirates. The Gram stain may reveal Gram-negative coccobacilli with polymorphonuclear leukocytes. Rapid diagnostic tests such as the direct immunofluorescence test for the presumptive identification of *Y. pestis* F1 antigen are of interest for the rapid management of patients with the suspicion of disease.[63] Serologic tests to detect antibodies to the F1 antigen by passive hemoagglutination assay or enzyme-linked immunosorbent assay methods are available. A fourfold increase in titer (or a single titer of 1:16 or more) may provide presumptive evidence of plague in culture-negative cases. Antibiotic treatment should be started on the basis of clinical suspicion, usually involving an aminoglycoside (streptomycin, gentamicin) and/or doxycycline or chloramphenicol.

Pulmonary infections present a particular risk for human epidemics owing to the contagiousness of the organism. Doxycycline (100 mg twice daily for 7 days) prophylaxis of family members of index cases is indicated within the standard 7-day maximum plague incubation period.

Paragonimiasis

Paragonimiasis is caused by a lung fluke, often *P. westermani*. Humans become infected through the ingestion of undercooked or raw crabs, crayfish, or their juices. The infection is endemic in SE Asia (including Thailand, the Philippines, Vietnam, China, and Taiwan), South and North America,[64] and Africa, with most cases being reported in Asia. The disease is well described, although rare, in travelers to endemic regions.[65] The incubation period may vary from one to several months after exposure.

The disease presents as a chronic bronchopneumonic process with productive cough, thoracic pain, and low-grade fever. The worms produce extensive inflammation and cavity formation, and the infection should be considered in individuals with nodular cavitating lung lesions, with rusty-brown bloody sputum. Acute paragonimiasis can present as pneumothorax as the worms invade the lung tissue. Diagnosis usually rests on clinical recognition and detection of the worms eggs in expectorated sputum. Treatment involves praziquantel. Prevention is based on avoiding eating raw crayfish and crabs.

Coccidioidomycosis and Histoplasmosis

Coccidioidomycosis and histoplasmosis are two fungal infections acquired by the respiratory route and often involve the respiratory system. Coccidioidomycosis is caused by inhalation of *Coccidioides immitis*, a dimorphic fungus found in dust and soil. The pathogen is present only in semi-arid regions of the Americas. Symptomatic disease develops in approximately 40% of individuals infected by *C. immitis*, presenting as a flu-like syndrome. The radiologic finding is often that of hilar pneumonia with lymphadenitis and pleural involvement. In a well-described outbreak of coccidioidomycosis in a 126-member church group traveling to Mexico, the average incubation period was 12 days (range 7–20 days); chest pain was present in 76% and cough in 66% of the affected travelers.[66] The diagnosis is serological, antibodies appear 1–3 weeks after the onset of symptoms.

Histoplasmosis is caused by infection with a soil-inhabiting dimorphic fungus, *Histoplasma capsulatum*. The agent is ubiquitous, but diffusion is higher in the tropical belt and the US. Outbreaks of acute histoplasmosis among travelers have been repeatedly reported.[67–69] The disease may evolve as a mild, spontaneously resolving condition, but severe and systemic disease may develop in immunocompromised patients. In an outbreak of histoplasmosis among college students from the US visiting Acapulco, 229 persons developed an acute febrile respiratory illness with cough, shortness of breath, chest pain, or headache.[70] Chest X-ray may show patchy infiltrates or interstitial pneumonia. Diagnosis may be extremely difficult unless the disease is considered in the differential diagnosis, and most cases are unrecognized and considered as bacterial bronchitis

or influenza. Confirmation of the disease usually involves a urine antigen assay, or comparison of acute- and convalescent-phase serum specimens.

Both fungal infections are sensitive to the azoles (fluconazole and itraconazole) and amphotericin-based preparations.

Tuberculosis

Tuberculosis (TB) is a widely distributed infection and a leading cause of human morbidity and mortality. Travel can increase the risk of tuberculosis, especially among individuals traveling to resource-limited settings, those visiting friends and relatives, those performing healthcare or service work overseas, and those traveling for extended periods. Most individuals who become infected with *Mycobacterium tuberculosis* do not become ill (i.e., do not develop the disease), and are diagnosed as having latent TB infection (LTBI), often on the basis of a skin test or interferon-γ-based assays.

TB Among Travelers from Low- to High-Endemicity Areas

There is mounting evidence of the association between travel and an increased risk for LTBI. Lobato first demonstrated that US children who had traveled abroad had a significantly higher probability of having a positive tuberculin skin test than children without a history of travel.[71] More recently, Cobelens et al. estimated the risk of acquiring *M. tuberculosis* infection among long-term (≥3 months) Dutch travelers to Africa, Asia, and Latin America as 3.3% per year. This rate is very similar to that of native populations in the visited countries, and much higher than the 0.01% yearly risk in The Netherlands.[72] Abubakar et al. recently provided the first evidence in the UK that travel to countries with high levels of TB infection may be an independent risk factor for acquiring LTBI. This effect was not mitigated by BCG vaccination.[73] A recent systematic review using tuberculin skin testing (TST) conversion as a surrogate for LTBI calculated the cumulative incidence of LTBI in long-term (median 11 months) travelers to be 2%, which is what could be expected among local populations in many developing countries.[74] Other factors identified for increased TB risk among travelers were: being a healthcare worker, a longer cumulative duration of travel, and a longer total time spent in TB-endemic countries.[72]

Air travel itself is not considered a major risk factor for transmission of tuberculosis: only a few cases of LTBI have been associated with exposure to an infectious traveler on a plane, and no cases of active infection have been linked.[75] The risk of TB transmission on ships[76] and trains[77] has also been described, but is similarly of little epidemiologic importance.

Active TB (as opposed to LTBI) was 16 times more likely to be reported in individuals seeking medical care at a GeoSentinel site among those born in low-income countries and who were now living in high-income countries and traveling to their region of birth to visit friends and relatives, than it was among those born and living in high-income countries and traveling to low-income countries to visit friends and relatives, and more than 60 times more common than it was among tourist travelers.[78] Despite this, the evidence of association between actual travel (as opposed to demographics of travels) and active TB (as opposed to LTBI) is sparse. In the most well-known report describing health-associated diseases, TB was not mentioned,[1] and TB was not present in a list of causes of mortality among American missionaries in Africa.[79] Jung and Banks[80] found the incidence rate of LTBI to be 1.283/1000 person/months of travel, and active TB 0.057/1000 person/months of travel among Peace Corps volunteers. These rates are significantly higher than in the general US population, but lower than those reported by Cobelens et al.[72]

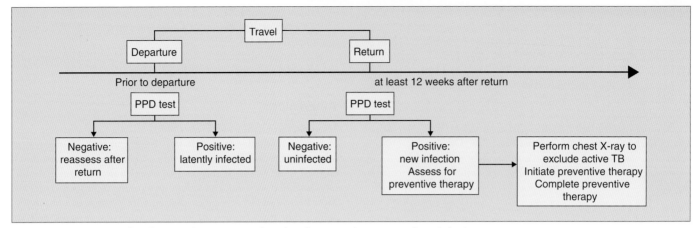

Figure 56.3 Prevention of TB disease in long-term travelers: identification and treatment of new infections.

Prevention guidelines state that persons with infectious TB should postpone air travel. Epidemiologic investigations for contacts of infectious passengers are indicated only within 3 months from exposure for passengers on travels of >8 h duration.[75] Travelers to high TB-endemic areas can employ behavioral modifications (individuals traveling to provide healthcare should use respiratory precautions in caring for patients with probable tuberculosis), and/or post-travel screening to assess for LTBI and evaluation for tuberculosis in individuals with a compatible disease (Fig. 56.3). A vaccine (BCG) is available but it is not protective in the adult population and is not routinely recommended.

Conclusion

Respiratory infections represent the third most frequent health problem for international travelers. The incidence is underestimated mainly because the majority of infections are mild and not incapacitating. Most are due to cosmopolitan agents, and 'tropical' and/or geographically restricted infections are rare. The RTI of perhaps the most significance to travelers is influenza. Travelers represent the primary vehicle of the yearly spread of influenza around the globe, and are critical to the global spread of new pandemics. Effective anti-influenza vaccines exist, and all travelers should receive yearly influenza immunization and be instructed in hand-washing and cough/sneeze hygiene. All travelers should also be up to date for other vaccines, including those that prevent RTIs, including measles, pneumococcal diseases, Hib, diphtheria, and pertussis. Clinicians caring for an ill returned traveler with an RTI should characterize the illness as upper or lower tract RTI, and consider the travel itinerary, exposure history, clinical manifestations, incubation period, and host-specific conditions.

References

1. Steffen R. Health risk for short term travelers. In: Steffen R, Lobel HO, Haworth J, et al, editors. Travel Medicine. Proceedings of the First Conference on International Travel Medicine. Berlin: Springer-Verlag; 1989. p. 27–36.
2. Freedman DO, Weld LH, Kozarsky PE, et al. Spectrum of disease and relation to place of exposure among ill returned travelers. N Engl J Med 2006;354:119–30.
3. Parola P, Soula G, Gazin P, et al. Fever in travelers returning from tropical areas: prospective observational study of 613 cases hospitalized in Marseilles, France, 1999–2003. Trop Med Infect Dis 2006;4:61–70.
4. Jernigan DB, Hofmann J, Cetron MS, et al. Outbreak of Legionnaires' disease among cruise ship passengers exposed to a contaminated whirlpool spa. Lancet 1996;275:545–7.
5. World Health Organization (WHO). Influenza A(H1N1) – update 50. June 17, 2009. Available from: http://www.who.int/csr/don/2009_06_17/en/index.html
6. Cobelens FGJ, Van Deutekom H, Draayer-Jansen IWE, et al. Risk of infection with mycobacterium tuberculosis in travelers to areas of high tuberculosis endemicity. Lancet 2000;356:461–5.
7. Dingle JH, Badger GF, Jordan Jr WS, et al. Illness in the Home: Study of 25 000 Illnesses in a Group of Cleveland Families, Cleveland: The Press of the Western Reserve University; 1969.
8. Kendrick MA. Study of illness among Americans returning from international travel; July 11–August 24, 1971 (preliminary data). J Infect Dis 1972;126:684–5.
9. Odolini S, Parola P, Gkrania–Klotsas E, et al. Travel-related imported infections in Europe, EuroTravNet 2009. Clin Microbiol Infect. 2011 Jun 10.
10. Schlagenhauf P, Chen LH, Wilson ME, et al. GeoSentinel Surveillance Network. Sex and gender differences in travel-associated disease. Clin Infect Dis 2010 Mar 15;50(6):826–32.
11. Mizuno Y, Kudo K. Travel-related health problems in Japanese travelers. Travel Med Infect Dis 2009 Sep;7(5):296–300. Epub 2009 Apr 16.
12. Cabada MM, Maldonado F, Mozo K, et al. Self-reported health problems among travelers visiting Cuzco: a Peruvian Airport survey. Travel Med Infect Dis 2009 Jan;7(1):25–9.
13. Leroy H, Arvieux C, Biziragusenyuka J, et al. A retrospective study of 230 consecutive patients hospitalized for presumed travel-related illness (2000–2006). Eur J Clin Microbiol Infect Dis 2008 Nov;27(11):1137–40.
14. Camps M, Vilella A, Marcos MA, et al. Incidence of respiratory viruses among travelers with a febrile syndrome returning from tropical and subtropical areas. J Med Virol 2008 Apr;80(4):711–5.
15. Luna LK, Panning M, Grywna K, et al. Spectrum of viruses and atypical bacteria in intercontinental air travelers with symptoms of acute respiratory infection. J Infect Dis 2007 Mar 1;195(5):675–9.
16. Leder K, Sundararajan V, Weld L, et al. Respiratory tract infections in travelers: a review of the GeoSentinel Surveillance Network. Clin Infect Dis 2003;36:399–406.
17. O'Brien D, Tobin S, Brown GV, et al. Fever in returned travelers: review of hospital admissions for a 3-year period. Clin Infect Dis 2001;33:603–9.
18. Matteelli A, Beltrame A, Saleri N, et al. Respiratory syndrome and respiratory tract infections in foreign-born and national travelers hospitalised with fever in Italy. J Travel Med 2005;12:190–6.
19. Hagmann S, Neugebauer R, Schwartz E, et al. for the GeoSentinel Surveillance Network. Illness in children after international travel: Analysis from the GeoSentinel Surveillance Network. Pediatrics 2010;125(5):e1072–80.
20. Gluckman SJ. Acute respiratory infections in a recently arrived traveler to your part of the world. Chest 2008;134:163–71.

21. Miller MA, Valway SE, Onorato IM. Tuberculosis risk after exposure on airplanes. Tuber Lung Dis 1996;77.

22. Kenyon TA, Valway SE, Ihle WW, et al. Transmission of multidrug-resistant Mycobacterium tuberculosis during a long airplane flight. NEJM 1996;334:933–8.

23. Zuckerman JN. TB or not TB: air travel and tuberculosis. Travel Med Infect Dis 2010;8:81–3.

24. Moser MR, Bender TR, Margolis HS, et al. An outbreak of influenza aboard a commercial airliner. Am J Epidemiol 1979 Jul;110(1):1–6.

25. Parkins KJ, Poets CF, O'Brien LM, et al. Effect of exposure to 15% oxygen on breathing patterns and oxygen saturation in infants: interventional study. BMJ 1998;316:887–94.

26. Dreake DE, Gray CL, Ludwig MR, et al. Descriptive epidemiology of injury and illness among cruise ship passengers. Ann Emerg Med 1999;33:67–72.

27. Edelstein P, Cetron MS. Sea, wind, and pneumonia. Clin Infect Dis 1999;29:39–41.

28. Cooke GS, Lalvani A, Gleeson FV, et al. Acute pulmonary schistosomiasis in travelers returning from Lake Malawi, sub-Saharan Africa. Clin Infect Dis 1999 Oct;29(4):836–9.

29. Schwartz E. Pulmonary schistosomiasis. Clin Chest Med 2002 Jun;23(2):433–43.

30. Nuorti JP, Whitney CG, MD for the ACIP Pneumococcal Vaccines Working Group. Updated Recommendations for Prevention of Invasive Pneumococcal Disease Among Adults Using the 23-Valent Pneumococcal Polysaccharide Vaccine (PPSV23). MMWR September 3, 2010;59(34).

31. Pickering LK, Baker CJ, Freed GL, et al. Immunization Programs for Infants, Children, Adolescents, and Adults: Clinical Practice Guidelines by the Infectious Diseases Society of America. Clinical Infectious Diseases 2009;49:817–40.

32. Grohskopf L, Uyeki T, Bresee J, et al. Prevention and Control of Influenza with Vaccines: Recommendations of the Advisory Committee on Immunization Practices (ACIP), 2011. MMWR August 26, 2011;60(33):1128–32.

33. Health and Safety Executive. The control of Legionellosis including Legionnaires' disease. London: Health and Safety Executive; 1991. p. 1–19.

34. Freedman DO, Kozarsky PE, Weld LH, et al. GeoSentinel: the global emerging infections sentinel network of the international society of travel medicine. J Travel Med 1999;6:94–8.

35. Jelinek T, Corachan M, Grobush M, et al. Falciparum malaria in European tourists to the Dominican Republic. Emerg Infect Dis 2000;6:537–8.

36. World Health Organisation. Cumulative number of reported probable cases of severe acute respiratory syndrome. Online. Available: www.who.int/csr/sars/country/en/index.html (accessed Sept 28, 2011).

37. Drosten C, Gurther S, Preiser W, et al. Identification of a novel coronavirus in patients with Severe Acute Respiratory Syndrome. N Engl J Med 2003;348:1967–76.

38. Ksiazek TG, Edman D, Goldsmith CS, et al. A novel coronavirus associated with severe acute respiratory syndrome. N Engl J Med 2003;348:1953–66.

39. Lee N, Hui D, Wu A, et al. A major outbreak of severe acute respiratory syndrome. N Engl J Med 2003;348:1986–94.

40. Poutamen SM, Low DE, Henrey B, et al. Identification of severe acute respiratory syndrome in Canada. N Engl J Med 2003;348:1995–2005.

41. Booth CM, Matukas LM, Tomlinson GA, et al. Clinical features and short-term outcomes of 144 patients with SARS in the Greater Toronto Area. JAMA 2003;289:1–9.

42. Centers for Disease Control and Prevention. Severe acute respiratory syndrome and coronavirus testing. United States 2003. Online. Available: www.cdc.gov/mmwr/preview/mmwrhtml/mm5214al.html

43. World Health Organisation. H5N1 avian influenza: Timeline of major events 14 July 2011. http://www.who.int/csr/disease/avian_influenza/H5N1_avian_influenza_update.pdf. Accessed on 28 Sept 2011.

44. World Health Organisation. Clinical management of human infection with avian influenza A (H5N1) virus. Updated advice 15 August 2007. Online. Available: http://www.who.int/influenza/resources/documents/ClinicalManagement07.pdf (accessed Sept 28, 2011).

45. Zane S, Uyeki T, Bodnar U, et al. Influenza in travelers, tourism workers, and residents in Alaska and the Yukon Territory, summer 1998 (poster). Presented at the 6th Conference of the International Society for Travel Medicine, Montreal, Canada, June 6–10, 1999.

46. Balkhy HH, Memish ZA, Bafaqeer S, et al. Influenza a common viral infection among Hajj pilgrims: time for routine surveillance and vaccination. J Travel Med 2004;11(2):82–6.

47. Surveillance for travel-associated Legionnaires disease: United States, 2005–2006. MMWR Morb Mortal Wkly Rep 2007;56:1261–1263.

48. Ricketts K, Joseph CA, Yadav R, on behalf of the European Working Group for Legionella Infections. Travel–associated Legionnaires' disease in Europe in 2008. Euro Surveill 2010;15(21):pii=19578. Available online: http://www.eurosurveillance.org/ViewArticle.aspx?ArticleId=19578.

49. Anonymous. Cluster of cases of Legionnaire's disease associated with a Bangkok hotel. Communicable Dis Report CDR Weekly 1999;9:147.

50. Den Boer JW, Yzerman EPF, Schellekens J, et al. A large outbreak of Legionnaires' disease at a flower show, the Netherlands, 1999. Am Infect Dis 2002;37–43.

51. World Health Organisation. Epidemiology, prevention and control of legionellosis: memorandum of a WHO meeting. Bull WHO 1990;68:155–64.

52. Currie BJ. Melioidosis: an important cause of pneumonia in residents of and travelers returned from endemic regions. Eur Respir J 2003;22:542–50.

53. Abbas M, Emonet S, Schrenzel J, et al. Melioidosis: a poorly known tropical disease. Rev Med Suisse 2011 May 11;7(294):1000, 1002–5.

54. Allworth AM. Tsunami lung: a necrotising pneumonia in survivors of the Asian tsunami. Med J Aust 2005 Apr 4;182(7):364.

55. Peetermans WE, Wijngaerden EV, Eldere JV, et al. Melioidosis brain and lung abscess after travel to Sri Lanka. Clin Infect Dis 1999;28:921–2.

56. Dharakul T, Anuntagool SS, Chaowagul N, et al. Diagnostic value of an antibody enzyme-linked immunosorbent assay using affinity-purified antigen in an area endemic for melioidosis. Am J Trop Med Hyg 1997;56:418–23.

57. Appassakij H, Silpojakul KR, Wansit R, et al. Diagnostic value of indirect hemoagglutination test for melioidosis in an endemic area. Am J Trop Med Hyg 1990;42:248–53.

58. Sejvar J, Bancroft E, Winthrop K, et al. Leptospirosis in "Eco-Challenge" athletes, Malaysian Borneo, 2000. Emerg Infect Dis 2003 Jun;9(6):702–7.

59. Leung V, Luong ML, Libman M. Leptospirosis: pulmonary hemorrhage in a returned traveler. CMAJ 2011 Apr 19;183(7):E423–7.

60. Montero-Tinnirello J, de la Fuente-Aguado J, Ochoa-Diez M, et al. Pulmonary hemorrhage due to leptospirosis. Med Intensiva. 2011 May 16.

61. WHO/HSE/EPR/2008.3. Interregional meeting on prevention and control of plague. Antananarivo, Madagascar 1 –11 April 2006. Online. Available: http://www.who.int/csr/resources/publications/WHO_HSE_EPR_2008_3w.pdf

62. World Health Organisation. Human plague in 1996. Wkly Epidemiol Rec 1998;47:366–9.

63. Chanteau S, Rabarijaona L, O'Brien T, et al. F1 antigenaemia in bubonic plague patients, a marker of gravity and efficacy of therapy. Trans R Soc Trop Med Hyg 1998;92:572–3.

64. Lane MA, Barsanti MC, Santos CA, et al. Human paragonimiasis in North America following ingestion of raw crayfish. Clin Infect Dis 2009 Sep 15;49(6):e55–61.

65. Guiard-Scmid JB, Lacombe K, Osman D, et al. La paragonimose: une affection rare á ne pas méconnaitre. Presse Med 1998;27:1835–7.

66. Cairns L, Blythe D, Kao A, et al. Outbreak of coccidioidomycosis in Washington State residents returning from Mexico. Clin Infect Dis 2000;30:61–4.

67. Morgan J, Cano MV, Feikin DR, et al. A large outbreak of histoplasmosis among American travelers associated with a hotel in Acapulco, Mexico, spring 2001. Am J Trop Med Hyg 2003;69:663–9.

68. Lyon GM, Bravo AV, Espino A, et al. Histoplasmosis associated with exploring a bat-inhabited cave in Costa Rica, 1998–1999. Am J Trop Med Hyg 2004;70:438–42.

69. Salomon J, Flament Saillour M, De Truchis P, et al. An outbreak of acute pulmonary histoplasmosis in members of a trekking trip in Martinique, French West Indies. J Travel Med 2003;10:87–93.

70. Centres for Diseases Control and Prevention. Outbreak of acute febrile respiratory illness among college students – Acapulco, Mexico, March, 2001. MMWR 2001;50:359–60.

71. Lobato MN, Hopewell PC. Mycobacterium tuberculosis infection from countries with a high prevalence of tuberculosis. Am J Respir Crit Care Med 1998;158:1871–5.

72. Cobelens FGJ, van Deutekom H, Draayer-Jansen IWE, et al. Association of tuberculin sensitivity in Dutch adults with history of travel to areas with a high incidence of tuberculosis. Clin Infect Dis 2001;33:300–4.

73. Abubakar I, Matthews T, Harmer D, et al. Assessing the effect of foreign travel and protection by BCG vaccination on the spread of tuberculosis in a low incidence country, United Kingdom, October 2008 to December 2009. Euro Surveill 2011;16(12):pii=19826. Available online: http://www.eurosurveillance.org/ViewArticle.aspx?ArticleId=19826

74. Freeman RJ, Mancuso JD, Riddle MS, Keep LW. Systematic review and meta-analysis of TST conversion risk in deployed military and long-term civilian travelers. J Travel Med 2010;17:233–42.

75. Tuberculosis and air travel: Guidelines for prevention and control' (http://www.who.int/tb/publications/2008/WHO_HTM_TB_2008.399_eng.pdf)

76. Houk VN, Baker JH, Sorensen K, et al. The epidemiology of tuberculosis infection in a close environment. Arch Environ Health 1968;16:26–50.

77. Moore M, Valvay SE, Ihle W, et al. A train passenger with pulmonary tuberculosis: evidence of limited transmission during travel. Clin Infect Dis 1999;28:52.

78. Leder K, Tong S, Weld L, et al. Illness in travelers visiting friends and relatives: a review of the Geosentinel Surveillance Network. Clin Infect Dis 2006;43:1185–93.

79. Frame JD, Lange DR, Frankenfield DL. Mortality trends of American missionaries in Africa, 1945–1985. Am J Trop Med Hyg 1992;46:686–90.

80. Jung P, Banks RH. Tuberculosis risk in US Peace Corps volunteers, 1996–2005. J Travel Med 2008;15:87–94.

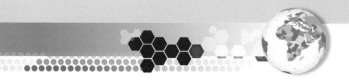

Appendix: Popular Destinations

Susanne M. Pechel and Hans D. Nothdurft

In this chapter you will find a tabular overview of 11 of the most popular short-term travel destinations worldwide. Emphasis is given on the prevailing malaria situation, on vaccination requirements, and on potential infectious and non-infectious health risks in the respective travel regions. The listings are not complete by far, but should help the reader be aware of the most important health risks and direct him or her to specific information in other chapters of this book.

As a precondition, the national recommendations in general immunization programs for children, adolescents and adults should always be followed. Not all of the vaccines mentioned in this overview are available or licensed everywhere. The listing of vaccinations available does not constitute a general recommendation for the respective region, but might help the traveler and the health advisor to come to the right decision.

All information given is based on the data provided by WHO, CDC, and DTG (see references).

Table A.1 Brazil	
Malaria situation	High risk in Acre, Rondõnia and Roraima.
	Lower risk in Amapà, Amazonas, Maranhao (W), Mato Grosso (N), Parà (not Belém City), Tocantins (W) and outskirts of Porto Velho, Boa Vista, Macapá, Manaus, Santarém, Maraba, Rio Branco, Cruzeiro do Sul.
	No malaria: Eastern coast including Fortaleza, Recife, Iguaçu and most city centres.
	Multidrug-resistant *P. falciparum* reported. *P. vivax* resistance to chloroquine reported.
Vaccination requirement	None
Vaccine-preventable diseases	Hepatitis A and B
	Influenza
	Typhoid fever
	Yellow fever
Other infectious health risks	Travelers' diarrhea and enteric parasites
	Chagas' disease
	Dengue fever
	Giardiasis
	Leishmaniasis
	Leptospirosis
	Schistosomiasis (northeast only)
Non-infectious health risks	Marine hazards

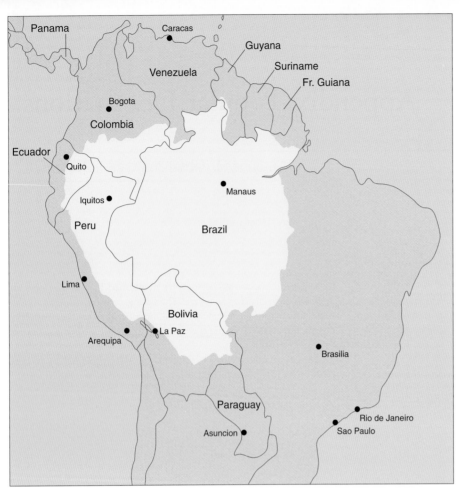

Figure A.1 Map of Amazon Basin.

Table A.2 Argentina	
Malaria situation	Minimal risk in the northern province of Salta. Occasional cases in Misiones (Department Iguazu) and Chaco. *P. vivax* 100% No malaria: all other parts of the country.
Vaccination requirements	None
Vaccine-preventable diseases	Hepatitis A and B Influenza Typhoid fever Yellow fever (Iguaçu Falls)
Other infectious health risks	Chagas" disease Dengue fever Brucellosis Leishmaniasis Travelers' diarrhea and enteric parasites
Non-infectious health risks	Animal-associated hazards

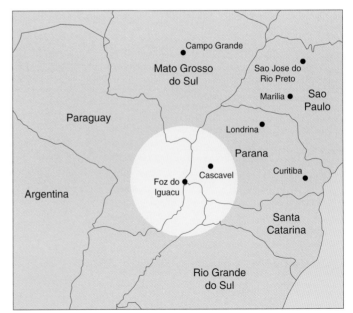

Figure A.2 Iguaçu Falls, Argentina, Brazil.

Table A.3 Peru

Malaria situation	Low risk in the whole country of Peru below 2000 m, mainly in Ayacucho, Junín, Loreto, Madre de Dios, Piura, Tumbes, San Martin, Puerto Maldonado and Iquitos. *P. falciparum* approx. 11%, P. vivax 89% No malaria: Lima, Cuzco, Macchu Picchu, Ayacucho, highland of the Andes and the coastline around Lima, Ica and Nazca
Vaccination requirements	None
Vaccine-preventable diseases	Hepatitis A and B Influenza Typhoid fever Yellow fever
Other infectious health risks	Bartonellosis Chagas' disease Dengue fever Leishmaniasis Brucellosis Plague Travelers' diarrhea and intestinal parasites
Non-infectious health risks	Altitude and Acute Mountain sickness Animal-associated hazards Trekking injuries Altitude sickness

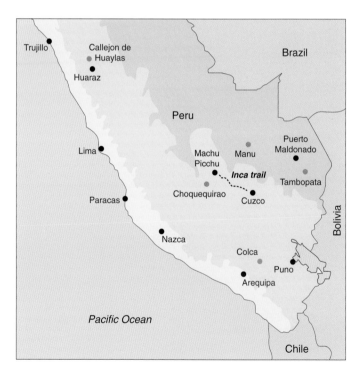

Figure A.3 Map of Inca Trail, Peru.

Table A.4 Caribbean Islands (Especially Cuba, Dominican Republic, Haiti)

Malaria situation	<u>Dominican Republic:</u> Low risk in the whole country, mainly in the western provinces (Azua, Bahoruco, Elias Pina, San Juan, and Dajabón) and La Altagracia (Punta Cana). No malaria: Santo Domingo and Santiago. P. falciparum 100% No chloroquine resistance reported. <u>Haiti:</u> Low risk in the whole country below altitude of 600m including cities. Minimal risk in Port-au-Prince *P. falciparum* 100% Chloroquine resistance recently reported. All other Caribbean islands free of malaria.
Vaccination requirements	<u>Dominican Republic, Cuba, Puerto Rico:</u> None <u>Haiti:</u> Yellow fever vaccination certificate is required from travelers coming from countries with yellow fever transmission.
Vaccine-preventable diseases	Cholera (Haiti, Dominican Republic only) Hepatitis A and B Influenza Typhoid fever
Other infectious health risks	Dengue fever Leishmaniasis Schistosomiasis (DR) Cutaneous larva migrans (especially Jamaica) Travelers' diarrhea very common (Cuba, DR and Haiti) and enteric parasites
Non-infectious health risks	Marine hazards Hurricanes & storms Ciguatera poisoning

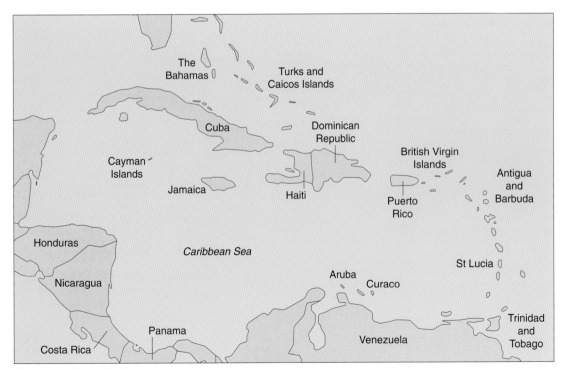

Figure A.4 Map of Caribbean Islands.

Table A.5 Mexico and Central American States

Malaria situation	Belize:
	Malaria risk varies within regions. It is moderate in Stan Creek and Toledo districts and low in Cayo, Corozal and Orange Walk
	No malaria: Belize City
	P. falciparum < 1%
	Costa Rica:
	Lower risk in Limon/Huetar Atlantica (Matina and Telemanca)
	Minimal risk in Puntarenas/Brunca, Alajuela/Huetar Norte (Los Chiles), Guanacaste/Chorotega and Heredia/Central Norte
	P. falciparum 2%
	No malaria: all cities and rest of the country
	El Salvador:
	Minimal risk in the provinces of Santa Ana, Ahuachapán and La Unión, *P. falciparum* 5–10%
	No malaria: rest of the country
	Guatemala:
	Low risk in the whole country below altitude < 100 m in Escuintla, Izabal, Alta Verapaz, Baja Verapaz, Chiquimula, Petén, Quiché, Suchitepéquez, and Zacapa. *P. falciparum* < 1%
	No malaria: Guatemala City, Antiqua, Lake Atitlan
	Honduras:
	Low risk in the whole country below altitude 1000 m, mainly in Gracias a Dios and Islas de la Bahia. *P. falciparum* 14%, P. vivax (85%) and mixed infections (1%).
	No malaria: Tegucigalpa and San Pedro Sula
	Mexico:
	Low risk in rural areas <1000 m altitude in southern border regions. Minimal risk in other areas. *P. falciparum* < 1%
	No malaria: larger cities, Yucatan, archeological sites
	Panama:
	Low risk in provinces along the Atlantic coast (Bocas del Toro) and in the border areas to Costa Rica and Colombia (Colon, Chiriquí, Darién, Ngobe Bugle, Panama, Kuna Yala , San Blas Islands and Veraguas). P. vivax 99%
	No malaria: Cities, rest of the country
Vaccination requirements	Mexico:
	None
	Guatemala, Costa Rica, Belize, Honduras, El Salvador, Panama:
	Yellow fever vaccination certificate is required from travelers (age-related) coming from countries with yellow fever transmission (Costa Rica and Honduras: also having transited more than 12 hours through the airport of countries with risk of yellow fever transmission).
Vaccine-preventable diseases	Hepatitis A and B
	Influenza
	Typhoid fever
	Yellow fever (East Panama)
Other infectious health risks	Leptospirosis (Costa Rica)
	Chagas' disease
	Dengue fever
	Bot fly (especially Belize)
	Leishmaniasis
	Travelers' diarrhea and enteric parasites
Non-infectious health risks	Diving disorders
	Marine hazards
	Ciguatera poisoning (especially Mexico)
	Security risk (Drug violence)

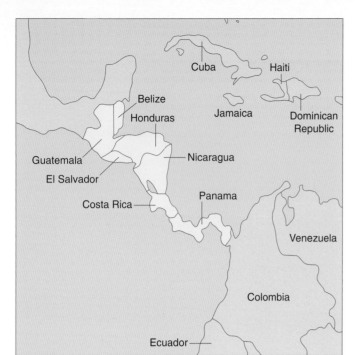

Figure A.5 Map of Central American States.

Table A.6 Southeast Asia (Cambodia, Laos, Thailand, Vietnam)	
Malaria situation	<u>Cambodia:</u> Low to moderate risk in the whole country, in all forested rural regions, including coastal areas. Minimal risk in the southern Mekong region. *P. falciparum* 66% No malaria: Pnomh Penh, Angkor Wat <u>Laos:</u> Low risk in the whole country. *P. falciparum* 97% No malaria: Vientiane <u>Thailand:</u> Low risk mainly towards the international borders, like in the northern border areas including golden triangle as well as in the southernmost provinces and coastal parts of the country, Khao Sok National Park and most of the islands (Ko Chang, Ko Mak, Ko Phangan, Ko Phi Phi, Ko Tao). *P. falciparum* 42% No malaria: Bangkok, Chanthaburi, Chiang Mai, Chiang Rai, Pattaya, Ko Phuket, Ko Samui and central areas of the northern part of the country <u>Vietnam:</u> Low risk in the whole country below 1500 m, mainly in the provinces of Gia Lai, Dak Lak, Kon Tum, Binh Phuoc, Dak Nong, Khanh Hoah, Quang Tri, Ninh Thuan, Quang Nam and Lai Chau Minimal risk in the Northeast and South of the country. *P. falciparum* 75–80% No malaria: Urban centres, Red River delta and coastline north of Nha Trang
Vaccination requirements	Yellow fever vaccination certificate is required from travelers (age-related) coming from countries with yellow fever transmission (Cambodia, Thailand: also having transited through countries with risk of yellow fever transmission).
Vaccine-preventable diseases	Cholera Hepatitis A and B Influenza Japanese Encephalitis Typhoid fever
Other infectious health risks	Avian influenza H5N1 Chikungunya Fever Dengue fever Leptospirosis Plague Schistosomiasis Monkey bites Scrub and marine typhus Travelers' diarrhea and enteric parasites
Non-infectious health risks	Diving disorders Marine hazards

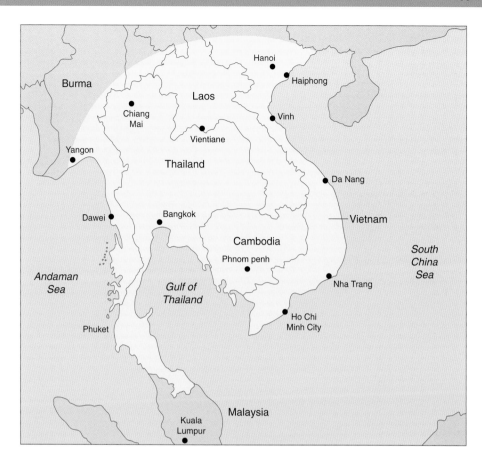

Figure A.6 Map of Southeast Asia (Cambodia, Laos, Thailand, Vietnam).

Table A.7 Bali and Surrounding Islands

Malaria situation	High risk in Irian Jaya and all islands east of Bali (including Lombok, Gili, Sumba, Sumbawa, Timor, Flores, Molukkes a.o.). Lower risk in the other parts of the country. No malaria: Big cities and tourist areas of Java and Bali. *P. falciparum* resistant to chloroquine and sulfadoxine–pyrimethamine reported. *P. vivax* resistant to chloroquine reported. Human *P. knowlesi* infection reported in the province of Kalimantan.
Vaccination requirement	Yellow fever vaccination certificate is required from travelers over 9 months of age arriving from countries with risk of yellow fever transmission.
Vaccine-preventable diseases	Hepatitis A and B Influenza Japanese Encephalitis Typhoid fever
Other infectious health risks	Avian influenza (H5N1) Dengue Leptospirosis Chikungunya Schistosomiasis (Sulawesi) Monkey bites Travelers' diarrhea and enteric parasites
Non-infectious health risks	Food poisoning from marine toxins Marine hazards.

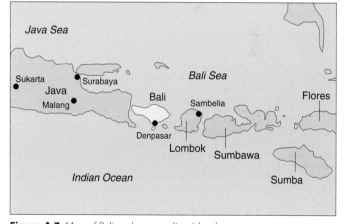

Figure A.7 Map of Bali and surrounding islands.

Table A.8 Indian Subcontinent	
Malaria situation	India: Low risk in the whole country at altitudes below 2000 m. Moderate risk of falciparum malaria and drug resistance in the north-eastern states, Andaman and Nicobar Islands, Chhattisgarh, Gujarat, Jharkhand, Karnataka, (without Bangalore), Madhya Pradesh, Maharasthra (without Mumbai, Nagpur, Nasik and Pune), Orissa and West Bengal (without Kolkata). Overall 40–50% of cases due to *P. falciparum*. *P. falciparum* resistance to chloroquine and sulfadoxine–pyrimethamine reported. No malaria: Areas above 2000 m in Himachal Pradesh, Jammu, Kaschmir, Sikkim, Arunchal Pradesh and the Lakkadives. Nepal: Low risk (mainly during rainy season) in the south of Terai districts (Bara, Dhanukha, Kapilvastu, Mahotari, Parsa, Rautahat, Rupendehi and Sarlahi including Royal Chitwan Park) bordering India predominantly *P. vivax*. *P. falciparum* resistant to chloroquine and sulfadoxine-pyrimethamine reported No malaria: Kathmandu, Pokhara, Northern Nepal Sri Lanka: Low risk in the whole country at altitudes below 1200 m. *P. falciparum* resistant to chloroquine and sulfadoxine–pyrimethamine reported. No malaria: Districts of Colombo, Galle, Gampaha, Kalutara, Matara and Nuwara Eliya
Vaccination requirement	Yellow fever vaccination certificate is required from travelers (age-related) arriving from countries with risk of yellow fever transmission.
Vaccine-preventable diseases	Cholera Hepatitis A and B Influenza Japanese Encephalitis Typhoid fever (very common)
Other infectious health risks	Chikungunya Dengue Leishmaniasis Tick-bite fever Travelers' diarrhea and enteric parasites
Non-infectious health risks	Motor vehicle accidents Marine hazards

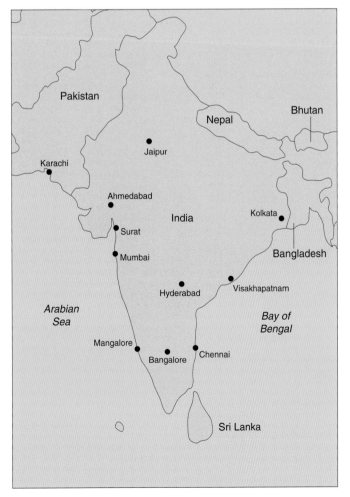

Figure A.8 Map of Indian subcontinent.

Table A.9 Eastern Mediterranean (Turkey, Cyprus)

Malaria situation	Cyprus: 　No malaria risk Turkey: 　Minimal risk in the southeast of the country (Diyarbakir, Mardin and Sanliurfa). *P. vivax* 100% 　No malaria: Tourist resorts in the west and southwest of the country.
Vaccination requirements	None
Vaccine-preventable diseases	Hepatitis A and B Influenza Typhoid fever
Other infectious health risks	Avian influenza (H5N1) Brucellosis Crimean-Congo hemorrhagic fever Leishmaniasis Travelers' diarrhea and enteric parasites
Non-infectious health risks	Marine hazards

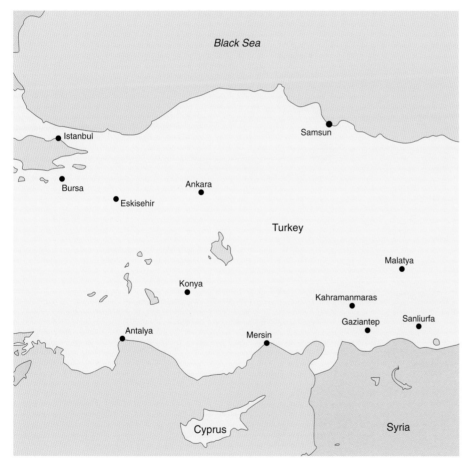

Figure A.9 Map of Eastern Mediterranean (Turkey, Cyprus).

Table A.10 Western Europe (Austria, Germany, Switzerland, Italy, France, Spain)

Malaria situation	No malaria risk
Vaccination requirements	None
Vaccine-preventable diseases	Hepatitis A and B
	Influenza
	Tick-borne encephalitis
Other infectious health risks	Brucellosis
	Avian influenza (H5N1)
	Leishmaniasis
	Lyme disease
	Anaplasmosis

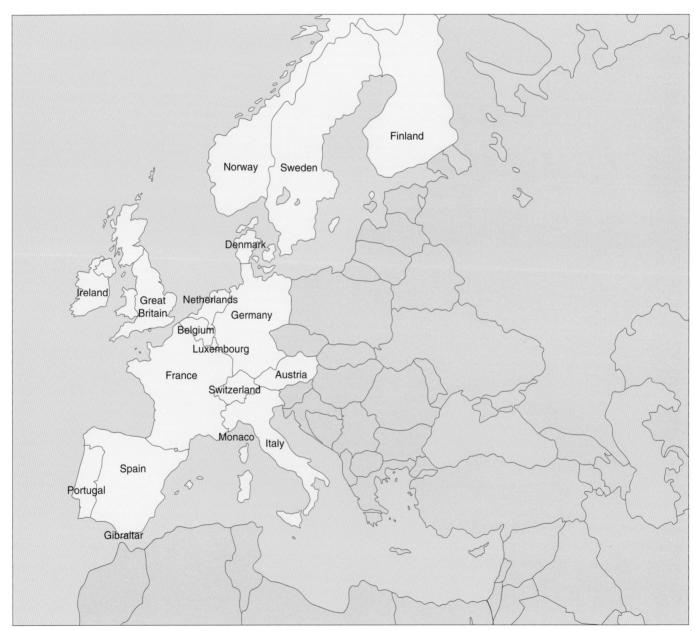

Figure A.10 Western Europe (Austria, Germany, Switzerland, Italy, France, Spain).

Table A.11 African Safaris

Malaria situation	<u>Kenya:</u> High risk in the whole country below 2500 m, including the cities. Minimal risk in Nairobi and in the highlands above 2500 m of Central, Eastern, Nyanza, Rift Valley and Western. *P. falciparum* > 99% Resistance to chloroquine and sulfadoxine-pyrimethamine reported <u>Tanzania:</u> High risk in the whole country below 1800 m, including cities and National Parks. Lower risk in altitudes between 1800 and 2500 m, in Dar es Salaam and Zansibar. *P. falciparum* > 99% Resistance to chloroquine and sulfadoxine-pyrimethamine reported <u>South Africa:</u> High risk in Mpumalanga (including Kruger National Park), Limpopo province (north and north-east) and north-eastern KwaZulu-Natal as far south as Tugela-River (including Tembe- and Ndumu wild parks). Minimal risk at Tugela River, Swartwater, Umfolozi and Hluhluwe parks. *P. falciparum* 58% *P. falciparum* resistance to chloroquine and sulfadoxine–pyrimethamine reported. No malaria: Cities and all the other parts of the country <u>Namibia:</u> High risk in Cubango and Kunene valley, Caprivi strip and the northern and northeastern regions of Oshana, Oshikoto, Omusati, Omaheke, Ohangwena and Otjozondjupa including Etosha pan. *P. falciparum* > 99% *P. falciparum* resistance to chloroquine and sulfadoxine–pyrimethamine reported No malaria: Cities, coastline and south of the country <u>Botswana:</u> High risk in the northern parts of the country: Boteti, Chobe, Northern Ghanzi, Kasane, Ngamiland, Okavango and Tutume districts. Lower risk in the eastern regions Bobirwa and Selebi-Phikwe. *P. falciparum* > 99%. *P. falciparum* resistance to chloroquine reported No malaria: Gaborone and southern parts of the country
Vaccination requirement	Yellow fever vaccination certificate is required from travelers (age-related) arriving from countries with risk of yellow fever transmission. (South Africa and Botswana: also having transited through the airport of countries with risk of yellow fever transmission).
Vaccine-preventable diseases	Hepatitis A and B Influenza Cholera Meningococcal disease Typhoid fever Yellow fever (Kenya)
Other infectious health risks	African sleeping sickness (Kenya and Tanzania only) African Tick-bite fever (especially South Africa) Chikungunya Dengue Leishmaniasis Rift valley fever Schistosomiasis Travelers' diarrhea and enteric parasites
Non-infectious health risks	Motor vehicle accidents Security risks (Nairobi)

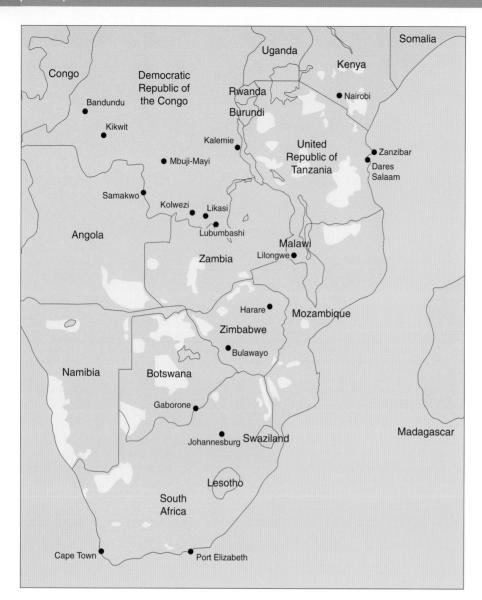

Figure A.11 Map of African safaris.

Table A.12 Mediterranean Africa

Malaria situation	**Egypt:** Mainly free of malaria. Very limited risk from June to October in El Fayum governorate (no indigenous cases reported since 1998). **Morocco and Tunisia:** No malaria risk
Vaccination requirement	**Egypt and Tunisia:** Yellow fever vaccination certificate is required from travelers over 1 year of age arriving from countries with risk of yellow fever transmission. **Morocco:** None
Vaccine-preventable diseases	Hepatitis A and B Influenza Meningococcal disease Typhoid fever
Other infectious health risks	Avian influenza (H5N1) Dengue Leishmaniasis Schistosomiasis Tick-bite fever Travelers' diarrhea and enteric parasites
Non-infectious health risks	Marine hazards

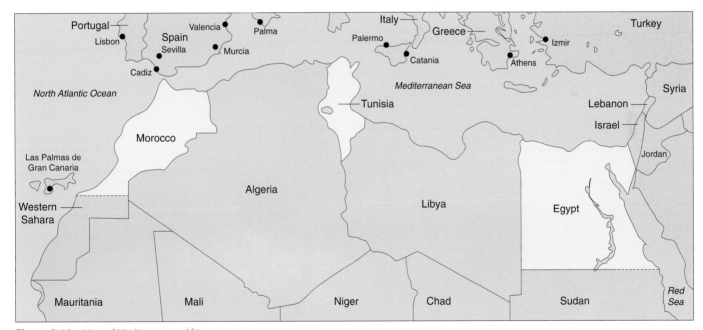

Figure A.12 Map of Mediterranean Africa.

References

1. CDC Health Information for International Travel 2012: The Yellow Book, Centers of Disease Control and Prevention, Atlanta/USA, 2012, ISBN 978 01 9 976901 8

2. International Travel and Health 2012, World Health Organization, 2012, Geneva/Switzerland, ISBN 9789241580472

3. Malaria prevention (Malariavorbeugung) 2012, German Society of Tropical Medicine and International Health (DTG), 2012, Hamburg/Germany, www.dtg.org

4. Travax enCompass www.travax.com

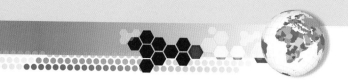

Index

NB: Page numbers in *italics* refer to boxes, figures and tables.

A

Abacavir *280*
Abdominal ultrasound 469
Academic institutions *27–29*
Acanthamoeba spp *38*
Acaris lumbricoides 473
Accidents 6–7, 33
  elderly 244
  mass gatherings 358–359
  motor vehicle 232–233, *233*
  pre-travel advice *32*
Acclimatization 383–384
Accreditation Canada International 344
Acetaminophen *221–223*, 427
Acetazolamide *221–223*
  high altitude 233–234, 364–367, *365*
Aciclovir *221–223*
Acquired immunodeficiency syndrome *see* HIV/
  AIDS
Actinobacillus infections 416–417
Acupressure *221–223*, 400
Acute coronary syndrome 259
Acute coryzal illness 511
Acute gastrointestinal disease (AGE) 351
Acute laryngitis 511
Acute mountain sickness (AMS)/high-altitude
  cerebral edema (HACE) 244, 363–367,
  366
  epidemiology 363–364
  pathophysiology 364
  presentation/diagnosis 364, *364*, *366*
  prevention 367, *367*
  treatment 364–367, *365–366*
Acute psychosis 335
Acute renal failure 174
Acute schistosomiasis (Katayama syndrome) 472,
  478, 481, 504
Adenovirus 181
Adjustment, U-curve hypothesis 310
Adolescents
  adolescent pertussis vaccine (Tdap) 126–127
  see also Pediatric/adolescent travelers
Adoption *see* International adoption
Adrenaline (epinephrine) 17
Advisory Committee of Immunization Practices
  (ACIP) 269–270
Aedes spp 57, 235–236, 413–414
  yellow fever vector 8, 102
Aedes aegypti 55, 57–59, 288, 480
  transmission 102, 479
Aedes albopictus 55, 480
Aerobacter aerogenes 428
Aeromedical evacuation 7
Aeromonas spp *38*, 201, 210, 423
Aerosolized red tide respiratory irritation
  (ARTRI) 430
Aerospace Medical Association (AsMA) 344,
  409–410
Africa, Mediterranean *535*, *535*
African safaris *533*, *534*

African scorpions (*Leiurus*), sting 419–420
African tick bite fever *498*
After-drop 387
Age
  diving medicine 373
  travelers' diarrhea (TD) 182, *183*
  yellow fever vaccine 109
AIDS *see* HIV/AIDS
Air Carrier Access Act (US) 249
Air travel
  diving before 377
  elderly 243
  physically disabled 252–253, *252*
  pre-existing disease 258–259, *258–259*
  pregnancy 220
Airborne disease 408–409
Aircraft cabin 405–412
  airborne disease 408–409
  cosmic radiation 407–408
  health problems 34
  humidity 407
  hypoxia 232
  overview 405, *406*
  ozone 407
  pesticides 408
  pressurized cabin 405–408, *406*
  see also Passenger health
Albendazole 208, *209*, *221–223*, 489–490
Alcohol withdrawal 446
Alcoholics Anonymous 440
Alcohol-related injuries 437
Allergies 152, *221–223*, 262
  eosinophilia 502, *502*
Alligators, mortality *415*
Allogeneic hematopoietic stem cell transplantation
  (allo-HSCT) 268
Alternative medications 229
Altitude
  pre-travel advice *32*
  sickness *221–223*
  see also High altitude
Amanita phalloides (death cap
  mushroom) 431–432
Amblyomma americanum 57–58
Amebiasis, invasive *471*, 472–473
Amebic colitis *199*
Amebic liver abscess *478*, 481
American Academy of Obstetrics and
  Gynecology 219
American Academy of Pediatrics 235–236
American Academy of Sleep Medicine
  (AASM) 243–244
  jet lag 392–394
American bark scorpion (*Centruroides*),
  sting 419–420
American College of Chest Physicians 452
American College of Emergency Physicians
  (ACEP) 350
American College of Obstetrics and
  Gynecology 220, 229
American Dental Association (ADA) 345

American Diabetes Association (ADA) 258, 261
American Medical Association (AMA) 344
American Society of Plastic Surgeons (ASPS) 345
American Society of Tropical Medicine and
  Hygiene (ASTMH) 15, 18, 23
American Travel Health Nurses Association
  (ATHNA) 15–16, 18, 23
Amitriptyline 427
Amnesic shellfish poisoning (ASP) *426*, 430–431
Amodiaquine 157
Amoxicillin *221–223*, 238, 515
  /clavulanic acid *221–223*, 268
  /sulbactam *221–223*
Amphetamines 394, *394*
Ampicillin 203, 480
Anaconda, mortality *415*
Analgesics 374
Ancylostoma braziliense 488
Ancylostoma duodenale *38*, 473
Anemia 174, 260
Anesthetic techniques 70
Angiostrongylus spp 507–508
Angiostrongylus cantonensis 481, 505
Animal attack injuries 415–417, *415*, *415*
  emergency care *417*
  infection 416–417, *418*, *418*
  prevention 416, *416*
  treatment 416, *418*
Animal contact, pediatric/adolescents 234
Anopheles spp 8, 236, 413–414
Antacids 152, *221–223*
Anthrax 120, 518
Antibiotics 215, *221–223*, 238
  resistance 203
  travelers' diarrhea (TD) 203–205, *204*
Anticoagulants 152–153
Anticonvulsants 374
Antidepressants 374, 445
Antiemetics 205, *221–223*
Antihistamines *221–223*, 236, 374
  motion sickness 402
Antimalarials *221–223*, 374
Antimicrobial agents 374
  travelers' diarrhea (TD) *192*, 194–195, *194*
Antimotility agents 205, 245
Anti-motion sickness agents 374
Antiparasitics *221–223*
Antipsychotics 374, 441
  atypical 441
Antiretroviral drugs 280–281
Antispasmodics 215
Antivirals *221–223*
Anxiety disorders 295, 311–312
Apidae stings 419
Appointments, travel clinics 16
AQUAMAT study 177
Arcobacter spp 201
Arcobacter butzleri 201
Argentina *524*, *524*
Aripiprazole, psychosis 441
Armodafinil 243–244, 394, *394*

Arrhythmias 387, 427
Artemether
  advantages/disadvantages *176*
  /lumefantine 169
  standby emergency treatment (SBET) *169*
Artemisinin 157
  advantages/disadvantages *176*
  combination therapies (ACTs) 164
Arterial gas embolism (AGE) 375–376
Arthropod bites 413–415, *494*
  dermatoses 494–495, *495*
  prevention 413–414, *414*
  treatment 414–415, *414*
  venomous 419–420
Ascaris spp, stool testing 319
Ascaris lumbricoides 38, 504
Asian tiger mosquito (*Aedes albopictus*) 55, 480
Aspirin *221–223*
Asplenia 260, 266–268
Asthma *221–223*, 369, 374
  eosinophilia 502, *502*
Astrovirus 181
Atazanavir *276*, 280
Atovaquone *280*
Atovaquone/proguanil (AP) 153–154
  advantages/disadvantages *176*
  adverse effects *146–147*
  children 237
  clinical utility score *147*
  dialysis 260
  efficacy 153–154
  elderly 244
  indications 154
  contraindications 154
  mode of action 153
  pregnancy *221–223*, 226, *226*
  resistance 140–141, *144*, 153–154
  standby emergency treatment (SBET) 169, *169*
  tolerability 154, 496
Atrax robustus bites 419
Atropine 427
Atropine sulfate diphenoxylate hydrochloride *221–223*
Automatic external defibrillator (AED) 411
Automobile travel 224
Avian influenza 517
Azithromycin 157, 245, 280, 286, 308
  pregnancy *221–223*, 226, 227
  travelers' diarrhea (TD) *192*, 195, 203, *204*, 205

B

Bacille Calmette–Guérin (BCG) vaccine 9, 132
Bacillus anthracis 518
Backpackers, medical kit 63–64
Bacteria
  travelers' diarrhea (TD) 181, 200–201
  persistent travelers' diarrhea (PTD) 209–210
Bacterial gastroenteritis 271
Balance 398, *399–400*
Balantidium coli 38
Bali 529, *529*
Banana spiders (*Phoneutria*) bite 419
Barbiturates 152
Bariatric tourism 345
Barometric pressure *363*
Barotrauma 375
  inner-ear 375
  middle ear 375
  preventing 375
  pulmonary 375–376
  sinus 375

Bartonella spp 416–417
Bears
  attacks *415*
  mortality *415*
Bed nets 236
Behavioral difficulties *311*
Behavioral strategies
  circadian rhythm *392*
  HIV/AIDS 274–275, *276*
  motion sickness *400*
Benzodiazepines 243–244, 394, 397, 441, 446
  motion sickness 400, 402
Benztropine, psychosis 441
Beverage recommendations *193*, 227
Biopesticide repellents *56*
BioUD (2-Undecanone) 57
Bipolar I disorder 442–444
  incidence 443
Bisacodyl *221–223*
Bismuth subsalicylate (BSS) *221–223*
  travelers' diarrhea (TD) 191, *192*, 194, *194*, 205
BiteBlocker 57
Bites
  venomous injuries *414*, 417–422
  non-venomous injuries 413–417
  see also Arthropod bites; Marine animal bites
Blastocystis spp 199–200
Blastocystis hominis 38, 182, 200, 203
Blindness 254
Blisters 338
Blood eosinophil count 469
Blood testing 214
Boat travel, pregnancy 220
  see also Cruise ships
Body temperature 381
  measurement sites 382
  measuring instruments 381–382
  monitoring 17, 381–382
  see also Temperature extremes
Botanical repellents 56–57, *56*
  vs DEET 56–58
Box jellyfish (*Chironex fleckeri*), venom 422
Boyle's Law 375
Bradycardia 426–427
Brainerd diarrhea 210
Branhamella catarrhalis, laryngitis 511
Brazil 523, *524*
Brazilian wandering spider (*Phoneutria nigriventer*) bite 419
Breastfeeding *221–223*, 228–229
  doxycycline 152
  drugs and 228
  immunizations 229
  malaria 228–229
  practicalities 229
  yellow fever vaccine 109
Brief psychotic disorder 442
British Lung Foundation 260
British Thoracic Society 452
Bronchodilators, inhaled *221–223*
Buclizine *401*
Buddy-care *see* Self-diagnosis/treatment
Burkholderia pseudomallei 477, 517–518
Burns 338
Business travelers *see* Corporate/executive travelers

C

Cabin humidity 220
Caffeine 394, *394*
Caiman, mortality *415*
Calcineurin inhibitors 269
Calcium channel blockers *221–223*

Campylobacter spp *38*, 187–188, 209, 227, 238
  detection, frequency 200
  HIV/AIDS 184, 279–280
  incidence 185, *187*
  post-infectious irritable bowel syndrome (PI-IBS) 211–212
  resistance 203, 205
  travelers' diarrhea (TD) 180–181, 200–201, 203, 205
Campylobacter jejuni 198–199, 210–211
  travelers' diarrhea (TD) 194–195, 199–201
Canada Transportation Act 249
Cancer chemotherapy 269, *271*
Canes 253
Cape buffalo, mortality *415*
Capnocytophaga spp 416–417
Capnocytophaga canimorsus 266–268, 416–417
Car travel 466
Carbamazepine 152
Cardiac problems 259–260, 369–370
Cardiopulmonary resuscitation (CPR) 411
Cardiovascular agents *374*
Cardiovascular problems 33, *259*
Care delivery, models 15–16, *15*, 312
Caribbean Islands 526, *526*
Cash, traveler's 465
Cefixime 227
Celiac serologies 214
Celiac sprue 212, *213*
Centers for Disease Control and Prevention (CDC) (US) 2, 13, 59
  atovaquone/proguanil (AP) 154
  CDC/WHO Safe Water System 44
  chlorine 44
  diarrhea 185
  guidelines for travelers 101
  immunization 76, 294
  information resources 17
  IR3535 55, 59
  malaria 135–136, 143, 163, 299
  medications 345–346
  mefloquine 150, 226
  picaridin 55–56, 59, 236
  pneumococcal vaccine 84
  rabies 118
  routine adult vaccines *82*
  training 15, 23
  traveler-oriented information 18
  Vaccine Information Statements (VIS) 18
  vaccines 75
  varicella 128
  Vessel Sanitation Program (VSP) 350
  websites 25–26
  yellow fever 107–108
Central American bullet ant (*Parapomera clavata*) 419
Central American States 527, *528*
Central nervous system (CNS) 481
Centruroides sting 419–420
Cephalosporins *221–223*
Cercarial dermatitis 495
Cerebral malaria 174
Certificate in Travel Health (CTH) 2
Cetirizine *221–223*
Chagas disease 274, *471*
Chancroid 499, *499*
Chemical repellents 53–56
Chemokine co-receptor antagonists 280, *280*
Chemoprophylaxis
  elderly 244
  HIV/AIDS 277–280, *280*
  travelers' diarrhea (TD) 191–193, 195, 279–280
  see also Malaria chemoprophylaxis
Chemotherapy, cancer 269, *271*
Chest X-rays 470

Chickenpox *see* Varicella (chickenpox) and herpes zoster vaccines
Chigger mites *52, 414*
Chikungunya (CHIK) fever *478,* 480
Chilblains 388
Children
  antibiotics 238
  development 295
  doxycycline 152
  expatriates 311–312
  growth standard charts (WHO) 293
  high altitude 370
  malaria prevention 157–158, 308
  safety seats 435–436
  standby emergency treatment (SBET) 169, *170*
  travelers' diarrhea (TD) 182–183, *183*
  see also Pediatric vaccines; Pediatric/adolescent travelers
Chlamydia spp 319, 511
Chlamydia trachomatis 499
Chlamydophila pneumoniae 515
Chloramphenicol 480
Chlordiazepoxide 446
Chlorine dioxide *39*
Chloroquine (CQ) 147–148
  advantages/disadvantages *39*
  breastfeeding 228–229
  children 237
  efficacy 147–148
  elderly 244
  HAART *280*
  indications 148
  contraindications 148
  mode of action 147
  neurological disease 262
  pregnancy *221–223,* 226, *226,* 228
  resistance 140, *144,* 147–148
  standby emergency treatment (SBET) 169, *169*
  tolerability 148
Chloroquine (CQ)-resistant *Plasmodium falciparum* (CRPf) 140, 147–148, 157, 176, 224–226, 237
Chloroquine (CQ)-resistant *Plasmodium vivax* (CRPv) 140, 144–145
Chloroquine (CQ)-sensitive *Plasmodium falciparum* 140
Chloroquine (CQ)-sensitive *Plasmodium vivax* 140
Chloroquine phosphate/sulfate *146–147*
Chloroquine/mefloquine (MQ)-resistant zones 145
Chloroquine/proguanil 147–148, *147,* 496
Chloroquine-resistant zones *144–147,* 145
Chloroquine-sensitive zones 145
Chlorpheniramine *221–223*
Cholera 9
Cholera vaccine *102,* 110–111
  adverse events (AE) *103–105,* 111
  dosing schedules *103–105,* 110–111
  drug/vaccine interactions 111
  HIV/AIDS *278–279*
  immune response 111
  indications 110
  contraindications 110
  pediatric *131*
  pregnancy *225*
  risks *106*
Cholestyramine 427
Chromobacterium spp 423
Chronic illness
  obstructive pulmonary disease (COPD) 260, 352, 369
  pediatric/adolescent travelers 234
  standby emergency treatment (SBET) 169, *170*
  travelers' diarrhea (TD) *see* Persistent travelers' diarrhea (PTD)

Chrysanthemum cinerariifolium 58
Chrysops (deer fly) 504
Chumakov Institute of Poliomyelitis and Viral Encephalitides 102
Ciguatera 338, 425–428, *426–427, 427,* 493
Ciguatoxin (CTX) 425, 427
Cimetidine *221–223*
Cinnarizine *401,* 402
Ciprofloxacin 228, 238, 480
  pregnancy *221–223,* 227
  travelers' diarrhea (TD) *194, 204*
Ciprofloxacin-resistant *Campylobacter* 203
Circadian rhythm *392*
Citronella 57
Citrus juice 47
Clarification techniques 40
Clarithromycin, pregnancy 227
Clavulanic acid *221–223,* 268
Clindamycin *221–223*
Clinics
  overseas 450–451, *451*
  see also Travel clinics
Clonorchis sinensis 38
Clonazepam 402
Clostridium difficile 214, 279
  travelers' diarrhea (TD) 199, 201, 210
Clothing 388, *388*
Coagulation-flocculation (C-F) technique *39, 40*
Coca leaf tea 366–367
Coccidioides immitis 519
Coccidioidomycosis 519
Cochliomyia hominivorax 492
Cochrane analysis 203, 402
Code of Practice for Access to Air Travel for Disabled People (UK) 249
Codeine *221–223*
Cognitive difficulties *311*
Cold
  adaptation 383
  stress 382–383, *383*
Cold injuries 386–389, *387–388*
  preventing 388–389, *388*
Colon, ulcers *199*
Colorectal cancer 212–213
Colostomies 262
Combined hepatitis A/B vaccine 35, *35,* 95–96
  accelerated schedules 96
  adverse events (AE) 96
  dosing schedules 95–96
  drug/vaccine interactions 96
  immune response 96
  indications 95
  contraindications 95
  pediatric 130
  precautions 95
  trade names *89*
Committee to Advise on Tropical Medicine and Travel (CATMAT) (Canada) 15, 139
Common cold, epidemiology 10
Communicable diseases 352
Compensation 328
Comprehensive resources *26*
Computers 17
Concentration *311*
Conception 157
Congestion *221–223*
Conjugate vaccines 125, 130, *131*
Conjunctivitis, differential diagnosis 175–176
Connective tissue disorders *502*
Constipation *221–223*
Consular information *27–29*
Consultations
  key suggestions 34
  pre-travel *see* Pre-travel consultation
Contaminated water 338

Contraceptives, oral 152
Controlled breathing, motion sickness 398
Convulsive disorders 262
Coral cuts 338
Cordylobia anthropophaga (tumbu fly) *492, 492, 492*
Coronary artery disease (CAD) 370, 374
Corporate/executive travelers 283–289
  costs, illness 284
  crisis management 286
  dignitary medicine 285
  employee perspective 285–287
  employer perspective 283–284
  environmental risks 286–287
  fitness 283–286
  healthy worker effect 284
  infectious disease, risk 288
  medical kit 64, 286, *287*
  medical threat assessment (MTA) 285–286, *285*
  overview 283
  practitioners, role 284
  pre-/post- travel health services 284
  special issues 287–288
Corticosteroids 265–266, *266–267*
Corynebacterium diphtheriae 511, 515
Coryzal syndrome *512,* 515
Cosmetic surgery 345
Cosmic radiation 407–408
Cosmopolitan dermatoses 493–496
Costs
  illness, corporate/executive travelers 284
  premature attrition 305
Co-trimoxazole 238
Cough *221–223*
Counseling
  expatriates 309
  international adoption 292
  standby emergency treatment (SBET) *168*
  transplant recipients 268–269
  vaccines 75
Country
  of origin, travelers' diarrhea (TD) 183
  specific databases *27–29*
Cramps, heat 385
C-reactive protein (CRP) 175
Creeping eruption 504
  diagnosis 496–497, *497*
Crime avoidance *see* Security issues
Crocodile, mortality *415*
Crohn's and Colitis Association (Australia) 262
Cruise Lines International Association (CLIA) 350, 352
Cruise Ship and Maritime Medicine Section (ACEP) 350
Cruise ships 349–356
  behavior 353, *354*
  health/sanitation/safety 350
  illness 350–352
  North Atlantic 349
  overview 349
  passengers/crew 349
  physically disabled 253
  preparation 352–353, *353*
  return 353
  vessel sanitation program (VSP) 350, *350*
Crutches 253
Cryptosporidium spp 37–38, 44, 351, 473
  detection, frequency 200
  disinfectants 46
  halogens 44, 47
  HIV/AIDS 184
  stool studies 214
  travelers' diarrhea (TD) 192–193, 199, 202, 203
Cryptosporidium hominis 202

Cryptosporidium parvum 38, 210
   HIV/AIDS 274–275
   travelers' diarrhea (TD) 182, 203–204, 209
Culex spp 111–112
Cultural differences 456–457
Cultural identity 297
Culture shock 309–312, *311*
Currency, local 465
Cutaneous gnathostomiasis 493
Cutaneous larva migrans (CLM) *490*, 504
   diagnosis 496–497
Cutter Lemon Eucalyptus Insect Repellent 57
Cyclizine *401*
Cyclospora cayetanensis 182, 210, 274, 473
   detection, frequency *200*
   travelers' diarrhea (TD) 202–204, *203*
   persistent travelers' diarrhea (PTD) 209, *209*
Cyclospora spp *38*, 44, 214
   travelers' diarrhea (TD) 182, 199, 202–203
Cymbopogon nardus 57
Cyproheptadine 427
Cystic fibrosis 369

D

Dapsone/pyrimethamine *226*
Darunavir *276, 280*
Death *see* Mortality
Death cap mushroom 431–432
Decade for Action for Road Safety 434
Decompression illness (DCI) 338, 376–377
   prevention 377
   treatment 377
Decompression sickness (DCS) 375–376
   types I/II 376
Decongestants *374*
Deep-vein thrombosis (DVT) 243, 286, 410, 449
DEET (*N,N*-diethyl-3methylbenzamide) 53–56, 236
   vs BioUD 57
   bites 413–414
   vs botanical repellents 56–58
   effectiveness 59
   formulation choice 54
   mosquito bites 143–144
   permethrin 58
   vs picaridin 55–56
   pregnancy *221–223*, 224
   registry 55
   safety/toxicity 54–55, *55*
   ticks 237
Dehydration *198*, 389
   kayaking/rafting 338
   pre-travel advice *32*
   voluntary 389
Delavirdine *276, 280*
Deloitte Center for Health Solutions 343–344
Dengue fever 235–236, 478, 479–480, *498*
   differential diagnosis 175–176
   epidemiology 10
   hemorrhagic (DHF) 479
   post-travel screening 472
Dengue shock syndrome (DSS) 479
Dental care 323
Dental problems 336, *336*
Dental tourism 345
Department of Global Alert and Response (WHO) 358
Department of Transportation (US) 220, 251–252
Depression *311*, 427
   major *see* Major depression
Dermacentor occidentalis 58
Dermacentor variabilis 57

Dermatitis
   cercarial 495
   marine life 495–496, *495*
Dermatobia hominis (human botfly) *492, 492, 492*
Dermatophytosis 494
Dermatoses *497*
   arthropod-related 494–495, *495*
   cosmopolitan 493–496
   diagnosed overseas 487
   diagnosed on return 487, *488*
   eosinophilia 503–504, *503*
   tropical 487–493
Desert environments 337
Destinations
   medical kits 63
   popular 523–535
Dexamethasone 221–223
   high altitude 233–234, 364–367, *365*
Dextroamphetamine *401*
Dextroamphetamine sulfate 402
Dextromethorphan 221–223
Diabetes mellitus 18, 260–261, 370–371, 374
Diabetes Monitor (ADA) 261
Dialysis 260
Diarrhea, incidence 37
   see also Persistent travelers' diarrhea (PTD); Travelers' diarrhea (TD)
Diarrheic shellfish poisoning (DSP) *426*, 430
Dicloxacillin 221–223
Didanosine *276, 280*
Dientamoeba fragilis 209, 214
Diet 388, *392*, 393
Diffuse cutaneous leishmaniasis (DCL) 490
Diffusely adhering *Escherichia coli* (DAEC) 200, *201*
Dignitary medicine 285
Dihydrofolate reductase (DHFR) 153
Diloxanide furoate 209
Dimenhydrinate 221–223
   motion sickness *401*, 402
Dinoflagellates 425–427, 430
Diphenhydramine 221–223, 236, 441
Diphenoxylate 205
Diphtheria 515
   vaccination 68, 80–81, 225, 278–279
Diphtheria, tetanus, pertussis (DTP) vaccine 9, 77–78, *78*, 82
   adverse effects 78, *81*
   ages/intervals *78*
   dosing schedules 78, *79–80*
   immune response, measures 78
   indications 77
   contraindications 77, *81*
   pediatric 126, *126–127*
   precautions 77–78
Diphyllobothrium latum 38
Diptera spp *492, 492*, 504
Dirofilaria spp 496–497
Dirofilaria immitis 473
Disabled travelers 249–255
   attendants 252
   developmental/cognitive impairment *250–251*, 254–255
   general advice 249, *250–251*
   hearing impairment 253
   legislation 249
   physical disability 252–253, *252*
   resources 27–29
   service animals 254, *254*
   speech impairment 253–254
   trip choice 249–252
   visual impairment 254
Diseases, information *27–29*
Disillusionment, U-curve hypothesis 309–310
Disinfectants 39, *41–43, 45, 46–47*

Disinfection, defined 38
   see also Water disinfection
Divers Alert Network (DAN) 18, 338, 373
Diving 373–379
   age 373
   common disorders 374–377, *374*
   fitness 373–374
   flying after 377
   hazards 378
   medical evaluation 373
   overview 373
   physics/physiological changes 374–375
   returning to 377, *377*
Division of Immunization (Canada) 20–21
Documentation
   travel health program 16–17, 20
   traveler *35*
   vaccines 75
Dopabutamine 427
Dopamine 427
Doxycycline 151–153
   adverse effects *146–147*
   children 237
   clinical utility score *147*
   dialysis 260
   efficacy 151
   HAART *280*
   contraindications 152–153
   mode of action 151
   neurological disease 262
   pregnancy 157, *221–223*, 226
   pulmonary infection 519
   resistance 140, *144*, 151
   ticks 237
   tolerability 151–152, 496
Dracunculus medinensis 38, 496–497
Dress, traveler's 465
Drowning 436–437
   kayaking/rafting 338
   phase-factor matrix *435*
   prevention 437
Drug-resistant malaria 140–141
Drugs
   hypersensitivity 502, *502*
   information sources *27–29*
Dry heat exchange 382
Duke-National University of Singapore 344
Dukoral vaccine 111

E

Earache 232
Eastern mediterranean *531, 531*
Echinococcus granulosus 38
Ectoparasites 502–503
Edema
   diagnosis 498
   heat 386
Education
   patient 18
   travelers' diarrhea (TD) 192–193, *193*
Edwardiella spp 423
Efavirenz *276, 280*
Elderly 241–247
   air travel, tips 243
   fitness 241–242
   general advice 241–243, *242*
   health insurance 242
   infections, travel-related 244–245
   medical conditions 243–244
   medical services, overseas 243
   medications 242–243
   risks 241, *242*

travel arrangements 242
trip choice 241
vaccine-preventable infections 245–246
Electrocardiogram (ECG) 259, 469
Electronic devices 465
email advice, travel clinics 22
forums 30
medical record (EMR) 15, 17–18
notifications/feeds 30
Elephant, mortality *415*
Emergencies
animal attack injuries *417*
in-flight 243, 410–411
medical kit (EMK) 411
oxygen, aircraft cabin 410
see also Standby emergency treatment (SBET)
Emerging diseases *27–29*
Emetrol *221–223*
Emotional difficulties *311*
Emtricitabine *280*
Encephalitis *478*
Encephalitozoon intestinalis 209
Endoscopic evaluation 214–215
End-stage renal disease (ESRD) 260
Enfuvirtide *280*
Entamoeba spp 182, 202
Entamoeba dispar 182, 209
screening 472–473
travelers' diarrhea (TD) 202
Entamoeba histolytica 38, *38*, 182, 305, 473, 481
incidence 185
stool testing 319, 472–473
travelers' diarrhea (TD) 202–204, *202*, 209
Enteric fever 298, *299*, *478*, 480
Enteric viruses *38*
Enteroaggregative (adherent) *Escherichia coli* (EAEC) 181, 187, 210, 238
detection, frequency *200*
incidence *187*
travelers' diarrhea (TD) 199–200, *201*
Enterobacteriaceae 209–210
Enterobius spp 502
Enterocytozoon bieneusi 209
Enterohemorrhagic *Escherichia coli* (EHEC) 181, 199–200, *201*
Enteroinvasive *Escherichia coli* (EIEC) 181, 199–200, *201*
Enteropathogenic *Escherichia coli* (EPEC) 181, 199–200, *201*
Enterotoxigenic *Escherichia coli* (ETEC) *38*, 179, 187–188, 209, 351
detection, frequency *200*
incidence 185, *187*
pregnancy 225, 227
travelers' diarrhea (TD) 181, 185, 199–200, *201*
vaccines 110, 194
Enterotoxinogenic *Bacteroides fragilis* (ETBF) 201
Environmental factors
assessment 382–383
health problems 10
respiratory tract infections (RTIs) *515*
Environmental Protection Agency (EPA) (US) 40, 57, 236
picaridin 55–56, 236
registration 43–44
Enzymatic phase, heatstroke 384
Eosinophilia 501–509
associated conditions *502*
asymptomatic 506
biology 501
causes 501–503
clinical syndromes 503–506
fever 482

patient evaluation 506–508, *507*
respiratory tract infections (RTIs) *515*
undiagnosed 508
Ephedrine *401*, 402
Epidemics 516–517
Epidemiology
bulletins *27–29*
cornerstones 5–6, *6*
Epinephrine (adrenaline) 17
Equipment, travel clinics 16–18
Erysipelothrix spp 423
Erysipelothrix rhusiopathiae 423
Erythromycin 216, *221–223*, 238
Escherichia coli 37–38, 227, 428
enterohemorrhagic (EHEC) 181, 199–200, *201*
enteroinvasive (EIEC) 181, 199–200, *201*
enteropathogenic (EPEC) 181, 199–200, *201*
Shiga toxin-producing (STEC) 200, *201*
travelers' diarrhea (TD) 185, 193, 199–200
see also Enteroaggregative (adherent) *Escherichia coli* (EAEC); Enterotoxigenic *Escherichia coli* (ETEC)
Ethical concerns, medical tourism 344
Ethnic groups 300–301, *301*
'E-thrombosis' 451
Etravirina 276, *280*
Eucalyptus 55, 57
European Aviation Safety Authority (EASA) 411
European Centre for Disease Prevention and Control (ECDC) 2, 17
European Economic Area (EEA) 460
European Health Insurance Card 460
European Union, international adoption 291
European Working Group for Legionella Infections (EWGLI) 516–517
Evacuation 459
aeromedical 7
insurance *330*
local 459
long-distance 459
medical 313
policies 312
Evaporative heat exchange 382
Examination, pre-travel 20
Executives *see* Corporate/executive travelers
Exercise 220–224, *392*, *393*
treadmill test (ETT) 370
Exercise-induced bronchospasm (EIB) 369
Exertional heatstroke (EHS) 384–385
Exhaustion, heat 385
Expatriates 305–316
children 311–312
culture shock 309–312, *311*
families 315
international care settings 312–313
medical assessment 306
pre-travel consultation 306–307, *306*, 309
preparation 307–309
psychological approach 306–307, 309, *314*/physical, combined 313, *313–314*
psychometric testing 307
reintegration 314–315
return 307–309, 313–315, *313–314*
risks 305
security issues 312
sending organization 306
Expedition Advisory Centre (Royal Geographical Society) 333
Expeditions 327–342
common disorders 333–339, *334*
desert environments 337
jungle/tropical environments 337–338
kayaking/rafting 338

mountaineering 335–337, *336*
polar environment 335, *335*
scuba diving 338–339
death overseas 340
difficult situations 339–340
liability 331–333
local healthcare 339
luxury 339
medical care, others 339–340
medical kit *65*, *66*, 331, *332*
overview 327
personal preparation 328–331, *329*
repatriation 340
return 341
risk assessment 328–331, *330*, *330–331*
safety/security 340
trip physician 327–329
websites *331*
Expertise 15
Eyeworm 504

F

Facilities, travel clinics 16–18
Factor V Leiden (FVL) 450, 452
Fasciola infection 505
Fasciola gigantica 496–497
Fasciola hepatica 38
Fatal injuries 433–434
Fatigue, chronic 427
Febrile rash 498, *498*, *498*
Federal Aviation Administration (FAA) 220, 261, 411
Fees, travel clinic 19
fee-for-service basis 19
types 19
Fever 383
causes 498, *498*
eosinophilia 506
Fever, returned travelers 475–486
causes 475, *476–477*
central nervous system (CNS) 481
clinical presentation 479–482
diagnostic work-up 482–483, *482*
epidemiology 475–477
hemorrhagic 481
history, travel/exposure 477
incubation period 478, *478*
information sources 483
laboratory studies 482–483
vs local residents 477
management 483, *483*
mode of exposure 478–479
persistent/relapsing 481–482
pre-travel vaccination 479
undifferentiated 479–481
Fidaxomicin 210
Filariasis *471*, 473, 506
Filter testing 43–44
Filtration technique *39–43*, 40–44, *41*
Finance, travel clinics 19
First Need filter 40
First-aid *see* Medical kits
Fit for Travel website 18
Fitness 32–33, 241–242
5HT4 agonist 216
Fleas *52*, *414*
Flies *52*
Fluconazole 286
Fludrocortisone acetate 427
Fluid consumption 389
Flunarizine 402
Fluoroquinolones 203, 244–245, 268, 279–280
travelers' diarrhea (TD) *192*, 194–195, *194*, 203–205, *204*

Fluoxetine 427, 445
Food and Drug Administration (FDA) 58, 75, 154, 224–226, 229, 394–395
Food recommendations 465
  hygiene 237
  pre-travel advice 32
  pregnancy 227
  travelers' diarrhea (TD) 193
Food/water safety issues, transplant recipients 268
Food-borne illness 351
  amnesic shellfish poisoning (ASP) 430–431
  ciguatera 425–428, 426–427, 427
  diarrheic shellfish poisoning (DSP) 426, 430
  mushroom poisoning 431–432, 431
  neurotoxic shellfish poisoning (NSP) 426, 430
  paralytic shellfish poisoning (PSP) 426, 430
  pufferfish (fugu) poisoning 426, 429–430, 429
  scombroid 426, 428–429, 428, 428
Foot injury 261
Foreign Affairs and International Trade Canada 460, 460
Foreigners' clinics 458
For-profit international healthcare organizations 458
Forward osmosis 43
Fosamprenavir 276, 280
Freezers, vaccine 17
Frostbite 335, 386, 388
  treatment 388
Fugu poisoning 426, 429–430, 429
Furazolidine 221–223
Fusion inhibitors (FI) 280, 280

G

Gabapentin 428
Gambierdiscus toxicus 425
Gamow Bag® 366, 366
Gastroenteritis, bacterial 271
Gastrointestinal disorders 33
  antidiarrheal medications 221–223
  cruise ships 351–352
  eosinophilia 505
  persistent travelers' diarrhea (PTD) 212–213
  pre-existing 261–262
Gender issues 182, 373
GeoSentinel Network (ISTM/CDC) 299, 305, 308, 321, 513
  fever 475
German consensus recommendations, SBET 163
Giardia spp 38, 44, 319
  travelers' diarrhea (TD) 192–193, 199–200, 203–204
Giardia intestinalis 38, 351
Giardia lamblia 214, 473
  travelers' diarrhea (TD) 182, 202
  persistent travelers' diarrhea (PTD) 208, 208
  detection, frequency 200
  incidence 185
Giardiasis 305
Gila monster, venom 422
Ginger 221–223
Ginkgo biloba 365, 367
Global Burden of Disease Study (WHO) 437
Global Dental Safety Organization for Safety and Asepsis Procedures 345
Global public health approach 434, 435
Gnathostoma spp 496–497, 504
Gnathostoma hispidum 493
Going on holiday with a lung condition (British Lung Foundation) 260
Good Samaritans, air travel 411
Government recommendations, sources of 27–29
Graft-versus-host disease (GVHD) 268
Granular-activated carbon (GAC) 40

Guaifenesin 221–223
Guide dogs 254, 254
Guiding Principles on Human Cell, Tissue and Organ Transplantation (WHO) 345
Guillain–Barré syndrome (GBS) 262
Gymnodinium breve 430
Gynecology 371

H

H₁ antagonists 429
Habituation, motion sickness 400
Haddon's event-phase matrix 434, 435
Haemagogus spp 8, 102
Haemophilus influenzae 511, 517
  type B 9, 68, 268, 278–279, 294–295
Hague Convention, international adoption 291
Hajj pilgrimage 8, 358, 358
Halofantrine 157, 169, 221–223
Halogens 39, 44–46, 45
  taste, improving 44–46
  toxicity 46
Halomonas spp 423
Haloperidol 441, 446
Hand luggage, medication 257
Harvard Medical School Dubai Center 344
Hastings Center Report 343
Hazardous waste supplies 17
Headache 427
  high altitude (HAH) 363
Healing see Medical tourism
Health Canada 55, 143
Health Care Guidelines for Cruise Ship Medical Facilities (ACEP) 350
Health Information for International Travel (CDC) (yellow book) 101, 137–139, 284
Health insurance see Insurance plans
Health risks see Risk
Healthcare see Overseas healthcare; Travel clinics
'Healthy migrant effect' 319
'Healthy worker effect' 284
Hearing impairment 253
Heat
  adaptation 383
  balance 382
  treatment, water disinfection 38–40, 39
Heat-related illness 384–386
  cramps 385
  edema 386
  exhaustion 385
  stress 382, 382
  syncope 385
Heatstroke 384–385
  classic 384
  clinical picture 384
  diagnosis 384
  differential diagnosis 384
  early presentation 384
  pathophysiology 384
  prevention 385
  prognosis 385
  treatment 384–385, 385
Helicobacter pylori 319
Helmets 436
Helminths 502, 503
Heloderma venom 422
Hematologic disorders 370
Hematological phase, heatstroke 384
Hematopoietic stem cell transplants 269, 271
Hemodialysis (HD) 260
Hemophilus B conjugate 225
Hemorrhagic fevers 481
Hemorrhoids 221–223
Henry's Law 375
Hepatic phase, heatstroke 384

Hepatitis A virus (HAV) 9, 38
  incubation period 478
  post-travel screening 470–472, 471
  risk 37
  visiting friends and relatives (VFR) 298, 302
Hepatitis A (HA) vaccine 68, 87–89, 92–94
  accelerated schedules 89
  adverse events (AE) 89
  dosing schedules 88–89, 88–89
  drug/vaccine interactions 89
  elderly 245
  estimated risk 95
  expatriates 307
  HIV/AIDS 275, 278–279
  immune response 89
  indications 87
  contraindications 87
  pediatric 126–127, 130, 131
  precautions 87–88
  pregnancy 225
  prevalence 88
  prevention see Immunoglobulin (Ig)
  trade names 89
  /typhoid combined 89, 92–94
  see also Combined hepatitis A/B vaccine
Hepatitis B virus 9
  incubation period 478
  migrant patients 318
  post-travel screening 470–472, 471
Hepatitis B vaccine (HBV) 68, 88–89, 90–95, 92–94
  accelerated schedules 91
  adverse events (AE) 95
  dosing schedules 88, 90–91
  drug/vaccine interaction 95
  elderly 245
  estimated risk 95
  expatriates 307
  HIV/AIDS 275, 278–279
  immune response 91–95
  indications 90
  contraindications 90
  pediatric 126–127, 128–129
  precautions 90
  prevalence 91
  trade names 89
  visiting friends and relatives (VFRs) 302
Hepatitis E virus 38, 227, 478
Herpes zoster see Varicella (chickenpox) and herpes zoster vaccines
High altitude 361–372
  acclimatization 361–362
  cardiac disease 259
  corporate/executive travelers 286–287
  cough 368
  diabetes 261
  diving 377
  environment 361–363, 363
  exercise 362
  headache (HAH) 363
  medical conditions, effects 368–371, 369
  pediatric/adolescents 232–234
  pregnancy 228
  pulmonary edema see High-altitude pulmonary edema (HAPE)
  -related conditions 368
  retinal hemorrhage (HARH) 368
  sickness, elderly 244
  sleep 362–363
  syndromes 363
  websites 361, 362
  see also Acute mountain sickness (AMS)/ high-altitude cerebral edema (HACE)

High altitude pulmonary edema (HAPE) *366, 366,* 367–368
  epidemiology 367
  pathophysiology 367
  presentation/diagnosis 367, *368*
  prevention *365,* 368
  treatment 367–368
High efficiency particulate (HEPA)
  filters 407–408
Highly active antiretroviral therapy
  (HAART) 273–274
  vaccines 275–277, *276, 280*
Hippopotamus, mortality *415*
Histoplasma capsulatum 519
Histoplasmosis 519
HIV/AIDS 184, 273–282
  behavioral precautions 274–275, *276*
  checklist *281*
  chemoprophylaxis 277–280, *280*
  control policies 308–309
  Cryptosporidium spp 202
  drug interactions 280–281
  eosinophilia 503
  expatriates 308–309
  health risks 274
  healthcare overseas 281
  humanitarian aid workers (HAW) 323
  incubation period *478*
  infections 9
  international adoption 292–293
  international borders 281
  migrant patients 318–319
  mortality/complications 7
  neurocysticercosis 274
  overview 273–274
  pre-travel advice 33, 274–281
  post-travel screening 470, *471*
  rebound 277, *278–279*
  Salmonella spp 201
  specific travel advice 18
  vaccination 74, 275–277, *278–279*
  visiting friends and relatives (VFR) 300
  see also Immunocompromised travelers
Hobo spider (*Tageneria*) bite 419
Honeybees (*Apidae*) stings 419
Honeymoon period, U-curve hypothesis
  309
Hookworm 473
  creeping eruption 496–497
  eosinophilia 504, 506–507
  urticaria 504
Hookworm folliculitis 489, *490*
Hookworm-related cutaneous larva migrans
  (HRCLM) 488–490, *488–490*
Hornets (*Vespidae*) stings 419
Hospital care, overseas 458
Hotels, security issues 465
Human botfly (*Dermatobia hominis*) 492, *492,*
  492
Human immunodeficiency virus *see* HIV/AIDS
Human papilloma virus (HPV) vaccine *80,*
  85–86
  dosing schedules 86
  indications *78, 82,* 85–86, 129
  contraindications 86, 129
  pediatric *127,* 129
  precautions 86
Humanitarian aid workers (HAW) 321–325
  diagnostics *324*
  morbidity 322–324, *322*
  mortality 321–322
  overview 321
  psychological evaluation *324–325*
  recommendations 324, *324–325*
  vaccinations *324*
Humidity, aircraft cabin 407

Hydration
  dehydration *see* Dehydration
  fluid consumption 389
  hypohydration 389
  hyponatremia 389
  isotonic fluids 389
  overhydration 389
  pre-travel advice *32*
  rehydration 389, *390*
Hydrocodone *221–223,* 365
Hydrocortisone suppositories *221–223*
Hydroxyzine 427
Hyena, mortality *415*
Hymenoptera 419
Hyperbaric chambers 366, *366*
Hypersensitivity 109, 152, 496
Hyperthermia 244
Hyperthermic phase, heatstroke 384
Hypoderma lineatum 492
Hypoglycemia 174, 388
Hypohydration 389
Hyponatremia 389
Hypotension 427
Hypothermia 244, 386–388, *386*
  complications 387–388
  diagnosis 387
  treatment 387
Hypoxia 361–362
  aircraft cabins 232
  -inducible factor (HIF) 362
  inhalation test (HIT) 260

I

Ibuprofen *221–223,* 419
Idiopathic inflammatory bowel disease (IBD)
  212
Idoquinol *221–223*
Illusory self-motion 397
Immersion foot 388
Immune globulins *225*
Immune response
  cholera vaccine 111
  combined hepatitis A/B vaccine 96
  diphtheria, tetanus, pertussis (DTP) 78
  hepatitis A (HA) vaccine 89
  hepatitis B vaccine (HBV) 91–95
  influenza vaccine 99
  Japanese encephalitis (JE) vaccine 113
  measles, mumps and rubella (MMR)
    vaccine 83
  meningococcal vaccine 114–115
  pneumococcal vaccine *79–80,* 85
  rabies vaccine 118
  tick-borne encephalitis (TBE) vaccine
    119–120
  typhoid fever vaccine 97
  varicella (chickenpox) and herpes zoster
    vaccines 84
  yellow fever vaccine 109
Immunity
  altered states 109
  immune status 277
  travelers' diarrhea (TD) 183, *184*
  vaccines 74
  see also Immunocompromised travelers
Immunization Action Coalition (IAC) 16
Immunizations
  active 67–69, *68–69*
  breastfeeding 229
  elderly 245
  expatriates 307
  humanitarian aid workers (HAW) *324*
  immune suppression *267*
  international adoption 294–295

  migrant patients 319
  passive 69–70
  pediatric/adolescent travelers 235
  pregnancy 224, *225*
  principles 67–76
  recommended 9
  regulatory/advisory 76
  required 8
  route 70–72
  routine 8–9, 245
  serologic testing 73–74
  underlying conditions *267*
  visiting friends and relatives (VFR) 301–302,
    302
  see also Vaccines
Immunocompromised travelers 74, 265–272
  additional considerations 270–271, *271*
  asplenic travelers 266–268
  cancer chemotherapy 269, *271*
  corticosteroids/tumor necrosis factor-α
    inhibitors 265–266, *266–267*
  overview 265, *267*
  rabies, lymphoma and 269–270
  see also HIV/AIDS; Transplant recipients
Immunoglobulin (Ig) 89–90
  administration 73
  adverse events (AE) 90
  dosing schedules 90
  drug/vaccine interaction 90
  indications 89–90
  contraindications 90
Impetiginization 488–489
Impetigo 493–494, *494*
Indian subcontinent 530, *530*
Indinavir *276, 280*
Infants
  doxycycline 152
  malaria chemoprophylaxis 157–158
  see also Pediatric vaccines; Pediatric/adolescent
    travelers
Infections
  animal attack 416–417, *418, 418*
  blood/tissue dwelling parasites 473–474
  control 17
  elderly 244–245
  eosinophilia 140, *502*
  marine 423, *423*
  respiratory *see* Respiratory tract infections
    (RTIs)
  Rickettsial 480
  systemic *198*
Infectious diseases 7
  corporate/executive travelers 288
  expatriates 308
  international adoption 294
  tropical *469*
Infectious Diseases Society of America (IDSA) 15,
  18
Inflammatory bowel disease (IBD) 262
  idiopathic 212
In-flight emergencies, elderly 243
Influenza 517
  aircraft cabin 409
  avian 517
  cruise ships 351
  H1N1 strain 409
  incubation period *478*
Influenza vaccine 68, 92–94, 98–99
  adverse events (AE) 99
  dosing schedules 88, 98–99
  estimated risk 95
  HIV/AIDS *278–279*
  immune response 99
  immunocompromised travelers 270
  indications 98
  contraindications 98

pediatric *126–127*, 128
precautions 98
pregnancy *225*
Information resources 16–18, 25–30
clinician 17–18
electronic forums/listservs 30
electronic notifications/feeds 30
journals 25, *26*
point-of-care destination resources 26–30, *27–29*
reference texts 25, *26*
websites 25–26, *27–29*
Injuries 433–438
aircraft travel 232
alcohol-related 437
animals *see* Animal attack injuries
cold *see* Cold injuries
cruise ships 352
elderly 244
fatal 433–434
global public health approach 434, *435*
non-fatal 434
overview 433
prevention 434, *435*
road traffic safety 435–436, *435–436*
water-related 436–437, *437*
Insects 51–61
habitat avoidance 51
insecticides 58
mosquitoes *see* Mosquitoes
pediatric/adolescent travelers 235–237, *236*
personal protection 51–59
physical protection 52–53, *52, 53–54*
repellents 53–58, *55–56, 221–223*
stimuli, attracting 51, *52*
treatment 236
Institut Pasteur Dakar 102
Institute of Medicine (US) 75
Insulin *374*
adjustment 261
Insurance plans 219–220, 257
elderly 242
expeditions 328, 333
international adoption 293
travel 19, 460–461, *460*
Integrase inhibitors 280, *280*
Interferon-γ release assay (IGRA) 470
International adoption 291–296
child development 295
ethical issues 291–292
health problems 293
immunization 294–295
infectious disease 294
medical preparation, carers/families 292–293, *292*
nutritional status 293–294
overview 291
pre-adoption evaluation 292
post-adoption consultation 293, *294*
pre-travel consultation, adoptees 293
social impact 295
International agencies *27–29*
International Air Transport Association (IATA) 409–410
International Association for Medical Assistance to Travelers (IAMAT) 18, 243, 258, 293, 339
International Certificate of Vaccination or Prophylaxis (ICVP) 17, 107
International Commission for Radiological Protection (ICRP) 408
International Committee of the Red Cross (ICRC) 321–322, 324
International Convention for Safety of Life at Sea (SOLAS) (IMO) 350

International Diabetes Federation 261
International Diploma of Mountain Medicine 337
International factors
adoption *see* International adoption
borders, HIV/AIDS 281
care settings, expatriates 312–313
International Headache Society 363
International Health Regulations (IHRs) (WHO) 101
International Maritime Organization (IMO) 350
International Narcotics Control Board (INCB) 64
International Porter Protection Group (IPPG) 333
International Sanitary Regulations (WHO) 350
International Social Service (Geneva), international adoption 291
International Society for Aesthetic Plastic Surgeons 345
International Society of Travel Medicine (ISTM) 2, 299, 339
travel clinics 13, 15–16, 18, 23, 352
Travel Medicine Forum 30
International SOS 243
International Travel and Health (WHO) 106, 139
Into Thin Air (Krakauer) 335
Intoxication, treatment 445–446
Intradermal route, vaccines 72, *73*
Intramuscular (IM) route, vaccines 70–71, *70, 71*
Iodine *221–223*
Iodine resins 44, *45*
Iodoquinol 209
IR3535 (ethyl-butylacetylaminoproprionate) 55
Iron supplementation 220
Irritable bowel syndrome (IBS) 195
post-infectious (PI-IBS) 211–212, *211*, 215, *215*
Isospora spp 199, 214
Isospora belli *38*, 473
HIV/AIDS 184, 274–275
travelers' diarrhea (TD) 182, 209
Isotonic fluids 389
Ivermectin 489–490
Ixodes dammini 58
Ixodes persulcatus 118
Ixodes ricinus 118, 132
Ixodes scapularis 57–58

J

Japanese encephalitis (JE) 9, *302*
HIV/AIDS 275, *278–279*
Japanese encephalitis (JE) vaccine *102, 106*, 111–113, *111*
adverse events (AE) 113
children 237
chimeric (JE-CV) 112
dosing schedules *102–105*, 112–113
drug/vaccine interactions 113
elderly 245
expatriates 307
immune response *103–105*, 113
inactivated cell-culture (IC51) 112
indications 112
contraindications 112
live attenuated (SA-14-14-2) 112
pediatric 131–132, *131*
pregnancy *225*
JE (Vero-cell) vaccination 68
Jet lag 34, 243–244, 287–288, 391–396
defined 391
effects 392
getting to sleep 393–394, *394*

physiology 391–392, *392*
staying awake 394–395, *394*
treatments 392–395, *394*
JEV (mouse brain) vaccination 68
Johns Hopkins Singapore International Medical Center 344
Joint Commission International (JCI) 344, 455
Journal of Travel Medicine 2
Journals 25, *26*
Jungle environments 337–338

K

Kaolin 238
Katayama syndrome (acute schistosomiasis) 472, *478*, 481, 504
Kayaking/rafting 338
Kissing bugs *52*
Klebsiella pneumoniae 428
Komodo dragon (*Varanus komodoensis*) bites 416–417

L

Laboratory test 468–469
Lactation, malaria chemoprophylaxis 157 *see also* Pregnancy
Lactobacillus GG 193, 205
Lamivudine *280*
Lancet 358
Language barriers 301
Lantana camara 57
Laryngitis *512*
diagnosis 515
Latent TB infection (LTBI) 519
Latrodectus bite 419
Laws 16
Legal issues
liability, expeditions 328, 331–333
restrictions, medical kits 64
travel clinics 18
vaccines 75
Legionella spp 351, 511, 513, 517
Legionella pneumophila type 1 517
Legionnaire's disease (legionellosis) 517
cruise ships 351
epidemiology 10
incubation period *478*
Leishmania spp 491
Leishmania braziliensis 490
Leishmania chagasi 274
Leishmania donovani 274
Leishmania infantum 274
Leishmania major 490
Leishmania mexicana 490
Leishmania tropica 490
Leishmaniasis
diffuse cutaneous (DCL) 490
epidemiology 10
expatriates 305
HIV/AIDS 274
incubation period *478*
localized cutaneous (LCL) 490–492, *490–491*
mucosal (ML) 490–491
post-travel screening *471*, 473
recurrent cutaneous (RCL) 490
Leptospira interrogans 518
Leptospirosis 475, *478*, 480–481, 518
Leukocytosis, differential diagnosis 176
Levofloxacin 268, 286, 308
travelers' diarrhea (TD) *194, 204*
Liability, expeditions 328, 331–333
Lice *52, 414*
Lidocaine 427
Light therapy 392–393

Limb lymphedema 493, *494*
Lions, mortality *415*
Lippia uckambensis 57
Listeria spp 227, 268
Listservs 18, 30
Liver disease 262
Liver enzymes, elevated *482*
Loa loa 473, 496–497, 504, 506
Local regulations 466
Localized cutaneous leishmaniasis (LCL)
490–492, *490–491*
Lodging, travelers' diarrhea (TD) 185
Loeffler's syndrome 504–505, *504*
vs acute schistosomiasis 504
Long-term travelers 158
Loperamide 205, 215, *221–223*, 238
Lopinavir *276*, *280*
Loratadine *221–223*
Lorazepam *401*, *402*, 441
Low molecular weight heparin (LMWH) 452
Lower respiratory tract infections (LRTIs)
511
Loxosceles bite 419, *419*
Lumefantrine 169, *169*
Lung disease 260
Lyme disease 237
Lymphangitis *see* Nodular lymphangitis
Lymphoma 269–270
Lyssavirus spp 116
see also Rabies

M

Magnesium 152
Magnesium sulfate 446
Maitotoxin 425
Major depression 444–445, *444*
diagnosis 444–445
incidence 444
treatment 445
Mal de débarquement syndrome (MDD) 397
Malabsorptive states, post-infectious 210–211,
211
MalaQuick 166–167
Malaria 135–142
breastfeeding 228–229
cardiac disease 259–260
chemotherapy 176–177, *176*
children 236–237
dialysis 260
differential diagnosis 175–176, *176*
'doctors delay' 176
drug-resistant 140–141
elderly 244
epidemiology 6, 8, *136–137*, 137–139,
138
expatriates 307–308
fever *478*, *479*
humanitarian aid workers (HAW) 322
immunity development 173
laboratory parameters 175
microscopic diagnosis 175
overview 135
phase-factor matrix *435*
post-travel screening *471*, 473
pregnancy 224–227
prevention 268
returned travelers 475
risk 135–137
self-diagnosis/treatment 163–172
species distribution 139–140, *139*
symptomatology 173–175
treatment 226–227
visiting friends and relatives (VFR) 299–300,
299, *299*, 302

Malaria chemoprophylaxis 143–162, 224–226,
226
algorithm *156*
approach 143–144
appropriate drugs 144
current drug regimes 147–155
drug resistance 144–145, *144*, *145*
early diagnosis/treatment 144
future directions 155–157
HIV/AIDS 277–279, *280*
illustrative cases 158–159
inappropriate drugs 157
neurologic disease 262
personal protection 143–144
risk assessment 143
special populations 157–158
tolerability 496
Malarone 262
Malassezia furfur 494
Mania 442–444, *443*
diagnosis 443
incidence 443
treatment 443–444
Mannitol 428
Mansonella ozzardi 506
Mansonella perstans 473, 506
Mansonella streptocerca 506
Maps, information sources 27–29
Maraviroc *280*
Marine animal bites/stings 422–423
dermatitis 495–496, *495*
infections 423, *423*
prevention 422–423
treatment *421*, 423
Marketing, travel health program 21–22, *21*
Mass Gathering Medicine (*Lancet* conference) 358
Mass gatherings 357–359
accidents 358–359
communicable disease 358
non-communicable disease 358–359
defined 357
management 357
planning 359
pre-travel consultation 359
risks 357
sizes 357
Measles 9
aircraft cabin 409
distribution of notification rate *82*
vaccination *68*, *225*, 278–279
Measles-mumps-rubella (MMR) vaccine 79–83,
79, *80*
adverse effects 81–83, *81*
dosing schedule 79–80, 81
exemplified immunization schedule *82*
immune response measures 83
indications *78*, 81, *82*
contraindications 81
pediatric *126–127*, 127
precautions 81
pregnancy 228
risks *81*
Meclizine *221–223*, *401*
Medical devices 253
Medical Information Form (MEDIF) (IATA) 409
Medical interview, post-travel 468, *469*
Medical kits 33, 63–66
aircraft 411
basic 65–66, *65*
caring for others 65
comprehensive 65, 66, *66*
contents 63–65, *64*, 457
corporate/executive travelers 286, *287*
emergency (EMK) 411
expeditions 65, 66, 328, 331, *332*
international adoption *292*

overview 63
packaging 64, *64*
pediatric/adolescent travelers 235, *235*
pregnancy 229
specialist providers *65*
Medical tourism 343–347
adverse effects/complications 346
bariatric tourism 345
cosmetic surgery 345
dental tourism 345
general considerations 344
growth 456
medications 345–346
reproductive tourism 345
transplant tourism 345
types 343–344, *344*
MedicAlert (US) 258
Medications 17
hand luggage 257
overseas 345–346
Mediterranean Africa *535*, *535*
Mefloquine (MQ) 148–151
advantages/disadvantages *39*
adverse events (AE) *146–147*, 149–150
breastfeeding 228–229
children 237
clinical utility score *147*
contraindications 150–151
dialysis 260
efficacy 148–149
HAART *280*
meta-analysis 149
mode of action 148
neurological disease 262
pregnancy *221–223*, 224–226, *226*, 228
resistance 140, *140*, 144, 148–149, 176
standby emergency treatment (SBET) 169, *169*
tolerability *145–146*, 149, 496
Melatonin 243–244, 393–394, *394*
Meliodosis 517–518
Memory difficulties *311*
Meningococcal disease *302*
Meningococcal meningitis 76
Meningococcal vaccine *68*, *102*, 113–115, *114*
adverse events (AE) *106*, 115
conjugate 130
dosing schedules *103–105*, 114
drug/vaccine interactions 115
immune response 114–115
indications 113–114
contraindications 114
pediatric *126–127*, 130, *131*
pregnancy 225
Mental health 323–324
Mercury preservatives 75
Methicillin-resistant *Staphylococcus aureus*
(MRSA) 493–494
Methicillin-sensitive *Staphylococcus aureus*
(MSSA) 493–494
Metoclopramide *221–223*
Metronidazole 208, *209*, 210, *221–223*, 227
Mexican beaded lizard (*Heloderma*), venom 422
Mexico *527*, *528*
Mexiletine 427
Microsporidium spp 184, 209
Migrant patients 317–320
core values/best practice 319–320
health evaluation 317–319
screening 317–319, *318*
Milk of magnesia *221–223*
Minnesota Immigrant Health Task
Force 319–320
Missionary clinics 460
Mobile phones 465
Mobility, health problems 34
Modafinil 243–244, 394, *394*

Models of care 312
Monkeys, bites *418*
Monoamine oxidase (MAO) inhibitors 440, 445
Morbidity 7–10
  expatriates 305, *306*
  humanitarian aid workers (HAW) 322–324,
    322
Morganella morganii 428
Mortality 6–7
  animal attacks *415*
  expatriates 305
  expeditions 340
  humanitarian aid workers (HAW) 321–322
Mosquitoes *32, 52*, 235–236
  bite relief 59
  deterrents *414*
  population reduction 58–59
Motion sickness 34, 233, 397–403
  adjunctive/new agents 402
  candidates 398
  defined 397–398
  elderly 243
  mechanism 398
  pediatric/adolescent travelers 233
  prevention/treatment 398–400, *401*, 402,
    403
  triggers 397–398
  vestibular (balance) system 398, *399–400*
Motor vehicles
  accidents 232–233, *233*
  health problems 34
Mountaineering 335–337, *336*
Mucosal leishmaniasis (ML) 490–491
Multiple sclerosis (MS) 262
Mumps 9
  vaccination *68*, 225
  see also Measles-mumps-rubella (MMR)
    vaccine
Musculoskeletal pains 427
Mushroom poisoning 431–432, *431*
Myasthenia gravis 262
Mycobacterium abscessus 346, 496
Mycobacterium marinum 423
Mycobacterium tuberculosis 9, 274, 408–409, 470,
  519
Mycoplasma spp 511
Mycoplasma genitalium 499
Mycoplasma pneumoniae 515
Myiasis 492, *492, 492*
Myocardial infarction 259

N

Naloxone 445
Naproxen *221–223*
Narcotics Anonymous 440
National AIDS Manual (NAM) 281
National Association for Colitis and Crohn's
  Disease (UK) 262
National Childhood Vaccine Injury Act (NCVIA)
  (US) 16, 18, 75
National Coordination Center for Traveler's
  Health Advice (LCR)
  (Netherlands) 14–15
National Travel Health Network and Centre
  (NaTHNaC) (UK) 2, 13, 17, 25–26
Necator americanus 473
Needle-free application, vaccines 72
Needlestick Prevention and Safety Act (US) 18
Neisseria menigitidis 8, 113, 481
  vaccines 268, 275–277, *278–279*
Nelfinavir *276, 280*
Neomycin 194
Neoplasm *502*
Neurocysticercosis 274, 473

Neurologic disease *259*, 262
  eosinophilia 505, *505*
  high altitude 370
  malaria prophylaxis 262
Neuropsychiatric disease, severe 262
Neuropsychiatric effects, mefloquine (MQ) 150
Neuropsychological problems 33
Neurotoxic shellfish poisoning (NSP) *426*, 430
Nevirapine *276, 280*
New Horizons (US Dept of
  Transportation) 251–252
Nicotinamide *394*
Nicotinamide adenine dinucleotide (Nadh) 395
Nifedipine 233–234, *365*, 427
Nitazoxanide 208–209, *209*
Nitrofurantoin *221–223*
Nitrogen narcosis 378
Nitzschia pungens 430–431
Nodular lymphangitis *491*
  diagnosis 498
Non-fatal injuries 434
Non-governmental organisations (NGOs) 321
  mortality pattern 322
Non-infectious health problems 7, 10
Non-ionizing radiation 408
Non-nucleoside reverse transcriptase inhibitor
  (NNRTI) 280, *280*
Non-steroidal anti-inflammatory drugs
  (NSAIDs) *221–223*, 419, 427
Non-typhoidal *Salmonellae* (NTS) 275
Non-venomous injuries 413–417
Norfloxacin *194, 204*
Norovirus (NoV) 38
  cruise ships 351–352
  detection, frequency *200*
  diarrhea 185
  incidence 185, *187*
  travelers' diarrhea (TD) 181, 201–202
Norwalk virus 181
Nucleoside reverse transcriptase inhibitor
  (NRTI) 280
Nucleotide reverse transcriptase inhibitor
  (NtRTI) 280, *280*
Nursing care, overseas 457
Nursing mothers see Breastfeeding
Nutritional status 293–294

O

Obstetrics 371
Ocimum americanum 57
Oestrus ovis 492
Ofloxacin *194*, 480
Olanzapine, psychosis 441
Older people see Elderly
Olympics 358
Omeprazole *221–223*
Onchocerca volvulus 473
Onchocerciasis 493, *494*
Ondansetron *221–223, 365*
Ophthalmologic conditions 371
Opioid intoxication 445
Oral poliovirus vaccine (OPV) 68
Oral rehydration solution (ORS) 227
Organizational support 313
Otitis media 515
Outbreaks, information sources 27–29
Outdoor activities 233–234
Overhydration 389
Overland groups 64
Overseas health care 455–462
  approach, critical differences 456–457
  assistance websites *27–29*
  categories 457–458, *457*

changes 455–456
  common conditions 456
  death 340
  elderly 243
  HIV/AIDS 281
  insurance 460–461, *460*
  medical tourism 456
  medications 345–346, 458–459
  overview 455, *456*
  pharmacy issues 458–459
  planning ahead *457*, 459–460, *459*
  pregnancy 219–224
  psychiatric disorders 450–451, *451*
  risks 456
  see also Evacuation; Medical kits
Overwhelming post-splenectomy infection
  (OPSI) 266–268
Oxygen
  dissociation curve of blood 405, *406*
  emergency, aircraft cabin 410
  resources *369*
Oxymetazoline *221–223*
Ozone, aircraft cabin 407

P

Packaging 64, *64, 65*
Panton Valentine leukocidine (PVL)-positive
  Staphylococcus aureus 493–494
Paraclinical tests 468–469
Paragonimiasis 519
Paragonimus spp 505
Paragonimus westermani 38, 519
Paralytic shellfish poisoning (PSP) *426*, 430
Parapomera clavata 419
ParaSight-F 166
Parasites
  migrant patients 319
  post-travel screening 472–474
  travelers' diarrhea (TD) 182
  persistent travelers' diarrhea (PTD) 208–209
Paromomycin 209, *209, 221–223*, 227
Paroxetine 445
Partial adjustment, U-curve hypothesis 310
Passenger health 409–411
  assessment criteria 409–410
  medical clearance 409
Pasteurella spp 416–417
Patent foramen ovale (PFO) 374
Patient education 18
Patient Group Directions (PGD) 15
Peace Corps volunteers (PCVs) 321
  mental health 324
  mortality 322
  tuberculosis (TB) 322
Pediatric vaccines 125–133, *126–127*
  accelerating 129, *129*
  conjugate 125
  intercurrent illness 126
  polysaccharide 125
  recommended 130
  required 129–130
  routine 126–129, *126–127, 129*
  specific considerations 125–126
  travel 129–132
Pediatric/adolescent travelers 219–230
  air travel 232
  chronic medical conditions 234
  immunization 235
  insect-borne diseases 235–237, *236*
  medical kit 235, *235*
  motion sickness 233
  motor vehicle accidents 232–233, *233*
  outdoor activities 233–234
  returned/immigrating 238–240

risk-taking behaviors 234, *235*
safety/comfort 231–235
schedules 232
travelers' diarrhea (TD) 237–238, *238*
Pelargonium citrosum Van Leenii 57
Pelodera strongyloides 496–497
Penicillin *221–223*, 515
Permethrin 58
Persistent travelers' diarrhea (PTD) 207–218
　bacteria 209–210
　clinical approach 213–216
　definitions/epidemiology 207–208
　gastrointestinal diseases 212–213
　history/physical examination 213–214, *213*
　laboratory work-up 214–215
　parasites 208–209
　pathogenetic mechanisms 208–213, *208*
　post-infectious processes 210–212
　therapy 215–216, *215*
　unknown pathogens 210
Personal security *see* Security issues
Pertussis vaccine *68*, 80
　adolescent (Tdap) 126–127
　adverse effects *81*
　pregnancy *225*
　see also Diphtheria, tetanus, pertussis (DTP)
　　vaccine
Peru *525*, *525*
Pesticides, aircraft cabin 408
Pharmacopeias *26*
Pharyngitis 511, *512*
　diagnosis 515
Phenothiazines *221–223*
Phenytoin 152, 402
Phoneutria spp 419
Phoneutria nigriventer bites 419
Photocatalytic disinfection *41–43*, 46
Photo-induced disorders 496
Photosensitivity 496
Phototherapy, adjusting circadian rhythm
　392
Physalia physalis sting 423
Physical difficulties *311*
Physical disability 410
　see also Disabled travelers
Physical examination, post-travel 468
Picaridin 55–56, *56*, 236, 413–414
Pigs, feral/wild, mortality *415*
Plague 518–519
　vaccine 121, *131*
Plasmodium spp 163, 473
Plasmodium falciparum 163
　atovaquone/proguanil (AP) 153–154, 226
　azithromycin 157
　business travelers 288
　chemoprophylactic drugs 144
　chloroquine (CQ) 147–148
　chloroquine (CQ)-resistant (CRPf) 140,
　　147–148, 176
　chloroquine (CQ)-sensitive 140
　distribution 139–140, *139*
　doxycycline 151, 153
　epidemiology 7–8
　expatriates 305
　fatality rate 136–137
　HIV/AIDS 279
　incubation period *478*
　indigenous populations 174–175
　mefloquine (MQ) 149
　mortality rate 173
　pediatrics 158
　pregnancy 157, 224, 308
　primaquine 154–155
　proguanil-resistant 147–148
　rapid diagnosis tests (RDTs) 164–165, *166*,
　　167

screening 473
severe manifestations, adults 173–174, *174*
standby emergency treatment (SBET) 168, 170
symptomatology 173–174
tafenoquine 155
transmission rate 137, *138*
visiting friends and relatives (VFRs) 299
Plasmodium knowlesi 173
Plasmodium malariae
　chemotherapy 176
　chloroquine (CQ) 147
　chloroquine (CQ)-resistant 140
　distribution 139–140, *139*
　mortality rate 173
　rapid diagnosis tests (RDTs) 166, *167*
　recurrence 175
Plasmodium ovale
　atovaquone/proguanil (AP) 154
　chemotherapy 176
　chloroquine (CQ) 147
　clinical presentation 175
　distribution 139–140, *139*
　doxycycline 151
　mortality rate 173
　primaquine 141, 154
　rapid diagnosis tests (RDTs) 166, *167*
　recurrence 175
Plasmodium vivax
　atovaquone/proguanil (AP) 154
　chemoprophylactic drugs 144
　chloroquine (CQ) 147
　chloroquine (CQ)-resistant (CRPv) 140
　chloroquine (CQ)-sensitive 140
　clinical presentation 175
　distribution 139–140, *139*
　doxycycline 151
　expatriates 305
　mortality rate 173
　pregnancy 224
　primaquine 141, 154–155
　rapid diagnosis tests (RDTs) 165–166, *166*,
　　167
　recurrence 174
　tafenoquine 155–156
　transmission rate *138*
Plesiomonas spp 210
Plesiomonas shigelloides *138*, 201, 428
Pneumococcal vaccine *68*, 80, 84
　adverse events (AE) *81*, 85
　dosing schedule 85
　immune response *79–80*, 85
　indications 84–85
　contraindications 85
　pediatric *126–127*, 128
　polysaccharide (PPV), elderly 245
　precautions 85
　pregnancy *225*
7-valent pneumococcal conjugate vaccine
　(PCV-7) 268
Pneumocystis jiroveci 279
Pneumonia 511, 515, 517
　causes *512*
Pneumothorax, spontaneous 374
Point-of-care destination resources 26–30, *27–29*
Poisonous animals *32*
Polar environments 335, *335*
Policies 16
Polio (poliomyelitis) 9
Polio (poliomyelitis) vaccine *68*, 92–94, 115–116,
　115
　accelerated schedules 116
　dosing schedules *103–105*, 116
　HIV/AIDS *278–279*
　indications 116
　contraindications 116
　pediatric *126–127*, 127–128

precautions 116
pregnancy *225*
risks *106*
Poliovirus 38
Polysaccharide vaccines 125
　pneumococcal (PPV) 245
23-valent polysaccharide vaccine (PPV-23) 267
Popular destinations 523–535
Portuguese Man o' War jellyfish (*Physalia physalis*),
　sting 423
Post-infectious irritable bowel syndrome
　(PI-IBS) 207, 210–211, *211*
Post-traumatic stress disorder (PTSD) 446
Potable, terminology defined 38
Potassium permanganate 47
PPD (purified protein derivative)
　conversion rate 322, *323*
　tests 83
Praziquantel *221–223*
Pre-existing disease 257–264
　air travel 258–259, *258–259*
　destination country 259
　general principles 257
　preparation 257–258, *258*
　return 259
　specific problems 259–262
Pregnancy 219–230
　alternative medications 229
　altitude 228
　doxycycline 152
　FDA use-in-pregnancy ratings *228*
　food/beverage precautions 227
　immunizations 224, *225*
　malaria 157, 224–227, 308
　medical care, overseas 219–224
　medical kit 229
　medications *221–223*, 228, 229
　planning 228
　pre-travel preparation 219–224, *220*
　standby emergency treatment (SBET) 169,
　　170
　yellow fever vaccine 109
Premature attrition, costs 305
Prescriptions 458
Pre-travel consultation 20, 31–36
　adoptees 293
　advice *32*, *34–35*, *35*, *35*
　components 32
　cruise ships 352–353, *353*
　discussion topics 33–34
　examination 20
　expatriates 309
　fitness 32–33
　function 63
　general considerations 33
　goals 31
　health problems, during/after 34
　health risks, analysis 33–34
　HIV/AIDS 274–281
　logistics/mechanics 31–32
　mass gatherings 359
　preventive measures 34
　questions *32*
　transplant recipients 268–269
　travelers' diarrhea (TD) 184–185
　visiting friends and relatives (VFR) 301–303
Pre-travel screening, expeditions 334–335
Primaquine 154–155
　adverse effects *146–147*
　children 237
　clinical utility score *147*
　efficacy 154–155
　HAART *280*
　indications 155
　contraindications 155
　mode of action 154

pregnancy 157, *221–223*, *226*
resistance 141, *144*, 154–155
tolerability 155
Primary eosinophilic disorders *502*
Probiotics *192*, 193
Procedures 16
Products, selling travel-related 19, *19*
Professional development, travel clinics 23
Professional societies *27–29*
Profitability, travel clinics 19–20
Proguanil
adverse effects *146–147*
breastfeeding 228–229
children 237
clinical utility score *147*
elderly 244
HAART *280*
pediatrics 158
pregnancy 157, *221–223*, 226
-resistant *Plasmodium falciparum*
147–148
Proguanil/chloroquine 147–148, *147*, 496
see also Atovaquone/proguanil (AP)
Promethazine *401*, 402
Prophylaxis *see* Chemoprophylaxis
Propranolol, psychosis 441
Protease inhibitors (PI) *280*, *280*
Protective measures 224
clothing *52*
see also Security issues
Protozoa *503*
non-pathogenic *214*
Prurigo 494, *495*
Pruritis 427
diagnosis 496, *497*
Pseudoephedrine *221–223*
Psychiatric disorders 439–447
clinical care, overseas 450–451, *451*
expeditions 334–335
high altitude 371
international travel 442–445
psychosis *see* Psychotic patient
screening, pre-travel 450
substance use *see* Substance use disorders
suicide *see* Suicidal patients
traumatic events 446
traveler typology 449
Psychological assessment 306–307
Psychological training 309
Psychometric testing 307
Psychotic patient 430
brief psychotic disorder 442
treatment 430
Psyllium hydrophilic muciloid *221–223*
Public transport 466
Pufferfish (fugu) poisoning *426*, 429–430, *429*
Pulmonary disorders 260
barotrauma 375–376
edema 174
embolism (PE) 243, 449–450
eosinophilia 504–505, *504*, 515
high altitude 369–370
hypertension (PHT) 370
respiratory tract infections (RTIs) *512*, 515
Purification, defined 38
PUTA (psychologically unfit to travel in Asia)
335
Pyemotes ventricosus 496–497
Pyodermas 493–494
Pyridoxine *221–223*
Pyrimethamine
advantages/disadvantages *39*
/dapsone *226*
standby emergency treatment (SBET) *169*
/sulfadoxine 157, 169, *221–223*
Python, mortality *415*

Q

Qinghaosu 157, 226–227
Qualifications 14–15, *14*
Quality Healthcare Advice Trent
Accreditation 344
Quarantine Stations (CDC) 350, 352
Quinacrine *209*
Quinidine *221–223*
Quinine 157, 176, 226
advantages/disadvantages *39*
standby emergency treatment (SBET) 169, *169*
/tetracycline 169
Quinine sulfate *221–223*
Quinolones *221–223*, 228

R

Rabies 9
humanitarian aid workers (HAW) 323
Lyssavirus spp 116
prophylaxis, lymphoma 269–270
visiting friends and relatives (VFRs) *302*
Rabies vaccine 68, *92–94*, 102, 116–118, *117*
accelerated schedules 118
adverse events (AE) 118
boosters 118
dosing schedules *103–105*, 117–118
drug/vaccine interactions 118
expatriates 307
HIV/AIDS *278–279*
immune response 118
indications 116
contraindications 117
pediatric 130–131, *131*
pre-exposure 116–118
post-exposure (PEP) 118
precautions 117
pregnancy *225*
risks *106*
Radiation exposure 220
Rafting 338
Raltegravir *280*
Ranitidine *221–223*
Rapid diagnostic tests (RDTs) 164–168
laboratory analysis 164–166, *167*
principle/availability 164, *165*, *165*
rationale 164
self-use 166–167, *167–168*
Recurrent cutaneous leishmaniasis (RCL) 490
Reference texts 25, *26*
Referrals, travel health program 21
Refrigerators, vaccine 17
Registration Eligibility Decision (RED) (EPA) 54
Regulations 16
local 466
Rehydration 389, *390*
Renal disease 260
Renal phase, heatstroke 384
Repatriation 313, 340
insurance 293, 328
Repel Lemon Eucalyptus Insect Repellent 57
Repellents, insect 53–58, *55–56*,
alternative 58
Reproductive tourism 345
Reptiles, venomous *414*, 420–422, *420–421*,
420, *422*
Resources 16
see also Information resources
Respiratory tract infections (RTIs) 511–522
causes/presentation 511, *512*
cruise ships 351
diagnosis *513*
environmental factors *515*
epidemics 516–517

epidemiology 512–513
management 513–515, *514*, *515*
manifestations/complications *513*
pre-existing *259*, 260
prevention 516, *516*
risk factors 513
transmission 513
tropical/geographically restricted 517–520
Resuscitation equipment 411
Revenue, travel clinic 19
Reverse culture shock 313, 324
Reverse osmosis 43
'Reverse squeeze', middle-ear barotrauma 375
Re-warming complications 387–388
Reye syndrome 205
Rhinoceros, mortality *415*
Rickettsia africae 480
Rickettsia australis 480
Rickettsia conorii 480
Rickettsia rickettsii 480
Rickettsia typhi 480
Rickettsial infections *478*, 480
Rifampin 244–245
Rifaximin 191, 215–216, 238, 245
travelers' diarrhea (TD) *192*, *194*, 195, *204*,
205
'Rights to care' 457
Risk 5
behavior 308
counseling, vaccines 75
Ritonavir *276*, *280*
Road traffic safety 435–436, *435–436*
Rotavirus
incidence 185, *187*
travelers' diarrhea (TD) 181, 202
vaccine, pediatric *126*, 129
Royal College of Nursing (UK) 18
Royal College of Obstetricians and
Gynaecologists 220
Royal College of Physicians and Surgeons
(Glasgow) 15
Royal Geographical Society
Expedition Advisory Centre 333
expedition mortality 330
RSS (really simple syndication) feeds 30
Rubella 9
vaccination 68, *225*
see also Measles-mumps-rubella (MMR) vaccine

S

Saccharomyces boulardii 205
Safety
children 231–235
cruise ships 350
expeditions 340
information sources *27–29*
seals, medication 458–459
see also Security issues
Saline nasal spray *221–223*
Salmeterol *365*
Salmonella spp 38, *38*, 227, 238, 351
detection, frequency *200*
HIV/AIDS 184, 275, 279–280
incidence 185, *187*
travelers' diarrhea (TD) 181, 185, 199, 201
persistent travelers' diarrhea (PTD) 209, 211
Salmonella enterica serotype *typhi* see *Salmonella typhi*
Salmonella enteritidis 268
Salmonella paratyphi 96–97, 175–176, 480
Salmonella typhi *38*, 96, 130, 175–176, 194,
275
enteric fever 480
risk 37

Salmonellosis 280
Sanitation 47, 350
Sanofi Pasteur, yellow fever vaccine 102
Saquinavir *276*, 280
Sarcoptes scabiei 496–497
Sarcoptes scabiei var. hominis 495
SARS (severe acute respiratory syndrome) 516–517
Saunas 383–384
Sawyer Biologic viral filter 40
Saxitoxin 430
Scabies *414*, 495
Scalp ringworm 494
Schistosoma spp 319, 473
Schistosoma haematobium 472, 508
Schistosoma mansoni 472
Schistosoma mekongi 481
Schistosomiasis
    acute (Katayama syndrome) 472, *478*, 481, 504
    eosinophilia 506
    epidemiology 10
    expatriates 305
    post-travel screening *471*, 472
Schizophrenia 442
    treatment 442
Science (magazine) 343
Scombroid *426*, 428–429, *428*, *428*
Scooters 252–253, *252*
Scopolamine 243
    motion sickness *401*, 402
Scopolamine hydrobromide *401*
Scorpions 419–420, *420*
Screening, pre-travel, psychiatric disorders 450
Screening, post-travel 467–474
    general 468–469
    medical history 467
    migrant patients 317–319, *318*
    specific 470–474, *471*
    targeted populations 468
    traveler selection/timing 467–468
Scuba diving 338–339
Sea-bather's eruption (sea lice) 495
Seasickness 352
Seatbelts 435–436
Security issues 463–466
    on arrival 464–465
    before departure 464, *464*
    car travel 466
    expatriates 312
    expeditions 340
    hotels 465
    information sources *27–29*
    local regulations 466
    mobile phones/electronic devices 465
    overview 463–464, *464*
    situational awareness 463, 465–466
    taxis/public transport 466
Sedation, children 232
Sedatives *374*, 394, *394*
Sedimentation 40
Selective serotonin reuptake inhibitors (SSRIs) 397, 445
Self-diagnosis/treatment 312, 457
    infectious diseases 308
    malaria 163–172, 308
    travelers' diarrhea (TD) 203–204
Septicemia, differential diagnosis 175–176
SEQUAMAT study 177
Serologic testing 73–74
Serotonin 3 (5HT3) antagonists 215
Sertraline 445
Service charges, travel clinics 16
Sexual contacts, pre-travel advice *32*

Sexually transmitted diseases (STDs) 33, 499, *499*
    elderly 245
    epidemiology 9–10
    expatriates 308
    HIV/AIDS 274
    post-travel screening 470
    risks 287
    visiting friends and relatives (VFR) 300
Shanchol vaccine 111
Sharks, mortality *415*
Shellfish poisoning
    amnesic (ASP) *426*, 430–431
    diarrheic (DSP) *426*, 430
    neurotoxic (NSP) *426*, 430
    paralytic (PSP) *426*, 430
Shiga toxin-producing *Escherichia coli* (STEC) 200, *201*
Shigella spp 38, *38*, 187–188, 238, 351
    detection, frequency *200*
    incidence 185, *187*
    risk 37
    travelers' diarrhea (TD) 181, 185, 201, 203
    persistent travelers' diarrhea (PTD) 209, 211
    vaccines 194
Shigella dysenteriae 201
Shigellosis *198*, 227
Ships, health problems 34
    see also Cruise ships
Shock, re-warming 387
Shoreland's Travax EnCompass 243
Short-notice travel, travel clinics 22–23
Sickle cell anemia 260
Sildenafil *365*
Silver *45*, 46
Sinusitis 515
Situational awareness 463, 465–466
Skin disorders 487–500
    cancer 269
    cosmopolitan dermatoses 493–496
    diagnosis 496–498, *496–497*
    eosinophilia 503–504, *503*
    epidemiology 487, *488*
    skin and soft tissue infections (SSTI) 493–494
    standing folds *198*
    tropical dermatoses 487–493
    see also Sexually transmitted diseases (STDs)
Skin protection, outdoor activities 233
Skin-So-Soft bath oil 55
Sleep
    high altitude 362–363
    schedule adjustment 392, *392*
Sleep-disordered breathing (SDB) 369
Small intestinal bacterial overgrowth (SIBO) 215
Smallpox 120–121
Snow blindness (UV keratitis) 368
Social impact, international adoption 295
Society for Accessible Travel and Hospitality 258, 260
Soft tissue involvement
    eosinophilia 503–504, *503*
    skin and soft tissue infections (SSTI) 493–494
Solar UV disinfection (SODIS) *39*, 46
Solid organ transplants 269, *270*
Sopite syndrome 398
Southeast Asia *528*, *529*
Special adult vaccines 101–124
    adverse events (AE) 102, *103–105*
    live 102
    overview 101–102, *102*
    practical considerations 102, *103–105*
    recommended 110–120
    required 102–110
    special circumstances 120–121
Specialized resource texts 26

Speech impairment 253–254
Spiders 419–420, *419*, *420*
Spirillum minus 416–417
Spiritual/philosophical difficulties *311*
Spirometra spp 504
Spirulina spp 496–497
Sport drinks 389
Standards, professional 16, 18
Standby emergency treatment (SBET) 163, 167–168
    counseling 168
    drug recommendations *165*, 169–170, *169*
    guidelines 168
    indications 168
    pregnancy/children/chronic illness 169, *170*
    principle/rationale 167–168
    rapid diagnosis tests (RDTs) and 166
    recommendations, balancing 169–170, *170–171*
Staphylococcus aureus 493–494, 517
    methicillin-resistant (MRSA) 493–494
    methicillin-sensitive (MSSA) 493–494
    Panton Valentine leukocidine (PVL)-positive 493–494
Stavudine 280
Stegomyia mosquito 8
Stema baths 383–384
Steroids, inhaled *221–223*
Stimulants 394–395
Stingray injuries 422–423
Stings
    marine animal 422–423
    venomous injuries 417–422
    non-venomous injuries 413–417
Stomach awareness 397–398
Stonefish sting *421*, 423, *423*
Stool studies 214, *214*
Streptobacillus monoliformis 416–417
Streptococcus spp 493–494
Streptococcus pneumoniae 84–85, 245
    respiratory tract infections (RTIs) 511, 515, 517
    vaccine 275–277, *278–279*
Streptococcus pyogenes, group A 493–494, 512–513, 515, 517
Stress 449–450
    briefing 309, *310*
    expatriates 305, *311*
    heat 382, *382*
Stressors 287
Strongyloides spp 270–271, 496–497, 504
    eosinophilia 504, 506–507
    hyperinfection syndrome 319
Strongyloides stercoralis 38, 274, 473, 496–497
Strongyloidosis 506
    post-travel screening *471*, 472
Subcutaneous nodules 504
Subcutaneous route, vaccines 70–72, *71*, *72*
Substance use disorders 445–446
    alcohol withdrawal 446
    international travel 445–446
    treatment 445–446
Sudden infant death syndrome (SIDS) 234
Suicidal patients 441–442
    assessment 441–442
    trauma 446
Sulbactam *221–223*
Sulfadoxine
    advantages/disadvantages *39*
    /pyrimethamine 157, 169, *221–223*
    standby emergency treatment (SBET) *169*
Sulfamethoxazole 194, 480
Sulfisoxazole *221–223*
Summary of Inspections of International Cruise Ships (CDC) 350

Sun exposure
 circadian rhythm adjustment *392, 393*
 kayaking/rafting 338
 pre-travel advice *32, 33*
Sunscreen 233
Supplies
 adverse events 17
 travel clinics 16–18
Support services 16
*Supporting staff responding to disasters:
 Recruitment, briefing and on-going
 care* (manual) 312
Suprachiasmatic nucleus (SCN) 391–392
Surveillance bulletins *27–29*
Sweating 382
Sydney funnel web spider (*Atrax robustus*)
 bite 419
Syncope, heat 385
Syphilis, post-travel screening *471*

T

Tachycardia 426
Tadalafil *365*
Tafenoquine 155–157
 efficacy 155–156
 indications 157
 contraindications 156
 resistance 155–156
 tolerability 156
Tageneria bite 419
Taxis 466
Telecommunications devices for the deaf
 (TDD) 253
Telemedicine 313, 411
Telephone advice, travel clinics 22
Teletypewriter (TTY) telephone 253
Temazepam 394
Temperature extremes 381–390
 acclimatization 383–384
 cold injuries 386–389, *387–388*
 heat-related illness 384–386
 thermoregulation 382–383
 see also Body temperature
Tenofovir *280*
Terrorist attacks 358
Tetanus vaccine 68, *80*
 adverse effects *81*
 HIV/AIDS *278–279*
 pregnancy *225*
 see also Diphtheria, tetanus, pertussis (DTP)
  vaccine
Tetracycline 203, 210, *221–223*, 228–229
 /quinine 169
Tetrodotoxin 429
Thermoregulation 382–383
Thimerosal 75
'Third Culture Kids' (TCKs) 315
Thromboembolic disease 243
Thrombophlebitis 220
Thrombosis *see* Venous thrombosis
Thymic disorder 109
Tick-borne diseases 237
Tick-borne encephalitis (TBE) vaccine 68, *102*,
 118–120, *119*
 adverse events (AE) 120
 criteria 119
 dosing schedules *103–105*, 119, *120*
 drug/vaccine interactions 120
 HIV/AIDS *278–279*
 immune response 119–120
 indications 119
 contraindications 119
 pediatric *131*, 132
 pregnancy *225*

Ticks *52*, 235
Tigers, mortality *415*
Tinea 494
Tinidazole 208, *209*
Tipranavir *280*
Tiredness *311*
Topical nasal decongestants *221–223*
Tourism *2, 2*
 medical kit 63–64
 see also Medical tourism
Toxoplasma gondii 275
Toxoplasmosis 227, 274
Training institutions *27–29*
Transplant recipients 268–269
 medication issues 269
 pre-travel counseling 268–269
 transplant tourism 345
 vaccination 269, *270–271*
Trauma 287, 337–338
Travel aids, general *27–29*
Travel clinics 13–24
 benefits *14*
 finance 19
 forms 18
 information resources 16–18
 legal issues 18
 management 22–23, *22*
 mid journey services 20
 off-site services 20
 organizing 16–18
 overview 13
 point-of-care destination resources 26–30,
  27–29
 professional development 23
 profitability 19–20
 short-notice travel 22–23
 standards, professional 16, 18
 telephone/email advice 22
 travel medicine, practice 13–14, *14,
  14*
 travel-related products, selling 19, *19*
 tuberculosis testing 19–20
 vaccines 16, 19–20
 visiting friends and relatives (VFR)
  301
Travel health program
 appointments 16
 brochures 22
 care delivery, models 15–16, *15*
 contract services 22
 costs 16
 documentation 16–17, 20
 examination, pre-travel 20
 expertise 15
 frequently asked questions 14–16
 internet/print/media 21
 laws/regulations/standards 16
 mailings 22
 marketing/promoting 21–22, *21*
 policies/procedures/resources 16
 post-trip evaluation 21
 qualifications 14–15, *14*
 reception staff 20
 referrals 21
 service charges 16
 service evaluation 21
 staff/administration issues 20
 starting 14–18
 support services 16
 vaccine adverse events (AE) 20–21
 word of mouth 21
 see also Pre-travel consultation
Travel Medicine Forum (ISTM) 30
Travel packages, meals 185
Travel type, medical kit 63–64
Travel warnings *27–29*

Travelers' diarrhea (TD) 7, *7*
 antibiotics 204–205, *204*
 antiemetic agents 205
 antimotility agents 205
 bacteria 181, 200–201
 chemoprophylaxis 191–193, 195, *195*
 chronic *see* Persistent travelers' diarrhea (PTD)
 clinical characteristics 179–180, *180*
 complications 198–199, *198–199*
 definition/spectrum 197–199, *198*
 differential diagnosis *198*, 199, *200*
 elderly 244–245
 environmental factors 184–185
 epidemiology 7–8, *7*, 179–190, *180*, 237–238
 etiology 180–181, *180*
 expatriates 308
 geographic region, risk 185, *186–187*
 history 179
 HIV/AIDS 279–280
 hosts at risk 180–184, *180*
 management 203–205, *204, 204*
 medical conditions, underlying 184
 military incidence 186–188, *187*
 parasites 182, 202–203
 pathogenic mechanisms *198*
 pediatric/adolescent travelers 237–238, *238*
 pregnancy 227
 prevention, impact 191
 prevention, strategies 191–195, *192*
 self-diagnosis/treatment 203–204
 signs/symptoms 197–198, *198*
 specific agents, clinical features 199–203, *200*
 systemic infections *198*
 treatment *221–223*, 227, 238
 viruses 181, 201–202
Traveler's Guide to Safe Dental Care (ADA) 345
TravelMed 30
TravelPlus program (US) 258
'Trench foot' (immersion foot) 388
Triage approach 307
Trichinella spp 508
Trichophyton rubrum 494
Trichuris spp 502
Trichuris trichiura 38, 473
Trimethoprim 194, *221–223*, 480
 /sulfamethoxazole combination (TMP/
  SMX) 194–195, 203–204, 209
Tripanavir 276
Tropical dermatoses 487–493
Tropical environments 337–338
Tropical sprue 210
TropNetEurope 299
True flies *414*
Trypanosoma cruzi 474
Trypanosoma gambiense 474
Trypanosoma rhodesiense 474
Trypanosomal chancre 493, *493*
Trypanosomiasis 10, 474
Tuberculin skin testing (TST) 470
Tuberculosis (TB) 132, 519–520
 aircraft cabin 408–409
 ethnic groups 300–301, *301*
 expatriates 308
 humanitarian aid workers (HAW) 322–323,
  323
 incubation period *478*
 low-high endemicity 519–520
 migrant patients 317–318
 post-travel screening 470, *471*
 prevention *520*
 testing clinics 19–20
 vaccination 68, *278–279*
Tumbu fly 492, *492, 492*
Tumor necrosis factor-α inhibitors 265–266,
 266–267
Tunga penetrans 492–493

Tungiasis 492–493, *493*
Ty21a oral typhoid vaccine 97
Typhoid (fever)
   post-travel screening *471*
   visiting friends and relatives (VFRs) *302*
Typhoid fever vaccine *68, 92–94,* 96–98, 261
   adverse events (AE) 97
   dosing schedules 97
   drug/vaccine interactions 98
   elderly 245–246
   estimated risk *95*
   HIV/AIDS *278–279*
   immune response 97
   indications 97
   contraindications 97
   pediatric 130, *131*
   precautions 97
   pregnancy *225*
   prevalence *96*
   trade names *89*

U

U-curve hypothesis 309–310
Ulcers *199,* 491, *491*
Ultraviolet (UV) radiation *39, 41–43,* 46
   keratitis (snow blindness) 368
Umrah pilgrimage 8
Unconjugated polysaccharide vaccines 69
Undersea and Hyperbaric Medicine Society
   (UHMS) 373–374
United Nations (UN) 321
   mortality pattern 322
   UNICEF 291
United States Coast Guard 350
University of Guelph, BiteBlocker study
   57
Upper respiratory infection (URI) *221–223*
Urinary tract infections 261
Urticaria 497–498, *498,* 504

V

Vaccinations
   clinics 16, 19–20
   supplies 17
   see also Vaccines
Vaccine Adverse Event Reporting System
   (VAERS) 18, 20–21
Vaccine Information Statements (VIS) 18
Vaccine-preventable disease (VPD) 6, 8–9
   corporate/executive traveler 288
   cruise ships 352
   elderly 245–246
   HIV/AIDS 275
Vaccines
   adverse events (AE) 20–21, *69,* 74, *74,* 81
   anesthetic techniques 70
   cardiac disease 259
   contraindications 74–75, *75*
   diabetes 261
   documentation/risk counseling 75
   elderly 245–246
   fever, returned travelers 479
   handling/administration 70
   HIV/AIDS 275–277
   immunocompromised travelers 74, *267,* 270,
     271
   immunology 67–74, *68*
   information sources *27–29*
   interchangeability 73–74
   intradermal route 72, *73*
   intramuscular (IM) route 70–71, *70, 71*
   killed 68–69
   legal issues 75

live 67–68
mercury preservatives 75
needle-free application 72
oral route 70, 72
pediatric *see* Pediatric vaccines
pulmonary disease 260
renal disease 260
risks *81*
route of administration 70–72
routine 77–100
simultaneous administration 72–73,
   73
special *see* Special adult vaccines
stocking/storing 75–76
subcutaneous route 70–72, *71, 72*
terminology *69*
transplant recipients 269, *270–271*
travelers' diarrhea (TD) 194
see also Immunizations
Vaccines for Children Program 18
Valaciclovir *221–223*
Valsalva's maneuver 406
Valuables, traveler's 465
Vancomycin 210
Varanus komodoensis bites 416–417
Varicella (chickenpox) and herpes zoster
   vaccines *68,* 83–85
   adverse events (AE) *81,* 84
   dosing schedules *79–80,* 84
   drug/vaccine interactions 84
   elderly 246
   immune response 84
   indications 83
   contraindications *81,* 83
   pediatric *126–127,* 128
   precautions 83
   pregnancy *225*
Varilrix 83
Varivax III 83
VARIVAX pregnancy registry 228
Vection 397
Venomous injuries *414,* 417–422
   animals, pre-travel advice *32*
   prevention 418, *418*
   sea creatures, scuba diving 338
   snakes, mortality *415*
Venous thromboembolism (VTE) 243
Venous thrombosis (VT) 449–453
   incidence/etiology 449
   mechanism 451–452
   overview 449
   passenger-related factors 450, *451*
   prevention 452
   recommendations 452
   risks 450, *450, 451*
   travel-related factors 450–451
Vesiculobullous lesions 488–489
Vespidae stings 419
Vessel sanitation program (VSP) 350, *350*
Vestibular (balance) system 398, *399–400*
Vi polysaccharide typhoid vaccine 97
Vibrio spp 181, 423
Vibrio carchariae 423
Vibrio cholerae 37, *38,* 110, 181, 194,
   201
Vibrio parahaemolyticus 181, 201, 423
Vibrio vulnificus 262, 423, *423*
Violin spider group (*Loxosceles*) bite 419,
   419
VIP clinics 458
Viruses 181, 201–202
Visiting friends and relatives (VFRs)
   297–304
   barriers to protecting 298
   defined 297
   epidemiology, travel 298–301

medical kit 64
pre-travel consultation 301–303
as risk group 297–298
screening 467
travelers 18
Visual impairment 254
Vitamin A 153
Voriconazole 269

W

Walkers 253
   barefoot *32*
Warsaw Convention 253
Water
   contaminated 338
   pre-travel advice *32*
   purification *221–223*
   sports 220, 233
Water disinfection 37–49
   chemical products *45*
   commercial devices *41–43*
   hygiene 237
   overview 37
   preferred technique 47, *47*
   pregnancy 227
   reaction 44
   sanitation 47
   treatment methods 38–47, *38*
Water-borne diseases 351
   etiology/risk 37, *38*
Water-related injuries 436–437, *437*
Websites 25–26, *27–29*
   altitude 361, *362*
   expeditions *331*
   oxygen resources 332, *369*
   security/risk *464*
West Nile Virus (WNV) 7
Western Europe *532, 532*
Wheelchairs 252–253, *252*
Widow spiders (*Latrodectus*) bite 419
Wilderness Medicine (Auerbach) 38,
   337
Wilderness travel, medical kit 64
Withdrawal, cultural adaptation *311*
Women, diving 373
World Health Assembly 345
World Health Organization (WHO)
   atovaquone/proguanil (AP) 154
   chlorine 44
   Collaborating Center (JCI) 455
   counterfeit medications 345–346
   cruise regulations 350
   diarrhea 37
   emergency care 437
   Global Burden of Disease Study 437
   health guidance 2, 13
   hepatitis B vaccination 90, 128–129
   HIV/AIDS 9–10
   immunization 76, 294
   influenza 409
   information resources 17, 139
   International Health Regulations (IHRs)
     101
   malaria 135, 137, 143
   mass gatherings 358
   measles-mumps-rubella (MMR) vaccine
     127
   mefloquine (MQ) 150
   nutrition 293
   pesticides 408
   polio 115, 127–128
   pregnancy 227
   rabies 116, 118
   road traffic accidents 433–435

SARS (severe acute respiratory syndrome) 516
smallpox 120
standby emergency treatment (SBET) 169
transplant tourism 345
traveler's thrombosis 449
tuberculosis (TB) 322, 408–409
vaccines 75
websites 25–26
yellow fever 8, 102, 106–109
World Recreational Scuba Training Council
        (RSTC) 373–374
World Report on Road Traffic Injury
        Prevention 434
World Tourism Organization 13–14, 437
WRIGHT (WHO Research Into Global Hazards
        of Travel) project 449–450, 452
Wuchereria bancrofti 473, 506

X

X-rays 470
d-Xylose testing, blood test 214

Y

Yellow fever (YF) 8, *302*
Yellow fever (YF) vaccine *68*, 76, 102, *102*
    adverse events (AE) *103–105*, 109–110
    breastfeeding 228–229
    children 129–130, *129*, *131*, 237
    dosing schedules *103–105*, 109
    drug/vaccine interactions 110
    elderly 246
    HIV/AIDS *278–279*
    immune response 109
    immunocompromised travelers 270
    indications 108–109
    contraindications 109
    pregnancy *225*
    recommendations 106–108, *107–108*
    risks *106*
Yersinia enterocolitica 38, 201, 210
Yersinia pestis 121, 518
Yersinia spp 199

Z

Zidovudine *280*
Zolpidem 243–244, *365*, *394*
Zostavax 83